AIDS

Etiology, Diagnosis, Treatment, and Prevention

AIDS

Etiology, Diagnosis, Treatment, and Prevention

Third Edition

Edited by

Vincent T. DeVita, Jr., M.D.
Benno C. Schmidt Chair in Clinical
  Oncology
Attending Physician and Member
Program of Molecular Pharmacology and
  Therapeutics
Memorial Sloan-Kettering Cancer Center
Professor of Medicine
Cornell University Medical College
New York, New York

Samuel Hellman, M.D.
Dean, Division of the Biological Sciences
  and The Pritzker School of Medicine
Vice President for the Medical Center
The University of Chicago
Chicago, Illinois

Steven A. Rosenberg, M.D., Ph.D.
Chief of Surgery
National Cancer Institute
Professor of Surgery
Uniformed Services University of the Health
  Sciences School of Medicine
Bethesda, Maryland

Dr. Rosenberg edited this book in his private capacity, and no official endorsement or support by the National Institutes of Health is intended or should be inferred.

Associate Editors

James Curran, M.D.
Director, Division of HIV/AIDS
National Center for Infectious Diseases
Centers for Disease Control
Atlanta, Georgia

M. Essex, D.V.M., Ph.D.
Chairman, Harvard AIDS Institute
Chairman, Department of Cancer Biology
Harvard School of Public Health
Mary Woodard Lasker Professor of Health
  Sciences
Harvard University
Boston, Massachusetts

Anthony S. Fauci, M.D.
Director, National Institute of Allergy and
  Infectious Diseases
Chief, Laboratory of Immunoregulation
National Institute of Allergy and Infectious
  Diseases
Director, Office of AIDS Research
National Institutes of Health
Bethesda, Maryland

Dr. Fauci edited this book in his private capacity, and no official endorsement or support by the National Institutes of Health is intended or should be inferred.

J.B. Lippincott Company / Philadelphia

With 73 contributors

Coordinating Editorial Assistant: Eileen Wolfberg
Indexer: Sandi King
Interior Designer: Charles Field
Cover Designer: William T. Donnelly
Production Manager: Janet Greenwood
Production Services: Carol Florence
Compositor: TAPSCO, Inc.
Printer/Binder: Courier Westford
Color Insert Printer: Princeton Polychrome Press

Third Edition

6 5 4 3 2

AIDS: etiology, diagnosis, treatment and prevention/edited by
    Vincent T. DeVita, Jr., Samuel Hellman, Steven A. Rosenberg.—3rd ed.
        p.   cm.
    Includes bibliographical references and index.
    ISBN 0-397-51229-5
    1. AIDS (Disease)   I. DeVita, Vincent T.   II. Hellman, Samuel.
III. Rosenberg, Steven A.
    [DNLM: 1. Acquired Immunodeficiency Syndrome.   WD 308 A28821]
RC607.A26A346   1992
616.97'92—dc20
DNLM/DLC
for Library of Congress   91-46702
                                                                 CIP

The authors and publisher have exerted every effort to ensure that drug
selection and dosage set forth in this text are in accord with current
recommendations and practice at the time of publication. However, in view of
ongoing research, changes in government regulations, and the constant flow of
information relating to drug therapy and drug reactions, the reader is urged to
check the package insert for each drug for any change in indications and
dosage and for added warnings and precautions. This is particularly important
when the recommended agent is a new or infrequently employed drug.

Contributors

Susan K. Aoki, M.D.
Staff Physician, Sacramento Medical
  Foundation Blood Center
Sacramento, California

David W. Archibald, D.M.D., D.Sc.
Associate Professor of Oral Pathology, University of
  Maryland Dental School
Baltimore, Maryland

James E. Balow, M.D.
Professor of Medicine, Uniformed Services University
  of the Health Sciences
Clinical Director, National Institute of Diabetes and
  Digestive and Kidney Diseases
Chief, Kidney Disease Section, National Institutes of
  Health
Bethesda, Maryland

David M. Bell, M.D.
Acting Chief, HIV Infections Branch, Hospital
  Infections Program
National Center for Infectious Diseases, Centers for
  Disease Control
Altanta, Georgia

Daniel R. Benson, M.D.
Professor of Orthopaedic Surgery, Chief of Spine
  Service
University of California at Davis
Sacramento, California

Ruth L. Berkelman, M.D.
Chief, Surveillance Branch, Division of HIV/AIDS
National Center for Infectious Diseases, Centers for
  Disease Control
Atlanta, Georgia

Dani P. Bolognesi, Ph.D.
James B. Duke Professor
Director, Center for AIDS Research
Duke University Medical Center
Durham, North Carolina

Stephen L. Boswell, M.D.
Instructor of Medicine, Harvard Medical School
Director of HIV Clinical Service, Massachusetts
  General Hospital
Boston, Massachusetts

William Breitbart, M.D.
Assistant Professor of Psychiatry, Cornell University
  Medical College
Assistant Attending Psychiatrist, Memorial Sloan-
  Kettering Cancer Center
New York, New York

Bruce J. Brew, M.D.
Senior Lecturer in Medicine, University of New South
  Wales
Consultant Physician and Lecturer, St. Vincent's
  Medical Centre
Sydney, Australia

Karina M. Butler, M.B., B.Ch., M.R.C.P.I.
Senior Staff Fellow, Pediatric Branch
National Cancer Institute
Bethesda, Maryland

Kathleen McMahon Casey, M.Ed., M.A., R.N.
HIV Care Program Manager
Critical Care America
New York, New York

Willard Cates, Jr., M.D., M.P.H.
Adjunct Professor of Epidemiology and Biostatistics
Emory University of School of Public Health
Adjunct Professor of Community Health and
  Preventive Medicine
Morehouse School of Medicine
Director, Division of Training
Epidemiology Program Office
Centers for Disease Control
Atlanta, Georgia

Susan Y. Chu, Ph.D.
Epidemiologist, Division of HIV/AIDS
National Center for Infectious Diseases, Centers for
  Disease Control
Atlanta, Georgia

Ruth I. Connor, Ph.D.
Research Fellow, Aaron Diamond AIDS Research
  Center
New York, New York

James Curran, M.D.
Director, Division of HIV/AIDS
National Center for Infectious Diseases
Centers for Disease Control
Atlanta, Georgia

Richard T. Davey, Jr., M.D.
Medical Officer, Section of Clinical and Molecular
  Retrovirology
National Institute of Allergy and Infectious Diseases
Warren G. Magnuson Clinical Center
National Institutes of Health
Bethesda, Maryland

Don C. Des Jarlais, Ph.D.
Deputy Director of Research, Narcotic and Drug
  Research, Inc.
Director of Research, Chemical Dependency Institute
Beth Israel Medical Center
New York, New York

M. Essex, D.V.M., Ph.D.
Chairman, Harvard AIDS Institute
Chairman, Department of Cancer Biology
Harvard School of Public Health
Mary Woodard Lasker Professor of Health Sciences
Harvard University
Boston, Massachusetts

Judith Falloon, M.D.
Senior Investigator, Critical Care Medicine
  Department
Warren G. Magnuson Clinical Center
National Institutes of Health
Bethesda, Maryland

Anthony S. Fauci, M.D.
Director, National Institute of Allergy and Infectious
  Diseases
Chief, Laboratory of Immunoregulation
National Institute of Allergy and Infectious Diseases
Director, Office of AIDS Research
National Institutes of Health
Bethesda, Maryland

Martin S. Favero, Ph.D.
Chief, Nosocomial Infections Laboratory Branch
Hospital Infections Program
National Center for Infectious Diseases
Centers for Disease Control
Atlanta, Georgia

Gerald Friedland, M.D.
Professor of Medicine and Public Director, AIDS
  Program
Yale University School of Medicine
New Haven, Connecticut

Samuel R. Friedman, Ph.D.
Principal Investigator, Narcotic and Drug Research,
  Inc.
New York, New York

Bruce G. Gellin, M.D., M.P.H.
Clinical Instructor in Public Health and Medicine,
  Cornell University Medical College
New York, New York

Julie Louise Gerberding, M.D., M.P.H.
Assistant Professor of Medicine, Infectious Diseases
University of California, San Francisco
Director, HIV Prevention Services
San Francisco General Hospital
San Francisco, California

Peter John Gomatos, M.D., Ph.D.
Infectious Disease Officer
Infectious Disease Service
Department of Medicine
Walter Reed Army Medical Center
Washington, DC

Lawrence O. Gostin, J.D.
Executive Director
American Society of Law and Medicine
Adjunct Professor of Health Law
Harvard School of Public Health
Assoc. Dir., World Health Org./Howard University
  Collaborative Center on Health Legislature
Boston, Massachusetts

William A. Haseltine, Ph.D.
Professor of Pathology, Harvard Medical School
Harvard School of Public Health
Chief, Division of Human Retrovirology
Dana-Farber Cancer Institute
Boston, Massachusetts

Barton F. Haynes, M.D.
Frederic M. Hanes Professor of Medicine
Department of Medicine
Duke University School of Medicine
Chief, Division of Rheumatology and Immunology
Department of Medicine
Duke University Medical Center
Durham, North Carolina

David K. Henderson, M.D.
Associate Director, Warren Grant Magnuson Clinical
    Center
National Institutes of Health
Bethesda, Maryland

Martin S. Hirsch, M.D.
Professor of Medicine, Harvard Medical School
Physician, Infectious Disease Unit
Massachusetts General Hospital
Boston, Massachusetts

David D. Ho, M.D.
Professor of Medicine and Microbiology, New York
    University School of Medicine
Director, Aaron Diamond AIDS Research Center
New York, New York

Jimmie C. Holland, M.D.
Wayne E. Chapman Chair in Psychiatric Oncology
Chief, Psychiatry Service, Memorial Sloan-Kettering
    Cancer Center
Professor of Psychiatry, Cornell University Medical
    College
New York, New York

Paul V. Holland, M.D.
Clinical Professor of Medicine, Division of
    Hematology/Oncology
University of California at Davis
Medical Director and Chief Executive Officer,
    Sacramento Medical Foundation Blood Center
Sacramento, California

Paul B. Jacobsen, Ph.D.
Assistant Professor of Psychology in Psychiatry,
    Cornell University Medical College
Assistant Attending Psychologist, Memorial Sloan-
    Kettering Cancer Center
New York, New York

Margaret I. Johnston, Ph.D.
Associate Director, Basic Research and Development
    Program
Division of Acquired Immunodeficiency Syndrome
National Institute of Allergy and Infectious Diseases
Bethesda, Maryland

G. D. Kelen, M.D., F.R.C.P.(C.), F.A.C.E.P.
Associate Professor
Director of Research
Residency Director
Emergency Medicine
Johns Hopkins University School of Medicine
Baltimore, Maryland

Robert Klein, M.D.
Associate Professor of Medicine and Epidemiology
    and Social Medicine
Albert Einstein College of Medicine
New York, New York
Division of Infectious Diseases
Montefiore Medical Center
Bronx, New York

Donald P. Kotler, M.D.
Associate Professor of Clinical Medicine, Columbia
    University College of Physicians and Surgeons
St. Luke's Roosevelt Hospital Center
New York, New York

Joseph A. Kovacs, M.D.
Senior Investigator, Critical Care Medicine
    Department
Clinical Center
National Institutes of Health
Bethesda, Maryland

H. Clifford Lane, M.D.
Chief, Section of Clinical and Molecular Retrovirology
Laboratory of Immunoregulation
National Institute of Allergy and Infectious Diseases
National Institutes of Health
Bethesda, Maryland

Alexandra M. Levine, M.D.
Professor of Medicine and Chief, Division of
    Hematology
University of Southern California School of Medicine
Deputy Clinical Director, Norris Cancer Hospital and
    Research Institute
Los Angeles, California

Stewart J. Levine, M.D.
Medical Staff Fellow, Critical Care Medicine
    Department
National Institutes of Health
Bethesda, Maryland

Alan R. Lifson, M.D., M.P.H.
Assistant Professor, Department of Epidemiology and
    Biostatistics
University of California School of Medicine
San Francisco, California

Jonathan M. Mann, M.D., M.P.H.
Professor of Epidemiology and International Health,
    Harvard School of Public Health
Director, International AIDS Center
Harvard AIDS Institute
Cambridge, Massachusetts

Ruthanne Marcus, M.P.H.
Assistant Chief, HIV Infections Branch
Hospital Infections Program
National Center for Infectious Diseases
Centers for Disease Control
Atlanta, Georgia

Henry Masur, M.D.
Chief, Critical Care Medicine Department
Warren G. Magnuson Clinical Center
National Institutes of Health
Bethesda, Maryland

John J. McGowan, Ph.D.
Director, Division of Extramural Activities
National Institute of Allergy and Infectious Diseases
National Institutes of Health
Bethesda, Maryland

Hindi T. Mermelstein-Lunzer, M.D.
Assistant Professor of Psychiatry, Health Science
   Center at Brooklyn School of Medicine
Brooklyn, New York
Fellow, Memorial Sloan-Kettering Cancer Center
Director, Psychiatric Oncology
Staten Island University Hospital
Staten Island, New York

Ronald T. Mitsuyasu, M.D.
Professor of Medicine, Division of
   Hematology and Oncology
UCLA Medical Center
Director, UCLA Center for Aids Research and
   Education (CARE)
Los Angeles, California

Alan Neaigus, Ph.D.
Project Director, Narcotic and Drug Research, Inc.
New York, New York

Donald W. Northfelt, M.D.
Assistant Clinical Professor of Medicine, Division of
   AIDS Activities/Oncology
Department of Medicine
San Francisco General Hospital
University of California
San Francisco, California

Thomas A. Peterman, M.D., M.Sc.
Chief, Viral Studies Section
Clinical Research Branch
Division of STD/HIV Prevention
National Center for Prevention Services
Centers for Disease Control
Atlanta, Georgia

Herbert B. Peterson, M.D.
Chief, Women's Health and Fertility Branch, Division
   of Reproductive Health
National Center for Chronic Disease Prevention and
   Health Promotion
Centers for Disease Control
Atlanta, Georgia

Philip A. Pizzo, M.D.
Chief of Pediatrics
Head, Infectious Diseases
National Cancer Institute
Bethesda, Maryland

Michael A. Polis, M.D., M.P.H.
Senior Investigator, AIDS Section
Critical Care Medicine Department
Senior Investigator
Warren G. Magnuson Clinical Center
National Institutes of Health
Bethesda, Maryland

Richard W. Price, M.D.
Professor of Neurology, University of Minnesota
   Medical School
Head, Department of Neurology
The University of Minnesota Hospital and Clinic
Minneapolis, Minneapolis

Douglas D. Richman, M.D.
Professor of Pathology and Medicine, University of
   California, San Diego
Chief, Virology Section
Director, Research Center for AIDS and HIV Infection
San Diego Veterans Affairs Medical Center
San Diego, California

David E. Rogers, M.D.
The Walsh McDermott University Professor of
   Medicine, Cornell University Medical College
Attending Physician
The New York Hospital
New York, New York

Martha F. Rogers, M.D.
Chief, Epidemiologic Studies Branch
Division of HIV/AIDS
National Center for Infectious Diseases
Centers for Disease Control
Atlanta, Georgia

Marian E. Roke, M.D.
Consultant Neurologist, Seymour Medical Clinic
Vancouver, British Columbia, Canada

Zeda F. Rosenberg, Sc.D.
Assistant to the Director, National Institute of Allergy
   and Infectious Diseases
National Institutes of Health
Bethesda, Maryland

Bijan Safai, M.D., D.Sc.
Professor of Medicine, Cornell University Medical
   College
Chief of Dermatology and Member, Memorial Sloan-
   Kettering Cancer Center
New York, New York

Robert T. Schooley, M.D.
Professor of Medicine
Head, Infectious Disease Division
University of Colorado Health Sciences Center
Denver, Colorado

Joseph Schwartz, M.D.
Dermatology Fellow, Memorial Sloan-Kettering
    Cancer Center
New York, New York

James Shelhamer, M.D.
Deputy Chief, Critical Care Medicine Department
National Institutes of Health
Bethesda, Maryland

Nicholas M. Stamatos, M.D., Ph.D.
Resident, Department of Medicine
Infectious Disease Service
Department of Medicine
Walter Reed Army Medical Center
Washington, DC

M. B. Vasudevachari, D.V.M., Ph.D.
Research Assistant Professor, Georgetown University
    School of Medicine
Washington, DC

Paul A. Volberding, M.D.
Professor of Medicine, University of California,
    San Francisco
Chief, AIDS Program and Medical Oncology
San Francisco General Hospital
San Francisco, California

Robert E. Walker, M.D.
Section of Clinical and Molecular Retrovirology
National Institute of Allergy and Infectious Diseases
National Institutes of Health
Bethesda, Maryland

Judith N. Wasserheit, M.D., M.P.H.
Chief, Sexually Transmitted Diseases Branch
National Institute of Allergy and Infectious Diseases
National Institutes of Health
Bethesda, Maryland

Seth L. Welles, Ph.D.
Department of Epidemiology
Harvard School of Public Health
Boston, Massachusetts

Preface

This is the third edition of AIDS. The first edition was published in 1985. Between these editions, substantial progress has been made in our understanding of the disease and, unfortunately, in the extent of the epidemic and its importance throughout the world. In order to deal with this explosion of knowledge, we asked Myron Essex, Anthony Fauci, and James Curran to serve as associate editors with us. These outstanding experts have helped in planning and organizing the book, as well as identifying appropriate experts to author the individual chapters. This edition is different from the previous ones, but still follows a similar scheme. Certain areas covered in the previous chapters have been expanded, and there are many new chapters. Even those chapters similarly named have been markedly changed both in subject matter and, frequently, in choice of author. Basic considerations have been reorganized to reflect the biological and molecular biological understanding of the virus and the immunologic aspects of HIV infection. The changing epidemiology of the disease is presented in a separate section of the book. The section on clinical manifestations of the disease has been expanded and focuses on both the disease itself and the infectious complications associated with it. A new section on treatment has been added recognizing the variety of potential strategies for the development of therapies. There are specific discussions of agents and of important approaches to HIV-positive patients and their families. A section of the book deals with strategies for prevention and how the major mechanisms of transmission should be addressed. Included in this section is a discussion of potential vaccines. Finally, a section has been added addressing HIV infection and the health care worker, a controversial but vital issue confronting society and medicine.

Much has changed since the last edition but not the importance of the disease. If anything, the epidemic proportions have become more apparent. We derive some confidence for success in the treatment of AIDS and in the wealth of information that has been provided since the last edition, but we are chastened by the enormity of the human dimension of this devastating disease. We hope that this book will serve as an important source of information in our efforts to deal with this dread disease.

Vincent T. DeVita, Jr.
Samuel Hellman
Steven A. Rosenberg

Contents

*Color figures for Chapters 11B and 12 will be found in Chapter 11B.

I

Basic Considerations

Origin of AIDS

Myron Essex

When a "new" infectious disease such as acquired immunodeficiency syndrome (AIDS) appears, the causative agent has to have existed previously under one of several possible circumstances. First, the etiologic agent may represent a more virulent mutant variant or recombinant of an organism that was either previously infecting the same population without causing disease or had a distinctly different profile of disease pathology. Second, the organism may have been introduced from a relatively isolated population of people who had developed a resistance to the lethality of the agent. Third, the organism may have been introduced to humans from another species. This third explanation seems highly likely for the human immunodeficiency virus type 2 (HIV-2), and increasingly likely for HIV-1. For either the second or third explanation of an origin for HIV, understanding how the human or nonhuman host evolved to resist the lethal effects of the virus may provide valuable clues for developing effective prevention and therapy techniques.

AIDS was first recognized as a new and distinct clinical entity in 1981.[1-3] The first cases were recognized because of an unusual clustering of diseases such as Kaposi's sarcoma and *Pneumocystis carinii* pneumonia in young homosexual men. Although such syndromes were occasionally observed in distinct subgroups of the population—such as older men of Mediterranean origin in the case of Kaposi's sarcoma, or severely impaired cancer patients in the case of *Pneumocystis carinii* pneumonia—the occurrence of these diseases in previously healthy young people was unprecedented. Because most of the first cases of this newly defined clinical syndrome involved homosexual men, it at first seemed logical that the cause of this syndrome might be related to a life-style habit unique to that population. In the 1960s and 1970s, the revolution in sexual permissiveness brought with it an enhanced societal acceptance of homosexuality. The development of commercial bathhouses and other outlets for homosexual contact increased promiscuity, and self-selected segments of the male homosexual population had increased numbers of sexual contacts. It is not surprising, then, that such factors as frequent exposure to sperm, rectal exposure to sperm, or amyl or butyl nitrate "poppers," which were used to enhance sexual performance, were considered potential causes of AIDS. Yet while it was apparent that AIDS was a new disease, most homosexual life-style habits had changed only in a relative sense.

AIDS cases were soon reported in other populations as well, including intravenous (IV) drug users[4] and hemophiliacs.[5-7] Although these groups were not necessarily exposed to amyl or butyl nitrate or to frequent contact with sperm, it was argued that they, like male homosexuals, may have been exposed to frequent immunostimulatory doses of foreign proteins and tissue antigens. Hemophiliacs used clotting factor preparations, which were prepared from the pooled blood of a huge number of donors, and IV drug users often used needles contaminated with small amounts of blood from previous users, thereby increasing their exposure to foreign tissue antigens. Even independent of clinical AIDS, asymptomatic hemophiliacs and IV drug users were often found to have inverted T-lymphocyte helper to suppressor ratios, as did AIDS patients and a proportion of asymptomatic homosexual men. However, for patients not infected with HIV, the increased T-cell ratios were more often due to an increase in the number of T-suppressor cells, as opposed to the decrease in T-helper cells seen in AIDS patients and HIV carriers with progressing disease. The increase in T-suppressor cells is presumably due to frequent antigenic stimulation.

Three new categories of AIDS patients were soon observed: blood transfusion recipients,[8,9] adults from central Africa,[10-12] and infants born to mothers who themselves had AIDS or were IV drug users.[13-15] The patients with transfusion-associated cases had received donations from an AIDS patient at least 3 years before showing symptoms.[8,9]

AN INFECTIOUS ETIOLOGY FOR AIDS

These and other developments discussed below made it clear that an infectious etiology for AIDS should be considered.[16] Several studies were soon initiated to determine seroprevalence rates for exposure to numerous microorganisms, especially viruses, and to compare exposure to given agents in AIDS patients and controls.[17] High on the list of candidate viruses were cytomegalovirus, because it was already associated with a less severe immunosuppression in kidney transplant patients; Epstein-Barr virus, presumably because it was a lymphotropic virus; and hepatitis B virus, because infection with this virus was known to occur at elevated rates in both homosexual men and recipients of blood or blood products. If a virus such as hepatitis B, Epstein-Barr, or cytomegalovirus were to be etiologically involved, it would presumably have to be a newly mutated or a recombinant genetic variant.

At the same time, my group,[18,19] Gallo and his colleagues,[20,21] and Montagnier and his colleagues[22] all independently postulated that a variant T-lymphotropic retrovirus might be the etiologic agent of AIDS. Among the most compelling reasons for this hypothesis was that the human T-lymphotropic retrovirus (HTLV), discovered by Gallo and his colleagues[23] in 1980, was the only human virus known to infect T-helper lymphocytes at that time. It was already clear that T-helper lymphocytes became impaired or were eliminated in clinical AIDS.[13,24–26]

There were other compelling reasons to consider an HTLV-related retrovirus. HTLV was known to be transmitted through the same routes as the etiologic agent of AIDS; sexual contact, with transmission apparently more efficient from males; transmission by blood; and transmission from mothers to newborns.[27] Among animal retroviruses, the lymphotropic feline leukemia virus was known to be a major cause of lethal immunosuppression in cats.[28] Even HTLV-I, which only causes leukemia or neurologic disease in a fraction of infected individuals, was known to cause a nonlethal immunosuppression.[29]

Attempts to detect a virus related to HTLV-I or HTLV-II[30] met with partial success. Although antibodies cross-reactive with HTLV-I and HTLV-related genomic sequences were found in a minority of AIDS patients,[18–20,22] the reactivity was weak, suggesting either the co-infection of AIDS patients with an HTLV, or the etiologic role of a distant, weakly reactive virus. Soon after, proof that the disease was linked to T-lymphotropic retroviruses was obtained by Gallo and his colleagues.[31–34] Further characterization of the agent—now termed human immunodeficiency virus type 1 (HIV-1)—revealed that it was only distantly related to HTLV

yet was the same as the isolate detected earlier by Montagnier and his colleagues.[22]

ORIGINS OF HUMAN RETROVIRUSES

HTLV, the first human retrovirus identified, was known to be present at elevated rates in regions such as southwestern Japan, the Caribbean basin, northern South America, and Africa, and at lower rates in most of North America and Europe. The theory that this virus originated in Africa was initially suggested by Gallo, who cited early reports of Africans in southwestern Japan.[35] Miyoshi and his colleagues then identified a virus related to HTLV in Asian monkeys.[36] This virus, designated simian T-cell leukemia virus (STLV), was later found in African monkeys and apes[37,38] and associated with lymphoproliferative diseases in captive macaques from Asia.[39]

Seroepidemiologic studies in Old World primates from both Asia and Africa revealed that more than 30 species of monkeys and apes had widespread infection with an STLV (Table 1–1).[40] However, on further molecular characterization it was recognized that the STLVs from Japanese macaques and related Asian species of primates were not as closely related to HTLV as were STLVs isolated from African primates such as chimpanzees and African green monkeys.[41] Thus, all isolates of HTLV—whether from Japanese, Caribbean, or African people—were highly related to African strains of STLV but not as highly related to Asian strains of STLV. This suggested that all HTLVs thus far identified evolved from a subgroup of STLVs present in Africa but not in Asia. It also suggested quite clearly that the STLV/HTLV family of retroviruses had been present in numerous species of Old World monkeys for some time before moving to humans from an African species of monkey or ape.

As a group, the HTLV/STLV viruses vary little from one isolate to another, while the HIV-1 viruses and the HIV-2/SIV group of viruses vary highly from one isolate to another.[42,43] Although the HIV-1 viruses appear to

Table 1–1. Retroviruses Related to HTLV and HIV in Subhuman Primates

Region	Species	HTLV	HIV-1	HIV-2
Africa	Chimpanzee	+	+	−
	Baboon	+	−	−
	Green monkey	+	−	+
	Mangabey	*	−	+
Asia	Macaque	+	−	−†
America	Marmoset	−	−	−

* Not known.
† Although the wild macaques examined have all been seronegative, monkeys in captivity are often infected with an SIV that is closely related to HIV-2.

cause AIDS or a related disease in a very high proportion of infected people, the HTLV/STLV viruses rarely cause lethal disease in people or monkeys.[44] SIVs appear non-virulent in their natural African monkey hosts.[44,45] HIV-2 appears less virulent than HIV-1 but is associated with some cases of AIDS.[46–48]

The high prevalence rates of infection with STLV in so many species of Old World monkeys also indicate that STLV only rarely causes lymphoma or other diseases under natural circumstances. Although it is unclear why STLV and HTLV are so limited in their pathogenicity, evolutionary pressure within the monkey species may have selected for a virus that was not highly virulent. An STLV of low virulence might then have been transmitted to humans, where it remained a virus of limited virulence.

Whereas substantial genetic variation is seen among different isolates of HIV-1, particularly in the envelope gene, the same degree of variation is not seen in HTLV. Presumably, the rate of genetic drift seen in retroviruses is related to their rate of replication. HIVs, as lenti-type retroviruses, have a greater ability to circumvent the usual rigid requirements for cell division of the retroviruses. The possibility of existing in episomal form and the presence of regulatory genes that allow a rapid increase in replication rate are properties not associated with simpler retroviruses. This replication potential, along with a reverse transcriptase that is substantially more error prone,[49] helps explain why genomic variation among HIVs is substantially greater than among other retroviruses.

While HIV-1 can replicate to high titers and be detected as free virus in serum or plasma, HTLV cannot. Because HTLV is apparently transmitted both between individuals and within the body only in a cell-associated manner, the rate of evolutionary diversion of this virus should be considerably less. Very different and more rapid evolutionary development would apparently occur in the case of HIV-1.

DIVERSION AMONG HUMAN LENTIRETROVIRUSES

Based on relatedness of nucleotide sequences and the diversion seen among HIVs, it has been estimated that HIV-1 and HIV-2 could have separated from each other as little as 40 to 50 years ago.[50] The first documented infection with HIV-1, based on antibody detection, occurred in 1959.[51]

Nucleotide sequence drift is most rapid in the *env* gene, where variation occurs at about three times the rate of that seen in the *pol* gene, with an intermediate rate for *gag*. The average differences between HIV-1 *env* sequences deviate at a rate of about 1% per year.[43] This suggests that differences between *env* sequences of random HIV-1 isolates in the United States may be about 15% as of 1992, and for African isolates 25% or

more. The higher degree of conservation observed among samples from clustered patients as compared to random donors in the same geographic area provided strong evidence for dental exposure.[52]

Env gene variations of 5% can be seen for viruses isolated from the same individual. Cultivation *in vitro* appears to initially select for more highly related strains and to diminish subsequent rates of diversion.[53–55] While this is compatible with the *in vivo* selection pressure that might be expected as a result of a host immune response, the clear type of immune selection observed for the equine infectious anemia lentivirus has not been observed.[56] Similarly, although HIV-1 viruses with a range of *in vitro* cytopathicity have been observed, the degree of cytopathicity *in vitro* has not been linked to virulence *in vivo*. It is thus not clear whether HIV-1 isolates with reduced cytopathic effect were selected for survival by host pressure.

Recombination between different HIV genomes has rarely been observed, either for different HIVs or between HIV-1 and HIV-2. This seems surprising, particularly for HIV-1/HIV-2 recombinants, which should be easier to detect.

Dual infections with HIV-1 and HIV-2 have been reported.[57,58] and, if accurately reflected by serotype analyses, would appear to be quite frequent.[59] If the apparent lack of recombinants is a true indication of the situation, it might reflect a highly effective system for host cell interference for replication.

HIVs may have more than 20 different message transcripts, especially because of the regulatory and accessory genes, which are usually doubly spliced and may present pieces of the same information in multiple transcripts.[60,61] These multiple transcripts do not appear to induce selection for recombinants or defective genomes. With HTLV-I, though, the leukemic cells often appear to select for deleted replication defective proviruses.[62]

ORIGIN OF HIV-1

Once HIV-1 was recognized as the cause of AIDS, it soon became apparent that this virus was new to human populations in the western hemisphere. If HIV-1 had been present in populations of people in Africa to the point of evolutionary equilibration, as seen with HTLV, it probably would have been limited to isolated tribes of people, and would represent a situation in which selection for host immunity rather than selection of an avirulent virus would have occurred. Such isolation seemed essential if evolutionary equilibration had occurred, because in both the United States and Haiti, blacks are just as likely as whites to develop clinical AIDS after exposure to HIV-1.

The possibility that HIV-1 or a related virus was present in human populations in central Africa at the same time or even before AIDS was diagnosed in the

United States seemed even more likely when what was apparently the same syndrome was reported in Africans who sought treatment in Europe. Subsequently, it was recognized that HIV-1 infection and clinical AIDS were rapidly spreading in central Africa (Table 1–2).

Serum samples collected from Africans at earlier periods were also examined for the presence of antibodies reactive with HIV-1. In some cases, the examination of stored samples suggested elevated rates of infection in Africa during the period 1965–1975. Subsequently it was revealed that most of those surveys were conducted with first-stage tests that were imperfect, and the reactors were mostly false positives, due either to contamination of the HIV antigen or to "sticky sera" containing antibodies that reacted nonspecifically because the sera had been repeatedly frozen and thawed and maintained under poor conditions.

While examining sera taken from Africa from 1955 to 1965, we found one antibody-positive sample that was clearly positive in a specific manner.[51] When tested by radioimmunoprecipitation, this sample contained high titers of antibodies that were reactive with virtually all the major antigens of HIV-1 detectable by this technique: gp160, gp120, p55, gp41, p27, p24, and p17. However, this sample represented only a rare positive reactor in a high-risk group of individuals exposed to venereal infections and AIDS-like illnesses in a region of central Africa that is now known to have high rates of infection with HIV-1. Yet only 1% or less of the individuals tested from what is now classified as a region of moderate to high prevalence—Kinshasa, Zaire—were positive, which suggests that the virus was then only rarely present in places that would now be classified as within the AIDS belt of Africa (see Table 1–2). Again,

this suggested that HIV-1 or a virus very similar to it recently moved to the cities of this region of Africa, and we could speculate that the virus had either moved from subhuman primates to people just prior to the mid-1950s or had been introduced to cities through the migration of a few resistant carriers from a previously isolated tribe or tribes. Population redistribution was occurring at that time, with movement of previously isolated people to newly expanding cities. Still, it seems unlikely that HIV-1 would have been present, as such, for many generations in isolated tribal regions. If this were so, we might expect to find Africans who show greater resistance to infection and disease development, owing to genetic evolution of the human species. In prospective studies conducted to date, exposed Africans appear to develop clinical AIDS and other signs and symptoms of HIV disease as rapidly as individuals in the United States or Europe.[63] Furthermore, as mentioned above, the degree of genomic variation seen in African isolates of HIV-1 is generally greater than that seen in isolates in Europe or the United States.

A virus that could be a progenitor of HIV-1 was recently isolated from a chimpanzee in central Africa.[64] This finding, combined with the knowledge that all HIV-1 viruses tested appear to be avirulent when inoculated into chimpanzees, is also compatible with a subhuman primate origin for HIV-1. Some African isolates of HIV-1 appear to be as close to the chimpanzee isolate as to other prototype strains of HIV-1.[65]

HIV-RELATED RETROVIRUSES OF MONKEYS

Soon after the recognition of clinical AIDS in people, several clinical reports described outbreaks of severe infections, wasting disease, and death in several colonies of Asian macaques housed at primate centers in the United States.[66,67] Such diseases were subsequently designated simian AIDS, or SAIDS. As in the case of human AIDS, numerous possible causes were considered. Following the recognition that SAIDS appeared to be of infectious origin, cytomegalovirus of monkeys was also considered as a possible etiologic agent.

We investigated the possibility that rhesus monkeys and related species with SAIDS housed at the New England Regional Primate Research Center might be infected with T-lymphotropic retroviruses related to HIV, because several other exogenous retroviruses had been found in subhuman primates, including the Mason-Pfizer type D virus of rhesus,[68] the gibbon ape leukemia virus,[69] and related simian sarcoma virus found in a wooly monkey,[70] and the recently described STLV in numerous Old World species.[36,39] Seroepidemiologic screening revealed that a proportion of the SAIDS monkeys had antibodies that cross-reacted with HIV,[71] while healthy rhesus monkeys had no such antibodies. Although the antibodies cross-reacted with core antigens of HIV-1, they showed only very weak cross-reactivity

Table 1–2. Estimates of Representative Seroprevalence Rates for HIV-1 and HIV-2 in Healthy Adults in West and Central Africa

Region	Country	Seropositivity Rate (%) HIV-1	Seropositivity Rate (%) HIV-2
Central Africa	Angola	1–5	1–5
	Burundi	>10	<1
	Congo	1–5	<1
	Kenya	5–10	<1
	Malawi	>10	<1
	Mozambique	1–5	1–5
	Uganda	>10	<1
	Zaire	5–10	<1
	Zambia	>10	<1
West Africa	Benin	<1	<1
	Burkina Faso	1–5	1–5
	Cape Verde	<1	1–5
	Guinea Bissau	<1	5–10
	Ivory Coast	5–10	1–5
	Senegal	<1	1–5

with the envelope antigens. However, the same antibody-positive rhesus sera reacted well with putative virus envelope antigens in reverse transcriptase–containing cultures of indicator human T4 cells cocultivated with buffy coat lymphocytes from antibody-positive monkeys.[71] Further characterization of the cultures revealed the presence of type C virus–like particles, and antigens detectable with antibodies from either SAIDS monkeys or people with AIDS. The sizes of the protein antigens detected by radioimmunoprecipitation were similar to those of HIV-1. This primate virus was named STLV-III because of its relationship to HIV-1 (which was then called HTLV-III and/or LAV), and later simian immunodeficiency virus, SIV, or SIV-2.[72] When SIV antigens were tested with sera from people with AIDS or healthy carriers, virtually all sera had antibodies to core antigens.

At the same time, studies were conducted with colonized rhesus monkeys with SAIDS, wild-caught and colony-maintained African green monkeys (*Cercopithicus aethiops*), and other African monkey species (see Table 1–1). These studies were undertaken because human AIDS, while clearly present in Africa, had not yet been found in people in Asia. In a serologic survey, 20% to 70% of different groups of wild-caught African green monkeys were found to be seropositive.[45,73] These included monkeys from the eastern region of sub-Saharan Africa—extending from Ethiopia to South Africa—and from Senegal, in the western region of sub-Saharan Africa. Wild-caught African green monkeys were seropositive even more often than colony-maintained animals of the same species. Although baboons were seronegative, species closely related to the African green monkey (also termed genons and vervets), such as the mangabey, the diana monkey, and the mona monkey, were also infected with an agent that was serologically related to SIV.

Unlike captive rhesus monkeys, whose SIV infection was associated with SAIDS, African green monkeys infected with SIV appeared to remain healthy. Captive African green monkeys infected with SIV, unlike macaques, revealed no disease symptoms. In addition, at least half of the healthy wild-caught African green monkeys showed evidence of exposure to SIV on the basis of antibodies. Although the possibility that SIV caused an unusual case of disease in this species could not be ruled out, especially if the disease occurred after reproductive life, it seemed clear that SIV was not closely linked to an immunosuppressive syndrome in African green monkeys as it was in macaques. It was clear, for example, that the African green monkey species was thriving despite the massive losses imposed by humans using it as a source of food.

As with STLV and HTLV, the possibility that SIV might cause disease rarely in African green monkeys in advanced age could not be ruled out. Yet it was clear that this species had evolved a resistance such that the virus did not cause severe disease as it did in rhesus monkeys, and as HIV-1 did in people. In the case of HTLV and STLV, it appeared that evolutionary adaptation had selected for a virus of low virulence. It is more difficult to postulate why SIV in African monkeys apparently does not cause disease, while a closely related virus does cause disease in macaques. In fact, since wild macaques do not appear to be infected with SIV, and because the virus is limited to a small set of African primates, it appears likely that the virus accidently infected captive rhesus monkeys quite recently. One possible explanation is that African species evolved to manifest immune resistance, while the virus itself retained its virulence and causes symptoms only when it infects a species with no previous experience with the virus, such as the macaque. This explanation is also compatible with the widespread distribution of the virus in a high proportion of African monkeys. However, it may seem surprising that a virus that had coexisted for this long with the African green monkey species was not widely distributed in more species of Old World primates. And in one species in which an SIV-related virus is present—humans in west Africa (see below)—this virus does not appear to be frequently associated with highly lethal disease.

More recent studies revealed that the SIV present in macaques and mangabeys is closest to the best characterized strains of HIV-2 from west African people. Whereas the macaque virus may have come from human materials experimentally inoculated into laboratory animals, the mangabey virus is more likely to be a potential source of infection in humans, because its range includes West Africa.[74] To date, however, most mangabey studies have been done with captive animals, sometimes also including animals that were inoculated with materials from macaques and/or people.

Recent studies also revealed that African green monkeys themselves have a number of subtypes of SIVs, depending on the superspecies of monkey and the geographic location.[75,76] As a group, these SIVs are more closely related to HIV-2 than to HIV-1.[43,76] Whether some green monkeys endemic to west Africa might also have a subtype of SIV that is even more highly related to HIV-2 remains to be determined. An SIV of a distinctly different type was recently identified in a mandrill, and it seems likely that new viruses in the spectrum of SIVs will be identified in other African monkeys.[77]

HIV-2

Because a relative of HIV-1—SIV—had been found in wild African primates and was only about 50% related to HIV-1 at the genomic level, it seemed logical that viruses more highly related to SIV might also be present in human populations. Serum samples from west African prostitutes were examined to determine if they had antibodies that were more highly cross-reactive with SIV than with HIV-1.[78] West Africa was chosen because at that time it was largely free of HIV-1 and clinical AIDS, and female prostitutes were selected because they are at high risk for infection with sexually transmitted viruses.

Through Western blot techniques, it became clear that a significant proportion of Senegalese prostitutes had antibodies that were highly reactive with all the major antigens of SIV detected by this technique.[46] These included the *gag*-encoded p24, the *pol*-encoded p64/53 and p34, and the *env* gene–encoded transmembrane protein p34. Yet when the same SIV antigens were reacted by Western blotting with sera from HIV-1–infected individuals of either European or central African origin with classic disease manifestations, little or no reaction was seen with the transmembrane protein. Because the transmembrane protein of SIV is usually smaller than the comparable protein of HIV-1, this is manifested as the loss of reactivity where it might be expected at gp41 and the acquisition of reactivity with gp32, the carboxy terminus peptide of the *env* gene of SIV.[46] The class of reactivity seen with serum samples from west African prostitutes was in fact virtually indistinguishable from that seen with serum samples from African monkeys or captive rhesus. Similar results were also obtained by radioimmunoprecipitation, except that this procedure readily detects the gp120 amino terminus *env* glycoprotein that is often missed by Western blotting. In this case, serum samples from the west African prostitutes reacted very well with the gp120 and gp160 of SIV, but reacted only infrequently and quite weakly with the gp120 and gp160 of HIV-1.[78]

With evidence that a virus more closely related to SIV than to HIV-1 was present in a number of Senegalese prostitutes, more extensive studies were undertaken to determine if the SIV-related virus was more widely distributed in Africa, particularly in west Africa. The screening of more than 2,000 high-risk individuals from central Africa, including many individuals with AIDS and other sexually transmitted diseases, revealed no evidence that HIV-2 was present in the same regions in which HIV-1 was rampant (see Table 1–2).[79] However, pockets of infection with HIV-2 were detected in Mozambique and Angola, which, though distant from west Africa, are often on the same trade routes as Guinea Bissau and Cape Verde, west African countries with some of the highest rates of infection.[80] Within Senegal, prevalence rates for HIV-2 are substantially higher in the southern region of Casamance, which borders Guinea Bissau, than in the northern region.[81]

Infection with HIV-2 is substantially higher in female prostitutes than in other population groups,[80] indicating that this virus is also sexually transmitted. However, HIV-2 appears to be transmitted less efficiently than HIV-1, by both perinatal and sexual transmission.[82] Analysis of circulating lymphocytes by PCR techniques reveals that most HIV-2–infected carriers have lower proportions of infected cells than HIV-1–infected carriers, and/or fewer copies of proviral genomes per infected cell.[83] As with the infrequently pathogenic HTLV-1, but not the highly virulent HIV-1,[81] the age-specific prevalence for HIV-2 increases with increasing age. This

presumably happens because relatively few HIV-2–infected people are lost from the population due to death.

These observations suggest that HIV-2 is less virulent than HIV-1. The relatively low proportion of HIV-2–infected individuals with immunosuppression-associated diseases that are endemic to their region, such as tuberculosis, supports this hypothesis.[80] However, case reports and cross-sectional studies have clearly revealed some cases of HIV-2–associated AIDS.[84–87] The apparent reduction in the number of cases of HIV-2–associated AIDS also led to suggestions that HIV-2 was introduced into people more recently than HIV-1; thus, most infected people would not yet be infected long enough to develop disease. This theory was recently ruled out, however, because older stored blood samples have shown antibodies to HIV-2,[88] and HIV-2 actually appears to have been present in Senegal much longer than HIV-1, even though disease rates are higher for HIV-1.[82,89]

A recently analyzed, prospective study of commercial sex workers in West Africa infected with HIV-1 and HIV-2 revealed that HIV-1–infected individuals developed AIDS about 12 times more frequently than HIV-2–infected individuals in the same cohort. HIV-2–infected people also had T4-lymphocyte values that were intermediate between the normal values of uninfected people and the much reduced numbers of T4 cells seen in HIV-1–infected people. Similar results were obtained following skin testing for anergy to purified protein derivative.

Although HIV-2 can also cause AIDS, it appears to be less virulent than HIV-1. Whether the lesser virulence arises from HIV-2 causing less severe disease after a longer induction period in most infected people, or no disease at all in most, remains to be determined.

CONCLUSIONS

A large family of HIV-related retroviruses is present in humans and monkeys in sub-Saharan Africa. All members of this family have the same complex genomic structure, share at least 40% to 50% homology, and infect T lymphocytes through the CD4 receptor.

Although both HIV-1 and HIV-2 appear to have entered the human population several decades ago, HIV-1 is more virulent than HIV-2. Numerous SIV-type viruses are present at high rates in African green monkeys, in which they appear to cause little or no disease. Although SIV in African green monkeys is more closely related to HIV-2 than to HIV-1, the viruses in mangabeys and macaques are the closest relatives of HIV-2. The macaque virus also appears to have originated from either a human or an African monkey source, as Asian primates show no evidence of natural infection. A chimpanzee virus, more related to HIV-1 than to HIV-2, was also identified in Africa. It seems likely that additional HIV progenitor viruses will be identified in African primates. Understanding how subhuman primates naturally resist disease from HIV-related viruses should facilitate the development of new ways to treat and prevent HIV disease in people.

REFERENCES

1. Gottlieb MS, Schroff R, Schanker HM et al: *Pneumocystis carinii* pneumonia and mucosal candidiasis in previously healthy homosexual men: Evidence of a new acquired cellular immunodeficiency. N Engl J Med 305:1425, 1981

2. Masur H, Michelis MA, Greene JB et al: An outbreak of community-acquired *Pneumocystis carinii* pneumonia: Initial manifestation of cellular immune dysfunction. N Engl J Med 305:1431, 1981

3. Seigal FP, Lopez C, Hammer GS et al: Severe acquired immunodeficiency in male homosexuals, manifested by chronic perianal ulcerative herpes simplex lesions. N Engl J Med 305:1439, 1981

4. Centers for Disease Control: Centers for Disease Control Task Force on Kaposi's sarcoma and opportunistic infections. N Engl J Med 306:248, 1982

5. Davis KC, Horsburgh CR Jr, Hasiba U et al: Acquired immunodeficiency syndrome in a patient with hemophilia. Ann Intern Med 98:284, 1983

6. Poon MC, Landay A, Prasthofer EF et al: Acquired immunodeficiency syndrome with *Pneumocystis carinii* pneumonia and *Mycobacterium avium-intracellulare* infection in a previously healthy patient with classic hemophilia: Clinical, immunologic, and virologic findings. Ann Intern Med 98:287, 1983

7. Elliot JL, Hoppes WL, Platt MS et al: The acquired immunodeficiency syndrome and *Mycobacterium avium-intracellulare* bacteremia in a patient with hemophilia. Ann Intern Med 98:290, 1983

8. Curran JW, Lawrence DN, Jaffe H et al: Acquired immunodeficiency syndrome (AIDS) associated with transfusions. N Engl J Med 310:69, 1984

9. Jaffe HW, Francis DP, McLane MF et al: Transfusion-associated AIDS: Serologic evidence of human T-cell leukemia virus infection of donors. Science 223:1309, 1984

10. Piot P, Quinn TC, Taelman H et al: Acquired immunodeficiency syndrome in a heterosexual population in Zaire. Lancet 2:65, 1984

11. Van de Perre P, Rouvroy D, Lepage P et al: Acquired immunodeficiency syndrome in Rwanda. Lancet 2:62, 1984

12. Clumeck N, Mascart Lemone F, de Maubeuge J et al: Acquired immune deficiency syndrome in black Africans. Lancet 1:642, 1983

13. Rubinstein A, Sicklick M, Gupta A et al: Acquired immunodeficiency with reversed T4/T8 ratios in infants born to promiscuous and drug-addicted mothers. JAMA 249:2350, 1983

14. Oleske J, Minnefor A, Cooper R Jr et al: Immune deficiency syndrome in children. JAMA 249:2345, 1983

15. Scott GB, Buck BE, Leterman JG et al: Acquired immunodeficiency syndrome in infants. N Engl J Med 310:76, 1984

16. Francis DP, Curran JW, Essex M: Epidemic acquired immune deficiency syndrome (AIDS): Epidemiologic evidence for a transmitted agent. JNCI 71:1, 1983

17. Rogers MF, Morens DM, Stewart JA et al: National case-control study of Kaposi's sarcoma and *Pneumocystis carinii* pneumonia in homosexual men: Part 2. Laboratory results. Ann Intern Med 99:151, 1983

18. Essex M, McLane MF, Lee TH et al: Antibodies to cell membrane antigens associated with human T-cell leukemia virus in patients with AIDS. Science 220:859, 1983

19. Essex M, McLane MF, Lee TH et al: Antibodies to human T-cell leukemia virus membrane antigens (HTLV-MA) in hemophiliacs. Science 221:1061, 1983

20. Gelmann EP, Popovic M, Blayney D et al: Proviral DNA of a retrovirus, human T-cell leukemia virus, in two patients with AIDS. Science 220:862, 1983

21. Gallo RC, Sarin PS, Gelmann EP et al: Isolation of human T-cell leukemia virus in acquired immune deficiency syndrome (AIDS). Science 220:865, 1983

22. Barre-Sinoussi F, Chermann J-C, Rey F et al: Isolation of T-lymphotropic retrovirus from a patient at risk for acquired immune deficiency syndrome (AIDS). Science 220:868, 1983

23. Poiesz BJ, Ruscetti FW, Gazdar AF et al: Detection and isolation of type C retrovirus particles from fresh and cultured lymphocytes of a patient with cutaneous T-cell lymphoma. Proc Natl Acad Sci USA 77:7415, 1980

24. Ammann AJ, Abrams D, Conant M et al: Acquired immune dysfunction in homosexual men: Immunologic profiles. Clin Immunol Immunopathol 27:315, 1983

25. Fahey JL, Prince H, Weaver M et al: Quantitative changes in T helper or T suppressor/cytotoxic lymphocyte subsets that distinguish acquired immune deficiency syndrome from other immune subset disorders. Am J Med 76:95, 1984

26. Lane HC, Masur H, Gelmann EP et al: Correlation between immunologic function and clinical subpopulations of patients with the acquired immune deficiency syndrome. Am J Med 78:417, 1985

27. Essex M: Adult T-cell leukemia/lymphoma: Role of a human retrovirus. JNCI 69:981, 1982

28. Essex M: Horizontally and vertically transmitted oncornavirus of cats. Adv Cancer Res 21:175, 1975

29. Essex M, McLane MF, Tachibana N et al: Seroepidemiology of HTLV in relation to immunosuppression and the acquired immunodeficiency syndrome. In Gallo RC, Essex M, Gross L (eds): Human T-cell Leukemia Viruses, p 355. Cold Spring Harbor, New York, Cold Spring Harbor Press, 1984

30. Kalyanaraman VS, Sarngadharan MG, Robert-Guroff M et al: A new subtype of human T-cell leukemia virus (HTLV-II) associated with a T-cell variant of hairy cell leukemia. Science 218:571, 1982

31. Popovic M, Sarngadharan MG, Read E et al: Detection, isolation, and continuous production of cytopathic retroviruses (HTLV-III) from patients with AIDS and pre-AIDS. Science 224:497, 1984

32. Gallo RC, Salahuddin SZ, Popovic M et al: Frequent detection and isolation of cytopathic retroviruses (HTLV-III) from patients with AIDS and at risk for AIDS. Science 224:500, 1984

33. Schupbach J, Popovic M, Gilden RV et al: Serological analysis of a subgroup of human T-lymphotropic retroviruses (HTLV-III) associated with AIDS. Science 224:503, 1984

34. Sarngadharan MG, Popovic M, Bruch L et al: Antibodies reactive with human T-lymphotropic retroviruses (HTLV-III) in the serum of patients with AIDS. Science 224:506, 1984

35. Gallo RC, Sliski AH, de Noronha CM et al: Origins of human T-lymphotropic viruses. Nature 320:219, 1986

36. Miyoshi I, Yoshimoto S, Fujishita M et al: Natural adult T-cell leukemia virus infection in Japanese monkeys. Lancet 2:658, 1982

37. Saxinger CW, Lange-Wantzin G, Thomsen K et al: Human T-cell leukemia virus: A diverse family of related exogenous retroviruses of humans and old world primates. In Gallo RC, Essex ME, Gross L (eds): Human T-cell Leukemia/Lymphoma Virus, p 323. Cold Spring Harbor, New York, Cold Spring Harbor Press, 1984

38. Guo HG, Wong-Staal F, Gallo RC: Novel viral sequences related to human T-cell leukemia virus in T cells of a seropositive baboon. Science 223:1195, 1984

39. Homma T, Kanki PJ, King NW Jr et al: Lymphoma in macaques: Association with exposure to virus of human T lymphotropic family. Science 225:716, 1984

40. Hayami M, Komuro A, Nozawa K et al: Prevalence of antibody to adult T-cell leukemia virus-associated antigens (ATLA) in Japanese monkeys and other nonhuman primates. Int J Cancer 33:179, 1984

41. Watanabe T, Seiki M, Hirayama Y et al: Human T-cell leukemia virus type I is a member of the African subtype of simian viruses (STLV). Virology 148:385, 1986

42. Alizon M, Wain-Hobson S, Montagnier L et al: Genetic variability of the AIDS virus: Nucleotide sequence analysis of two isolates from African patients. Cell 46:63, 1986

43. Myers G, Pavlakis GN: Evolutionary potential of complex retroviruses. In Wagner RR, Fraenkel-Cowat H (eds): Viruses. The Retroviridae (J Levy, ed). New York, Plenum Press, in press

44. Essex M, Kanki P: Origins of the AIDS virus. Sci Am 259: 64, 1988

45. Kanki PJ, Kurth R, Becker W et al: Antibodies to simian T-lymphotropic virus type III in African green monkeys and recognition of STLV-III viral proteins by AIDS and related sera. Lancet 1:1330, 1985

46. Barin F, Mboup S, Denis F et al: Serological evidence for a virus related to simian T-lymphotropic retrovirus III in residents of West Africa. Lancet 2:1387, 1985

47. Clavel F, Mansinho K, Charmaret S et al: Human immunodeficiency virus type 2 infection associated with AIDS in West Africa. N Engl J Med 316:1180, 1987

48. Marlink RG, Ricard D, Mboup S et al: Clinical, hematologic, and immunologic cross-sectional evaluation of individuals exposed to human immunodeficiency virus type 2 (HIV-2). AIDS Res Hum Retroviruses 4:137, 1988

49. Bebenek K, Abbotts J, Roberts JD et al: Specificity and mechanisms of error-prone replication by human immunodeficiency virus-1 reverse transcriptase. J Biol Chem 264:16948, 1989

50. Smith TF, Srinivasan A, Schochetman G et al: The phylogenetic history of immunodeficiency viruses. Nature 333: 573, 1988

51. Nahmias AJ, Weiss J, Yao X et al: Evidence for human infection with an HTLV-III/LAV-like virus in Central Africa, 1959. Lancet 1:1278, 1986

52. MMWR, Jan 18, 1991, p 21

53. Goodenow M, Huet T, Saurin W et al: HIV-1 isolates are rapidly evolving quadrispecies: Evidence for viral mixtures and preferred nucleotide substitutions. J AIDS 2:344, 1989

54. Balfe P, Simmonds P, Ludlam CA et al: Concurrent evolution of human immunodeficiency virus type 1 in patients infected from the same source: Rate of sequence change

and low frequency of inactivating mutations. J Virol 64: 6221, 1990

55. Delassus S, Cheynier R, Wain-Hobson S: Evolution of the HIV-1 *nef* and LTR sequences over a four year period *in vivo* and *in vitro*. J Virol 65:225, 1991

56. Issel CJ, Montelaro RC, Foil LD: Virology of equine retroviruses. In Salzman LA (ed): Animal Models of Retrovirus Infection and Their Relationship to AIDS, p 95. Orlando, Fla, Academic Press, 1986

57. Rayfield M, de Cock K, Heyward W et al: Mixed human immunodeficiency virus (HIV) infection in an individual: Demonstration of both HIV type 1 and type 2 proviral sequences by using polymerase chain reaction. J Infect Dis 158:1170, 1988

58. Evans LA, Odehouri K, Thomson-Honnebier G et al: Simultaneous isolation of HIV-1 and HIV-2 from an AIDS patient. Lancet 2:1389, 1988

59. Denis F, Barin F, Gershy-Damet G et al: Prevalence of human T-lymphotropic retroviruses type III (HIV) and type IV in Ivory Coast. Lancet 1:408, 1987

60. Schwartz S, Felber BK, Benko DM et al: Cloning and functional analysis of multiply spliced mRNA species of human immunodeficiency virus type 1. J Virol 64:2519, 1990

61. Schwartz S, Felber BK, Fenyo E et al: Env and vpu proteins of human immunodeficiency virus type 1 are produced from multiple bicistronic mRNAs. J Virol 64:5448, 1990

62. Korber B, Okayama A, Donnelly R et al: PCR analysis of defective human T-cell leukemia virus type 1 (HTLV-I) proviral genomes in adult T cell leukemia. J Virol 65: 5471, 1991

63. Mann JM, Bila K, Colebunders RL et al: Natural history of human immunodeficiency virus infection in Zaire. Lancet 2:707, 1986

64. Huet T, Cheynier R, Meyerhaus A et al: Genetic organization of a chimpanzee lentivirus related to HIV-1. Nature 345:356, 1990

65. de Leys R, Vanderborght B, Haesevelde MV et al: Isolation and partial characterization of an unusual human immunodeficiency retrovirus from two persons of West-Central African origin. J Virol 64:1207, 1990

66. Letvin NL, Eaton KA, Aldrich WR et al: Acquired immunodeficiency syndrome in a colony of macaque monkeys. Proc Natl Acad Sci USA 80:2718, 1983

67. Henrickson RV, Maul DH, Osborn KG et al: Epidemic of acquired immunodeficiency in rhesus monkeys. Lancet 1:338, 1983

68. Chopra HC, Mason MM: A new virus in a spontaneous mammary tumor of a rhesus monkey. Cancer Res 30:2081, 1970

69. Kawakami TG, Huff SD, Buckley PM et al: C-type virus associated with gibbon lymphosarcoma. Nature New Biol 235:170, 1972

70. Theilen GH, Gould D, Fowler M et al: C-type virus in tumor tissue of a woolly monkey (*Lagothrix* spp.) with fibrosarcoma. JNCI 47:881, 1971

71. Kanki PJ, McLane MF, King NW Jr et al: Serologic identification and characterization of a macaque T-lymphotropic retrovirus closely related to human T-lymphotropic retroviruses (HTLV) type III. Science 228:1199, 1985

72. Biberfeld G, Brown F, Esparza J et al: WHO working group on characterization of HIV-related retroviruses: Criteria for characterization and proposal for a nomenclature system. AIDS 1:189, 1987

73. Kanki PJ, Alroy J, Essex M: Isolation of T-lymphotropic

retrovirus related to HTLV-III/LAV from wild-caught African green monkeys. Science 230:951, 1985

74. Hirsch VM, Olmsted RA, Murphey-Corb M et al: An African primate lentivirus (SIV) closely related to HIV-2. Nature 339:389, 1989

75. Johnson PR, Fornsgaard A, Allan J et al: Simian immunodeficiency viruses from African green monkeys display unusual genetic diversity. J Virol 64:1086, 1990

76. Allan JS, Short M, Taylor ME et al: Species-specific diversity among simian immunodeficiency viruses from African green monkeys. J Virol 65:2816, 1991

77. Tsujimoto H, Hasegawa A, Maki N et al: Sequence of a novel simian immunodeficiency virus from a wild-caught African mandril. Nature 341:539, 1989

78. Kanki PJ, Barin F, Mboup S et al: New human T-lymphotropic retrovirus related to Simian T-lymphotropic virus type III$_{AGM}$ (STLV-III$_{AGM}$). Science 232:238, 1986

79. Kanki PJ, Allan J, Barin F et al: Absence of antibodies to HIV-2/HTLV-4 in six central African nations. AIDS Res Hum Retroviruses 3:317, 1987

80. Kanki PJ, Mboup S, Ricard D et al: Human T-lymphotropic virus type 4 and the human immunodeficiency virus in west Africa. Science 236:827, 1987

81. Kanki PJ, Marlink R, Siby T et al: Biology of HIV-2 infection in west Africa. In Papas T (ed): Gene Regulation and AIDS, p 255. Houston, Texas, Portfolio Publishing Company of Texas, 1990

82. Kanki PJ, Mboup S, Marlink R et al: Prevalence of human immunodeficiency virus type 2 (HIV-2) and human immunodeficiency virus type 1 (HIV-1) in west African female prostitutes (Submitted)

83. Korber B, Kanki P, Barin F et al: Genetic and antigenic variability in different HIV-2 viral isolates. In Chermann J-C, Barre-Sinoussi F (eds): IVth International Conference on AIDS Associated Cancers in Africa, p 170. Paris, France, FRAMACOM, 1989

84. Poulsen AG, Aaby P, Fredericksen K et al: Prevalence of and mortality from human immunodeficiency virus type-2 in Bissau, west Africa. Lancet 1:827, 1989

85. Naucler A, Albino P, da Silva AP et al: HIV-2 infection in hospitalized patients in Bissau, Guinea-Bissau, AIDS 5:301, 1990

86. Romieu I, Marlink R, Kanki P et al: HIV-2 Link to AIDS in West Africa. J AIDS 3:220, 1990

87. Le Guenno BM, Barabe P, Griffet PA et al: HIV-2 and HIV-1 AIDS cases in Senegal: Clinical patterns and immunological perturbations. J AIDS 4:421, 1991

88. Kawamura M, Yamazaki S, Ishikawa K et al: HIV-2 in west Africa in 1966. Lancet 1:385, 1989

89. Marlink R, Kanki PJ, Mboup S et al: Reduced virulence of HIV-2 compared to HIV-1 (Submitted)

2

Etiology of AIDS: Biology of Human Retroviruses

Ruth I. Connor   *David D. Ho*

The human immunodeficiency virus (HIV), previously known as lymphadenopathy-associated virus (LAV), human T-cell lymphotropic virus type III (HTLV-III), or AIDS-related virus (ARV), is an RNA virus that belongs to the lentivirus family of nononcogenic, cytopathic retroviruses.[1] HIV shares morphologic, biologic, and molecular properties with prototypic animal lentiviruses, including visna virus, caprine arthritis encephalitis virus, and equine infectious anemia virus.[2–5] Like HIV in humans, these viruses cause slow progressive wasting disorders, including neurodegeneration, that are often fatal.[6,7] On the basis of viral protein cross-reactivity and sequence similarity, HIV-1 is very closely related to the primate retrovirus, simian immunodeficiency virus (SIV).[8–11] SIVmac causes a form of simian AIDS in captive macaques, whereas SIV sooty mangabey (SIVsm) and African green monkey (SIVagm) are nonpathogenic in their respective hosts.[12,13] HIV-1 also shares sequence homology and serologic reactivity with another group of human T-cell lymphotropic retroviruses referred to as HIV-2, which were first isolated from west Africans.[14–16] HIV-2 is clearly associated with immunodeficiency and a clinical syndrome similar to AIDS[17,18]; however, it may be less pathogenic than HIV-1.

The HIV-1 virion is slightly more than 100 nm in diameter and on electron microscopy appears as a dense cylindrical core surrounded by a lipid envelope (Fig. 2–1A). The virion core is comprised of structural proteins encoded by the HIV-1 *gag* gene, the RNA genome, and virally encoded enzymes, including reverse transcriptase and integrase, which are required for efficient viral replication (Fig. 2–1B). The RNA genome is approximately 10 kilo-base pairs in length and is characterized by the presence of two flanking long terminal repeat (LTR) sequences as well as genes encoding core

proteins (*gag*), reverse-transcriptase/protease/endonuclease enzymes (*pol*), and envelope glycoproteins (*env*) (Fig. 2–2). Unlike other nonprimate retroviruses, the HIV-1 genome contains at least six additional genes, three of which (*tat, rev, nef*) are believed to function in the regulation of virus replication.

LIFE CYCLE

The CD4 Receptor

Mature T lymphocytes can be divided into two subsets on the basis of selective expression of either CD4 or CD8 surface glycoproteins.[19] T lymphocytes bearing CD8 interact with a broad range of cells expressing class I major histocompatibility complex (MHC) gene products, while CD4+ T lymphocytes associate with a more restricted group of cells bearing class II MHC molecules.[20,21] Interaction of CD4− and CD8-bearing cells with specific MHC gene products is essential in the maturation and efficient activation of T lymphocytes, and in shaping the T-cell repertoire during thymic development.[22] Within the framework of the immune system, CD4+ cells recognize peptide antigens through a T-cell receptor (TCR) in the context of class II MHC expressed on the antigen-presenting cell. It is postulated that CD4 serves as an adhesion molecule, binding a nonpolymorphic region of class II antigens and thereby stabilizing the MHC class II–TCR complex.[23,24] However, interaction with CD4 on the cell surface has been shown to trigger signal transduction through the p56[lck] tyrosine kinase,[25] suggesting a more active role for CD4 in the regulation of T-cell activation.

Evidence that CD4 also serves as the cellular receptor for HIV-1 was first suggested by the selective and

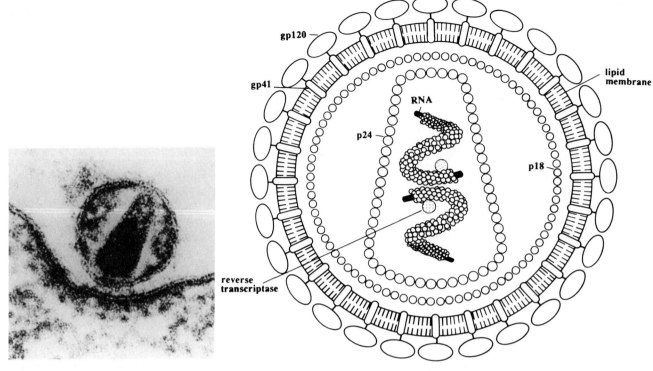

Figure 2–1. (**A**) An electron micrograph of the HIV-1 virion. The characteristic dark, cylindrical core is surrounded by a lipid envelope, which is acquired as the virion buds from the surface of an infected cell. (Photo courtesy of H. Gelderblom.) (**B**) A schematic diagram of the components of the HIV-1 virion, including the envelope glycoproteins (gp120 and gp41), the nucleocapsid proteins (p24 and p18), the RNA genome and associated reverse transcriptase (Modified from Gallo RC, Montagnier L: AIDS in 1988. Scient Amer 4:41, 1988).

progressive depletion of CD4+ T lymphocytes in patients with acquired immunodeficiency syndrome (AIDS), indicating a specific tropism of the virus for cells bearing the CD4 surface antigen.[26] Consistent with this possibility, monoclonal antibodies (mAb) to CD4 were shown to block cell infection, indicating the in-

volvement of CD4 in some part of the viral replication cycle.[27–29] In addition, treatment of uninfected cells with anti-CD4 mAb inhibited their binding to HIV-1–infected cells and blocked the formation of multinucleated giant cells or syncytia.[27] Antibodies to CD4 were also shown to block infection of susceptible cells with a pseudotype

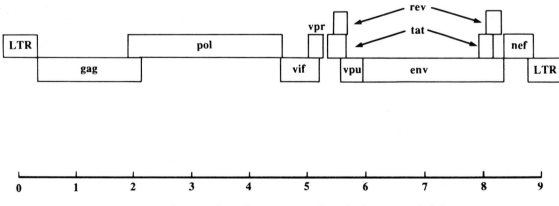

Figure 2–2. HIV-1 genome. The gene length is expressed on the bottom in kilobases.

of vesicular stomatitis virus–bearing HIV-1 envelope antigens,[27] indicating the specific interaction of CD4 with viral proteins. Definitive evidence of the role of CD4 as the receptor for HIV-1 was obtained by the successful coprecipitation of a receptor-virus complex consisting of the CD4 molecule and a 110-kilodalton (kD) viral protein.[30]

The mature CD4 protein is a 55-kD molecule composed of four tandem immunoglobulin-like extracellular regions (designated V1 through V4), a transmembrane region, and a cytoplasmic segment.[31] The availability of the gene encoding CD4 has enabled a more detailed examination of the interaction of this molecule with specific viral proteins and allowed further determination of its role in the pathogenesis of AIDS. Studies by Maddon et al[32] demonstrate that the introduction of the gene encoding CD4 and subsequent expression of this molecule on the surface of both lymphoid and nonlymphoid human cells is sufficient to render them susceptible to infection with HIV-1. Moreover, virus was shown to bind specifically to transformed cells expressing CD4, indicating that HIV-1 interaction with cell-surface CD4 represents an initial event in the viral life cycle. This view was supported by the discovery that a soluble, truncated form of CD4 lacking the transmembrane and cytoplasmic regions could effectively block virus attachment to the cell and inhibit both virus replication and syncytia formation.[33–38] Interestingly, however, murine cells transfected with the gene encoding human CD4 were able to bind HIV-1 but remained refractory to infection, an observation which suggested that additional factors may be required for viral entry.[32]

Delineation of the site on CD4 involved in HIV-1 binding was initially carried out using a panel of anti-CD4 mAb to block HIV infection and syncytia formation.[39] By this method, a binding domain was identified and defined by a cluster of mAb including Leu-3a. Phenotypic analysis of CD4 expressed on nonhuman primate cells also identified a single, consistently conserved epitope recognized by Leu-3a.[40] The ability of a truncated, soluble form of CD4 (sCD4) containing only the first two N-terminal immunoglobulin-like domains to block HIV-1 infection in susceptible target cells suggested that the domain involved in viral binding was located within this region of the CD4 molecule.[37,41]

The generation of specific mutations in the CD4 molecule has allowed more definitive mapping of the residues involved in HIV-1 recognition.[42–44] Studies by Peterson and Seed[42] identified several point mutations in the cDNA encoding CD4 that resulted in amino acid substitutions which restricted or destroyed the capacity of HIV-1 to interact with CD4. These changes were localized to an eight-residue segment in a portion of the molecule corresponding to the CD4 V1 domain. The importance of the V1 domain in HIV-1 binding was substantiated in studies using human/mouse chimeric CD4 proteins.[45,46] Although human and mouse CD4 share moderate sequence homology, murine CD4 fails to bind HIV-1 gp120. Chimeric molecules containing both human and mouse sequences were used to identify the amino terminal immunoglobulin-like domain of human CD4 as critical for gp120 binding.[45] Subsequent studies revealed that substitution of as few as three nonconserved murine residues into the corresponding position of the human CD4 molecule was sufficient to abolish binding of HIV-1 gp120.[46] These residues were located within the V1 domain of CD4, with some contribution from the V2 domain. In studies by Arthos et al,[47] the V1 domain when expressed as a soluble, truncated derivative of CD4 was found to compete as efficiently as the entire extracellular segment for high-affinity binding to gp120. Consistent with earlier studies, mutational analysis identified a single site (residues 41 to 55) within the V1 domain containing determinants involved in gp120 binding.

The V1 domain of CD4 shares both amino acid and structural homology with the immunoglobulin κ light chain variable domain.[31] The location of two cysteine residues, separated by 67 amino acids, suggests the formation of an intrachain disulfide bond characteristic of variable region domains.[42,47] Exposure of sCD4 to conditions that disrupt the proper tertiary structure of the molecule results in loss of binding activity,[48,49] which suggests that the HIV-1 binding site on CD4 is conformationally determined. Mutations in regions of CD4 outside the V1 domain have been shown to decrease gp120 binding[44,46]; however, these changes may be attributable to indirect effects on the V1 domain as a result of more global conformational disruption, rather than to direct involvement of these regions in formation of the gp120 binding site.

Monoclonal antibodies that bind to regions of CD4 more proximal to the cell membrane have been shown to block infection and cell fusion without affecting virus binding.[50,51] One possibility is that these antibodies interfere with a step after binding but before virus entry, possibly as a result of steric interference with the fusogenic regions of the HIV-1 envelope glycoproteins. Mutations within the V1 region of CD4 have also been shown to disrupt syncytia formation without interfering with virus binding,[52] indicating that attachment of the virion to the target cell surface and subsequent membrane fusion events may be independently mediated by spatially distinct sites within the V1 domain of CD4. It is clear from these and other studies that CD4 may participate directly in both HIV-1 binding to the cell surface and membrane fusion; however, in most cases, the nature and extent of the domains involved in mediating these functions have yet to be fully defined.

Role of HIV-1 Envelope Glycoproteins

BINDING TO CD4

Attachment of HIV-1 requires successful interaction between CD4 expressed on the surface of the target cell and the viral envelope glycoprotein, gp120. As for other retroviruses, the envelope glycoproteins of HIV-1 are synthesized as a precursor polypeptide (gp160) that is subsequently glycosylated and cleaved to yield the external protein gp120 and the transmembrane protein gp41.[53-57] These envelope proteins are incorporated into the outer lipid bilayer of the virion in a typical spike-and-knob configuration, resulting in a pentamer-hexamer pattern of clustering with an estimated total of 72 protrusions per virion.[58-60] HIV-1 gp120 and gp41 are encoded by the *env* gene, which exhibits a high degree of sequence diversity among different isolates of HIV-1.[61,62] Despite this divergence, several highly conserved regions of the molecule have been identified and are believed to play an important role in virus binding to the CD4 receptor. Studies by Lasky *et al*[63] initially localized potential CD4 binding sites to the C-terminal fourth conserved region of gp120. Monoclonal antibodies to an epitope within this domain blocked the high-affinity (10^{-9} M) interaction between CD4 and gp120, which suggested that this region may be directly involved in HIV-1 binding to CD4. Mapping studies using anti-gp120 mAb[64-66] and site-directed mutagenesis[67,68] have since confirmed the importance of the C-terminal region of gp120 in CD4 binding and have identified the direct association of specific residues. In studies by Olshevsky *et al*,[68] single amino acid changes within the constant regions C2, C3, and C4 of HIV-1 gp120 were found to reduce CD4 binding without causing global conformational disruption of the molecule. Although spatially distinct, these residues may be brought together by the proper tertiary folding of the molecule to form a conformationally dependent binding site (Fig. 2–3).[69,70] These studies raise the possibility that the CD4 binding site on gp120 is more complex than was previously believed, possibility involving the direct association of multiple discontinuous determinants.

FUSION AND ENTRY

As part of the mature virion, gp120 remains associated with the transmembrane protein gp41 through noncovalent interactions mediated by hydrophobic regions at both ends of the gp120 molecule.[71] This heterodimeric complex is generated by the intracellular cleavage of the precursor protein gp160 during virus maturation. As has been shown for other enveloped viruses, tryptic cleavage of integral membrane proteins is a critical step in mediating subsequent fusion between viral and host cell membranes (reviewed by White *et al*[72]). Mutations that alter the endoproteolytic cleavage site of HIV-1 gp160 result in the production of mature virions that are morphologically indistinguishable from wild-type virus but are no longer infectious.[73,74] Characteristic of both orthomyxoviruses and paramyxoviruses, fusogenic activity is triggered by the generation of a novel N-terminal region on the transmembrane glycoprotein subunit following endoproteolytic cleavage.[72] Similar mechanisms may govern the entry of HIV-1 into susceptible target cells and may also mediate the cytopathic fusion of HIV-1 infected and uninfected cells. Indeed, mutations affecting the hydrophobic N-terminus of the

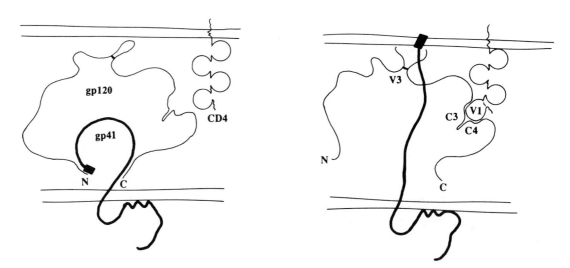

Figure 2–3. gp120/gp41 association and interaction with CD4. The CD4 molecule is shown at the top extending from the cell, and the lower structure shows the globular gp120 associated with the transmembrane gp41; C, carboxy terminus; N, amino terminus. The darkened block at the N-terminus of gp41 represents the fusion domain of gp41. In the second panel, the constant regions C3 and C4 of gp120 are shown interacting with the V1 domain of CD4, followed by a conformational change, cleavage of the V3 loop, activation of the fusion domain, and subsequent insertion into the cell membrane.

HIV-1 transmembrane glycoprotein gp41 have been shown to disrupt membrane fusion, altering not only viral entry but also affecting syncytia formation.[75-77]

Several studies have now identified a second domain necessary for fusion and infection located within a region of gp120 corresponding to the third variable region (V3). The V3 region forms a loop based on the presence of Cys residues at positions 301 and 336, and is the principal region involved in the induction of type-specific antibodies that neutralize HIV-1.[78-81] Although most of the amino acids of the V3 loop are extremely variable between different strains of HIV-1, a Gly-Pro-Gly-Arg sequence at the tip of the loop is highly conserved and forms the binding site for antibodies that block HIV-1 infection and inhibit the fusion of infected cells.[82,83] Studies by Freed et al[84] using site-directed mutagenesis demonstrated that single amino acid changes within the V3 loop region greatly reduced or abolished the ability of HIV-1 envelope glycoproteins to mediate syncytia formation, suggesting the importance of this region in a step leading to virus fusion. The precise nature of V3 involvement in virus-mediated fusion is not known; however, recent studies indicate that conserved sequences at the tip of the V3 loop contain sites that are sensitive to proteolytic cleavage.[85] Enhancement of cell fusion by proteolytic cleavage of envelope glycoproteins has been documented for other retroviruses,[86] including ecotropic murine retrovirus,[87] raising the possibility that additional cleavage of gp120 by cell surface proteinases may play a similar role in mediating HIV-1 fusion events.

Successful entry of HIV-1 is dependent on the introduction of the viral nucleocapsid core into the cytoplasm of susceptible target cells. Based on the appearance of virus particles within endosomal compartments, initial studies suggested that HIV-1 was internalized as a result of endocytosis of the receptor–virus complex into intracellular vesicles.[88] This pathway is utilized by several enveloped viruses, notably orthomyxoviruses, and is dependent on the low pH of acidic endosomes for efficient viral entry. However, compelling evidence now indicates that HIV-1 entry occurs by direct fusion of viral and host cell membranes.[89,90] In studies by Stein et al,[89] neutralization of the acidic pH in endosomal compartments with lysosomotropic agents failed to inhibit HIV-1 nucleocapsid entry into the cytoplasm of treated cells, making it unlikely that the entry process is dependent on a low pH environment. In further studies by Maddon et al,[90] mutant CD4 molecules that were restricted in their ability to undergo internalization had, when expressed on the surface of HeLa cells, the same capacity to mediate HIV-1 entry and infection. Mouse–human CD4 chimeras with only the amino terminal residues of human CD4 were also found to be capable of mediating infection,[45] as were truncated CD4 molecules lacking the cytoplasmic domain.[91] Overall, the weight of evidence supports the view that HIV-1 entry occurs through direct fusion of viral and host cell membranes in a manner that is pH independent and does not require endocytosis of the CD4 receptor.

Viral Replication in Infected Cells

Following binding and internalization, the HIV-1 virion is rapidly uncoated and a single-strand complementary DNA is generated from the HIV-1 genomic RNA using the virus-encoded reverse transcriptase (Fig. 2–4). A second strand of DNA is then synthesized, yielding a double-stranded DNA copy of the original HIV-1 RNA genome. After translocation to the nucleus, the viral DNA is inserted into host cell chromosome by the virus-encoded integrase. As with other cytopathic retroviruses, much of the newly synthesized viral DNA can remain in an unintegrated form in the host cell cytoplasm. In other retroviral systems, the accumulation of unintegrated DNA has been associated with superinfection and cell death in vitro, and this mechanism has been suggested to play a role in the cytopathicity of HIV-1.[92-94] However, in studies by DeRossi et al,[95] transfection of full-length HIV-1 DNA into CD4-negative cells resulted in virion production and accumulation of unintegrated DNA without concomitant cell death, which suggests that other mechanisms must be involved in HIV-1–mediated cytopathology.

Regulation of HIV-1 replication is dependent on the complex and coordinate interaction of a wide range of viral and host cell factors. Activation of the host cell, mediated by exogenous antigens, mitogens, or select cytokines, is required for the successful completion of HIV-1 integration and expression of proviral DNA.[96,97] In quiescent cells, HIV-1 replication is arrested during reverse transcription, resulting in the generation of an incomplete replicative intermediate that is labile within the cell.[97] Once integrated, the proviral DNA may remain latent in the absence of cellular activation, with restriction of the replication cycle. However, upon cellular activation, a number of host transcriptional factors are induced that bind recognition sites within the HIV-1 enhancer element, resulting in the induction of viral transcription. Expression of genes encoding viral regulatory proteins mediates, through integrated feedback mechanisms, the transcriptional enhancement of all viral genes, including the late expression of genes encoding the virion structural proteins. Following translation, viral proteins are subject to posttranslational processing, including cleavage, glycosylation, myristilation, and phosphorylation. Assembly of the virion core composed of HIV-1 RNA, modified viral proteins, and enzymes takes place at the plasma membrane. Mature virions are formed by budding through the cell membrane, during which time they acquire an outer lipid bilayer containing the external and transmembrane envelope glycoproteins.

DIVERSITY

HIV-1 replication, like that of other retroviruses, is subject to a high rate of mutation,[98,99] leading to the generation of considerable genetic diversity among different HIV-1 isolates (Fig. 2–5). Mutations are introduced into the HIV-1 genome during reverse transcription at an

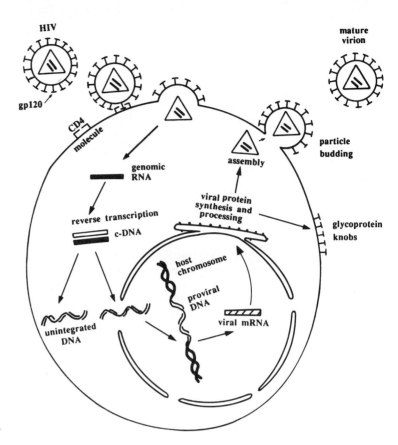

Figure 2-4. HIV-1 replication cycle.

estimated frequency as high as 10^{-4} per base, or approximately one mismatch per genome per replication cycle.[98] Additional factors including duplications, insertions, deletions, and recombination events increase the probability of genomic heterogeneity.[100] On the basis of restriction enzyme mapping[101-103] and DNA sequence analysis,[104-107] a broad range of diversity has been reported among different isolates of HIV-1. Independent isolates from geographically distinct areas have been found to differ by as much as 26% of amino acid residues in the envelope sequence.[108]

The distribution of sequence differences is not uniform throughout the viral genome.[61,109-111] As illustrated in studies by Starcich *et al*,[61] changes in the nucleotide sequence of *env* are much more prevalent than sequence changes in other viral genes. A comparison of two HIV-1 isolates from the United States revealed differences of 11.4% in the nucleotide sequence of *env*, while regions of *gag* differed by only 5.6% in nucleotide sequence. Changes within *env* were characterized by in-frame deletions, insertions, and/or duplications, in contrast to changes seen in the more conserved *gag* and *pol*, which were largely single point mutations. In addition, single nucleotide changes in *env* frequently occurred in the first or second codon position, resulting in nonsilent amino acid substitutions. Changes in the third codon position in *env* were also associated with

amino acid changes, whereas third codon changes in *gag* were almost always silent.

Interspersed between the hypervariable regions of *env* are other more conserved areas, including 18 highly conserved cysteine residues.[70,112] Based on the predicted secondary structure and hydrophilicity pattern, the hypervariable regions of the extracellular envelope glycoprotein have features characteristic of antigenic epitopes.[61] For other lentiviruses, sequence diversity in the *env* region has been linked to changes in antigenicity.[113-115] It is unclear whether antigenic variants of HIV-1 may arise as a result of similar *env* gene diversity; however, nucleotide sequence analysis of the hypervariable regions of the *env* gene indicates frequent amino acid substitutions in regions involved in recognition by neutralizing antibodies and cytotoxic T cells.[116] Moreover, the inability of type-specific antibodies from a given individual to neutralize homologous viral isolates suggests that genetically and antigenically distinct variants may arise *in vivo,* possibly in response to immunologically driven selective pressures.

Several lines of evidence support the evolution of genetic diversity *in vivo.*[117,118] In one study, isolates of HIV-1 were derived sequentially from several individuals over a 1- or 2-year period. Serial isolates derived from one patient were shown by restriction enzyme analysis to be more closely related to each other than

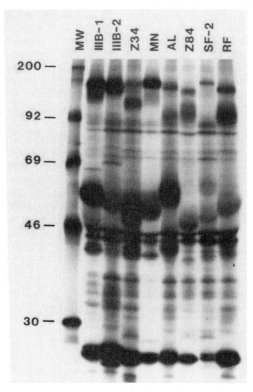

Figure 2–5. Diversity among different isolates of HIV-1 illustrated by radioimmunoprecipitation assay.

forms. Strikingly, similar changes were not observed among virus populations isolated after short-term passage in peripheral blood mononuclear cells (PBMC), suggesting that *in vitro* culture may select for virus populations that are not representative of those found *in vivo*.

The significance of genetic diversity in HIV-1 infection is not fully understood. Isolates of HIV-1 with divergent biologic activities have been identified, which suggests that genotypic changes may influence the overall functional properties of the virus.[120,121] The emergence of HIV-1 variants that are more cytopathic *in vitro* and replicate efficiently in a wider range of susceptible cells has been shown to correlate with disease progression in infected individuals.[122] Studies indicate that HIV-1 isolated from the PBMC of asymptomatic patients replicates slowly, producing only low levels of virus after prolonged culture.[123–125] By contrast, HIV-1 isolated from patients with advanced-stage disease replicates rapidly, producing high levels of virus in infected cells. The successful propagation of slow-growing virus isolates in cells transfected with the HIV-1 transactivating regulatory gene, *tat,* suggests a possible defect at the level of transcription.[126] Although DNA sequence analysis of the HIV-1 *tat* gene in sequential HIV-1 isolates has failed to identify positive selection for more efficient *tat* activity,[119] the possibility remains that sequence diversity in other regions of the HIV-1 genome may alter replicative capacity and cytopathicity, giving rise to genotypic variants with increased pathogenicity *in vivo*. A recent report by Kestler *et al*[127] indicates that strong selective pressures may operate *in vivo* for maintenance of a functionally active *nef* gene. While deletion of *nef* has been found to have no effect on virus replication *in vitro,*[128–130] *nef* was required for maintenance of high virus loads during the course of persistent infection in rhesus monkeys infected with SIVmac. *In vivo,* mutants defective for *nef* were rapidly replaced by functional forms of *nef,* which suggested that *nef* may play a critical role in the virus's life cycle and may contribute to pathogenicity by allowing the virus to persist at high levels within the host.[127]

The presence of HIV-1 variants with distinct biologic properties is further supported by analysis at the clonal level. Studies using biologic clones of HIV-1, derived by limiting dilution of PBMC from an infected individual, indicate variability among different clones with respect to replication kinetics, cytopathicity, and target cell tropism (R. I. Connor, unpubl. data). Additional studies using infectious molecular clones derived from HIV-1 isolates containing multiple virus genotypes further suggest an inherent diversity of biologic activities. Consistent with previous observations, Groenik *et al*[131] found differences in syncytium-inducing capacity and T-cell line tropism among molecular clones of HIV-1 derived from single isolates. Interestingly, the ability to induce syncytia and T-cell tropism, which were coupled in the parental isolates, were found to be discernible properties at the clonal level. Based on these find-

to isolates derived from other individuals, differing by as little as one restriction site over a 1-year period.[117] Moreover, the pattern of restriction fragments generated from isolates from several different patients indicated the presence within each isolate of a mixture of highly related yet distinct viral genomes. Direct sequencing and comparison of the predominant viral clones for three serial isolates suggested that these viruses had evolved in parallel from a common progenitor.[117] Further studies into the nature and extent of genetic variation during chronic infection have also revealed a large number of related yet distinguishable genotypic variants in serial viral isolates.[118]

In conjunction with the high rate of sequence mutation and accumulating evidence of genotypic diversity within serial isolates, this observation suggests that HIV-1 may rapidly and continuously evolve *in vivo* as a heterogeneous population of related yet distinct variants. Studies by Meyerhans *et al*[119] using direct sequence analysis of polymerase chain reaction (PCR)-amplified and molecularly cloned regions of the HIV-1 *tat* gene identified genotypic changes occurring in four sequential virus isolates. A complex interplay of HIV-1 variants, referred to as quasi-species, was characterized by abrupt fluctuations over time of dominant and minor virus

ings, it seems likely that HIV-1 isolates contain a mixture of multiple virus genotypes which, depending on the nature and extent of genetic diversity, may contribute to shaping the overall biologic phenotype of the virus. Studies aimed at elucidating the sequence diversity of HIV-1 variants with divergent biologic activities may help identify specific determinants that give rise to altered biologic activity and may provide evidence for the evolution of more pathogenic molecular variants *in vivo.*

CYTOPATHICITY

The high replicative capacity of certain HIV-1 isolates appears to correlate with the induction of cytopathic changes *in vitro.* Studies by Tersmette *et al*[132–134] demonstrate that virus isolates from patients with AIDS and AIDS-related complex (ARC) replicate to high titer and induce syncytia formation in PBMC more readily than certain slow-growing isolates obtained from asymptomatic patients. The most rapid progression to AIDS and the lowest survival rate following diagnosis were observed in individuals with high-replicating, syncytium-inducing HIV-1 isolates. Moreover, a significant correlation was found between the mean replicative rate of HIV-1 isolates and the rate of CD4+ cell decrease. Overall, the recovery of high-replicating, syncytium-inducing isolates was associated with a rapid loss of CD4+ cells and the development of ARC or AIDS.

The generation of syncytia with progression to cell death is a characteristic feature of T cells infected with HIV-1 *in vitro* (Fig. 2–6). A single infected cell expressing high levels of HIV-1 envelope glycoproteins on its surface may successfully mediate fusion with many uninfected CD4+ cells, leading to the formation of short-lived, multinucleated giant cells. The recruitment of large numbers of uninfected CD4+ T cells in the formation of syncytia may represent one mechanism of HIV-1–induced cytopathology and may explain in part the profound depletion of CD4+ cells associated with end-stage disease.

The mechanism of HIV-1–induced syncytia formation is not fully understood. Processes similar to those involved in the fusion of the virus envelope with the target cell membrane during virus entry may operate in mediating cell-cell fusion and syncytia formation. It is clear from early studies that the induction of cell fusion is directly associated with the HIV-1 envelope glycoproteins.[135,136] Expression of HIV-1 envelope glycoproteins by transfection of the *env* gene,[136] or infection with recombinant vaccinia virus[135] in the absence of other HIV-1 structural or regulatory proteins, was shown to be sufficient to induce syncytia formation in susceptible CD4+ cell lines. Syncytium formation did not occur in cell lines lacking CD4, and could be blocked by certain anti-CD4 mAb,[137] indicating that at least part of the specificity of HIV-1–induced cytopathology is governed by interaction with CD4.

The introduction of specific mutations into the genes encoding HIV-1 envelope glycoproteins has allowed functional mapping of the regions involved in syncytia formation.[73,74] Mutations within the cleavage site of the glycoprotein precursor gp160 dramatically decrease syncytium formation *in vitro,* indicating that cleavage of gp160 is an important step in the activation of envelope fusion activity.[74] As with other enveloped retroviruses, this site represents a highly conserved region, which emphasizes its importance in virus processing and suggests the possible maintenance of a structure-function relationship in the activation of virus-cell and cell-cell fusion. Cleavage of gp160 by host cell proteases produces the external glycoprotein gp120, which contains the receptor-binding domain, and the transmembrane glycoprotein gp41, which anchors the complex in the cell membrane. The N-terminal region of gp41, which is generated following cleavage, contains a region composed almost entirely of hydrophobic amino acids.[138] Similar regions are found within the transmembrane envelope proteins of both orthomyxoviruses and paramyxoviruses and have been implicated in mediating virus membrane fusion (reviewed by White *et al*[77]). Several studies have now shown that specific mutations introduced into the N-terminus of HIV-1 gp41 abrogate membrane fusion and syncytia formation.[75–77] In one study, amino acid substitutions were identified throughout the first 31 residues of the N-terminus of gp41, which affected fusion activity without altering the processing and expression of envelope glycoproteins or CD4 receptor binding,[77] suggesting that these events may be independently mediated by different regions of the molecule.

HIV-1 gp41 also contains a second hydrophobic region that spans the membrane and anchors the envelope glycoproteins. In recent studies by Helseth *et al,*[139]

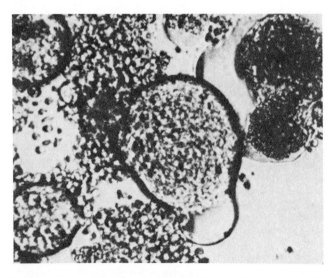

Figure 2–6. HIV-1 infected CD4+ lymphoblastoid cell culture showing syncytia formation. (Photo courtesy of N. Yamamoto.)

changes within and proximal to this region resulted in mutants that were defective for syncytia formation and virus replication. Mutations within the transmembrane region had no effect on the levels of envelope glycoprotein expression or CD4 binding. It seems likely, based on these studies, that the binding of HIV-1 gp120 to CD4 occurs independently of membrane fusion activity and that the subsequent initiation of cell fusion may involve interaction of both the N-terminus and transmembrane hydrophobic regions of gp41.

The cytopathic effects of HIV-1 infection in CD4+ cells *in vivo* may not be limited to the induction of syncytia formation. Normal peripheral blood lymphocytes are often killed *in vitro* without evidence of cell-cell fusion. One possibility is that "autofusion" may occur, involving different parts of the plasma membrane of a single infected cell. This in turn may result in permeability changes that would be lethal to the cell. "Single cell killing" is typical of many field isolates cultured *in vitro*. The possibility that additional mechanisms may be operating in the induction of viral cytopathicity has been suggested by several studies,[140–150] although the significance and relative contribution of each of these processes remain somewhat controversial. It is suggested that high-level virus replication may take over normal cellular synthetic processes, interfering with the synthesis, degradation, transport, and processing of cellular mRNA and proteins.[140] Alternatively, the accumulation of high levels of unintegrated HIV-1 DNA may alter the permeability of the cell membrane,[141] while intracellular complexing of CD4-gp120 may lead to reduced CD4 mRNA and protein in infected cells.[142] Other proposed mechanisms of HIV-induced cytopathicity involve altered second messenger production, resulting in changes in signal transduction,[143] and the autoimmune destruction of infected cells by HIV-1–specific cytotoxic T cells[144–146] and by antibody-dependent cytotoxic mechanisms.[147–150] The role of each or any of these processes in mediating HIV cytopathology remains to be determined.

TROPISM

Human T lymphocytes and monocyte-macrophages are thought to be the primary cells involved in HIV-1 infection, reflecting the preferential tropism of HIV-1 for cells bearing the CD4 molecule on their surface. While all strains of HIV-1 appear to grow well in primary T lymphocytes, only some isolates are able to replicate efficiently in macrophages or in immortalized T-cell lines.[151] In particular, HIV isolated from the brain tissue of infected individuals can be distinguished from virus isolated from the peripheral blood based on the ability of brain-derived isolates to replicate in macrophage cultures.[152] Infected cells found within brain tissue frequently include macrophages and related microglial cells,[153] suggesting that differential tropism may arise as a result of *in vivo* selection. Primary isolates of HIV-1

derived from short-term culture in PBMC frequently display a similar pattern of restricted cell tropism and replicate poorly if at all in established T-cell lines. By contrast, most commonly used laboratory isolates, such as HIV-1IIIB, are extremely well adapted for growth in T-cell lines as a result of continuous long-term culture under conditions that promote selection for replicative efficiency.

Factors that determine the efficiency of infection and replication and ultimately cell tropism may be linked to many stages within the virus replication cycle, including binding and entry, synthesis of viral DNA, integration into the host cell genome, transcription of viral mRNA, translation, and assembly of mature virions. In studies by Kim *et al*,[154] various stages of the HIV-1 life cycle were examined to determine the factors that contribute to virus tropism. Virus replication was evaluated in monocyte and T-cell lines, both of which express the CD4 receptor. Variation in the level of CD4 expression has been suggested to influence the susceptibility of certain cells to infection with HIV-1[155]; however, the correlation between infectivity and CD4 expression is not absolute. In the study by Kim and co-workers, the monocyte cell line U937 was found to have a higher percentage of CD4+ cells than the H9 T-cell line but was much less susceptible to infection with the HIV-1 W13 strain. Poor growth of this virus in U937 cells was not a result of deficiencies at the level of gene expression, based on the efficiency of LTR activity and levels of viral RNA expression. Differences were observed, however, in the amount of unintegrated linear HIV-1 DNA measured shortly after infection of U937 and H9 cells. This points to factors in the initial stages of infection, presumably involving virus entry and/or reverse transcription. Direct assessment of the amount of virion genomic RNA measured soon after infection indicated that 5- to 10-fold higher amounts of HIV-1 were entering H9 cells than U937 cells, suggesting that the major block in infection of U937 cells occurred at the level of entry before initiation of reverse transcription. This finding was supported in studies by Cann *et al*[156] using a molecularly cloned isolate of HIV-1, termed HIV-1JR-CSF. This isolate was directly cloned after only limited culture in PBMC without adaptation in cell lines. Restricted replication of HIV-1JR-CSF in T-cell lines was traced to inefficient entry of the virus, which could be overcome when proviral DNA from HIV-1JR-CSF was directly transfected into the previously nonpermissive cells.

Entry of HIV-1 into a target cell is dependent on interaction of the viral envelope glycoproteins with CD4 expressed on the cell surface. It is clear from several studies that the HIV-1 *env* gene contains determinants that can affect virus pathogenicity, including tropism and host cell range.[157,158] Cordonnier *et al*[159] identified a single amino acid change at position 425 of the envelope glycoprotein gp120 that abolished the ability of HIV-1 to infect U937 cells but had no effect on infectivity of T-cell lines or activated peripheral blood lymphocytes. In efforts to further map regions within the *env* gene that confer selective tropism, several groups have utilized recombinant viruses generated by exchanging regions of the *env* gene between HIV-1 isolates with distinct tropisms.[160–162] In early studies by Liu *et al*,[160] recombinant viruses derived from a molecularly cloned peripheral blood isolate (HIV-1SF2) that contained the *env* gene from a CNS-derived isolate (HIV-1SF128A) displayed the parental HIV-1SF128A tropism for macrophages, clearly indicating that all the necessary determinants for macrophage tropism lay within this region. A comparison of the *env* genes of the two parental isolates revealed 91.1% nucleotide sequence homology and 85.1% amino acid homology. Changes consisted of substitutions, deletions, and insertions and occurred primarily within the hypervariable regions (V1, V2, and V4) and CD4 binding domain of gp120, and the fusion domain of gp41. By exchanging progressively smaller fragments in the generation of recombinant viruses, several groups have now identified determinants that confer macrophage tropism within a segment of the *env* gene encoding the V3 domain of gp120.[161,162] Studies by Takeuchi *et al*[163] have since demonstrated that a single amino acid change at position 311 of HIV-1 gp120, which falls within the V3 loop, is sufficient to account for the expanded host cell range of a variant HIV-1 isolate. The significance of the V3 region of the *env* gene in determining cell tropism is currently not known, but this domain (amino acids 298 to 327) is clearly distinct from the CD4 binding site as defined by Lasky *et al*[63] (amino acids 397 to 439) and Olshevsky *et al*.[68] Mutations within this region have been shown to significantly reduce infectivity without affecting virus binding, which suggests that efficient entry of HIV-1 into macrophages may be determined by postbinding events and may involve interaction with sites contained within the V3 loop.

Regions within the HIV-1 *env* gene have also been shown to correlate with infection in established T-cell lines. In contrast to the relatively small region of gp120 that determines macrophage tropism, recent mapping studies have identified a larger overlapping region of 321 amino acids that is required for efficient viral replication in the Hut78 T-cell line.[162] This region encompasses the V1, V2, V3, and V4 hypervariable regions and the CD4 binding site of gp120, and, by virtue of its extended size, may reflect the presence of multiple, discontinuous determinants. In addition to T-cell tropism, elements within this region code for the regulatory genes *tat* and *rev*, which may play a role in determining the kinetics and level of replication in T-cell lines. Consistent with this possibility, HIV-1 isolates exhibiting increased replication kinetics and high cytopathicity have also been shown to acquire an expanded host cell range. In studies by Schuitemaker *et al*,[164] syncytium-inducing isolates of HIV-1 could be distinguished from non-syncytium-inducing isolates on the basis of their transmissibility to various T-cell and monocytoid cell lines. Rapidly growing, cytopathic isolates readily infected the H9 T-cell line, while noncytopathic isolates were unable to establish infection.

Although a hallmark of HIV-1 infection is the se-

lected tropism of the virus for cells bearing the CD4 antigen, accumulating evidence suggests that HIV-1 may also infect *in vitro* a variety of cells that express no detectable CD4, including neuronal cells, glial cells, endothelial cells, oligodendrocytes, astrocytes, muscle cells, colorectal cells, B cells, and bone marrow progenitor cells (Table 2–1).[165–171] Entry and replication of HIV-1 in these cells *in vitro* is frequently inefficient, and the mechanisms that govern infection of CD4− cells are currently unknown. One possibility raised by several studies suggests that an expanded host cell range may result from phenotypic mixing in cells infected with more than one virus. So-called pseudotype viruses commonly arise during viral assembly in which envelope glycoproteins are exchanged between two unrelated replication-competent enveloped viruses. The resulting virions display a mosaic of envelope glycoproteins. Formation of pseudotype viruses in doubly infected cells has been demonstrated for several enveloped viruses,[172,173] and recent studies indicate that HIV-1 may also form pseudotypes in cells infected with xenotropic murine leukemia virus (MLV),[174] amphotropic MLV (A-MLV),[175,176] vesicular stomatitis virus,[27,32,177] herpes simplex virus,[177] and human T-cell leukemia virus (HTLV).[178,179] HIV-1 pseudotypes formed with these viruses frequently acquire an expanded host cell range that includes various CD4− cells. Although to date pseudotype viruses have not been demonstrated in HIV-1–infected individuals, the frequency of multiple infection with HTLV, cytomegalovirus (CMV), Epstein-Barr virus, human herpes 6,[180–183] and other viruses during the course of HIV infection suggests that pseudotypes may arise and may account in part for the spread of HIV-1 to CD4− cells.

In vitro, low-level persistent infection with HIV-1 has been documented in a number of CD4− cells lines.[184–188] In studies by Cao *et al*,[184] productive HIV-1 infection was established in five different hepatoma cell lines that were negative for both CD4 protein and mRNA.

Table 2–1. Cells Susceptible to HIV-1 Infection

IN VITRO

CD4+ T lymphocytes[26]
Monocyte/macrophages[152,196,200]
Microglia[166]
Bone marrow CD34+ precursor cells[168]
Monocytic and T-cells lines[151, 155]
Glioma and neuroblastoma cell lines[187, 188]
Tumor cell lines from colon[165] and liver[184]

IN VIVO

CD4+ T lymphocytes[240]
Monocyte/macrophages[152,153,170,193,196,200,247]
Epithelial langerhans' cells[201,234,235,239]
Follicular dendritic cells[243, 244]
Brain endothelial cells[193]
Microglia, astroglia, oligodendroglia[193,255]
Undefined cells in the retina, cervix, and colon[189–192]

Infection in these cell lines was not blocked by anti-CD4 mAb or by sCD4, suggesting a CD4-independent route of infection. Similar findings have been reported using CD4− cells of fibroblastoid,[185] glial,[167,168,186,187] rhabdosarcoma,[167] and neuronal[188] origin. *In vivo,* there is also evidence of expanded tropism in tissues and cells that are not known to be CD4+. HIV-1 infection has been documented in many nonlymphoid tissues, including colon, rectum, duodenum, cervix, retina, and brain.[189–193] Cumulatively, these studies raise the possibility that HIV-1 infection in certain cell types may occur through pathways independent of CD4, perhaps by interaction with a second, as yet unidentified receptor.

INFECTION OF MONONUCLEAR PHAGOCYTES

Within the peripheral blood, infected CD4+ T lymphocytes form a primary reservoir for HIV-1.[194,195] Virus can be readily identified in purified populations of peripheral blood T cells derived from HIV-1–infected individuals by coculture methods, *in situ* hybridization, immunofluorescent staining, and gene amplification.[194] Evidence that HIV-1 may also infect cells of macrophage lineage was provided in early studies by Ho *et al*[196] in which HIV-1 was directly recovered from peripheral blood monocyte-macrophages of infected patients. The finding that HIV-1 could be isolated from monocytes but not T cells of infected individuals during acute infection suggested that these cells may be involved in the early stages of disease as well as during fulminant infection.[197] In other studies, virus-producing mononuclear phagocytes were identified within primary cultures of brain tissue from an AIDS patient,[152] and HIV-1 proteins were found associated with follicular dendritic cells within the lymph node germinal centers,[198] observations suggesting that within certain tissues HIV-1 may preferentially infect cells of macrophage lineage. Since that time, cells having morphologic and growth properties characteristic of monocyte-macrophages have been associated with virus expression in the brain, lung, and skin.[199–201] The possibility that monocyte-macrophages may be productively infected was further substantiated by the finding that monocytes could support HIV-1 replication *in vitro*[196] and that infection could be blocked by antibodies to the CD4 receptor.[202]

In studies by Gartner *et al*,[152] virus isolates recovered from the brain and lung tissues of AIDS patients were found to replicate efficiently *in vitro* and displayed a higher tropism for macrophages than for T cells. In contrast to T-cell infection, virus production from infected macrophages was persistent and occurred in the absence of significant cell proliferation. The ability to replicate efficiently in monocyte-macrophages is a characteristic feature of lentivirus infections.[203,204] Prototypic animal lentiviruses, including visna virus and caprine arthritis-encephalitis virus, establish persistent infection within the host that is characterized by slow but progressive development of immunosuppressive, inflammatory, or degenerative diseases. These viruses exhibit a strong tropism for cells of macrophage lineage, although virus replication is restricted by the state of cellular differentiation.[204] Levels of virus production are initially low within circulating monocytes. However, as the cells enter the tissues and begin to differentiate, the rate of virus replication increases dramatically. By controlling the rate of viral replication, infected monocyte-macrophages serve as reservoirs for the dissemination of infection to target tissues such as the lung and CNS.

Control of HIV-1 replication within infected mononuclear phagocytes is similarly influenced by factors that govern the state of cellular differentiation and/or activation. Cytokines that play a critical role in the regulation of immune responses *in vivo* have been shown *in vitro* to alter the level of HIV-1 gene expression in infected monocyte-macrophages. Granulocyte-macrophage colony-stimulating factor (GM-CSF), which stimulates the maturation and differentiation of granulocyte and monocyte bone marrow precursor cells, was found to alternately increase HIV-1 replication in primary monocyte-macrophages[205] and to decrease reverse transcription and viral antigen expression in the chronically infected promonocyte cell line, U937.[206] In studies by Koyanagi *et al,*[207] large increases in HIV-1 production were observed following treatment of primary monocyte-macrophages with three hematopoietic growth factors—GM-CSF, macrophage colony-stimulating factor (M-CSF), and interleukin-3 (IL-3), which suggested that factors that induce macrophage growth and differentiation may increase virus replication in infected cells. In the same study, HIV-1 replication was enhanced in infected cells by interferon-γ (IFN-γ), a potent activator of macrophage function. Interestingly, increases in HIV-1 replication were observed only when the cells were treated with IFN-γ before infection; treatment with IFN-γ after infection resulted in a decrease in HIV-1 production. In other studies, treatment of uninfected macrophages with either IFN-α, IFN-β, or IFN-γ was found to reduce the formation of proviral DNA and restrict productive infection with HIV-1.[208,209] Discrepancies in the observed effects of certain cytokines, such as GM-CSF and IFN-γ, suggest that additional factors, including the target cell, virus strain, and cytokine concentration, may be critical in determining the overall effect of these factors on the regulation of HIV-1 gene expression.

In vivo, most cytokines function as part of a complex network that governs the regulation of immune responses (reviewed by Balkwill and Burke[210]). The production and activity of these factors are coordinately controlled through integrated feedback mechanisms. In this regard, many cytokines are known to function in an autocrine/paracrine manner to modulate the state of differentiation or activation of other immune cells. In particular, production of TNF-α by activated macrophages results in recruitment of additional macrophages and further activation of inherent cytotoxic activity. During chronic disease, production of both TNF-α and interleukin-1 (IL-1) by activated macrophages has been associated with systemic effects in the induction of fever and cachexia. Increased levels of TNF-α have been noted in the sera of AIDS patients, which might explain in part the prominant symptoms of fever and wasting in these patients.[211] Although purified monocytes from HIV-1–infected patients[212,213] and monocytic cells infected with HIV-1 in vitro[214] have been shown to produce increased levels of TNF-α on stimulation by exogenous factors, these findings remain somewhat controversial.

In turn, TNF-α and IL-1 have each been shown to upregulate the expression of viral genes in HIV-1–infected T cells,[215–217] while TNF-α, alone and in concert with IL-6, was found to increase HIV-1 production from infected monocytic cells.[218] Synthesis of IL-6 is inducible in many cell types, including mononuclear phagocytes and T cells, and plays an important role in the differentiation of B cells into plasma cells.[219,220] Elevated levels of IL-6 have been found in the serum of HIV-1–infected individuals,[221] which may contribute to the polyclonal B-cell activation observed in AIDS patients.

Clearly, the mechanisms that govern HIV-1 replication in infected mononuclear phagocytes are not fully understood. Several studies indicate that HIV-1 gene expression may be upregulated in vitro during monocyte differentiation or activation by exogenous stimuli, including phorbol esters and various cytokines.[205–209,222,223] Many of these factors have been shown to stimulate LTR-driven RNA transcription in HIV-1–infected T cells through induction of the nuclear factor NF-κB.[224–227] In particular, phorbol myristate acetate (PMA), IL-1, and TNF-α have been found to stimulate viral transcription by inducing an NF-κB-like protein that binds to enhancer regions within the HIV-1 LTR.[215,227,228] In monocytes, increases in HIV gene expression mediated through induction of NF-κB have been linked to cellular differentiation,[229] which suggests that NF-κB activity in these cells may be developmentally regulated. In other studies, treatment of monocyte cell lines with the bacterial endotoxin, lipopolysaccharide (LPS), was found to stimulate HIV-1 LTR activity through the induction of NF-κB-like DNA binding factors.[230] In contrast to transcriptional induction of HIV-1 expression, IL-6 has been shown to induce HIV-1 expression by alternative mechanisms. In studies by Poli et al,[218] treatment of both acutely and chronically infected monocytic cells with IL-6 stimulated the expression of HIV-1 proteins and increased reverse transcriptase activity without significantly increasing the levels of HIV-1 RNA, indicating that IL-6 may act posttranscriptionally to alter expression of HIV-1.

Tissue Distribution of Infected Monocyte-Macrophages

HIV-1 replication and assembly within infected macrophages occurs at both the plasma and cytoplasmic membranes, in contrast to HIV-1–infected T lymphocytes, where viral assembly is almost exclusively confined to the plasma membrane.[231,232] Ultrastructural studies indicate that HIV-1 assembly in macrophages is strongly associated with elements of the Golgi apparatus, where viral particles can be seen within vacuoles concentrated in the perinuclear region.[232] In chronically infected macrophages, replication is predominantly intravacuolar, leading to large accumulations of intracytoplasmic viral particles. Paradoxically, these chronically infected cells release only low levels of mature viral progeny, despite the relatively high frequency of infected cells detected in vitro. Moreover, infected macrophages in culture are relatively resistant to HIV-1–induced cytopathic effects and, unlike T lymphocytes, are rarely associated with the formation of multinucleated giant cells. The ability to sustain low-level persistent infection while harboring large numbers of viral particles has led many to suggest that infected macrophages may serve as reservoirs for the persistence and dissemination of HIV in vivo.[231–233]

SKIN

Examination of tissue samples from AIDS patients has shown virus present in infected cells of macrophage lineage in the skin, lymphatic tissues, lungs, spinal cord, and brain. Within the skin, epidermal Langerhans cells appear to be a predominant target for infection with HIV-1.[201,234,235] In vitro, human epithelial Langerhans cells are easily infected with HIV-1, and the virus released into culture supernatants has been shown to infect heterologous PBMC.[236] The possibility that these cells may also be infected in vivo was suggested by the demonstration of reduced numbers of Langerhans cells in skin samples from AIDS patients.[237] Although immunohistochemical analysis of skin samples from HIV-1–infected patients failed to demonstrate the presence of HIV-1 in these cells,[238] subsequent studies using antibodies to HIV-1 core proteins (p17 and p24) identified viral antigens associated with Langerhans cells in skin biopsies from seven of 40 HIV-1 seropositive individuals.[201] Ultrastructural analysis has confirmed the presence of HIV particles and budding virus associated with Langerhans cells in the skin and oral mucosa.[239]

LYMPH NODES

The presence of Langerhans cells in the skin and mucous membranes has suggested they may serve as early targets for HIV-1 infection, and may subsequently disseminate the virus to regional lymph nodes.[235] The first isolate of HIV-1 (then termed LAV) was derived in 1983 from the lymph node tissue of a patient suffering from persistent generalized lymphadenopathy.[240] HIV-1 particles have since been directly demonstrated in the lymph nodes of HIV-1 seropositive patients[241,242] and have been associated in these tissues with CD4-bearing follicular dendritic cells.[243] In studies by Cameron et al,[244] viral replication in follicular dendritic cells was found to correlate with reduced antibody titers and progressive follicular destruction in patients with or at risk for AIDS.

LUNGS

The development of AIDS is frequently associated with severe pulmonary complications resulting from opportunistic infection by a variety of pathogens, most commonly *Pneumocystis carinii*. A large percentage of pediatric AIDS patients also suffer from pulmonary complications caused by infiltration of lymphocytes and plasma cells into the peribronchial and interstitial spaces of the lung (lymphocytic interstitial pneumonitis, LIP). In early studies, identification of HIV-1 RNA in the lung tissue of patients with AIDS-related LIP by *in situ* hybridization techniques,[245] and virus isolation from bronchoalveolar lavage fluid,[246] suggested that HIV-1 may play a role in mediating pulmonary dysfunction. In studies by Salahuddin *et al,*[200] pulmonary macrophages from both AIDS patients and normal donors were found to be susceptible to HIV-1 infection *in vitro.* Moreover, spontaneous production of HIV-1 was detected in primary pulmonary macrophage cultures from AIDS patients, suggesting that these cells may be targets for infection *in vivo.*[200] Although infected macrophages do not appear to undergo significant cytopathology in vitro, HIV-1–induced defects in functional activity, in particular defense against intracellular pathogens, may increase the likelihood of opportunistic infections. In addition, infected pulmonary macrophages expressing viral antigens have been shown to be targets for lysis by HIV-specific cytotoxic T lymphocytes, and may be responsible for the induction of inflammatory reactions in the lungs of HIV-1–infected individuals.[247]

CENTRAL NERVOUS SYSTEM

Involvement of the central nervous system (CNS) in HIV-1 infection is characterized by a number of distinct neurologic syndromes including subacute encephalitis, vacuolar myelopathy, aseptic meningitis, and peripheral neuropathy (reviewed by Price *et al*[248]). Considerable evidence now indicates that macrophages within the brain and CNS are a primary target for HIV-1 infection. Ultrastructural analysis of these tissues has shown viral particles accumulated within cytoplasmic vacuoles and budding from the plasma membrane of infected macrophages.[249] In early studies, HIV-1 DNA and RNA were detected in the brains of infected patients,[250] and virus was subsequently isolated from the brain and CNS[196,251] of patients suffering from neurologic syndromes associated with AIDS. In studies by Gabuzda *et al,*[153] HIV-1 antigens were identified in cells resembling monocyte-macrophages in the brain tissue of neurosymptomatic AIDS patients. Using *in situ* hybridization techniques and immunohistochemical staining, Koenig and associates also identified macrophages as the predominant

cell type in the brain producing HIV-1.[170] Several additional *in situ* studies have since confirmed this initial conclusion,[252,253] including a report by Wiley *et al,*[193] who also noted HIV-1 infection of cerebral endothelial cells and, in one severe case of AIDS dementia complex, rare involvement of neurons and glial cells. Consistent with this finding, primary cultures of microglial cells, in addition to immortalized glioma and neuroblastoma cell lines, have been shown to support HIV-1 replication *in vitro.*[166,186–188]

The detection of HIV-1 DNA in brain tissue and the recovery of infectious virus from the brain and CSF strongly suggest that HIV-1 may have a causal role in the neurologic dysfunction associated with AIDS. Although the precise mechanisms for HIV-1–mediated pathology in the CNS are not well understood, several possibilities have been raised by recent studies (Fig. 2–7). HIV-1 isolates derived from the brain and CNS have been shown to replicate efficiently in macrophage and glioma cell cultures *in vitro.* Although with low frequency, infection of endothelial cells, oligodendrocytes, and astrocytes has also been reported.[254,255] Conceivably, direct cytotoxicity of these cells may arise as a result of infection and replication of the virus. Alternatively, expression of viral antigens on the surface of infected cells may indirectly make them targets for cytotoxic T cells.[256] HIV-1 infection may also interfere with the "luxury functions" of neural cells, without apparent cytotoxicity. Although *in situ* studies indicate a limited degree of neural cell involvement *in vivo* (particularly of neurons), recent data support direct infection of neuronal cells *in vitro.* In studies by Li *et al,*[188] HIV-1 infection was established in a cell line of neuroectodermal origin that expressed no detectable CD4 protein or mRNA. Entry of the virus was not blocked by selected anti-CD4 mAb (OKT4A, Leu-3a), indicating that infection in certain neurons may occur independently of CD4, possibly through interaction of the virus with an alternate receptor.

Despite the relatively low cytopathic effects of HIV-1 infection in PBMC and other tissue macrophages, infected macrophages in the brain are frequently associated with the formation of multinucleated giant cells. In studies by Koenig *et al,*[170] both mononuclear and multinuclear macrophages in the brain tissue of infected patients were shown to be actively synthesizing viral RNA and producing progeny virions. In patients with AIDS dementia complex, the amount of HIV-1 detected in the CNS has in some cases exceeded that detected in the blood or other tissues.[196,251] Considerable genetic diversity has been noted among different isolates of HIV-1 which may give rise to viruses with altered biologic characteristics and increased pathogenicity *in vivo.* Isolates of HIV-1 that rapidly replicate to high titer have been associated with expanded tropism and increased cytopathicity in T-cell lines *in vitro.* This altered biologic phenotype is believed to correlate with increased virulence in the host. Certain isolates of HIV-1, particularly those recovered from brain tissue and cerebrospinal

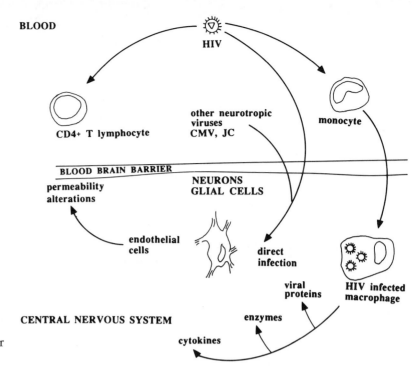

BLOOD

HIV

CD4+ T lymphocyte

other neurotropic
viruses
CMV, JC

monocyte

BLOOD BRAIN BARRIER

permeability
alterations

NEURONS
GLIAL CELLS

endothelial
cells

direct
infection

viral
proteins

HIV infected
macrophage

CENTRAL NERVOUS SYSTEM

enzymes

cytokines

Figure 2–7. Possible mechanisms for HIV-1 induced pathology in the CNS.

fluid, display preferential tropism for cells of macrophage lineage. In studies by Koyanagi *et al,*[257] HIV-1 recovered from the brain tissue of a patient with AIDS dementia complex was found to replicate preferentially in primary macrophage cultures. By contrast, virus isolated from the cerebrospinal fluid of the same patient replicated only in primary glial cells, which suggests that specific patterns of tropism may arise within distinct sites in the CNS. Moreover, this suggests that certain neurotropic strains of HIV-1 may be more prone to attack cells of the CNS, which may have implications for the development of neurologic dysfunction within the host.

Infection of macrophages and related microglia with HIV-1 may also result in neuropathologic changes by indirect mechanisms. Differentiation and activation of infected macrophages *in vivo* may trigger the release of specific cytokines or proteolytic enzymes that are toxic to endothelial cells, astrocytes, or neurons. This process may in turn cause a breakdown of the blood-brain barrier or dysfunction of the adjacent brain parenchyma. In particular, TNF-α, produced by activated macrophages, has been shown to have multiple effects on neural cells *in vitro,* including decreased proliferation of glioma-derived cell lines and cytotoxicity.[258] Oligodendrocyte necrosis, myelin dilatation, and demyelination have also been shown to occur when spinal cords were exposed to TNF-α *in vitro.*[259] HIV-1 infection of monocytes *in vitro* has been shown to augment TNF-α production, and increased levels of TNF-α have been demonstrated in the serum of infected patients, which may indirectly contribute to the neurologic dysfunction and destruction associated with AIDS dementia.

In addition, HIV-1 gp120, which may be shed from virions or infected cells *in vivo,* has been shown *in vitro* to have neurotoxic effects. Low concentrations of HIV-1 gp120 were shown to be toxic to mouse hippocampal neurons.[260] This cytotoxic effect was blocked by anti-CD4 antibody (OKT4A) and by vasoactive intestinal peptide. These studies suggest that HIV-1 gp120 may cause nervous system damage by competing with the endogenous neurotropic activity of vasoactive intestinal peptide. Other investigators have reported the neurotoxic effect of HIV-1 envelope glycoproteins on chick dorsal-root ganglion neurons in culture.[261] HIV-1 gp120 was found to have partial sequence homology with neuroleukin, a factor that promotes the survival of certain neurons *in vitro.*[261–263] Neurotoxicity was suggested to result from interference of neuroleukin by HIV-1 gp120; however, the discovery that neuroleukin was indistinguishable from glucophosphoisomerase,[264,265] an enzyme in the glycolytic pathway, has raised doubts about the role of this factor in the development of AIDS-related neuropathology.

Co-infection with other viruses, in particular CMV and JC virus, has also been suggested to play a role in the pathogenesis of AIDS dementia complex.[266–268] These viruses are found with high frequency in immunocompromised patients, including those with AIDS, and may have direct or indirect effects on the neurologic disease induced by HIV-1. Co-infection of glial or neuronal cells with either virus may increase HIV-1 replication through transactivation of HIV-1 LTR by heterologous viral regulatory proteins.[269] Alternatively, infection with CMV may indirectly elicit immune responses leading to an influx of macrophages which may be targets for HIV-1 infection. Macrophages already infected with HIV-1 may also be recruited to the brain, increasing the overall viral burden in the CNS.

HIV-1 INFECTION OF HEMATOPOIETIC PROGENITOR CELLS

Individuals infected with HIV-1 frequently have hematologic abnormalities, including neutropenia, anemia, granulocytopenia, and thrombocytopenia.[270-277] Such abnormalities are believed to result from suppression of bone marrow hematopoiesis, leading to deficiencies in the development of one or more blood cell lineages.[278-280] Abnormalities in bone marrow hematopoiesis may arise as a result of direct effects of HIV-1 on progenitor cells or on the accessory cells that support the growth and differentiation of precursor cells. The possible role for accessory cells (in particular macrophages and T lymphocytes) in suppression of bone marrow hematopoiesis has been suggested by several *in vitro* studies done using both human and primate cell systems.[281,282] In studies by Wantanabe *et al,*[282] replication of SIVmac in macrophages isolated from the bone marrow of infected rhesus monkeys was shown to inhibit progenitor cell growth and colony formation *in vitro.* Other studies suggest that disturbances in certain T-cell subsets and the production of inhibitory factors by accessory cells may also adversely affect hematopoiesis in the bone marrow.[283-285]

In patients with thrombocytopenia, evidence of HIV-1 infection has been found in megakaryocytes, myelocytes, and myelomonocytes,[286] which suggests that direct infection of progenitor cells may account for hematologic abnormalities in certain cases. However, the possibility that infected hematopoietic progenitor cells are a major reservoir for HIV-1 in the bone marrow remains controversial. *In vitro,* purified populations of normal bone marrow cells expressing the CD34 antigen have been shown to support HIV-1 replication.[168] A small percentage of cells in the bone marrow express CD34, including hematopoietic progenitors that give rise to all cell lineages.[287,288] Steinburg and colleagues[280] demonstrated reduced *in vitro* growth of erythroid, granulocyte-macrophage, and T-lymphocyte colonies following infection of normal bone marrow–derived cells with HIV-1, suggesting a direct causal role for the virus in mediating suppression of hematopoiesis.

The possibility that bone marrow progenitor cells may also be infected with HIV-1 *in vivo* was suggested by several studies that demonstrated decreased *in vitro* growth of progenitor cells isolated from HIV-1–infected individuals.[276-278] In studies by Donahue *et al,*[279] macrophage-depleted bone marrow cells from AIDS and ARC patients did not differ from those of healthy seronegative donors in the ability to generate granulocyte-macrophage, erythroid, or multilineage colonies in response to stimulation with recombinant GM-CSF.

However, antibodies present in the serum of HIV-1–infected patients were found to suppress colony formation from progenitors of ARC/AIDS patients but not from normal individuals. Suppression of hematopoietic colony formation was also observed with rabbit antiserum to HIV-1 gp120. Although still considered controversial, these results suggest that progenitor cells may be infected with HIV-1 *in vivo,* and that growth and differentiation of cells expressing viral antigens may be inhibited directly or indirectly by antibody-mediated immune mechanisms.

Despite considerable *in vitro* evidence indicating that CD34+ progenitor cells may be targets for HIV-1 infection, several recent studies have failed to demonstrate HIV-1 DNA in purified populations of CD34+ cells from HIV-1–infected individuals.[289,290] Using sensitive PCR methods to amplify specific viral sequences, von Laer *et al*[289] reported the absence of detectable HIV DNA in CD34+ progenitor cells from symptomatic HIV-1 seropositive patients. Using similar PCR methods, Davis and colleagues[290] also failed to detect HIV DNA in CD34+ cells from six of seven asymptomatic HIV-infected individuals and four of four patients with ARC or AIDS. Moreover, no HIV-1 DNA was detected in samples of granulocyte-macrophage–derived colonies from any of the HIV-1–infected patients, indicating that macrophage progenitors are not a significant source of HIV-1 in the bone marrow. By contrast, the frequency of detection of HIV-1 DNA in bone marrow–derived CD3+T lymphocytes from patients with ARC or AIDS suggests that these cells may be the main site of HIV-1 infection, although this has yet to be confirmed.

Although HIV-1 infection is frequently associated with the development of hematologic abnormalities, the role of HIV-1 in mediating suppression of hematopoiesis and the underlying pathogenic mechanisms are often difficult to delineate. Secondary infection with other viruses and therapy for AIDS or other opportunistic infections may contribute to abnormalities in hematopoiesis independently or in concert with HIV-1. Both CMV and hepatitis B virus (HBV) have been shown to affect the growth of normal bone marrow precursors *in vitro,* and may contribute to bone marrow suppression in immunocompromised AIDS patients.[291,292] In addition, significant blood cell abnormalities, including anemia, leukopenia, and neutropenia, have been reported in a majority of HIV-1 seropositive individuals receiving zidovudine, especially those patients with more advanced disease.[293]

QUANTITATION AND *IN VIVO* INFECTION

In vivo, the course of infection with HIV-1 may be governed by complex interactions between the virus and the host immune system. Although little is known of the dynamics of HIV-1 replication within an infected individual, it is reasonable to suggest that immune mechanisms may be elicited that contribute to the restriction of viral replication and the establishment of latent infection. Initial infection with HIV-1 is characterized by the onset of acute illness, and in the short period prior to seroconversion, virus may be detected in the cerebrospinal fluid, PBMC, and plasma.[294-297] High levels of infectious HIV-1 have recently been demonstrated in both the plasma and PBMC of infected individuals during primary infection (Fig. 2–8), suggesting that the viral burden may be more extensive than was previously thought. Rapid declines in the amount of free and cell-associated virus were observed at seroconversion, suggesting the development within the host of effective immune responses capable of limiting viral replication.[297]

Questions concerning the relationship between virus burden and immunologic status in HIV-1–infected individuals have been posed by several groups.[194,298-300] In early studies, *in situ* hybridization and immunofluorescent staining were used to determine the frequency of cells expressing viral mRNA and surface proteins, respectively.[298] Based on these studies it was suggested that the frequency of circulating PBMC infected with HIV-1 *in vivo* was low (roughly 1 in 10⁵ PBMC). However, these techniques may underestimate the viral burden *in vivo,* since a proportion of latently infected cells may contain HIV-1 DNA yet express no detectable viral RNA or proteins. Indeed, recent studies now indicate that levels of HIV-1 in the blood and plasma of infected individuals are much higher than was previously estimated.[299] Using PCR techniques capable of detecting HIV-1 proviral DNA, Simmonds *et al*[300] determined the average frequency of PBMC carrying HIV-1 provirus to be 1 in 8,000 cells. The frequency was lower in asymptomatic patients (1 in 6,000 to 1 in 80,000 cells) but higher (1 in 770 to 1 in 3,300 cells) in AIDS patients. In studies by Schnittman *et al,*[194] HIV-1 DNA was detected in enriched populations of peripheral blood CD4+ T lymphocytes, but rarely in the enriched monocyte fractions, an observation which suggested that CD4+ T cells may be the predominant viral reservoir within the peripheral blood. The frequency of CD4+ T cells containing HIV-1 DNA was estimated to be at least 1 in 100 cells in patients with AIDS, while in asymptomatic patients the frequency ranged from 1 in 100 to 1 in 100,000 cells.

The low frequency of HIV-1 DNA detected in peripheral blood monocytes implies that only a small number of these cells are infected *in vivo.* This finding remains controversial, in light of additional studies that suggest that monocytes may play a more prominent role as a viral reservoir in the peripheral blood. In studies by McElrath *et al,*[301] HIV-1 DNA was detected with high frequency (74%) by PCR in purified monocyte populations from HIV-1 seropositive individuals. Several groups have successfully cultured HIV-1 from blood monocytes, and in studies by Schrier *et al,*[302] HIV-1 antigens were readily detected in culture supernatants of monocyte-derived macrophages from infected patients. Recently, HIV-1 was detected in monocytes from nine of nine symptomatic patients with the use of sensitive end-point dilution culture methods (H. Yoshiama, unpubl. data). Quantitation of virus titers indicated that in four of nine cases, the level of HIV-1 in monocytes exceeded that in peripheral blood lymphocytes. Although these findings suggest that the frequency of infected

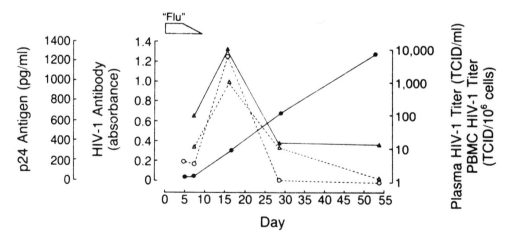

Figure 2–8. Sequential changes in HIV-1 antibody titers (solid circles) and p24 antigen concentrations (open circles) measured in plasma for a single patient during primary infection, and titers of infectious HIV-1 in plasma (open triangles) and peripheral blood mononuclear cells (solid triangles). "Flu" denotes a mononucleosis-like syndrome. (From Daar E, Moudgil T, Meyer RD et al: Transient high levels of viremia in patients with primary human immunodeficiency virus type 1 infection. N Eng J Med 324:961, 1991)

monocytes may be greater than previously estimated, it is not clear whether HIV-1 infection in these cells is latent *in vivo,* and if not, what percentage of cells may actively express the virus.

In a high proportion of peripheral blood leukocytes, HIV-1 proviral DNA has been shown to be replication competent,[303] an observation consistent with the high recovery rate of infectious virus from plasma and PBMC of infected patients at all stages of disease.[299] While data derived from PCR studies indicate that the proportion of infected PBMC within the peripheral circulation may be low, the titers of infectious virus detected in plasma and PBMC by coculture methods indicate a much higher degree of HIV-1 viremia. In studies by Ho *et al,*[299] HIV-1 was recovered from 100% of infected individuals at all stages of disease. The titers of infectious virus in the plasma increased with disease progression, with mean levels of 30, 3,500, and 3,200 tissue culture infectious doses (TCID) per milliliter for asymptomatic, ARC, and AIDS patients respectively. The frequency of infected PBMC increased from 1 in 50,000 cells for asymptomatic patients to approximately 1 in 400 cells for patients with AIDS or ARC. The high rate of virus recovery from the plasma of HIV-1 seropositive individuals indicates that HIV-1 replication within the host is not completely latent, and that circulating antibodies are insufficient to neutralize HIV-1 *in vivo.*

It is clear that protective immunity does not persist following primary infection with HIV-1, and evidence of increasing virus burden appears coincident with disease progression in infected individuals (Fig. 2–9). Progression to AIDS is marked by an increasing frequency of infected cells and elevated levels of plasma viremia. The mechanisms that govern the persistence of HIV within the host and ultimately the transition from latent to fulminant infection are not known. It is likely that multiple factors, including the virus inoculum, the site of infection, and the immune status of the host, have bearing on the course of disease.[304] Based on our knowledge to date, several additional factors may contribute to this process. Increased sequence diversity coupled with the high mutation rate of specific HIV-1 genes may allow the virus to evade immune surveillance and persist within the host. The emergence of genotypic variants with altered biologic activities, including increased replication rates, cytopathicity, and expanded tropism, may increase the overall pathogenicity of the virus. In addition, infection of cells of the macrophage lineage, which appear relatively resistant to HIV-1–mediated cytopathology, may provide a reservoir for dissemination of HIV-1 to multiple sites in the body, including the brain and CNS. Other factors such as concomitant infection with other viruses, disruption of cytokine regulatory networks, and infection of hematopoietic progenitor cells may contribute to eventual immune dysfunction. In the face of increasing virus burden, decreases in CD4+ T cells may result directly from HIV-1–mediated cytopathicity or indirectly through

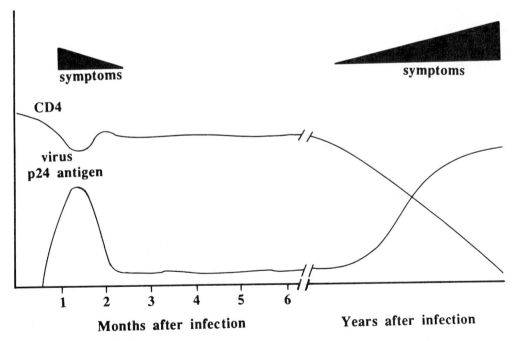

Figure 2–9. Changes in CD4-cell count and viral antigen levels during the course of HIV-1 infection. (Modified from Clark SJ, Saag MS, Decker WD et al: High titers of cytoplasmic virus in the plasma of patients with symptomatic primary HIV-1 infection. N Eng J Med 324:954, 1991)

autoimmune mechanisms. The profound immuno-suppression and opportunistic disease characteristic of HIV-1 infection and AIDS are consistent with the central role these cells play in the induction of immune responsiveness and regulation of immune function *in vivo*.

REFERENCES

1. Chiu I-M, Yaniv A, Dahlberg JE et al: Nucleotide sequence evidence for the relationship of AIDS retrovirus to lentiviruses. Nature 317:366, 1985
2. Gonda, MA, Wong-Staal F, Gallo RC et al: Sequence homology and morphologic similarity of HTLV-III and visna virus, a pathogenic lentivirus. Science 227:173, 1985
3. Sonigo P, Alizon M, Staskus K et al: Nucleotide sequence of the visna lentivirus: Relationship to the AIDS virus. Cell 42:369, 1985
4. Nathanson N, Georgsson G, Palsson PA et al: Experimental visna in Islandic sheep: The prototype lentivirus infection. Rev Infect Dis 7:75, 1985
5. Stephens RM, Casey JW, Rice NR: Equine infectious anemia virus gag and pol genes: Relatedness to visna and AIDS virus. Science 231:589, 1986
6. Narayan O, Cork LC: Lentiviral diseases of sheep and goats: Chronic pneumonia, leukoencephalomyelitis and arthritis. Rev Infect Dis 7:89, 1985
7. Cheevers WP, McGuire TC: Equine infectious anemia virus: Immunopathogenesis and persistence. Rev Infect Dis 7:83, 1985
8. Daniel MD, Letvin NL, King NW et al: Isolation of T-cell tropic HTLV-III-like retrovirus from macaques. Science 228:1201, 1985
9. Kanki PJ, McLane MF, King NW Jr et al: Serologic identification and characterization of a macaque T-lymphotropic retrovirus closely related to HTLV-III. Science 228:1199, 1985
10. Chakrabarti L, Guyader M, Alizon M et al: Sequence of simian immunodeficiency virus from macaque and its relationship to other human simian retroviruses. Nature 328:543, 1987
11. Fukasawa M, Miura T, Hasequawa A et al: Sequence of simian immunodeficiency virus from African green monkey, a new member of HIV/SIV group. Nature 333:457, 1988
12. Letvin NL, Daniel MD, Sehgal PK et al: Induction of AIDS-like disease in macaque monkeys with T-cell tropic retrovirus STLV-III. Science 230:71, 1985
13. Fultz P, McClure HM, Anderson DC et al: Isolation of a T-cell lymphotropic retrovirus from naturally infected sooty mangabey monkeys (*Cercocebus atys*). Proc Natl Acad Sci USA 83:5286, 1986
14. Clavel F, Guetard D, Brun-Vezinet F et al: Isolation of a new human retrovirus from West African patients with AIDS. Science 233:343, 1986
15. Clavel F, Guyader M, Guetard D et al: Molecular cloning and polymorphism of the human immunodeficiency virus type 2. Nature 324:691, 1986
16. Guyander M, Emerman M, Sonigo P et al: Genome organization and transactivation of the human immunodeficiency virus type 2. Nature 326:662, 1987
17. Clavel F, Mansinho K, Chamaret S et al: Human immunodeficiency virus type 2 infection associated with AIDS in West Africa. N Engl J Med 316:1180, 1987
18. Brun-Vezinet F, Rey MA, Katlama C et al: Lymphadenopathy-associated virus type 2 in AIDS and AIDS-related complex: Clinical and virological features in four patients. Lancet 1:128, 1987
19. Reinherz E, Schlossman SF: The differentiation and function of human T lymphocytes. Cell 19:821, 1980
20. Engleman EG, Benike C, Grumet C et al: Activation of human T lymphocyte subsets: Helper and suppressor/cytotoxic T cells recognize and respond to distinct histocompatibility antigens. J Immunol 127:2124, 1981
21. Meuer SC, Schlossman SF, Reinherz E: Clonal analysis of human cytotoxic T lymphocytes T4+ and T8+ effector T cells recognize products of different major histocompatibility complex regions. Proc Natl Acad Sci USA 79:4395, 1982
22. Robey E, Axel R: CD4: Collaborator in immune recognition and HIV infection. Cell 60:697, 1990
23. Gay D, Maddon P, Sekaly R et al: Functional interaction between human T-cell protein CD4 and the major histocompatibility complex HLA-DR antigen. Nature 328:626, 1987
24. Doyle C, Strominger JL: Interaction between CD4 and class II MHC molecules mediates cell adhesion. Nature 330:256, 1987
25. Marth JD, Peet R, Krebs EG et al: A lymphocyte-specific protein-tyrosine kinase gene is rearranged and overexpressed in the murine T cell lymphoma LSTRA. Cell 43:393, 1985
26. Klatzmann D, Barre-Sinoussi F, Nugeyre MT et al: Selective tropism of lymphadenopathy associated virus (LAV) for helper-inducer T lymphocytes. Science 225:59, 1984
27. Dalgleish AG, Beverley PCL, Clapham PR et al: The CD4 (T4) antigen is an essential component of the receptor for the AIDS retrovirus. Nature 312:763, 1984
28. Klatzmann D, Champagne E, Chamaret S et al: T-lymphocyte T4 molecule behaves as the receptor for human retrovirus LAV. Nature 312:767, 1984
29. McDougal JS, Mawle A, Cort SP et al: Cellular tropism of the human retrovirus HTLV-III/LAV: I. Role of T-cell activation and expression of the T4 antigen. J Immunol 135:3151, 1985
30. McDougal JS, Kennedy MS, Sligh JM et al: Binding of HTLV/LAV to T4+ T cells by a complex of the 110 K viral protein and the T4 molecule. Science 231:382, 1986
31. Maddon PJ, Littman DR, Godfrey M et al: The isolation and nucleotide sequence of a cDNA encoding the T cell surface protein T4: A new member of the immunoglobulin gene family. Cell 42:93, 1985
32. Maddon PJ, Dalgleish AS, McDougal JS et al: The T4 gene encodes the AIDS virus receptor and is expressed in the immune system and the brain. Cell 47:333, 1986
33. Smith DH, Byrn RA, Marsters SA et al: Blocking of HIV-1 infectivity by a soluble, secreted form of the CD4 antigen. Science 238:1704, 1987
34. Fisher RA, Bertonis JM, Meier W et al: HIV infection is blocked in vitro by recombinant soluble CD4. Nature 331:76, 1988
35. Hussey RE, Richardson NE, Kowalski M et al: A soluble CD4 protein selectively inhibits HIV replication and syncytia formation. Nature 331:78, 1988
36. Deen KC, McDougal JS, Inacker R et al: A soluble form of CD4 (T4) protein inhibits AIDS virus replication. Nature 331:81, 1988
37. Traunecker A, Luke W, Karjalainen K: Soluble CD4 mol-

ecules neutralize human immunodeficiency virus type 1. Nature 331:84, 1988

38. Clapham PR, Weber JN, Whitby D et al: Soluble CD4 blocks the infectivity of diverse strains of HIV and SIV for T cells and monocytes but not for brain and muscle cells. Nature 337:368, 1989

39. Sattentau QJ, Dalgleish AG, Weiss RA: Epitopes of the CD4 antigen and HIV infection. Science 234:1120, 1986

40. McClure MO, Sattentau QJ, Beverley PCL: HIV infection of primate lymphocytes and conservation of the CD4 receptor. Nature 330:487, 1987

41. Berger EA, Fuerst TR, Moss B: A soluble recombinant polypeptide comprising the amino-terminal half of the extracellular region of the CD4 molecule contains an active binding site for human immunodeficiency virus. Proc Natl Acad Sci USA 85:2357, 1988

42. Peterson A, Seed B: Genetic analysis of monoclonal antibody and HIV binding sites on the human lymphocyte antigen CD4. Cell 54:65, 1988

43. Mizukami T, Fuerst TR, Berger EA et al: Binding region for human immunodeficiency virus (HIV) and epitopes for HIV-blocking monoclonal antibodies of the CD4 molecule defined by site-directed mutagenesis. Proc Natl Acad Sci USA 85:9273, 1988

44. Brodsky MH, Warton M, Myers RM et al: Analysis of the site in CD4 that binds to the HIV envelope glycoprotein. J Immunol 144:3078, 1990

45. Landau NR, Warton M, Littman DR: The envelope glycoprotein of the human immunodeficiency virus binds the immunoglobulin-like domain of CD4. Nature 334:159, 1988

46. Clayton LK, Hussey RE, Steinbrich R et al: Substitution of murine for human CD4 residues identifies amino acids critical for HIV-gp120 binding. Nature 335:363, 1988

47. Arthos J, Deen KC, Chaikin MA et al: Identification of the residues in human CD4 critical for the binding of HIV. Cell 57:469, 1989

48. McDougal JS, Nicholson JKA, Cross GD et al: Binding of the human retrovirus HTLV III/LAV/HIV to the CD4 (T4) molecule: Conformation dependence, epitope mapping, antibody inhibition, and potential for idiotypic mimicry. J Immunol 137:2937, 1986

49. Ibegbu CC, Kennedy MS, Maddon PJ et al: Structural features of CD4 required for binding to HIV. J Immunol 142:2250, 1989

50. Healy D, Dianda L, Moore JP et al: Novel anti-CD4 monoclonal antibodies separate human immunodeficiency virus infection and fusion of CD4+ cells from virus binding. J Exp Med 172:1233, 1990

51. Celada F, Cambiaggi C, Maccari J et al: Antibody raised against soluble CD4-rgp120 complex recognizes the CD4 moiety and blocks membrane fusion without inhibiting CD4-gp120 binding. J Exp Med 172:1143, 1990

52. Camerini D, Seed B: A CD4 domain important for HIV-mediated syncytium formation lies outside the virus binding site. Cell 60:747, 1990

53. Robey WG, Safai B, Oroszlan S et al: Characterization of envelope and core structural gene products of HTLV-III with sera from AIDS patients. Science 228:593, 1985

54. Veronese FD, DeVico AL, Copeland TD et al: Characterization of gp41 as the transmembrane protein coded by the HTLV III/LAV envelope gene. Science 229:1402, 1985

55. Chakrabarti S, Robert-Guroff M, Wong-Staal F et al: Expression of the HTLV III envelope gene by a recombinant vaccinia virus. Nature 320:535, 1986

56. Hu SL, Kosowski SG, Dalrymple JM: Expression of AIDS virus envelope gene in recombinant vaccinia viruses. Nature 320:537, 1986

57. Willey RL, Bonifacino JS, Potts BJ et al: Biosynthesis, cleavage, and degradation of the human immunodeficiency virus type 1 envelope glycoprotein gp160. Proc Natl Acad Sci USA 85:9580, 1988

58. Gelderblom HR, Hausmann EHS, Ozel M et al: Fine structure of human immunodeficiency virus (HIV) and immunolocalization of structural proteins. Virology 156:171, 1987

59. Takahashi I, Takama M, Ladhoff AM et al: Envelope structure model of human immunodeficiency virus type 1. J AIDS 2:136, 1989

60. Ozel M, Pauli G, Gelderblom HR: The organization of the envelope projections on the surface of HIV. Arch Virol 100:255, 1988

61. Starcich BR, Hahn BH, Shaw GM et al: Identification and characterization of conserved and variable regions in the envelope gene of HTLV III/LAV, the retrovirus of AIDS. Cell 45:637, 1986

62. Willey RL, Rutledge RA, Dias S et al: Identification of conserved and divergent domains within the envelope gene of the acquired immune deficiency syndrome retrovirus. Proc Natl Acad Sci USA 83:5038, 1986

63. Lasky LA, Nakamura G, Smith DH et al: Delineation of a region of the human immunodeficiency virus type 1 gp120 glycoprotein critical for interaction with the CD4 receptor. Cell 50:975, 1987

64. Linsley PS, Ledbetter JA, Kinney-Thomas E et al: Effect of anti-gp120 monoclonal antibodies on CD4 receptor binding by the env protein of human immunodeficiency virus type 1. J Virol 62:3695, 1988

65. Dowbenko D, Nakamura G, Fennie C et al: Epitope mapping of the human immunodeficiency virus type 1 gp120 with monoclonal antibodies. J Virol 62:4703, 1988

66. Sun, N-C, Ho DD, Sun CRY et al: Generation and characterization of monoclonal antibodies to the putative CD4-binding domain of human immunodeficiency virus type 1 gp120. J Virol 63:3579, 1989

67. Cordonnier A, Riviere Y, Montagnier L et al: Effects of mutations in hyperconserved regions of the extracellular glycoprotein of human immunodeficiency virus type 1 on receptor binding. J Virol 63:4464, 1989

68. Olshevsky U, Helseth E, Furman C et al: Identification of individual human immunodeficiency virus type 1 gp120 amino acids important for CD4 receptor binding. J Virol 64:5701, 1990

69. Fennie C, Lasky LA. Model for intracellular folding of the human immunodeficiency virus type 1 gp120. J Virol 63:639, 1989

70. Tschachler E, Buchow H, Gallo RC et al: Functional contribution of cysteine residues to the human immunodeficiency virus type 1 envelope. J Virol 64:2250, 1990

71. Helseth E, Olshevsky U, Furman C et al: Human immunodeficiency virus type 1 gp120 envelope glycoprotein regions important for association with the gp41 transmembrane glycoprotein. J Virol 65:2119, 1991

72. White J, Kielian M, Helenius A: Membrane fusion proteins of enveloped animal viruses. Q Rev Biophys 16:151, 1983

73. McCune JM, Rabin LB, Feinberg MB et al: Endoproteolytic cleavage of gp160 is required for the activation of human immunodeficiency virus. Cell 53:55, 1988

74. Freed EO, Meyers DJ, Risser R: Mutational analysis of the cleavage sequence of the human immunodeficiency virus

type 1 envelope glycoprotein precursor gp160. J Virol 63: 4670, 1989

75. Kowalski M, Potz J, Basiripour L et al: Functional regions of the envelope glycoprotein of human immunodeficiency virus type 1. Science 237: 1351, 1987

76. Kowalski M, Bergeron L, Dorfman T et al: Attenuation of human immunodeficiency type 1 cytopathic effect by a mutation affecting the transmembrane envelope glycoprotein. J Virol 65:281, 1991

77. Freed EO, Myers DJ, Risser R: Characterization of the fusion domain of the human immunodeficiency virus type 1 envelope glycoprotein gp41. Proc Natl Acad Sci USA 87:4650, 1990

78. Goudsmit J, Debouck C, Meloen RH et al: Human immunodeficiency virus type 1 neutralizing epitope with conserved architecture elicits early type-specific antibodies in experimentally infected chimpanzees. Proc Natl Acad Sci USA 85:4478, 1988

79. Javaherian K, Langlois AJ, McDanal C et al: Principle neutralizing domain of the human immunodeficiency virus type 1 envelope protein. Proc Natl Acad Sci USA 86:6768, 1989

80. Matsushita S, Robert-Guroff M, Rusche J et al: Characterization of a human immunodeficiency virus neutralizing monoclonal antibody and mapping of the neutralizing epitope. J Virol 62:2107, 1988

81. Parker TJ, Clark ME, Langlois AJ et al: Type-specific neutralization of the human immunodeficiency virus with antibodies to env-encoded peptides. Proc Natl Acad Sci USA 85:1932, 1988

82. Rusche JR, Javaherian K, McDanal C et al: Antibodies that inhibit fusion of human immunodeficiency virus-infected cells bind a 24-amino acid sequence of the viral envelope gp120. Proc Natl Acad Sci USA 85:3198, 1988

83. Skinner MA, Langlois AJ, McDanal CB et al: Neutralizing antibodies to an immunodominant envelope sequence do not prevent gp120 binding to CD4. J Virol 62:4195, 1988

84. Freed EO, Myers DJ, Risser R: Identification of the principal neutralizing determinant of human immunodeficiency virus type 1 as a fusion domain. J Virol 65:190, 1991

85. Clements GJ, Price-Jones MJ, Stephans PE et al: The V3 loops of the HIV-1 and HIV-2 surface glycoproteins contain proteolytic cleavage sites: A possible function in viral fusion? AIDS Res Hum Retroviruses 7:3, 1991

86. Anderson KB, Skov H: Retrovirus-induced cell fusion is enhanced by protease treatment. J Gen Virol 70:1921, 1989

87. Anderson KB: Cleavage fragments of the retrovirus surface protein gp70 during virus entry. J Gen Virol 68:2193, 1987

88. Pauza CD, Price TM: Human immunodeficiency virus infection of T cells and monocytes proceeds via receptor-mediated endocytosis. J Cell Biol 107:959, 1988

89. Stein BS, Gowda SD, Lifson JD et al: pH-independent entry into CD4-positive T cells via virus envelope fusion to the plasma membrane. Cell 49:659, 1987

90. Maddon PJ, McDougal JS, Clapham PR et al: HIV infection does not require endocytosis of its receptor CD4. Cell 54: 865, 1988

91. Bedinger P, Moriarty A, von Borstel RC et al: Internalization of human immunodeficiency virus does not require the cytoplasmic domain. Nature 334:162, 1988

92. Weller SK, Joy AE, Temin HM: Correlation between cell killing and massive second-round superinfection by members of some subgroups of avian leukosis virus. J Virol 33:494, 1980

93. Keshet E, Temin HM: Cell killing by spleen necrosis virus is correlated with a transient accumulation of spleen necrosis virus DNA. J Virol 31:376, 1979

94. Levy JA, Kaminsky LS, Marrow WJW et al: Infection by the retrovirus associated with the acquired immunodeficiency syndrome: Clinical, biological and molecular features. Ann Intern Med 103:694, 1985

95. DeRossi A, Franchini G, Aldovini A et al: Differential response to the cytopathic effects of human T-cell lymphotropic virus type III (HTLV III) superinfection in T4+ (helper) and T8+ (suppressor) T-cell clones transformed by HTLV-I. Proc Natl Acad Sci USA 83:4297, 1986

96. Gowda SD, Stein BS, Mohagheghpour N et al: Evidence that T cell activation is required for HIV-1 entry in CD4+ lymphocytes. J Immunol 142:773, 1989

97. Zack JA, Arrigo SJ, Weitsman SR et al: HIV-1 entry into quiescent primary lymphocytes: Molecular analysis reveals a labile, latent viral structure. Cell 61:213, 1990

98. Dougherty JP, Temin HM: Determination of the rate of base-pair substitution and insertion mutations in retrovirus replication. J Virol 62:2817, 1988

99. Leider JM, Palese P, Smith FI: Determination of the mutation rate of a retrovirus. J Virol 62:3084, 1988

100. Coffin JM: Genetic variation in AIDS viruses. Cell 46:1, 1986

101. Wong-Staal F, Shaw GM, Hahn BH et al: Genomic diversity of human T-lymphotropic virus type III. Science 229:759, 1985

102. Shaw GM, Hahn BH, Arya SK et al: Molecular characterization of human T-cell leukemia (lymphotropic) virus type III in the acquired immune deficiency syndrome. Science 226:1165, 1984

103. Benn S, Rutledge R, Folks T et al: Genomic heterogeneity of AIDS retroviral isolates from North America and Zaire. Science 230:949, 1985

104. Ratner L, Haseltine W, Patarca R et al: Complete nucleotide sequence of the AIDS virus HTLV III. Nature 313:277, 1985

105. Wain-Hobson S, Sonigo P, Danos O et al: Nucleotide sequence of the AIDS virus LAV. Cell 40:9, 1985

106. Sanchez-Pescador R, Power MD, Barr PJ et al: Nucleotide sequence and expression of an AIDS-associated retrovirus (ARV-2). Science 227:484, 1985

107. Muesing MA, Smith DH, Cabradilla CD et al: Nucleic acid structures and expression of the human AIDS/lymphadenopathy retrovirus. Nature 313:430, 1985

108. Alizon M, Wain-Hobson S, Montagnier L et al: Genetic variability of the AIDS virus: Nucleotide sequence analysis of two isolates from African patients. Cell 46:63, 1986

109. Hahn BH, Gonda MA, Shaw GM et al: Genomic diversity of the AIDS virus HTLV-III: different viruses exhibit greatest divergence in their envelope genes. Proc Natl Acad Sci USA 82:4813, 1985

110. Rabson A, Martin MA: Molecular organization of the AIDS retrovirus. Cell 40:477, 1985

111. Ratner L, Gallo RC, Wong-Staal F: HTLV-III, LAV, and ARV are variants of the same AIDS virus. Nature 313:636, 1985

112. Gregory TJ, Leonard CK, Riddle L et al: Disulfide bond assignment and characterization of N-linked glycosylation sites in recombinant HIV-1 type IIIB gp120 produced in CHO cells. J Cell Biochem Suppl 14D:151, 1990

113. Clements JE, Pederson FS, Narayan O et al: Genomic changes associated with antigenic variation of visna virus

during persistent infection. Proc Natl Acad Sci USA 77: 4454, 1980

114. Montelaro RC, Parelch B, Orrego A et al: Antigenic variation during persistent infection by equine infectious anemia virus, a retrovirus. J Biol Chem 259:10539, 1984

115. Salinovich O, Payne SL, Montelaro RC et al: Rapid emergence of novel antigenic and genetic variants during persistent infection. J Virol 57:71, 1986

116. Simmonds P, Balfe P, Ludham CA et al: Analysis of sequence diversity in hypervariable regions of the external glycoprotein of human immunodeficiency virus type 1. J Virol 64:5840, 1990

117. Hahn BH, Shaw GM, Taylor ME et al: Genetic variation in HTLV-III/LAV over time in patients with AIDS or at risk for AIDS. Science 231:1548, 1986

118. Saag MS, Hahn BH, Gibbons J et al: Extensive variation of human immunodeficiency virus type-1 in vivo. Nature 334:440, 1988

119. Meyerhans A, Cheynier R, Albert J et al: Temporal fluctuations in HIV quasispecies in vivo are not reflected by sequential HIV isolations. Cell 58:901, 1989

120. Fisher AG, Ensoli B, Looney D et al: Biologically diverse molecular variants within a single HIV-1 isolate. Nature 334:444, 1988

121. Sakai K, Dewhurst S, Ma X et al: Differences in cytopathicity and host cell range among infectious molecular clones of human immunodeficiency virus type 1 simultaneously isolated from an infected individual. J Virol 62: 4078, 1988

122. Cheng-Meyer C, Seto D, Tateno M et al: Biologic features of HIV-1 that correlate with virulence in the host. Science 240:80, 1988

123. Asjo B, Morfeldt-Manson L, Albert J et al: Replicative capacity of human immunodeficiency virus from patients with varying degrees of severity of HIV infection. Lancet 2:660, 1986

124. Fenyo EM, Morfeldt-Manson L, Chiodi F et al: Distinct replicative and cytopathic characteristics of human immunodeficiency virus isolates. J Virol 62:4414, 1988

125. Fenyo EM, Albert J, Asjo B: Replicative capacity, cytopathic effect and cell tropism of HIV. AIDS 3(suppl 1):S5, 1989

126. Asjo B, Albert J, Chiodi F et al: Improved tissue culture technique for production of poorly replicating human immunodeficiency virus strains. J Virol Methods 19:191, 1988

127. Kestler HW, Ringler DJ, Mori K et al: Importance of the nef gene for maintenance of high virus loads and for the development of AIDS. Cell 65:651, 1991

128. Luciw PA, Cheng-Meyer C, Levy JA: Mutational analysis of the human immunodeficiency virus: The orf-B region down regulates virus replication. Proc Natl Acad Sci USA 84:1434, 1987

129. Terwilliger E, Sodrowski JG, Rosen CA et al: Effects of mutations within the 3' orf open reading frame region of the human T-cell lymphotropic virus type III (HTLV III/LAV) on replication and cytopathicity. J Virol 60:754, 1986

130. Fisher AG, Ensoli B, Ivanoff L et al: The sor gene of HIV-1 is required for efficient virus transmission in vitro. Science 237:888, 1987

131. Groenik M, Fouchier RAM, De Goede REY et al: Phenotypic heterogeneity in a panel of infectious molecular human immunodeficiency virus type 1 clones derived from a single individual. J Virol 65:1968, 1991

132. Tersmette M, De Goede REY, Al BJM et al: Differential syncytium-inducing capacity of human immunodeficiency virus isolates: Frequent detection of syncytium-inducing isolates in patients with acquired immunodeficiency syndrome (AIDS) and AIDS-related complex. J Virol 62:2026, 1988

133. Tersmette M, Gruters RA, DeWolf F et al: Evidence for a role of virulent human immunodeficiency virus (HIV) variants in the pathogenesis of acquired immunodeficiency syndrome: Studies on sequential HIV isolates. J Virol 63:2118, 1989

134. Tersmette M, Lange JMA, DeGoede REY et al: Association between biological properties of human immunodeficiency virus variants and risk for AIDS and AIDS mortality. Lancet 1:983, 1989

135. Lifson JD, Feinberg MB, Reyes GR et al: Induction of CD4-dependent cell fusion by the HTLV-III/LAV envelope glycoprotein. Nature 323:725, 1986

136. Sodrowski J, Goh WC, Rosen C et al: Role of the HTLV III/LAV envelope in syncytium formation and cytopathicity. Nature 322:470, 1986

137. Lifson JD, Reyes GR, McGrath MS et al: AIDS retrovirus induced cytopathology: Giant cell formation and involvement of CD4 antigen. Science 232:1123, 1986

138. Gallaher WR: Detection of a fusion peptide sequence in the transmembrane protein of human immunodeficiency virus. Cell 50:327, 1987

139. Helseth E, Olshevsky U, Gabuzda D et al: Changes in the transmembrane region of the human immunodeficiency virus type 1 gp41 envelope glycoprotein affect membrane fusion. J Virol 64:6314, 1990

140. Koga Y, Lindstrom E, Fenyo EM et al: High levels of heterodisperse RNAs accumulate in T-cells infected with human immunodeficiency virus and normal thymocytes. Proc Natl Acad Sci USA 85:4521, 1988

141. Leonard R, Zagury D, Desportes I et al: Cytopathic effect of human immunodeficiency virus in T4 cells is linked to the last stage of virus infection. Proc Natl Acad Sci USA 85:3570, 1988

142. Hoxie JA, Alpers JD, Rackowski JL et al: Alterations in T4 (CD4) protein and mRNA synthesis in cells infected with HIV. Science 234:1123, 1986

143. Gupta S, Vayuvegula B: Human immunodeficiency virus–associated changes in signal transduction. J Clin Immunol 7:486, 1987

144. Walker BD, Chakrabarti S, Moss B et al: HIV-specific cytotoxic T lymphocytes in seropositive individuals. Nature 328:345, 1897

145. Walker BD, Flexner C, Paradis TJ et al: HIV-1 reverse transcriptase is a target for cytotoxic T lymphocytes in infected individuals. Science 240:64, 1988

146. Koenig S, Earl P, Powell D et al: Group-specific, major histocompatibility complex class I-restricted cytotoxic responses to human immunodeficiency virus I (HIV-1) envelope proteins by cloned peripheral blood T cells from an HIV-1 infected individual. Proc Natl Acad Sci USA 85: 8638, 1988

147. Rook AH, Lane HC, Folks T et al: Sera from HTLV-III/LAV antibody-positive individuals mediate antibody-dependent cellular cytotoxicity against HTLV-III/LAV infected T cells. J Immunol 138:1064, 1987

148. Ojo-Amaize EA, Nishanian P, Keith DE Jr et al: Antibodies to human immunodeficiency virus in human sera induce cell-mediated lysis of human immunodeficiency virus-infected cells. J Immunol 139:2458, 1987

149. Ljunggren K, Bottiger B, Biberfeld G et al: Antibody-dependent cellular cytotoxicity-inducing antibodies

against human immunodeficiency virus. J Immunol 139: 2263, 1987

150. Blumberg R, Paradis T, Hartshorn KL et al: Antibody-dependent cell-mediated cytotoxicity against cells infected with the human immunodeficiency virus. J Infect Dis 156:878, 1987

151. Evans LA, McHugh TM, Stiltes DP et al: Differential ability of human immunodeficiency virus isolates to productively infect human cells. J Immunol 138:3415, 1987

152. Gartner S, Markovitz P, Markovitz DM et al: The role of mononuclear phagocytes in HTLV-III/LAV infection. Science 223:215, 1986

153. Gabuzda DH, Ho DD, de la Monte SM et al: Immunohistochemical identification of HTLV-III antigen in the brains of patients infected with AIDS. Ann Neurol 20:289, 1986

154. Kim S, Ikeuchi K, Groopman J et al: Factors affecting cellular tropism of human immunodeficiency virus. J Virol 64:5600, 1990

155. Asjo B, Ivhed I, Gidlund M et al: Susceptibility to infection by the human immunodeficiency virus (HIV) correlates with T4 expression in a parental monocytoid cell line and its subclones. Virology 157:359, 1987

156. Cann AJ, Zack JA, Go AS et al: Human immunodeficiency virus type 1 T-cell tropism is determined by events prior to provirus formation. J Virol 64:4735, 1990

157. Cheng-Meyer C, Quiroga M, Tung JW et al: Viral determinants of human immunodeficiency virus type 1 T-cell or macrophage tropism, cytopathicity and CD4 antigen modulation. J Virol 64:4390, 1990

158. York-Higgins D, Cheng-Meyer C, Bauer D et al: Human immunodeficiency virus type 1 cellular host range, replication, and cytopathicity are linked to the envelope region of the viral genome. J Virol 64:4016, 1990

159. Cordonnier A, Montagnier L, Emerman M: Single amino-acid changes in HIV envelope affect viral tropism and receptor binding. Nature 340:571, 1989

160. Liu ZQ, Wood C, Levy JA et al: The viral envelope gene is involved in macrophage tropism of a human immunodeficiency virus type 1 strain isolated from brain tissue. J Virol 64:6148, 1990

161. O'Brien WA, Koyanagi Y, Namazie A et al: HIV-1 tropism for mononuclear phagocytes can be determined by regions of gp120 outside the CD4-binding domain. Nature 348:69, 1990

162. Shioda T, Levy JA, Cheng-Meyer C: Macrophage and T cell-line tropism of HIV-1 are determined by specific regions of the envelope gp120 gene. Nature 349:167, 1991

163. Takeuchi Y, Akutsu M, Murayama K et al: Host range mutant of human immunodeficiency virus type 1: Modification of cell tropism by a single point mutation at the neutralization epitope in the env gene. J Virol 65:1710, 1991

164. Schuitemaker H, Kootstra NA, De Goede REY et al: Monocytotropic human immunodeficiency virus type 1 (HIV-1) variants detectable in all stages of HIV-1 infection lack T-cell line tropism and syncytium-inducing ability in primary T-cell culture. J Virol 65:356, 1991

165. Adachi A, Koenig S, Gendelman HE et al: Productive, persistent infection of human colorectal cell lines with human immunodeficiency virus. J Virol 61:209, 1987

166. Cheng-Meyer C, Rutka JT, Rosenblum ML et al: Human immunodeficiency virus can productively infect cultured human glial cells. Proc Natl Acad Sci USA 84:3526, 1987

167. Clapham PR, Weber JN, Whitby D et al: Soluble CD4 blocks the infectivity of diverse strains of HIV and SIV for T cells and monocytes but not for brain and muscle cells. Nature 337:368, 1989

168. Folks TM, Kessler SW, Orenstein JM et al: Infection and replication of HIV-1 in purified progenitor cells of normal human bone marrow. Science 242:919, 1988

169. Harouse JM, Kunsch C, Hartle HT et al: CD4-independent infection of human neural cells by human immunodeficiency virus type 1. J Virol 63:2527, 1989

170. Koenig S, Gendelman H, Orenstein J et al: Detection of AIDS virus in macrophages in brain tissue from AIDS patients with encephalopathy. Science 233:1089, 1986

171. Monroe JE, Calender A, Mulder C: Epstein-Barr virus-positive and -negative B cell lines can be infected with human immunodeficiency virus types 1 and 2. J Virol 62:3497, 1988

172. Zavada J: Viral pseudotypes and phenotypic mixing. Arch Virol 50:1, 1976

173. Boettiger D: Animal virus pseudotypes. Prog Med Virol 25:37, 1979

174. Lusso P, di Marzo Veronese F, Ensoli B et al: Expanded HIV-1 cellular tropism by phenotypic mixing with murine endogenous retroviruses. Science 247:848, 1990

175. Chesebro B, Buller R, Portis J et al: Failure of human immunodeficiency virus entry and infection in CD4-positive brain and skin cells. J Virol 64:215, 1990

176. Spector DH, Wade E, Wright DA et al: Human immunodeficiency virus pseudotypes with expanded cellular and species tropism. J Virol 64:2298, 1990

177. Zhu Z, Chen SSL, Huang AS: Phenotypic mixing between human immunodeficiency virus and vesicular stomatitis virus or herpes simplex virus. J AIDS 3:215, 1990

178. Clapham P, Nagy K, Weiss RA: Pseudotypes of human T cell leukemia virus types 1 and 2: Neutralization by patients' sera. Proc Natl Acad Sci USA 81:2886, 1984

179. Landau NR, Page KA, Littman DR: Pseudotyping with human T-cell leukemia virus type 1 broadens the human immunodeficiency virus host range. J Virol 65:162, 1991

180. Lee H, Swanson P, Shorty VS et al: High rate of HTLV-II infection in seropositive I.V. drug abusers in New Orleans. Science 244:471, 1989

181. Fiala M, Cone LA, Chang C et al: Cytomegalovirus viremia increases with progressive immune deficiency in patients with HTLV-III. AIDS Res 2:175, 1986

182. Raffi F, Boudart D, Billaudel S: Acute co-infection with human immunodeficiency virus (HIV) and cytomegalovirus. Ann Intern Med 112:234, 1990

183. Salahuddin SZ, Ablashi DV, Markham PD et al: Isolation of a new virus, HBLV, in patients with lymphoproliferative disorders. Science 234:596, 1986

184. Cao Y, Freidman-Kien AE, Huang Y et al: CD4-independent, productive human immunodeficiency virus type 1 infection of hepatoma cell lines in vitro. J Virol 64:2553, 1990

185. Tateno M, Gonzalez-Scarano F, Levy JA: Human immunodeficiency virus can infect CD4-negative fibroblastoid cells. Proc Natl Acad Sci USA 86:4287, 1989

186. Chiodi F, Fuerstenberg S, Gidlund M et al: Infection of brain-derived cells with human immunodeficiency virus. J Virol 61:1244, 1987

187. Dewhurst S, Sakai K, Bresser J et al: Persistent productive infection of human glial cells by human immunodeficiency virus (HIV) and by infectious molecular clones of HIV. J Virol 61:3774, 1987

188. Li XL, Moudgil T, Vinters HV et al: CD4-independent,

productive infection of a neuronal cell line by human immunodeficiency virus type 1. J Virol 64:1383, 1990

189. Nelson JA, Wiley CA, Reynolds-Kohler C et al: Human immunodeficiency virus detected in bowel epithelium from patients with gastrointestinal symptoms. Lancet 1: 259, 1988

190. Moyer MP, Huot RI, Ramirez A et al: Infection of human gastrointestinal cells by HIV-1. AIDS Res Hum Retroviruses 6:1409, 1990

191. Pomerantz RJ, Kuritzkes DR, de la Monte SM et al: Infection of the retina by human immunodeficiency virus type 1. N Engl J Med 317:1643, 1987

192. Pomerantz RJ, de la Monte SM, Donegan SP et al: Human immunodeficiency virus (HIV) infection of the uterine cervix. Ann Intern Med 108:321, 1988

193. Wiley CA, Schrier RD, Nelson JA et al: Cellular localization of human immunodeficiency virus infection within the brains of acquired immune deficiency syndrome patients. Proc Natl Acad Sci USA 83:7089, 1986

194. Schnittman SM, Psallidopoulos MC, Lane HC et al: The reservoir for HIV-1 in human peripheral blood is a T cell that maintains expression of CD4. Science 245:305, 1989

195. McElrath MJ, Pruett JE, Cohn ZA: Mononuclear phagocytes of blood and bone marrow: Comparative roles as viral reservoirs in human immunodeficiency virus type 1 infections. Proc Natl Acad Sci USA 86:675, 1989

196. Ho DD, Rota TR, Hirsh MS: Infection of monocyte/macrophages by human T lymphotropic virus type III. J Clin Invest 77:1712, 1986

197. Popovic M, Gartner S: Isolation of HIV-1 from monocytes but not T lymphocytes. Lancet 2:916, 1987

198. Tenner-Racz K, Racz P, Dietrich M et al: Altered follicular dendritic cells and virus-like particles in AIDS and AIDS-related lymphadenopathy. Lancet 1:105, 1985

199. Gartner S, Markovits P, Markovitz DM et al: Virus isolation from and identification of HTLV-III/LAV-producing cells in brain tissue from a patient with AIDS. JAMA 256:2365, 1986

200. Salahuddin SZ, Rose RM, Groopman JE et al: Human T lymphotropic virus type III infection of human alveolar macrophages. Blood 68:281, 1986

201. Tschaler E, Groh V, Popovic M et al: Epidermal Langerhans' cells: A target for HTLV-III/LAV infection. J Invest Dermatol 88:233, 1987

202. Collman R, Godfrey B, Cutilli J et al: Macrophage-tropic strains of human immunodeficiency virus type 1 utilize the CD4 receptor. J Virol 64:4468, 1990

203. Narayan O, Wolinsky JS, Clements JE et al: Slow virus replication: The role of macrophages in the persistence and expression of visna viruses of sheep and goats. J Gen Virol 59:345, 1982

204. Gendelman HE, Narayan O, Kennedy-Stoskopf S et al: Tropism of sheep lentiviruses for monocytes: Susceptibility to infection and virus gene expression increase during maturation of monocytes to macrophages. J Virol 58: 67, 1986

205. Perno C-F, Yarochan R, Cooney DA et al: Replication of human immunodeficiency virus in monocytes: Granulocyte/macrophage colony stimulating factor (GM-CSF) potentiates virus production yet enhances the antiviral effect mediated by 3'-azido-2',3'-dideoxythymidine (AZT) and other dideoxynucleoside congeners of thymidine. J Exp Med 169:933, 1989

206. Hammer SM, Gillis JM, Groopman JE et al: In vitro mod-

ification of human immunodeficiency virus infection by granulocyte-macrophage colony-stimulating factor and γ-interferon. Proc Natl Acad Sci USA 83:8734, 1986

207. Koyanagi Y, O'Brien WA, Zhao JQ et al: Cytokines alter production of HIV-1 from primary mononuclear phagocytes. Science 241:1673, 1988

208. Kornbluth RS, Oh PS, Munis JR et al: The role of interferons in the control of HIV replication in macrophages. Clin Immunol Immunopathol 54:200, 1990

209. Kornbluth RS, Oh PS, Munis JR et al: Interferons and bacterial lipopolysaccharide protect macrophages from productive infection by human immunodeficiency virus in vitro. J Exp Med 169:1137, 1989

210. Balkwill FR, Burke F: The cytokine network. Immunol Today 10:299, 1989

211. Lahdevirta J, Maury CPJ, Teppo A-M et al: Elevated levels of circulating cachectin/tumor necrosis factor in patients with acquired immunodeficiency syndrome. Am J Med 85:289, 1988

212. Roux-Lombard P, Modoux C, Cruchaud A et al: Purified blood monocytes from HIV-1 infected patients produce high levels of TNF-α and IL-1. Clin Immunol Immunopathol 50:374, 1989

213. Voth R, Rossol S, Klein K et al: Differential gene expression of IFN-α and tumor necrosis factor-α in peripheral blood mononuclear cells from patients with AIDS related complex and AIDS. J Immunol 144:970, 1990

214. Molina J-M, Scadden DT, Byrn R et al: Production of tumor necrosis factor α and interleukin 1β by monocytic cells infected with human immunodeficiency virus. J Clin Invest 84:733, 1989

215. Osborn L, Kunkel S, Nabel GJ: Tumor necrosis factor α and interleukin 1 stimulate the human immunodeficiency virus enhancer by activation of the nuclear factor NFκB. Proc Natl Acad Sci USA 86:2336, 1989

216. Folks TM, Clouse KA, Justement J et al: Tumor necrosis factor α induces expression of human immunodeficiency virus in a chronically infected T-cell clone. Proc Natl Acad Sci USA 86:2363, 1989

217. Israel N, Hazan U, Alcami J et al: Tumor necrosis factor stimulates transcription of HIV-1 in human T lymphocytes, independently and synergistically with mitogens. J Immunol 143:3956, 1989

218. Poli G, Bressler P, Kinter A et al: Interleukin 6 induces human immunodeficiency virus expression in infected monocytic cells alone and in synergy with tumor necrosis factor α by transcriptional and post-transcriptional mechanisms. J Exp Med 172: 151, 1990

219. Kishimoto T: The biology of interleukin-6. Blood 74:1, 1989

220. Wong GG, Clark SC: Multiple actions of interleukin 6 within a cytokine network. Immunol Today 9:137, 1988

221. Breen EC, Rezai AR, Nakajima K et al: Infection with HIV is associated with elevated IL-6 levels. J Immunol 144: 480, 1990

222. Pauza CD, Galindo J, Richman DD: Human immunodeficiency virus infection of monoblastoid cells: Cellular differentiation determines the pattern of virus replication. J Virol 62:3558, 1988

223. Folks TM, Justement J, Kinter A et al: Characterization of a promonocyte clone chronically infected with HIV and inducible by 13-phorbol-12-myristate acetate. J Immunol 140:1117, 1988

224. Siekevitz M, Josephs SF, Dukovich M et al: Activation of

the HIV-1 LTR by T cell mitogens and the trans-activator protein of HTLV-I. Science 238:1575, 1987

225. Tong-Starksen SE, Luciw PA, Peterlin BM: Human immunodeficiency virus long terminal repeat responds to T-cell activation signals. PNAS 84:6845, 1987

226. Harada S, Koyanagi Y, Nakashima H et al: Tumor promoter, TPA, enhances replication of HTLV-III/LAV. Virology 154:249, 1986

227. Nabel G, Baltimore D: An inducible transcription factor activates expression of human immunodeficiency virus in T cells. Nature 326:711, 1987

228. Duh EJ, Maury WJ, Folks TM et al: Tumor necrosis factor α activates human immunodeficiency virus type 1 through induction of nuclear factor binding to the NF-κB sites in the long terminal repeat. Proc Natl Acad Sci USA 86:5974, 1989

229. Griffin GE, Leung K, Folks TM et al: Activation of HIV gene expression during monocyte differentiation by induction of NF-κB. Nature 339:70, 1989

230. Pomerantz RJ, Feinberg MB, Trono D et al: Lipopolysaccharide is a potent monocyte/macrophage-specific stimulator of human immunodeficiency virus type 1 expression. J Exp Med 172:253, 1990

231. Gendelman HE, Orenstein JM, Baca LM et al: The macrophage in the persistence and pathogenesis of HIV infection. AIDS 3:475, 1989

232. Orenstein JM, Meltzer MS, Phipps T et al: Cytoplasmic assembly and accumulation of human immunodeficiency virus types 1 and 2 in recombinant human colony-stimulating factor-1-treated human monocytes: An ultrastructural study. J Virol 62:2578, 1988

233. Roy S, Wainberg MA: Role of the mononuclear phagocyte system in the development of acquired immunodeficiency syndrome (AIDS). J Leukotrienes Biol 43:91, 1988

234. Braathen LR, Ramirez G, Kunze ROF et al: Langerhans' cells as primary target cells for HIV infection. Lancet 2:1094, 1987

235. Niedecken H, Lutz G, Bauer R et al: Langerhans' cell as primary target and vehicle for transmission of HIV. Lancet 2:519, 1987

236. Ramirez G, Braathen LR, Kunze ROF et al: In vitro infection of human epidermal Langerhans' cells with HIV (abstr). Presented at the 9th International Conference on Lymphatic Tissues and Germinal Centres in Immune Reactions, Oslo, Norway, 1987

237. Belsito DV, Sanchez MR, Baer RL et al: Reduced Langerhans' cell Ia antigen and ATPase activity in patients with the acquired immunodeficiency syndrome. N Engl J Med 310:1279, 1984

238. Kanitakis J, Marchacd C, Su H et al: Immunohistochemical study of normal skin of HIV-1 infected patients shows no evidence of infection of epidermal Langerhans' cells by HIV. AIDS Res Hum Retroviruses 5:293, 1989

239. Rappersberger K, Gartner S, Schenk P et al: Langerhans' cells are an actual site of HIV-1 replication. Intervirology 29:185, 1988

240. Barre-Sinoussi F, Chermann JC, Rey F et al: Isolation of a T-lymphotropic retrovirus from a patient at risk for acquired immune deficiency syndrome (AIDS). Science 220:868, 1983

241. Baroni CD, Pezzella F, Mirolo M et al: Immunohistochemical demonstration of p24 HTLV-III major core protein in different cell types within lymph nodes from patients with lymphadenopathy syndrome (LAS). Histopathology 10:5, 1986

242. Le Tourneau A, Audouin J, Diebold J et al: LAV-like viral particles in lymph node germinal centers in patients with the persistent lymphadenopathy syndrome and the acquired immunodeficiency syndrome–related complex: An ultrastructural study of 30 cases. Hum Pathol 17:1047, 1986

243. Armstrong JA, Horne R: Follicular dendritic cells and virus-like particles in AIDS-related lymphadenopathy. Lancet 2:370, 1984

244. Cameron PU, Dawkins RL, Armstrong JA et al: Western blot profiles, lymph node ultrastructure and viral expression in HIV-1 infected patients: A correlative study. Clin Exp Immunol 68:465, 1987

245. Chayt KJ, Harper ME, Merselle LM et al: Detection of HTLV-III RNA in lungs of patients with AIDS and pulmonary involvement. JAMA 256:2356, 1986

246. Ziza, J-M, Brun-Vezinet F, Venet A et al: Lymphadenopathy-associated virus isolated from bronchoalveolar lavage fluid in AIDS-related complex with lymphoid interstitial pneumonitis. N Engl J Med 313:183, 1985

247. Plata, F, Autran B, Martins LP et al: AIDS virus-specific cytotoxic T lymphocytes in lung disorders. Nature 328:348, 1987

248. Price RW, Brew B, Sidtis J et al: The brain in AIDS: Central nervous system HIV-1 infection and AIDS dementia complex. Science 239:586, 1988

249. Orentstein JM, Janotta F: Human immunodeficiency virus and papova virus infections in acquired immunodeficiency syndrome: An ultrastructural study of three cases. Hum Pathol 19:350, 1988

250. Shaw GM, Harper ME, Hahn BH et al: HTLV-III infection in brains of children and adults with AIDS encephalopathy. Science 227:177, 1985

251. Levy JA, Shimabukuro J, Hollander H et al: Isolation of AIDS-associated retroviruses from cerebrospinal fluid and brains of patients with neurological symptoms. Lancet 2:586, 1985

252. Vazeux R, Brousse N, Jarry A et al: AIDS subacute encephalitis. Identification of HIV-infected cells. Am J Pathol 126:403, 1987

253. Pumarola-Sune T, Navia BA, Cordon-Cardo C et al: HIV antigen in the brains of patients with the AIDS dementia complex. Ann Neurol 21:490, 1987

254. Stoler MH, Eskin TA, Benn S et al: Human T-cell lymphotropic virus type III infection of the central nervous system: A preliminary in situ analysis. JAMA 256:2360, 1986

255. Gyorkey F, Melnick JL, Gyorkey P: Human immunodeficiency virus in brain biopsies of patients with AIDS and progressive encephalopathy. J Infect Dis 155:870, 1987

256. Sethi KK, Naher H, Stroehmann I: Phenotypic heterogeneity of cerebrospinal fluid-derived HIV-specific and HLA-restricted cytotoxic T-cell clones. Nature 335:178, 1988

257. Koyanagi Y, Miles S, Mitsuyasu RT et al: Dual infection of the central nervous system by AIDS viruses with distinct cellular tropisms. Science 236:819, 1987

258. Rutka JT, Giblin JR, Berens ME et al: The effects of human recombinant tumor necrosis factor on glioma-derived cell lines: Cellular proliferation, cytotoxicity, morphological and radioreceptor studies. Int J Cancer 47:573, 1988

259. Selmaj KW, Raine CS: Tumor necrosis factor mediates myelin and oligodendrocyte damage in vitro. Ann Neurol 23:339, 1988

260. Brennerman DE, Westbrook GL, Fitzgerald SP et al: Neuronal cell killing by the envelope protein of HIV and its prevention by vasoactive intestinal peptide. Nature 335:639, 1988

261. Lee MR, Ho DD, Gurney ME: Functional interaction and partial sequence homology between human immunodeficiency virus and neuroleukin. Science 237:1047, 1987

262. Gurney ME, Heinrich SP, Lee MR et al: Molecular cloning and expression of neuroleukin, a neurotropic factor for spinal and sensory neurons. Science 234:566, 1986

263. Gurney ME, Apatoff BR, Spear GT et al: Neuroleukin: A lymphokine product of lectin-stimulated T cells. Science 234:574, 1986

264. Chaput M, Claes V, Portetelle D et al: The neurotropic factor neuroleukin is 90% homologous with phosphohexose isomerase. Nature 332:454, 1988

265. Faik P, Walker JI, Redmill AA et al: Mouse glucose-6-phosphate isomerase and neuroleukin have identical 3' sequences. Nature 332:455, 1988

266. Wiley CA, Nelson JA: Role of human immunodeficiency virus and cytomegalovirus in AIDS encephalitis. Am J Pathol 133:73, 1988

267. Nelson JA, Reynolds-Kohler C, Oldstone MB et al: HIV and HCMV coinfect brain cells in patients with AIDS. Virology 165:286, 1988

268. Wiley CA, Grafe M, Kennedy C et al: Human immunodeficiency virus (HIV) and JC virus in acquired immunodeficiency syndrome (AIDS) patients with progressive multifocal leukoencephalopathy. Acta Neuropathol (Berl) 76:338, 1988

269. Gendelman HE, Phelps W, Feigenbaum L et al: Transactivation of the human immunodeficiency virus long terminal repeat sequence by DNA viruses. Proc Natl Acad Sci USA 83:9759, 1986

270. Castella A, Croxson TS, Mildvan et al: The bone marrow in AIDS: A histologic, hematologic and microbiological study. Am J Clin Pathol 84:424, 1985

271. Lake JP, Lee S, Spira S: Bone marrow findings in AIDS patients. Am J Clin Pathol 81:799, 1984

272. Perkocha LA, Rodgers GM: Hematologic aspects of human immunodeficiency virus infection: Laboratory and clinical considerations. Am J Hematol 29:94, 1988

273. Schneider DR, Picker LJ: Myelodysplasia in the acquired immunodeficiency syndrome. Am J Clin Pathol 84:144, 1982

274. Treacy M, Lai L, Costello C et al: Peripheral blood and bone marrow abnormalities in patients with HIV related diseases. Br J Haematol 65:289, 1987

275. Zon LI, Arkin C, Groopman JE: Hematologic manifestations of the human immunodeficiency virus (HIV). Br J Haematol 66:251, 1987

276. Bagnara GP, Zauli G, Giovannini M et al: Early loss of circulating hemopoietic progenitors in HIV-1 infected subjects. Exp Hematol 18:426, 1990

277. Ganser A: Abnormalities of hematopoiesis in the acquired immunodeficiency syndrome. Blut 56:49, 1988

278. Stella CC, Ganser A, Hoelzer D: Defective in vitro growth of the hemopoietic progenitor cells in the acquired immunodeficiency syndrome. J Clin Invest 80:286, 1987

279. Donahue RE, Johnson MM, Zon LI et al: Suppression of in vitro hematopoiesis following human immunodeficiency virus infection. Nature 326:200, 1987

280. Steinberg HN, Crumpacker CS, Chatis PA: In vitro suppression of normal human bone marrow progenitor cells by human immunodeficiency virus. J Virol 65:1765, 1991

281. Leiderman IZ, Greenberg ML, Adelsberg BR et al: A glycoprotein inhibitor of in vitro granulopoiesis associated with AIDS. Blood 70:1257, 1987

282. Wantanabe M, Ringler DJ, Nakamura M et al: Simian immunodeficiency virus inhibits bone marrow hematopoietic progenitor cell growth. J Virol 64:656, 1990

283. Cunningham-Ruddles S, Michelis MA, Masur LJ: Serum suppression of lymphocyte activation in vitro in acquired immunodeficiency disease. J Clin Immunol 3:156, 1983

284. Laurence J, Gottlieb AB, Kunkel HG: Soluble suppressor factors in patients with acquired immune deficiency syndrome and its prodrome: Elaboration in vitro by T lymphocyte-adherent cell interactions. J Clin Invest 72:2072, 1983

285. Lunardi-Iskandar Y, Nuyeyre MT, Georgoulias V et al: Replication of the human immunodeficiency virus 1 and impaired differentiation of T cells after in vitro infection of bone marrow immature T cells. J Clin Invest 83:610, 1989

286. Zucker-Franklin D, Cao Y: Megakaryocytes of human immunodeficiency virus-infected individuals express viral RNA. Proc Natl Acad Sci USA 86:5595, 1989

287. Sutherland HJ, Eaves CJ, Eaves AC et al: Characterization and partial purification of human marrow cells capable of initiating long-term hematopoiesis in vitro. Blood 74:1563, 1989

288. Andrews RG, Singer JW, Bernstein ID: Precursors of colony-forming cells in humans can be distinguished from colony-forming cells by expression of the CD33 and CD34 antigens and light scatter properties. J Exp Med 169:1721, 1989

289. von Laer D, Hufert FT, Fenner TE et al: CD34+ hematopoietic progenitor cells are not a major reservoir of the human immunodeficiency virus. Blood 76:1281, 1990

290. Davis BR, Schwartz DH, Marx JC et al: Absent or rare human immunodeficiency virus infection of bone marrow stem/progenitor cells in vivo. J Virol 65:1985, 1991

291. Sing CK, Ruscetti FW: Preferential suppression of myelopoiesis in normal human bone marrow cells after in vitro challenge with human cytomegalovirus. Blood 75:1965, 1973

292. Zeldis JB, Mugishima H, Steinberg HN et al: In vitro hepatitis B infection of human bone marrow cells. J Clin Invest 78:411, 1986

293. Richman DD, Fischl MA, Grieca MH et al: The toxicity of azidothymidine (AZT) in the treatment of patients with AIDS and AIDS-related complex: A double blind, placebo-controlled trial. N Engl J Med 317:192, 1987

294. Gaines H, Albert J, von Sydow M et al: HIV antigenaemia and virus isolation from plasma during primary HIV infection. Lancet 1:1317, 1987

295. Albert J, Gaines H, Sonnerborg et al: Isolation of human immunodeficiency virus (HIV) from plasma during primary HIV infection. J Med Virol 23:67, 1987

296. Goudsmit J, de Wolf F, Paul DA et al: Expression of human immunodeficiency virus antigen (HIV-Ag) in serum and cerbrospinal fluid during acute and chronic infection. Lancet 2:177, 1986

297. Daar ES, Moudgil T, Meyer RD et al: Transient high levels of viremia in patients with primary human immunodeficiency virus type 1 infection. N Engl J Med 324:961, 1991

298. Harper ME, Marselle LM, Gallo RC et al: Detection of lymphocytes expressing human T-lymphotropic virus type III in lymph nodes and peripheral blood from infected individual by in situ hybridization. Proc Natl Acad Sci USA 83:772, 1986

299. Ho DD, Moudgil T, Alam M: Quantitation of human im-

munodeficiency virus type 1 in the blood of infected persons. N Engl J Med 321:1621, 1989

300. Simmonds P, Balfe P, Peutherer JF et al: Human immunodeficiency virus-infected individuals contain provirus in small numbers of peripheral mononuclear cells and at low copy numbers. J Virol 64:864, 1990

301. McElrath MJ, Steinman RM, Cohn ZA: Latent HIV-1 infection in enriched populations of blood monocytes and T cells from seropositive patients. J Clin Invest 87:27, 1991

302. Schrier RD, McCutchan JA, Venable JC et al: T-cell induced expression of human immunodeficiency virus in macrophages. J Virol 64:3280, 1990

303. Brinchmann JE, Albert J, Vartdal F: Few infected CD4+ T cells but a high proportion of replication-competent provirus copies in asymptomatic human immunodeficiency virus type 1 infection. J Virol 65:2019, 1991

304. McCune JM: HIV-1: The infective process in vivo. Cell 64:351, 1991

3

The Molecular Biology of HIV-1

William A. Haseltine

The life cycle of the human immunodeficiency virus type 1 (HIV-1), a small RNA virus, lies at the heart of the acquired immunodeficiency syndrome (AIDS) pandemic. The spread of the disease is primarily determined by the infectious properties of this virus. Progressive lethal degeneration of the immune and central nervous systems results from long-term chronic replication of this virus. The details of the virus's life cycle and structure permit it to escape clearance by the immune system and render it resistant to vaccines. Ultimately our ability to control the AIDS pandemic, already destined to claim more than 50 million lives, will depend on our ability to interrupt the life cycle of this virus. The present review summarizes briefly our current understanding of this virus. Opportunities for intervention will be highlighted.

THE HIV-1 LIFE CYCLE: AN OVERVIEW

The life cycle of HIV-1 can be divided into two phases, establishment of infection and productive infection (Fig. 3–1). Infection of a target cell is established *via* a set of virus–cell interactions that include binding of the virus to the cell surface, fusion of the virus and cell membranes, entry of the virus capsid into the cytoplasm, conversion of the viral RNA to DNA, and entry of the viral DNA into the nucleus. Once the viral DNA enters the nucleus, infection is established. The viral DNA may be integrated into the host DNA or may form stable circles. Once integration has occurred, the progeny of the infected cell will also be infected.

Expression begins when viral DNA is transcribed into RNA by the host polymerase II. The viral RNA is processed by splicing and exported to the cytoplasm, where it is translated into viral protein. The virus capsid, which assembles on the inner surface of the membrane, incorporates full-length viral RNA into the newly formed particles. New viruses are made as the virus buds through a region of the cell membrane. The outer surface protein of the virus, located on the surface of the cell membrane, becomes associated with the nascent virus particles during the budding process.

Replication of the virus is controlled by host cell as well as by viral genes. The state of differentiation and activation of the infected cell may determine the rate of each step in the virus's life cycle. Additionally, some of the proteins specified by the virus affect the rate of accumulation of the primary RNA transcript in the nucleus, the processing and export of the viral transcripts, and the rate of assembly and budding of the virus particles. The role of some of the viral genes in replication remains to be defined.

The following description summarizes the current state of knowledge of each step of the replication cycle.

ESTABLISHMENT OF INFECTION

Attachment and Entry

THE HIV-1 ENVELOPE GLYCOPROTEIN

Binding of the virus to the target cell and fusion of the virus and cell membranes is mediated by the virus-specified envelope glycoprotein.[1-6] This protein is located on the surface of the virus particle as well as on the surface of virus-producing cells. Because the binding and fusion reactions are the initial step in the virus's life cycle, and because the virus envelope glycoprotein is located on the surface of the virus particle and infected cells, it is a preferred target for antiviral drugs and vaccines.

BIOSYNTHESIS OF THE ENVELOPE GLYCOPROTEIN

The envelope glycoprotein is made late in the life cycle from singly spliced messenger RNA (see Fig. 3–1). The envelope mRNA is bicistronic and specifies both the

Figure 3–1. Schematic diagram of the retrovirus life cycle. Establishment (left): Steps of establishment are: (1) Virus binding to a cell receptor. (2) Penetration of a cell membrane. (3) Provirus synthesis. (4) Migration of the provirus to the nucleus. (5) Integration. Expression (right): Steps of virus expression include: (1) Transcription of proviral DNA by cellular RNA polymerase II. (2) Messenger RNA processing. (3) Messenger RNA transport and genomic RNA transport. (4) Synthesis of viral proteins. (5) Assembly of virion particle. (6) Budding and maturation of the virus particles.

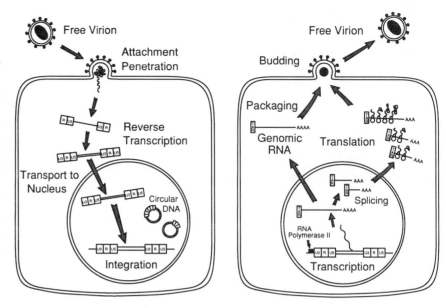

vpu and *env* proteins. The *env* protein is made as a single 856-amino acid polypeptide, gp160.[7,8] The nascent *env* protein is directed to the rough endoplasmic reticulum *via* an amino terminal signal sequence. The *env* protein precursor is anchored to the rough endoplasmic reticulum *via* an approximately 40-amino acid transmembrane region.[9–11] Folding and dimer formation of the *env* precursor protein occur in the endoplasmic reticulum.[12,13] Cleavage of the gp160 precursor into the gp120 and gp41 subunits probably occurs in a post-endoplasmic reticulum compartment.[13–16] The gp160 precursor is directed to the Golgi apparatus, where it is heavily modified by the addition of branched sugar chains.[17,18] Over half of the final molecular weight of the envelope glycoprotein is derived from such additions. The branched sugar side chains are trimmed by a variety of cellular enzymes, including α-glucosidases, and additional sugar molecules are added to these side chains as the protein transits the Golgi apparatus.[17]

The precursor protein is cleaved at two adjacent sites by cellular proteases into an amino terminal fragment, designated gp120, that is destined to be located entirely on the surface of the virus particle, and gp41, which is a transmembrane protein.[14,19,20] The cleavage event is thought to occur in the trans-Golgi compartment. At or about the time that the protein is deposited on the surface of the cell, tetramers of the envelope glycoprotein form.[12,21,22] A number of drugs inhibit biosynthesis of the *env* protein. These include brefeldin A, which blocks protein transport from the endoplasmic reticulum to the Golgi apparatus, tunicamycin, which prevents addition of branched sugars to the nascent protein, and inhibitors of the α-glucosidase and mannosidases, which trim the sugar side chains.[23] Most of these drugs are highly toxic to the host cells. The ex-

ceptions are inhibitors of the α-glucosidases, some of which are currently being tested for clinical efficacy.

gp120-CD4 BINDING

Binding of the virus to cells occurs *via* high-affinity interactions between gp120 and the CD4 molecule located on the surface of the subset of lymphocytes.[1–3] Most of the binding studies have been done using monomeric gp120. The initial binding constant of laboratory isolates of the gp120-CD4 is approximately 2×10^{-9} M.[24] However, after 30 minutes at 25° C or higher the dissociation constant of gp120 increases considerably, to about 2×10^{-10} M, presumably because of an induced-fit rearrangement of gp120 and CD4. The affinity of the gp120 of most primary HIV-1 isolates for CD4 is often two orders of magnitudes less than that of the laboratory strains.

The region of CD4 recognized by gp120 has been mapped using a set of anti-CD4 monoclonal antibodies and by mutagenesis. The region is located between amino acids 40 and 82. Antibodies to this region block gp120 binding to CD4 and also block infection. X-ray crystallographic analysis of the amino terminal domains of this CD4 protein reveals that the gp120 binding region protrudes from the surface of CD4 as a discrete structure.

Fine structure mutation mapping as well as secondary structure analysis of gp120 has defined the binding site on gp120 for CD4. The gp120-CD4 binding site is formed from four noncontiguous regions of gp120 amino acids brought into continuity by the secondary and tertiary structure of the protein.[9,24,25] According to one hypothesis, the CD4 binding region is located in a pocket of gp120. The bottom of the pocket is hydrophobic and interacts with the hydrophobic amino acids that protrude from the surface of CD4. The surface of the binding pocket is hydrophilic and also contains three positively charged amino acids. A mutation in any one of the three charged amino acids substantially reduces the affinity of gp120 for CD4. It is thought that these charged amino acids interact with the oppositely charged amino acids at the base of the CD4 binding region.

INFECTION OF CD4-NEGATIVE CELLS

HIV-1 binds nonspecifically to a variety of cell types. Several experiments indicate that some cell types that do not express CD4 can be infected.[26] It is possible that nonspecific binding of some cell types may trigger virus–cell membrane fusion events in the absence of CD4 binding.

FUSION

Entry of the virus into cells requires fusion of the virus and cell membranes.[4] Fusion is mediated by the *env* protein itself.[23,24] A short sequence of hydrophobic amino acids located at the amino terminus of gp41 specifies the fusion function.[27] Mutations of these fusion regions result in envelope glycoproteins that are either partially or wholly defective for fusion.[9] Activation of the fusion region requires cleavage of the envelope glycoprotein precursor at a site immediately amino terminal to this hydrophobic amino acid sequence.[19,20]

The biochemical details of this fusion reaction are not known. Some cells that express surface CD4 fuse readily with HIV-1. However, some cells that express abundant surface CD4 are resistant to HIV-1 infection as a consequence of a defect in the membrane fusion reaction.[26,28] Host cell factors that determine the ability of the HIV-1 envelope to mediate membrane-to-membrane fusion after CD4 binding are not understood. A much more detailed knowledge of the fusion reaction is required before specific antifusion drugs can be designed.

It is not clear whether virus–cell membrane fusion is sufficient to initiate infection. It is conceivable that an additional set of interactions between virus and host proteins is needed before penetration of the capsid into the cytoplasm can occur. This possibility was highlighted by the observation that viruses which carry envelope glycoproteins deleted for the intracytoplasmic region of gp41 show a severe defect in infectivity, despite the demonstrated ability of such mutant envelope glycoproteins to mediate membrane-to-membrane fusion (Gabuzda and Sodroski, unpubl. observ.).[9]

Conversion of RNA to DNA

SYNTHESIS OF VIRAL DNA

The process of conversion of viral DNA to RNA is central to the life cycle of HIV-1. During this process the duplex viral genome is converted to a single double-stranded DNA form.[29-31] The reaction relies on the concerted activity of the viral DNA polymerase and ribonuclease H. Both of these enzymes are packaged in multiple copies within the virus particle.

DNA synthesis is initiated by elongation of a cellular tRNA, which in the case of HIV-1 is a tRNA lysine annealed to a site near the 5′ end of the viral genome (Fig. 3–2).[32,33] The tRNA associates with the viral RNA during packaging of the viral genome into the virus particle. Elongation of the nascent DNA strand occurs to the end of the viral genome, yielding a 630-nucleotide-long DNA fragment called minus strong stop DNA.[34] This fragment retains the tRNA covalently bound to its 5′ terminus. The viral ribonuclease H degrades the RNA annealed to the 3′ end of the minus strong stop DNA, permitting this DNA to anneal to a complementary sequence at the 3′ end of the second RNA genome.[30,35] Elongation proceeds to the end of the second strand, producing a full-length minus strand copy of the viral genome. The RNA opposite the newly formed DNA is selectively degraded by the action of the viral ribonuclease H in two locations, one near a polypurine track, located near the 3′ end of the RNA genome, and a second site located near the center of the viral genome.[36,37] The RNA fragment lo-

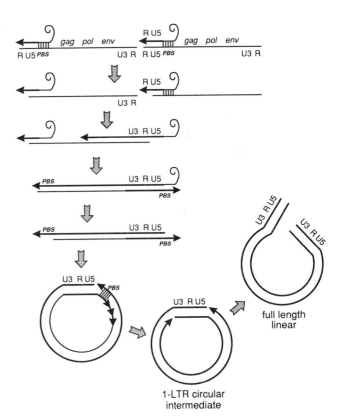

Figure 3–2. Mechanism of viral DNA synthesis. Viral RNA is drawn as thin lines, whereas the newly synthesized DNA is drawn as thick lines.

cated at the 3′ end serves to initiate DNA synthesis of the plus strand. The 3′ end of the RNA copies the minus strong stop DNA and continues to copy the initiating tRNA attached to the minus strong stop through the site where it is annealed through the primer binding site of the tRNA.[30] The tRNA is then degraded by the action of the viral ribonuclease H, revealing a DNA sequence complementary to primer binding site at the opposite end of the minus strand. Annealing of these two regions results in the formation of a circular DNA intermediate.[38,39] The final step of proviral DNA occurs when the viral DNA polymerase displaces the 3′ end of the plus strand and copies the remaining sequence. The result is a full-length linear DNA molecule that contains a long terminal redundancy (LTR) at either end. This reaction occurs entirely in the cytoplasm.

Many details of this reaction remain obscure. The viral proteins that remain associated with the viral genome during the process of conversion of viral RNA to DNA are unknown. It is unknown whether cytoplasmic proteins facilitate this reaction. The basic for selective degradation of RNA by the viral ribonuclease H is also unknown. The means by which the DNA polymerase displaces the minus strand as a final step in the synthesis of the viral DNA is unknown.

The rate of conversion of viral RNA to DNA is reported to depend on the type of cell infected and on the state of activation of the cell. For example, conversion of viral RNA to DNA occurs within the first 2 to 6 hours upon infection of replicating CD4+ T-cell lines.[40,41] However, this process takes place over a much longer period, 1 to 2 days, upon infection of primary monocyte and macrophage cultures. It has been reported that following infection of nonstimulated primary T cells, viral DNA synthesis is arrested before synthesis of the first, minus strand DNA is complete.[42] It is also reported that this incomplete replicative intermediate has a half-life of less than 1 day.[42] Accordingly, it is postulated that infection of resting T cells by HIV-1 is self-limiting.

INHIBITORS OF VIRAL DNA SYNTHESIS

Synthesis of viral DNA may be inhibited by a variety of dideoxynucleosides and dideoxynucleoside analogues.[43-48] Such drugs are active as triphosphorylated intermediates.[49,50] They are incorporated into the elongating DNA chain. The viral DNA polymerase does not contain a 3′ exonuclease activity. Once incorporated, such dideoxynucleosides terminate DNA polymerization.[49,50]

Variation of HIV-1 constitutes a potential barrier to long-term treatment with such dideoxynucleoside analogues. Virus strains readily mutate to resistance to the most commonly used drug, azothymidine (AZT).[51] Resistance occurs *via* alteration of specific amino acids in the viral DNA polymerase.[52]

Recently a family of benzodiazepine analogues has been identified that inhibits the DNA polymerase activity of HIV-1.[53] Such drugs are currently being tested for clinical activity. The basis for the activity of these drugs is not known.

BIOSYNTHESIS OF VIRAL DNA POLYMERASE AND RIBONUCLEASE H

The viral DNA polymerase and ribonuclease H are synthesized as part of an extended polypeptide from full-length viral RNA.[30] Synthesis of these two proteins requires that a −1 frameshift event occur between the first and second long open reading frames of the viral genome.[54-56] Such frameshift events occur at a ratio of 1:20. Therefore the ratio of *gag* and *gag* to *pol* precursors is approximately 20:1 in the infected cells.

It is likely that the *gag/pol* precursors form a dimer during particle assembly, as all of the viral proteins specified by the second long open reading frame, including the viral protease, DNA polymerase, ribonuclease H, and integrase proteins, form stable dimers as isolated purified proteins. Furthermore, structural studies of the retroviral protease indicate that this protein is active only as a dimer.[57-59] It is likely that the *gag/pol* precursor dimers become associated with the budding capsid *via* interactions with the amino terminal *gag* residues, which contain self-assembly determinants.[60-61]

During the budding process the viral protease is activated and cleaves to the *gag* precursor and to multiple proteins. The DNA polymerase and ribonuclease H proteins are initially cleaved into a 65-kilodalton protein. A subsequent slow cleavage event cuts the 65-kD homodimer into a 65-kD and 51-kD heterodimer.[62-65] This heterodimer is the active form of DNA polymerase present in the mature HIV-1 particle.[64,66] The heterodimer contains both DNA polymerase and ribonuclease H activities. A 15-kD ribonuclease H protein has also been purified from virus particles. The 15-kD ribonuclease H forms a stable dimer. The 15-kD ribonuclease H protein is not active by itself. Ribonuclease H activity of this protein is restored by addition of the 51-kD form of the viral polymerase.[67] The structure of the ribonuclease H protein has been determined by x-ray crystallography.[68] No drugs that inhibit the ribonuclease H activity have been described. Inhibitors of this reaction should inhibit HIV-1 replication.

Integration and Circularization of Viral DNA

After synthesis in the cytoplasm, the viral DNA migrates to the nucleus. The process by which the viral DNA enters the nucleus is unknown. In replicating cells the viral DNA may gain access to the nucleus as the nuclear membrane dissolves and reforms during cell division. HIV-1 also productively infects nondividing cells such as monocytes, macrophages, and dendritic cells.[69,70] The means by which viral DNA gains access to the nuclei of such cells is unknown.

Once the viral DNA reaches the nucleus, it may either integrate into the host cell DNA or circularize.[30] Both the integrated and circular forms of DNA are stable in the cell that is initially infected. However, only the integrated DNA replicates as the cells divide. Consequently, in the absence of reinfection, circular viral DNA forms are diluted from the population. It has been reported that stable circular DNA forms may persist in infected noncycling CD4+ T cells, in contrast to the report cited above.

THE INTEGRATION REACTION

Integration of HIV-1 occurs by covalent joining of the ends of the viral DNA with host DNA. The viral DNA is inserted between a five-base repeat of the host sequence, and the terminal two nucleotides of the virus DNA are deleted at the junction of the host and viral sequences.[71,72] No preferred chromosome or site of integration into the host nuclear DNA has been detected.

Integration in vitro   The HIV-1 integration reaction can be mimicked *in vitro,* either using a preintegration complex purified from the cytoplasm of newly infected cells[13] or using the purified virus-specified integrase protein and synthetic DNA substrates containing specific terminal LTR sequences.[32,73,74]

The preintegration complex purified from the cytoplasm of newly infected cells has a sedimentation velocity of approximately 80S.[41] The particle contains full-length linear viral DNA molecules. The particle also contains the 31-kD viral integrase protein.[75] No other virus proteins are stably associated with the preintegration complex in detectable amounts.[75] It is not known whether the preintegration particle also contains proteins specified by the infected cell.

Incubation of the preintegration complex with target DNA molecules results in rapid quantitative integration.[41] The reaction occurs in the absence of added nucleoside triphosphates. The sequence of the junction of the virus and host DNA is the same as that observed in natural infections, with a five-nucleotide repeat of the host DNA sequence and a two-base deletion at the termini of the linear viral DNA.[76,77] Studies of the reactions of purified HIV-1 integrase protein and synthetic double-stranded DNA oligonucleotide sequences at the termini of linear viral DNA have also been done.[73,74]

For most retroviruses, the *cis*-acting DNA sequences necessary for proper integration *in vivo* are limited to inverted repeats present at the termini of the linear viral DNA molecule.[78,79] For HIV-1, these inverted repeats are short, most likely consisting of only four base pairs at each terminus.[62,63] Other sequences outside of the short inverted repeats most likely play a role in HIV-1 integration, as the purified HIV-1 integrase appears to recognize the sequence of the 3′ terminus of linear viral DNA more efficiently than it recognizes the 5′ terminus.[74]

The purified integrase protein makes a specific endonucleolytic cleavage to remove two nucleotides from the 3′ end of a duplex DNA oligonucleotide which mimics one of the termini of linear viral DNA.[73,74] The purified integrase protein also cleaves target DNA randomly and covalently joins the 5′ end of the nick generated in oligonucleotide to the 3′ end of the target molecule.[74] The reaction with the purified enzyme mimics the integration reaction that occurs at one end of the viral DNA.

The Integrase Protein   The integrase protein is made from the same precursor as the DNA polymerase and ribonuclease H proteins. The integrase protein comprises the carboxy terminus of this precursor. It is cleaved from the precursor by the viral protease late in virus particle maturation. The 31-kD protein is present in multiple copies in the virus particle. The purified integrase protein forms a stable dimer.

In summary, the integrase protein of HIV-1 contains multiple activities. It specifically recognizes sequences at the HIV-1 viral DNA termini, and it possesses both specific and nonspecific endonuclease activities. The protein also is capable of joining viral and target DNA sequences. No specific inhibitors of this enzyme have been described. Inhibitors of the integration reaction should inhibit virus replication in most cell types.

CIRCULARIZATION

Linear as well as circular forms of DNA can be detected in the nuclei of CD4+ T-cell lines shortly after infection.[40,41] However, the linear DNA forms disappear rapidly, whereas the circular forms are stable for many days. At least three types of circular DNA forms are present within the nuclei of cells infected with retroviruses.[30] The majority of the circular DNA forms contain one LTR. The linear sequences of the viral genes are not permuted in such circles.

The second most abundant type of circles present in the nucleus of infected cells contain two LTRs. The viral genes are not permuted in these circles. Such circles appear to form by end-to-end joining of the full-length linear DNA. The sequence at the junction of the two-LTRs does not contain a deletion of the terminal CA dinucleotide.

The nuclei of infected cells contain a second type of two-LTR circles. The sequence of the viral genes of this class of two-LTR circles is permuted. Some of the sequences have undergone an inversion with respect to one another as well. The termini of the LTRs present in these circles are deleted for the terminal CA dinucleotide. These circles presumably arise as a result of an autointegration and strand exchange reaction. An autointegration event without strand exchange should also give rise to a population of smaller one-LTR circles of heterogeneous length. Such circles have also been detected in the nuclei of infected cells.

It is possible that the one-LTR circles and the nonpermuted two-LTR circles serve as a substrate for RNA transcription in resting cells. For example, visna virus is reported to replicate well in nonreplicating choroid plexus cells in the absence of detectable levels of integrated viral DNA. It is conceivable that the stable circular DNA present in the nuclei of infected noncycling cells serves as a template for RNA synthesis.

In vitro *Circle Formation*   It has recently become possible to mimic all three types of circle formation *in vitro.*[41a] Cytoplasmic extracts of uninfected cells contain an activity that converts the viral DNA purified from the cytoplasm of newly infected cells into one-LTR circles. The cellular activity presumably promotes homologous recombination between the terminally redundant ends of the viral DNA. This cellular activity requires nucleoside triphosphate. Viral DNA present in the purified preintegration complex is also a suitable substrate for this cellular activity.

Nonpermuted two-LTR circles can also be made on incubation of a viral DNA purified from the cytoplasm of newly infected cells with either purified T4 DNA ligase or extracts from uninfected cells. This reaction is very inefficient. However, if the termini of the viral DNA are made blunt-ended by incubation with a viral DNA polymerase and triphosphate precursors, the efficiency of formation of two-LTR circles by the purified DNA ligase or by extracts of uninfected cells is increased dramatically. This observation indicates that the majority of viral DNA present in the cytoplasm does not contain blunt ends. Viral DNA present in the preintegration complex is also a suitable substrate for circularization, provided that the termini have been made blunt. The formation of two-LTR circles by this means requires adenosine triphosphate.

In the absence of target DNA and nucleoside triphosphates, the DNA present in the cytoplasmic extracts or in the purified preintegration complex is stable to incubation at 37° C for several hours. However, addition of any of the four deoxyribo- or ribonucleotide triphosphates to the cytoplasmic extracts or a purified preintegration complex results in efficient autointegration reactions in the absence of target DNA. The presence of a nucleoside triphosphate is absolutely required for the autointegration reaction.

These experiments indicate that upon entry into the nucleus, viral DNA is subject to four completing reactions (Fig. 3–3): integration into the host cell DNA, autointegration, end-to-end ligation, and homologous recombination of the terminally redundant sequences. Factors that affect each of these reactions may affect the outcome of the infection.

EXPRESSION OF INFECTION

Early Stage of Virus Expression

SYNTHESIS OF VIRAL RNA

The first step in the expression of virus in the infected cell is transcription of RNA from the duplex form of viral DNA in the nucleus of the cell. The initial product of the completed transcription reaction is a full-length linear RNA molecule that extends from the 5′ end of the R region in the 5′ LTR to the 3′ end of the R region in the 3′ LTR (Fig. 3–4). The primary RNA transcript contains a 5′ TAR structure and a 3′ terminal poly A, as is typical of many eukaryotic RNA mRNAs. Only one strand of the viral DNA is transcribed, the sense strand. This strand can be translated to yield virus proteins. Two copies of the full-length primary transcript are incorporated into each budding virus particle. These primary

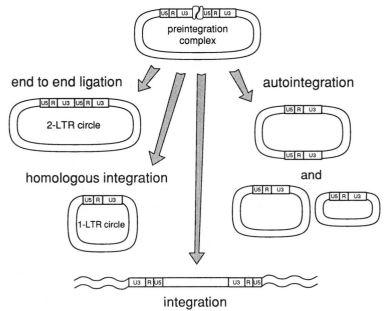

Figure 3–3. Structures of the viral DNA forms found in an infected cell. The viral preintegration complex, formed in the cytoplasm of the cell shortly after infection, contains linear viral DNA and the viral integrase protein. The preintegration complex moves to the nucleus, where several reactions can occur. Some of the linear viral DNA integrates into the host genome to form the provirus. In addition, 1-LTR circles, simple 2-LTR circles, and circular products of autointegration can be found among the unintegrated viral DNA forms in the nucleus. The asterisks on the autointegration products denote the new LTR-target junctions formed by the autointegration reaction.

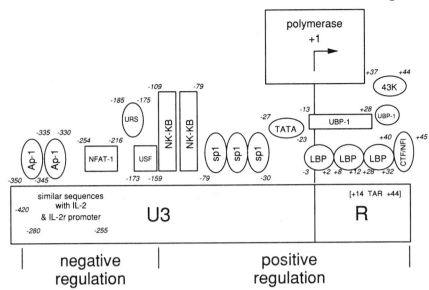

Figure 3–4. The relative location and similarity of some of the sequences in the LTR to consensus sequences, which are known to bind cellular proteins, raise the possibility that these proteins also regulate HIV-1 proviral LTR-directed RNA transcription. The location of the negative regulatory gene and the NRE is not shown.

transcripts form a stable dimer and constitute the genome of the virus particle.

The full-length primary transcripts contain multiple splice sites. More than 30 different spliced forms of viral RNA have been identified in the nucleus of infected cells. The full-length and spliced mRNAs are transported to the cytoplasm where they serve to direct the synthesis of the virus proteins.

CELLULAR CONTROL OF VIRAL RNA EXPRESSION

Synthesis of the full-length primary transcripts of the virus's genetic information is controlled by cellular and viral factors. In some cells, such as resting primary CD4+ T cells, no viral RNA can be detected in the cells despite the presence of detectable amounts of integrated viral DNA in the cell population.[80] In this cell type, synthesis of viral RNA depends on stimulation of T cells.[81] The requirements for RNA synthesis in other types of infected cells, such as monocytes, macrophages, T helper, and dendritic cells, are not known.

Viral RNA is made by the cellular enzyme RNA polymerase II. Sequences located near the site of RNA initiation control the rate of initiation of this enzyme. Some of these sequences exert a positive effect on transcription initiation, others negatively regulate transcription initiation. These sequences, located very near the site of RNA initiation, include the TATAA sequences and the SP1 sequences, and are required for RNA transcription and for viral replication.[82] The tandemly repeated sequence 5' to the SP1 binding site acts as an inducible enhancer in T cells. These sequences bind the activated NF-κB transcription factor.[83,84] The activation of viral RNA synthesis that occurs on stimulation of T cells by nonspecific mitogens can be attributed, at least in part, to the ability of the activated NF-κB to stimulate transcription initiation.

LTR sequences 5' to the enhancer repress RNA initiation. These sequences are called the *negative regulatory element* (NRE).[85] Two sequences within the NRE, one that binds the previously identified cellular protein USF and a second that binds a protein present in activated T cells, designated an NFAT-1 like sequence,[85] contribute to the negative effect of transcription initiation.[86] The absence of detectable viral RNA in T cells that contain integrated viral DNA may be due in part to binding by these sequences of cellular proteins that are active in the nuclei of resting cells. Such proteins may either be inactivated or displaced on stimulation of T cells. No function has been assigned to the AP-1 binding sites of the 5' end of the LTR.[87]

The viral enhancer also increases the rate of virus gene expression in primary cells, including mixed peripheral blood lymphocyte (PBL) cultures, CD4+ T cells, monocytes and macrophages, and dendritic cells. The NRE region negatively affects virus replication in Jurkat cells, T cells, monocytes, and dendritic cells.[71] Cellular proteins also bind to sequences located 3' to the site of RNA initiation. Cellular proteins identified that bind to these sequences include the UBP-1 and LBP sequences.[88,89] The role of these proteins in transcription initiation has not been established. Deletion of these sequences does not reduce the rate of HIV-1 LTR RNA initiation measured in the absence of viral proteins.

THE TRANSACTIVATOR

A virus-specified regulatory gene called the transactivator (*tat*)[90–95] controls the rate of primary transcript synthesis and may also control the efficiency with which the viral transcripts are translated into protein[94–96] (see Fig. 3–7).

The transactivator gene contains two coding exons.

The *tat* mRNA is made by joining a short exon located near the central region of the genome to a sequence near the 3′ end of the *env* gene. The *gag, pol, vif,* and most of the *vpr* sequences are deleted from the 5′ part of the message, whereas the *vpt, vpu,* and most of the *env* sequences are removed from the 3′ part of the *tat* mRNA. The *tat* mRNAs contain initiation codons for *rev* and for *nef.* However, the site of translation initiation at the *tat* initiation codon is so strong that the initiation codons of *rev* and *nef,* also present in this mRNA, do not function.[97]

A 16-kD *tat* protein is made by translation of the doubly spliced RNA. A smaller 15-kD *tat* protein is made from a singly spliced RNA from which the *gag, pol,* and *vif* sequences have been removed by splicing but which retains sequences 3′ to the first coding exon of *tat.* The 15-kD protein is also a transactivator. This arrangement permits *tat* to be made both in the presence and in the absence of *rev* activity, an activity that suppresses the splicing event that removes the *vpu* and *env* sequences.

Tat is critical for virus replication.[98,99] In the absence of *tat,* very little viral RNA accumulates. Some experiments indicate that *tat* increases the rate of RNA initiation.[100-105] Other experiments indicate that *tat* increases the ability of RNA polymerase II to elongate short transcripts that terminate prematurely following efficient transcription initiation.[106-110]

The *tat* protein binds to a short region at the 5′ end of the nascent RNA strand.[104,111-114] This region is designated a *transactivator response sequence* (TAR).[84] TAR forms a stable hairpin loop.[105,115] A stretch of basic amino acids of the *tat* protein specifically recognizes a short trinucleotide bulge region in the context of the TAR stem-loop structure.[113,114,116,117]

The *tat* protein binds to TAR as a consequence of the specific interaction between the basic amino acid regions and the RNA nucleotides (Fig. 3–5).[107,113,117-122]

The loop region of TAR is required for *tat* activity. Several cellular proteins that specifically recognize the loop sequence in the context of a stable stem-loop structure have been identified.[113-126] Cellular proteins have also been identified that bind to the upper part of the stem region of TAR. The role of these cellular proteins in transactivation has not yet been defined.

At least two different cellular proteins that bind to the *tat* protein have also been described. One of these proteins, the product of the TBP-1 gene, is a member of a conserved family of cellular proteins.[127] Proteins with substantial similarity of sequence to TBP-1 are found in diverse species, including yeast and *Xenopus.* One member of this family of proteins represses RNA elongation in yeast.

Several experiments indicate that sequences in the promoter affect *tat* activity. Substitution of sequences within the TF-IIB initiation factor binding region reduces *tat* activity without necessarily reducing the rate of promoter-directed RNA synthesis.

These experiments provide the basis for a hypothesis for *tat* action. According to this hypothesis, *tat* pro-

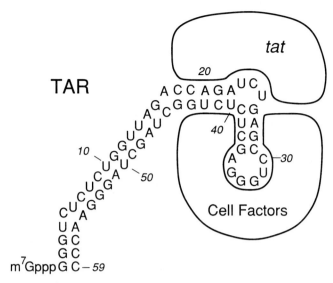

Figure 3–5. Binding of *tat* and cellular proteins to TAR RNA. The primary and secondary structures of TAR RNA of the HIV-1 HXB2 strain are shown.

tein and cellular proteins bind to the nascent RNA *via* the TAR sequence. This RNA protein structure interacts with the complex of transcription initiation factors and RNA polymerase II at the site of initiation and increases the processive character of the RNA II polymerase, which initiates subsequent rounds of RNA synthesis. This hypothesis explains most of the observations regarding *tat* activity. It does not provide an explanation for reports that under some conditions, *tat* increases the translation efficiency of TAR-initiated RNA.

Viruses defective for *tat* do not replicate in CD4+ T-cell lines or in primary blood lymphocytes. Some benzodiazepine derivatives inhibit the *tat* activity of HIV-1 as well as the *tat* activities of the related viruses, HIV-2 and simian immunodeficiency virus (SIV). The family of benzodiazapine analogues that inhibit *tat* activity do not inhibit viral DNA polymerase. The anti-*tat* benzodiazapines may be useful in the treatment of HIV-1 infections.

THE REGULATOR OF VIRION PROTEIN EXPRESSION

The primary transcript of HIV-1 is transformed by splicing into more than 30 distinct smaller RNA species, each one of which encodes one or more proteins.[97] The primary transcript contains two major and at least three minor 5′ (donor) splice sites. The primary transcript also contains at least seven major as well as several minor 3′ (acceptor) splice sites.[97] Cellular splicing components recognize these sequences and alter the primary viral RNA transcript. The virus-specified regulatory protein, the regulator of virion protein expression (*rev*), selectively regulates accumulation of unspliced, singly spliced, and multiply spliced viral RNAs.

In the absence of *rev* function, multiply spliced

mRNAs exit the nucleus where they are translated.[128–132] The *gag, pol, vif,* and most *vpr* sequences, as well as the *vpt, vpu,* and most of the *env* sequences, are deleted from the mRNAs that exit the nucleus for translation in the absence of *rev* function. These short, multiply spliced RNAs have the capacity to encode functional *tat, rev,* and *nef* proteins. The proteins that appeared in the virus particle, the capsid proteins, the replicative genes, *vpr,* and the envelope glycoprotein are made from sequences that are spliced out of the mRNAs and that can be translated in the absence of *rev.* For this reason, *rev* is essential for synthesis of virus particles.[133]

The rev *Protein*   The *rev* protein is specified by two coding exons.[110,134] The 5' coding exon overlaps the 3' end of the first coding exon of *tat,* and the second coding exon overlaps the 3' coding exon of the *tat* and *env* coding sequences. The first coding exon of *rev* is preceded by two splice sites located between the initiation codons of *tat* and *rev.* Deletion by splicing of the *tat* initiation codon from the *rev* message permits utilization of the weaker *rev* initiation codon. Both *tat* and *rev* share common 5' and 3' splice sites that join the first and second coding exons. Sequences essential for *rev* function are located entirely within the second coding exon.

The rev *Responsive Element*   A sequence located in the 3' end of the *env* gene is essential for *rev* function.[135] This sequence is called the *rev* responsive element (RRE) (Fig. 3–6). The sequence forms a complex of stem-loop structure.[129] A high-affinity binding site for *rev* protein is formed by a short stem-loop structure that forms within the large loop of the RRE stem-loop struc-ture.[136–139] This smaller stem-loop structure forms a high-affinity binding site for *rev.*[140–144] A basic sequence within the *rev* protein specifically recognizes this site.[145] *Rev* protein binding to the RRE is cooperative.[146] Multiple *rev* proteins bind to the RRE, possibly nucleated by *rev* binding to the high-affinity *rev* binding site.[141,146,147] Cellular proteins that bind to the RRE have also been identified.[148] The function of such proteins in *rev* activity is unknown.

cis-*Acting Repressive Sequences*   *Rev* function is necessitated by the existence of sequences, located within genes, that encode the structural proteins, including *gag, pol,* and *env.*[149] These sequences, designated *cis*-acting repressive sequences (CRS), prevent translation of viral RNA which carries these sequences in the absence of a functional *rev* interaction with an RRE element located on the same RNA strand (Fig. 3–7).

The primary function of the CRS sequences is to retain RNA in the nucleus. It is likely that the CRS sequences function by binding to cellular proteins. Some of the cellular proteins that bind to CRS and that retain the RNA in the nucleus may be part of the splicing complex. Other types of CRS elements may also exist.

Under some experimental conditions, normal amounts of full-length and singly spliced viral mRNAs accumulate in the nucleus of cells in the absence of *rev* function.[129,131] However, these RNA species are not exported to the cytoplasm for translation. In other experiments, full-length RNA appears to be unstable in the absence of *rev* function.[150,151] It has been proposed that the CRS elements recognize components of the cellular splicing apparatus and that the interaction of *rev* with

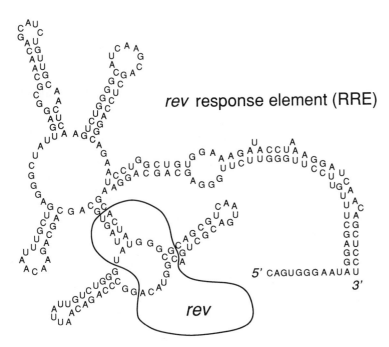

rev response element (RRE)

Figure 3–6.   Binding of the HIV-1 *rev* protein to RRE RNA. The RRE RNA of HIV-1 HXB2 strain is shown.

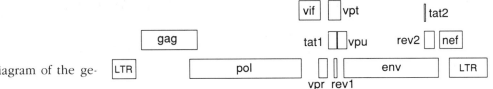

Figure 3–7. Schematic diagram of the genome of HIV-1.

RRE on the same RNA species displaces the cellular splicing components from the viral RNA, permitting export of the viral mRNA from the cytoplasm.

Whatever the detailed mechanism of *rev* action, this regulatory pathway is remarkable in several respects. *Rev* binding to RRE can overcome the effect of viral CRS elements as well as the effect of defective 3′ and 5′ splice sites introduced into the introns of heterologous mRNAs such as globin RNA.[152] The RRE element is also unusual as it can function from a distance of at least several thousand nucleotides from the site of CRS repression.

A hypothesis that explains most of the observations regarding *rev* function is that *rev* binding to RRE permits rapid export of RNA from the nucleus regardless of its association with splicing factors or other cellular proteins that act to retain it within the nucleus. This hypothesis does not explain the observation that overproduction of RNA containing CRS elements in the absence of *nef* may sometimes result in cytoplasmic accumulation of RNA that is not present in polysomes. It is possible that nuclear export and polysome association are usually coupled.[153]

The *rev* protein is a suitable target for antiviral drugs, as it is essential for virus replication. There appears to be a linear relationship between the amount of *rev* protein and the amount of virus structural proteins made. For this reason, inhibition of *rev* activity should inhibit virus replication. A synthetic oligonucleotide complementary to *rev* has been shown to inhibit virus replication.

tnv

The HIV-1 IIIB and BRU strains produce a variant of the *tat* and *rev* proteins. This protein is made from an mRNA that includes the first coding exon of *rev* spliced to a small exon in *env*, which in turn is spliced to the second coding exon of *tat* and *rev*.[154,155] A fusion protein, designated the *tnv* protein, is made from the mRNA. The amino terminus of the fusion protein comprises the amino specified by the first coding exon of *tat*. The central region of the *tnv* protein is comprised of a short sequence of *env*-derived amino acids. The carboxy terminus of this protein is specified by the second coding exon of *rev*. The *tnv* protein has almost full *tat* activity and has a low but detectable level of *rev* activity.[154,155] The *tnv* protein is not required for replication of HIV-1 IIIB strains. A mutation in the 5′ splice site at the 3′ end of the *env* coding exon which eliminates *tnv* protein

expression does not reduce the rate of virus replication in CD4+ T-cell lines. The *tnv* protein is not made by most strains of HIV-1. It is unlikely that the *tnv* protein plays an important role in HIV-1 replication.

nef

A third viral protein made early in infection is the product of the 3′ open reading frame that begins 3′ to the envelope coding sequence and overlaps most of the U3 region of the 3′ LTR.[84,156,157] This open reading frame specifies a 25- to 27-kD protein designated the *nef* protein.[158,159] The protein is myristylated at the amino terminus[158] and is located primarily in the cytoplasm of the infected cells.[160]

The 3′ splice site of the *nef* messenger RNA is the same as that which is used as the acceptor for the second coding exons of *tat* and *rev*. The *nef* initiation codon is the first methionine codon of this mRNA (Fig. 3–8).[91] The *nef* protein is not required for viral replication in cell culture.[161,162] Many strains of HIV-1, isolated after multiple passage in cell culture, as well as many cultured isolates of the related HIV-2 and SIV viruses are defective for *nef* expression. It is likely that *nef*-defective viruses replicate more rapidly in cell culture than do the *nef*+ viruses.[161–163]

There is some evidence that *nef* may be required for efficient replication during natural infections. It is reported that *nef*− mutants of SIV of macaque origin do not replicate to high titers and do not induce disease on injection into susceptible monkeys. Moreover, stop codons introduced into the SIV *nef* revert to wild-type on growth of the virus in the monkeys.[164]

The phenotype observed for HIV-1 *nef* depends both on the cells and on the *nef* allele used. The *nef* of the BH8 provirus isolate, a derivative of the HIV-1 IIIB strain, retards the growth of the virus in CD4+ T Jurkat cells, at least in the context of the HXB2 provirus (a provirus also derived from the HIV-1 IIIB isolate).[162] In contrast, the ELI *nef* allele obtained from the provirus of the HIV-1 ELI strain accelerates the growth of the virus in Jurkat cells in the context of the same provirus. Moreover, the ELI *nef* allele is required for initiation of low multiplicity of infection of primary CD4+ T cells and monocyte-macrophage cultures, in the context of the HXB2 provirus. The BH8 allele does not permit virus to initiate low multiplicity infection in these primary cell types in the context of the HXB2 provirus. Mutations of the ELI *nef* allele in this context eliminate

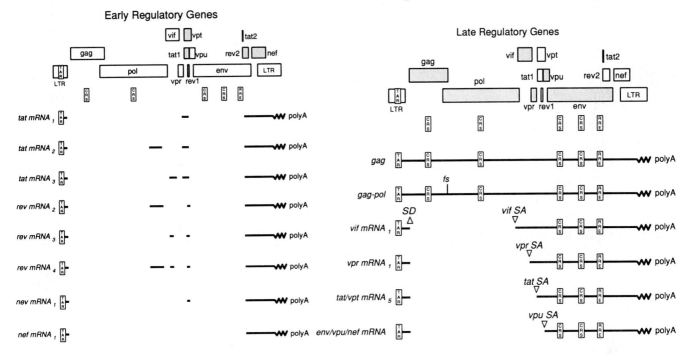

Figure 3–8. Messenger RNA synthesis.

the ability of these viruses to initiate low multiplicities of infection in the primary cell types.

It is likely that repeated passage of primary HIV-1 isolates in culture results in inactivation of *nef* function, either by introduction of obvious premature termination codon or by introduction of subtle missense mutations that inactivate *nef* function. According to this hypothesis, the phenotype of ELI *nef,* the allele that permits virus to initiate low multiplicity infection of a variety of primary cell types, reflects the most important feature of this gene.

Some *nef* alleles are reported to decrease the rate of HIV-1 LTR-initiated transcription of heterologous genes.[165,166] The initial observations were disputed as some researchers found that sequences of the viral LTR located on the same plasmid as the *nef* plasmid could themselves compete for transcription initiation factors required for HIV-1 LTR transcription initiation.[167–169]

The *nef* protein is reported to have both GTP binding and GTPase activities.[170] These reports have also been disputed.[171] The *nef* protein is phosphorylated.[172] It is clear that further work is needed to understand the role of this gene in HIV-1 infections.

Late Stage of Virus Expression

The function of the *rev* protein divides the expression phase of the virus life cycle into two stages—an early stage of expression, in which multiple spliced mRNAs are translated, and a late phase, in which full-length and singly spliced mRNAs are translated. During the early stage of expression, only regulatory proteins are made. The central event in transition from early to late stages of the expression phase is accumulation of the functional *rev* protein. Accumulation of *rev* protein is in turn dependent on synthesis of full-length mRNA, which serves as a precursor to the *rev* mRNA. Synthesis of full-length mRNA is itself dependent on the function of *tat*. The expression of *tat* is dependent on the synthesis of small amounts of primary transcript by the unaided HIV-1 promoter. The cascade of regulatory events required for the late stage of viral expression helps to account for regulated synthesis of virus RNA in natural infections.

ASSEMBLY OF THE CAPSID PRECURSOR

The virus capsid assembles in precursor form at the inner surface of the plasma membrane.[173–175] Membrane association requires amino terminal modification by myristylation of the capsid and capsid-replicative enzyme precursors. Inhibitors of the myristylation reaction inhibit virus replication and may be useful as antiviral drugs.[176,177]

The capsid precursor and the capsid-replicative enzyme precursors co-assemble into virus particles. Assembly, budding, and maturation of the capsid occur in the absence of the envelope glycoprotein.[178] The process of budding of virus from the membrane is not well understood. In some retroviruses mutants in the amino terminal region of the capsid precursor are competent for assembly but defective for budding through the plasma membrane.[179,180]

Release of the virus particle from the surface of the cell may be a rate-limiting step in virus maturation. Premature truncation of amino acids from the capsid precursor results in assembly and budding of virus particles. However, such particles are not efficiently released from the cell surface.[181] The virus particles remain attached to the surface via a tether (Fig. 3–9). The budded virus particle and the tether are both sheathed in a membrane derived from the plasma membrane. Tethered immature virus particles are also evident on examination of cells infected with wild-type virus.[182]

The envelope glycoprotein, deposited on the exterior surface of the plasma membrane, assembles onto the virus particles during the budding process. The basis for the association between the budding virus capsid and envelope glycoprotein is not known. However, normal human CD4 can also be efficiently incorporated into another retrovirus, that of the avian leahosis virus.

The virus genomic RNA is captured by the assembling capsid precursor polyprotein. The viral RNA contains a sequence that is required for efficient incorporation of the genomic RNA into virus particles.[183–185] This sequence is called the packaging sequence, or Psi sequence. The Psi sequence is located on the viral RNA in the vicinity of the site of initiation of the capsid precursor near the 5′ end of the molecule.[183–185] Part of the Psi sequence is removed from all spliced mRNAs. For this reason, only full-length viral RNAs are incorporated into budding particles.

A sequence near the carboxy terminus of the capsid precursor is required for efficient encapsidation of the genomic viral RNA.[184–186] This sequence contains two clusters of a cysteine and histidine domain that is conserved among retroviruses. Mutations that alter cysteine or histidine residues in these domains markedly reduce encapsidation of the viral RNA.[184,186] Mutants in the viral RNA or in the capsid precursor that prevent passaging of the viral genome do not interfere with virus assembly and budding. Virus capsids devoid of viral RNA do assemble and bud from the surface of cells transfected by such mutants, but have been reported to show abnormalities in core structure.[184,185]

The details of RNA passaging and assembly are not understood. Only two copies of the viral RNA are incorporated per virus particle, despite the existence of multiple binding sites for viral RNA within the assembling particle.[187] During the packaging process, the tRNA primer becomes tightly associated with the viral RNA.[188]

Inhibitors of this complex process should have antiviral properties. The complex process of assembly lends itself to inhibition. Inhibition of capsid precursor assembly, of budding, of release of budding particles, and of genome capture by the assembling virus should inhibit virus replication. Co-expression of capsid precursors defective for assembly has been shown to interfere with virus replication.[189]

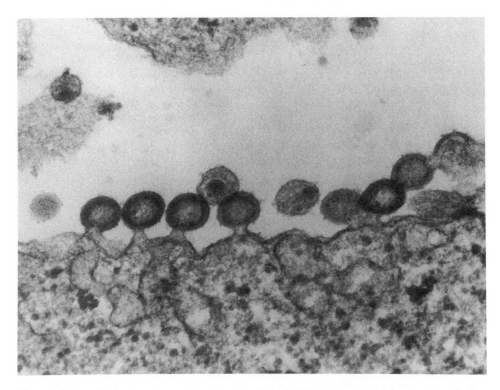

Figure 3–9. Scanning electron micrographs of HIV-1 virus particles accumulating at the surface of the COS-7 cells transfected with p6 mutant proviruses.

PROTEOLYTIC ACTIVATION OF VIRUS INFECTIVITY

The capsid and capsid enzyme precursor proteins are processed into mature forms by a virally specified protease enzyme. The capsid precursors are ultimately cleaved into four major polypeptides. The myristylated amino terminal polypeptide p17 remains associated with the membrane surface after cleavage.[190] This protein is called the matrix protein. The sequences carboxy terminal to p17, which specify the major core protein, are not associated with the membrane of the mature virus particle. The major core protein is initially cleaved to a 25-kD protein. This protein in turn is processed to a 24-kD form in a late cleavage event.[191] The major capsid protein forms a cone-shaped or tubular structure around the ribonucleoprotein that contains the viral RNA.[190] The inner virus core is very likely to contain virus-replicative enzymes, including DNA polymerase, RNAse H, and integrase.

The carboxy terminal region of the capsid precursor is cleaved into two smaller proteins, a 9-kD and a 6-kD protein. The 9-kD protein contains the sequences that bind to the viral RNA.[186,187] This protein is called the nucleocapsid protein. Sequences of the 6-kD protein are required for release of the virus particle from the surface of the infected cell.[181]

The sequences that specify the viral protease are also present in the capsid-replicative enzyme precursor. The protease itself is cleaved from the precursor by action of the viral protease to yield a 10-kD monomer.[192] The viral protease also cleaves the replicative enzyme precursors into 65- and 31-kD DNA polymerase and integrase proteins.[63,193] Very late in maturation the 65-kD homodimer is cleaved to the 65–51-kD active form of the viral DNA polymerase–ribonuclease H enzyme.

The viral protease is active as a homodimer.[194] The three-dimensional structure of this viral protease has been determined by x-ray crystallography.[195,196] The active site of the protease is created by association of two aspartic acids.[196,197] Each monomer of the enzyme contains a single aspartic acid. For this reason, dimerization is required for the creation of an active protease. The specificity of proteolytic cleavage appears to be determined mainly by the primary amino acid sequence as well as by the tertiary structure of the substrate.[198,199]

The means by which the protease is activated in the assembled virus particle is not known. It is possible that the capsid-replicative enzyme precursors in the assembled virus form homodimers. The dimeric form of the precursor protease might cleave an adjacent precursor. Alternatively, it may be possible for the homodimer to initiate an autocleavage event whereby the protease is freed from the precursor. Proteolytic cleavage of the capsid and capsid-replicative enzyme is required for virus replication.[200,201] Viruses defective for protease assemble and bud from the surface.[173,201] However, the assembled virus particles are not capable of initiating a second round of infection. It is thought that the defect of protease either prevents penetration of a cell following binding and fusion or prevents completion of the process of reverse transcription. The viral protease is sensitive to inhibition by transition state analogues of the natural substrate.[202–206] The peptide-like inhibitors contain a tetrahedral atom, usually a carbon atom, in the position of the cissile bond. Many of the inhibitors tried to date do not have favorable pharmacologic properties. However, several inhibitors that demonstrate preferential inhibition of viral rather than cellular proteases are currently being evaluated for clinical efficacy as antiviral drugs.

The Late Regulatory Genes

Three viral proteins not previously identified in other retroviruses are made late in infection from singly spliced mRNAs—the products of *vif, vpr,* and *vpu.* The singly spliced mRNAs accumulate late in infection as a consequence of *rev* function.

vif

The longest of the mRNA species specifies the 23-kD *vif* protein.[207,208] *Vif* is located immediately 3′ to the *pol* open reading frame. The *vif* protein is found in the cytoplasm of infected cells. The *vif* protein is not exported into supernatant fluids and is not incorporated into mature virus particles. Virus protein synthesis, viral capsid assembly, and virus budding appear to be normal in *vif*-defective viruses.

Viruses defective for *vif* show a selective defect for initiation of infection in some established cell lines.[209,210] The titer of *vif*+ and *vif*− viruses may differ by more than 1,000-fold when assayed on some established CD4+ cell lines. The titer of the same two virus stocks may be high and indistinguishable when assayed on other CD4+ cell lines. The basis for the selective defect in replication is not known. It is speculated that *vif* may increase the specific infectivity of HIV-1 in natural body fluids.

The basis for the selective defect in replication in *vif*− viruses is not known. It has been reported, but not confirmed, that *vif* may act as a protease to remove carboxy terminal amino acids from the envelope transmembrane glycoprotein.[211]

vpr

The *vpr* protein is also made from its own mRNA, which accumulates late in the laboratory virus's life cycle.[212] Viruses defective for the *vpr* protein initiate new rounds of infection much more slowly than do their nondefective counterparts.[213,214]

The *vpr* protein is incorporated in multiple copies into the mature virus particle.[215,216] With the exception of the envelope glycoprotein, *vpr* is the only viral protein found highly associated with the mature virus particle that is not covalently linked to the *gag* precursor. It is not known how the *vpr* protein becomes associated with the mature virus particle. *Vpr* produced by an independent gene can be incorporated in *trans* into a *vpr*-defective virus particle.

Vpr protein acts to increase the rate of RNA transcription from cellular and viral promoters.[215] The *vpr* protein stimulates the HIV-1 LTR initiation by threefold. It is possible that the *vpr* protein, carried into the infected cell by the virus particle, increases the initial basal rate of transcription of the provirus. In the absence of *tat*, very few full-length primary transcripts of viral RNA accumulate. It is possible that *vpr*-mediated activation of early rounds of viral transcription increases the rate of accumulation of the viral RNA, permitting synthesis of the first *tat* proteins, which are necessary for subsequent stages in expression of the virus's genetic information.

vpu

The *vpu* protein is made from the same mRNA as is the envelope glycoprotein. The mRNA accumulates late in the virus's life cycle. The initiation codon of *vpu* is used with about the same frequency as is the *env* AUG codon on the same mRNA in *in vitro* translation reactions.

The *vpu* protein is a 15- to 20-kD protein that is located in the cytoplasm of the infected cell.[217–219] The *vpu* protein is not found to be associated with the mature virus particle. There is some evidence that *vpu* may be located within the Golgi apparatus.

Vpu affects the efficiency of assembly and budding of virus particles.[220,221] The same amount of capsid and envelope proteins are made in the presence and absence of *vpu*. However, *vpu* increases the amount of virus capsid proteins released into the supernatant fluid, at least in some cell types. In some cases, *vpu* increases the ratio of released to cell-associated viral proteins by 10-fold or more.

It has been reported that *vpu* affects envelope glycoprotein processing. In one case, it has been reported that *vpu* increases the amount of envelope glycoprotein that reaches the surface of the cell and decreases the amount of *env* protein degraded intercellularly (Karn, Babson College Meeting Report). A second report indicates that *vpu* may help dissociate the envelope glycoprotein CD4 complex formed within the Golgi apparatus. It is not clear how the effects of *vpu* on the envelope precursor can affect assembly and budding of capsid proteins, as these two processes appear to be independent.

vpt

A fourth virus protein may also be made late in infection. All strains of HIV-1 contain a conserved open reading frame, T, overlapping the first coding exons of *tat, rev,* and the *vpu* open reading frame. *In vitro* transcription translation of mRNA from this region results in synthesis of a 15-kD *tat* protein and a 21-kD *tat*-T fusion protein designated the *vpt* protein.[222] The *vpt* protein arises from a −1 frameshift event that occurs near the amino terminus of the *tat* protein. The *vpt* protein made in cells is stable. A mutant that contains a fourth frameshift between the *tat* and T open reading frames produces a detectable amount of a stable *vpt* protein when *tat* is provided in *trans*. The ratio between the 15-kD *tat* protein and *vpt* protein made in *in vitro* transcription translation reactions is 20:1. The function of the *vpt* protein is not known. The *vpt* protein has neither *tat* nor *rev* activity. The function of the *vpt* protein is not known.

SUMMARY

The complex nature of the life cycle of HIV-1 in infected people can be partially understood in terms of the complex nature of the virus itself. People infected by AIDS are infected for life. Lifelong infection is a consequence of the insertion of viral genetic material into the host cell, a fundamental property of all retroviruses, including HIV-1.

Despite chronic infection, few of the cells sensitive to infection, the CD4+ T cells, are found to be infected during the early years of infection. Low levels of infection of this population may reflect inefficient conversion of viral RNA to DNA in the cytoplasm of resting T cells. Infection of this population may be self-limiting.

Mitogenic stimulation of PBLs of infected patients is required to observe prolific replication. Low levels of virus expression from unstimulated populations of infected primary lymphocyte cells are a consequence of the requirement for activation of transcription factors. Mitogenic stimulation of T cells activates transcription factors necessary for viral RNA expression.

Virus infection continues in infected people despite a continuing antiviral immune response. The virus eludes the immune response by several strategies. In some cells virus DNA is present but no viral proteins are made. Such cells are invisible to the immune system. In other cells regulatory proteins but not structural proteins are made, a consequence of low levels of virus transcription and consequently low levels of *tat* and *rev* protein. Such cells should also be largely invisible to the immune system. Virus particles that are produced are coated by an envelope glycoprotein. The envelope glycoprotein is shielded from the immune system by a heavy coating of carbohydrates, which are not recognized as foreign by the immune system. Those regions of the envelope glycoprotein which are exposed are not sensitive to inhibition by antiviral antibodies. Moreover, antigenic epitopes of the virus vary during the course of replication. Rapid variation in the primary nucleic acid of protein sequences is a result of multiple mistakes introduced into the viral genome during the course of replication.

HIV-1 is transmitted sexually. Sexual transmission can be understood, at least in part, by the activity of three viral genes active late in the virus's life cycle. Together these three genes—*vif, vpr,* and *vpu*—increase the amount of virus produced by infected cells, increase the specific infectivity of the virus, and increase the rate of events that occur early in infection.

HIV-1 is vulnerable to drugs that inhibit replication of all states of its complex life cycle. Therapy using combinations of drugs that act at different stages of the life cycle should permanently suppress virus replication. Curative therapy of AIDS is a realistic and attainable goal.

Acknowledgments: Work was supported by NIH grants AI 24845 (NCDDG), AI 24755, AI 29873, AI 28193, and AI 28691. The author thanks Chris Farnet, Dana Gabuzda, Heinrich Gottlinger, Karl Kalland, Yichen Lu, Ernest Terwilliger, and Emmanuel Zazopolous for helpful comments.

REFERENCES

1. Dalgleish AG, Beverley PC, Clapham PR et al: The CD4 (T4) antigen is an essential component of the receptor for the AIDS retrovirus. Nature (London) 312:763, 1984
2. Klatzmann D, Champagne E, Chamaret S et al: T-lymphocyte T4 molecule behaves as the receptor for human retrovirus LAV. Nature (London) 312:767, 1984
3. McDougal JS, Mawle A, Cort SP et al: Cellular tropism of the human retrovirus HTLV III/LAV: I. Role of T cell activation and expression of the T4 antigen. J Immunol 135:3151, 1985
4. Stein B, Gonda S, Lifson J et al: pH-independent HIV entry into CD4-positive T cells via virus envelope fusion to the plasma membrane. Cell 49:659, 1987
5. Sodroski JG, Goh WC, Rosen C et al: Role of the HTLV-III/LAV envelope in syncytium formation and cytopathicity. Nature 322:470, 1986
6. Lifson JD, Feinberg MB, Reyes GR et al: Induction of CD4-dependent cell fusion by the HTLV/III LAV envelope glycoprotein. Nature 323:725, 1986
7. Allen JS, Colligan JE, Darin F et al: Major glycoprotein antigens that induce antibodies in AIDS patients are encoded by HTLV-III. Science 228:1091, 1985
8. Robey WG, Safai B, Oroszian S et al: Characterization of envelope and core structural gene products of HTLV-III with sera from AIDS patients. Science 225:593, 1985
9. Kowalski M, Potz J, Basiripour L et al: Functional regions of the envelope glycoprotein of human immunodeficiency virus type 1. Science 237:1351, 1987
10. Berman P, Nunes W, Hattar O: Expression of membrane-associated and secreted variants of gp160 of human immunodeficiency virus type 1 in vitro and in continuous cell lines. J Virol 62:3135, 1988
11. Haffar O, Dowbenko D, Berman P: Topogenic analysis of the human immunodeficiency virus type 1 envelope glycoprotein, gp160, in microsomal membranes. J Cell Biol 107:1677, 1988
12. Earl P, Doms R, Moss B: Oligomeric structure of the human immunodeficiency virus type 1 envelope glycoprotein. Proc Natl Acad Sci USA 87:648, 1990
13. Earl P, Moss B, Doms R: Folding, interaction with GRP78-BiP, assembly and transport of the human immunodeficiency virus type 1 envelope protein. J Virol 65:2047, 1991
14. Willey R, Bonifacino J, Potts B et al: Biosynthesis, cleavage and degradation of the human immunodeficiency virus 1 envelope glycoprotein gp160. Proc Natl Acad Sci USA 85:9580, 1988
15. Dewar R, Vasudevachari M, Natarajan V, Silzmann N: Biosynthesis and processing of human immunodeficiency virus type 1 envelope glycoproteins: Effect of monensin on glycosylation and transport. J Virol 63:2452, 1989
16. Stein B, Englemann E: Intracellular processing of gp160 HIV-1 envelope precursors. J Biol Chem 265:2640, 1990
17. Kozarsky K, Penman M, Basiripour L et al: Glycosylation and processing of the human immunodeficiency virus type 1 envelope protein. J AIDS 2:163, 1989
18. Matthews TJ, Weinhold KJ, Lyerly HK et al: Interaction between the human T-cell lymphotropic virus type IIIB envelope glycoprotein gp120 and the surface antigen CD4: Role of carbohydrate in binding and cell fusion. Proc Natl Acad Sci USA 53:55, 1987
19. McCune JM, Rabin LB, Feinberg MB et al: Endoproteolytic cleavage of gp160 is required for activation of human immunodeficiency virus. Cell 53:55, 1988
20. Freed E, Myers D, Risser R: Mutational analysis of the cleavage sequence of the human immunodeficiency virus type 1 envelope glycoprotein precursor gp160. J Virol 63:4670, 1989
21. Pinter A, Honnen W, Tilley S et al: Oligomeric structure of gp41, the transmembrane protein of human immunodeficiency virus type 1. J Virol 63:2674, 1989
22. Schawaller M, Smith C, Skehel J, Wiley D: Studies with cross-linking reagents on the oligomeric structure of the env glycoprotein of HIV. Virology 172:367, 1989
23. Walker B, Chakrabarti S, Moss B et al: HIV-specific cytotoxic T lymphocytes in seropositive individuals. Nature 328:345, 1987
24. Lasky LA, Nakamura G, Smith DH et al: Delineation of a region of the human immunodeficiency virus type 1 gp120 glycoprotein critical for interaction with the CD4 receptor. Cell 50:975, 1987
25. Olshevsky UE, Helseth E, Furman C et al: Identification of individual HIV-1 gp120 amino acids important for CD4 receptor binding. J Virol 64:5701, 1990
26. Maddon PJ, Dalgleish AG, McDougal JS et al: Cell 47:333, 1986
27. Gallaher WR: Detection of a fusion peptide sequence in the transmembrane protein of human immunodeficiency virus. Cell 50:327, 1987
28. Chesebro B, Buller R, Portis J, Wehrly K: Failure of human immunodeficiency virus entry and infection in CD4-positive human brain and skin cells. J Virol 64:215, 1990
29. Varmus H: Retroviruses. Science 240:1427, 1988
30. Varmus HE, Swanstrom R: Replication of retroviruses. In Weiss R, Teich N, Varmus H, Coffin J (eds): RNA Tumor Viruses, p 369. Cold Spring Harbor, New York, Cold Spring Harbor Laboratory, 1982
31. Varmus HE, Swanstrom R: Replication of retroviruses. In Weiss R, Teich N, Varmus H, Coffin J (eds): RNA Tumor Viruses, 2nd ed, p 74. Cold Spring Harbor, New York, Cold Spring Harbor Laboratory, 1985
32. Starcich B, Ratner L, Josephs SF et al: Characterization of long terminal repeat sequences of HTLV-III. Science 227:538, 1985
33. Meusing M, Smith D, Cabradilla C et al: Nucleic acid structure and expression of the human AIDS retrovirus. Nature 313:450, 1985
34. Coffin JM, Haseltine WA: Terminal redundancy and the

origin of replication of Rouse sarcoma virus RNA. Proc Natl Acad Sci USA 74:1908, 1977

35. Panganiban AT, Fiore D: Ordered interstrand and intrastrand DNA transfer during reverse transcription. Science 241:1064, 1988

36. Finston WI, Champoux JJ: RNA primed initiation of Moloney murine leukemia virus plus strands by reverse transcriptase *in vitro*. J Virol 51:26, 1984

37. Charman P, Clavel F: A single-stranded gap in human immunodeficiency virus unintegrated linear DNA defined by a central copy of the polypurine tract. J Virol 65:2415, 1991

38. Galboa E, Mitra SW, Goff S, Baltimore D: A detailed model of reverse transcription and tests of crucial aspects. Cell 18:93, 1979

39. Junghans RP, Boone LR, Skalka AM: Products of reverse transcription in avian retrovirus analyzed by electron microscopy. J Virol 43:544, 1982

40. Kim S, Byrn R, Groopman J, Baltimore D: Temporal aspects of DNA and RNA synthesis during human immunodeficiency virus infections: Evidence for differential gene expression. J Virol 63:3708, 1989

41. Farnet CM, Haseltine WA: Integration of human immunodeficiency virus type 1 DNA *in vitro*. Proc Natl Acad Sci USA 87:4164, 1990

41a. Farnet C, Haseltine WA: The circularization of human immunodeficiency virus type 1 (HIV-1) DNA in vitro. 1991 (in press)

42. Zack JA, Arrigo SA, Weitsman SR et al: HIV-1 entry into quiescent primary lymphocytes: Molecular analysis reveals a labile latent viral structure. Cell 61:213, 1990

43. Furman PA, Barry DW: Spectrum of antiviral activity and mechanism of action of zidovudine. Am J Med 85(suppl 2A):176, 1988

44. Mitsuya H, Weinhold KJ, Furman PA et al: 3'-Azido-3'-deoxythimidine (BW A509U): An antiviral agent that inhibits the infectivity and cytopathic effect of human T-lymphotropic virus type III lymphadenopathy-associated virus in vitro. Proc Natl Acad Sci USA 82:7096, 1985

45. Mitsuya H, Broder S: Inhibition of in vitro infectivity and cytopathic effect of human T-lymphotropic virus type III/lymphadenopathy associated virus (HTLV III/LAV) by 2'-3'-dideoxynucleosides. Proc Natl Acad Sci USA 83:1911, 1986

46. Ahluwalin G, Conney DA, Mitsuya H et al: Initial studies in the cellular pharmacology of 2',3'-dideoxyinosine, an inhibitor of HIV infectivity. Biochem Pharmacol 36:3797, 1987

47. Balzarini J, Kang GJ, Dalal M et al: The anti-HTLV III (anti-HIV) and cytotoxic activity of 2',3'-didehydro-2',3'-dideoxyribonucleosides. Mol Pharmacol 32:162, 1987

48. Lin TS, Schinazi RF, Prusoff WM: Potent and selective in vitro activity of 3'-deoxythymidine-2'-ene (3'-deoxy-2'-3'-didehydrothymidine) against human immunodeficiency virus. Biochem Pharmacol 36:2713, 1987

49. Furman PA, Fyfe JA, St Clair MH et al: Phosphorylation of 3'-azido-3'-deoxythymidine and selective interaction of the 5'-triphosphate with HIV reverse transcriptase. Proc Natl Acad Sci USA 83:8333, 1986

50. St Clair MH, Richards CA, Spector T et al: 3'-Azido-3'-deoxythymidine triphosphates as an inhibitor and substrate of purified human immunodeficiency virus reverse transcriptase. Antimicrob Agents Chemother 31:1972, 1987

51. Larder BA, Darby G, Richman DD: HIV with reduced sensitivity to zidovudine (AZT) isolated during prolonged therapy. Science 243:1731, 1989

52. Larder BA, Kemp SD: Multiple mutations in HIV-1 reverse transcriptase confer high-level resistance to zidovudine (AZT). Science 246:1155, 1989

53. Pauwels R, Andries K, Desmyter J et al: Potent and selective inhibition of HIV-1 replication in vitro by a novel series of TIBO derivatives. Nature 343:470, 1990

54. Jacks T, Varmus HE: Expression of the Rouse sarcoma virus pol gene by ribosomal frameshifting. Science 230:1237, 1985

55. Wilson W, Braddock M, Adams SE et al: HIV expression strategies: Ribosomal frameshifting is directed by a short sequence in both mammalian and yeast systems. Cell 55:1159, 1988

56. Jacks T, Power MD, Masiarz FR et al: Characterization of ribosomal frameshifting in HIV-1 gag-pol expression. Nature 231:280, 1988

57. Miller M, Jaskolski M, Mohana Rao JK et al: Crystal structure of a retroviral protease proves relationship to aspartic protease family. Nature 337:576, 1989

58. Navia MA, Fitzgerald PMD, McKeever BM et al: Three-dimensional structure of aspartyl protease from human immunodeficiency virus HIV-1. Nature 337:615, 1989

59. Weber IT, Miller M, Jaskolski M et al: Molecular modeling of the HIV-1 protease and its substrate binding site. Science 243:928, 1989

60. Dickson C, Eisenmann R, Fan H et al: Protein biosynthesis and assembly. In Weiss RA, Teich N, Varmus HE, Coffin JM (eds): RNA Tumor Viruses, p 513. Cold Spring Harbor, New York, Cold Spring Harbor Laboratory, 1982

61. Dickson E, Eisenmann R, Fan H: Protein synthesis and assembly. In Weiss RA, Teich N, Varmus HE, Coffin JM (eds): RNA Tumor Viruses, 2nd ed, p 135. Cold Spring Harbor, New York, Cold Spring Harbor Laboratory, 1985

62. Veronese FDM, Copeland TD, Devico AL et al: Characterization of highly immunogenic p66/p51 as the reverse transcriptase of HTLV III/LAV. Science 231:1289, 1986

63. Lightfoote MM, Coligan JE, Folks TM et al: Structural characterization of reverse transcriptase and endonuclease polypeptides of the acquired immunodeficiency syndrome retrovirus. J Virol 60:771, 1986

64. Lowe DM, Atiken A, Bradley C et al: HIV-1 reverse transcriptase: Crystallization and analysis of domain structure by limited proteolysis. Biochemistry 27:8884, 1988

65. Muller B, Restle T, Weiss S et al: Co-expression of the subunits of the heterodimer of HIV-1 reverse transcriptase in *Escherichia coli*. J Biol Chem 264:13975, 1989

66. Schatz O, Cramme FV, Gruninger-Leitch F, LeGrice SFJ: Point mutations in conserved amino acid residues within the C-terminal domain of HIV-1 reverse transcriptase specifically repress RNAse H function. FEBS Lett 257:311, 1989

67. Hostomsky Z, Hostomska Z, Hudson GO et al: Reconstitution in vitro of RNAse H activity by using purified N-terminal and C-terminal domains of human immunodeficiency virus type 1 reverse transcriptase. Proc Natl Acad Sci USA 88:1148, 1991

68. Davies JF, Hostomska Z, Hostomsky Z et al: Crystal structure of the ribonuclease H domain of HIV-1 reverse transcriptase. Science 252:88, 1991

69. Gartner S, Markovits P, Markovitz DM et al: The role of mononuclear phagocytes in HTLV III/LAV infection. Science 233:215, 1986

70. Langhoff E, Terwilliger EF, Bos HJ et al: Replication of HIV-1 in primary dendritic cell cultures. Proc Natl Acad Sci USA 88:998, Sept 1991

71. Muesing MA, Smith DH, Cabradilla CD et al: Nucleic acid structure and expression of the human AIDS/lymphade-nopathy retrovirus. Nature 313:450, 1985

72. Bushman FD, Fujiwara T, Craigie R: Retroviral DNA integration directed by HIV integration protein in vitro. Science 249:1555, 1990

73. Sherman PA, Fyfe JA: Human immunodeficiency virus integration protein expressed in *Escherichia coli* possesses selective DNA cleaving activity. Proc Natl Acad Sci USA 87:5119, 1990

74. Bushman FD, Craigie R: Activities of human immunodeficiency virus (HIV) integration protein in vitro: Specific cleavage and integration of HIV DNA. Proc Natl Acad Sci USA 88:1339, 1991

75. Farnet CM, Haseltine WA: Determination of the viral proteins present in the HIV-1 preintegration complex. J Virol 65:1910, 1991

76. Ellison V, Abrams H, Roe T et al: Human immunodeficiency virus integration in a cell-free system. J Virol 64:2711, 1990

77. Myrick K, Farnet CM, Haseltine WA: An integration based retroviral cloning strategy illustrates correct in vitro insertion of HIV-1 DNA. J Virol (in press)

78. Colicelli J, Goff SP: Mutants and pseudorevertants of Moloney murine leukemia virus with alterations at the integration site. Cell 42:573, 1985

79. Colicelli J, Goff SP: Sequence and spacing requirements of a retrovirus integration site. J Mol Biol 199:47, 1988

80. Schinittman SM, Psallidopoulos MC, Lane HC et al: The reservoir for HIV-1 in human peripheral blood is a T cell that maintains expression of CD4. Science 245:305, 1989

81. Folks T, Powell DM, Lightfoote MM, Benn S, Martin MA, Fauci AS. Induction of HTLV-III/LAV from a nonvirus-producing T-cell line: Implications for latency. Science 231:600, 1986

82. Harrich D, Garcia J, Wu F et al: Role of SP1-binding domains in in vitro transcriptional regulation of the human immunodeficiency virus type 1 long terminal repeat. J Virol 63:2585, 1989

83. Nabel G, Baltimore D: An inducible transcription factor activates expression of human immunodeficiency virus in T cells. Nature (London) 326:711, 1987

84. Rosen CA, Sodroski JG, Haseltine WA: The location of *cis*-acting regulatory sequences in the human T cell lymphotropic virus type III (HTLV-III/LAV) long terminal repeat. Cell 41:813, 1985

85. Shaw JP, Utz PJ, Durand DB et al: Identification of a putative regulator of early T cell activation genes. Science 241:202, 1988

86. Lu Y, Touzijian N, Stenzel M et al: Identification of *cis*-acting repressive sequences within the negative regulatory element of human immunodeficiency virus type 1. J Virol 64:5226, 1990

87. Franza BR Jr, Rauscher FJ III, Josephs SF, Curran T: The *fos* complex and *fos*-related antigens recognize sequence elements that contain AP-1 binding sites. Science 239:1150, 1988

88. Wu FK, Garcia JA, Harrich D, Gaynor RB: Purification of the human immunodeficiency virus type 1 enhancer and TAR binding proteins EBP-1 and UBP-1. EMBO J 7:2117, 1988

89. Jones KA, Luciw PA, Duchange N: Structural arrangements of transcription control domains within the 5′-untranslated leader regions of the HIV-1 and HIV-2 promoters. Genes Dev 2:1101, 1988

90. Sodroski J, Patarca R, Rosen C et al: Location of the *trans*-activating region of the genome of the human T-cell lymphotropic virus type III. Science 229:74, 1985

91. Arya SK, Guo C, Josephs SF, Wong-Staal F: *Trans*-activator of human T-lymphotropic virus type 3 (HTLV-III). Science 229:69, 1985

92. Gendelman HE, Phelps WA, Feigenbaum L et al: Trans-activation of the human immunodeficiency virus long terminal repeat sequence by DNA viruses. Proc Natl Acad Sci USA 83:759, 1986

93. Peterlin BM, Luciw PA, Barr PJ, Walker MD: Elevated levels of mRNA can account for the trans-activation of human immunodeficiency virus. Proc Natl Acad Sci USA 83:9734, 1986

94. Cullen BR: *Trans*-activation of human immunodeficiency virus occurs via a biomodal mechanism. Cell 46:973, 1986

95. Wright CM, Felber BK, Paskalis H, Pavlakis GN: Expression and characterization of the *trans*-activator of HTLV-III/LAV virus. Science 234:988, 1986

96. Rosen CA, Sodroski JG, Goh WC et al: Post transcriptional regulation accounts for the *trans*-activation of the human T lymphotropic viruses type III (HTLV-III/LAV). Nature 319:555, 1986

97. Schwartz S, Felber BK, Benko DM et al: Cloning and functional analysis of multiple spliced mRNA species of human immunodeficiency virus. J Virol 64:2519, 1990

98. Dayton AL, Sodroski JG, Rosen CA et al: The *trans*-activator gene of the human T-cell lymphotropic virus type III is required for replication. Cell 44:941, 1986

99. Fisher AG, Feinberg MB, Joseph SF et al: *Trans*-activator gene of HTLV-III as essential for virus replication. Nature 320:367, 1986.

100. Rice AP, Matthews MB: Transcriptional but not translational regulation of HIV-1 by the *tat* gene product. Nature 332:551, 1988

101. Jeang KT, Shank PR, Kumar A: Transcriptional activation of homologous viral long terminal repeats by the human immunodeficiency virus type 1 of the human T-cell leukemia virus type 1 tat proteins occurs in the absence of a de novo protein synthesis. Proc Natl Acad Sci USA 65:8291, 1988

102. Laspia MF, Rice AP, Mathews MB: HIV-1 *tat* protein increases transcriptional initiation and stabilizes elongation. Cell 59:283, 1989

103. Laspia MF, Rice AP, Mathews MB: Synergy between HIV-1 tat and adenovirus E1A is principally due to stabilization of transcriptional elongation. Genes Dev 4:2397, 1990

104. Roy S, Delling U, Chen C-H et al: A bulge structure in HIV-1 TAR RNA is required for tat binding and tat-mediated trans-activation. Genes Dev 4:1365, 1990

105. Jacobvits A, Smith DS, Jakobvits EB, Capon DJ: A discrete element 3′ of human immunodeficiency virus 1 (HIV-1) and HIV-2 mRNA initiation sites mediates transcriptional activation by an HIV *trans* activator. Mol Cell Biol 8:2555, 1988

106. Kao S-Y, Calman AF, Luciw PA, Peterlin BM: Anti-termination of transcription within the long terminal repeat of HIV-1 by *tat* product. Nature 330:489, 1987

107. Selby MJ, Bain ES, Luciw PA, Peterlin BM: Structure, sequence, and position of the stem-loop in *tar* determine

transcriptional elongation by *tat* through the HIV-1 long terminal repeat. Genes Dev 3:547, 1989

108. Toohey MG, Jones KA: In vitro formation of short RNA polymerase II transcripts that terminate within the HIV-1 and HIV-2 promoter-proximal downstream regions. Genes Dev 3:265, 1989

109. Marciniak RA, Cainan BJ, Frankel AD, Sharp PA: HIV *tat* protein *trans*-activates transcription *in vitro*. Cell 63:791, 1990

110. Feinberg MB, Jarrett RF, Aldovini A et al: HTLV-III expression and production involve complex regulation at the levels of splicing and translation of viral RNA. Cell 46:807, 1985

111. Müller WEB, Okamoto T, Reuter P et al: Functional characterization of tat protein from human immunodeficiency virus. J Biol Chem 265:3803, 1990

112. Dingwall C, Ernberg I, Gait MJ et al: Human immunodeficiency virus 1 tat protein binds trans-activation-responsive region (TAR) RNA *in vitro*. Proc Natl Acad Sci USA 86:6925, 1989

113. Weeks KM, Ampe C, Schultz SC et al: Fragments of the HIV-1 tat protein specifically bind TAR RNA. Science 249:1281, 1990

114. Cordingley MG, La Femina RL, Callahan PL et al: Sequence-specific interaction of tat protein and tat peptides with the transactivation-responsive sequence element of human immunodeficiency virus type 1 *in vitro*. Proc Natl Acad Sci USA 87:8985, 1990

115. Muesing MA, Smith DH, Capon DJ: Regulation of mRNA accumulation by a human immunodeficiency virus *trans*-activator protein. Cell 48:691, 1987

116. Dingwall C, Ernberg I, Gait MJ et al: HIV-1 *tat* protein stimulates transcription by binding to a U-rich bulge in the stem of the TAR RNA structure. EMBO J 9:4145, 1990

117. Roy S, Parkin NT, Rosen C et al: Structural requirements for *trans* activation of human immunodeficiency virus type 1 long terminal repeat-directed gene expression by *tat*: Importance of base pairing, loop sequence, and bulges in the *tat*-responsive sequence. J Virol 64:1402, 1990

118. Calnan BJ, Tidor B, Biancalana S et al: Arginine-mediated RNA recognition: The arginine fork. Science 252:1167, 1991

119. Berkhout B, Jeang K-T: *trans* activation of human immunodeficiency virus type 1 is sequence specific for both the single-stranded bulge and loop of the *trans*-acting-responsive hairpin: A quantitative analysis. J Virol 63:5501, 1989

120. Berkhout B, Gatignol A, Rabson AB, Jeang K-T: TAR-independent activation of the HIV-1 LTR: Evidence that *tat* requires specific regions of the promoter. Cell 62:757, 1990

121. Feng S, Holland EC: HIV-1 *tat trans*-activation requires a loop sequence within TAR. Nature 334:165, 1988

122. Garcia JA, Harrich D, Soultanakis E et al: Human immunodeficiency virus type 1 LTR TATA and TAR region sequences required for transcriptional regulation. EMBO J 8:765, 1989

123. Gatignol A, Kumar A, Rabson A, Jeang K-T: Identification of cellular proteins that bind to the human immunodeficiency virus type 1 trans-activation-responsive TAR element RNA. Proc Natl Acad Sci USA 86:7828, 1989

124. Gaynor R, Soultanakis E, Kuwabara M et al: Specific binding of a HeLa cell nuclear protein to RNA sequences in the human immunodeficiency virus transactivating region. Proc Natl Acad Sci USA 86:4858, 1989

125. Marciniak RA, Garcia-Lanco MA, Sharp PA: Identification and characterization of the HeLa nuclear protein that specifically binds to the trans-activation-response (TAR) element of human immunodeficiency virus. Proc Natl Acad Sci USA 87:2624, 1990

126. Gatignol A, Buckler-White A, Berkhout B, Jeang K-T: Characterization of a human TAR RNA-binding protein that activates the HIV-1 LTR. Science 251:1597, 1991

127. Nelbock P, Dillon PJ, Perkins A, Rosen CA: A cDNA for a protein that interacts with the human immunodeficiency virus *tat* transactivator. Science 248:1650, 1990

128. Malim MH, Hauber J, Fenrick R, Cullen BR: Immunodeficiency virus rev trans-activator modulates the expression of the viral regulatory genes. Nature 335:181, 1988

129. Malim MH, Hauber J, Les Y et al: The HIV-1 *rev trans*-activator acts through a structured target sequence to activate export of unspliced viral mRNA. Nature 338:254, 1989

130. Hammarskjöld M-L, Heimer J, Hammarskjöld B et al: Regulation of human immunodeficiency virus *env* expression by the *rev* gene product. J Virol 63:1959, 1989

131. Emerman M, Vazeux R, Peden K: The *rev* gene product of the human immunodeficiency virus affects envelope-specific RNA localization. Cell 57:1155, 1989

132. Hadzopoulou-Cladaras M, Felber BK, Cladaras C et al: The *rev* (*trs/art*) protein of human immunodeficiency virus type 1 affects viral mRNA and protein expression via *cis*-acting sequence in the *env* region. J Virol 63:1265, 1989

133. Terwilliger E, Burghoff R, Sia R et al: The *art* gene product of the human immunodeficiency virus is required for replication. J Virol 62:655, 1988

134. Sodroski JG, Goh WC, Rosen C et al: A second post-transcriptional *trans*-activator gene required for HTLV-III replication. Nature 321:412, 1986

135. Dayton AI, Terwilliger EF, Potz J et al: *Cis*-acting sequences responsive to the *rev* gene product of the human immunodeficiency virus. J AIDS 1:441, 1988

136. Cochrane AW, Chen C-H, Rosen CA: Specific interaction of a human immunodeficiency virus *rev* protein with a structured region in the *env* mRNA. Proc Natl Acad Sci USA 87:1198, 1990

137. Heaphy S, Dingwall C, Ernberg I et al: HIV-1 regulator of virion expression (*rev*) protein binds to an RNA stem-loop structure located within the *rev*-responsive element region. Cell 60:685, 1990

138. Kjems J, Brown M, Chang DD, Sharp PA: Structural analysis of the interaction between the human immunodeficiency virus *rev* protein and the *rev* response element. Proc Natl Acad Sci USA 88:683, 1991

139. Solomin L, Felber BK, Pavlakis GN: Different sites of interaction for *rev, tev,* and *rex* proteins within the *rev*-responsive element of human immunodeficiency virus type 1. J Virol 64:6010, 1990

140. Zapp ML, Green MR: Sequence-specific RNA binding by the HIV-1 *rev* protein. Nature 342:714, 1989

141. Daly TJ, Rusche JR, Malone TE, Frankel AD: Circular dichroism studies of the HIV-1 *rev* protein and its specific RNA binding site. Biochemistry 129:9791, 1990

142. Dayton ET, Powell DM, Dayton AI: Functional analysis of CAR, the target sequence for *rev* protein of HIV-1. Science 246:1625, 1989

143. Olsen HS, Nelbock P, Cochrane AW, Rosen CA: Secondary structure is the major determinant for interaction of HIV *rev* protein RNA. Science 247:845, 1990

144. Malim MH, Tiley LS, McCarn DF et al: HIV-1 structural gene expression requires binding of the *rev trans*-activator to its RNA target sequence. Cell 60:675, 1990

145. Malim MH, Bohnlein S, Hauber J, Cullen BR: Functional dissection of the HIV-1 *rev trans*-activator derivation of the *trans*-dominant repressor of *rev* function. Cell 58:205, 1989

146. Malim MH, Cullen BR: HIV-1 structural gene expression requires the binding of multiple rev monomers to the viral RRE: Implications for HIV-1 latency. Cell 85:241, 1991

147. Olsen HE, Cochrane AW, Dillon PJ et al: Interaction of the human immunodeficiency virus type 1 *rev* protein with structured region in *env* mRNA is dependent upon multimer formation mediated through a basic stretch of amino acids. Genes Dev 1:1357, 1990

148. Vaishnav YN, Vaishnav M, Wong-Staal F: Identification and characterization of a nuclear factor that specifically binds to the rev response element (RRE) of human immunodeficiency virus type 1 (HIV-1). New Biol 3:142, 1991

149. Rosen CA, Terwilliger E, Dayton A et al: Intragenic *cis*-acting *art* gene-responsive sequences of the human immunodeficiency virus. Proc Natl Acad Sci USA 85:2071, 1988

150. Felber BK, Drysdale CM, Pavlakis GN. Feedback regulation of human immunodeficiency virus type 1 expression by the *rev* protein. J Virol 64:3734, 1990

151. Lu X, Heimer J, Rekosh D, Hammarskjöld M-L: U1 small nuclear RNA plays a direct role in the formation of a rev-regulated human immunodeficiency virus *env* mRNA that remains unspliced. Proc Natl Acad Sci USA 87:7598, 1990

152. Chang DD, Sharp PA: Regulation by HIV *rev* depends upon recognition of splice sites. Cell 59:789, 1989

153. Arrigo SJ, Chen ISY: Rev is necessary for translation but not cytoplasmic accumulation of HIV-1 *vif, vpr,* and *env/vpu* 2 RNAs. Genes Dev 5:808, 1991

154. Salfeld J, Gottlinger HG, Sia R et al: A tripartite HIV-1 *tat-env-rev* fusion protein. EMBO J 9:965, 1990

155. Benko DM, Schwartz S, Pavlakis GN, Felber BK: A novel human immunodeficiency virus type 1 protein, *tev,* shares sequences with *tat, env,* and *rev* proteins. Virology 64:2505, 1990

156. Ratner L, Haseltine W, Patarca R et al: Complete nucleotide sequence of the AIDS virus, HTLV-III. Nature 313:277, 1985

157. Wain-Hobson S, Sonigo P, Danos O et al: Nucleotide sequence of the AIDS virus, LAV. Cell 40:9, 1985

158. Allan JS, Coligan JE, Lee T-H et al: A new HTLV-III/LAV encoded antigen detected by antibodies from AIDS patients. Science 230:810, 1985

159. Arya SK, Gallo RC: Three novel genes of human T-lymphotropic virus type III: Immune reactivity of their products with sera from acquired immune deficiency syndrome patients. Proc Natl Acad Sci USA 83:2209, 1988

160. Franchini G, Robert-Guroff M, Ghrayeb J et al: Cytoplasmic localization of the HTLV-III 3′ orf protein in cultured T cells. Virology 155:539, 1986

161. Luciw PA, Cheng-Meyer C, Levy JA: Mutational analysis of the human immunodeficiency virus: The orf-E region down-regulates virus replication. Proc Natl Acad Sci USA 84:1434, 1987

162. Terwilliger E, Sodroski JG, Rosen CA, Haseltine WA: Effects of mutations within the 3′ orf open reading frame region of human T-cell lymphotropic virus type III (HTLV-III/LAV) on replication and cytopathogenicity. J Virol 60:754, 1986

163. Cheng-Mayer C, Iannello P, Shaw K et al: Differential effects of nef on HIV replication: Implications for viral pathogenesis in the host. Science 246:1629, 1989

164. Kestler III HW, Ringler DJ, Mori K et al: Importance of the nef gene for maintenance of high virus loads for the development of AIDS. Cell 65:651, 1991

165. Ahmad N, Venkatesan S: Nef protein of HIV-1 is a transcriptional repressor of HIV-1 LTR. Science 241:1481, 1985

166. Niederman TMJ, Thielan BJ, Ratner L: Human immunodeficiency virus type 1 negative factor is a transcriptional silencer. Proc Natl Acad Sci USA 86:1128, 1989

167. Bachelerie F, Alcami J, Hazan U et al: Constitutive expression of human immunodeficiency virus (HIV) nef protein in human astrocytes does not influence basal or induced HIV long terminal repeat activity. J Virol 64:3059, 1990

168. Hammes SR, Dixon EP, Malim MH et al: Nef protein of human immunodeficiency virus type 1: Evidence against its role as a transcriptional inhibitor. Proc Natl Acad Sci USA 86:9549, 1989

169. Kim S, Ikeuchi K, Byrn R et al: Lack of negative influence on viral growth by the nef gene of human immunodeficiency virus type 1. Proc Natl Acad Sci USA 86:9544, 1989

170. Guy B, Kieny M-P, Riviere Y et al: HIV F/3′ orf encodes a phosphorylated GTP-binding protein resembling an oncogene product. Nature 330:266, 1987

171. Kaminchik J, Bashan N, Pinchasi D et al: Expression and biochemical characterization of human immunodeficiency virus type 1 nef gene product. J Virol 64:3447, 1990

172. Guy B, Riviere Y, Dott K et al: Mutational analysis of the HIV nef protein. Virology 176:413, 1990

173. Gottlinger HG, Sodroski JG, Haseltine WA: Role of capsid precursor processing and myristylation in morphogenesis and infectivity of human immunodeficiency virus type 1. Proc Natl Acad Sci 86:5781, 1989

174. Bryant M, Ratner L: Myristylation-dependent replication and assembly of human immunodeficiency virus 1. Proc Natl Acad Sci USA 87:523, 1990

175. Pal R, Reitz MS Jr, Tschachler E et al: Myristoylation of *gag* proteins of HIV-1 plays an important role in virus assembly. AIDS Res Hum Retroviruses 6:721, 1990

176. Bryant ML, Heuckeroth RO, Kimata JT et al: Replication of human immunodeficiency virus 1 and Moloney murine leukemia virus is inhibited by different heteroatom-containing analogs of myristic acid. Proc Natl Acad Sci USA 86:8655, 1989

177. Bryant ML, Ratner L, Duronio RJ et al: Incorporation of 12-methoxydodecanoate into the human immunodeficiency virus 1 gag polyprotein precursor inhibits its proteolytic processing and virus production in a chronically infected human lymphoid cell line. Proc Natl Acad Sci USA 88:2055, 1988

178. Ratner L, Heyden NV, Garcia J et al: Formation of noninfectious HIV-1 virus particles lacking a full-length envelope protein. AIDS Res Hum Retrovirus 7:287, 1991

179. Rhee SS, Hunter E: Myristylation is required for intracellular transport but not for assembly of D-type retrovirus capsids. J Virol 61:1045, 1987

180. Rhee SS, Hunter E: Amino acid substitutions within the matrix protein of type D retroviruses affect assembly, transport and membrane association of a capsid. EMBO J 10:535, 1991

181. Gottlinger HG, Dorfman T, Sodroski JG, Haseltine WA: Effect of mutations affecting the p6 *gag* protein on human

immunodeficiency virus particle release. Proc Natl Acad Sci USA 88:3195, 1991

182. Katsumoto T, Hattori N, Kurimura T: Maturation of human immunodeficiency virus, strain LAV, in vitro. Intervirology 27:148, 1987

183. Lever A, Gottlinger H, Haseltine W, Sodroski J: Identification of a sequence required for efficient packaging of human immunodeficiency virus type 1 RNA into virions. J Virol 63:4085, 1989

184. Aldovini A, Young RA: Mutations of RNA and protein sequences involved in human immunodeficiency virus type 1 packaging result in production of noninfectious virus. J Virol 64:1920, 1990

185. Clavel F, Grenstein JM: A mutation of human immunodeficiency virus with reduced RNA packaging and abnormal particle morphology. J Virol 64:5230, 1990

186. Gorelick RJ, Nigida SM Jr, Bess JW Jr et al: Noninfectious human immunodeficiency virus type 1 mutants deficient in genomic RNA. J Virol 64:3207, 1990

187. Darlix J-L, Gabus C, Nugeyre M-T et al: *Cis* elements and *trans*-acting factors involved in the RNA dimerization of the human immunodeficiency virus HIV-1. J Mol Biol 216:680, 1990

188. Kleiman L, Gaudry S, Soulerice F et al: Incorporation of tRNA into normal and mutant HIV-1. Biochem Biophys Res Commun 174:1272, 1991

189. Trono D, Feinberg MB, Baltimore D: HIV-1 gag mutants can dominantly interfere with the replication of the wild-type virus. Cell 59:113, 1989

190. Gelderblom HR, Hausmann EHS, Ozel M et al: Fine structure of human immunodeficiency virus (HIV) and immunolocalization of structural proteins. Virology 156:171, 1987

191. Tritch RJ, Cheng Y-SE, Yin FH, Erickson-Vitanen S: Mutagenesis of protease cleavage sites in the human immunodeficiency virus type 1 gag polyprotein. J Virol 65:922, 1991

192. Debouck C, Gorniak JG, Strickler JE et al: Human immunodeficiency virus protease expressed in *Escherichia coli* exhibits autoprocessing and specific maturation of the gag precursor. Proc Natl Acad Sci USA 84:8903, 1987

193. Mous J, Heimer EP, Le Grice SFJ: Processing protease and reverse transcriptase from human immunodeficiency virus type 1 polyprotein in *Escherichia coli*. J Virol 62:1433, 1988

194. Nutt RF, Brady SF, Darke PL et al: Chemical synthesis and enzymatic activity of a 99-residue peptide with a sequence proposed for the human immunodeficiency virus protease. Proc Natl Acad Sci USA 85:7129, 1988

195. Navia MA, Fitzgerald PMD, McKeever BM et al: Three-dimensional structure of aspartyl protease from human immunodeficiency virus HIV-1. Nature 337:615, 1989

196. Wlodawer A, Miller M, Jaskolski M et al: Conserved folding in retroviral proteases: Crystal structure of a synthetic HIV-1 protease. Science 245:616, 1989

197. Lapatto R, Blundell T, Hemmings A, et al: X-ray analysis of HIV-1 proteinase at 2.7 Å resolution confirms structural homology among retroviral enzymes. Nature 342:299, 1989

198. Tomasselli AG, Hui JO, Sawyer TK et al: Interdomain hydrolysis of a truncated *Pseudomonas* exotoxin by the human immunodeficiency virus-1 protease. J Biol Chem 265:408, 1990

199. Tomasselli AG, Hui JO, Sawyer TK et al: Specificity and inhibition of proteases from human immunodeficiency virus 1 and 2.

200. Kohl NE, Emini EA, Schleif WA et al: Active human immunodeficiency virus protease is required for viral infectivity. Proc Natl Acad Sci USA 85:4686, 1988

201. Peng C, Ho BK, Chang TW, Chang NT: Role of human immunodeficiency virus type 1-specific protease in core protein maturation and viral infectivity. J Virol 63:2550, 1989

202. Dreyer GB, Metcalf BW, Tomaszek TA Jr et al: Inhibition of human immunodeficiency virus 1 protease *in vitro*: Rational design of substrate analogue inhibitors. Proc Natl Acad Sci USA 86:9752, 1989

203. Roberts NA, Martin JA, Kinchington D et al: Rational design of peptide-based HIV proteinase inhibitors. Science 248:558, 1990

204. Meek TD, Lambert DM, Dreyer GB et al: Inhibition of HIV-1 protease in infected T-lymphocytes by synthetic peptide analogues. Nature 343:90, 1990

205. McQuade TJ, Tomasselli AG, Lui L et al: A synthetic HIV-1 protease inhibitor with antiviral activity arrests HIV-like particle maturation. Science 247:454, 1990

206. Ashorn P, McQuade TJ, Thaisrivongs S et al: An inhibitor of the protease blocks maturation of human and simian immunodeficiency virus and spread of infection. Proc Natl Acad Sci USA 87:7472, 1990

207. Lee TH, Coligan JE, Allan JS et al: A new HTLV-III/LAV protein encoded by a gene found in cytopathic retroviruses. Science 231:1546, 1986

208. Kan NC, Franchini G, Wong-Staal F et al: Identification of HTLV-III/LAV sor gene product and detection of antibodies in human sera. Science 231:1553, 1986

209. Fisher AG, Ensoli B, Ivanoff I et al: The sor gene of HIV-1 is required for efficient virus transmission in vitro. Science 237:888, 1987

210. Strebel K, Daugherty D, Cohen D et al: The HIV 'A' (sor) gene product is essential for virus infectivity. Nature 328:728, 1987

211. Guy B, Geist M, Dott K et al: A specific inhibitor of cysteine proteases impairs a vif-dependent modification of human immunodeficiency virus type 1 env protein. J Virol 65:1325, 1991

212. Wong-Staal F, Chanda PK, Ghrayeb J: Human immunodeficiency virus: The eighth gene. AIDS Res Hum Retroviruses 3:33, 1987

213. Cohen EA, Terwilliger EF, Jalinoos Y et al: Identification of HIV-1 vpr product and function. J AIDS 3:11, 1990

214. Ogawa K, Shibata R, Kiyomasum T et al: Mutational analysis of the human immunodeficiency virus vpr open reading frame. J Virol 63:4110, 1989

215. Cohen EA, Dehni G, Sodroski JG, Haseltine WA: Human immunodeficiency virus *vpr* product is a vinon-associated regulatory protein. J Virol 64:3097, 1990

216. Yu XF, Matsuda M, Essex M, Lee TH: Open reading frame vpr of simian immunodeficiency virus encodes a virion-associated protein. J Virol 64:5688, 1990

217. Cohen EA, Terwilliger EF, Sodroski JG, Haseltine WA: Identification of a protein encoded by the vpu gene of HIV-1. Nature 344:532, 1988

218. Strebel K, Klimkait T, Martin MA: A novel gene of HIV-1, vpu, and its 16 kilodalton product. Science 241:1221, 1988

219. Matsuda Z, Chou MJ, Matsuda M et al: Human immunodeficiency virus type 1 has an additional coding sequence

in the central region of the genome. Proc Natl Acad Sci USA 85:6968, 1988

220. Terwilliger EF, Cohen EA, Lu YC et al: Functional role of human immunodeficiency virus type 1 vpu. Proc Natl Acad Sci USA 86:5163, 1989

221. Klimkait T, Strebel K, Hoggan MD et al: The human im-munodeficiency virus type 1-specific protein vpu is required for efficient virus maturation and release. J Virol 64:621, 1990

222. Henikoff S, Keene M, Fechtel K, Fristrom J: Gene within a gene: Nested Drosophila genes encoded unrelated proteins on opposite DNA strands. Cell 44:33, 1986

4

Immunopathogenesis of HIV Infection

Zeda F. Rosenberg   *Anthony S. Fauci*

In the last 10 years, the acquired immunodeficiency syndrome (AIDS) has evolved from an obscure constellation of opportunistic diseases in a handful of previously healthy homosexual men to a significant cause of morbidity and mortality in the United States and throughout the world. By the end of 1990, more than 160,000 cases of AIDS had been reported in the United States alone. AIDS is the end result of infection with the human immunodeficiency virus (HIV), a novel human pathogen that is a member of the lentivirus subgroup of retroviruses. It has been estimated that approximately 1 million people are presently infected with HIV in the United States, and nearly 10 million are infected worldwide.[1]

This chapter reviews the remarkable amount of information that has accumulated over the last 10 years concerning the immunologic defects in HIV infection and the mechanisms that HIV may use to inhibit immune function. In addition, this chapter examines the role that HIV may play in the neurologic abnormalities that occur during HIV infection. Lastly, we explore the phenomenon of clinical and microbiologic latency and the pathways involved in the activation of HIV expression and the deterioration of immune function.

IMMUNOLOGIC ABNORMALITIES IN HIV INFECTION

When AIDS was first recognized in 1981 in a group of previously healthy homosexual men,[2–4] it was clear that the constellation of specific opportunistic diseases was occurring because of a profound defect in immune function. On close examination, the primary abnormality was identified as a significant loss of the helper/inducer subset of T lymphocytes known as CD4+ T cells.[5] Because the CD4+ T cell plays a focal role in the regulation of virtually all human immune responses that are mediated by B cells, monocyte-macrophages, cytotoxic T cells, suppressor T cells, and natural killer (NK) cells, the eradication of CD4+ T cells results in a global immune suppression that renders the individual susceptible to a host of opportunistic diseases.[6] In addition to CD4+ T-cell–dependent functions, HIV may also directly affect the function of other immune competent cells such as B cells and monocyte-macrophages (see below).

T-Cell Defects

The reduction in the number of CD4+ T cells during HIV infection directly affects several CD4+ T-cell–dependent immunologic reactions such as delayed-type hypersensitivity, mitogen-induced lymphocyte blast transformation, and cytotoxic T-lymphocyte (CTL) activity.[5,7,8] The importance of CD4+ T cells in mitogen-induced responses has been shown in experiments in which peripheral blood mononuclear cells (PBMC) from AIDS patients were reconstituted with CD4+ T cells so that the proportion of CD4+ T cells was identical in both AIDS patient cultures and control cultures. The restoration of CD4+ T cells in the AIDS patient cultures resulted in a restoration of the mitogen-induced blast responses to control levels but not in a restoration of antigen-specific responses.[9] A reduction in the number of CD4+ T cells also resulted in a reduction in the level of specific cytokines secreted by CD4+ T cells. In this regard, it has been shown that the defective CD8+ CTL

61

activity in AIDS patients can be augmented by the addition of exogenous interleukin-2 (IL-2) to the culture.[8]

However, certain defects in CD4+ T-cell function in AIDS patients cannot be explained on the basis of declining CD4+ T-cell levels and appear to result from an intrinsic defect in the remaining CD4+ T cells. For example, it was shown early in the AIDS epidemic that CD4+ T cells from patients with AIDS were impaired in their ability to induce immunoglobulin secretion from B cells and to respond to alloantigens.[10–12] It was subsequently demonstrated that during HIV infection, CD4+ T cells responded abnormally to a wide range of soluble antigens, including tetanus toxoid, *Cryptococcus neoformans,* and influenza, and that this defect was observed at all stages of HIV disease, including the asymptomatic phase, before CD4+ T-cell levels had dropped significantly.[13–16] The contribution of defective antigen-presenting cells to the impaired antigen-specific responses was ruled out by studies of antigen-specific responses in identical twins, one of whom had AIDS and the other of whom was HIV negative. With the use of antigen-presenting cells from the uninfected twin in coculture with CD4+ T cells from the infected twin, it was shown that defects in antigen-specific CD4+ T-cell responses were due to the CD4+ T cells alone.[17]

Other defects in CD4+ T-cell function during HIV infection have also been observed.[18] Several investigators have shown that T-cell cloning efficiency and colony formation is defective in HIV-infected individuals. Defective expression of IL-2 receptors, antigen- and mitogen-induced IL-2 production, and depressed HLA-restricted cytotoxic T-cell responses have been reported. Some of these defects may result from inhibitory factors that are present in the sera of HIV-infected individuals at all stages of infection. For example, sera from AIDS patients have been shown to suppress *in vitro* lymphocyte activation of T cells from uninfected individuals.

B-Cell Defects

In addition to the depletion of CD4+ T cells, HIV-infected individuals exhibit abnormalities in other limbs of the immune system. Although many of these abnormalities are caused by the relative absence of CD4+ T cells, T cell–independent immune function may also be affected during HIV infection. In HIV infection, B-cell function is severely impaired. B cells from HIV-infected individuals appear to be in a state of chronic activation.[10,19,20] The majority of AIDS patients exhibit spontaneous B-cell proliferation, increased hemolytic plaque-forming cells, and hypergammaglobulinemia. Recent data have indicated that a substantial proportion of these activated B cells are specific for HIV epitopes.[21] Although B cells in HIV infection are spontaneously hyperactive, they also exhibit an intrinsic defect in induced B-cell responses, such as antigen- and mitogen-induced immunoglobulin secretion, at all stages of infection.[10,19,22]

Monocyte/Macrophage Defects

In contrast to T and B cells, monocyte-macrophages appear to function relatively normally during HIV infection. In this regard, superoxide anion release, tumoricidal activity, intracellular antimicrobicidal activity, fungicidal activity, antibody-dependent cellular cytotoxicity (ADCC), response to interferon-γ, and production of tumor necrosis factor (TNF) are preserved in HIV-infected individuals. In addition, the role of monocyte-macrophages as antigen-presenting cells is maintained at a normal level.[18,23] Nonetheless, certain functional defects of monocyte-macrophages have been observed, including impaired chemotaxis, Fc receptor function, C3 receptor–mediated clearance, and monocyte-dependent T-cell proliferation.[18,24] However, because chronically ill patients often manifest impaired monocyte-macrophage function, it is unclear what proportion of these defects are specific to HIV infection. It is also not known whether tissue-specific monocyte-macrophages such as lung or brain macrophages exhibit distinct functional abnormalities.

Other Immunologic Defects

A functional defect in natural killer (NK) cells has been observed in HIV-infected individuals. Specifically, NK cells from HIV-infected individuals display depressed cytotoxic capabilities that can be restored to normal levels by the addition of IL-2, certain mitogens, or calcium ionophore.[23] Thus, it appears that these NK cells are unable to be activated when in contact with a target. However, once the defective NK cells are activated, they can readily perform cytolysis. More recently, it has been demonstrated that the CD16+/CD8+ NK cell population is selectively depleted in HIV infection, beginning early in the course of disease.[25] In fact it has been demonstrated that NK cells can be infected with HIV *in vitro.*[26]

Other immunologic abnormalities that have been reported in HIV-infected individuals include elevated levels of acid labile interferon-α, α_1-thymosin, β_2-microglobulin, and neopterin.[27,28] Levels of β_2-microglobulin and neopterin, substances that are produced during immune activation, are positively correlated with disease progression in HIV-infected individuals.[29,30] In addition, increases in circulating immune complexes have been reported in AIDS patients.[31]

PATHOGENIC MECHANISMS OF HIV INFECTION

Following the discovery of HIV in 1983,[32–34] seroepidemiologic studies revealed that all patients with AIDS and many individuals at risk for AIDS had been infected with HIV. However, initial attempts to isolate HIV from the peripheral blood of seropositive individuals were not always successful. In addition, *in situ* hybridization and immunofluorescence analyses of circulating lymphocytes of HIV-infected individuals showed that only between 1 in 10,000 to 1 in 100,000 cells expressed HIV RNA or viral protein.[35,36] As a result, it was difficult to envision how such a low level of HIV expression in the peripheral blood could account for the dramatic decline in CD4+ T-cell counts in AIDS patients.

However, with the aid of polymerase chain reaction (PCR) techniques, investigators have shown that a much higher proportion of T cells in the peripheral blood of HIV-infected individuals is infected with HIV than was previously found. PCR analysis has shown that approximately 1% of CD4+ T cells in patients with AIDS contain HIV DNA, while during the earlier stages of HIV disease, between 0.01% and 1% of CD4+ T cells are positive for HIV DNA.[36–38] In experiments designed to quantify the level of infectious HIV in the peripheral blood and plasma, it was found that AIDS patients harbored HIV in titers approximately two logs higher than those found in asymptomatic individuals.[39,40] In addition, the frequency of HIV-infected cells has been shown to be 5- to 10-fold higher in lymphoid tissues than in the peripheral blood of HIV-infected individuals.[40a]

A direct correlation between an increase in viral burden, CD4+ T-cell decline, and the development of AIDS has been shown in studies that examined the frequency of HIV DNA in CD4+ T cells from HIV-infected individuals who were either asymptomatic and clinically stable or manifesting progression to AIDS.[37,41,42] It was found that the frequency of HIV-infected CD4+ T cells rose during disease progression and remained relatively constant within a period of clinical stability. The increase in viral burden was also positively associated with a decline in CD4+ T-cell counts.

The clear relationship between viral burden and CD4+ T-cell decline, and the death of CD4+ T cells following HIV infection *in vitro*,[33,34,43] suggest that infection with HIV directly results in cell death. If it is assumed that direct infection of CD4+ T cells by HIV results in the loss of these cells, it is unclear why the production of new CD4+ T cells is unable to replenish the supply. This lack of CD4+ T-cell regeneration is also seen in patients whose HIV titers have declined during treatment with antiretroviral therapy. One explanation for the lack of CD4+ T-cell regeneration is that the CD4+ T-cell precursors in the thymus and bone marrow are also infected by HIV (Table 4-1). In this regard, HIV infection of thymic precursor cells has recently been demonstrated.[44] In addition, it has been shown by some investigators that HIV can infect CD34+ bone marrow progenitor cells *in vitro*[45,46] and can inhibit erythroid, granulocyte-macrophage, and T-cell colony formation.[46] Although several laboratories have failed to detect HIV infection of bone marrow precursor cells *in vivo*,[47–49] it was recently found that HIV DNA was present in the CD34+ bone marrow progenitor cells in approximately half of a group of patients with advanced HIV infection (S. Stanley *et al*, unpubl. observ.).

Table 4–1. Indirect Evidence Suggesting T-Cell Precursor Pool Dysfunction and/or Depletion of HIV-Infected Individuals

---

Early in the course of HIV infection, the frequency of infected CD4+ T cells is extremely low, yet counts progressively decline, suggesting that the precursor pool cannot regenerate mature CD4+ T cells.

Even with effective immunosuppression of HIV replication in patients receiving antiretroviral drugs, CD4+ T-cell counts often increase only marginally and virtually never return to normal levels.

Thymuses of HIV-infected individuals have been shown to be architecturally disrupted or destroyed.

CD4+ T Cell Cytopathicity

A number of mechanisms have been proposed to explain a direct cytopathic effect of HIV on the CD4+ T cell, including disruption of the cell membrane by large numbers of budding virions and interference with cellular metabolic functions because of viral requirements for RNA and protein synthesis.[18] In other retroviral systems, it has been observed that the accumulation of unintegrated viral DNA in the cytoplasm of the cell is associated with cytopathicity.[50,51] In HIV infection, large amounts of unintegrated viral DNA have been detected (Fig. 4–1).[52] During HIV infection of a CD4+ T-cell line, reinfection of cells is required to reach high levels of unintegrated viral DNA, which in turn are associated with cell death.[53]

Other proposed mechanisms of HIV-induced CD4+ T-cell killing involve the role of the HIV envelope glycoprotein. The HIV envelope glycoprotein binds with high affinity to the CD4 molecule that is present on the surface of certain types of human cells, particularly CD4+ T cells and monocyte-macrophages.[54,55] In experiments in which CD4+ and CD4− monocytoid cell lines were transfected with plasmids containing the HIV envelope gp160, the CD4+ transfected cells exhibited a cytopathic effect. Because the pores of the nuclear membrane of the CD4+ transfectants were filled with gp160-CD4 complexes, it is thought that the cytopathicity was due to the inhibition of the transport of molecules between the nucleus and cytoplasm.[56] Studies with recombinant HIV viruses have demonstrated that the ability of HIV to induce cytopathicity is determined by the *env* region of the viral genome.[57] In addition, it has recently been shown that the transmembrane envelope glycoprotein is important for HIV-induced cell killing, because a mutation in the gp41 amino terminal region led to reduced cell killing while the levels of viral protein and replication were unaffected.[58] Production of cytopathic *env* proteins may be one mechanism by which the presence of high levels of unintegrated viral DNA leads to cell death, because it has been shown

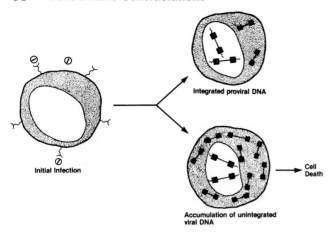

Figure 4–1. The accumulation of unintegrated HIV DNA in HIV-infected cells.

that unintegrated viral DNA can serve as template for the manufacture of HIV *env* and core proteins.[59]

There are several pathways by which CD4+ T cells may be eliminated during HIV infection that do not result from direct HIV-induced cell killing. For example, the binding of HIV envelope glycoproteins that are expressed on the surface of an HIV-infected cell to CD4 receptors on the surface of many uninfected T4 cells can result in the formation of multinucleated giant cells or syncytia.[18] Although syncytia form readily during *in vitro* HIV infection and cells die within days after formation, it is not known what role, if any, syncytia may play *in vivo* in the pathogenesis of HIV infection. In addition, it is known that single HIV-infected cells die without syncytia formation, that substantial HIV replication can occur in the absence of syncytia formation, and that not all cell cultures with substantial numbers of syncytia experience significant cytopathicity.[18]

Autoimmune mechanisms may also play an important role in the pathogenesis of HIV infection. The binding of free HIV envelope glycoproteins (gp120) to CD4 molecules on the surface of uninfected CD4+ T cells may convert these cells into targets for immune-mediated destruction.[60] *In vitro*, CD4+ T cells may also function as antigen-presenting cells and become targets for lysis by cytotoxic CD4+ T lymphocytes following presentation of processed gp120.[61,62] In addition, it has been found that HIV-infected humans have circulating CD8+ CTL that can lyse uninfected CD4+ T cells.[63] Because these CTL have not been found in HIV-infected chimpanzees, it has been hypothesized that the absence of HIV-induced disease in chimpanzees may be due to the absence of CD4+ T-cell–specific CTL.[63] Another potential pathway for autoimmune-mediated destruction of bystander CD4+ T cells involves antibodies that may cross-react with the class II major histocompatibility complex (MHC) antigens. Insofar as both gp120 and

class II MHC bind to CD4, it is possible that antibodies directed against gp120 can cross-react with class II MHC molecules and result in the destruction of uninfected cells.[64]

Immunologic Impairment Without Cell Death

The existence of HIV-induced impairment of T-cell function in otherwise viable cells was recognized early in the AIDS epidemic. Impairment of T-cell responses to soluble antigens has been observed in all stages of HIV infection and spanning a wide range of CD4+ T-cell numbers.[18] Indeed, impairment of antigen-specific responses to tetanus toxoid and poliovirus have been observed as early as 3 months after seroconversion.[65] Impairment of antigen-specific responses in HIV infection may be due to a selective depletion of antigen-specific CD4+ T cells. One group of investigators has found that memory cells are selectively depleted in a group of HIV-infected asymptomatic individuals with normal numbers of CD4+ T cells.[66] However, during later stages of HIV infection, when naive T cells are also depleted, loss of T-cell responsiveness is due primarily to intrinsic defects in T-cell activation via the T-cell receptor (TCR)/CD3 complex.[67] PCR analysis of HIV infection of CD4+ T cell subsets *in vivo* has revealed that memory CD4+ T cells are preferentially infected with HIV, with memory cells harboring HIV DNA at a level 4- to 10-fold higher than that found in naive cells.[68] In a related animal model, simian immunodeficiency virus (SIV) infection in macaques, it has been shown by PCR analysis that SIV exclusively infects a subset of CD4+ T cells that contain both actively proliferating cells and resting memory cells.[69]

Because the CD4 molecule is intimately involved in antigen-specific responses by virtue of its role as ligand to the class II MHC complex, inhibition of antigen-specific responses could occur if HIV infection resulted in alterations in CD4 expression. Although HIV-infected CD4+ T cells *in vivo* express CD4,[36] HIV-induced downregulation of CD4 expression in T cells has been observed *in vitro*.[70,71] A decrease in surface CD4 expression in HIV-infected monocytic cells has also been observed.[72] One mechanism by which CD4 expression is downregulated in HIV-infected cells *in vitro* involves the intracellular complexing of gp160 envelope glycoproteins with CD4 and the subsequent prevention of CD4 delivery to the cell surface (Fig. 4–2).[73,74] In contrast to HIV-infected CD4+ T cells, HIV infection of monocytic cells does not result in a decrease in CD4 mRNA, and thus depressed CD4 expression presumably occurs via a posttranscriptional event.[72]

Another molecule that has been shown to be reduced following HIV infection *in vitro* is the TCR/CD3 complex.[75] The lack of surface expression of the TCR/CD3 molecules, which is thought to be caused by a defect in the transcription of the CD3 γ chain gene, could

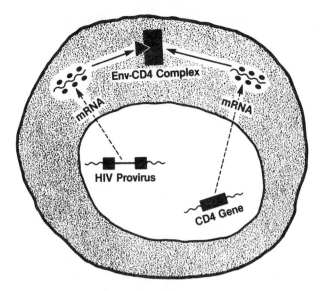

Figure 4–2. Complexing of HIV-envelope glycoprotein and CD4 molecule within an HIV-infected cell.

easily affect the ability of the infected cell to respond immunologically. It has also been shown that as the level of HIV protein synthesis rises during acute HIV infection *in vitro,* the level of cellular protein synthesis markedly declines.[76]

In vitro exposure of CD4+ T cells to several HIV proteins, including gp120, gp41, and p24, also results in suppression of cell function (reviewed by Rosenberg and Fauci[18]).[77,78] HIV gp120 binding to the CD4 receptor could inhibit the interaction between CD4 and class II MHC molecules that is essential for antigen-specific responses. The inhibition of antigen-specific T-cell proliferation by soluble gp120 has been shown to be blocked by soluble CD4, which suggests that suppression of responses results from the interaction of gp120 with surface CD4.[79] This interaction may disrupt the normal cellular signal transduction pathways.[80–82] In this regard, it has been found that suppression of mitogen- or antigen-induced T-cell activation by inactivated HIV or soluble envelope glycoproteins occurs early in the activation process at the level of the initiation of inositol phospholipid metabolism.[81,82]

A soluble suppressor factor has also been recognized in cell-free supernatants of unstimulated PBMC from HIV-infected individuals and *in vitro* infected CD4+ T cells. This suppressive factor shares antigenic determinants with a murine retroviral transmembrane protein, p15E, that has been shown to have immunosuppressive properties.[83] In addition to their potential role in CD4+ T-cell cytopathicity (see above), autoantibodies to CD4+ T cells may also play a role in CD4+ T-cell suppression.[84]

Role of Monocyte-Macrophages in HIV Infection

There exists a large body of data on HIV infection of macrophages *in vitro* and the identification and isolation of HIV from circulating monocytes as well as tissue-specific macrophages in the lung and brain (reviewed by Rosenberg and Fauci[18]). It has been observed that the characteristics of monocyte-macrophage infection differ from those of CD4+ T-cell infection. First, in contrast to HIV infection of CD4+ T cells, HIV-infected monocyte-macrophages exhibit little or no cytopathicity.[85] In addition, depending on the state of differentiation of the cell, HIV-infected monocyte-macrophages can express HIV in a restricted manner, with little or no detectable virus released into the extracellular environment. However, virus production may occur intracellularly, with viral particles budding into and accumulating within intracytoplasmic vesicles.[85–87] Because HIV-infected monocyte-macrophages that exhibit predominantly intracellular viral production do not express HIV antigens on the cell surface, these infected cells can be sheltered from HIV-specific immune responses and function as ideal reservoirs of infection.

Examination of circulating monocytes for the presence of HIV DNA has generated conflicting results. Several groups of researchers have determined that there exists *in vivo* a low frequency of HIV-infected circulating monocytes.[88,89] However, it has also been reported that the level of HIV-infected monocytes in the peripheral blood is nearly identical to that of circulating CD4+ T cells.[38] Although the frequency of infected blood monocytes may be important in HIV pathogenesis, HIV infection of tissue-specific macrophages may play an even greater role. In this regard, it has been shown that once monocytoid cells begin to differentiate, they are more readily infectible by HIV and produce higher levels of HIV. Chronically HIV-infected monocytoid cells that are induced to differentiate by exposure to differentiating agents such as hydroxyvitamin D_3 exhibit a marked enhancement in HIV production.[90] Similarly, acute HIV infection of a promyelocytic cell line was greatly facilitated following exposure of the cells to hydroxyvitamin D_3, retinoic acid, or tissue plasminogen activator.[91] In addition, primary monocytes that were cultured in the presence of macrophage colony-stimulating factor, a cytokine that induces monocyte differentiation, were greater than 400-fold more susceptible to HIV infection than monocytes cultured in medium alone.[92]

The role of HIV-infected monocyte-macrophages in HIV pathogenesis is not clear at present. However, the results of several studies suggest that infected monocyte-macrophages may play an important role in the spread of HIV *in vivo.* For example, it has been shown *in vitro* that monocytes from HIV-infected individuals could be induced to express HIV following contact with activated T cells.[93] In addition, a monocytoid cell line infected with HIV and producing virus only intracellularly can transmit HIV to T cells by cell-cell contact.[87] Thus, *in vivo* T cell–macrophage interactions that occur during normal immune responses could result in the activation of HIV expression in latently infected macrophages and the transmission of HIV to activated CD4+ T cells. Alternatively, these interactions could result in the transmission of HIV from infected CD4+ T cells to activated macrophages. As will be discussed in greater detail below, it is becoming increasingly apparent that classic immunologic reactions can enhance HIV replication and dissemination throughout the body.

Variations in Host Cell Tropism

HIVs isolated from infected individuals display both genetic variations as well as differences in host cell range.[94–97] Changes in host cell range in HIV isolates from the same individual over time have also been observed.[98,99] These studies have suggested that the emergence of viral isolates that can replicate more efficiently in a broad range of T and monocytoid cell lines in addition to PBMC is associated with progression to AIDS.[98,100,101] Certain strains of HIV replicate with higher efficiency in monocyte-macrophages than in CD4+ T cells, while other strains replicate preferentially in CD4+ T cells.[85,96]

The relevance of these findings to the pathogenesis of HIV infection is unclear at present because *in vitro* monocytotropic viruses can originate from CD4+ T cells *in vivo*.[102] In studies of the determinants of T-cell versus monocyte-macrophage tropism of HIV, it has been found that once HIV has entered the host cell and reverse transcription is initiated, viral replication occurs to the same extent in both monocyte-macrophages and T cells.[103] Thus, the restriction in cell tropism appears to occur at the level of viral binding and entry into the cell and does not appear to involve the sequences in the HIV long terminal repeat (LTR).[104]

This observation is consistent with studies that implicate the HIV envelope as the major determining factor in viral tropism.[105] When *env* regions of HIVs that differed in host range were exchanged, the limited host range of a particular HIV isolate could be expanded.[57] This result was also observed by exchanging the *env* region between exclusively T-cell tropic and macrophage tropic strains of HIV.[106] It has been suggested that the determination of host range by the HIV envelope may be due to a wide variation in envelope-specific affinities for CD4 between diverse HIV isolates.[107] However, several groups have found that HIV tropism for cells of the monocyte-macrophage lineage appears to reside in a region of the HIV envelope that is outside of the CD4 binding domain.[106,108,109] A recent study has shown that the difference in host range between a prototypic HIV isolate and a variant HIV with a wider host range is due to a single point mutation in the *env* gene.[110]

HIV Infection of Diverse Cell Types

Because of the high-affinity binding of HIV gp120 to the CD4 receptor, presumably any cell in the body that expresses surface CD4 can be infected by HIV. In the immune system, antigen-presenting cells such as dendritic cells and Langerhans cells express CD4 and have been shown to be infected by HIV *in vivo*[111,112] and *in vitro*.[113] By *in situ* hybridization, between 3% and 21% of dendritic cells in the peripheral blood expressed HIV, a range that is 30- to 200-fold higher than that observed in lymphocytes and monocytes.[112] A decrease in the number and function of Langerhans and dendritic cells has also been observed in HIV-infected individuals.[112,114]

An extensive record of cells and cell lines that can be infected by HIV either *in vitro* or *in vivo* has been compiled since HIV was first discovered. This list includes CD4+ cells and cell lines such as transformed human B cells, colorectal cells, glioma cells, neuroretinal cells, and cervical cells.[18] Infection of human lung, foreskin, and embryo fibroblastoid cell lines, osteoblasts, epithelial cells, and primary fibroblasts has been reported.[115–117] While neither surface nor cytoplasmic expression of CD4 could be detected in these cells, infection could be blocked by monoclonal antibodies to CD4, suggesting the presence of very low levels of CD4 expression.

Reports of HIV infection of cells that did not express the CD4 receptor and could not be blocked by monoclonal antibodies against CD4 or by soluble CD4 itself have recently appeared.[118,119] These cells include neuroblastoma cells, a human mesenchymal rhabdomyosarcoma-derived cell line, fibroblastoid cell lines, fetal neural cells, primary human chondrocyte cells, NK cells, synovial cells, hepatoma cell lines, and foreskin fibroblasts.[26,115,117,120] These observations raise the possibility that HIV may rarely utilize other cellular receptors to gain entry into the cell. In this regard, it has been demonstrated that gp120 can bind to both serum and macrophage-associated human lectins in a manner that is oligosaccharide-mediated and CD4-independent.[121] It has been hypothesized that the binding of serum lectins to virion gp120 would make the virus sticky and allow the binding of HIV to a variety of cell surface structures. It is not known whether this binding occurs *in vivo* or if it is sufficient to permit HIV infection.

Other mechanisms for HIV entry into CD4− cells involve the formation of pseudotype virions that contain the HIV genome within the envelope of a virus that can infect CD4− cells. In this regard, it has been found that pseudotyping of HIV with murine retroviruses greatly expanded the host range of HIV.[122] In an experimental system that may have relevance to the *in vivo* situation in which individuals are infected with both HIV and HTLV-1, pseudotyping of HIV with HTLV-1 allowed for HIV infection of CD4− cells such as CD8+ T cells, B-lymphoid cells, epithelial cells, and skeletal muscle cells.[123,124] Infection of CD8+ cells has also been observed *in vitro* in experiments in which CD8+ cells were cocultured with HIV-infected CD4+ cells.[125]

The role of HIV infection of non-immune system cells in the pathogenesis of HIV-induced disease is not known at present. Because a large number of miscellaneous clinical manifestations, including gastrointestinal (GI) symptoms and bone marrow abnormalities, are present during HIV infection, it has been hypothesized that HIV infection of cells other than CD4+ T cells and monocyte-macrophages may play a role. For example, insofar as human megakaryocytes are able to take up HIV when cocultured with infected CD4+ T cells,[126] it is possible that certain platelet abnormalities in HIV-infected individuals may be caused by the presence of HIV within these cells. Regarding the role of HIV in renal and GI abnormalities, HIV has been observed in the renal epithelium of patients with HIV-associated nephropathy and in the enterochromaffin cells in the rectal mucosa.[127,128] More recently, HIV infection of primary cultures of human ileal and colonic epithelium has also been reported.[129]

Neuropsychiatric Manifestations

One common manifestation of HIV infection is a broad spectrum of neurologic abnormalities, a syndrome that has been termed *AIDS encephalopathy* or *AIDS dementia complex.*[130] Although a number of opportunistic infections and neoplasms may affect neurologic function in HIV-infected individuals, AIDS dementia complex occurs frequently in patients in the absence of other known causes of central nervous system (CNS) defects.[131] In an effort to understand the pathogenesis of HIV-induced CNS disease, researchers have studied the brain for evidence of HIV infection. HIV DNA, RNA, and infectious virus have been detected in brain tissue from AIDS patients. HIV has also been isolated from the cerebrospinal fluid (CSF) of HIV-infected individuals early in the course of infection and even in individuals without clinically apparent CNS disease.[18]

Although there have been isolated reports of HIV infection of capillary endothelial cells, astrocytes, and oligodendroglial cells, it is generally thought that HIV preferentially infects cells of the monocyte-macrophage lineage in the brain.[18] In this regard, during HIV infection of primary cultures of adult human brain containing a mixture of astrocytes and microglial cells, only the microglial cells became infected.[132] HIV infection of brain microglial cells *in vitro* was shown to be dependent on the CD4 receptor and often resulted in syncytia formation which led to cell death.[133] Only an *in vitro*–adapted macrophage tropic strain of HIV and not a T-lymphotropic strain infected these primary brain cultures. Recently, expression of HIV RNA has been detected in spinal cords of HIV-infected patients with vacuolar myelopathy and was found to be localized to areas of macrophage infiltration.[134]

The role of HIV-infected monocyte-macrophages in the pathogenesis of neurologic disease has not been precisely delineated. One indirect mechanism of HIV-induced neuropathogenesis involves the production of soluble factors by HIV-infected macrophages that affect either HIV replication or neuronal cell function.[135] It has been shown that monocytes secrete a number of cytokines following exposure to neuropeptides.[136] One such cytokine, IL-6, which acts on a variety of cells including neural cells, is found in the CSF of patients with advanced HIV disease and in higher concentrations than in early HIV infection.[137] IL-6 is produced by astrocytes in response to another cytokine, TNF-α.[138] As will be discussed below, both TNF-α and IL-6 can augment the expression of HIV in chronically infected promonocytic cells, and because astrocytes are activated in areas of inflammation or injury, their proximity to HIV-infected macrophages may result in the enhancement of HIV replication in the brain.[139] HIV-infected mononuclear phagocytes have also been shown to secrete toxic factors that destroy chick and rat neurons in culture[140] and cause damage in human brain aggregates.[141]

Another mechanism by which HIV may disrupt neurologic function is by blocking the binding of neurotropic factors. It has been hypothesized that HIV gp120 interferes with the binding of neurotropic factors such as neuroleukin or neuropeptide transmitters such as vasoactive intestinal peptide.[18] Alternatively, HIV proteins may be directly toxic to neuronal cells. Exposure of mammalian central neurons to gp120 results in increased intracellular free calcium levels and neuronal injury.[142] The observed neurotoxicity could be inhibited by anti-gp120 antibodies or by calcium channel antagonists but not by anti-CD4 antibodies,[142,143] which suggests that gp120-induced neuronal injury is not mediated by gp120-CD4 binding. In addition, another HIV protein, *tat,* has been shown to be a potent and lethal neurotoxic agent in mice.[144]

A potential autoimmune response may also be responsible for the neuronal dysfunction observed in AIDS. It has recently been discovered that astrocytes share a common immunologic determinant with a peptide from the HIV transmembrane glycoprotein, gp41 and that antibodies against this determinant have been found in the CSF of some AIDS patients.[145]

CLINICAL LATENCY TO ACTIVE DISEASE

Because of the diverse array of pathogenic mechanisms by which HIV may impair human immune and neurologic function and render the host susceptible to opportunistic infections and neoplasms, it is puzzling why the development of AIDS occurs over such a long and variable time frame. From the time of initial infection with HIV, a median of 10 to 11 years elapses before the onset of AIDS.[146] In recent years, the events that take place following initial infection with HIV are becoming increasingly clear. As the number of HIV-infected individuals rises, prospective cohort studies have revealed that the majority of infected individuals experience an acute symptomatic illness within 2 to 4 weeks following infection.[147] During this acute illness, total lymphocyte counts are depressed, including those of CD4+ and CD8+ T-cell subsets and B cells, and HIV p24 antigen levels are high.[148] At the time of seroconversion, CD8+ cells increase, B cells return to relatively normal levels, CD4+ T cells rebound but not to normal levels, and serum HIV p24 antigen levels decline, suggesting that the primary immune response to HIV infection is able to suppress HIV replication.[147]

Following the development of an anti-HIV immune response, the asymptomatic phase of HIV infection ensues. During the asymptomatic phase, the level of CD4+ T cells gradually declines. In some individuals, CD4+ T-cell numbers drop precipitously just prior to the development of AIDS,[149] whereas in others, CD4+ T-cell numbers continue their linear rate of decline to a level that allows the development of opportunistic infections and neoplasms.[150] Undoubtedly, CD4+ T cells are being slowly destroyed during this period. As is discussed below, the rate of CD4+ T-cell destruction may be related to events that occur during the normal functioning of the human immune system.

HIV Expression and T-Cell Activation

One of the primary requirements for isolation of HIV from PBMC in culture involves the mitogenic activation of uninfected target T cells.[151] Although quiescent T cells can be infected by HIV *in vitro,* reverse transcription of the viral genomic RNA to full-length double-stranded DNA is incomplete and virus production does not occur unless the cells are subsequently activated.[152] Thus, one role for mitogenic activation of HIV-infected T cells may be the induction of specific cellular factors that are necessary for the completion of reverse transcription.

It has been previously demonstrated that antigenic stimulation of peripheral blood lymphocytes also results in enhanced HIV replication.[153,154] Recently it was found that stimulation of primary T-cell blasts with purified protein derivative resulted in an enhancement in HIV LTR-driven gene expression.[155] In addition, exposure of cloned human T cells transiently transfected with HIV-LTR-CAT plasmids to tetanus toxoid resulted in transactivation of the HIV LTR.[156] Physiologic concentrations of bacterial lipopolysaccharide (LPS) that are achievable *in vivo* have also been shown to effectively stimulate HIV-LTR-CAT constructs in transfected monocytoid cell lines but not T-cell lines, as well as HIV expression in chronically HIV-infected monocytoid cells.[157]

The mechanism by which mitogens and certain antigens upregulate HIV expression is the same one that is used by the cell during T-cell activation to upregulate IL-2 and IL-2 receptor gene expression. The regulation of gene expression during T-cell activation occurs via the induction of cellular factors (*e.g.,* NF-κB) that bind to specific sequences in the enhancer region of the IL-2 and IL-2 receptor genes.[158,159] Because these NF-κB binding sequences are also present in the HIV LTR, ex-

posure of HIV-infected cells to mitogens or antigens and the subsequent induction of NF-κB results in the binding of NF-κB to the HIV enhancer and initiation of mRNA transcription.[157,160]

There is also recent evidence that T-cell activation signals that do not involve mitogens or the antigen-receptor complex may also result in stimulation of HIV expression. It has been shown that stimulation of the CD28 accessory molecule induces both the HIV LTR- and NF-κB-driven gene expression.[161]

Regulation of HIV Expression by Heterologous Viruses

HIV-infected individuals are often infected by a number of other viral pathogens whose replicative processes may include the induction of cellular proteins that facilitate viral gene transcription. Because infection by these heterologous viruses may affect HIV replication, a number of studies have examined the role of heterologous viruses in the upregulation of HIV expression and found that herpes simplex virus (HSV) type 1, cytomegalovirus (CMV), Epstein–Barr virus (EBV), adenovirus, hepatitis B virus (HBV), human herpes virus (HHV) type 6, pseudorabies virus, and human T-cell leukemia virus (HTLV) type I can enhance HIV replication.[18,162,163] It has recently been shown that an EBV early gene product can synergize with the HIV *tat* gene product in the activation of the HIV LTR.[164] Although many of these studies used transfection assays to measure induction of HIV LTR–induced gene expression, it was also demonstrated that co-infection of cells by HIV and HSV-1,[165] CMV,[166] HHV-6,[167] or HSV-2[168] resulted in increased HIV replication. The mechanisms of heterologous virus–induced enhancement of HIV expression have been shown to involve the induction of a variety of cellular DNA-binding proteins that interact with several distinct sites in the HIV LTR, including the Spl transcription factor binding sites.[169–171] Recent studies on HHV-6 suggest an additional pathway by which infection with heterologous viruses may affect HIV replication and disease progression. It has been found that HHV-6 induces CD4 expression in CD8+ T cells and thus renders these cells susceptible to infection by HIV.[172]

Not all heterologous viral genes enhance HIV expression. In fact, it has recently been reported that the *rep* protein from adeno-associated virus can downregulate HIV LTR–driven CAT expression as well as the replication of an HIV proviral clone.[173] In this regard, there has been one report that co-infection with HHV-6 suppressed HIV replication but enhanced cell killing.[174]

Role of Cytokines in the Regulation of HIV Expression

A considerable body of data has been gathered over the past several years on the role that physiologic inductive signals, in the form of cytokines secreted during normal immune responses, may play in the activation of HIV expression and hence contribute to the conversion of a clinically asymptomatic HIV infection to AIDS.[175]

Using both primary cells and HIV-infected cell lines, a number of investigators have shown that TNF-α and IL-6 can enhance HIV replication during both acute HIV infection and in chronically infected monocytic cells, and, in the case of TNF-α, in T cells.[176–180] It has also been demonstrated that granulocyce-macrophage colony-stimulating factor (GM-CSF) and IL-3 can augment HIV expression in monocytes.[181] Exposure of chronically infected monocytic cells to either TNF-α and IL-6 or TNF-α and GM-CSF resulted in a synergistic increase in HIV expression.[175] These data are consistent with the observation that TNF-α and IL-6 also synergize in the induction of T-cell growth.[182] The synergy between TNF-α and IL-6 in the induction of HIV expression is physiologically relevant, because TNF-α induces the expression of IL-6 *in vivo*.[183]

It has been shown that TNF-α can activate the HIV LTR and that this activation is the result of the induction of NF-κB.[156,179,184] Metabolically, cytokine-mediated induction of HIV expression has been shown to involve the activation of protein kinase C, which may in turn activate NF-κB-like transcription factors.[185] In the case of IL-6– and GM-CSF–induced upregulation of HIV expression, posttranscriptional mechanisms appear to be more important for virus induction (Poli and Fauci, unpubl. observ.) (Fig. 4–3).[178]

Analogous to their *in vivo* functions, studies suggest that TNF-α and IL-6 function in an autocrine or paracrine manner to induce HIV expression.[178,186] In this regard, endogenous TNF-α has been shown to play a role in the constitutive expression of HIV *in vitro*.[186] Although several studies have failed to detect an increase in TNF-α, IL-6, or GM-CSF production following infection of monocyte-macrophages by HIV,[187,188] the majority of studies have demonstrated that TNF-α and IL-6 expression is elevated in HIV-infected cells.[179,189,190] The production of TNF-α by *in vitro* HIV-infected monocytoid cells suggests that the interaction between HIV-infected monocytes and T cells *in vivo* may result in enhanced spread of HIV in the T-cell population.[179] It has recently been shown that memory CD4+ T cells and not naive CD4+ T cells produce IL-6.[191] Because memory CD4+ T cells are preferentially infected by HIV *in vivo*,[68] it is possible that IL-6 production may act in an autocrine or paracrine manner during infection of CD4+ T cells.

Elevated levels of TNF-α have been observed in sera from AIDS patients.[192] Mononuclear cells from AIDS patients exhibit an increased half-life of TNF-α mRNA.[193] Alveolar macrophages and, to a lesser extent, peripheral blood monocytes from HIV-infected patients with active *P. carinii* pneumonia exhibited markedly elevated TNF-α production as compared to peripheral blood monocytes from HIV-infected patients without *P. carinii* pneumonia.[199] TNF-α has been shown to be selectively concentrated in the pleural fluid of patients with tuberculous pleuritis.[195]

Analyses of IL-6 levels in the serum of HIV-infected individuals have engendered a wide range of results. Mean serum levels of IL-6 bioactivity were found to be abnormally elevated in early HIV infection but not in uninfected individuals or in those with AIDS.[189] Other

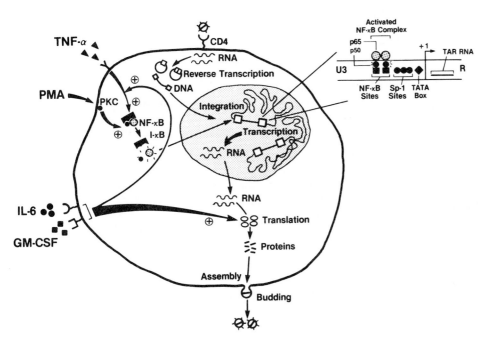

Figure 4–3. Mechanisms of cytokine-mediated induction of HIV expression in monocyte/macrophages.

investigators have found that serum IL-6 levels are elevated early in HIV infection, are higher in patients with AIDS-related complex, and are highest in AIDS patients.[190] In addition, individuals infected with monocytotropic strains of HIV had higher serum IL-6 levels than individuals infected with T-cell tropic strains of HIV, consistent with the fact that monocytes and not T cells produce high levels of IL-6 *in vitro*.[189] However, other investigators have found no increase in serum IL-6 in HIV-infected individuals.[196] As mentioned earlier, IL-6 has been detected in the CSF of the majority of HIV-infected individuals in advanced stages of disease.[137] IL-6 activity is found in the CSF of patients with early-stage disease, albeit at lower concentrations that in late-stage disease. IL-6 has also been found to be produced by Kaposi's sarcoma cells and is required for optimal growth of these cells.[197]

Further *in vivo* relevance of cytokine-induced enhancement of HIV expression is derived from studies which showed that TNF-α and IL-6 are produced by activated B cells from HIV-infected patients in levels that are sufficient to induce the expression of HIV in chronically infected cell lines and in autologous T cells.[198] Exposure of the *in vivo* activated B cells to HIV gp120 resulted in amplification of the secretion of both cytokines. It has also recently been shown that IL-6 is involved in sustaining the spontaneous B-cell activation observed in HIV-infected individuals.[196] Thus, the activation of B cells, as well as the activation and/or HIV infection of T cells and monocyte-macrophages, can cause an upregulation in the production of cytokines that are capable of increasing HIV replication. Although relatively few data are available on the production of GM-CSF during HIV infection, studies on the use of GM-CSF *in vivo* as a therapeutic agent showed that, consistent with *in vitro* observations, serum p24 antigen levels increased briefly following exposure to GM-CSF.[199]

TNF-α induction of HIV expression may be the underlying factor in other circumstances in which HIV replication is enhanced. For example, secondary infection of HIV-infected monocytoid cells by paramyxovirus increased the steady-state level of TNF-α mRNA by 5- to 10-fold.[179] Thus, one of the mechanisms by which heterologous viral infections may upregulate HIV expression is *via* TNF-α–induced expression of HIV. Likewise, *in vitro* differentiation of monocyte-macrophages by hydroxyvitamin D_3 and subsequent augmentation of HIV expression was associated with an increase in expression of TNF-α receptors.[90] In addition, antibody to TNF-α could inhibit HIV production in these cells.

As our knowledge about the ways in which HIV infection is transformed from a chronic asymptomatic infection to AIDS increases, it is hoped that therapeutic strategies can be developed that favor the maintenance of the clinically latent state. Because cytokines function within a complex network that comprises both positive and negative regulation of lymphocyte activation, it was of interest to determine if any of the known human cytokines could inhibit HIV replication directly or interfere with cytokine induction of HIV expression. Transforming growth factor (TGF)-β is a cytokine that is known to have immunosuppressive properties[200] and can regulate immune functions in an autocrine manner.[201] One study has found that TGF-β suppresses by both transcriptional and posttranscriptional pathways the constitutive as well as induced expression of HIV in chronically infected cells.[202] In contrast, others have reported that TGF-β augments acute viral infection in human PBMC and that antibodies to TGF-β blocked cocaine-induced enhancement of HIV expression.[203]

Another strategy for pharmacologic modulation of HIV expression involves drugs that can counter the HIV-inductive effects of cytokines and may result in a lower viral burden and a slower decline in CD4+ T cells. One such compound, N-acetyl-L-cysteine (NAC), has been shown to inhibit both PMA and TNF-α induction of HIV expression in acutely and chronically infected cell lines and PBMC.[204,205] NAC increases the level of intracellular glutathione that is required for the destruction of reactive oxidative intermediates (ROIs). Because ROIs are produced by both PMA and TNF-α, it is thought that NAC interferes with the action of PMA and TNF-α by scavenging the excess ROIs.[204] It is also likely that NAC suppresses HIV infection by mechanisms independent of glutathione (G. Poli and A. S. Fauci, unpubl. observ.).

SUMMARY

The ability of HIV to utilize the CD4 receptor as the initial step in viral replication has resulted in its ingress into the immune system. Like the majority of viral pathogens, once HIV has established itself within the CD4+ T cells and monocyte-macrophages, it is able to usurp host regulatory mechanisms to its own advantage. However, in the case of HIV, the principal function of the host cells is that of immune protection. Thus, HIV may survive and flourish in the face of and because of ongoing immunoregulatory functions. Clearly, many unanswered questions concerning the pathogenesis of HIV infection remain, specifically regarding the precise mechanisms of HIV-induced CD4+ T-cell destruction and the role of HIV in neurologic disease and other clinical manifestations. However, sufficient knowledge exists to suggest that the development of therapeutic strategies that would impede the replication and spread of HIV during acute infection as well as the activation of HIV expression during the asymptomatic phase could significantly prolong the lives of HIV-infected individuals.

REFERENCES

1. Centers for Disease Control: HIV prevalence estimates and AIDS case projections for the United States: Report based upon a workshop. MMWR 39:1, 1990

2. Seigal FP, Lopez C, Hammer GS et al: Severe acquired immunodeficiency in male homosexuals, manifested by chronic perianal ulcerative herpes simplex lesions. N Engl J Med 305:1439, 1981

3. Masur H, Michelis MA, Greene JB et al: An outbreak of community-acquired *Pneumocystis carinii* pneumonia: Initial manifestation of cellular immune dysfunction. N Engl J Med 305:1431, 1981

4. Gottlieb MS, Schroff R, Schanker HM et al: *Pneumocystis carinii* pneumonia and mucosal candidiasis in previously healthy homosexual men: Evidence of a new acquired cellular immunodeficiency. N Engl J Med 305:1425, 1981

5. Ammann AJ, Abrams D, Conant M et al: Acquired immune dysfunction in homosexual men: Immunologic profiles. Clin Immunol Immunopathol 27:315, 1983

6. Bowen DL, Lane HC, Fauci AS: Immunopathogenesis of the acquired immunodeficiency syndrome. Ann Intern Med 103:704, 1985

7. Lane HC, Fauci AS: Immunologic abnormalities in the acquired immunodeficiency syndrome. Annu Rev Immunol 3:477, 1985

8. Rook AH, Masur H, Lane HC et al: Interleukin-2 enhances the depressed natural killer and cytomegalovirus-specific cytotoxic activities of lymphocytes from patients with the acquired immune deficiency syndrome. J Clin Invest 72:398, 1983

9. Fauci AS, Masur H, Gelmann EP et al: NIH Conference: The Acquired Immunodeficiency Syndrome. An update. Ann Intern Med 102:800, 1985

10. Lane HC, Masur H, Edgar LC et al: Abnormalities of B-cell activation and immunoregulation in patients with the acquired immunodeficiency syndrome. N Engl J Med 309:453, 1983

11. Gupta S, Safai B: Deficient autologous mixed lymphocyte reaction in Kaposi's sarcoma associated with deficiency of Leu-3+ responder T cells. J Clin Invest 71:296, 1983

12. Gupta S, Gillis S, Thornton M, Goldberg M: Autologous mixed lymphocyte reaction in man: XIV. Deficiency of the autologous mixed lymphocyte reaction in acquired immune deficiency syndrome (AIDS) and AIDS related complex (ARC). In vitro effect of purified interleukin-1 and interleukin-2. Clin Exp Immunol 58:395, 1984

13. Lane HC, Depper JM, Greene WC et al: Qualitative analysis of immune function in patients with the acquired immunodeficiency syndrome: Evidence for a selective defect in soluble antigen recognition. N Engl J Med 313:79, 1985

14. Giorgi JV, Fahey JL, Smith DC et al: Early effects of HIV on CD4 lymphocytes in vivo. J Immunol 138:3725, 1987

15. Hoy JF, Lewis DE, Miller GG: Functional versus phenotypic analysis of T cells in subjects seropositive for the human immunodeficiency virus: A prospective study of in vitro responses to *Cryptococcus neoformans*. J Infect Dis 158:1071, 1988

16. Shearer GM, Salahuddin SZ, Markham PD et al: Prospective study of cytotoxic T lymphocyte responses to influenza and antibodies to human T lymphotropic virus-III in homosexual men: Selective loss of an influenza-specific, human leukocyte antigen-restricted cytotoxic T lymphocyte response in human T lymphotropic virus-III positive individuals with symptoms of acquired immunodeficiency syndrome and in a patient with acquired immunodeficiency syndrome. J Clin Invest 76:1699, 1985

17. Fauci AS: AIDS: Immunopathogenic mechanisms and research strategies. Clin Res 35:503, 1987

18. Rosenberg ZF, Fauci AS: The immunopathogenesis of HIV infection. Adv Immunol 47:377, 1989

19. Pahwa SG, Quilop MT, Lange M et al: Defective B-lymphocyte function in homosexual men in relation to the acquired immunodeficiency syndrome. Ann Intern Med 101:757, 1984

20. Ammann AJ, Schiffman G, Abrams D et al: B-cell immunodeficiency in acquired immune deficiency syndrome. JAMA 251:1447, 1984

21. Amadori A, Zamarchi R, Ciminale V et al: HIV-1-specific B cell activation: A major constituent of spontaneous B cell activation during HIV-1 infection. J Immunol 143:2146, 1989

22. Edelman AS, Zolla-Pazner S: Response of mononuclear cells from HIV-infected patients to B-cell mitogens: Correlation with immunological and clinical features of disease progression. AIDS 4:859, 1990

23. Rosenberg ZF, Fauci AS: Immunology of AIDS: Approaches to understanding the immunopathogenesis of HIV infection. Res Clin Lab 19:189, 1989

24. Ennen J, Seipp I, Norley SG, Kurth R: Decreased accessory cell function of macrophages after infection with human immunodeficiency virus type 1 in vitro. Eur J Immunol 20:2451, 1990

25. Mansour I, Doinel C, Rouger P: CD16+ NK cells decrease in all stages of HIV infection through a selective depletion of the CD16+ CD8+ CD3− subset. AIDS Res Hum Retroviruses 6:1451, 1990

26. Chehimi J, Bandyopadhyay S, Prakash K et al: In vitro infection of natural killer cells with different human immunodeficiency virus type 1 isolates. J Virol 65:1812, 1991

27. Koenig S, Fauci AS: AIDS: Immunopathogenesis and immune response to the human immunodeficiency virus. In DeVita VT Jr, Hellman S, Rosenberg SA (eds): AIDS: Etiology, Diagnosis, Treatment, and Prevention, ed 2, p 61. Philadelphia, JB Lippincott, 1988

28. Melmed RN, Taylor JM, Detels R et al: Serum neopterin changes in HIV-infected subjects: Indicator of significant pathology, CD4 T cell changes, and the development of AIDS. J AIDS 2:70, 1989

29. Fahey JL, Taylor JM, Detels R et al: The prognostic value of cellular and serologic markers in infection with human immunodeficiency virus type 1. N Engl J Med 322:166, 1990

30. Hofmann B, Wang YX, Cumberland WG et al: Serum beta 2-microglobulin level increases in HIV infection: Relation to seroconversion, CD4 T-cell fall and prognosis. AIDS 4:207, 1990

31. McDougal JS, Hubbard M, Nicholson JK et al: Immune complexes in the acquired immunodeficiency syndrome (AIDS): Relationship to disease manifestation, risk group, and immunologic defect. J Clin Immunol 5:130, 1985

32. Barre-Sinoussi F, Chermann JC, Rey F et al: Isolation of a T-lymphotropic retrovirus from a patient at risk for acquired immune deficiency syndrome (AIDS). Science 220:868, 1983

33. Gallo RC, Salahuddin SZ, Popovic M et al: Frequent detection and isolation of cytopathic retroviruses (HTLV-III) from patients with AIDS and at risk for AIDS. Science 224:500, 1984

34. Levy JA, Hoffman AD, Kramer SM et al: Isolation of lymphocytopathic retroviruses from San Francisco patients with AIDS. Science 225:840, 1984

35. Harper ME, Marselle LM, Gallo RC, Wong-Staal F: Detection of lymphocytes expressing human T-lymphotropic

virus type III in lymph nodes and peripheral blood from infected individuals by in situ hybridization. Proc Natl Acad Sci USA 83:772, 1986

36. Schnittman SM, Psallidopoulos MC, Lane HC et al: The reservoir for HIV-1 in human peripheral blood is a T cell that maintains expression of CD4. Science 245:305, 1989

37. Simmonds P, Balfe P, Peutherer JF et al: Human immunodeficiency virus–infected individuals contain provirus in small numbers of peripheral mononuclear cells and at low copy numbers. J Virol 64:864, 1990

38. McElrath MJ, Steinman RM, Cohn ZA: Latent HIV-1 infection in enriched populations of blood monocytes and T cells from seropositive patients. J Clin Invest 87:27, 1991

39. Ho DD, Moudgil T, Alam M: Quantitation of human immunodeficiency virus type 1 in the blood of infected persons. N Engl J Med 321:1621, 1989

40. Coombs RW, Collier AC, Allain JP et al: Plasma viremia in human immunodeficiency virus infection. N Engl J Med 321:1626, 1989

40a. Pantaleo G, Graziosi C, Butini L et al: Lymphoid organs function as major reservoirs for human immunodeficiency virus. Proc Natl Acad Sci USA 88:9838, 1991

41. Schnittman SM, Greenhouse JJ, Psallidopoulos MC et al: Increasing viral burden in CD4+ T cells from patients with human immunodeficiency virus (HIV) infection reflects rapidly progressive immunosuppression and clinical disease. Ann Intern Med 113:438, 1990

42. Genesca J, Wang RY, Alter HJ, Shih JW: Clinical correlation and genetic polymorphism of the human immunodeficiency virus proviral DNA obtained after polymerase chain reaction amplification. J Infect Dis 162:1025, 1990

43. Klatzmann D, Barre-Sinoussi F, Nugeyre MT et al: Selective tropism of lymphadenopathy associated virus (LAV) for helper-inducer T lymphocytes. Science 225:59, 1984

44. Schnittman SM, Denning SM, Greenhouse JJ et al: Evidence for susceptibility of intrathymic T-cell precursors and their progeny carrying T-cell antigen receptor phenotypes TCR alpha beta + and TCR gamma delta + to human immunodeficiency virus infection: A mechanism for CD4+ (T4) lymphocyte depletion. Proc Natl Acad Sci USA 87:7727, 1990

45. Folks TM, Kessler SW, Orenstein JM et al: Infection and replication of HIV-1 in purified progenitor cells of normal human bone marrow. Science 242:919, 1988

46. Steinberg HN, Crumpacker CS, Chatis PA: In vitro suppression of normal human bone marrow progenitor cells by human immunodeficiency virus. J Virol 65:1765, 1991

47. von Laer D, Hufert FT, Fenner TE et al: CD34+ hematopoietic progenitor cells are not a major reservoir of the human immunodeficiency virus. Blood 76:1281, 1990

48. Molina JM, Scadden DT, Sakaguchi M et al: Lack of evidence for infection of or effect on growth of hematopoietic progenitor cells after in vivo or in vitro exposure to human immunodeficiency virus. Blood 76:2476, 1990

49. Davis BR, Schwartz DH, Marx JC et al: Absent or rare human immunodeficiency virus infection of bone marrow stem/progenitor cells in vivo. J Virol 65:1985, 1991

50. Keshet E, Temin HM: Cell killing by spleen necrosis virus is correlated with a transient accumulation of spleen necrosis virus DNA. J Virol 31:376, 1979

51. Weller SK, Joy AE, Temin HM: Correlation between cell killing and massive second-round superinfection by members of some subgroups of avian leukosis virus. J Virol 33:494, 1980

52. Shaw GM, Hahn BH, Arya SK et al: Molecular characterization of human T-cell leukemia (lymphotropic) virus type III in the acquired immune deficiency syndrome. Science 226:1165, 1984

53. Pauza CD, Galindo JE, Richman DD: Reinfection results in accumulation of unintegrated viral DNA in cytopathic and persistent human immunodeficiency virus type 1 infection of CEM cells. J Exp Med 172:1035, 1990

54. Dalgleish AG, Beverley PC, Clapham PR et al: The CD4 (T4) antigen is an essential component of the receptor for the AIDS retrovirus. Nature 312:763, 1984

55. Klatzmann D, Champagne E, Chamaret S et al: T-lymphocyte T4 molecule behaves as the receptor for human retrovirus LAV. Nature 312:767, 1984

56. Koga Y, Sasaki M, Nakamura K et al: Intracellular distribution of the envelope glycoprotein of human immunodeficiency virus and its role in the production of cytopathic effect in CD4+ and CD4− human cell lines. J Virol 64:4661, 1990

57. York-Higgins D, Cheng-Mayer C, Bauer D et al: Human immunodeficiency virus type 1 cellular host range, replication, cytopathicity are linked to the envelope region of the viral genome. J Virol 64:4016, 1990

58. Kowalski M, Bergeron L, Dorfman T et al: Attenuation of human immunodeficiency virus type 1 cytopathic effect by a mutation affecting the transmembrane envelope glycoprotein. J Virol 65:281, 1991

59. Stevenson M, Haggerty S, Lamonica CA et al: Integration is not necessary for expression of human immunodeficiency virus type 1 protein products. J Virol 64:2421, 1990

60. Weinhold KJ, Lyerly HK, Stanley SD et al: HIV-1 GP120-mediated immune suppression and lymphocyte destruction in the absence of viral infection. J Immunol 142:3091, 1989

61. Lanzavecchia A, Roosnek E, Gregory T et al: T cells can present antigens such as HIV gp120 targeted to their own surface molecules. Nature 334:530, 1988

62. Siliciano RF, Lawton T, Knall C et al: Analysis of host-virus interactions in AIDS with anti-gp120 T cell clones: Effect of HIV sequence variation and a mechanism for CD4+ cell depletion. Cell 54:561, 1988

63. Zarling JM, Ledbetter JA, Sias J et al: HIV-infected humans, but not chimpanzees, have circulating cytotoxic T lymphocytes that lyse uninfected CD4+ cells. J Immunol 144:2992, 1990

64. Ziegler JL, Stites DP: Hypothesis: AIDS is an autoimmune disease directed at the immune system and triggered by a lymphotropic retrovirus. Clin Immunol Immunopathol 41:305, 1986

65. Teeuwsen VJ, Siebelink KH, de Wolf F et al: Impairment of in vitro immune responses occurs within 3 months after HIV-1 seroconversion. AIDS 4:77, 1990

66. van Noesel CJ, Gruters RA, Terpstra FG et al: Functional and phenotypic evidence for a selective loss of memory T cells in asymptomatic human immunodeficiency virus–infected men. J Clin Invest 86:293, 1990

67. Gruters RA, Terpstra FG, De Jong R et al: Selective loss of T cell functions in different stages of HIV infection: Early loss of anti-CD3-induced T cell proliferation followed by anti-CD3-induced cytotoxic T lymphocyte generation in AIDS-related complex and AIDS. Eur J Immunol 20:1039, 1990

68. Schnittman SM, Lane HC, Greenhouse J et al: Preferential infection of CD4+ memory T cells by human immunodeficiency virus type 1: Evidence for a role in the selective

T-cell functional defects observed in infected individuals. Proc Natl Acad Sci USA 87:6058, 1990

69. Willerford DM, Gale MJ Jr, Benveniste RE et al: Simian immunodeficiency virus is restricted to a subset of blood CD4+ lymphocytes that includes memory cells. J Immunol 144:3779, 1990

70. Folks T, Benn S, Rabson A et al: Characterization of a continuous T-cell line susceptible to the cytopathic effects of the acquired immunodeficiency syndrome (AIDS)-associated retrovirus. Proc Natl Acad Sci USA 82:4539, 1985

71. Hoxie JA, Haggarty BS, Rackowski JL et al: Persistent non-cytopathic infection of normal human T lymphocytes with AIDS-associated retrovirus. Science 229:1400, 1985

72. Geleziunas R, Bour S, Boulerice F et al: Diminution of CD4 surface protein but not CD4 messenger RNA levels in monocytic cells infected by HIV-1. AIDS 5:29, 1991

73. Crise B, Buonocore L, Rose JK: CD4 is retained in the endoplasmic reticulum by the human immunodeficiency virus type 1 glycoprotein precursor. J Virol 64:5585, 1990

74. Jabbar MA, Nayak DP: Intracellular interaction of human immunodeficiency virus type 1 (ARV-2) envelope glycoprotein gp160 with CD4 blocks the movement and maturation of CD4 to the plasma membrane. J Virol 64:6297, 1990

75. Willard-Gallo KE, Van de Keere F, Kettmann R: A specific defect in CD3 gamma-chain gene transcription results in loss of T-cell receptor/CD3 expression late after human immunodeficiency virus infection of a CD4+ T-cell line. Proc Natl Acad Sci USA 87:6713, 1990

76. Agy MB, Wambach M, Foy K, Katze MG: Expression of cellular genes in CD4 positive lymphoid cells infected by the human immunodeficiency virus, HIV-1: Evidence for a host protein synthesis shut-off induced by cellular mRNA degradation. Virology 177:251, 1990

77. Ruegg CL, Strand M: Inhibition of protein kinase C and anti-CD3-induced Ca2+ influx in Jurkat T cells by a synthetic peptide with sequence identity to HIV-1 gp41. J Immunol 144:3928, 1990

78. Nong Y, Kandil O, Tobin EH et al: The HIV core protein p24 inhibits interferon-gamma-induced increase of HLA-DR and cytochrome b heavy chain mRNA levels in the human monocyte-like cell line THP1. Cell Immunol 132:10, 1991

79. Manca F, Habeshaw JA, Dalgleish AG: HIV envelope glycoprotein, antigen specific T-cell responses, and CD4. Lancet 335:811, 1990

80. Horak ID, Popovic M, Horak EM et al: No T-cell tyrosine protein kinase signalling or calcium mobilization after CD4 association with HIV-1 or HIV-1 gp120. Nature 348:557, 1990

81. Cefai D, Debre P, Kaczorek M et al: Human immunodeficiency virus-1 glycoproteins gp120 and gp160 specifically inhibit the CD3/T cell-antigen receptor phosphoinositide transduction pathway. J Clin Invest 86:2117, 1990

82. Hofmann B, Nishanian P, Baldwin RL et al: HIV inhibits the early steps of lymphocyte activation, including initiation of inositol phospholipid metabolism. J Immunol 145:3699, 1990

83. Laurence J, Kulkosky J, Dong B et al: A soluble inhibitor of T lymphocyte function induced by HIV-1 infection of CD4+ T cells: Characterization of a cellular protein and its relationship to p15E. Cell Immunol 128:337, 1990

84. Weimer R, Daniel V, Zimmermann R et al: Autoantibodies against CD4 cells are associated with CD4 helper defects

in human immunodeficiency virus-infected patients. Blood 77:133, 1991

85. Gartner S, Markovits P, Markovitz DM et al: The role of mononuclear phagocytes in HTLV-III/LAV infection. Science 233:215, 1986

86. Gendelman HE, Orenstein JM, Martin MA et al: Efficient isolation and propagation of human immunodeficiency virus on recombinant colony-stimulating factor 1-treated monocytes. J Exp Med 167:1428, 1988

87. Mikovits JA, Raziuddin, Gonda M et al: Negative regulation of human immune deficiency virus replication in monocytes: Distinctions between restricted and latent expression in cells. J Exp Med 171:1705, 1990

88. Psallidopoulos MC, Schnittman SM, Thompson LM 3d et al: Integrated proviral human immunodeficiency virus type 1 is present in CD4+ peripheral blood lymphocytes in healthy seropositive individuals. J Virol 63:4626, 1989

89. Spear GT, Ou CY, Kessler HA et al: Analysis of lymphocytes, monocytes, and neutrophils from human immunodeficiency virus (HIV)-infected persons for HIV DNA. J Infect Dis 162:1239, 1990

90. Locardi C, Petrini C, Boccoli G et al: Increased human immunodeficiency virus (HIV) expression in chronically infected U937 cells upon in vitro differentiation by hydroxyvitamin D3: Roles of interferon and tumor necrosis factor in regulation of HIV production. J Virol 64:5874, 1990

91. Kitano K, Baldwin GC, Raines MA, Golde DW: Differentiating agents facilitate infection of myeloid leukemia cell lines by monocytotropic HIV-1 strains. Blood 76:1980, 1990

92. Kalter DC, Nakamura M, Turpin JA et al: Enhanced HIV replication in macrophage colony-stimulating factor-treated monocytes. J Immunol 146:298, 1991

93. Schrier RD, McCutchan JA, Venable JC et al: T-cell-induced expression of human immunodeficiency virus in macrophages. J Virol 64:3280, 1990

94. Wong-Staal F, Shaw GM, Hahn BH et al: Genomic diversity of human T-lymphotropic virus type III (HTLV-III). Science 229:759, 1985

95. Saag MS, Hahn BH, Gibbons J et al: Extensive variation of human immunodeficiency virus type 1 in vivo. Nature 334:440, 1988

96. Evans LA, McHugh TM, Stites DP, Levy JA: Differential ability of human immunodeficiency virus isolates to productively infect human cells. J Immunol 138:3415, 1987

97. Cloyd MW, Moore BE: Spectrum of biological properties of human immunodeficiency virus isolates. Virology 174:103, 1990

98. Cheng-Mayer C, Seto D, Tateno M, Levy JA: Biologic features of HIV-1 that correlate with virulence in the host. Science 240:80, 1988

99. Sakai K, Dewhurst S, Ma XY, Volsky DJ: Differences in cytopathogenicity and host cell range among infectious molecular clones of human immunodeficiency virus type 1 simultaneously isolated from an individual. J Virol 62:4078, 1988

100. Tersmette M, Gruters RA, de Wolf F et al: Evidence for a role of virulent human immunodeficiency virus (HIV) variants in the pathogenesis of acquired immunodeficiency syndrome: Studies on sequential HIV isolates. J Virol 63:2118, 1989

101. Balachandran R, Thampatty P, Enrico A et al: Human immunodeficiency virus isolates from asymptomatic ho-

mosexual men and from AIDS patients have distinct biologic and genetic properties. Virology 180:229, 1991

102. Massari FE, Poli G, Schnittman SM, Psallidopoulos MC et al: In vivo T lymphocyte origin of macrophage-tropic strains of HIV. Role of monocytes during in vitro isolation and in vivo infection. J Immunol 144:4628, 1990

103. Kim S, Ikeuchi K, Groopman J, Baltimore D: Factors affecting cellular tropism of human immunodeficiency virus. J Virol 64:5600, 1990

104. Pomerantz RJ, Feinberg MB, Andino R, Baltimore D: The long terminal repeat is not a major determinant of the cellular tropism of human immunodeficiency virus type 1. J Virol 65:1041, 1991

105. Cheng-Mayer C, Quiroga M, Tung JW et al: Viral determinants of human immunodeficiency virus type 1 T-cell or macrophage tropism, cytopathogenicity, and CD4 antigen modulation. J Virol 64:4390, 1990

106. Liu ZQ, Wood C, Levy JA, Cheng-Mayer C: The viral envelope gene is involved in macrophage tropism of a human immunodeficiency virus type 1 strain isolated from brain tissue. J Virol 64:6148, 1990

107. Ivey-Hoyle M, Culp JS, Chaikin MA et al: Envelope glycoproteins from biologically diverse isolates of immunodeficiency viruses have widely different affinities for CD4. Proc Natl Acad Sci USA 88:512, 1991

108. O'Brien WA, Koyanagi Y, Namazie A et al: HIV-1 tropism for mononuclear phagocytes can be determined by regions of gp120 outside the CD4-binding domain. Nature 348:69, 1990

109. Shioda T, Levy JA, Cheng-Mayer C: Macrophage and T cell-line tropisms of HIV-1 are determined by specific regions of the envelope gp120 gene. Nature 349:167, 1991

110. Takeuchi Y, Akutsu M, Murayama K et al: Host range mutant of human immunodeficiency virus type 1: Modification of cell tropism by a single point mutation at the neutralization epitope in the env gene. J Virol 65:1710, 1991

111. Tschachler E, Groh V, Popovic M et al: Epidermal Langerhans cells—a target for HTLV-III/LAV infection. J Invest Dermatol 88:233, 1987

112. Macatonia SE, Lau R, Patterson S et al: Dendritic cell infection, depletion and dysfunction in HIV-infected individuals. Immunology 71:38, 1990

113. Patterson S, Knight SC: Susceptibility of human peripheral blood dendritic cells to infection by human immunodeficiency virus. J Gen Virol 68:1177, 1987

114. Dreno B, Milpied B, Bignon JD et al: Prognostic value of Langerhans cells in the epidermis of HIV patients. Br J Dermatol 118:481, 1988

115. Werner A, Winskowsky G, Cichutek K et al: Productive infection of both CD4+ and CD4− human cell lines with HIV-1, HIV-2 and SIVagm. AIDS 4:537, 1990

116. Mellert W, Kleinschmidt A, Schmidt J et al: Infection of human fibroblasts and osteoblast-like cells with HIV-1. AIDS 4:527, 1990

117. Ikeuchi K, Kim S, Byrn RA et al: Infection of nonlymphoid cells by human immunodeficiency virus type 1 or type 2. J Virol 64:4226, 1990

118. Clapham PR, Weber JN, Whitby D et al: Soluble CD4 blocks the infectivity of diverse strains of HIV and SIV for T cells and monocytes but not for brain and muscle cells. Nature 337:368, 1989

119. Tateno M, Gonzalez-Scarano F, Levy JA: Human immunodeficiency virus can infect CD4-negative human fibroblastoid cells. Proc Natl Acad Sci USA 86:4287, 1989

120. Cao YZ, Friedman-Kien AE, Huang YX et al: CD4-independent, productive human immunodeficiency virus type 1 of hepatoma cell lines in vitro. J Virol 64:2553, 1990

121. Larkin M, Childs RA, Matthews TJ et al: Oligosaccharide-mediated interactions of the envelope glycoprotein gp120 of HIV-1 that are independent of CD4 recognition. AIDS 3:793, 1989

122. Canivet M, Hoffman AD, Hardy D et al: Replication of HIV-1 in a wide variety of animal cells following phenotypic mixing with murine retroviruses. Virology 178:543, 1990

123. Lusso P, Lori F, Gallo RC: CD4-independent infection by human immunodeficiency virus type 1 after phenotypic mixing with human T-cell leukemia viruses. J Virol 64:6341, 1990

124. Landau NR, Page KA, Littman DR: Pseudotyping with human T-cell leukemia virus type I broadens the human immunodeficiency virus host range. J Virol 65:162, 1991

125. De Maria A, Pantaleo G, Schnittman SM et al: Infection of CD8+ T lymphocytes with HIV: Requirement for interaction with infected CD4+ cells and induction of infectious virus from chronically infected CD8+ cells. Proc Natl Acad Sci USA 146:2220, 1991

126. Zucker-Franklin D, Seremetis S, Zheng ZY: Internalization of human immunodeficiency virus type I and other retroviruses by megakaryocytes and platelets. Blood 75:1920, 1990

127. Cohen AH, Sun NC, Shapshak P, Imagawa DT: Demonstration of human immunodeficiency virus in renal epithelium in HIV-associated nephropathy. Mod Pathol 2:125, 1989

128. Levy JA, Margaretten W, Nelson J: Detection of HIV in enterochromaffin cells in the rectal mucosa of an AIDS patient. Am J Gastroenterol 84:787, 1989

129. Moyer MP, Huot RI, Ramirez A Jr et al: Infection of human gastrointestinal cells by HIV-1. AIDS Res Hum Retroviruses 6:1409, 1990

130. Price RW, Brew B, Sidtis J et al: The brain in AIDS: Central nervous system HIV-1 infection and AIDS dementia complex. Science 239:586, 1988

131. Navia BA, Price RW: The acquired immunodeficiency syndrome dementia complex as the presenting or sole manifestation of human immunodeficiency virus infection. Arch Neurol 44:65, 1987

132. Watkins BA, Dorn HH, Kelly WB et al: Specific tropism of HIV-1 for microglial cells in primary human brain cultures. Science 249:549, 1990

133. Jordan CA, Watkins BA, Kufta C, Dubois-Dalcq M: Infection of brain microglial cells by human immunodeficiency virus type 1 is CD4 dependent. J Virol 65:736, 1991

134. Weiser B, Peress N, La Neve D et al: Human immunodeficiency virus type 1 expression in the central nervous system correlates directly with extent of disease. Proc Natl Acad Sci USA 87:3997, 1990

135. Fauci AS: The human immunodeficiency virus: Infectivity and mechanisms of pathogenesis. Science 239:617, 1988

136. Lotz M, Vaughan JH, Carson DA: Effect of neuropeptides on production of inflammatory cytokines by human monocytes. Science 241:1218, 1988

137. Laurenzi MA, Siden A, Persson MA et al: Cerebrospinal fluid interleukin-6 activity in HIV infection and inflammatory and noninflammatory diseases of the nervous system. Clin Immunol Immunopathol 57:233, 1990

138. Benveniste EN, Sparacio SM, Norris JG et al: Induction

and regulation of interleukin-6 gene expression in rat astrocytes. J Neuroimmunol 30:201, 1990

139. Vitkovic L, Kalebic T, de Cunha A, Fauci AS: Astrocyte-conditioned medium stimulates HIV-1 expression in a chronically infected promonocyte clone. J Neuroimmunol 30:153, 1990

140. Giulian D, Vaca K, Noonan CA: Secretion of neurotoxins by mononuclear phagocytes infected with HIV-1. Science 250:1593, 1990

141. Pulliam L, Herndier BG, Tang NM, McGrath MS: Human immunodeficiency virus-infected macrophages produce soluble factors that cause histological and neurochemical alterations in cultured human brain. J Clin Invest 87:503, 1991

142. Dreyer EB, Kaiser PK, Offermann JT, Lipton SA: HIV-1 coat protein neurotoxicity prevented by calcium channel. Science 248:364, 1990

143. Kaiser PK, Offermann JT, Lipton SA: Neuronal injury due to HIV-1 envelope protein is blocked by anti-gp120 antibodies but not by anti-CD4 antibodies. Neurology 40:1757, 1990

144. Sabatier JM, Vives E, Mabrouk K et al: Evidence for neurotoxic activity of tat from human immunodeficiency virus type 1. J Virol 65:961, 1991

145. Yamada M, Zurbriggen A, Oldstone MBA, Fujinami RS: Common immunologic determinant between human immunodeficiency virus type 1 gp41 and astrocytes. J Virol 65:1370, 1991

146. Rutherford GW, Lifson AR, Hessol NA et al: Course of HIV-I infection in a cohort of homosexual and bisexual men: An 11 year follow up study. Br Med J 301:1183, 1990

147. Tindall B, Cooper DA: Primary HIV infection: Host responses and intervention strategies. AIDS 5:1, 1991

148. Gaines H, von Sydow MA, von Stedingk LV et al: Immunological changes in primary HIV-1 infection. AIDS 4:995, 1990

149. Kaplan JE, Spira TJ, Fishbein DB et al: A six-year follow-up of HIV-infected homosexual men with lymphadenopathy: Evidence for an increased risk for developing AIDS after the third year of lymphadenopathy. JAMA 260:2694, 1988

150. Phillips AN, Lee CA, Elford J, Janossy G et al: Serial CD4 lymphocyte counts and development of AIDS. Lancet 337:389, 1991

151. Rosenberg ZF, Fauci AS: Induction of expression of HIV in latently or chronically infected cells. AIDS Res Hum Retroviruses 5:1, 1989

152. Zack JA, Arrigo SJ, Weitsman SR et al: HIV-1 entry into quiescent primary lymphocytes: Molecular analysis reveals a labile, latent viral structure. Cell 61:213, 1990

153. Margolick JB, Volkman DJ, Folks TM, Fauci AS: Amplification of HTLV-III/LAV infection by antigen-induced activation of T cells and direct suppression by virus of lymphocyte blastogenic responses. J Immunol 138:1719, 1987

154. Zack JA, Cann AJ, Lugo JP, Chen IS: HIV-1 production from infected peripheral blood T cells after HTLV-I induced mitogenic stimulation. Science 240:1026, 1988

155. Horvat RT, Wood C: HIV promoter activity in primary antigen-specific human T lymphocytes. J Immunol 143:2745, 1989

156. Hazan U, Thomas D, Alcami J et al: Stimulation of a human T-cell clone with anti-CD3 or tumor necrosis factor induces NF-kappa B translocation but not human immunodeficiency virus 1 enhancer-dependent transcription. Proc Natl Acad Sci USA 87:7861, 1990

157. Pomerantz RJ, Feinberg MB, Trono D, Baltimore D: Lipopolysaccharide is a potent monocyte/macrophage-specific stimulator human immunodeficiency virus type 1 expression. J Exp Med 172:253, 1990

158. Bohnlein E, Lowenthal JW, Siekevitz M et al: The same inducible nuclear proteins regulates mitogen activation of both the interleukin-2 receptor-alpha gene and type 1 HIV. Cell 53:827, 1988

159. Greene WC, Bohnlein E, Ballard DW: HIV-1, HTLV-1 and normal T-cell growth: transcriptional strategies and surprises. Immunol Today 10:272, 1989

160. Nabel G, Baltimore D: An inducible transcription factor activates expression of human immunodeficiency virus in T cells. Nature 326:711, 1987

161. Gruters RA, Otto SA, Al BJM et al: Non-mitogenic T cell activation signals are sufficient for induction of human immunodeficiency virus transcription. Eur J Immunol 21:167, 1991

162. Bohnlein E, Siekevitz M, Ballard DW et al: Stimulation of the human immunodeficiency virus type 1 enhancer by the human T-cell leukemia virus type I tax gene product involves the action of inducible cellular proteins. J Virol 63:1578, 1989

163. Levrero M, Balsano C, Natoli G et al: Hepatitis B virus X protein transactivates the long terminal repeats of human immunodeficiency virus types 1 and 2. J Virol 64:3082, 1990

164. Mallon R, Borkowski J, Albin R et al: The Epstein-Barr virus BZLF1 gene product activates the human immunodeficiency virus type 1 5′ long terminal repeat. J Virol 64:6282, 1990

165. Albrecht MA, DeLuca NA, Byrn RA et al: The herpes simplex virus immediate-early protein, ICP4, is required to potentiate replication of human immunodeficiency virus in CD4+ lymphocytes. J Virol 63:1861, 1989

166. Casareale D, Fiala M, Chang CM et al: Cytomegalovirus enhances lysis of HIV-infected T lymphoblasts. Int J Cancer 44:124, 1989

167. Lusso P, Ensoli B, Markham PD et al: Productive dual infection of human CD4+ T lymphocytes by HIV-1 and HHV-6. Nature 337:370, 1989

168. Kucera LS, Leake E, Iyer N et al: Human immunodeficiency virus type 1 (HIV-1) and herpes simplex virus 2 (HSV-2) can coinfect and simultaneously replicate in the same human CD4+ cell: Effect of coinfection on infectious HSV-2 and HIV-1 replication. AIDS Res Hum Retroviruses 6:641, 1990

169. Laurence J: Molecular interactions among herpesviruses and human immunodeficiency viruses. J Infect Dis 162:338, 1990

170. Barry PA, Pratt-Lowe E, Peterlin BM, Luciw PA: Cytomegalovirus activates transcription directed by the long terminal repeat of human immunodeficiency virus type 1. J Virol 64:2932, 1990

171. Rando RF, Srinivasan A, Feingold J et al: Characterization of multiple molecular interactions between human cytomegalovirus (HCMV) and human immunodeficiency virus type 1 (HIV-1). Virology 176:87, 1990

172. Lusso P, DeMaria A, Malnati M et al: Induction of CD4 and susceptibility to HIV-1 infection in human CD8+ T lymphocytes by human herpesvirus 6. Nature 349:533, 1991

173. Antoni BA, Rabson AB, Miller IL et al: Adeno-associated virus rep protein inhibits human immunodeficiency virus type 1 production in human cells. J Virol 65:396, 1991

174. Carrigan DR, Knox KK, Tapper MA: Suppression of human immunodeficiency virus type 1 replication by human herpesvirus-6. J Infect Dis 162:844, 1990

175. Rosenberg ZF, Fauci AS: Immunopathogenic mechanisms of HIV infection: Cytokine induction of HIV expression. Immunol Today 11:176, 1990

176. Folks TM, Clouse KA, Justement J et al: Tumor necrosis factor-alpha induces the expression of the human immunodeficiency virus from a chronically infected T cell clone. Proc Natl Acad Sci USA 86:2365, 1989

177. Tsunetsugu-Yokota Y, Honda M: Effect of cytokines on HIV release and IL-2 receptor alpha expression in monocytic cell lines. J AIDS 3:511, 1990

178. Poli G, Bressler P, Kinter A et al: Interleukin 6 induces human immunodeficiency virus expression in monocytic cells alone and in synergy with tumor necrosis factor alpha by transcriptional and post-transcriptional mechanisms. J Exp Med 172:151, 1990

179. Lacoste J, D'Addario M, Roulston A et al: Cell-specific differences in activation of NF-kappa B regulatory elements of human immunodeficiency virus and beta interferon promoters by tumor necrosis factor. J Virol 64:4726, 1990

180. Mellors JW, Griffith BP, Ortiz MA et al: Tumor necrosis factor-alpha/cachectin enhances human immunodeficiency virus type 1 replication in primary macrophages. J Infect Dis 163:78, 1991

181. Schuitemaker H, Kootstra NA, van Oers MH et al: Induction of monocyte proliferation and HIV expression by IL-3 does not interfere with anti-viral activity of zidovudine. Blood 76:1490, 1990

182. Kuhweide R, Van Damme J, Ceuppens JL: Tumor necrosis factor-alpha and interleukin-6 synergistically induce T cell growth. Eur J Immunol 20:1019, 1990

183. Zhang YH, Lin JX, Vilcek J: Interleukin-6 induction by tumor necrosis factor and interleukin-1 in human fibroblasts involves activation of a nuclear factor binding to a kappa B-like sequence. Mol Cell Biol 10:3818, 1990

184. Latham PS, Lewis AM, Varesio L et al: Expression of human immunodeficiency virus long terminal repeat in the human promonocyte cell line U937: Effect of endotoxin and cytokines. Cell Immunol 129:513, 1990

185. Kinter AL, Poli G, Maury W et al: Direct and cytokine-mediated activation of protein kinase C induces human immunodeficiency virus expression in chronically infected promonocytic cells. J Virol 64:4306, 1990

186. Poli G, Kinter A, Justement JS et al: Tumor necrosis factor alpha functions in an autocrine manner in the induction of human immunodeficiency virus expression. Proc Natl Acad Sci USA 87:782, 1990

187. Molina JM, Schindler R, Ferriani R et al: Production of cytokines by peripheral blood monocytes/macrophages infected with human immunodeficiency virus type 1 (HIV-1). J Infect Dis 161:888, 1990

188. Molina JM, Scadden DT, Amirault C et al: Human immunodeficiency virus does not induce interleukin-1, interleukin-6, or tumor necrosis factor in mononuclear cells. J Virol 64:2901, 1990

189. Birx DL, Redfield RR, Tencer K et al: Induction of interleukin-6 during human immunodeficiency virus infection. Blood 76:2303, 1990

190. Honda M, Kitamura K, Mizutani Y et al: Quantitative analysis of serum IL-6 and its correlation with increased levels of serum IL-2R in HIV-induced diseases. J Immunol 145:4059, 1990

191. Kasahara Y, Miyawaki T, Kato K et al: Role of interleukin 6 for differential responsiveness of naive and memory CD4+ T cells in CD2-mediated activation. J Exp Med 172:1419, 1990

192. Wright SC, Jewett A, Mitsuyasu R, Bonavida B: Spontaneous cytotoxicity and tumor necrosis factor production by peripheral blood monocytes from AIDS patients. J Immunol 141:99, 1988

193. Voth R, Rossol S, Klein K et al: Differential gene expression of IFN-alpha and tumor necrosis factor-alpha in peripheral blood mononuclear cells from patients with AIDS related complex and AIDS. J Immunol 144:970, 1990

194. Krishnan VL, Meager A, Mitchell DM, Pinching AJ: Alveolar macrophages in AIDS patients: Increased spontaneous tumour necrosis factor-alpha production in *Pneumocystis carinii* pneumonia. Clin Exp Immunol 80:156, 1990

195. Barnes PF, Fong SJ, Brennan PJ et al: Local production of tumor necrosis factor and IFN-gamma in tuberculosis pleuritis. J Immunol 145:149, 1990

196. Amadori A, Zamarchi R, Veronese ML et al: B cell activation during HIV-1 infection: II. Cell-to-cell interactions and cytokine requirement. J Immunol 146:57, 1991

197. Miles SA, Rezai AR, Salazar-Gonzalez JF et al: AIDS Kaposi sarcoma-derived cells produce and respond to interleukin 6. Proc Natl Acad Sci USA 87:4068, 1990

198. Rieckmann P, Poli G, Kehrl JH, Fauci AS: Activated B lymphocytes from human immunodeficiency virus–infected individuals induce virus expression in infected T cells and a promonocytic cell line, U1. J Exp Med 173:1, 1991

199. Pluda JM, Yarchoan R, Smith PD et al: Subcutaneous recombinant granulocyte-macrophage colony-stimulating factor used as a single agent and in an alternating regimen with azidothymidine in leukopenic patients with severe human immunodeficiency virus infection. Blood 76:463, 1990

200. Kehrl JH, Wakefield LM, Roberts AB et al: Production of transforming growth factor-beta by human T lymphocytes and its potential role in the regulation of T cell growth. J Exp Med 163:1037, 1986

201. Lucas C, Bald LN, Fendly BM, Mora-Worms M et al: The autocrine production of transforming growth factor-beta 1 during lymphocyte activation: A study with a monoclonal antibody-based ELISA. J Immunol 145:1415, 1990

202. Poli G, Kinter A, Justement JS et al: Transforming growth factor β suppresses human immunodeficiency virus expression and replication in infected cells of the monocyte/macrophage lineage. J Exp Med 173:589, 1991

203. Peterson PK, Gekker G, Chao CC et al: Cocaine potentiates HIV-1 replication in human peripheral blood mononuclear cell cocultures: Involvement of transforming growth factor-beta. J Immunol 146:81, 1991

204. Roederer M, Staal FJ, Raju PA et al: Cytokine-stimulated human immunodeficiency virus replication is inhibited by N-acetyl-L-cysteine. Proc Natl Acad Sci USA 87:4884, 1990

205. Kalebic T, Kinter A, Poli G et al: Suppression of human immunodeficiency virus expression in chronically infected monocytic cells by glutathione, glutathione ester, and N-acetylcysteine. Proc Natl Acad Sci USA 88:986, 1991

5

Immune Responses to HIV Infection

Barton F. Haynes

The immune response to the human immunodeficiency virus (HIV) is determined by many complex factors. First, the extraordinary host-virus interactions that lead to the pathogenesis of AIDS induce profound functional host immune defects beginning soon after infection with HIV.[1] Prominent forms of HIV-induced immune dysfunction include defects in T- and B-cell responses to specific antigens, polyclonal hypergammaglobulinemia, enhanced autoantibody and immune complex formation, dysregulated cytokine production, decreased natural killer (NK) cell activity, and defective monocyte and dendritic cell function.[1-4] Thus, at the time when the host immune system begins to mount an anti-HIV immune response designed to neutralize free HIV and eliminate HIV-infected cells, many of the cellular components of the immune responses are being adversely affected by HIV. Second, evidence suggests that the route of HIV infection,[5] the amount of HIV in the inoculum, the pathogenic potential of a given HIV strain,[6] and host genetic factors[7] may modify the host response to HIV. Third, evidence is accruing that some components of an immune response to HIV may either enhance HIV infectivity or, in some circumstances, may be directly responsible for clinical manifestations of the disease.[8-11] Finally, the remarkable ability of HIV to mutate genome sequences and change the primary amino acid sequence of HIV proteins produces an effective mechanism with which HIV may evade otherwise effective antiviral immune responses.[12-15]

Because of lack of an acceptable animal model for HIV infection, and because the attack rate of acquired immunodeficiency syndrome (AIDS) may approach 100% of those infected with HIV, the nature of the immune responses that may protect against HIV infection remains unknown. Nonetheless, several recent studies

in chimpanzees have provided evidence that anti-*env* neutralizing antibodies may protect subjects from a challenge with cell-free HIV.[16-18] Because HIV infection in humans most often occurs *via* transfer of cell-associated HIV, many investigators have proposed that anti-HIV cellular responses are also likely to be important for prevention or control of HIV infection.[11] What follows is a summary of recent studies that have mapped various types of anti-HIV immune responses during progressive stages of HIV infection.

ANTIBODY RESPONSES TO HIV

Recent studies have documented the immunologic and virologic events that occur during acute HIV infection.[6,19-28] Acute HIV infection frequently manifests as an influenza- or mononucleosis-like syndrome, with fever, adenopathy, pharyngitis, rash, myalgias, and anthralgias common symptoms. Abnormal results on liver function tests, hepatosplenomegaly, encephalopathy, and neuropathy occur less commonly.[6] Five to 10 days after HIV infection, there is rapid rise in serum *gag* p24 protein levels, a rise in serum infectious HIV levels, a rise in circulating HIV infected CD4+ T cells, and a transient decrease in total circulating CD4+ T cells.[6,28] Circulating infectious virus levels peak from 10 to 20 days following HIV infection and fall precipitiously coincident with an increase in the level of anti-HIV antibodies (Table 5-1) and resolution of initial clinical symptoms.[6] In recently infected individuals with high-titer plasma viremia, HIV isolates are replication-competent and highly cytopathic.[6] Thus, virus with high replicative potential may commonly be transmitted by sexual routes in these individuals and may account for

Table 5–1. Antibody Responses to HIV During HIV Infection

Antibody Specificity	Comment	References
Anti-HIV neutralizing antibody	Type (isolate-specific) antibodies are against V3 loop of gp120 aa 303–38; group-specific (cross-neutralize many isolates) antibodies against carbohydrate and/or conformational determinants; onset 2–4 weeks after primary HIV infection; present throughout course of HIV infection; found in serum, CSF, urine	16–18, 30–57
Antibodies that bind to NK cells and monocytes *via* FcR and sensitize FcR+ cells to kill gp120+ cells *via* antibody dependent cellular cytotoxicity (ADCC)	ADCC anti-HIV antibodies bind to multiple epitopes of gp120 and gp41 HIV *env* protein; present in the highest levels in early stages of HIV infection; levels decrease as AIDS develops; found in serum and CSF	58–70
Anti-p24 HIV *gag* antibodies	Rise after initial HIV antigenemia of acute HIV infection decreases; stay elevated until ARC/AIDS develops; fall in anti-p24 antibody levels heralds rise in HIV antigenemia and onset of AIDS	6, 22, 26, 28, 53
Anti-*nef* HIV antibodies	Rise before antibodies to other structural proteins after seroconversion; decrease prior to onset of AIDS	72, 76
Anti-*rev, vpr, vpu* protease and *tat* HIV antibodies	Present in variable numbers of patients; decrease prior to development of AIDS in some studies	71, 73, 74, 75
Anti-HIV enhancing antibodies	Antibodies against epitopes of HIV gp41 that promote HIV infectivity *in vitro;* presence has been correlated with progression to AIDS	8–10

ARC = AIDS-related complex; FcR = receptor for the Fc portion of IgG.

their clinical symptoms and rapid seroconversion.[6] Infection of others with smaller amounts of HIV, or with less virulent or defective HIV strains, could explain reports of prolonged virus-positive, antibody-negative periods in individuals with subclinical primary HIV infection.[29]

Anti-HIV Neutralizing Antibodies

Neutralizing antibodies inhibit the infectivity of free HIV or HIV-infected cells and have been proposed to be one component of a salutary or protective anti-HIV immune response.[16–18,30–33] Human serum anti-HIV neutralizing antibodies have been identified that are either isolate (type)-specific (*i.e.,* neutralize only one isolate or related isolates)[30,34–37] or are group-specific (*i.e.,* neutralize many types of HIV isolates, regardless of the degree of primary sequence diversity).[33,38,39] To date, the epitopes to which most anti-HIV neutralizing antibodies bind have been located on envelope gp120 or gp41 proteins.[30–37,40–42] Animal studies have suggested that neutralizing epitopes may be present on HIV core proteins as well,[43] although most naturally occurring HIV neutralizing antibodies are against envelope proteins.[142] Type-specific HIV neutralizing antibodies bind to the third hypervariable region of HIV *env* gp120.[34–37,42,44,45] Because the region to which the predominant species of type-specific neutralizing antibodies bind (gp120 *env* aa 303–338) is flanked by cysteine residues that join in

a disulfide bond to form a loop structure, this region is called the gp120 V3 loop.[42,45] Antibodies against the V3 loop region have been postulated to inhibit HIV infection by preventing cleavage of gp120, thus preventing a necessary conformational change in gp120 required for entry of HIV into the cell or required for infected cell fusion.[46–48] Although the regions of HIV proteins to which group-specific HIV neutralizing antibodies bind are not known, recent data suggest that they may be conformational[49,50] or carbohydrate in nature.[51] After HIV infection, type-specific neutralizing antibodies appear in serum, followed by more broadly reactive, group-specific anti-HIV neutralizing antibodies.[38,39] Serum neutralizing antibody levels begin to rise 2 to 4 weeks after primary HIV infection[15,38,39] and peak during the asymptomatic phase of HIV infection.[31–33,52–54] Most studies have demonstrated that anti-HIV neutralizing antibodies are present in the symptomatic stages of AIDS-related complex (ARC) and AIDS, although frequently at lower levels than during the asymptomatic stages of HIV infection.[31,33,52–57]

Antibodies That Promote Antibody-Dependent Cellular Cytotoxicity of HIV-Infected Cells

Anti-gp160 antibodies in the serum and cerebrospinal fluid of HIV-infected subjects have been demonstrated that bind to IgG Fc receptor (R)–bearing NK cells *via* antibody Fc region and sensitize IgG FcR+ cells to kill HIV gp160-expressing, or gp120-coated, target cells.[58–65] Peripheral blood monocytes from AIDS patients can also mediate ADCC of HIV-infected cells.[66]

Although ADCC antibodies have been described against p24 *gag* proteins, most studies have found serum anti-HIV ADCC antibodies to react with either HIV gp120 or gp41 *env* proteins.[60–63,67,68] Anti-HIV antibodies that mediate ADCC of gp120- or gp41-expressing target cells arise soon after infection with HIV, are predominantly of the IgG1 subclass, and are present throughout all stages of HIV infection, although ADCC antibody levels decrease somewhat with the onset of AIDS.[58–62,69,70]

Anti-*gag* Antibodies

Anti-p24 antibodies appear within the first 2 weeks of acute HIV infection.[6,22,26,28,53] A rise in p24 antibody levels correlates well with the precipitous fall in infectious HIV antigenemia that occurs as the symptoms of acute HIV infection subside.[6,28] Antibodies to HIV p24 *gag* proteins rise to their highest levels during the asymptomatic seropositive stage and then fall to generally undetectable levels with the onset of AIDS.[6,22,26,28] Antibodies against the p17 *gag* protein of HIV have been reported to neutralize HIV and to cross-react with the thymic hormone thymosin $\alpha1$.[43]

Antibodies to Other HIV Proteins

Antibodies to HIV *rev, nef, tat, vpu, vpr,* and HIV protease proteins have been reported in variable percentages of HIV patients.[71–75] Antibodies to *nef* proteins have been found in HIV-infected subjects who were otherwise HIV seronegative.[76] In general, levels of antibody to all of these HIV proteins decrease as HIV infection progresses to AIDS.[71–75]

Antibodies That Enhance HIV Infection *in vitro*

Robinson *et al* have described antibodies in AIDS patient sera that augment rather than inhibit HIV infectivity *in vitro*.[8,9] HIV-enhancing antibodies have been shown to bind to epitopes in *env* gp41.[9] Interestingly, the presence of HIV-enhancing antibodies has been correlated with progression of HIV infection to AIDS.[10]

T-LYMPHOCYTE RESPONSES TO HIV

Cellular T-lymphocyte responses are essential for the control of numerous viral infections. CD4+ T-helper cell responses are required for both induction of B-cell antibody production and for induction of other T-cell responses. In HIV infection, anti-HIV T-helper cell responses, major histocompatibility (MHC) class I and MHC class II anti-HIV cytotoxic T-lymphocytes (CTL), and non-MHC-restricted CD8+ T-cell anti-HIV activities have been identified (Table 5–2).

T-Helper Cell Epitopes of HIV Proteins

A number of MHC class II–restricted T-helper cell epitopes of HIV proteins have been identified that are recognized by both HIV-infected humans and immunized animals.[77,78] Although T-helper cell epitopes have been found in many HIV proteins, including *env, gag,* and *pol,*[77,78] a few of these epitopes are immunodominant in that they are frequently recognized by T cells of infected humans or immunized animals.[77] Moreover, although these epitopes are clearly presented to CD4+ T-helper cells in the context of polymorphic MHC class II molecules, many of the HIV T-helper epitopes can be presented by more than one MHC class II type.[77,78] For example, Cease and colleagues have identified two immunodominant T-cell epitopes on the gp120 mole-

Table 5–2. T-Lymphocyte Responses to HIV During HIV Infection

Type of T-Lymphocyte Response	Comment	References
T cell proliferative response to HIV *env* gp120	High in asymptomatic seropositive subjects; decrease with onset of AIDS	77, 78, 80
Class I–restricted anti-HIV *env* and *gag* CTL	High in asymptomatic seropositive subjects; decreases with onset of AIDS; precursors of this type of CTL are also present in noninfected subjects	11, 81–89
Class II–restricted anti-HIV CTL	Precursors present in noninfected, infected, and gp160-immunized subjects	81, 91, 92
CD8+ anti-HIV T cells that suppress HIV reverse transcriptase (RT) *in vitro*	CD8+ T cell suppressor of HIV RT production and infection mediated by secreted factors from CD8 cells; non-MHC restricted; activity decreases with progression to AIDS	96, 97

cule, termed T1 and T2.[79] T cells of 85% of HIV-infected subjects recognize and secrete interleukin-2 (IL-2) in response to one of the two peptides *in vitro*.[77] Proliferative responses to HIV gp120 *in vitro* are highest in asymptomatic seropositive subjects and decrease with the onset of AIDS.[80]

Anti-HIV MHC-Restricted CTL

MHC class I–restricted CTL have been demonstrated against *gag, env, nef,* and *pol* HIV proteins.[11,81-88] Remarkably, anti-HIV class I–restricted CTL in asymptomatic HIV-seropositive subjects circulate in extraordinary frequency, on the order of 10 to 20 CTL precursors per 10^4 peripheral blood mononuclear cells (PBMC).[89] This level is sufficiently high to allow the detection of anti-HIV CTL in suspensions of fresh peripheral blood T cells—a measurement not possible when CTL are measured against other infectious agents such influenza viruses.[11,81,82] In influenza and other human infectious diseases, the CTL precursor frequency is lower than that for HIV, and *in vitro* expansion of CTL precursors in the presence of HIV antigen has been necessary to detect CTL.[90] Class I–restricted anti-HIV CTL are highest in frequency in peripheral blood during the asymptomatic seropositive stage and fall to low or nondetectable levels in AIDS.[89]

Precursors of class II MHC–restricted CTL have been identified in peripheral blood of HIV-infected subjects[91] and in noninfected subjects who have been immunized with recombinant HIV gp160.[92]

Recently the remarkable observation was made that precursors of both MHC class I[89] and MHC class II–restricted CTL[93] are present in the peripheral blood of *uninfected* normal subjects, and that prior to infection, normal subjects appear to be already "primed" to respond to HIV proteins and generate "memory" CTL responses.[11] Interestingly, of MHC-restricted CTL detected in fresh peripheral blood, all have been restricted by MHC class I antigens.[81] MHC class II–restricted CTL have only been detected following repeated *in vitro* stimulation with viral antigen.[91] Thus, anti-HIV CTL precursors that are MHC class I restricted are present at a frequency of 1 to 5 per 10^4 PBMC in HIV-*uninfected* subjects, rise in frequency to 10 to 20 per 10^4 PBMC in asymptomatic HIV-infected subjects, proliferate in response to HIV proteins, and can be expanded and cloned *in vitro*.[11,81,89] As HIV infection progresses to AIDS, the number of MHC class I–restricted CTL decreases.[11,81,94]

Reasons for the loss of MHC-restricted anti-HIV CTL effector function in AIDS patients are at present unknown. It has been proposed that a combination of factors such as a decrease in CD4 T-helper function and IL-2 production, HIV infection of antigen-presenting cells leading to immune dysfunction and destruction, and HIV infection of generative hematopoietic microenvironments may contribute to decreases in HIV-

specific CTL.[11,81,94] Recently it was demonstrated that the effector cytolytic mechanisms of CD8+ CTL in AIDS patients are intact, but that there is a defect in the ability of clonal expansion of anti-HIV CTL precursors.[94] Finally, one study has demonstrated that HIV-infected humans have CD8+ CTL that are capable of killing *uninfected* CD4+ target cells in an MHC-restricted manner.[95]

CD8+ T Cells That Suppress HIV Replication by Secretion of Soluble Factors

CD8+ T-lymphocytes from HIV-infected individuals have been observed to inhibit HIV replication in naturally infected CD4+ cells *in vitro*.[96] This antiviral activity is not mediated by NK cells, is not HLA restricted, and is dependent on the number of CD8+ cells present.[96,97] This type of anti-HIV activity is not mediated through target cell killing, but rather is mediated *via* CD8+ cell secretion of soluble anti-HIV factors.[97-99] Recent studies by Mackewicz *et al* have demonstrated that the gradual decrease of CD8+ T cell antiviral activity over time may be related to progression to AIDS in HIV-infected individuals.[97]

NON-T-CELL–MEDIATED ANTI-HIV CELLULAR IMMUNE RESPONSES

Non-T-cell–mediated immunity, such as is mediated by NK and other FcR+ cells that directly kill virally infected cells or that mediate ADCC (Table 5–3), is potentially very important as an anti-HIV immune response, because these forms of immunity can eliminate virally infected cells in a non-MHC-restricted fashion and do not require a memory T-cell response for effector cell induction.[61,81] Thus, devising ways of augmenting or inducing NK responses against HIV-infected allogeneic cells and/or against malignant cells that arise in the context of AIDS are important areas of research. The role that anti-HIV NK and ADCC activation play in the maintenance of the asymptomatic HIV-seropositive state are unknown. However, recent data have demonstrated decreases in both anti-HIV ADCC and NK effector cell function with progression to AIDS, thus suggesting a pathophysiologic link to the development of AIDS.[58-69]

Although monocytes in AIDS patients have been shown to have a chemotactic defect,[100] monocytes from asymptomatic seropositive subjects have been shown to mediate ADCC against HIV-coated target cells[66] and to mediate monocyte tumoricidal activity *in vitro*—a potential mechanism of immune response against Kaposi's sarcoma and other tumors that occur in AIDS.[100,101]

Immune Responses to HIV in Children

Most current HIV infections in children in the United States occur perinatally.[102] Interestingly, vertical trans-

Table 5–3. Non-T Cell Anti-HIV Cellular Immune Responses

Type of Cellular Responses	Comment	References
Antibody-dependent cellular cytotoxicity (ADCC) mediated by natural killer (NK) cells	Antibodies capable of sensitizing IgG FcR+ NK cells present in high levels in asymptomatic HIV-seropositive subjects; decreased ADCC activity in AIDS due to decrease in NK cell function and decrease in level of anti-HIV ADCC antibodies	58–70, 88
Monocyte-mediated ADCC against HIV-infected cells	Present in peripheral blood monocytes of HIV-infected subjects	66
Monocyte-mediated tumoricidal activity	Present in AIDS patients; ? relevance to control of Kaposi's sarcoma in AIDS	101
NK cell cytotoxic activity for HIV-infected cells	Present early in HIV infection; decreases as AIDS develops; decrease in NK activity related in part to lack of IL-2 production needed for NK cell activation	88, 122, 123

mission of HIV has been correlated with the absence of maternal high-affinity maternal antibodies to the V3 loop of gp120.[103] Most infants born to HIV-positive mothers will passively acquire maternal anti-HIV antibody *in utero,* which may persist up to 15 to 18 months postnatally.[102] In this situation, the polymerase chain reaction (PCR) assay for HIV proviral PNA sequences has been used to detect HIV infection and to distinguish the truly infected infant from the uninfected infant with passively acquired HIV antibody.[104] In children under 12 months of age, AIDS frequently occurs in the presence of higher T-cell levels (500–1,000 cells/mm^3) than are seen in adults with AIDS.[2] However, in older infants and children, anti-HIV immune responses and progressive immune defects that develop over the course of HIV infection are similar to those seen in adults.[2]

PATHOGENIC VERSUS SALUTARY ANTI-HIV IMMUNE RESPONSES

Because of the observations that CD4+ T cells, human monocytes, macrophages, dendritic cells, and Langerhans cells are all capable of infection by HIV *in vivo,* numerous investigators have suggested that one component of the pathogenesis of the immune dysfunction in HIV infection might be immune-mediated damage of HIV-infected T cells and antigen-presenting cells.[11,93,105–108] Moreover, gp120 *env* protein exists in a cell-free soluble form, and it has been proposed that anti-HIV antibody and cellular responses can damage uninfected CD4+ cells that have soluble gp120 bound to the cell surface.[109,110] As mentioned earlier, the presence of enhancing antibody against HIV *env* gp41 has been associated with progressive HIV infection.[8–10] At present it is difficult to determine if anti-HIV immune responses are salutary, destructive, or both. There is reason to speculate that at least in the case of anti-HIV CTL, both salutary and destructive anti-HIV immune responses occur.[11,81] That HIV-specific antibody responses and anti-HIV CTL responses decrease in the wake of

progression to AIDS is suggestive that these immune responses promote the asymptomatic HIV-seropositive state. On the other hand, there is increasing evidence for the involvement of HIV-specific CTL in HIV-induced pulmonary inflammatory disease, CNS disease, and lymphadenitis.[11,81] For example, high numbers of anti-HIV CTL have been isolated from the lungs of HIV-infected patients with lymphocytic alveolitis that are capable of killing HIV-infected macrophages.[111,112] Moreover, the presence of anti-HIV CTL capable of killing a variety of types of HIV-infected antigen-presenting cells in lymph nodes, bone marrow, and thymus supports the notion that, over time, anti-HIV CTL that originally keep HIV infection in check by killing virus-infected cells, by continued killing of antigen-presenting cells and other immune types, could gradually promote progressive immune system dysfunction.[11,81,108]

OVERVIEW OF THE HOST IMMUNE RESPONSE TO HIV

Figure 5–1 summarizes the time course of select types of anti-HIV immune responses in progressive stages of HIV infection. In acute HIV infection, an early plasma viremia of extremely infectious HIV is controlled by the appearance of anti-HIV antibody.[6] Similarly, relatively high numbers of circulating HIV-infected cells are cleared by the onset of the appearance of anti-HIV CD8+ CTL and by NK cells and macrophages mediating anti-HIV ADCC.[11,61,81] It is thought that the asymptomatic phase of HIV infection is maintained by high levels of HIV-neutralizing (and possibly anti-p24) antibodies, anti-HIV MHC-restricted CD8+ CTL, and anti-HIV ADCC-mediated by NK cells and macrophages. Declines in CD4+ T cells, serum anti-p24 antibody levels, anti-MHC class I–restricted CD8+ CTL, and ADCC effector cell function coincident with rises in serum p24 antigen levels and the reappearance of infectious HIV in plasma and PB cells herald the onset of AIDS.[6,11,28,61,81,113,114]

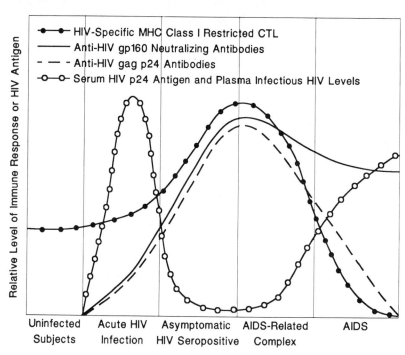

Figure 5–1. Course over time of levels of HIV-specific MHC class I–restricted CTL, anti-HIV gp160 neutralizing antibodies, anti-HIV *gag* p24 antibodies, and p24 antigen and plasma infectious HIV levels.

A central and critical question remains as to why this highly coordinated and multifaceted anti-HIV immune response does not control HIV infection. The answer to this question is not known but likely is related in part to the ability of HIV to be spread *via* cell-cell fusion, the use of the CD4 molecule as the HIV receptor, and the ability of HIV to rapidly mutate *env* and structural protein sequences.

HIV mutants have been isolated from single patients over time that have become resistant to circulating HIV-neutralizing antibodies.[13,15] In other viral systems, CTL-resistant virus mutants have also arisen over time.[115] Moreover, anti-HIV immune responses may fail owing to the inability of effector cells and antigen-presenting cells to contact HIV-infected cells without themselves becoming infected by HIV. Finally, it is likely that the regenerative lymphoid microenvironments such as bone marrow and thymus ultimately fail, owing to infection of nurturing bone marrow and thymus stromal cells[105–108,116] and to HIV infection of lymphoid and myeloid precursors themselves.[117–121] Identification of novel ways of stimulating elevated levels of salutary anti-HIV immune responses either prior to HIV infection or in the early stages of HIV infection remains a high priority of AIDS research.

REFERENCES

1. Fauci AS: The human immunodeficiency virus: Infectivity and mechanisms of pathogenesis. Science 239:617, 1988
2. Stiehm ER, Wara DW: Immunology of HIV. In Pizzo PA, Wilfert CM (eds): Pediatric AIDS: The Challenge of HIV Infection in Infants, Children, and Adolescents, p 95. Baltimore, Williams & Wilkins, 1991
3. Edelman AS, Zolla-Pazner S: AIDS: A syndrome of immune dysregulation, dysfunction, and deficiency. FASEB 3:22, 1989
4. Sattentau QJ: HIV infection and the immune system. Biochem Biophys Acta 989:255, 1989
5. Weiss SH, Goedert JJ, Gartner S et al: Risk of human immunodeficiency virus (HIV-1) infection among laboratory workers. Science 239:68, 1988
6. Clark SJ, Saag MS, Decker WD et al: High titers of cytopathic virus in plasma of patients with symptomatic primary HIV-I infection. N Engl J Med 324:954, 1991
7. Itescu S, Brancato LJ, Buxbaum J et al: A diffuse infiltrative CD8 lymphocytosis syndrome in human immunodeficiency virus (HIV) infection: A host immune response associated with HLA-DR5. Ann Intern Med 112:3, 1990
8. Robinson WE, Montefiori DC, Mitchell WM et al: Antibody-dependent enhancement of human immunodeficiency virus type 1 (HIV-1) infection *in vitro* by serum from HIV-1 infected and passively immunized chimpanzees. Proc Natl Acad Sci USA 86:4710, 1989
9. Robinson WE, Kawamura T, Gorny MK et al: Human monoclonal antibodies to the human immunodeficiency virus type I (HIV-1) transmembrane glycoprotein gp41 enhance HIV-1 infection *in vitro*. Proc Natl Acad Sci USA 87:3815, 1990
10. Homsy J, Meyer M, Levy JA: Serum enhancement of human immunodeficiency virus (HIV) infection correlates with disease in HIV-infected individuals. J Virol 64:1437, 1990
11. Plata F, Dadaglio G, Chenciner N et al: Cytotoxic T lymphocytes in HIV-induced disease: Implications for therapy and vaccination. Immunodefic Rev 1:227, 1989
12. Reitz MS, Wilson C, Naugle C et al: Generation of a neutralization-resistant variant of HIV-I is due to selection for a point mutation in the envelope gene. Cell 54:57, 1988

13. McKeating JA, Gow J, Goutsmit J et al: Characterization of HIV-I neutralization escape mutants. AIDS 3:777, 1989

14. Masuda T, Matsushita S, Kuroda MJ et al: Generation of neutralization-resistant HIV-I *in vitro* due to amino acid interchanges of third hypervariable env region. J Immunol 145:3240, 1990

15. Albert J, Abrahamsson B, Nagy K et al: Rapid development of isolate-specific-neutralizing antibodies after primary HIV-I infection and consequent emergence of virus variants which resist neutralization by autologous sera. AIDS 4:107, 1990

16. Berman PW, Gregory TJ, Riddle L et al: Protection of chimpanzees from infection by HIV-I after vaccination with recombinant glycoprotein gp120 but not gp160. Nature 345:622, 1990

17. Emini EA, Nara PL, Schleif WA et al: Antibody-mediated *in vitro* neutralization of human immunodeficiency virus type 1 abolishes infectivity for chimpanzees. J Virol 64:3674, 1990

18. Girard M, Kieny MP, Pinter A et al: Immunization of chimpanzees confers protection against challenge with human immunodeficiency virus. Proc Natl Acad Sci USA 88:542, 1991

19. Cooper DA, Gold J, MacLean P et al: Acute AIDS retrovirus infection. Lancet 1:537, 1985

20. Ho DD, Sarngadharan MG, Resnick L et al: Primary human T lymphotropic virus type III infection. Ann Intern Med 103:880, 1985

21. Goudsmit J, de Wolf F, Paul DA et al: Expression of human immunodeficiency virus antigen (HIV-Ag) in serum and cerebrospinal fluid during acute and chronic infection. Lancet 2:177, 1986

22. Allain J-P, Lauvian Y, Paul DA, Senn D: Serological markers in early stages of human immunodeficiency virus infection in hemophiliacs. Lancet 2:1233, 1986

23. Gaines H, Albert J, von Sydow M et al: HIV antigenemia and virus isolation from plasma during primary HIV infection. Lancet 1:1317, 1987

24. Albert J, Gaines H, Sonnerborg A et al: Isolation of human immunodeficiency virus (HIV) from plasma during primary HIV infection. J Med Virol 23:67, 1987

25. Wall RA, Denning DW, Amos A: HIV antigenemia in acute HIV infection. Lancet 1:566, 1987

26. Paul DA, Falk LA, Kessler HA et al: Correlation of serum HIV antigen and antibody with clinical status in HIV-infected patients. J Med Virol 22:357, 1987

27. von Sydow M, Gaines H, Sonnerborg A et al: Antigen detection in primary HIV infection. Br Med J 296:238, 1988

28. Daar ES, Moudgil T, Meyer RD, Ho DD: Transient high levels of viremia in patients with primary human immunodeficiency virus type 1 infection. N Engl J Med 324:961, 1991

29. Imagawa DT, Lee MH, Wolinsky SM et al: Human immunodeficiency virus type 1 infection in homosexual men who remain seronegative for prolonged periods. N Engl J Med 320:1458, 1989

30. Matthews TJ, Langlois AJ, Robey WG et al: Restricted neutralization of divergent human T-lymphotropic virus type III isolates by antibodies to the major envelope glycoprotein. Proc Natl Acad Sci USA 83:9709, 1986

31. Weiss RA, Clapham RP, Cheingsong-Popov R et al: Neutralization of human T-lymphotropic virus type III by sera of AIDS and AIDS-risk patients. Nature 316:69, 1985

32. Robert-Guroff M, Brown M, Gallo RC: HTLV-III-neutralizing antibodies in patients with AIDS and AIDS-related complex. Nature 316:72, 1985

33. Weiss RA, Clapham PR, Weber JN et al: Variable and conserved neutralization antigens of human immunodeficiency virus. Nature 324:572, 1986

34. Putney SD, Matthews TJ, Robey WG et al: HTLV-III/LAV-neutralization antibodies to an *E. coli*-produced fragment of the virus envelope. Science 234:1392, 1986

35. Palker TJ, Clark ME, Langlois AJ et al: Type-specific neutralization of the human immunodeficiency virus with antibodies to env-encoded synthetic peptides. Proc Natl Acad Sci USA 85:1932, 1988

36. Rusche JR, Javaherian K, McDanal C et al: Antibodies that inhibit fusion of human immunodeficiency virus–infected cells bind a 24 amino acid sequence of the viral envelope gp120. Proc Natl Acad Sci USA 85:3198, 1988

37. Goudsmit J, Debouck C, MeLeon RH et al: Human immunodeficiency virus type 1 neutralization with conserved architecture elicts early type-specific antibodies in experimentally infected chimpanzees. Proc Natl Acad Sci USA 85:4478, 1988

38. Nara PL, Robey WG, Arthur LV et al: Persistent infection of chimpanzees with human immunodeficiency virus: Serological responses and properties of reisolated viruses. J Virol 61:3173, 1987

39. Goudsmit J, Thiriart C, Smit L et al: Temporal development of cross-neutralization between HTLV-IIIB and HTLV-IIIRF in experimentally infected chimpanzees. Vaccine 6:229, 1986

40. Ho DD, Sarngadharan MG, Hirsh MS et al: Human immunodeficiency virus neutralizing antibodies recognize several conserved domains on the envelope glycoproteins. J Virol 61:2024, 1987

41. Weiss RA, Clapham PR, McClure MO et al: Human immunodeficiency viruses: Neutralization and receptors. J AIDS 1:536, 1988

42. Putney SD, Javaherin K, Rusche J et al: Features of the HIV envelope and development of a subunit vaccine. In Putney SD, Bolognesi DP (eds): AIDS Vaccine: Basic Research and Clinical Trials, p 3. New York, Marcel Dekker, 1989

43. Sarin PS, Sun DK, Thornton AH et al: Neutralization of HTLV-III/LAV replication by antiserum to thymosin α1. Science 232:1135, 1986

44. Palker TJ, Matthews TJ, Langlois AJ et al: Polyvalent human immunodeficiency virus synthetic immunogen comprised of envelope gp120 T helper cell sites and B cell neutralization epitopes. J Immunol 142:3612, 1989

45. Javaherian K, Langlois AJ, McDanal C et al: Principal neutralizing domain of the human immunodeficiency virus type 1 envelope protein. Proc Natl Acad Sci USA 86:6768, 1989

46. Hattori T, Koito A, Takasuki K et al: Involvement of tryptase-related cellular protease(s) in human immunodeficiency virus type 1 infection. FEBS Lett 248:48, 1989

47. Kido H, Fukutomi A, Katanuma N: A novel membrane-bound serine esterase in human T4+ lymphocytes immunologically reactive with antibody inhibiting syncytia induced by HIV-I. J Biol Chem 265:21979, 1990

48. Clements GJ, Price-Jones MJ, Stephens PE et al: The V3 loops of the HIV-1 and HIV-2 surface glycoproteins contain proteolytic cleavage sites: A possible function in viral fusion? AIDS Res Hum Retroviruses 7:3, 1991

49. Profy AT, Salinas PA, Eckler LI et al: Epitopes recognized

by the neutralizing antibodies of an HIV-1 infected individual. J Immunol 144:4641, 1990

50. Back NKT, Thiriart C, Delers A et al: Association of antibodies blocking HIV-1 gp160-sCD4 attachment with virus neutralizing activity in human sera. J Med Virol 31:200, 1990

51. Hansen JS, Clausen H, Nielsen C et al: Inhibition of HIV infection *in vitro* by anti-carbohydrate monoclonal antibodies: Peripheral glycosylation of HIV envelope glycoprotein gp120 may be a target for virus neutralization. J Virol 64:2833, 1990

52. Weber JN, Weiss RA, Robert C et al: Human immunodeficiency virus infection in two cohorts of homosexual men: Neutralizing sera and association of anti-gag antibody with prognosis. Lancet 1:119, 1987

53. Sei Y, Tsang PH, Chu FN et al: Inverse relationship between HIV-1 p24 antigenemia, anti-p24 antibody and neutralizing antibody response in all stages of HIV-1 infection. Immunol Lett 20:223, 1989

54. Alesi DR, Ajello D, Lupo G et al: Neutralizing antibody and clinical status of human immunodeficiency virus (HIV)–infected individuals. J Med Virol 27:7, 1989

55. Boucher CAB, de Wolf F, Houweling JTM et al: Antibody response to a synthetic peptide covering a LAV-1/HTLV-IIIB neutralization epitope and disease progression. AIDS 3:71, 1989

56. Berkower I, Smith GE, Giri C, Murphey D: Human immunodeficiency virus 1: Predominance of a group-specific neutralizing epitope that persists despite genetic variation. J Exp Med 170:1681, 1989

57. Katzenstein DA, Vujcil LK, Latif A et al: Human immunodeficiency virus neutralizing antibodies in sera from North Americans and Africans. J AIDS 3:810, 1990

58. Lyerly HK, Matthews TJ, Langlois AJ et al: Human T-cell lymphotropic virus IIIB glycoprotein (gp120) bound to CD4 determinants on normal lymphocytes and expressed by infected cells serves as a target for immune attack. Proc Natl Acad Sci USA 84:4601, 1987

59. Ojo-Amaize EA, Nishanian P, Keith DE et al: Antibodies to human immunodeficiency virus in human sera induce cell-mediated lysis of human immunodeficiency virus-infected cells. J Immunol 139:2458, 1987

60. Weinhold KJ, Lyerly HK, Matthews TJ et al: Cellular anti-gp120 reactivities in HIV-1 seropositive individuals. Lancet 1:902, 1988

61. Tyler DS, Lyerly HK, Weinhold KJ: Anti-HIV-1 ADCC. AIDS Res Hum Retroviruses 5:557, 1989

62. Tyler DS, Stanley SD, Nastala CA et al: Alterations in antibody-dependent cellular cytotoxicity during the course of HIV infection. J Immunol 144:3375, 1990

63. Tyler DS, Stanley SD, Zolla-Pazner S et al: Identification of sites within gp41 that serve as target for antibody-dependent cellular cytotoxicity by using human monoclonal antibodies. J Immunol 145:3276, 1990

64. Ljunggren K, Chiodi F, Broliden PA et al: HIV-1 specific antibodies in cerebral spinal fluid mediate cellular cytotoxicity and neutralization. AIDS Res Hum Retroviruses 5:629, 1989

65. Emskoetter T, Laer DV, Veismann S, Ermer M: HIV-specific antibodies, neutralizing activity and ADCC in the cerebrospinal fluid of HIV-infected patients. J Neuroimmunol 24:61, 1989

66. Jewett A, Giorgi JV, Bonavida B: Antibody dependent cellular cytotoxicity against HIV-coated target cells by peripheral blood monocytes from HIV seropositive asymptomatic patients. J Immunol 145:4065, 1990

67. Koup RA, Sullivan JL, Levine PH et al: Antigenic specificity of antibody-dependent cell-mediated cytotoxicity directed against human immunodeficiency virus in antibody positive sera. J Virol 63:584, 1989

68. Tanneau F, McChesney M, Lopez O et al: Primary cytotoxicity against the envelope glycoprotein of human immunodeficiency virus-1: Evidence for antibody dependent cellular cytotoxicity *in vivo*. J Infect Dis 162:837, 1990

69. Ljunggren K, Karlson A, Fenyo EM et al: Natural and antibody-dependent cytotoxicity in different clinical stages of human immunodeficiency virus type 1 infection. Clin Exp Immunol 75:184, 1989

70. Ojo-Amaize E, Nishanian PG, Heitjan DF et al: Serum and effector-cell antibody-dependent cellular cytotoxicity (ADCC) activity remains high during human immunodeficiency virus (HIV) disease progression. J Clin Immunol 9:454, 1989

71. Reiss P, DeRonde A, Lange JMA et al: Low antigenicity of HIV-1 rev: rev-specific antibody response of limited value as correlate of rev gene expression and disease progression. AIDS Res Hum Retroviruses 5:621, 1989

72. Reiss P, de Ronde A, Lange JMA et al: Antibody response to the viral negative factor (nef) in HIV-1 infection: A correlate of levels of HIV-1 expression. AIDS 3:227, 1989

73. Boucher CAB, DeJager MH, Debouck C et al: Antibody response to human immunodeficiency virus type 1 protease according to risk group and disease stage. J Clin Microbiol 27:1577, 1989

74. Reiss P, Lange JMA, de Ronde A et al: Antibody response to viral proteins U (vpu) and R (vpr) in HIV-1-infected individuals. J AIDS 3:115, 1990

75. Reiss P, Lange JMA, de Ronde A et al: Speed of progression to AIDS and degree of antibody response to accessory gene products of HIV-1. J Med Virol 30:163, 1990

76. Ameisen JC, Guy B, Lecocq JP et al: Persistent antibody response to the HIV-1 negative regulatory factor in HIV-1 infected seronegative persons. N Engl J Med 320:251, 1989

77. Clerici M, Stocks NI, Zajac RA et al: Interleukin-2 production used to detect antigenic peptide recognition by T-helper lymphocytes from asymptomatic HIV-seropositive individuals. Nature 339:383, 1989

78. Schrier RD, Gnann JW, Landes R et al: T cell recognition of HIV synthetic peptides in a natural infection. J Immunol 142:1166, 1989

79. Cease KB, Margaut H, Cornette JL et al: Helper T cell antigenic site identification in the acquired immunodeficiency syndrome virus gp120 envelope protein and induction of immunity in mice to the native protein using a 16-residue synthetic peptide. Proc Natl Acad Sci USA 84:4249, 1987

80. Torseth JW, Berman PW, Merigan TC: Recombinant HIV structural proteins detect specific cellular immunity *in vitro* in infected individuals. AIDS Res Hum Retroviruses 4:23, 1988

81. Walker BD, Plata F: Cytotoxic T lymphocytes against HIV. AIDS 4:177, 1990

82. Walker BD, Chakrabarti S, Moss B et al: HIV-specific cytotoxic T lymphocytes in seropositive individuals. Nature 328:345, 1987

83. Nixon DF, Townsend ARM, Elvin JG et al: HIV-I gag-specific cytotoxic T lymphocytes defined with recombi-

nant vaccinia virus and synthetic peptides. Nature 336:484, 1988

84. Clerici M, Lucey DR, Zajac RA et al: Detection of cytotoxic T lymphocytes specific for synthetic peptides of gp160 in HIV-seropositive individuals. J Immunol 146:2214, 1991

85. Hosmalin A, Cleric M, Houghten R et al: An epitope in human immunodeficiency virus 1 reverse transcriptase recognized by both mouse and human cytotoxic T lymphocytes. Proc Natl Acad Sci USA 87:2344, 1990

86. Koenig S, Fuerst TR, Wood LV et al: Mapping the fine specificity of a cytolytic T cell response to HIV-1 nef protein. J Immunol 145:127, 1990

87. Koup RA, Sullivan JL, Levine PH et al: Detection of major histocompatibility complex class I restricted HIV-specific cytotoxic T lymphocytes in the blood of infected hemophiliacs. Blood 73:1909, 1989

88. Riviere P, Tanneau-Salvadori F, Regnault A et al: Human immunodeficiency virus–specific cytotoxic responses of seropositive individuals: Distinct types of effector cells mediate killing of targets expressing gag and env proteins. J Virol 63:2270, 1989

89. Hoffenbach A, Langlade-Demoyen P, Dadaglio G et al: Unusually high frequencies of HIV-specific cytotoxic T lymphocytes in humans. J Immunol 142:452, 1989

90. Morrison LA, Braciale VL, Braciale TJ: Distinguishable pathways of viral antigen presentation to T lymphocytes. Immunol Res 5:294, 1986

91. Sethi KK, Naher H, Strehmann I: Phenotypic heterogeneity of cerebrospinal fluid-derived HIV-specific and HLA-restricted cytotoxic T cell clones. Nature 335:178, 1988

92. Orentas RJ, Hildreth JEK, Obah E et al: Induction of CD4+ human cytolytic T cell specific for HIV infected cells by a gp160 subunit vaccine. Science 248:1234, 1990

93. Siliciano RF, Lawton T, Knall C et al: Analysis of host-virus interactions in AIDS with anti-gp120 T cell clones: Effect of HIV sequence variation and a mechanism for CD4+ cell depletion. Cell 54:561, 1988

94. Pantaleo G, DeMaria A, Koenig S et al: CD8+ T lymphocytes of patients with AIDS maintain normal broad cytolytic function despite the loss of human immunodeficiency virus–specific cytotoxicity. Proc Natl Acad Sci USA 87:4818, 1990

95. Zarling JM, Ledbetter JA, Sias J et al: HIV-infected humans, but not chimpanzees, have circulating cytotoxic T lymphocytes that lyse uninfected CD4+ cells. J Immunol 144:2992, 1990

96. Walker CM, Moody DJ, Stites DP, Levy JA: CD8+ lymphocytes can control HIV infection *in vitro* by suppressing virus replication. Science 234:1563, 1986

97. Mackewicz CE, Ortega HW, Levy JA: CD8+ cell anti-HIV activity correlates with the clinical state of the infected individual. J Clin Invest 87:1462, 1991

98. Laurence J, Gottlieb AB, Kunkel HG: Soluble suppressor factors in patients with acquired immune deficiency syndrome and its prodrome. J Clin Invest 12:2072, 1983

99. Siegel JP, Djeu JY, Stocks NI et al: Sera from patients with the acquired immunodeficiency syndrome inhibit production of interleukin-2 by normal lymphocytes. J Clin Invest 75:1957, 1985

100. Smith PD, Ohura K, Masur H et al: Monocyte function in the acquired immune deficiency syndrome: Defective chemotaxis. J Clin Invest 74:2121, 1984

101. Kleinerman ES, Ceccorulli LM, Zwelling LA et al: Activation of monocyte-mediated tumoricidal activity in patients with acquired immunodeficiency syndrome. J Clin Oncol 3:1005, 1985

102. Rogers MF, Ou CY, Kilbourne B, Schochet MAN: Advances and problems in the diagnosis of HIV infection in infants. In Pizzo PA, Wilfert CM (eds): Pediatric AIDS: The Challenge of HIV Infection in Infants, Children and Adolescents, p 159. Baltimore, William & Wilkins, 1991

103. DeVosh Y, Calvelli TA, Wood DG et al: Vertical transmission of human immunodeficiency virus is correlated with the absence of high affinity/avidity maternal antibodies to the gp120 principal neutralizing domain. Proc Natl Acad Sci USA 87:3445, 1990

104. Rogers MF, Ou CY, Rayfield M et al: Use of the polymerase chain reaction for early detection of the proviral sequences of human immunodeficiency virus in infants born of seropositive mothers. N Engl J Med 320:1649, 1989

105. Tschachler E, Groh V, Popovic M et al: Epidermal Langerhan's cells: A target for HTLV-III/LAV infection. J Invest Dermatol 88:233, 1987

106. Macatonia SE, Patterson S, Knight SC: Suppression of immune responses by dendritic cells infected with HIV. Immunology 67:285, 1989

107. Laman JD, Claassen E, Von Rooijen N, Boersma WMJ: Immune complexes on follicular dendritic cells as a target for cytotoxic cells in AIDS. AIDS 3:543, 1989

108. Macatonia SE, Lau R, Patterson S et al: Dendritic cell infection, depletion and dysfunction in HIV infected individuals. Immunology 71:38, 1990

109. Weinhold KJ, Lyerly HK, Stanley SD et al: HIV-I-mediated immune suppression and lymphocyte destruction in the absence of viral infection. J Immunol 142:3091, 1989

110. Manca F, Habeshaw JA, Dalgleish AG: HIV envelope glycoprotein, antigens specific T-cell responses and soluble CD4. Lancet 335:811, 1990

111. Guillon JM, Autran B, Devis M et al: HIV-related lymphocytic alveolitis. Chest 94:1264, 1988

112. Autran B, Joly P, Guillon JM et al: T cell mediated cytotoxicity against HIV in seropositive patients: A physicopathological approach. Res Immunol [Ann Inst Pasteur] 140:103, 1989

113. O'Shea S, Cordery M, Barrett WY et al: HIV excretion patterns and specific antibody responses in body fluids. J Med Virol 31:291, 1990

114. Schnittman SM, Greenhouse JJ, Psallidopoulos MC et al: Increasing viral burden in CD4+ T cells from patients with HIV infection reflects rapidly progressive immunosuppression and clinical disease. Ann Intern Med 113:438, 1990

115. Pircher H, Moskophidis D, Rohrer U et al: Viral escape by selection of cytotoxic T cell-resistant virus variants *in vivo*. Nature 346:629, 1990

116. Numazaki K, Bai XQ, Goldman H et al: Infection of cultured human thymic epithelial cells by human immunodeficiency virus. Clin Immunol Immunopathol 51:185, 1989

117. Schnittman SM, Denning SM, Greenhouse JJ et al: Evidence for susceptibility of intrathymic T cell precursors and their TCRαβ+ and TCRγδ+ progeny to human immunodeficiency virus infection: A mechanism for T4 (CD4) lymphocyte depletion. Proc Natl Acad Sci USA 87:7727, 1990

118. DeRossi A, Calabro ML, Panozzo M et al: *In vitro* studies of HIV-1 infection in thymic lymphocytes: A putative role

of the thymus in AIDS pathogenesis. AIDS Res Hum Retroviruses 6:287, 1990

119. Tremblay M, Numazaki K, Goldman H, Wainberg MA: Infection of human thymic lymphocytes by HIV-1. J AIDS 3:356, 1990

120. Lewis SH, Reynolds-Kohler C, Fox HE, Nelson JA: HIV-1 in trophoblastic and villous Hofbauer cells and haematological precursors in eight week fetuses. Lancet 335: 565, 1990

121. Folks TM, Kessler SW, Orenstein JM et al: Infection and replication of HIV-1 in purified progenitor cells of normal human bone marrow. Science 242:919, 1988

122. Bonavida B, Katz J, Gottlieb M: Mechanism of defective NK cell activity in patients with acquired immunodeficiency syndrome (AIDS) and AIDS-related complex. J Immunol 137:1157, 1986

123. Mansour I, Doinel C, Rouger P: CD16+ NK cells decrease in all stages of HIV infection through a selective depletion of the CD16+ CD8+ CD3+ subset. AIDS Res Hum Retroviruses 6:1451, 1990

II

Epidemiology

6

Global Aspects of the HIV Epidemic

Jonathan M. Mann   *Seth L. Welles*

The early history of the human immunodeficiency virus (HIV) pandemic (pre-1981) remains obscure. Despite individual case reports of apparent HIV infection and disease from the 1960s, the substantial and worldwide spread of HIV appears to have started in the mid- to late-1970s.[1-4]

Following the reports of Kaposi's sarcoma[5,6] and *Pneumocystis carinii* pneumonia[7,8] among young, previously healthy homosexual men in California and New York, epidemiologists rapidly determined the routes of HIV transmission,[9] well before the etiologic agent was first identified. The development by epidemiologists of the information required by public health authorities for comprehensive and rational prevention guidelines, by early 1983, represents a public health triumph. That no additional or unsuspected routes of transmission have since been discovered is further testimony to the power of epidemiology as a science in the service of public health.

At the start of the second decade of work against the pandemic, both the accomplishments and limitations of the global epidemiology of HIV and acquired immunodeficiency syndrome (AIDS) should be acknowledged. In the past several years, important changes have occurred on two levels. First, the epidemic has evolved and expanded, both in geographic and in societal terms. Second, epidemiologists' understanding and conceptualization of the pandemic has evolved, owing both to changes in the pandemic and to building on earlier work. This chapter discusses the evolving global aspects of the HIV epidemic by considering first the development of case definitions and surveillance and then the global geography of HIV/AIDS.

CASE DEFINITIONS AND SURVEILLANCE

The original case definition, developed by the Centers for Disease Control (CDC) in 1981,[10] was revised twice, in 1985 and again in 1987.[11,12] For international purposes, in 1985 the World Health Organization (WHO) decided to propose two definitions of AIDS. First, the CDC (CDC/WHO) definition was recommended for those countries with the technical infrastructure required for its full utilization. Then, for other areas, particularly in Africa, where HIV testing and reliable diagnostic methods to confirm opportunistic infections and malignancies were frequently unavailable, a clinical case definition was proposed, based exclusively on signs and symptoms.

The first clinical definition, developed in late 1985 during a workshop in Bangui, Central African Republic, and subsequently known as the Bangui definition, was found to be fairly specific in African countries when HIV seroprevalence exceeded several percentage points.[13-15] However, the increasing availability of HIV serologic testing, the low specificity of the clinical definition in many countries, and the disappointingly low specificity of the pediatric variant of the Bangui definition all led to a decrease in its use.

In 1989 a new definition was proposed for Latin America and the Caribbean that reflected further experience with HIV disease and its manifestations in this region and combined features of both the CDC/WHO definition and the Bangui definition.[16]

Therefore, at present, there is no uniform, globally

applicable AIDS case definition. The CDC definition has been criticized for failure to include certain conditions, among them active pulmonary tuberculosis, other causes of death among injectable drug users, and gynecologic conditions such as cervical intraepithelial neoplasia, vaginal candidiasis, and pelvic inflammatory disease. More recently, the CDC developed a proposal to base the AIDS case definition on the CD4 cell count (pers. commun., James Curran, M.D., June 18, 1991). With the limited availability of reliable CD4 testing capability worldwide, this would likely result in the coexistence of four AIDS case definitions: the Bangui definition, the Caracas (Caribbean) definition, the current WHO/CDC definition based on indicator diseases, and a laboratory-based CD4 definition.

AIDS case surveillance is complicated not only by these persisting definitional complexities but also by problems of incomplete and delayed reporting.[17] The completeness of AIDS case reporting is adversely affected by logistic problems, a lack of a tradition of disease reporting to public health authorities in many areas, and personal or political secretiveness.[18] AIDS case reporting in the developing world, particularly in Africa, has been estimated to be only 10% to 20% complete.[18] Finally, the limited contribution of AIDS case reporting to an accurate understanding of the current status of the HIV epidemic remains a point of substantial misunderstanding.

Efforts to develop estimates of HIV seroprevalence have proceeded through several stages. Initial reports from virtually all countries involved seroprevalence studies from convenience samples, such as blood donors,[19] women attending prenatal clinics,[20,21] military recruits,[22] small groups of accessible commercial sex workers[23,24] and homosexual men,[25,26] and clients of sexually transmitted disease clinics.[23,27,28] These data were rapidly recognized to be of limited generalizability because of selection and participation bias. For example, whereas all military recruits could be tested for HIV status, knowledge that such testing (with its substantial personal and societal consequences) would be performed could motivate prospective recruits to avoid military service.[29] In addition, when HIV testing was proposed on a voluntary basis, those most likely to be HIV infected tended to refuse testing.[30] Thus, whereas voluntary prenatal testing has had high acceptability in Sweden, several studies on people attending prenatal and sexually transmitted disease clinics in the United States have documented a severalfold greater seroprevalence among those who refused voluntary testing (in these studies, blood from refusers was tested in an anonymous, unlinked manner).[30] Therefore, although longitudinal follow-up of large convenience sample populations has been useful, initial national seroprevalence estimates based on convenience sample surveys tended to be too high and required subsequent downward adjustment.[31]

A second approach, intended to avoid the bias of convenience samples, was to perform national serosurveys based on probability sampling. Two countries, Rwanda and Uganda, have completed such surveys. In Rwanda,[32] a modified cluster design was used, based on immunization coverage survey methodology. In this survey, only 1.6% of urban residents and 2.6% of rural residents refused to allow blood to be drawn. The survey fieldwork was completed in 10 days, the total cost was less than $50,000, and the results were published in 1989. In contrast, the Uganda national survey[33] required at least one year to complete and results were unavailable or unpublished for several years, although an estimate of 1 million HIV-infected Ugandans in mid-1989 was published in Ugandan newspapers. In the United States, feasibility studies for a national seroprevalence survey confirmed that the combination of participation bias and cost militated strongly against this approach.

Although individual reporting of HIV infections is mandatory or promoted in various countries, these reports appear to be of marginal value for projecting the size of the HIV-infected population. More recently, efforts to develop national seroprevalence estimates have been based on "families of surveys," as is done in the United States,[34] on back-calculations from reported AIDS cases,[35] or on extrapolations from the large number of available convenience sample surveys.[36] More recently, the development and application of targeted surveillance strategies has tended to replace the earlier effort at estimating the numbers of HIV-infected people in an entire population. Sentinel surveillance, in which specific groups are routinely sampled,[36] lot quality analysis, intended to detect if a predetermined HIV seroprevalence has yet occurred, and unlinked anonymous screening are examples of such approaches.[37,38] Cohort studies, while extremely useful for evaluating incidence rate and the impact of intervention programs, may not provide generalizable data.

In summary, the development of local, national, and international estimates of the numbers of HIV-infected people is essential for projecting future needs for care and support. However, generic problems in determining national prevalence, especially for a "moving target," are compounded by the profound personal and societal implications of HIV infection and the associated logistic, legal and ethical issues. At present a combination of approaches—the "family of surveys" concept—seems best adapted to providing reasonable estimates for health and social service planning purposes. Targeted surveillance strategies that take into account the practical objective and utility of the data to be collected are increasingly emphasized.

THE GLOBAL GEOGRAPHY OF HIV/AIDS

In mid-1991, WHO estimates that approximately 10 million people are HIV-infected worldwide.[39] HIV infections are far from uniformly distributed. Of the HIV-infected people, at least 6 million are in Africa, at least

2 million in the Americas, 1 million in Asia and Oceania, and 0.5 million in Europe. Of the 10 million, over 6 million are men and slightly under 4 million are women. Approximately 75% of HIV infections are estimated to have been heterosexually transmitted (with a 4:1 heterosexual to homosexual ratio), 10% are linked with injectable drug use, 10% have been perinatally transmitted, and the remaining 5% have been transmitted through contact with infected blood, principally in therapeutic settings (transfusions, administration of clotting factor to people with hemophilia, reuse of needles and other invasive equipment in formal and informal health care systems).

As of June 1, 1991, a cumulative total of 366,455 AIDS cases had been reported officially to WHO from 162 countries, including 52 countries in Africa, 45 in the Americas, 37 in Asia and Oceania, and 28 in Europe.[40] Only 18 countries or territories continue to report zero AIDS cases (one country each in Africa and Europe and 16 countries in Asia and Oceania). However, the actual cumulative number of adults who have developed AIDS is estimated to exceed 1 million; and as approximately 500,000 children are also thought to have developed AIDS, the cumulative global total of people with AIDS is at least 1.5 million.[41]

Three general features of the global epidemic of HIV/AIDS merit attention: HIV infection continues to spread in already affected areas; HIV is spreading, sometimes quite rapidly, to and within areas that were apparently unaffected or little affected by the pandemic; and as the epidemic matures in a specific community or country, it becomes more societally complex. Together, these features emphasize the general theme of differentiation: the HIV/AIDS pandemic has become an extremely complex mosaic composed of thousands of smaller epidemics, with sometimes independent but often interdependent dynamics.

The spread of HIV in already affected areas can be readily illustrated. In Abidjan, Côte d'Ivoire, HIV seroprevalence increased from about 1% in 1987 to over 7% by early 1991.[42] In Honduras, surveys among women commercial sex workers documented an increase in HIV prevalence from 20% to 45% from 1989 to 1990.[43]

The extension of the HIV pandemic to previously unaffected or little affected geographic areas has been most dramatic and is best documented in Southeast Asia. In Thailand in late 1987, approximately 1% of injectable drug users in Bangkok were HIV infected[44]; by 1990, a median of 32% of injectable drug users nationwide had become infected.[45] In the mid-1980s, HIV infections among women commercial sex workers in Bangkok were rarely reported; in mid-1990, nationwide surveys documented a median seroprevalence of nearly 10%.[45] Thus, with an estimate of 400,000 HIV-infected people,[39] in less than 5 years the HIV epidemic in Thailand has become approximately ten times larger than the HIV epidemic in the United Kingdom. Also, national averages can conceal dramatic developments at a local level. For example, in the northern Thai city of Chiengrai, the

proportion of women commercial sex workers who were HIV infected increased from 1% in October 1988 to 64% in June 1990.[45] Therefore, as already demonstrated among injectable drug users in New York City[46] and Milan,[47] among male homosexuals in San Francisco,[48] and among commercial sex workers in Nairobi[49] and Kigali,[50] an extremely high HIV seroincidence (exceeding 10% annually) can occur in any population group when the virus is present and the behaviors transmitting infection are sufficiently prevalent and intense.

The third theme of differentiation involves the epidemic's tendency to become societally complex within each population group. For example, while HIV seroprevalence in rural sub-Saharan Africa was generally less than 1% (with dramatic exceptions such as the Kagera region of Tanzania, or the Rakai district of Uganda), HIV is now spreading widely in rural Africa. In Côte d'Ivoire, 5% of rural adult residents are now HIV infected,[51] and the HIV seroprevalence among pregnant women in rural Zaire is estimated at 4%.[52]

Regardless of which risk-behavior group may be initially infected, HIV spreads to other populations. For example, in many areas of Latin America, homosexual men were initially most severely affected; however, by the mid-1980s, an increasing proportion of AIDS cases involved women.[53] For example, in Mexico, the male-to-female sex ratio of AIDS cases was 16:1 in 1985, but it had declined to 4:1 in 1990.[54] Increased awareness of the widespread distribution of risk behaviors for HIV transmission (only about 1 million of the estimated 5 million injectable drug users worldwide are thus far HIV infected, and the WHO recently estimated that 250 million new sexually transmitted infections occur each year worldwide),[39] combined with the long infectious period of HIV, suggests that HIV will eventually reach most if not all human communities and that within each community, the epidemiology of infection will become more complex over time.

The Americas

All of the 45 countries in the Americas have reported at least one case of AIDS to the Pan American Health Organization (PAHO/WHO); as of January 31, 1991, a total of 192,616 cases had been reported, of which 157,525 (82%) were from the United States.[55]

NORTH AMERICA

In the United States, approximately 1 million people are estimated to be HIV infected. As of May 1, 1991, 171,876 AIDS cases had been reported to WHO.[56] As of January 1, 1991, almost 100,000 people with AIDS had died[55]; by 1989, AIDS had become the second leading cause of death among U.S. men ages 20 to 45 years, and in 1991, AIDS is expected to become the fifth leading cause of death among U.S. women in the same age group.[35] Major features of the epidemic in the United

States, including its evolving racial/ethnic, socioeconomic, and risk-behavior profile, are presented elsewhere in this book.

In Canada, as of May 6, 1991, a total of 4,885 AIDS cases had been reported to the Federal Centre for AIDS, of which 4,826 (98.8%) were in adults; of these, 4,579 (94.9%) were in men.[57] In contrast to the United States, among adult men with AIDS, 83% reported homosexual/bisexual activity, 4% reported both homosexual/bisexual activity and injectable drug use, and only 1% reported injectable drug use as their sole risk factor.[57] Among Canadian women with AIDS, heterosexual activity was the major risk behavior, accounting for 69% of infections, while injectable drug use was reported by only 6%. Even when women from pattern II countries are excluded from the analysis, heterosexual activity remains the major risk behavior, accounting for 51% of HIV-infected women with an identified risk factor.[57] The national cumulative AIDS case rate is 186.3 per million, with provincial rates ranging from a high of 300.2 per million (British Columbia) to a low of 23.1 per million (Prince Edward Island); nevertheless, 70% of AIDS cases are reported from Ontario and Quebec provinces. As in the United States, the rate of increase in new AIDS cases has declined since 1987.

LATIN AMERICA AND THE CARIBBEAN

PAHO estimates that approximately 1 million people are HIV infected in Latin America and the Caribbean, of whom at least 150,000 are women.[55] According to these figures, one in every 125 men and one in every 500 women ages 15 to 49 years in Latin America and the Caribbean are estimated to be HIV infected.

In these areas, the largest proportion of reported AIDS cases is from Brazil (43%), followed by Mexico (17%), the Latin Caribbean (12%; Cuba, Dominican Republic, Haiti), the Andean area (9%; Bolivia, Colombia, Ecuador, Peru, Venezuela); the Caribbean (8%); the Central American isthmus (6%); and the southern cone (4%; Argentina, Chile, Paraguay, Uruguay).[58] Highest AIDS case rates (per 100,000 population) are found in the small islands (e.g., the 1989 rates were 68.6 for the Bahamas, 61.4 for Bermuda, and 15.3 for the Barbados).[59]

In the Caribbean, through December 1990, the largest transmission category was "other/unknown" (46%), which reflects societal pressure and concerns about stigmatization. Heterosexual transmission accounted for 32%, homosexual or bisexual contact for 17%, perinatal transmission for 5%, blood (transfusion and people with hemophilia) for 0.5%, and injectable drug use for only 0.1%. In contrast, in North America, 58% of AIDS cases are attributed to homosexual or bisexual transmission, 21% to injectable drug use, 10% to "other/unknown," 5% to heterosexual contact, 3% to blood, and 1% to perinatal transmission.[55]

In the Caribbean, a major shift in the risk category of AIDS cases has been reported, away from a predominance of homosexual/bisexual transmission in the early 1980s.[59,60] By mid-1986, the proportion of AIDS cases attributable to heterosexual transmission exceeded the proportion associated with homosexual/bisexual transmission, and reached 65% in 1989 (compared with 13% in 1985).[59] Thus, in Haiti, the male-female ratio of AIDS cases declined from 3:1 in 1983 to 1.5:1 in 1990.[60] Accordingly, an increasing proportion of AIDS cases in the Caribbean are in women (36% of AIDS cases in 1989 in the Dominican Republic).[59]

In Mexico, 6,510 AIDS cases had been reported to WHO as of May 1, 1991.[56] As in Canada, injectable drug use accounts for only about 1% of AIDS cases among adults.[53] As of January 1991, 43% of AIDS cases in men involved homosexuals, 28% involved bisexuals, and 16% involved heterosexuals. As previously mentioned, the proportion of men among Mexican AIDS cases has been rapidly declining, from a 25:1 ratio in 1984 to 4:1 in 1990; overall, the male-female sex ratio of Mexican AIDS cases for the years 1983–1990 was 6:1.[54] Finally, blood transfusion has accounted for 7% of AIDS cases among men and 66% of AIDS cases among women.[54] Studies in Mexico City had documented HIV seroprevalence levels of up to 7% among paid blood donors.[61]

In Latin America the epidemiologic picture is more complex. Whereas in most if not all countries, the initial AIDS cases were identified in homosexual or bisexual men, varying contributions of injectable drug use, receipt of blood products, and heterosexual contact can be identified. In Brazil, among men with AIDS, the proportion attributed to homosexual transmission decreased from 89% in the years 1980–1984 to 78% in 1985–1988, while transmission related to injectable drug use increased during the same period from 1% to 9%.[59,62] In 1985–1989, injectable drug use was the largest single factor associated with AIDS among women (38% of total). In some areas of Argentina, Brazil, and Uruguay, 20% to 50% of injectable drug users are HIV infected.[55]

In summary, the epidemiologic situation in the Americas is extremely complex, and evolving steadily from a predominance of homosexual transmission toward an increasing role for heterosexual transmission, with a variable contribution from injectable drug use.

Europe

An estimated 500,000 people are HIV infected in Europe, or one in 200 men and one in 1,400 women ages 15 to 49 years. As of December 31, 1990, a cumulative total of 47,481 AIDS cases from 31 countries had been reported to WHO, representing a 51% increase over the number of cases in the previous year. Five countries—France, Italy, Spain, Germany, and the United Kingdom—have accounted for 81% (38,571) of all European cases. The highest cumulative incidence is in Switzerland (242.9 per 1 million population), followed by France (234.1), Spain (192.6), Italy (143), and Denmark (139.9). The male-female ratio of European AIDS cases is 5.9:1.[63]

The major epidemiologic patterns reflect north-south and east-west differences. In northern Europe, the large majority of AIDS cases is associated with homosexual/bisexual behavior (*e.g.,* 67% of AIDS cases in Norway, 72% in Sweden, 76% in Denmark). However, in southern European countries like Italy and Spain, the majority of AIDS cases is linked with injectable drug use (66% and 64%, respectively). Countries in between, such as France, where 20% of cases is associated with injectable drug use), Switzerland (35%), and Austria (28%), occupy an intermediate position along this axis.[63] The "band" of high HIV seroprevalence among injectable drug users extends from northern Spain, through southern France and northern Italy, to Switzerland, Austria, and Yugoslavia. In Europe, the relative proportion of AIDS cases associated with injectable drug use in relation to AIDS cases transmitted by homosexual/bisexual contact has been evolving rapidly; in 1983, only six (2%) of 295 AIDS cases were linked exclusively to injectable drug use, while in 1989, 4,532 (36%) of 12,654 cases were linked to injectable drug use. In the first 6 months of 1990, the number of new AIDS cases among injectable drug users slightly exceeded the number of new AIDS cases associated with homosexual/bisexual transmission.[63]

Of all European AIDS cases, 97% have been reported from western Europe. Albania is the only European country that has not yet reported a single AIDS case; cumulative case rates in central and Eastern Europe, with the exception of Romania, range from zero to 7.3 per 1 million population, compared with a median of 71 cases per 1 million population in western Europe (range, 15.1 to 242.9 per 1 million). In 1989, of the estimated 500,000 HIV-infected persons in Europe, only about 10,000 were thought to be in Eastern or central Europe.[63] Despite these low estimates, several Eastern or central European countries conducted large-scale mandatory screening programs. For example, from January 1987 through January 1990, over 47 million HIV screening tests were performed in the Soviet Union, resulting in the identification of 429 HIV-infected Soviet citizens. Rates of HIV seropositivity of one per 2 million blood donors and one per 1.2 million pregnant women were found in these surveys.[64]

However, HIV infection is present, and increasing, in Eastern and central European countries. For example, in Poland, no cases of HIV seropositivity were found among injectable drug users in 1986–1987; the first HIV-infected injectable drug user was identified in August 1988. However, by 1989, 10% of injectable drug users examined in Warsaw were HIV infected.[42] Similarly, 39% of injectable drug users in Belgrade during 1986–1987[65] and 6.8% in Zagreb were HIV infected in 1989.[66] In addition, the dramatic outbreaks of HIV infection among infants and children in Romania (1,094 pediatric AIDS cases reported from Romania as of December 31, 1990),[63] and the Elista nosocomial epidemic, involving nine hospitals and at least 200 children in the Soviet Union,[67] serve as reminders of the ongoing vulnerability to HIV infection associated with inadequate quality of medical care services.

Finally, the proportion of AIDS cases associated with heterosexual transmission in Europe has increased steadily, from 6.9% in 1987 to 9.3% in 1990. Heterosexual transmission is the designated transmission category, for a cumulative total of 6% of AIDS cases among men and 28% among women.[63]

Africa

Africa has only 8% of the world's population but accounts for about 55% to 60% of HIV infections among adults; approximately 75% of adults who have developed AIDS are Africans. At least 6 million people are HIV infected in Africa, with a roughly equal sex distribution; in sub-Saharan Africa, one in every 35 men and women ages 15 to 49 years is HIV infected.[68]

Behind these general statistics, however, lies extraordinary diversity among and within countries throughout the continent.

First, HIV is spreading within low prevalence countries. In Nigeria, where an estimated 500,000 people are now HIV infected, the seroprevalence rate among women commercial sex workers increased from 3% in 1988 to 10% to 12% in 1990–1991, and among Nigerian blood donors from zero in 1987 to 1.5% in 1990.[69] Similarly, in the Republic of South Africa, where infection in black Africans was thought to be rare in the mid-1980s, studies in Natal found an increase in HIV seroprevalence from 1987 to 1990: from 0.4% to 2.1% among healthy women, from 2.4% to 4% among sexually transmitted disease clinic attendees, and from 1.3% to 8.5% among women commercial sex workers.[70] In addition, although 45,000 to 63,000 black South Africans were thought to be HIV infected at the end of 1989, the estimate had risen to 317,000 to 446,000 by the end of 1991.[71] As another example, seroprevalence among adult blood donors in Yaounde, the Cameroon, increased from 0.36% in 1987 to 1.0% in 1989.[72]

Second, while important exceptions exist to the general rule that HIV seroprevalence is higher in urban than rural areas (*e.g.,* the Kagera region of Tanzania and the Rakai district in Uganda), there is widespread evidence that HIV is spreading rapidly in rural areas of Africa.[33] In Côte d'Ivoire, where an estimated 400,000 persons are now HIV infected, HIV-1 seroprevalence among rural adult residents was 2.8%,[51] a level higher than that documented in the city of Abidjan in 1986.[73] Among healthy blood donors in rural northeastern Zaire, HIV seroprevalence increased from 2.8% in 1989 to 5.8% in 1990.[74] In rural Tanzania, HIV seroprevalence among pregnant women was 3.1% in 1988, but rose to 7.5% in 1990.[75] While some rural areas, even in heavily affected countries like Tanzania, are still relatively less affected—the seroprevalence among prenatal women in southeastern Tanzania is 0.4%,[76] and there was a sustained low seroprevalence of 0.9% in rural northern Zaire from 1976 to 1986[77]—levels of HIV prevalence in rural areas are generally increasing. In Bas-Zaire province, HIV seroprevalence in 1989–1990 was 7.6% among residents of large towns, 4.0% among small town dwellers, and 2.0% in rural villages.[52] Overall, the rural epidemic is advancing, although still several years behind the urban epidemic.

Third, HIV seroprevalence is clearly increasing in some areas but appears to be stable or stabilizing in other areas. For example, in Dar es Salaam, seroprevalence among pregnant women increased from 3.6% in 1986 to 8.9% in 1989.[78] In Lusaka, Zambia, HIV prevalence has increased to 25% among prenatal clinic attendees, to 17% among blood donors, and to 55% among attendees at sexually transmitted disease clinics.[79] In Kampala, HIV prenatal seroprevalence increased from 10% in 1985 to over 30% in 1990[80]; similarly, in Lilongwe, Malawi, 3% of pregnant women were HIV infected in 1986, but 18% were infected in 1989.[81]

Against this background of steady and often dramatic increases in the scope and intensity of HIV infection, the reports of stable seroprevalence or seroincidence are striking. In Kinshasa, Zaire, from 1987 to 1990, HIV seroincidence among employees of two large businesses and their spouses has remained at 0.6% or less, and HIV seroprevalence in several large, well-studied populations in Kinshasa has remained stable, at 4% to 6% since 1984.[82] Similarly, in Kananga, Zaire, HIV seroprevalence among prenatal clinic attendees and blood donors has remained stable, at low levels (1% to 3%).[83]

Further evidence of the extreme diversity of the HIV epidemic in Africa is found in the ratios of men and women HIV infected and ill. In Uganda, among 15- to 19-year-olds, infected women predominate by a factor of 2.5–6:1,[84] and in Yaounde, the Cameroon, HIV prevalence appears higher among women than men.[85] In contrast, in Abidjan (Côte d'Ivoire), even after differential hospitalization rates have been corrected for, the male-female ratio of AIDS cases is 2.5:1.[86] Analysis of these evolving patterns within the HIV epidemic in Africa has only started; in the next several years, it may be possible to identify and understand the biologic and societal bases of different trends in HIV spread and distribution in Africa. In the meanwhile, the increasingly obvious differentiation of the HIV epidemic in Africa should again caution those wishing to generalize about "African AIDS" or "African behaviors."

Asia and Oceania

The HIV/AIDS epidemic in Australia and New Zealand resembles the situation in northern Europe; the large majority of AIDS cases (2,494 and 229, respectively) are among homosexual or bisexual men.[87] For example, from 1982 to 1988, 88% of Australian AIDS cases were in the homosexual/bisexual transmission category, compared with only 1% of AIDS cases which were related exclusively to injectable drug use.[88]

Excluding Australia and New Zealand, the Southeast Asian and western Pacific countries reported a total of 778 cases to WHO as of May 1, 1991.[56] Japan reported the largest number of AIDS cases (374); all other countries in these regions reported a cumulative total of fewer than 100 AIDS cases.

In Japan, the first AIDS case was reported in March 1985. As of June 30, 1990, 285 AIDS cases had been reported; 93% of the cases were Japanese. Seventy-three percent of the reported AIDS cases had occurred in persons with hemophilia who had received imported blood products. Serosurveys among Japanese with hemophilia found 35% to be HIV infected. Homosexual men account for 14% of AIDS cases; HIV seroprevalence surveys among Japanese homosexual men in 1985–1987 found 1.8% to be HIV infected. In Japan, of 27 million blood donors, 44 (one per 613,000) were HIV infected; of these, 33 (75%) were from the Tokyo area. Limited serosurveys among injectable drug users in Matsumoto found no evidence of HIV infection. As of mid-1990, the official estimate was that 3,000 Japanese were HIV infected.[89]

In India, the first report of an indigenously acquired HIV infection was in 1986, among women commercial sex workers in the Madras area (Tamil Nadu).[90] Only 60 AIDS cases had been officially reported from India to WHO as of May 1, 1991.[56] However, serosurveys have been carried out among women commercial sex workers, men attending sexually transmitted disease clinics, and blood donors. In Madras, HIV seroprevalence among women commercial sex workers in 1985–1986 was approximately 10%; by 1990, it had reached 30%. Similarly, in Bombay, while the seroprevalence among women commercial sex workers was 2% in 1988, it had reached 30% in 1990. HIV seroprevalence among "promiscuous" men attending sexually transmitted disease clinics in Madras, Vellore, and Bombay increased from approximately 1% in 1986 to 10% in 1990.[91] In Bombay, HIV seroprevalence among paid blood donors in 1989 was 1.2%.[92] Finally, in the state of Manipur, located adjacent to Myanmar and the "Golden Triangle" heroin-producing areas, HIV seroprevalence among local injectable drug users increased dramatically, from 1% in 1988 to over 50% in 1990.[91,93] The precise size of the HIV epidemic in India is unknown, but a heterosexually transmitted epidemic is well underway; in contrast to heterosexual transmission in North America and Europe, the Southeast Asian heterosexual pattern is not linked closely with injectable drug use.

A broadly similar pattern has emerged in Thailand, where in a few years HIV/AIDS has progressed from a marginal issue to a national crisis. As of May 1, 1990, 94 AIDS cases had been reported to WHO[56]; estimates of the total number of HIV-infected Thais range from 85,000 to 100,000 (official)[94] to 300,000 to 400,000 (unofficial). Surveys in June 1989 in 14 provinces, which were extended to 73 provinces in June 1990, documented an increase in median seroprevalence among women commercial sex workers from 3.5% to 9.8%, and of men STD clinic attendees from zero to 2.5%. Seroprevalence among injectable drug users in Thailand reached a median of 32% in mid-1990,[94] while focal surveys in Bangkok have found an HIV prevalence exceeding 45% among injectable drug users.

In summary, the HIV/AIDS situation in Asia and Oceania remains volatile and dynamic. The speed of HIV spread in Thailand and the potential extent of HIV infection in India surprised many domestic and international observers. Although very low seroprevalence levels remain characteristic of most surveyed populations in Indonesia and the Philippines, conditions facilitating spread clearly exist; WHO estimates that by the mid-1990s, the number of HIV-infected Asians will exceed the number of HIV-infected people in the industrialized countries.

GLOBAL CLASSIFICATION SYSTEMS

In 1987, WHO developed a system of global epidemiologic patterns, dividing the world into three regions—I, II, and III.[95,96] The patterns were based on the temporal spread of HIV and on the major risk-behavior groups affected.

Pattern I involved areas in which extensive spread of HIV started in the late 1970s or early 1980s. In pattern I areas, sexual transmission occurred predominantly through homosexual or bisexual contact, although heterosexual transmission also occurred. By 1987, transmission through transfusion of blood and blood products was not a route of ongoing exposure to HIV; parenteral transmission in pattern I areas therefore involved principally sharing of injection equipment among injectable drug users. Finally, as the male-female ratio of HIV infections in pattern I areas averaged about 10:1, relatively little perinatal transmission was occurring. Pattern I areas included North America, western Europe, South Africa, Australia, and New Zealand.

Pattern II involved areas in which extensive HIV spread also started in the late 1970s and early 1980s. However, in pattern II areas, sexual transmission occurred predominantly through heterosexual contact, although homosexual transmission also occurred. By 1987, safety of blood for transfusion had not been achieved, so that HIV infections were continuing to be transmitted through this route. However, in pattern II areas, injectable drug use was virtually absent. Finally, as approximately equal numbers of men and women were affected, substantial perinatal transmission was occurring. Pattern II areas included sub-Saharan Africa and parts of the Caribbean.

Pattern III involved areas in which HIV was not introduced until the early to mid-1980s. In pattern III areas, while all routes of HIV transmission might be documented, numbers of HIV-infected or ill people were relatively small. Initial HIV infections or AIDS cases often occurred among homosexual or bisexual men who had had contact with men from other geographic areas, or in persons receiving blood or blood products (people with hemophilia) imported from pattern I countries. Pattern III initially included Latin America, north Africa, Eastern Europe, the Middle East, and Asia and Oceania (except for Australia and New Zealand).

Then, in 1988–1989, a new pattern was developed to describe Latin America and parts of the Caribbean. The designation of this pattern as I/II reflected a major evolution in these regions from predominantly homosexual/bisexual transmission toward an increasing proportion of heterosexual transmission.[97]

The pattern system was useful for several purposes. First, the framework emphasized the fundamental unity of the pandemic, characterized by universally occurring, yet quite limited, modes of transmission. Second, the patterns provided a baseline from which evolution of the pandemic could be described. Third, the system furnished epidemiologists and policy-makers with a framework and a vocabulary to help make the global epidemic and the regional specificities readily comprehensible.

From the beginning, WHO cautioned that these patterns were oversimplifications of a complex and dynamic reality. Nevertheless, by 1991, the framework's value has diminished markedly as a descriptive and conceptual instrument. Given the enormous increase in epidemiologic information as well as the evolution of the pandemic, the term "pattern III" no longer usefully incorporates epidemiologic situations as dramatically diverse as those in Thailand, India, the Philippines, and Indonesia. Yet Thailand, with extensive heterosexual and injectable drug use–related transmission, does not fit neatly into either pattern I (transmission predominantly related to injectable drug use) or pattern II (predominantly heterosexual transmission). Meanwhile, pattern I/II areas now include countries with predominantly heterosexual transmission (Trinidad and Tobago, Dominican Republic) and with predominantly homosexual/bisexual transmission (Peru). Pattern I includes countries whose epidemic is currently dominated by infections among injectable drug users, with perinatal transmission and spread to sexual partners (Italy, Spain), as well as countries with dominant homosexual/bisexual transmission (Norway, Sweden).

The major conceptual disadvantages of the existing framework are that it no longer provides an epidemiologically useful insight into present and short-term projected epidemiologic conditions and that it institutionalizes a dual message of compartmentalization and stability. A new conceptual framework is clearly required that will help improve understanding of the continuing evolution of the epidemic at community, national, and, when relevant, international levels. In addition, the inevitably static impression conveyed by the existing framework may exacerbate the pervasive tendency to denial of present epidemiologic realities, self-labeling of a country as "pattern III" being interpreted as implying safety from the pandemic.

Alternative categorization schemes can be suggested, and should be developed. For example, epidemiologic data on the distribution of HIV infection could be combined with information on the prevalence of risk behaviors to derive a population-based "vulnerability" assessment. This classification approach would have the advantage of linking the evolving epidemic with the scope and effectiveness of efforts to prevent infection.

SUMMARY AND CONCLUSIONS

The HIV/AIDS pandemic has challenged epidemiology in several respects. Since the discovery of AIDS in 1981, epidemiology has provided critical information on routes of transmission (and, of equal importance, on how HIV is *not* transmitted), and on the evolving status of the HIV/AIDS pandemic. The urgency of responding to a new global epidemic, combined with media interest unprecedented in intensity and duration, has often placed epidemiologic information, and epidemiologists, at the center of public attention. In turn, this central role may have contributed to a strengthening of awareness of epidemiology for the general public, policy-makers, and health professionals. In addition, the epidemiologic study of HIV/AIDS has brought the communities of communicable and chronic disease epidemiologists closer together. The time scale of HIV disease, the lengthy period of potential infectiousness, and the chronic nature of the behaviors involved in HIV transmission were more typical of chronic than traditional communicable disease experience; accordingly, HIV study required extensive use of logistic regression analysis, mathematical modeling, and other techniques for study of chronic disease.

The study of HIV/AIDS has also brought epidemiologists into close interaction with communities of affected people and has challenged the status quo of epidemiologic practice. For example, issues have arisen regarding consent for participation in epidemiologic studies, methods to ensure data confidentiality, and the responsibility of researchers to participants when study results are available. At the international level, "safari" or "parachute" research has been strongly criticized. This type of research involves expatriates who do not develop genuine collaboration with local investigators and who ignore their responsibility for research capability strengthening.

In summary, even as epidemiology has provided critical information for responding to the HIV/AIDS pandemic, the status quo of its own performance has been challenged.

REFERENCES

1. Pape J, Liautaud B, Thomas F et al: Characteristics of acquired immunodeficiency syndrome (AIDS) in Haiti. N Engl J Med 309:945, 1983
2. Malebranche R, Arnoux E, Guerin JM et al: Acquired immunodeficiency syndrome with severe gastrointestinal manifestations in Haiti. Lancet 2:873, 1983
3. Clumeck N, Sonnet J, Taelman H et al: Acquired immunodeficiency syndrome in African patients. N Engl J Med 310:492, 1984
4. Nzilambi N, DeCock KM, Forthal DM et al: The prevalence of infection with human immunodeficiency virus over a 10-year period in rural Zaire. N Engl J Med 318:276, 1988
5. Centers for Disease Control: Kaposi's sarcoma and *Pneumocystis* pneumonia among homosexual men—New York City and California. MMWR 30:305, 1981
6. Friedman-Kien AE: Disseminated Kaposi's sarcoma syndrome in young homosexual men. J Am Acad Dermatol 5:468, 1981
7. Centers for Disease Control: *Pneumocystis* pneumonia—Los Angeles. MMWR 30:250, 1981
8. Gottlieb MS, Schroff R, Schanker HM et al: *Pneumocystis carinii* pneumonia and mucosal candidiasis in previously healthy homosexual men: Evidence of a new acquired cellular immunodeficiency. N Engl J Med 305:1425, 1981
9. Jaffe HW, Keewhan C, Thomas PA et al: National case-control study of Kaposi's sarcoma and *Pneumocystis carinii* pneumonia in homosexual men: Part 1. Epidemiologic results. Ann Intern Med 99:145, 1983
10. Centers for Disease Control: Case definition of acquired immunodeficiency syndrome. MMWR 30:250, 1981
11. Centers for Disease Control: Revision of the case definition of acquired immunodeficiency syndrome for national reporting. MMWR 34:373, 1985
12. Centers for Disease Control: Revision of the CDC surveillance case definition for acquired immunodeficiency syndrome. MMWR 36(1S):1, 1987
13. World Health Organization Workshop on AIDS in Central Africa. Bangui, Central African Republic, Oct 22–24, 1985
14. Colebunders R, Francis H, Izaley L: Evaluation of a clinical case-definition of acquired immunodeficiency syndrome in Africa. Lancet 2:492, 1987
15. Widy-Wirski R, Berkley S, Downing R: Evaluation of the WHO clinical case definition for AIDS in Uganda. JAMA 260:3286, 1988
16. Pan American Health Organization: Working group on AIDS case definition. Epidemiol Bull PAHO 10:9, 1990
17. Harris JE: Reporting delays and the incidence of AIDS. JASA 85:915, 1990
18. Chin J: Global estimates of AIDS cases and HIV infections: 1990. AIDS 4(suppl 1):S277, 1990
19. Liskin L: Population Reports, vol 14, 1986, p L193
20. Melbye M, Njelesani EK, Bayley A et al: Evidence for heterosexual transmission and clinical manifestations of human immunodeficiency virus infection and related conditions in Lusaka, Zambia. Lancet 2:1113, 1986
21. Kanki P, M'Boup S, Ricard D et al: Human T-lymphotropic virus type 4 and human immunodeficiency virus in West Africa. Science 236:827, 1987
22. Burke DS, Brundage JF, Redfield RR et al: Human immunodeficiency virus infections among civilian applicants for United States military service, October 1985 to March 1986. N Engl J Med 317:132, 1986
23. Kreiss JK, Koech D, Plummer FA et al: AIDS virus infection in Nairobi prostitutes: Spread of the epidemic to east Africa. N Engl J Med 314:414, 1986
24. Van de Perre P, Carael M, Robert-Guroff M et al: Female prostitutes: A risk group for infection with human T-cell lymphotropic virus type III. Lancet 2:524, 1985
25. Goedert JJ, Biggar RJ, Winn DM et al: Determinants of

retrovirus (HTLV-III) antibody and immunodeficiency conditions in homosexual men. Lancet 2:711, 1984

26. Winkelstein W, Lyman DM, Padian N et al: Sexual practices and risk of infection by the human immunodeficiency virus: The San Francisco Men's Health Study. JAMA 257: 321, 1987

27. Simonsen JN, Cameron W, Gakinya MN et al: Human immunodeficiency virus infection among men with sexually transmitted diseases. N Engl J Med 319:274, 1988

28. Quinn TC, Glasser D, Cannon RO et al: Human immunodeficiency virus infection among patients attending clinics for sexually transmitted diseases. N Engl J Med 318:197, 1988

29. Centers for Disease Control: Trends in human immunodeficiency virus among civil applicants for military service—United States, October 1985—March 1988. MMWR 37:1, 1988

30. Hull HF, Bettinger CJ, Gallaher MM et al: Comparison of HIV-antibody prevalence in patients consenting and declining HIV-antibody testing in an STD clinic. JAMA 260: 935, 1988

31. Centers for Disease Control: Human immunodeficiency virus infection in the United States: A review of current knowledge. MMWR 36(suppl 6):1, 1987

32. Rwandan HIV Seroprevalence Study Group: Nationwide community-based serological survey of HIV-1 and other human retrovirus infections in a central African country. Lancet 1:941, 1988

33. AIDS Control Programme, Ministry of Health, Uganda: AIDS surveillance report, first quarter, 1990

34. Pappaioanou M, Dondero TJ, Petersen LR et al: The family of HIV seroprevalence surveys: Objectives, methods, and uses of sentinel surveillance for HIV in the United States. Public Health Rep 105:113, 1990

35. Centers for Disease Control: HIV prevalence estimates and AIDS case projections for the United States: Report based upon a workshop. MMWR 39/RR-16:1, 1990

36. Centers for Disease Control: Protocol: Sentinel hospital surveillance system for HIV infection. RFP 200-88-0623 (P). Atlanta, Centers for Disease Control, 1986

37. Novick LF, Berns D, Stricof R et al: HIV seroprevalence in newborns in New York State. JAMA 261:1745, 1989

38. Kelen GD, DiGiovanna T, Bisson L et al: Human immunodeficiency virus infection in emergency department patients. JAMA 262:516, 1989

39. Chin J: Present and future dimensions of the HIV/AIDS pandemic. Plenary presentation, 7th International Conference on AIDS, Florence, June 17, 1991

40. World Health Organization; WHO update: AIDS cases reported. Geneva, Global Programme on AIDS, June 1, 1991

41. World Health Organization, Office of Information: In point of fact; no. 74. Geneva, World Health Organization, May 1991

42. World Health Organization: Current and future dimensions of the HIV/AIDS pandemic—a capsule summary. WHO/GPA/RES/SFI/91.4. Geneva, April 1991

43. Quinn TC, Narain JP, Zacarias RK: AIDS in the Americas: A public health priority for the region. AIDS 4:709, 1990

44. Des Jarlais DC, Choopanya K, Wenston J et al: Risk reduction and stabilization of HIV seroprevalence among drug injectors in New York City and Bangkok, Thailand (abstr M.C.1). Presented at the 7th International Conference on AIDS, Florence, Italy, June 17, 1991

45. Division of Epidemiology, Ministry of Public Health, Thailand: HIV/AIDS situation and surveillance in Thailand. Sept 15, 1990

46. Des Jarlais DC, Friedman SR, Novick DM et al: HIV-1 infection among intravenous drug users in Manhattan, New York City, from 1977 through 1987. JAMA 261:1008, 1989

47. Nicolosi A, Musicco M, Saracco A et al: Incidence and risk factors of HIV infection: A prospective study of seronegative drug users from Milan and northern Italy, 1987–1989. Epidemiology 1:453, 1990

48. Stevens CE, Taylor PE, Zang EA et al: Human T-cell lymphotropic virus type III infection in a cohort of homosexual men in New York City. JAMA 255:2167, 1986

49. Piot P, Plummer FA, D'Costa LJ et al: Retrospective seroepidemiology of AIDS virus infection in Nairobi populations. J Infect Dis 155:1108, 1987

50. Van de Perre P, Clumeck N, Carael M et al: Female prostitutes: A risk group for infection with human T-cell lymphotropic virus type III. Lancet 2:524, 1985

51. Benoit SN, Gershy-Damet GM, Coulibaly A et al: Seroprevalence of HIV infection in the general population of the Côte d'Ivoire, West Africa. J AIDS 3:1193, 1990

52. Green SDR, Nganga N, Nganzi M et al: Seroprevalence of HIV-1 and HIV-2 infection in pregnancy in rural Zaire (abstr. T.P.E.24). Presented at the 5th International Conference on AIDS in Africa, Kinshasa, Zaire, Oct 11, 1990

53. Valdespino JL, Izazola JA, Rico B: AIDS in Mexico: Trends and projections. Bull Pan Am Health Organ 23:20, 1989

54. Mexico Ministry of Health: Boletin Mensual SIDA/ETS, no. 4, 1990, p 1017

55. Pan American Health Organization/World Health Organization: AIDS surveillance in the Americas, Feb 28, 1991

56. World Health Organization: Weekly Epidemiologic Record, vol 66, p 125, May 1991

57. Health and Welfare Canada, Federal Centre for AIDS: Surveillance update: AIDS in Canada, May 6, 1991

58. World Health Organization: Update: AIDS cases reported to Surveillance, Forecasting and Impact Assessment Unit (SFI). Office of Research (RES), Global Programme on AIDS, Feb 1, 1991

59. Quinn TC, Narain JP, Zacarias RK: AIDS in the Americas: A public health priority for the region. AIDS 4:709, 1990

60. Pape JW, Johnson WD: Epidemiology of AIDS in the Caribbean. Bailliere Clin Trop Med Commun Dis 3:31, 1988

61. Pan American Health Organization: Prevention of HIV transmission through blood and blood products: Experiences in Mexico. In: AIDS: Profile of an Epidemic, p 159. Washington, DC, Pan American Health Organization, Office of Organisation Mondiale de la Sante, 1989

62. Brazil Ministerio da Saude: AIDS Boletim Epidemiologico 1989. Ano II, no. 9. Semana Epidemiologica 9 a 13/1989

63. European Centre for the Epidemiological Monitoring of AIDS: AIDS surveillance in Europe. Quarterly report no. 28, Dec 31, 1990

64. George AM, Gromyko A: The way forward. Presented at the meeting on AIDS national programme support initiative for Eastern European countries, Feb 27 to March 1, 1990. World Health Organization Regional Programme on AIDS, ICP/GPA 097 2113s

65. Cobic P, Keserovic N, Radovanovic Z et al: HIV-1 and HTLV-1 infections among intravenous drug abusers in Belgrade, Yugoslavia. J AIDS 3:1197, 1990

66. Burek V, Maretic T, Zrinscak J et al: Prevalence of HIV infection in Yugoslavia and trends from 1985–89 (abstr F.C.553). Presented at the 6th International Conference on AIDS, San Francisco, June 22, 1990

67. Pokrovsky VV, Eramova IJ, Kuznetsova II et al: Nosocomial transmission of human immunodeficiency virus in Elista, USSR. Central Research Institute of Epidemiology, Moscow, and Regional and Global Programme on AIDS, World Health Organization, 1989

68. World Health Organization, Global Programme on AIDS: Current and future dimensions of the HIV/AIDS pandemic: A capsule summary. Geneva, World Health Organization, September 1990

69. Harry TO, Gashau W, Ekenna O et al: Growing threat of HIV infection in a low prevalence area (abstr T.P.E.21). Presented at the 5th International Conference on AIDS in Africa, Kinshasa, Zaire, Oct 11, 1990

70. Windsor IM: Surveillance of HIV infection in Natal-Kwazulu, South Africa (abstr T.O.B.6). Presented at the 5th International Conference on AIDS in Africa, Kinshasa, Zaire, Oct 11, 1990

71. Padayachee GN, Schall R: The current extent, short-term forecasts, and a long-term assessment of the HIV epidemic among the black population in South Africa (abstr T.P.E.13). Presented at the 5th International Conference on AIDS in Africa, Kinshasa, Zaire, Oct 11, 1990

72. Kaptue L, Zekeng L, Monny LM et al: Blood donor data as a monitor of HIV-1 trend in Yaounde (abstr T.P.E.40). Presented at the 5th International Conference on AIDS in Africa, Kinshasa, Zaire, Oct 11, 1990

73. Sato PA, Chin J, Mann JM: Review of AIDS and HIV infection: Global epidemiology and statistics. AIDS 3(suppl 1):S301, 1989

74. Knight P, Lusi KM: HIV seroprevalence among healthy blood donors in northeastern Zaire (abstr T.P.E.23). Presented at the 5th International Conference on AIDS in Africa, Kinshasa, Zaire, Oct 11, 1990

75. Hemed Y, Minja F, Nagele E et al: The use of HIV sentinel surveillance for the Mbeye regional AIDS programme: A 5-year experience (abstr T.O.B.5). Presented at the 5th International Conference on AIDS in Africa, Kinshasa, Zaire, Oct 11, 1990

76. Petry U, Kingu H, Sally K, Schedel I: Remarkably low prevalence of HIV-antibodies among pregnant women in southeastern Tanzania (abstr T.P.E.19). Presented at the 5th International Conference on AIDS in Africa, Kinshasa, Zaire, Oct 11, 1990

77. Nzilambi N, DeCock KM, Forthal DN et al: The prevalence of infection with human immunodeficiency virus over a 10 year period in rural Zaire. N Engl J Med 318:276, 1988

78. Urassa E, Mhalu FS, Mbena E et al: Prevalence of HIV-1 infection among pregnant women in Dar es Salaam, Tanzania (abstr T.P.E.22). Presented at the 5th International Conference on AIDS in Africa, Kinshasa, Zaire, Oct 11, 1990

79. Tembo G, van Praag E, Mutambo H, Kanyama J: Sentinel surveillance of HIV infection in Zambia (abstr T.P.E.28). Presented at the 5th International Conference on AIDS in Africa, Kinshasa, Zaire, Oct 11, 1990

80. Guay L, Mmiro F, Ndugwa C et al: Perinatal outcome in HIV-infected women in Uganda (abstract Th.C.42). Presented at Sixth International Conference on AIDS, San Francisco, June 21, 1990

81. Liomba NG, Guertler L, Eberle J et al: Comparison of the age distribution of anti-HIV-1 and anti-HBC in an urban population from Malawi (abstr W.G.O.29). Presented at the 5th International Conference on AIDS, Montreal, June 4, 1989

82. Mokwa K, Batter V, Behets F et al: Prevalence of sexually transmitted diseases in childbearing women in Kinshasa, Zaire, associated with HIV infection (abstr W.C.3251). Presented at the 7th International Conference on AIDS, Florence, Italy, June 1991

83. Brown R, Kawunda K: Sero-surveillance of HIV infection in Kananga, Zaire (abstr T.P.E.35). Presented at the 5th International Conference on AIDS in Africa, Kinshasa, Zaire, Oct 11, 1990

84. Berkley S, Naamara W, Okware S et al: AIDS and HIV infection in Uganda. Are more women infected than men? AIDS 4:1237, 1990

85. Kaptue L, Zekeng L, Monny LM et al: Blood donor data as a monitor of HIV-1 trend in Yaounde (abstr T.P.E.40). Presented at the 5th International Conference on AIDS in Africa, Kinshasa, Zaire, Oct 11, 1990

86. DeCock KM, Odehouri K, Moreau J et al: Rapid emergence of AIDS in Abidjan, Ivory Coast. Lancet 2:408, 1989

87. AIDS. NZ Med J, Dec 12, 1990

88. Solomon PJ, Wilson SR, Swanson CE, Cooper DA: Predicting the course of AIDS in Australia. Med J Aust 153:386, 1990

89. Japan Ministry of Health and Welfare: National AIDS control programme in Japan, Dec 31, 1990

90. Jacob JT, George BP, Jayakumari H, Simoes EAF: Prevalence of HIV infection in risk groups in Tamil Nadu, India. Lancet 1:160, 1989

91. Ramachandran P: Sentinel surveillance for HIV infection. CARC Calling 4:25, 1991

92. Fortnightly report from the HIV Serosurveillance Centers of Indian Council of Medical Research, Jan 31, 1989

93. Naik TN, Sarkar S, Singh HL et al: Intravenous drug users. A new high-risk group for HIV infection in India. AIDS 5:117, 1991

94. Thailand Ministry of Public Health, Division of Epidemiology: HIV/AIDS situation and surveillance in Thailand, Sept 15, 1990

95. Mann JM, Chin J, Piot P, Quinn T: The international epidemiology of AIDS. Sci Am 256:82, 1988

96. Chin J, Mann JM: Global patterns and prevalence of AIDS and HIV infection. AIDS 2(suppl 1):S247, 1988

97. Sato PA, Chin J, Mann JM: Review of AIDS and HIV infection: Global epidemiology and statistics. AIDS 3(suppl 1):S301, 1989

7

Epidemiology of HIV in the United States

Susan Y. Chu   *Ruth L. Berkelman*   *James W. Curran*

In 1981, the first cases of acquired immunodeficiency syndrome (AIDS) were reported from Los Angeles in five young homosexual men. A decade later, more than 161,000 cases of AIDS had been reported in the United States. Human immunodeficiency virus (HIV) infection is having a startling effect on mortality in young adults. By 1988, HIV/AIDS was the third leading cause of death in all men ages 25 to 44 years and the eighth leading cause of death among women ages 25 to 44 years,[1] and those rankings are rising (Fig. 7–1 and 7–2). The impact of HIV/AIDS on mortality is particularly devastating in certain areas. By 1988, in San Francisco, Los Angeles, and New York City, HIV/AIDS was the leading cause of death among young adult men; in New York State and New Jersey, HIV/AIDS was the leading cause of death in black women of reproductive age.[2] Because of the large number of persons infected and continuing transmission, the number of cases and the mortality from HIV infection will continue to increase into the forseeable future.

New patterns are emerging in the AIDS epidemic. HIV infection is expanding into different population subgroups and new geographic areas. Homosexual and bisexual men still account for the majority of AIDS cases in the United States, but more and more reported cases are associated directly or indirectly with intravenous (IV) drug use. Cases of AIDS associated with heterosexual transmission are increasing most rapidly (Fig. 7–3).[3] These trends are particularly alarming because these exposure groups show little evidence of reduction in rates of transmission of HIV. One effect has been an increase in the number of women and children affected by the AIDS epidemic. In addition, the geographic circle of HIV infection is expanding, with relatively more cases being reported from outside large coastal cities, from the central region of the country, and from smaller cities and rural communities.[4,5]

One pattern has remained constant throughout the epidemic—the disproportionately high rates of HIV/AIDS among black and Hispanic men, women, and children, who are overrepresented in nearly every transmission category.[6] The disproportionate AIDS rates for blacks and Hispanics primarily reflect the much higher rates of AIDS in black and Hispanic IV drug users, their sexual partners, and infants. The disparity by race/ethnicity is greatest in the northeastern and southeastern states, reflecting the high prevalence of HIV infection in IV drug–using populations in these areas.[7]

SURVEILLANCE OF AIDS AND HIV INFECTIONS IN THE UNITED STATES

From 1981 through February 1991, 167,803 cases of AIDS in the United States were reported to the Centers for Disease Control (CDC);[8] 106,361 (63%) persons were reported to have died, including over 80% of those diagnosed before 1987 (Fig. 7–4). All 50 states require reporting of AIDS to state health departments, which in turn report these cases, without names, to the CDC. The surveillance case definition was initially developed before the etiology of HIV was known. Revisions of the definition in 1985 and 1987 broadened the list of conditions reportable as AIDS, including presumptively diagnosed diseases (*e.g., Pneumocystis carinii* pneumonia and Kaposi's sarcoma), and placed greater emphasis on HIV testing as a component of diagnosis.[9,10] The 1987 revision was undertaken to more accurately reflect the magnitude and distribution of serious HIV morbidity in the United States and resulted in a substantial increase

Figure 7–1. Leading causes of death among men 25 to 44 years of age, United States, 1981–1989. (Data source: National Vital Statistics—Final data for 1981–1988; provisional data for HIV infection/AIDS for 1989. National Center for Health Statistics: Advance report of final mortality statistics, 1988. Monthly Vital Statistics Report 39 (7, suppl), 1990, and National Center for Health Statistics: Annual summary of births, marriages, divorces, and deaths: United States, 1989 (provisional data). Monthly Vital Statistics Report 38 (13), 1990)

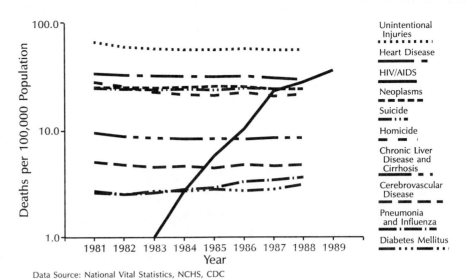

Data Source: National Vital Statistics, NCHS, CDC

Figure 7–2. Leading causes of death among women 25 to 44 years of age, United States, 1981–1989. (Data source: National Vital Statistics—Final data for 1981–1988; provisional data for HIV infection/AIDS for 1989. National Center for Health Statistics: Advance report of final mortality statistics, 1988. Monthly Vital Statistics Report 39 (7, suppl), 1990, and National Center for Health Statistics: Annual summary of births, marriages, divorces, and deaths: United States, 1989 (provisional data). Monthly Vital Statistics Report 38 (13), 1990)

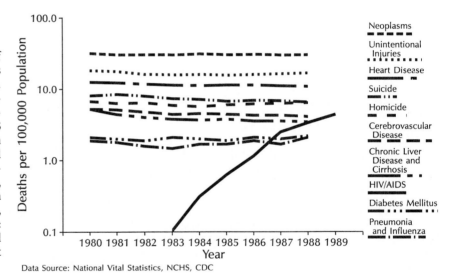

Data Source: National Vital Statistics, NCHS, CDC

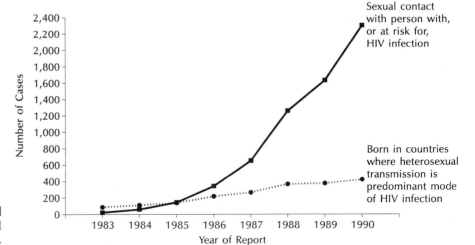

Figure 7–3. AIDS cases infected with HIV through heterosexual contact, United States, 1981–1990.

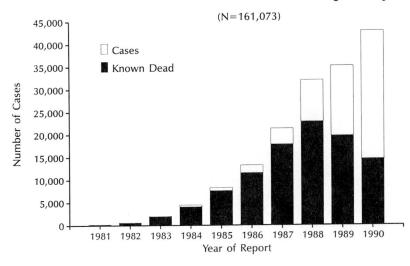

Figure 7–4. AIDS cases and known deaths, by year of report, United States, 1981–1990.

in reported cases.[11] In addition, persons meeting only the new criteria are more likely to be female, black, Hispanic, or IV drug users than are persons meeting the earlier definitions.[12] Reporting of AIDS is quite complete; a comparison of AIDS reports to death certificates in seven areas found that completeness of reporting ranged from 85% to 90% for the years 1986 through early 1989.[13,14] Completeness of reporting of AIDS cases, however, varies by geographic location and patient population.

Because AIDS develops years after infection with HIV, the epidemiology of reported AIDS cases reflects the pattern of HIV infections that occurred several years earlier. Surveys of HIV seroprevalence give a more current picture of the emerging patterns of HIV infection. Monitoring of trends in HIV infection is especially important in the context of rapidly changing infection rates. National estimates of the prevalence of HIV infection have been based primarily on back-calculation from AIDS case incidence and natural history data; in addition,

HIV seroprevalence studies of various special populations (*e.g.,* blood donors, civilian applicants to the military, and newborn infants) have lent confidence to these estimates.[15] Based on these data and on statistical modeling, the U.S. Public Health Service has estimated that approximately 1 million persons were infected with HIV in the United States by the end of 1989. Of the approximately 1 million persons currently infected, AIDS has been diagnosed in no more than 10%, but about 60% of infected persons may have CD4+ counts below 500/mm^3,[16] a level at which therapy and close medical follow-up are recommended.[16]

HOMOSEXUAL/BISEXUAL MEN

Most (59%) reported AIDS cases in the United States occur among homosexual or bisexual men without a history of IV drug use; 7% have occurred in male homosexual or bisexual IV drug users (Table 7–1).[8] Among

Table 7–1. AIDS Cases in Adults/Adolescents by Exposure Category and Sex, Reported Through February 1991, United States

Exposure Category	Males No.	Males (%)	Females No.	Females (%)	Total No.	Total (%)
Male homosexual/bisexual contact	97,687	(66)	—	—	97,687	(59)
Intravenous (IV) drug use (heterosexual)	27,854	(19)	8,301	(51)	36,155	(22)
Male homosexual/bisexual and IV drug use	10,916	(7)	—	—	10,916	(7)
Hemophilia/coagulation disorder	1,400	(1)	34	(0)	1,434	(1)
Heterosexual contact	3,553	(2)	5,354	(33)	8,907	(5)
Receipt of blood transfusion, blood components, or tissue	2,319	(2)	1,468	(9)	3,787	(2)
Other/Undetermined	4,841	(3)	1,173	(7)	6,014	(4)
Total	148,570	(100)	16,330	(100)	164,900	(100)

these populations, the proportion that is white has remained relatively stable at approximately 72%. However, the risk of AIDS in exclusively homosexual men is 1.3 and 1.7 times higher among black and Hispanic men than among white men; for bisexual men with AIDS, the differential is greater (3.6 and 2.5 times higher in blacks and Hispanics, respectively, than in white men).[6]

Cases diagnosed among homosexual and bisexual men continued to increase through 1990, but not as rapidly as in previous years; this slowing in the rate of increase was apparent earliest in New York City, Los Angeles, and San Francisco.[17] Possible reasons include a decline in the incidence of HIV infection, perhaps due to the effectiveness of prevention programs; the effect of treatments that delay progression of HIV disease; migration out of large metropolitan areas before diagnosis; and a decrease in the completeness of reporting.[18] The declines were much greater than could be explained by saturation of infection in the members of the population at highest risk and likely resulted, at least in part, from true changes in behavior patterns in much of the gay male population. Declines in the prevalence of syphilis, gonorrhea, and amebiasis in gay men in the early 1980s also suggest that high-risk sexual behaviors have declined.[19-21]

This plateauing in AIDS incidence among homosexual and bisexual men is not uniform across the country. The incidence continues to increase in certain metropolitan areas, among them Atlanta, Dallas, and Detroit.[18] Nor is the plateauing uniform across racial and ethnic groups. The incidence among homosexual and bisexual black and Hispanic men is increasing more rapidly than among homosexual and bisexual white men, especially in areas outside of New York City and Los Angeles.[18]

Recent evidence suggests that some men do not maintain safe sex practices[22-24] and that young homosexual men continue to engage in high-risk sexual behaviors and have high seroconversion rates.[25-27] Efforts to prevent further expansion of the epidemic of HIV among homosexual and bisexual men must be maintained, with an emphasis on reaching those at greatest risk, including adolescent and minority men who have sex with men.

INTRAVENOUS DRUG USERS

Through February 1991, 47,071 cases of AIDS among IV drug users had been reported in the United States, representing 29% of all cases in adults (see Table 7–1).[8] Of these, 10,916 (23%) occurred in homosexual or bisexual men. Fifty-one percent of women with AIDS and 26% of men with AIDS were IV drug users. Although cases of AIDS among IV drug users have been reported from every state in the United States, rates vary markedly by area, with the highest rates reported from Puerto Rico, New Jersey, New York, the District of Columbia, and Florida.[7] AIDS cases from these five areas represent 62% of all cases of AIDS in IV drug users.

The rate of AIDS associated with IV drug use in 1988 was 18 and 14 times higher among blacks and Hispanics, respectively, than among whites.[7] Except for the western states, where rates for whites, blacks, and Hispanics were similar, this difference by race or ethnicity was observed in all regions of the country and was greatest in the Northeast. IV drug use–associated AIDS cases accounted for 16% of all AIDS cases in whites, 53% in blacks, 56% in Hispanics, 6% in Asians/Pacific Islanders, and 29% in American Indians/Alaskan Natives.[7] Among Hispanics, IV drug use–associated cases primarily occur in persons of Puerto Rican ethnicity, by birth or ancestry.[28,29]

Seroprevalence studies of IV drug users in drug treatment programs also show wide variation in rates by geographic area. In 1988 and 1989, seroprevalence surveys in 65 drug treatment centers in 27 cities reported HIV seroprevalence rates ranging from 0% to 48%.[30] The highest seroprevalence rates for IV drug users in treatment were reported from Newark, NJ (43%), and New York City (34%). In some areas (New York City,[31,32] New Jersey,[33] San Francisco,[34,35] and Detroit[36]), the HIV seroprevalence among IV drug users has leveled off at high rates (40% to 50%), although rates of infection remain high, especially among black and Hispanic IV drug users.[36-38] Outside the Northeast, seroprevalence among IV drug users in treatment is lower; for example, it is 3% in Los Angeles, 8% in San Francisco, 11% in Atlanta, and 0% in Seattle.[31] Differences in infection rates remain incompletely explained but may be related to differences in access to drug treatment,[39,40] differences in needle-sharing practices, or other factors.[41] The explosive HIV epidemics in IV drug users in other cities in the United States and other countries (*e.g.,* Thailand, Italy, Scotland) indicate the serious potential for rapid spread into low prevalence areas.

The epidemiology of drug abuse is changing. Data on IV drug users suggest that most persons who inject heroin began use in the mid-1960s to mid-1970s.[42] Increasingly, cocaine and other drugs are being used IV; these drugs are often injected more frequently and are associated with increased needle-sharing.[43,44] In addition, drugs that are not injected may play an indirect role in HIV transmission. "Crack" cocaine use has been identified as a risk factor for the transmission of HIV infection and syphilis in recent epidemiologic studies in the United States.[45] Although the use of crack is not a mode of HIV transmission, the tendency of those who use crack to engage in unsafe sexual activity with multiple partners, including selling sex for money or drugs, increases the potential for sexual HIV transmission.[46-49]

WOMEN

In the United States, the number of AIDS cases reported in women has steadily increased. By February 1991, 16,330 cases of AIDS had been reported in women age 13 years or older; of these, 55% were reported since

January 1989. In 1990, women accounted for 12% of all reported cases in adults (see Table 7–1).[8]

Black and Hispanic women represent 73% of all U.S. women reported with AIDS; the cumulative incidence rates are 13 and 8 times higher for black and Hispanic women, respectively, than for white women.[50] However, the racial/ethnic disparity varies markedly by state, and these rates largely reflect the disproportionate numbers of black and Hispanic women with AIDS reported from the Northeast and Puerto Rico. Among Hispanics, the incidence is higher among those born in Puerto Rico than elsewhere, especially among IV drug users.

The regional distribution of AIDS cases in women is also changing. Earlier in the epidemic, before 1987, most women with AIDS were reported from large urban areas in the Northeast (65%).[51] However, there are increasing numbers of AIDS cases attributed to heterosexual transmission outside the Northeast and in more rural areas, particularly in the southeastern states.[5] AIDS in women is also expanding into smaller communities. Between 1985 and 1989, the proportion of women with AIDS in the United States reported from smaller communities (less than 1 million population) increased from 25% to 36% of the total.[51]

Unlike men, among whom the majority of cases are attributed to same-gender sexual contact, most cases in women—51%—have been attributed to IV drug use. However, this trend is gradually changing, with an increasing proportion of AIDS cases in women attributed to heterosexual transmission—from 15% in 1983 to 34% in 1990. Between 1989 and 1990, cases attributed to heterosexual contact increased 41%, faster than in any other transmission category (Table 7–2).[52] This is the only exposure category in which women with AIDS outnumber men (see Table 7–1). Moreover, women with AIDS are twice as likely as men with AIDS to be reported without an established risk factor. Many of these cases may represent unrecognized heterosexual transmission.[53]

Most heterosexual contact cases in women are related to sexual contact with an infected IV drug user (63%).[8] Ten percent of women with heterosexually acquired AIDS reported sexual contact with a bisexual man. The remaining heterosexual contacts were with persons with hemophilia (1%), transfusion recipients (2%), persons born in countries where heterosexual contact is the primary means of HIV transmission (*i.e.,* African and Caribbean countries; 12%), and persons with an unspecified risk for HIV infection (12%).

The larger number of reported heterosexually acquired AIDS cases among women may be related to several factors,[54,55] including the following: (1) A greater number of men are infected with HIV, and therefore a woman is more likely than a man to encounter an infected partner. (2) Male-female transmission of HIV may be more efficient than female-male transmission.[56] (3) Women may be less likely to practice "safe sex" because they may be less aware of their risk for HIV infection or less able to assert themselves and insist on protective sexual practices.[57]

Other data indicate that heterosexual spread of HIV will continue to increase, particularly among inner-city indigent populations.[3] Since 1985, gonorrhea, syphilis, and chancroid have been increasing at epidemic rates among urban minority populations in the United States.[22,58] To the extent that certain sexually transmitted diseases are risk factors for sexual transmission of HIV,[59,60] the higher incidence of such diseases may contribute to the higher incidence of AIDS in these groups.[22] In addition, sexual activity among adolescent women (15 to 19 years of age) is increasing. The National Survey of Family Growth showed an accelerated increase through the 1970s and 1980s in the proportion of adolescent women having premarital sexual intercourse,[61] with first sexual experiences occurring at younger ages. Among those 15 years of age, the proportion who had premarital sex increased from 4.6% in 1970 to 25.6% in 1988.[61] Younger age at first sexual intercourse was associated with a greater number of sex partners, increasing the risk for sexually transmitted infections, including HIV. Women are reported with AIDS at younger ages than men; approximately one fourth of women with AIDS were 20 to 29 years old at the time of diagnosis. Many were probably infected as teenagers.

Seroprevalence data on HIV infection in women predict increasing numbers of AIDS cases in the coming years. In an ongoing national survey measuring seroprevalence of HIV among women delivering infants in the United States, residual blood specimens routinely collected for metabolic screening of newborn infants are tested for HIV antibody.[62] Because maternal antibodies cross the placenta during pregnancy, a positive test indicates HIV infection in the mother. As of September 1990, survey data were available from 38 states and the District of Columbia. Rates varied markedly by state, with the highest HIV seroprevalence in New York (5.8 per 1,000), the District of Columbia (5.5 per 1,000), New Jersey (4.9 per 1,000), and Florida (4.5 per 1,000). Based on these data, an estimated 1.5 per 1,000 women delivering infants in 1989 in the United States were infected with HIV. If HIV prevalence in all reproductive-age women is the same as in childbearing women, then as many as 80,000 reproductive-age women were living with HIV in the United States in 1989.[62]

Smaller serosurveys have found pockets of very high rates of infection. In a 1-year study of births, seroprevalence rates as high as 2% to 4% were reported in New York City areas with high rates of drug use.[63] Serosurveys in 54 drug treatment centers in 28 cities also confirmed the strong association between HIV infection and IV drug use among women.[64] Seroprevalence rates for women in drug treatment programs ranged from 0% to 44.6%, with a median of 3.7%. Serosurveys of 85 sexually transmitted disease clinics in 31 cities reported a substantially lower median seroprevalence rate for women not reporting IV drug use (0.8%);[65] however, rates as high as 12.3% and 6.4% were reported from sexually

Table 7–2. Characteristics of Reported Persons with AIDS by Year of Report, and Percent Change (1989–1990)

Characteristic	1990			% Change, 1989 to 1990†
	Reported cases	(%)	Rate*	
SEX				
Male	38,082	(87.9)	30.9	5.9
Female	5,257	(12.1)	4.1	17.4
RACE/ETHNICITY				
White	22,342	(51.6)	11.8	2.5
Black	13,186	(30.4)	42.5	12.0
Hispanic	7,322	(16.9)	31.9	13.3
Asian/Pacific Islander	260	(0.6)	3.8	−8.8
American Indian/Alaskan Native	71	(0.2)	4.0	23.1
REGION (OF U.S.)				
Northeast	13,572	(31.3)	26.7	−2.2
Midwest	4,068	(9.4)	6.8	12.7
South	14,331	(33.1)	16.8	14.9
West	9,624	(22.2)	18.2	3.3
U.S. territories	1,744	(4.0)	46.2	31.0
POPULATION SIZE				
<100,000	2,781	(6.4)	4.7	8.8
100,000–499,999	4,270	(9.9)	9.1	12.7
500,000–999,999	4,293	(9.9)	12.5	12.2
≥1,000,000	31,995	(73.8)	28.4	5.5
EXPOSURE GROUP				
Homosexual/bisexual men	23,738	(54.8)	—	5.2
Intravenous drug users				
Women/heterosexual men	10,018	(23.1)	—	7.9
Homosexual/bisexual men	2,295	(5.3)	—	−2.7
Persons with hemophilia				
Adult/adolescent	340	(0.8)	—	−2.9
Child	31	(0.1)	—	16.7
Transfusion recipients				
Adult/adolescent	866	(2.0)	—	−1.0
Child	39	(0.1)	—	−2.6
Heterosexual contact	2,289	(5.3)	—	40.9
Born in Pattern II country‡	422	(1.0)	—	−10.1
Perinatal transmission	681	(1.6)	—	7.8
No identified risk	2,620	(6.0)	—	—
Total	43,339	(100.0)	17.2	7.2

* Rate per 100,000 population.
† Based on date of diagnosis, adjusted for reporting delay.
‡ Persons born in countries where heterosexual transmission predominates.

transmitted disease clinics in Miami and New York City, respectively.[66]

Ten percent of women with heterosexually acquired AIDS were infected from sexual contact with a bisexual man.[8] In contrast to rates of AIDS in women due to sexual contact with an IV drug user, rates due to sexual contact with a bisexual man vary less by state. Nationwide the rate of AIDS in women due to sex with a bisexual man is 7 times lower than the rate for AIDS due to sex with an IV drug user; however, in some states where HIV seroprevalence in IV drug users is low, sexual contact with bisexual men accounts for a substantial proportion of cases of heterosexually acquired AIDS in women (CDC, unpublished data).

Two instances of female-to-female sexual transmission of HIV have been reported.[67,68] In a review of AIDS cases in women who reported sexual contact with other women only (*n* = 79), 95% were IV drug users and 5%

Table 7–3. AIDS Cases in Children Less Than 13 Years Old, by Exposure Category, Reported Through February 1991, United States

Exposure Category	No.	(%)
Hemophilia/coagulation disorder	145	(5)
Perinatally acquired (mother's exposure):		
IV drug use	1,212	(42)
Sex with IV drug user	504	(17)
Sex with bisexual male	52	(2)
Born in Pattern II country*	219	(8)
Other heterosexual contact	141	(5)
Transfusion recipient	49	(2)
Other/undetermined	256	(9)
Receipt of blood transfusion, blood components, or tissue	255	(9)
Undetermined	70	(1)
Total	**2,903**	**(100)**

* Persons born in countries where heterosexual transmission predominates.

had a history of a blood transfusion, but no cases were attributed to female-to-female sexual transmission of HIV.[69] These data suggest that, as with other sexually transmitted infections, the frequency of female-to-female HIV transmission is very low.

HIV transmission through intravaginal insemination with unprocessed and processed donor semen has been reported,[70–72] although data on the magnitude of the risk are conflicting.[73] No safe procedures to remove HIV from semen have been found; therefore, insemination with semen from HIV-infected men is not recommended under any circumstances, and all semen donors should be screened for HIV infection.[72,74]

INFANTS AND CHILDREN

Through February 1991, 2,903 children less than 13 years of age had been reported to have AIDS (Table 7–3). AIDS in children is primarily a disease of infants and toddlers, with 70% of cases diagnosed in children less than 3 years old. Most (84%) children with AIDS were infected perinatally; 9% had received contaminated blood components, and 5% were infected in the course of treatment for hemophilia or other coagulation disorder.[8] With routine HIV antibody screening of the blood supply since 1985, the proportion of pediatric cases associated with HIV-contaminated blood or blood products will continue to decrease, and mother-to-child transmission will account for an increasing proportion of new infections in the United States (Fig. 7–5).

Because most children acquired HIV infection from their mother, the racial/ethnic and geographic distribution of children with AIDS parallels that of women with AIDS. Fifty-nine percent of perinatally acquired AIDS cases are among black children and 26% are in Hispanic children; cumulative AIDS incidence rates among black and Hispanic children are respectively 21 and 13 times the incidence rate in white children.[75] Of the mothers, 42% were reported to be IV drug users and 32% were sexual partners of infected men, of whom most (56%) were IV drug users. Most cases in children are reported from New York, Florida, New Jersey, Puerto Rico, Washington, DC, and California.[75]

There are other less common but important modes of HIV transmission in children. A number of case reports have clearly demonstrated postpartum transmission in infants who were breast-fed; where milk substitutes are readily available, women infected with HIV are discouraged from breast-feeding.[76] In developing countries, where breast-feeding is associated with improved child survival and safe and effective alternatives are lacking, the World Health Organization continues to consider the benefits of breast-feeding to outweigh

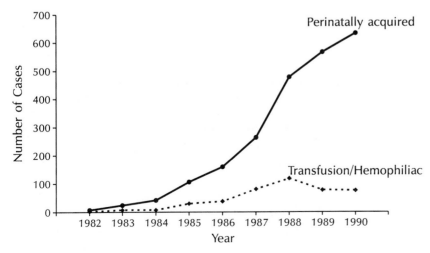

Figure 7–5. AIDS cases in children by exposure category, United States, 1981–1990.

the risks for most HIV-infected mothers. Pediatric HIV infection can also result from child sexual abuse.[77,78] Although transmission through sexual abuse of minors is rare, evaluations of children who have been sexually abused should include consideration of HIV transmission.[79]

Seroprevalence data have provided estimates of the number of infected infants in the United States. Based on the national survey measuring seroprevalence of HIV among women delivering infants in the United States, an estimated 6,079 women with HIV infection gave birth in the United States in 1989.[62] If we assume a perinatal transmission rate of 30%, approximately 1,800 (one in every 2,200) infants acquired HIV infection in 1989. This number is three times the number of children reported with perinatally acquired AIDS in 1989, predicting a much higher number of pediatric AIDS cases in the coming years.[75] Because of the particular needs of HIV-infected children and their families, the resources that will be required reach well beyond medical care costs, often including foster care for both HIV-infected and non-HIV-infected children.[80]

Although the highest number of childhood deaths from AIDS occur in the first year of life, the impact of HIV/AIDS as a cause of death has been most striking in the 1- to 4-year-old age group,[81] and particularly in the Northeast. By 1988, in New York State, HIV/AIDS was the first and second leading cause of death respectively in Hispanic and black children aged 1 to 4 years, accounting for 15% and 16% of all deaths in these age-race groups.[82] Because of the large number of women of childbearing age already infected, the mortality from HIV in infants and young children will undoubtedly rise.

BLOOD AND BLOOD PRODUCTS

Through February 1991, 5,621 (5,221 adults, 400 infants and children) persons had been reported as acquiring HIV infection and developing AIDS through receipt of blood or blood products in the United States. Of these, 28% had a history of hemophilia or other coagulation disorder and 72% were infected through transfusion of infected products.

The proportion of AIDS patients with a history of hemophilia or other coagulation disorder has remained relatively stable over time at 1% to 2%. The number of cases associated with transfusions, representing 2% of all cases in 1990, has leveled off in adults and is declining in children. HIV antibody screening of all blood donations, instituted in 1985, and heat treatment of factor concentrates, begun in 1984, have vastly reduced the risk of HIV transmission through blood components and virtually eliminated transmission from clotting factors. Virtually all newly reported cases associated with transfusion of infected blood or blood products reflect transmission from products received before screening for HIV antibody was available.[83] Because infected persons do not have antibody detectable by routinely used HIV screening tests until about 3 months after infection, there remains a small but finite risk of HIV infection from a blood transfusion. Estimates range from 1 in 36,000 to 1 in 153,000,[82,84–86] a risk that should decrease with improvements in donor deferral methods. This very low risk should not deter persons who need blood from receiving a transfusion.[82]

HEALTH CARE SETTINGS

Although HIV infection in health care workers results primarily from risk behaviors outside the health care setting, exposure to HIV-infected blood poses a definite occupational risk for health care and laboratory workers.[87–89] As of December 31, 1990, the CDC had been notified of 24 health care workers in the United States who had seroconverted following a documented occupational exposure to HIV-infected blood; another 16 health care workers were reported in whom HIV infection was thought to be occupationally acquired but seroconversion after a specific incident could not be documented (CDC, unpublished data). The best estimates of risk come from prospective studies. An analysis combining results from 14 prospective studies estimated the risk of transmission associated with percutaneous exposure to blood from an HIV-infected patient as 0.3% per exposure.[90] Although HIV infection following mucous membrane or extensive skin exposures to HIV-infected blood or concentrated virus has been reported in a few instances, the risk of these types of exposures is much lower than the risk of a needlestick exposure.[91,92]

In 1990–1991, three cases consistent with transmission of HIV to patients from a dentist during an invasive procedure were reported.[93] These cases were the first reported cases of transmission from a health care worker to patients, and although the precise risk for HIV transmission to patients from invasive procedures is not known, it is very low. Many professional groups, including the American Medical Association, the American Dental Association, and the CDC, have issued guidelines to prevent transmission of HIV and other blood-borne pathogens during exposure-prone invasive procedures.

HIV-2

A second human immunodeficiency virus, HIV-2, was first described in west Africans with AIDS in 1986.[94] HIV-2 is closely related to HIV-1, and the spectrum of disease and modes of transmission are thought to be similar to those of HIV-1.[95] Most cases have been reported among persons born in west Africa, though well-documented cases have been reported from Europe and North America. Eighteen persons with HIV-2 infection in the United States have been reported to the CDC; all of the 15 for whom historical information was available had recently emigrated from west Africa, had had sexual contact with west Africans, or had traveled to west Africa.[96,97] In sev-

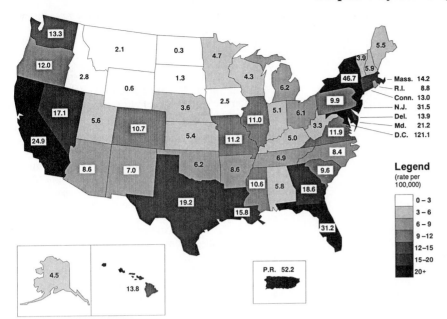

Mass. 14.2
R.I.   8.8
Conn. 13.0
N.J. 31.5
Del. 13.9
Md.   21.2
D.C. 121.1

Legend
(rate per
100,000)

0 – 3
3 – 6
6 – 9
9 –12
12 –15
15 –20
20+

Figure 7–6. AIDS annual incidence rates per 100,000 population, for cases reported in 1990, United States.

eral large blood donor surveys conducted in the United States, no donors with HIV-2 infection were detected.[96,98,99] As of 1991, HIV-2 infection remained rare in the United States, with nearly all cases detected in persons from west Africa.

CONCLUSION

Reported cases of AIDS continued to increase in the United States throughout the 1980s; between 1989 and 1990, the number of cases reported increased by 23%.[53] Because of the large number of persons already infected and the continuing high rates of transmission, the morbidity and mortality from HIV infection and AIDS will also continue to increase into the forseeable future. Long-term commitments of both science and society are needed to prevent further sexual, perinatal, and drug abuse–related transmission of HIV.

REFERENCES

1. Centers for Disease Control: Mortality attributable to HIV infection/AIDS—United States, 1981–1990. MMWR 40:41, 1991
2. Chu SY, Buehler JW, Berkelman RB: Impact of the human immunodeficiency virus on mortality in women of reproductive age. JAMA 264:225, 1990
3. Holmes KK, Karon JM, Kreiss J: The increasing frequency of heterosexually acquired AIDS in the United States, 1983–1988. Am J Public Health 80:858, 1990
4. Gardner LI, Brundage JF, Burke DS et al: Evidence for spread of the human immunodeficiency virus epidemic into low prevalence areas of the United States. J AIDS 2: 521, 1989
5. Berkelman R, Fleming P, Green T et al: The epidemic in

6. Selik RM, Castro KG, Pappaioanou M: Racial/ethnic differences in the risk of AIDS in the United States. Am J Public Health 78:1539, 1988
7. Centers for Disease Control: Update: Acquired immunodeficiency syndrome associated with intravenous-drug use—United States, 1988. MMWR 38:165, 1989
8. Centers for Disease Control: HIV/AIDS Surveillance Report, March 1991, pp 1–22
9. Centers for Disease Control: Revision of the case definition of acquired immunodeficiency syndrome for national reporting—United States. MMWR 34:373, 1985
10. Centers for Disease Control: Revision of the CDC surveillance case definition of acquired immunodeficiency syndrome. MMWR 36 (suppl 1S):1S, 1987
11. Berkelman RL, Heyward WL, Stehr-Green JK, Curran JW: Epidemiology of human immunodeficiency virus infection and acquired immunodeficiency syndrome. Am J Med 86: 761, 1989
12. Selik RM, Buehler JW, Karon JM et al: Impact of the 1987 revision of the case definition of acquired immunodeficiency syndrome in the United States. J AIDS 3:73, 1990
13. Buehler JW, Berkelman RL, Stehr-Green J, Leary L: Completeness of AIDS surveillance, United States (abstr). Presented at the Sixth International AIDS Conference, San Francisco, June 1990
14. Buehler JW, Devine OJ, Berkelman RL, Chevarley F: Impact of the human immunodeficiency virus epidemic on mortality trends in young men, United States. Am J Public Health 80:1080, 1990
15. Centers for Disease Control: Estimates of HIV prevalence and AIDS cases: Summary of a workshop, October 31–November 1, 1989. MMWR 39:110, 1990
16. National Institutes of Health: State-of-the-Art Conference on Azidothymidine Therapy for Early HIV Infection. Am J Med 89:335, 1990

AIDS in intravenous drug users and their heterosexual partners in the Southeastern United States (abstr). Presented at the Sixth International Conference on AIDS, San Francisco, June 1990

17. Karon JM, Berkelman RL: The geographic diversity of AIDS incidence trends in homosexual/bisexual men in the United States. J AIDS (in press)

18. Centers for Disease Control: Update: Acquired immuno-deficiency syndrome—United States, 1989. MMWR 39:81, 1990

19. Centers for Disease Control: Declining rates of rectal and pharyngeal gonorrhea in males—New York City. MMWR 33:295, 1984

20. Sorvillo FJ, Lieb L, Mascola L, Waterman SH: Declining rates of amebiasis in Los Angeles County: A sentinel for decreasing immunodeficiency incidence? Am J Public Health 79:1563, 1989

21. Aral SO, Holmes KK: Sexually transmitted diseases in the AIDS era. Sci Am 264:62, 1991

22. Adib M, Joseph J, Ostrow D: Relapse in safer sexual practices among homosexual men: Two year follow-up from the Chicago MACS (abstr). Presented at the Sixth International Conference on AIDS, San Francisco, June 1990

23. O'Reilly KR, Higgins DL, Galavotti C, Sheridan J, for the CDC AIDS Community Demonstration Projects: Relapse from safer sex among homosexual men: Evidence from four cohorts in the AIDS Community Demonstration Projects (abstr). Presented at the Sixth International Conference on AIDS, San Francisco, June 1990

24. Stall R, Ekstrand M, Pollack L et al: Relapse from safer sex: The next challenge for AIDS prevention efforts. J AIDS 3:1181, 1990

25. Hays RB, Kegeles SM, Coates TJ: High HIV risk-taking among young gay men. AIDS 4:901, 1990

26. Kingsley LA, Bacellar H, Zhou S et al: Temporal trends in HIV seroconversion: A report from the Multicenter AIDS Cohort Study (MACS) (abstr). Presented at the Sixth International Conference on AIDS, San Francisco, June 1990

27. Kellogg TA, Marelich WD, Wilson MJ et al: HIV prevalence among homosexual and bisexual men in the San Francisco Bay Area: Evidence of infection among young gay men (abstr). Presented at the Sixth International Conference on AIDS, San Francisco, June 1990

28. Selik RM, Castro KG, Pappaioanou M, Buehler JW: Birthplace and the risk of AIDS among Hispanics in the United States. Am J Public Health 79:836, 1989

29. Menendez BS, Drucker E, Vermund SH et al: AIDS mortality among Puerto Ricans and other Hispanics in New York City, 1981–1987. J AIDS 3:644, 1990

30. Allen DM, Onorato IM, Sweeney PA et al: Seroprevalence of HIV infection in intravenous drug users (IVDUs) in the United States (abstr). Presented at the Sixth International Conference on AIDS, San Francisco, June 1990

31. DesJarlais DC, Friedman SR, Novick DM et al: HIV-1 infection among intravenous drug users in Manhattan, New York City, from 1977 to 1987. JAMA 261:1008, 1989

32. Stoneburner RL, Chiasson MA, Weisfuse IB, Thomas PA: The epidemic of AIDS and HIV-1 infection among heterosexuals in New York City (editorial). AIDS 4:99, 1990

33. Green TA, Karon J, Stehr-Green J: Changes in U.S. AIDS incidence trends (abstr). Presented at the Sixth International Conference on AIDS, San Francisco, June 1990

34. Watters JK, Cheng Y, Segal M et al: Epidemiology and prevention of HIV in intravenous drug users in San Francisco, 1986–1989 (abstr). Presented at the Sixth International Conference on AIDS, San Francisco, June 1990

35. Moss AR, Bachetti P, Osmond D et al: Seroconversion for HIV in intravenous drug users in treatment, San Francisco,

1985–1990 (abstr). Presented at the Sixth International Conference on AIDS, San Francisco, June 1990

36. Ognjan A, Markowitz N, Pohlod D et al: HIV-1 and HTLV-1 infections in IVDUs in Detroit, 1985–1989 (abstr). Presented at the Fifth International Conference on AIDS, Montreal, June 1989

37. Wiebel W, Lampinen T, Chene D, Stevko B: HIV-1 seroconversion in a cohort of street intravenous drug users in Chicago (abstr). Presented at the Sixth International Conference on AIDS, San Francisco, June 1990

38. Steger KA, Zawacki A, Allen D et al: Antibody to HIV-1 in intravenous drug users entering methadone treatment programs in Boston (abstr). Presented at the Sixth International Conference on AIDS, San Francisco, June 1990

39. Watters JK, Lewis DK: HIV infection, race, and drug-treatment history (letter). AIDS 4:697, 1990

40. Centers for Disease Control: Risk behaviors for HIV transmission among IVDUs not in drug treatment—U.S., 1987–1989. MMWR 39:273, 1990

41. Hahn RA, Onorato IM, Jones TS, Dougherty J: Prevalence of HIV infection among intravenous drug users in the United States. JAMA 261:2677, 1989

42. Kozel NJ, Adams EH: Epidemiology of drug abuse: An overview. Science 234:970, 1986

43. Chaisson RE, Bacchetti P, Osmond D et al: Cocaine use and HIV infection in intravenous drug users in San Francisco. JAMA 261:561, 1989

44. Weiss SH: Links between cocaine and retroviral infection (editorial). JAMA 261:607, 1989

45. Miller HG, Turner CF, Moses LE (eds): AIDS, The Second Decade. Washington, DC, National Academy Press, 1990

46. Minkoff HL, McCalla S, Delke I et al: The relationship of cocaine use to syphilis and human immunodeficiency virus infections among inner city parturient women. Am J Obstet Gynecol 163:521, 1990

47. National Research Council: AIDS: Sexual Behavior and Intravenous Drug Use. Washington, DC, National Academy Press, 1989

48. Fullilove RE, Fullilove MT, Bowser BP, Gross SA: Risk of sexually transmitted disease among black adolescent crack users in Oakland and San Francisco, Calif. JAMA 263:851, 1990

49. Wolfe H, Vranizan KM, Gorter RG et al: Crack use and related risk factors in IVDUs in San Francisco (abstr). Presented at the Sixth International Conference on AIDS, San Francisco, June 1990

50. Ellerbrock TV, Bush TJ, Chamberland ME et al: Epidemiology of women with AIDS in the United States, 1981–1990: A comparison with heterosexual men with AIDS. JAMA (in press)

51. Fleming PL, Gwinn M, Oxtoby MJ: Epidemiology of HIV infection. In Yogev R, Connor E (eds): HIV in Infants and Pregnant Women: A System-Oriented Approach. St Louis, Mosby–Year Book, (in press)

52. Centers for Disease Control: Update: Acquired immuno-deficiency syndrome—United States, 1990. MMWR (in press)

53. Castro KG, Lifson AR, White CR et al: Investigations of AIDS patients with no previously identified risk factors. JAMA 259:1338, 1988

54. Guinan ME, Hardy A: Epidemiology of AIDS in women in the United States, 1981 through 1986. JAMA 257:2039, 1987

55. Wenstrom KD, Gall SA: HIV infection in women. Obstet Gynecol Clin North Am 16:627, 1989

56. Padian N, Shiboski S, Jewell N: The relative efficiency of female-to-male HIV sexual transmission (abstr). Presented at the Sixth International Conference on AIDS, San Francisco, June 1990

57. Stein ZA: HIV prevention: The need for methods women can use. Am J Public Health 80:460, 1990

58. Rolfs RT, Nakashima AK: Epidemiology of primary and secondary syphilis in the United States, 1981 through 1989. JAMA 264:1432, 1990

59. Holmberg SD, Horsburgh CR, Ward JW, Jaffe HW: Biologic factors in the sexual transmission of human immunodeficiency virus. J Infect Dis 160:116, 1989

60. Alexander NJ: Sexual transmission of human immunodeficiency virus: Virus entry into the male and female genital tract. Fertil Steril 54:1, 1990

61. Centers for Disease Control: Premarital sexual experience among adolescent women—United States, 1970–1988. MMWR 39:929, 1991

62. Gwinn M, Pappaioanou M, George JR et al: Prevalence of HIV infection in childbearing women in the United States. JAMA 265:1704, 1991

63. Novick LF, Berns D, Stricof R et al: HIV seroprevalence in newborns in New York State. JAMA 261:1745, 1989

64. Allen DM, Onorato IM, Sweeney PA et al: Seroprevalence of HIV infection in intravenous drug users (IVDUs) in the United States (abstr). Presented at the Sixth International Conference on AIDS, San Francisco, June 1990

65. McCray E, Onorato IM et al: HIV seroprevalence in clients attending sexually transmitted disease (STD) clinics in the United States, 1988–1990

66. Centers for Disease Control: The National HIV Seroprevalence Surveys. Summary of results: Data from serosurveillance activities through 1989. Rockville, MD, National AIDS Information Clearinghouse, 1990

67. Marmor M, Weiss LR, Lyden M et al: Possible female-to-female transmission of human immunodeficiency virus (letter). Ann Intern Med 105:969, 1986

68. Monzon OT, Capellan JMB: Female-to-female transmission of HIV (letter). Lancet 2:40, 1987

69. Chu SY, Buehler JW, Fleming PL, Berkelman RL: Epidemiology of reported cases of AIDS in lesbians, United States 1980–1989. Am J Public Health 80:1380, 1990

70. Stewart GJ, Tyler JP, Cunningham AL et al: Transmission of human T-cell lymphotropic virus type III (HTLV-III) by artificial insemination by donor. Lancet 2:581, 1985

71. Chaisson MA, Stoneburner RL, Joseph SC: Human immunodeficiency virus transmission through artificial insemination. J AIDS 3:69, 1990

72. Centers for Disease Control: HIV-1 infection and artificial insemination with processed semen. MMWR 39:249, 1990

73. Eskenazi B, Pies C, Newstetter A et al: HIV serology in artificially inseminated lesbians. J AIDS 2:187, 1989

74. Centers for Disease Control: Semen banking, organ and tissue transplantation, and HIV antibody testing. MMWR 37:57, 1988

75. Oxtoby MJ: Perinatally acquired human immunodeficiency virus infection. Pediatr Infect Dis J 9:609, 1990

76. Oxtoby MJ: Human immunodeficiency virus and other viruses in human milk: Placing the issues in broader perspective. Pediatr Infect Dis J 7:825, 1988

77. Fuller AK, Bartucci RJ: HIV transmission and childhood sexual abuse (letter). JAMA 259:2235, 1988

78. Gutman LT, St Claire KK, Weedy C et al: Human immunodeficiency virus transmission by child sexual abuse. Am J Dis Child 145:137, 1991

79. U.S. Department of Health and Human Services: Report of the Surgeon General's Workshop on Children with HIV Infection and Their Families, April 6–9, 1987. DHHS publication No. HRS-D-MC 87-1, 1987

80. Parrott RH: Childhood human immunodeficiency virus infection: The spectrum of costs. J AIDS 4:122, 1991

81. Kilbourne BW, Buehler JW, Rogers MF: AIDS as a cause of death in children, adolescents, and young adults (letter). Am J Public Health 80:499, 1990

82. Chu SY, Buehler JW, Oxtoby MJ, Kilbourne BW: Impact of the human immunodeficiency virus on mortality in children, United States. Pediatrics 87: 1991

83. Ward JW, Holmberg SD, Allen JR et al: Transmission of human immunodeficiency virus (HIV) by blood transfusions screened as negative for HIV antibody. N Engl J Med 318:473, 1988

84. Cohen ND, Munoz A, Reitz BA et al: Transmission of retrovirus by transfusion of screened blood in patients undergoing cardiac surgery. N Engl J Med 320:1172, 1989

85. Cumming PD, Wallace EL, Schoor JB, Dodd RY: Exposure of patients to human immunodeficiency virus through the transfusion of blood components that test anti-body negative. N Engl J Med 321:941, 1989

86. Busch M, Eble B, Heilbron D, Vyas G: Risk associated with transfusion of HIV-antibody-negative blood (letter). N Engl J Med 322:850, 1990

87. Marcus R, Kay K, Mann J: Transmission of human immunodeficiency virus (HIV) in health-case settings worldwide. Bull WHO 67:577, 1989

88. Henderson DK: HIV-1 in the health-care setting. In Mandell GL, Douglas RG Jr, Bennett JE (eds). Principles and Practice of Infectious Disease, 3rd ed. New York, Churchill Livingstone, 1990

89. Ciesielski C, Bell D, Chamberland M et al: When a house officer gets AIDS (reply). N Engl J Med 322:1156, 1990

90. Henderson DK, Fahey BJ, Willy M et al: Risk of occupational transmission of human immunodeficiency virus type 1 (HIV-1) associated with clinical exposures. Ann Intern Med 113:740, 1990

91. Centers for Disease Control: Update: Acquired immunodeficiency syndrome and human immunodeficiency virus infection among health-care workers. MMWR 37:229, 1988

92. Centers for Disease Control: Guidelines for prevention of transmission of human immunodeficiency virus and hepatitis B virus to health-care and public-safety workers. MMWR 38 (No. S-6), 1989

93. Centers for Disease Control: Update: Transmission of HIV infection during an invasive dental procedure—Florida. MMWR 40:21, 1991

94. Clavel F, Guetard D, Brun-Vezinet F et al: Isolation of a new human retrovirus from West Africa patients with AIDS. Science 233:343, 1986

95. Clavel F, Mansinko K, Chamaret S et al: Human immunodeficiency virus type 2 infection associated with AIDS in West Africa. N Engl J Med 316:1180, 1987

96. O'Brien TR, Schable CA, Polon C et al: HIV-2 infections in the United States (abstr). Presented at the Sixth International Conference on AIDS, San Francisco, June 1990

97. Centers for Disease Control: Surveillance for HIV-2 infection in blood donors—United States, 1987–1989. MMWR 39:829, 1990

98. Centers for Disease Control: AIDS due to HIV-2 infection—New Jersey. MMWR 37:33, 1988

99. Onorato I, Schable C, McCray G et al: Sentinel surveillance for HIV-2 infection in clinical setting, United States, 1988–1990 (abstr). Presented at the Sixth International Conference on AIDS, San Francisco, June 1990

8

Transmission of the Human Immunodeficiency Virus

Alan R. Lifson

This chapter reviews the ways in which the human immunodeficiency virus (HIV) is and is not transmitted. HIV is transmitted through three primary routes: sexual contact with an infected person, significant exposures to infected blood or blood products (including needles shared among intravenous [IV] drug users), and perinatally from an infected mother to her child. It is necessary for both HIV-infected and uninfected individuals to be aware of how HIV is transmitted to help prevent new infections from occurring. It is equally important for all individuals to be aware of how HIV is not transmitted to avoid unnecessary fears and actions.

TRANSMISSION THROUGH SEXUAL CONTACT

Male-to-Male Transmission

In the United States, 66% of all adults with acquired immunodeficiency syndrome (AIDS) are men who reported a history of sexual contact with another man; this includes the 7% of adult AIDS patients who reported both male homosexual contact and a history of IV drug use.[1] The proportion of cases due to male homosexual contact may vary in different geographic areas. For example, 95% of adults with AIDS in San Francisco reported a history of sexual contact with another man; this figure includes the 9% of adult AIDS patients who reported both male homosexual contact and a history of IV drug use.[2] In many other countries, the majority of AIDS cases also are in homosexual and bisexual men. For example, in northern European countries, including Denmark, the former Federal Republic of Germany, the Netherlands, Norway, Sweden, and the United Kingdom,

at least 70% of AIDS cases have occurred in homosexual or bisexual men.[3]

Early in the AIDS epidemic, many studies of homosexual and bisexual men associated HIV infection with receptive anal intercourse and multiple sexual partners.[4-9] For example, one analysis of a San Francisco cohort considered sexual practices with nonsteady partners, defined as persons with whom the subject had a sexual relationship lasting no longer than 2 days; in this analysis, the risk of HIV seroconversion was related to the number of nonsteady partners who ejaculated into the subject's rectum.[6] Several studies also suggested that practices potentially resulting in rectal trauma, such as douching, may be associated with an increased likelihood of HIV transmission.[4,5]

Although receptive anal intercourse may be associated with the greatest risk, seroconversion has been anecdotally reported among homosexual and bisexual men who denied receptive anal intercourse and reported insertive anal intercourse.[10,11] Anecdotal reports have also suggested HIV seroconversion due to receptive oral intercourse.[11-14] For example, one recent report described seroconversion for HIV antibody occurring in two homosexual men who reported no anal intercourse for 5 years or longer and multiple episodes of receptive oral intercourse with ejaculation.[12] Risk factors facilitating transmission through such exposures have not been conclusively identified. Therefore, receptive oral intercourse, even if associated with a lower risk of HIV infection than practices such as unprotected anal intercourse, should not be considered risk free.

One brief report hypothesized that two gay men seroconverted for HIV after insertive fellatio.[14] Several commentators noted that this report would have been more convincing if additional information had been provided about sexual practices during and prior to the period in which seroconversion occurred.[15,16] For example, since HIV infection may occur a number of weeks before seroconversion, it would have been important to know the last time these men were exposed to semen during any sexual contact (including receptive fellatio). As described below, HIV transmission through exposure to saliva, although theoretically possible, has not been conclusively documented.

Male-to-Female and Female-to-Male Transmission

Although the relative efficiency of transmission continues to be evaluated, both male-to-female and female-to-male transmission have been well documented. In the United States, 34% of adult women and 3% of adult men with AIDS are thought to have acquired HIV infection through heterosexual contact.[1] Although representing a minority of all AIDS cases, the proportion due to heterosexual contact has been slowly increasing over time.[17] Worldwide, heterosexual transmission may account for the great majority of HIV infections. The World Health Organization has described a pattern of transmission for much of Africa and increasingly certain Latin American countries, in which most cases of AIDS occur in heterosexuals and the ratio of infected males to females is approximately 1:1.[18] Heterosexual transmission may play an increasing role in many other parts of the world as well. For example, one recent study reported increasing rates of HIV infection among prostitutes in Bombay, India.[19]

Studies conducted early in the epidemic identified HIV in the semen of HIV-infected persons.[20] HIV has also been cultured from cell-free seminal fluid.[21] Infection with HIV after exposure to semen through artificial insemination has been documented.[22] HIV has also been recovered from cervical and vaginal secretions of HIV-infected women.[23,24]

Although anal intercourse may be associated with an increased risk of male-to-female transmission of HIV,[25] most HIV infections resulting from heterosexual contact have occurred among those who reported only vaginal intercourse.[26,27] For example, one study evaluated sexual partners of individuals with transfusion-associated HIV infections;[26] of ten women thought to have been infected through sexual contact with their husbands, only one reported a history of receptive anal intercourse.

There has been one report hypothesizing female-to-male transmission through oral-genital contact.[28] In this report, an HIV-infected man retrospectively reported as his only risk fellatio and cunnilingus with a female prostitute who used IV drugs. Several commentators noted that this report would have been more convincing if the prostitute had been contacted to verify

this information, or if her HIV infection status had been known.[29,30]

Female-to-Female Transmission

Researchers have described a small number of cases of HIV infection among women who reported sexual contact with other women.[31,32] In at least one report suggesting possible female-to-female transmission,[31] two women who practiced digital, oral-genital, and oral-anal contact were exposed to vaginal blood as a result of their sexual practices and menstruation. In an analysis of U.S. surveillance data,[33] of those women with AIDS who reported sexual relations only with a female partner, 95% reported a history of IV drug use; the remaining 5% acquired HIV infection through receipt of blood or blood products. Therefore, although female-to-female transmission of HIV appears to be a very rare event, HIV infection can occur among lesbian women because of other exposures.

Sexually Transmitted Diseases and HIV Transmission

A number of studies have suggested that HIV transmission may be facilitated by other sexually transmitted diseases associated with genital ulcers, such as herpes, syphilis, or chancroid. For example, among homosexual and bisexual men, HIV infection has been associated with prior syphilis and herpes simplex type 2 infection.[34,35] A number of studies of both man and women from Africa have also implicated genital ulcer disease as a risk for heterosexual transmission of HIV.[36–38] One possible mechanism by which genital ulcers may facilitate HIV transmission is by increasing susceptibility in the uninfected partner through disruption of the skin or mucosal lining. HIV has also been directly isolated from genital ulcers, as shown in one study of seropositive Nairobi prostitutes.[39] Therefore, genital ulcer disease may also be a risk factor for virus transmission by increasing the infectiousness of the seropositive partner.

Recent studies from Africa have also described nonulcerative sexually transmitted diseases as possibly promoting heterosexual transmission. For example, gonorrhea and *Chlamydia* infections were identified as risk factors for HIV infection among female prostitutes in Zaire.[40] Possibly these findings are due to cervicitis, either because of an increased number of target cells or because of cervical changes that increase the likelihood of HIV infection. Another report on women attending a sexually transmitted disease clinic in Kenya reported an association between cervical ectopy and HIV infection,[41] again suggesting that changes in the integrity of the cervix may increase susceptibility to HIV infection.

Whether other sexually transmitted diseases may

also facilitate HIV transmission is currently being evaluated. For example, one report of pregnant women in Malawi found an association of HIV infection with a history of genital warts[42]; the possible role of genital warts in facilitating HIV transmission will need to be confirmed by additional studies.

Nonetheless, it is clear that for many reasons, control of sexually transmitted diseases is integrally related to preventing the spread of HIV. The World Health Organization has indicated that prevention of sexually transmitted diseases may help reduce sexual transmission of HIV, and *vice versa*.[43]

Other Factors Facilitating Sexual Transmission

Several studies have suggested that sexual transmission is more likely to occur when the HIV-infected partner is immunosuppressed with advanced HIV disease (AIDS or AIDS-related conditions) or has a low CD4+ lymphocyte count.[44,45] Possibly this reflects a greater viral burden and an increased number of virus-infected cells, increasing the likelihood of transmission to a seronegative partner.

Genital trauma and exposure to blood during intercourse were discussed in several studies from Uganda and Malawi as factors possibly facilitating HIV transmission.[46,47] Such exposures included genital bleeding due to sex, and traditional vaginal preparations that may result in vaginal wall ulceration or bleeding.

Studies of men with sexually transmitted diseases from Kenya found that uncircumcised men were more frequently infected with HIV, even after controlling for a history of genital ulcers,[37] while studies of men from a sexually transmitted disease clinic in New York City did not identify an association between HIV infection and lack of circumcision.[48] Lack of circumcision may be more important as a risk factor in certain settings, and should be evaluated in additional epidemiologic studies. Studies of prostitutes from Nairobi have identified an association between HIV infection and the use of oral contraceptives.[49] This association will also need to be evaluated by additional studies.

Condoms

Although not foolproof, condoms play a major role in reducing transmission of HIV as well as many other sexually transmitted diseases.[50,51] Recommendations for condoms include the use of latex (rather than natural membrane) condoms and the use of only water-based lubricants.[50] The ingredients in some commercially available spermicides have been shown in the laboratory to inactivate HIV.[52] Although guidelines discuss the possible beneficial effect of spermicides in people who also use condoms during vaginal intercourse (for example, in the event of condom leakage), spermicides alone are not recommended to prevent HIV transmission.

TRANSMISSION THROUGH EXPOSURE TO INFECTED BLOOD, BLOOD PRODUCTS, OR TISSUE

Transmission through exposure to HIV-infected blood or blood products has been documented in three major settings: among recipients of blood or certain blood products, among persons with hemophilia who received clotting factor concentrates, and among IV drug users exposed to contaminated needles and syringes. Some health care personnel have also seroconverted after parenteral or mucous membrane exposure to HIV-infected blood. Several reports have also described HIV infection after tissue transplantation, or after unusual exposures to blood.

Blood Transfusions and Tissue Transplantation

In the United States, 2% of adults and 9% of children with AIDS are thought to have acquired HIV infection through receipt of a blood transfusion or blood components.[1] Studies suggest that the likelihood of HIV infection after transfusion with HIV-infected blood is high; for example, in one study 90% of recipients of HIV-positive blood were infected.[53] The very great majority of people infected through blood transfusions received blood before blood banks instituted HIV antibody testing and donor deferral programs to protect against HIV transmission. A small number of individuals have become infected since these mechanisms were instituted, typically because they received blood from a person who became HIV infected shortly before donation[54]; in such situations, there may have been insufficient time for the donor to develop antibodies before the blood was screened. According to one study, the risk of contracting HIV through receipt of a unit of blood that tests negative for HIV antibody is approximately 26 per million[54]; other studies have suggested even lower risks.[55] In some developing countries, lack of screening programs for blood continues to result in HIV transmission.

Several reports have described HIV infection after tissue transplantation, including infection in recipients of kidney, liver, and bone grafts.[56-58] In one of these reports, the cadaveric organ donor was screened for HIV antibody by EIA and found to be negative; this result appears to have been a false negative because of the large number of transfusions (56 units of blood and blood components) the patient had received before serum was collected for testing.[57]

Persons with Hemophilia or Other Coagulation Disorders

In the United States, 1% of adults and 5% of children with AIDS have hemophilia or other coagulation disorders.[1] Seroprevalence surveys have suggested a high prevalence of HIV infection among persons with hemophilia.[59] The great majority of HIV-infected persons with coagulation disorders received IV clotting factor before protective measures such as heat treatment of clotting factor concentrates and screening of blood and plasma were instituted. A few reports have described individuals who seroconverted for HIV while using concentrates that were dry-heated at lower temperatures (such as 60° C) for 24 to 30 hours.[60] Guidelines for the treatment of persons with hemophilia and recommendations for treating clotting factor concentrates to maximally inactivate HIV have been developed.[60,61]

Intravenous Drug Users

In the United States, 19% of adult men with AIDS are heterosexual men who reported a history of IV drug use; an additional 7% are homosexual or bisexual men who also reported IV drug use.[1] Of adult women with AIDS, 51% reported a history of IV drug use; an additional 21% reported sexual contact with an IV drug user. Of children with AIDS, 59% were born to mothers who were known to be either IV drug users or sexual partners of IV drug users. Therefore, IV drug users directly or indirectly may have a substantial impact on the spread of HIV infection.

HIV infection in IV drug users may in part be due to sexual transmission; for example, in one study of drug users from New York City, HIV antibody was associated by multivariate analysis with a higher number of sex partners who also used IV drugs.[62] However, among IV drug users an important mode of HIV transmission also is the sharing of needles and syringes already used by other drug users.[63] Studies of IV drug users in New York City also found HIV infection to be associated with the percentage of drug injections that took place in "shooting galleries."[62] Among persons who share needles, the practice of "booting" (washing out any drug left in the syringe with the user's own blood while the syringe needle is still in the vein) may increase the amount of blood in the contaminated apparatus to which the next user is exposed.[64] Several strategies to reduce transmission among IV drug users are being evaluated; these include bleach distribution, needle exchange, and drug treatment programs, including methadone maintenance programs.[65]

Several studies have discussed cocaine use as a risk factor for HIV infection. In one study of drug users from San Francisco, IV cocaine use significantly increased the risk of HIV infection.[66] The authors of this study suggested that cocaine use may be associated with a number of practices that increase the risk of HIV infection, such as more frequent injections, sharing of injection equipment, frequenting shooting galleries, and "booting."

Transmission in the Health Care Setting

A number of reports have described HIV infection in health care personnel after parenteral exposures to HIV-infected blood.[67-69] One prospective study of health care workers exposed parenterally to the blood of HIV-infected patients reported a seroprevalence rate in recipients of these exposures of approximately 0.5%.[67,68] In a second study, the risk for occupational transmission after a percutaneous injury was estimated to be approximately 0.6%; an analysis of all available studies by these authors resulted in an estimated seroconversion rate of approximately 0.3% per exposure.[69]

There have also been a few reports of health care workers infected after HIV-infected blood came in contact with skin which may have been broken (for example, due to dermatitis or chapping) or with mucous membranes.[70] Another report described HIV seroconversion in a mother who provided nursing care for her child with HIV infection.[71] In that report, the mother had repeated and extensive contact with the child's blood and body excretions (which sometimes contained blood); although she was not aware of open wounds or dermatitis, she did not wear gloves and often did not wash her hands immediately after these exposures.

Data from prospective studies suggest that the risk of HIV infection after exposure of skin or mucous membranes is much less than the risk of HIV infection after needlestick exposures.[68,69] For example, in one study of 136 health care workers who received 2,712 cutaneous exposures to blood from HIV-infected patients, no seroconversions occurred; an analysis of all available data by the authors identified no seroconversions in 668 health care personnel who received 1,051 mucous membrane exposures.[69]

To further reduce the risk of occupational transmission of HIV, the U.S. Public Health Service has issued guidelines recommending that health care workers follow universal blood and body fluid precautions, dispose of needles and other sharp objects properly, and follow other prudent infection control measures.[72] These guidelines also help protect against other blood-borne infectious agents, such as hepatitis B virus. HIV infection has also been described in laboratory workers exposed to concentrated virus preparations.[73,74] Guidelines have been developed for persons working with the virus in laboratory situations.[74]

One unresolved issue is whether zidovudine taken prophylactically after occupational exposures reduces the likelihood of HIV infection, and if so, to what extent.[75] Although some institutions have offered zidovudine as postexposure prophylaxis, there are diverse opinions among physicians about the use of zidovudine in this setting; data from both animal and human studies are not conclusive regarding the efficacy of zidovudine for prophylaxis after occupational exposure to HIV.[76] HIV infection after zidovudine prophylaxis has been described,[77,78] which suggests that such prophylaxis does not offer complete protection.

Health care workers involved in invasive procedures may experience percutaneous injuries and theoretically expose patients to their blood. One recent report described HIV infection in five patients without established risk factors who had invasive procedures performed by an HIV-infected dentist.[79] DNA sequence analysis showed that the HIV strains in these patients were similar (although not identical) to each other and to the HIV strain in the dentist. However, the exposure that may have resulted in viral transmission to these patients could not be conclusively identified. Among the possibilities are contamination of dental instruments with blood due to poor infection-control precautions; therefore, the precise mode of HIV transmission in this case is uncertain. To evaluate the possibility of HIV transmission from infected health care providers to their patients, several retrospective studies have evaluated patients of HIV-infected surgeons. In one such study, of 616 patients tested for HIV antibody, only one patient, an IV drug user whose medical history suggested that he may already have been infected at the time of surgery, was positive.[80] It is unknown what proportion of these patients were exposed to HIV-infected blood; however, these studies suggest that the likelihood of transmission from an HIV-infected health care worker to his or her patients is very low.

Nosocomial transmission of HIV through both unscreened blood products or unsterile needles has been previously described. For example, transfusions as well as unsterile needles used for injections were reported as sources of nosocomial HIV transmission to children in Romania.[81] In some countries, medical injections may be administered in certain dispensaries that reuse needles and syringes without adequate sterilization, thereby increasing the risk of HIV transmission.[82]

Unusual Exposures to Blood

HIV transmission has been suggested in a few reports involving unusual exposures to blood. One report described a 32-year-old man involved in a motor vehicle accident in Rwanda; during the accident, he received multiple lacerations and was covered with the blood of similarly injured and bleeding passengers.[83] A second report described HIV infection in a heterosexual male who frequently assaulted homosexual men, getting large amounts of blood on himself and frequent small lacerations on his hands; however, since he also reported an episode of IV drug use, the mode of transmission is less certain.[84] Both of these reports describe unusual exposures to blood but do not suggest new modes of HIV transmission.

Transmission from infected infants to their mothers, possibly through exposure to blood, was suggested in one report from the Soviet Union.[85] The children, who were presumed to have been infected through unsterile syringes, had stomatitis that resulted in bleeding. Mothers who breast-fed these children had nipple cracks, which may have facilitated transmission. The risk of such child-to-mother transmission would not be a major issue for most HIV-infected children, who have acquired HIV perinatally from already infected mothers; the possibility of such transmission could be further evaluated in settings where children are infected through exposures such as unscreened blood products or unsterile needles.

TRANSMISSION FROM AN INFECTED MOTHER TO HER CHILD

Of those children with AIDS in the United States, 84% have a mother who is either known to be infected with HIV or is a member of high-risk group.[1] As the number of HIV-infected women with AIDS increases throughout the world, this mode of transmission will account for an increasing number of HIV-infected children.

Several prospective studies of mothers with AIDS or other evidence of HIV infection have suggested rates of HIV transmission in the range of 15% to 40%, although transmission rates above and below this figure have been reported.[86-89] The identification of maternal factors increasing or decreasing the likelihood of HIV transmission may help to explain differences in transmission rates. Such factors may include the mother's stage of HIV infection and her degree of immunodeficiency. For example, maternal factors in one study that influenced the likelihood of transmission included a low CD4+ lymphocyte count, the presence of p24 antigen, and a high replication rate of HIV in culture.[90] One report suggested that maternal antibody to gp120 may affect the likelihood of HIV transmission[86]; the possibility that antibodies to specific viral components may reduce the likelihood of perinatal transmission requires additional evaluation.

Several lines of evidence suggest that intrauterine transmission of HIV occurs. HIV was isolated from a 20-week-old fetus[91] in one study. In a second study, HIV antigen and nucleic acid were identified in tissue from three fetuses aborted at 8 weeks; HIV was also identified in maternal trophoblastic cells and embryonic blood cell precursors.[92] Whether additional HIV transmission may also occur at the time of birth (for example, through exposure to blood during vaginal delivery) and, if so, to what extent, is uncertain. Because several investigators have reported HIV-infected children born by cesarean section, it cannot be concluded that this method of delivery prevents HIV transmission.[93]

One controversial issue is the role of breast-feeding in HIV transmission. HIV has been isolated in cell-free breast milk from HIV-infected women.[94] Virus transmission shortly after birth has been implicated in one report of a child born to a mother who acquired HIV infection from a postpartum blood transfusion; because she breast-fed the child for 6 weeks, HIV infection through breast feeding may have occurred.[95] Two other cases suggesting postnatal transmission through breast-feeding have also been reported.[96] The risk of transmission through breast-feeding has not been defined. Because of the possibility of postnatal transmission to a child who may not yet be infected, the U.S. Public Health Service has recommended that HIV-infected women avoid breast feeding.[97] However, other scientists and public health officials conclude that the many health-promoting benefits of breast-feeding may outweigh the risk of HIV transmission, particularly in developing countries.[98]

HOW HIV IS NOT TRANSMITTED

Casual and Household Contact

HIV has been isolated from several other body fluids, such as tears[99] and saliva.[100] This has raised questions as to whether casual contact with these fluids, such as in the home, office, or school, can result in HIV transmission. Laboratory studies indicate that HIV is much less frequently recovered from saliva than from blood, and that saliva may contain components that inhibit HIV infectivity.[100,101] Although one report described isolation of HIV from urine,[102] a second investigation of 48 seropositive individuals (several of whom had abnormal urine sediment and two of whom had HIV nephropathy) found urine specimens from all subjects to be negative for HIV by culture.[103]

As summarized in several reviews,[104,105] many studies in the United States and Europe have evaluated the risk of nonsexually transmitted HIV infection in over 700 household or boarding school contacts of persons infected with HIV. Household members had a variety of interactions with these infected persons, in some cases helping the infected person to bathe, dress, or eat; household members also shared a variety of household items and facilities. Some of these exposures probably resulted in contact with the saliva or other bodily secretions of the infected patients. None of these studies has found serologic or virologic evidence of HIV transmission among household members who lacked other risks for infection. For example, one study evaluated household contacts of 90 patients with AIDS.[106] In some cases, these contacts shared the bed, toilet, or bath/shower, as well as items such as combs, towels, eating utensils, plates, and glasses. Of 206 contacts (155 children and 51 adults) without other risk factors for HIV infection, no contact was HIV infected.

Another study found no HIV infection in 89 household contacts of 25 children with HIV infection.[107] Most of the infected children in this study were pre-school-aged and shared many items (such as toys and eating utensils) likely to be soiled with saliva or other bodily fluids. A third study[108] evaluated hemophiliac and non-hemophiliac children living together in a French boarding school. All children had close casual contact, in some cases for several years. Although about half of the children with severe hemophilia were found to be infected with HIV, no seroconversion was observed among 70 children without hemophilia.

If HIV is not transmitted by casual contact in households (where exposures are repeated and may be prolonged), it would be even less likely to occur in the workplace. Public Health Service guidelines for persons who share the same work environment state that workers known to be infected with HIV should not be restricted from work because they are infected, nor should they be restricted from using telephones, office equipment, toilets, showers, eating facilities, or water fountains.[109]

Studies of AIDS patients whose risk history is undetermined suggest several major reasons for having "no identified risk."[110,111] Many of these are individuals in whom no risk information is available; the subject may have died or been lost to follow-up before a detailed risk-history evaluation could be performed. Other subjects may have refused to discuss their risk-history information or may have denied a history of high-risk sexual or drug use practices to the interviewer for personal, social, or other reasons. For children with HIV infection, the risk history of the mother may be unknown. Sexually active heterosexual persons may not know if their sexual partner was HIV infected or a member of a high-risk group. In several analyses, of those subjects initially reported with an undetermined risk who were subsequently interviewed or in whom other follow-up information was obtained, most were reclassified.

Insects

Current laboratory and epidemiologic data continue to provide no support for arthropod transmission of HIV. Virus transmission through insects could theoretically occur through either biologic transmission (in which virus infects and multiplies inside the insect) or mechanical transmission (in which virus is spread on the mouthparts of the insect). With respect to biologic transmission, in one study HIV replication was not detected in bedbugs after either blood meals or intra-abdominal inoculation; and HIV replication was not detected in mosquitoes after intrathoracic inoculation.[112] Other studies have shown that HIV does not replicate in cell lines derived from arthropods.[113]

With respect to mechanical transmission, although HIV was cultured in one study from bedbugs (but not mosquitoes) up to 4 hours after engorging on blood containing high concentrations of HIV, bedbugs were unable to transmit HIV from infected to uninfected blood during interrupted feeding experiments.[114] In part this may be due to the extremely small amount of blood on the mouthparts of such insects.[115]

If arthropod transmission of HIV occurred, one would expect to see an increased incidence of HIV infection among household contacts who do not have established risk factors; as previously mentioned, no evidence for such transmission exists. Also, one might expect HIV infection in young children and elderly persons exposed to biting insects. The hypothesis of arthropod transmission was specifically evaluated in a community-based seroprevalence study in the town of Belle Glade, Florida.[116] Although 6% of persons ages 18 to 39 years had HIV antibody, no HIV infection was found in 138 children ages 2 to 10 years or in 131 persons aged 60 years or older. Blood samples were also tested for antibodies to five arboviruses as an index of exposure to mosquitoes; antibodies to one or more of these arboviruses did not significantly correlate with antibody to HIV.

REFERENCES

1. Centers for Disease Control: HIV/AIDS Surveillance Report, October 1991, pp 1–18
2. San Francisco Department of Public Health: AIDS Monthly Surveillance Report, October 1991, pp 1–8
3. Centers for Disease Control: Update: Acquired immunodeficiency syndrome—Europe. MMWR 39:850, 1990
4. Moss AR, Osmond D, Bacchetti P et al: Risk factors for AIDS and HIV seropositivity in homosexual men. Am J Epidemiol 125:1035, 1987
5. Winkelstein W, Lyman DM, Padian N et al: Sexual practices and risk of infection by the human immunodeficiency virus: The San Francisco Men's Health Study. JAMA 257:321, 1987
6. Darrow WW, Echenberg DF, Jaffe HW et al: Risk factors for human immunodeficiency virus (HIV) infections in homosexual men. Am J Public Health 77:479, 1987
7. Mayer KH, Ayotte D, Groopman JE et al: Association of human T lymphotropic virus type III antibodies with sexual and other behaviors in a cohort of homosexual men from Boston with and without generalized lymphadenopathy. Am J Med 80:357, 1986
8. Stevens CE, Taylor PE, Zang EA et al: Human T-cell lymphotropic virus type III infection in a cohort of homosexual men in New York City. JAMA 255:2167, 1986
9. Kingsley LA, Detels R, Kaslow R et al: Risk factors for seroconversion to human immunodeficiency virus among male homosexuals: Results from the Multicenter AIDS Cohort Study. Lancet 1:345, 1987
10. Lifson AR, O'Malley PM, Hessol NA et al: Recent HIV seroconverters in a San Francisco cohort of homosexual/bisexual men: Risk factors for new infection (abstr W. A. P. 46). Presented at the Fifth International Conference on AIDS, Montreal, June 4–9, 1989
11. Detels R, English P, Visscher BR et al: Seroconversion, sexual activity and condom use among 2915 HIV seronegative men followed for up to 2 years. J AIDS 2:77, 1989
12. Lifson AR, O'Malley PM, Hessol NA et al: HIV seroconversion in two homosexual men after receptive oral intercourse with ejaculation: Implications for counselling concerning safe sexual practices. Am J Public Health 80:1509, 1990
13. Mayer KH, DeGruttola V: Human immunodeficiency virus and oral intercourse. Ann Intern Med 107:428, 1987
14. Rozenbaum W, Gharakhanian S, Cardon B et al: HIV transmission by oral sex. Lancet 1:1395, 1988
15. Dassey DE: HIV and orogenital transmission. Lancet 2:1023, 1988
16. Detels R, Visscher B: HIV and orogenital transmission. Lancet 2:1023, 1988
17. Centers for Disease Control: Update: AIDS and human immunodeficiency virus infection in the United States: 1988 update. MMWR 38(suppl S-4):1, 1989
18. Mann JM, Chin J, Piot P, Quinn T: The international epidemiology of AIDS. Sci Am Oct:82, 1988
19. Bhave GG, Wagle UD, Tripathi SP, Seth GS: HIV serosurveillance in promiscuous females of Bombay, India (abstr F.C.612). Presented at the Sixth International Conference on AIDS, San Francisco, June 20–24, 1990
20. Ho DD, Schooley RT, Rota TR et al: HTLV-III in the semen and blood of a healthy homosexual man. Science 226:451, 1984
21. Levy JA: Human immunodeficiency viruses and the pathogenesis of AIDS. JAMA 261:2997, 1989
22. Chiasson MA, Stoneburner RL, Joseph SC: Human immunodeficiency virus transmission through artificial insemination. J AIDS 3:69, 1990
23. Vogt MW, Witt DJ, Craven DE et al: Isolation of HTLV III/LAV from cervical secretions of women at risk for AIDS. Lancet 1:525, 1986
24. Wofsy C, Cohen J, Hauer L et al: Isolation of AIDS-associated retrovirus from genital secretions of women with antibodies to the virus. Lancet 1:527, 1986
25. Padian N, Marquis L, Francis DP et al: Male-to-female transmission of human immunodeficiency virus. JAMA 258:788, 1987
26. Peterman TA, Stoneburner RL, Allen JR et al: Risk of human immunodeficiency virus transmission from heterosexual adults with transfusion-associated infections. JAMA 259:55, 1988
27. Laga M, Taelman H, Van der Stuyft P et al: Advanced immunodeficiency as a risk factor for heterosexual transmission of HIV. AIDS 3:361, 1989
28. Spitzer PG, Weiner NJ: Transmission of HIV infection from a woman to a man by oral sex. N Engl J Med 320:251, 1989
29. Chamberland ME, Conley LJ, Buehler JW: Unusual modes of HIV transmission (letter to ed). N Engl J Med 321:1476, 1989
30. Weiss SH: Unusual modes of HIV transmission (letter to ed). N Engl J Med 321:1476, 1989
31. Marmor M, Weiss LR, Lyden M et al: Possible female-to-female transmission of human immunodeficiency virus. Ann Intern Med 105:969, 1986
32. Monzon OT, Capellan JM: Female-to-female transmission of HIV. Lancet 2:40, 1987
33. Chu SY, Buehler JW, Fleming PL, Berkelman RL: Epidemiology of reported cases of AIDS in lesbians, United States 1980–89. Am J Public Health 80:1380, 1990
34. Holmberg SD, Stewart JA, Gerber AR et al: Prior herpes simplex virus type 2 infection as a risk factor for HIV infection. JAMA 259:1048, 1988
35. Stamm WE, Handsfield HH, Rompalo AM et al: The association between genital ulcer disease and acquisition of HIV infection in homosexual men. JAMA 260:1429, 1988
36. Greenblatt RM, Lukehart SA, Plummer FA et al: Genital ulceration as a risk factor for human immunodeficiency virus infection. AIDS 2:47, 1988
37. Simonsen JN, Cameron DW, Gakinya MN et al: Human immunodeficiency virus infection among men with sex-

ually transmitted diseases: Experience for a center in Africa. N Engl J Med 319:274, 1988

38. Plummer F, Cameron W, Simonsen N et al: Cofactors in male-female transmission of HIV (abstr 4554). Presented at the Fourth International Conference on AIDS, Stockholm, June 12–16, 1988

39. Kreiss JK, Coombs R, Plummer F et al: Isolation of human immunodeficiency virus from genital ulcers in Nairobi prostitutes. J Infect Dis 160:380, 1989

40. Laga M, Nzila N, Manoka AT et al: Non ulcerative sexually transmitted diseases (STD) as risk factors for HIV infection (abstr Th.C.97). Presented at the Sixth International Conference on AIDS, San Francisco, June 20–24, 1990

41. Moss GB, Clemetson D, D'Costa LJ et al: Association of cervical ectopy with heterosexual transmission of human immunodeficiency virus: Results of a study of couples in Nairobi, Kenya. J Infect Dis 164:588, 1991

42. Chiphangwi J, Dallabetta G, Saah A et al: Risk factors for HIV-1 infection in pregnant women in Malawi (abstr Th.C.98). Presented at the Sixth International Conference on AIDS, San Francisco, June 20–24, 1990

43. World Health Organization: Global Programme on AIDS and Programme of STD. Consensus statement from consultation on sexually transmitted diseases as a risk factor for HIV transmission. J AIDS 2:248, 1989

44. Osmond D, Bacchetti P, Chaisson RE et al: Time of exposure and risk of HIV infection in homosexual partners of men with AIDS. Am J Public Health 78:944, 1988

45. Laga M, Taelman H, Van der Stuyft P et al: Advanced immunodeficiency as a risk factor for heterosexual transmission of HIV. AIDS 3:361, 1989

46. Dallabetta G, Miotti P, Chiphangwi J et al: Vaginal tightening agents as risk factors for acquisition of HIV (abstr Th.C.574). Presented at the Sixth International Conference on AIDS, San Francisco, June 20–24, 1990

47. Hellmann NS, Nsubuga P, Mbidde EK, Desmond-Hellmann S: Specific heterosexual risk behaviors and HIV seropositivity in a Uganda STD clinic (abstr Th.C.578). Presented at the Sixth International Conference on AIDS, San Francisco, June 20–24, 1990

48. Chiasson MA, Stoneburner RL, Lifson AR et al: Risk factors for human immunodeficiency virus type 1 (HIV-1) infection in patients at a sexually transmitted disease clinic in New York City. Am J Epidemiol 131:208, 1990

49. Simonsen JN, Plummer FA, Ngugi EN et al: HIV infection among lower socioeconomic strata prostitutes in Nairobi. AIDS 4:139, 1990

50. Centers for Disease Control: Condoms for prevention of sexually transmitted diseases. MMWR 37:133, 1988

51. Rietmeijer CAM, Krebs JW, Feorino PM, Judson FN: Condoms as physical and chemical barriers against human immunodeficiency virus. JAMA 259:1851, 1988

52. Hicks DR, Martin LS, Getchell JP et al: Inactivation of HTLV-III/LAV-infected cultures of normal human lymphocytes by nonoxynol-9 in vitro. Lancet 2:1422, 1985

53. Donegan E, Stuart M, Niland JC et al: Infection with human immunodeficiency virus type 1 (HIV-1) among recipients of antibody-positive blood donations. Ann Intern Med 113:733, 1990

54. Ward JW, Holmberg SD, Allen JR et al: Transmission of human immunodeficiency virus (HIV) by blood transfusions screened as negative for HIV antibody. N Engl J Med 318:473, 1988

55. Cumming PD, Wallace EL, Schorr JB, Dodd RY: Exposure of patients to human immunodeficiency virus through the transfusion of blood products that test antibody negative. N Engl J Med 321:941, 1989

56. Kumar P, Pearson JE, Martin DH et al: Transmission of human immunodeficiency virus by transplantation of a renal allograft, with development of the acquired immunodeficiency syndrome. Ann Intern Med 106:244, 1987

57. Centers for Disease Control: Human immunodeficiency virus transmitted from an organ donor screened for HIV antibody—North Carolina. MMWR 36:306, 1987

58. Centers for Disease Control: Transmission of HIV through bone transplantation: Case report and public health recommendations. MMWR 37:597, 1988

59. Centers for Disease Control: Human immunodeficiency virus infection in the United States: A review of current knowledge. MMWR 36(suppl S-6):1, 1987

60. Centers for Disease Control: Safety of therapeutic products used for hemophilia patients. MMWR 37:441, 1988

61. Pierce GF, Lusher JM, Brownstein AP et al: The use of purified clotting factor concentrates in hemophilia: Influence of viral safety, cost and supply on therapy. JAMA 261:3434, 1989

62. Schoenbaum EE, Hartel D, Selwyn PA et al: Risk factors for human immunodeficiency virus infection in intravenous drug users. N Engl J Med 321:874, 1989

63. Sasse H, Salmaso S, Conti S, First Drug User Multicenter Study Group: Risk behaviors for HIV-1 infection in Italian drug users: Report from a multicenter study. J AIDS 2:486, 1989

64. Hoffman PN, Larkin DP, Samuel D: Needlestick and needleshare—the difference. J Infect Dis 160:545, 1989

65. Brickner PW, Torres RA, Barnes M et al: Recommendations for control and prevention of human immunodeficiency virus (HIV) infection in intravenous drug users. Ann Intern Med 110:833, 1989

66. Chaisson RE, Bacchetti P, Osmond D et al: Cocaine use and HIV infection in intravenous drug users in San Francisco. JAMA 261:561, 1989

67. Centers for Disease Control: Update: Acquired immunodeficiency syndrome and human immunodeficiency virus infection among health-care workers. MMWR 37:229, 1988

68. Marcus R, CDC Cooperative Needlestick Surveillance Group: Surveillance of health care workers exposed to blood from patients infected with the human immunodeficiency virus. N Engl J Med 319:1118, 1988

69. Henderson DK, Fahey BJ, Willy M et al: Risk for occupational transmission of human immunodeficiency virus type 1 (HIV-1) associated with clinical exposures: A prospective evaluation. Ann Intern Med 113:740, 1990

70. Centers for Disease Control: Update: Human immunodeficiency virus infections in health-care workers exposed to blood of infected patients. MMWR 36:285, 1987

71. Centers for Disease Control: Apparent transmission of human T-lymphotropic virus type III/lymphadenopathy-associated virus from a child to a mother providing health care. MMWR 35:76, 1986

72. Centers for Disease Control: Guidelines for prevention of transmission of human immunodeficiency virus and hepatitis B virus to health-care and public safety workers. MMWR 38(no. S-6):1, 1989

73. Weiss SH, Goedert JJ, Gartner S et al: Risk of human immunodeficiency virus (HIV-1) infection among laboratory workers. Science 239:68, 1988

74. Centers for Disease Control: 1988 agent summary statement for human immunodeficiency virus and report on

laboratory-acquired infection with human immunodeficiency virus. MMWR 37(suppl S-4):1, 1988

75. Henderson DK, Gerberding JL: Prophylactic zidovudine after occupational exposure to the human immunodeficiency virus: An interim analysis. J Infect Dis 160:321, 1989

76. Centers for Disease Control: Public Health Service statement on management of occupational exposure to human immunodeficiency virus, including considerations regarding zidovudine postexposure use. MMWR 39(no. RR-1):1, 1990

77. Looke DFM, Grove DI: Failed prophylactic zidovudine after needlestick injury. Lancet 335:1280, 1990

78. Lange JMA, Boucher CAB, Hollack CEM et al: Failure of zidovudine prophylaxis after accidental exposure to HIV-1. N Engl J Med 322:1375, 1990

79. Centers for Disease Control: Update: Transmission of HIV infection during invasive dental procedures—Florida. MMWR 40:377, 1991

80. Mishu B, Schaffner W, Horan JM et al: A surgeon with AIDS: Lack of evidence of transmission to patients. JAMA 264:467, 1990

81. Beldescu N, Apetrei R, Calumfirescu A: Nosocomial transmission of HIV in Romania (abstr Th.C.104). Presented at the Sixth International Conference on AIDS, San Francisco, June 20–24, 1990

82. Mann JM, Francis H, Davachi F et al: Risk factors for human immunodeficiency virus seropositivity among children 1–24 months old in Kinshasa, Zaire. Lancet 2:654, 1986

83. Hill DR: HIV infection following motor vehicle trauma in Central Africa. JAMA 261:3282, 1989

84. Carson P, Goldsmith JC: "Gay bashing" as possible risk for HIV infection. Lancet 337:731, 1991

85. Pokrovsky VV, Kuznetsova I, Eramova I: Transmission of HIV-infection from an infected infant to his mother by breast-feeding (abstr Th.C.48). Presented at the Sixth International Conference on AIDS, San Francisco, June 20–24, 1990

86. Goedert JJ, Mendez H, Drummond JE et al: Mother-to-infant transmission of human immunodeficiency virus type 1: Association with prematurity or low anti-gp120. Lancet 2:1351, 1989

87. Hira SK, Kamanga J, Bhat GJ et al: Perinatal transmission on HIV-1 in Zambia. Br Med J 299:1250, 1989

88. Halsey NA, Boulos R, Holt E et al: Transmission of HIV-1 infections from mothers to infants in Haiti: Impact on childhood mortality and malnutrition. JAMA 264:2088, 1990

89. European Collaborative Study: Children born to women with HIV-1 infection: Natural history and risk of transmission. Lancet 337:253, 1991

90. Boue F, Pons JC, Keros L et al: Risk for HIV 1 perinatal transmission vary with the mother's stage of HIV infection (abstr Th.C.44). Presented at the Sixth International Conference on AIDS, San Francisco, June 20–24, 1990

91. Jovaisas E, Koch MA, Schafer A et al: LAV/HTLV-III in 20-week fetus. Lancet 2:1129, 1985

92. Lewis SH, Reynolds-Kohler C, Fox HE, Nelson JA: HIV-1 in trophoblastic and villous Hofbauer cells, and haematologic precursors in eight-week fetuses. Lancet 335:565, 1990

93. Lifson AR, Rogers MF: Vertical transmission of human immunodeficiency virus. Lancet 2:337, 1986

94. Thiry L, Sprecher-Goldberger S, Jonckheer T et al: Isolation of AIDS virus from cell-free breast milk of three healthy virus carriers. Lancet 2:891, 1985

95. Ziegler JB, Cooper DA, Johnson RO, Gold J: Postnatal transmission of AIDS-associated retrovirus from mother to infant. Lancet 1:896, 1985

96. Colebunders R, Kapita B, Nekwei W et al: Breastfeeding and transmission of HIV. Lancet 2:1487, 1988

97. Centers for Disease Control: Recommendations for assisting in the prevention of perinatal transmission of human T-lymphotropic virus type III/lymphadenopathy-associated virus and acquired immunodeficiency syndrome. MMWR 34:721, 1985

98. Nicoll A, Killewo JZJ, Mgone C: HIV and infant feeding practices: Epidemiological implications for sub-Saharan African countries. AIDS 4:661, 1990

99. Fujikawa LS, Salahuddin SZ, Palestine AG et al: Isolation of human T-lymphotropic virus type III from the tears of a patient with the acquired immunodeficiency syndrome. Lancet 2:529, 1985

100. Ho DD, Byington RE, Schooley RT et al: Infrequency of isolation of HTLV-III virus from saliva in AIDS. N Engl J Med 313:1606, 1985

101. Fox PC, Wolff A, Yeh CK et al: Saliva inhibits HIV-1 infectivity. JADA 116:635, 1988

102. Levy JA, Kaminsky LS, Morrow WJW et al: Infection by the retrovirus associated with the acquired immunodeficiency syndrome: Clinical, biological and molecular features. Ann Intern Med 103:694, 1985

103. Skolnik PR, Kosloff BR, Bechtel LJ et al: Absence of infectious HIV-1 in the urine of seropositive viremic subjects. J Infect Dis 160:1056, 1989

104. Lifson AR: Do alternate modes for transmission of human immunodeficiency virus exist? JAMA 259:1353, 1988

105. Gershon RRM, Vlahov D, Nelson KE: The risk of transmission of HIV-1 through non-percutaneous, non-sexual modes: A review. AIDS 4:645, 1990

106. Friedland G, Kahl P, Saltzman B et al: Additional evidence for lack of transmission of HIV infection by close interpersonal (casual) contact. AIDS 4:639, 1990

107. Rogers MF, White CR, Sanders R et al: Lack of transmission of human immunodeficiency virus from infected children to their household contacts. Pediatrics 85:210, 1990

108. Berthier A, Chamaret S, Fauchet R et al: Transmissibility of human immunodeficiency virus in haemophiliac and non-haemophiliac children living in a private school in France. Lancet 2:598, 1986

109. Centers for Disease Control: Recommendations for preventing transmission of infection with human T-lymphotropic virus type III/lymphadenopathy-associated virus in the workplace. MMWR 34:681, 1985

110. Castro KG, Lifson AR, White CR et al: Investigations of AIDS patients with no previously identified risk factors. JAMA 259:1338, 1988

111. Lifson AR, Rogers MF, White C et al: Unrecognized modes of transmission of HIV: Acquired immunodeficiency syndrome in children reported without risk factors. Pediatr Infect Dis 6:292, 1987

112. Webb PA, Happ CM, Maupin GO et al: Potential for insect transmission of HIV: Experimental exposure of *Cimex hemipterus* and *Toxorhynchites amboinensis* to human immunodeficiency virus. J Infect Dis 160:970, 1989

113. Srinivasan A, York D, Bohan C: Lack of HIV replication in arthropod cells. Lancet 2:1094, 1987

114. Jupp PG, Lyons SF: Experimental assessment of bedbugs (*Cimex lectularius* and *Cimex hemipterus*) and mosquitoes (*Aedes aegypti formosus*) as vectors of human immunodeficiency virus. AIDS 1:171, 1987

115. Miike L: AIDS-related issues: Do insects transmit AIDS? Staff paper 1. Washington, DC, Health Program, Off of Technol Assessment, US Congress, Sept 1987

116. Castro KG, Lieb S, Jaffe HW et al: Transmission of HIV in Belle Glade, Florida: Lessons for other communities in the United States. Science 239:193, 1988

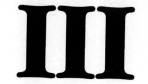

Clinical Manifestations

9

Clinical Spectrum of HIV Disease

Paul A. Volberding

Throughout the history of medicine several diseases have been recognized for the insight they can provide to the observant physician. Tuberculosis and syphilis are examples of complex, multisystem diseases that continue to challenge and instruct many disciplines of medical scientists and practitioners. The challenges posed by infection with the human immunodeficiency virus (HIV) alone would support its inclusion in such lists of instructive medical diseases. These challenges, combined with the problems caused by the complicating opportunistic infections and cancers associated with HIV infection, make the study of HIV disease uniquely able to shed light on many facets of the basic biology of human disease. In addition, HIV, because of the era in which the epidemic has appeared, affords unparallelled insight into the social and political forces surrounding Western science and medicine.

Several factors account for the interest in, and concern about, the HIV epidemic. The epidemic is large, it continues to spread rapidly, particularly in the developing world, and it is caused by currently noncurable infection with an extraordinarily high case fatality rate. In the United States, HIV-related deaths are already the second leading cause of mortality in men between the ages of 25 and 44 years, and rates in women are rapidly escalating as well. The impact of the epidemic on our health care system is already substantial. The care of patients with acquired immunodeficiency syndrome (AIDS) disproportionately affects the public health care sector, which is already overburdened and underfunded.

Yet the HIV epidemic has begun to have positive effects on the health care system. This epidemic has dramatically advanced our knowledge of retrovirology and human immunobiology, particularly through the use of the new scientific tools of molecular biology; HIV research has thereby validated the substantial prior investments made in this technology. Clearly, these scientific benefits will further our understanding of diseases beyond AIDS. Health care consumers and providers who are involved in the battle against AIDS communicate more directly than occurs in most disease settings. Already this close relationship has expedited drug evaluation and approval processes, benefits that should also apply in many other settings.

Among the many issues raised by the HIV epidemic, the clinical spectrum of the disease process begun by HIV infection commands immediate attention. For clinicians involved in the care of people affected by HIV, an understanding of the full spectrum of the manifestations of HIV infection is central to providing comprehensive and expert care. For the medical scientist and biologist, this understanding might afford new insights into the pathogenesis of HIV disease, an area that might, in turn, open avenues to the development of successful therapeutics.

This chapter reviews from a broad perspective the array of problems that develop in patients infected with HIV. We consider the pathogenesis of HIV infection and its associated opportunistic diseases, and review the natural history of these disorders. In this context, we review laboratory markers of the disease process and how they can reflect the natural history of the disease and its response to treatment. We also consider variations in HIV disease in various subpopulations. Lastly, we will speculate on how the knowledge of the natural history and spectrum of disease can influence a treatment plan for the HIV-infected patient.

PATHOGENESIS OF HIV DISEASE AND ITS RELATIONSHIP TO CLINICAL MANIFESTATIONS

HIV can infect and replicate in a wide variety of human cells. Infection of lymphocytes expressing the cell surface antigen, CD4, is the most studied and best understood.[1] In these CD4+ cells, HIV first attaches by an interaction between the large projecting viral glycoprotein, gp120, and a binding site on the CD4 cell surface antigen.[2-5] Although HIV may infect cells by other receptors,[6] it is thought that the interaction between the virus and the CD4 receptor is the most common and important mechanism.

After attachment to the CD4 receptor, the viral membrane fuses with that of the cell, and the viral nuclear contents are inserted into the host cell cytoplasm. This fusion is thought to be mediated by the viral antigen p41, which, along with gp120, comprises the gp160 viral antigen. Once inside the cytoplasm, the HIV genome is transcribed from single RNA strands to double-stranded DNA copies through the action of the HIV-specific enzyme, reverse transcriptase. This DNA, now coding for the HIV genome, is taken into the host cell nucleus and integrated into the host DNA through the action of a second HIV enzyme, integrase. Either immediately or after a dormant or "latent" period, the HIV genome (existing during latency as a provirus within the host genome) is activated to produce HIV gene products. Along with this activation, the HIV genome produces a third enzyme, protease, which clips long protein products into smaller subunits; these subunits are then further processed and, in the case of glycoproteins, glycosylated, to form the components of intact virions that assemble in the cytoplasm. HIV virions then bud from the surface of the cell. During budding, the virus acquires a lipid bilayer envelope from the host cell. This membrane contains host cell–derived antigens of major histocompatibility (MHC) class I and II structure. Following budding, viral protease continues to process the mature virion; myristelation of internal core proteins also continues. Intact virions are either released into the fluid surrounding the cell or passed directly to another cell by cell-cell contact.

The pathogenicity of HIV in infected CD4-bearing T lymphocytes is far from completely understood.[7] There is no doubt that HIV infection of such cells can lead to cell death. It is easily demonstrated by *in vitro* culturing of CD4+ lymphocytes with HIV that the majority of cells are destroyed within several weeks, although it is not known precisely how this cytotoxicity occurs. HIV infection can lead to the formation of giant multinucleated cells (syncytia), and this may explain the gradual reduction in CD4+ populations *in vivo.*[8] Another possibility is that HIV is directly cytotoxic, perhaps through the accumulation of viral gene products. In this area, most research has focused on the possible deleterious intracellular effect of gp120 or of large concentrations of nonintegrated viral DNA. Still another speculation is that HIV causes a programmed cell death—a poptosis even in uninfected cells.

Another interesting and still controversial aspect of the pathogenesis of HIV infection has to do with the relationship between the relative proportion of host cells infected with the virus and the degree of immune dysfunction. Early studies, using techniques now recognized to be insensitive, suggested that between one in 10,000 and one in 100,000 peripheral CD4+ T lymphocytes were HIV infected.[9] This led some to question whether the infection of such a small proportion of cells could explain the severe, progressive immune depletion associated with HIV disease. Studies using more sensitive techniques have recently demonstrated that as many as one in 100 peripheral CD4+ T lymphocytes are HIV infected, and that an even higher fraction of cells found in lymphocyte deposits in tissue (for example, in lymph nodes and spleen) are HIV infected. The high number of CD4+ cells infected with HIV, combined with the effect of HIV infection on the production of lymphokines and cytokines, may be sufficient to explain the mechanism of HIV-induced immune deterioration.

Although HIV infection may be most efficient in CD4 surface antigen–bearing cells, recent evidence suggests that cells expressing little or none of this antigen may also be susceptible to infection.[10,11] Other cell surface antigens may, it could be speculated, act as viral receptors, although with less avidity than do CD4 antigens. Little is known about this question, but it may be an important one, because infection of non-CD4+ cells may help explain some of the protean clinical manifestations of HIV disease. The degree of toxicity in these other cells is much less understood than for CD4+ lymphocytes. Macrophages, monocytes, and dendritic cells for example, may be chronically infected and may produce new virus without being destroyed.[12-15] Although HIV replication rates may be somewhat lower than in the lymphocyte, such cell populations may be a large and important reservoir, capable of harboring the virus and carrying it to various organs and to other cell types. Infection of monocytes and other cells within the central nervous system (CNS) may explain HIV-related encephalopathy.[16] Similarly, HIV has been demonstrated to infect cells within the gastrointestinal (GI) tract, perhaps causing the very frequent problems of HIV-induced enteropathy, wasting, and diarrhea.[17] Very little, however, is known about the biology of HIV infection of non-CD4+ cells and whether it is central to the pathogenesis of HIV disease or merely a coincident infection. Also, HIV disease is associated with many other end-organ consequences without, as yet, any firm explanation of the nature of these problems. For example, HIV infection has been associated with adrenal dysfunction,[18] with myocardial dysfunction,[19] and with neuropathy,[20,21] without direct infection of these organs. Although more sensitive techniques might demonstrate direct infection, conversely, these clinical problems may reflect infiltration by HIV-infected macrophages or may result from circulating products of HIV infection, including lymphokines and cytokines. These circulating factors may have distant and widespread effects.

The relationship between the degree of HIV-induced immune deficiency, as reflected in a decreasing number of CD4+ cells in the peripheral blood, and the development of specific disease processes is a subject of considerable ongoing research. It is clear that some disease manifestations are a direct consequence of immune deficiency; with others this association is much less clear. Perhaps best illustrating one pole of this dichotomy is the opportunistic infection, cytomegalovirus (CMV) retinitis. Subclinical infection with CMV is nearly ubiquitous in homosexual men with HIV disease. Yet even in this group, the reactivation of CMV infection with resulting retinal involvement is seldom seen until the CD4+ cell population in the peripheral blood is severely depleted, typically below 50 cells/mm³.[22] This opportunistic infection thus seems to represent a reactivation that is normally prevented by an intact immune response.

Illustrating the opposite relationship between CD4+ cell count and disease development is Kaposi's sarcoma, an HIV-associated malignancy that was recognized in the earliest days of the epidemic. Kaposi's sarcoma tends to be much less closely related to the degree of immune deficiency[23]: the median CD4+ cell count at the time of diagnosis of Kaposi's sarcoma is greater than 300 cells/mm³.[24] Furthermore, the incidence of Kaposi's sarcoma does not seem to increase substantially with a further decline in CD4+ cell count and instead is seen across the entire spectrum of CD4+ cell depletion. Therefore, when considering the etiology of Kaposi's sarcoma, we are less drawn to the role of immune deficiency or immune surveillance *per se,* but rather are inspired to look at other possibilities, including the direct effects of HIV or other viral infection.

The clinical relevance of the relationship of a specific opportunistic disease to the level of immune deficiency is clear. Monitoring the level of CD4+ cell counts allows us to predict, with increasing accuracy, an individual's risk for those opportunistic infections that are directly related to the level of immune deficiency.[23,25–29] As effective antibiotics are available, they can then be used prophylactically to prevent or delay the onset of a particular opportunistic disease. This strategy is, of course, much less likely to be successful for diseases that do not have such a direct relationship to a measurable degree of immune deficiency.

A final aspect of pathogenesis important to clinicians has to do with the incidence and clinical behavior of illnesses in the HIV-infected patient that are not causally related to HIV infection. Numerous examples of such illnesses can be cited. In some, the diagnosis may be complicated by the coincident HIV infection; in others, the clinical course may be affected by the HIV infection; in yet others, management may be complicated. For example, syphilis—especially neurosyphilis—may be more difficult to diagnose in the setting of HIV infection.[30,31] Serologic tests may be false negative, possibly owing to a blunted immune reaction to infection. If true, it might be anticipated that more cases of advanced syphilis will be encountered, which may give the impression that the clinical course of syphilis is accelerated by coincident HIV infection when it may in fact be due to delays in diagnosis.

The diagnosis of Hodgkin's disease is not more difficult in the patient with HIV infection, nor is the incidence of this cancer apparently increased in the epidemic of HIV.[32] However, some evidence indicates that the clinical presentation and clinical course of Hodgkin's disease may be influenced by coincident HIV infection. Compared with disease in age- and sex-matched controls, Hodgkin's disease in the HIV-infected patient is more likely to be of the mixed cellularity cell type, to be advanced in disease stage, and to be symptomatic at presentation.[33,34] Hodgkin's disease in the HIV-infected person may be less responsive to standard chemotherapy.[35]

Lastly, the treatment of diseases not directly related to HIV infection may be complicated by this infection. Again, Hodgkin's disease and other cancers are good illustrations. Reduced bone marrow reserve, a common feature of HIV infection, may be caused by direct infection of marrow progenitor cells.[36,37] This in turn can limit the ability of the marrow to tolerate cytotoxic chemotherapy and must be considered in the management of such patients. Also, HIV infection decreases tolerance to a number of drugs (particularly with regard to cutaneous rashes associated with the use of many antibiotics), which may complicate the management of otherwise non-HIV-related infectious diseases.

NATURAL HISTORY OF HIV DISEASE

In contrast to the difficulties confronting clinicians earlier in the HIV epidemic, we now have a substantial body of information that allows us to follow and predict with some accuracy the clinical course of patients with HIV infection. Understanding this natural history is of immediate and substantial significance to the clinicians and clinical investigators. Similar to the value in understanding the life cycle of HIV itself, the ability to accurately stage and predict the future clinical course of the HIV-infected patient allows us to plan, apply, and follow medical interventions that might ultimately improve patient outcome.

We now know that HIV infection induces a disease process that is continuous and progressive. Earlier in the epidemic, when we knew little about this process, we developed a terminology to help impart a sense of order. For example, the term ''acquired immunodeficiency syndrome,'' or AIDS, was developed, followed later by the concept of AIDS-related complex, or ARC. AIDS was defined as the appearance of certain dramatic and often life-threatening infections or cancers; ARC denoted a combination of less urgent signs and symptoms, accompanied by a measurable depletion of immune competence. Both of these concepts were essential to our understanding of the new disease we were encountering. Although imprecise by today's level of understanding, these clinical groupings allowed us to track the course of the epidemic and anticipate much about the transmission of the etiologic agent even before it was identified. The understanding that patients with a less immediately life-threatening form of the disease, namely ARC, often progressed to full-blown AIDS made it apparent, even early in the epidemic, that whatever the etiologic agent was, it probably had a rather prolonged period of subclinical infection. This assumption of a prolonged disease process, beginning before overt clinical symptoms could be detected, was supported by a variety of other studies, including studies of immune abnormalities in populations at high risk for AIDS. For example, evaluations of the ratios of CD4+ to CD8+ T lymphocytes demonstrated that many apparently healthy homosexual men had abnormal immune function.[38,39] In fact, a considerable part of clinical attention early in the epidemic, before HIV diagnostic tests were available, was devoted to the problems faced by the "worried well"—those people who were thought to be at some risk for AIDS, based on their behaviors. As we learned more about the natural history of the disease process, and as tests to diagnose HIV infection and more accurately measure the immune effects of this infection became available, we recognized the need to revise some of our earlier concepts. This led to a gradual abandonment of ARC as a useful diagnostic term. Even AIDS as an identifiable entity has lost much of its clinical meaning. Instead, we increasingly appreciate that HIV infection is, itself, a disease that can be staged using laboratory tests that estimate the degree of associated immune deficiency. We now know that there is a single, continuous disease process beginning with the initial exposure to the infectious agent and terminating in the advanced forms of immune deficiency, with death resulting from the complex interactions between the HIV infection itself and the secondary opportunistic infections and malignancies.[40,41]

The arbitrary separation of patients into discrete diagnostic groupings can cause problems, and we should be cautious with our terminology. Nevertheless, it can be useful to separate the continuous process of HIV disease into several phases, each of which has its own working definition, clinical and laboratory features, and medical intervention implications. Therefore, the following discussion considers separately the syndrome of acute retroviral infection, the period of asymptomatic HIV disease, the periods of early and late symptomatic disease, and, last, advanced disease, in which mortality rates increase rapidly. It must be stressed that these phases are not demarcated clearly. Rather, individual patients pass nearly imperceptibly from one to the next; and in many patients, even patients in the advanced stages of HIV disease, periods of relative lack of symptoms can alternate with periods of increasing symptomatology. Central to the subsequent discussion is the role of laboratory markers in staging the disease process. For each phase of disease, we will consider how these markers vary and how they might be used clinically in monitoring the disease course or the effect of medical intervention (Table 9–1).

HIV Transmission

A detailed review of the modes of HIV transmission is beyond the scope of this chapter; however, an awareness of the routes of infection is important for the clinician. Indeed, one of the main obligations of the physician managing patients with HIV disease is to be able to speak with confidence about transmission in order to play a role in HIV prevention.[42] In addition, issues of HIV transmission are directly important as they relate to the health care provider's own risk of acquiring the infection

Table 9–1. Stages of HIV Disease

Stage and Clinical Features	Typical Duration	CD4+ Cell Range (cells/mm³)
Acute retroviral syndrome (Brief mononucleosis-like illness)	1–2 wk	1,000–500
Asymptomatic (No symptoms or signs other than lymphadenopathy)	10+ yr	750–500
Early Symptomatic (Non-life-threatening infections, chronic or intermittent symptoms)	0–5 yr	500–100
Late symptomatic (Increasingly severe symptoms, life-threatening infections, cancers)	0–3 yr	200–50
Advanced (Increasing hazard of death, less transferrable "opportunistic" infections)	1–2 yr	50–0

in the course of patient care, or of transmitting the virus to patients if the provider is infected.

HIV is transmitted through limited types of exposure. No current evidence supports respiratory transmission of this virus. Direct inoculation of fluid containing the virus seems essential, although instances of transcutaneous infection, either through the exposure of infected blood to mucous membranes or broken skin or the exposure of highly concentrated laboratory cultures of HIV to the unbroken skin, have been reported.[43] Much more common is the transmission of HIV disease by unprotected sexual intercourse, and by the direct inoculation of contaminated blood or blood products.

The likelihood of transmission following different types of exposure varies widely. The probability appears to be less affected by the biology of the person exposed to the contaminated material than by the titer of virus in the contaminated material, the amount inoculated, and the route of inoculation. On one end of the spectrum are persons who receive transfusions of HIV-infected blood. Here, regardless of the recipient's age or health, HIV infection follows with near certainty.[44,45] On the other hand, a single unprotected sexual exposure to HIV is much less likely to result in successful transmission. The precise risk of transmission following such an exposure is difficult to estimate but probably ranges from 1 in 100 to 1 in 1,000.[46] Risks are probably higher for the receptive partner in unprotected anal intercourse with an infected partner than for a woman engaging in unprotected vaginal intercourse with an infected male partner.[47] The risk of parenteral inoculation is also difficult to estimate.[48,49] This risk is likely to vary depending on the viral titer of the inoculant and the amount inoculated. It is estimated that the titer of free HIV in the plasma is less than $10^{0.5}$ TCID/ml in the early stages of disease, but may be as high as 10^3 TCID/ml in patients with more severe immune deficiency.[50–52] Also, the volume of the inoculate appears to influence the likelihood of transmission. Health care workers exposed from cutaneous puncture wounds by surgical needles, for example, have a severalfold lower risk of infection than persons similarly injured from hollow needles, which carry substantially more blood. Similarly, infection across unbroken skin has not been reported, except in one laboratory worker exposed to extremely concentrated virus stocks.[53]

The transmission of HIV to the newborn infants of HIV-infected women is of great concern, and in this area the data are increasing.[54–56] Early estimates suggested that as many as 50% to 70% of children born to HIV-infected women would be infected. More recent studies, however, estimate this risk to be between 17% and 30%.[57] Transmission appears to take place most commonly *in utero,* although documented cases of transmission after birth are reported,[58] including cases of infection through breast milk.[59] Interestingly, *in utero* transmission of HIV may be less common in women with specific antibodies to HIV.[55] In one study, women with antibodies to a specific region of HIV were much less likely to transmit the virus to their offspring than women lacking these antibodies. This information has given some hope for the development of vaccines, as these women may have a relatively protective immune response to HIV.

Acute Retroviral Infection

Following HIV exposure, the first step in the disease process is a successful "take" of the inoculated virus in the new host. Whether the initial infection occurs through cell-free virions or through HIV-infected inoculated cells is not known, but may be important in efforts to abort infection after inoculation. Successful infection may be followed by a brief and self-limited symptom complex. This symptom complex, called the *acute retroviral syndrome,* has been described in the prospective studies of Cooper et al[60] and has been retrospectively identified in many patients with HIV disease. Based on closely observed cases of occupational exposure to HIV in health care workers[61] and in cohorts of homosexual men, it is now estimated that this acute syndrome may be more common than was previously thought—perhaps occurring in 90% of cases. Often, because of the physician's lack of awareness and the rather nonspecific nature of its presentation, the syndrome is misdiagnosed as influenza or infectious mononucleosis.[62–65] Generally, the acute retroviral syndrome begins approximately 1 to 3 weeks (range, 5 days to 3 months) after initial infection and lasts for 1 to 2 weeks. Fevers, pharyngitis, headache, malaise, and a diffuse cutaneous erythematous rash are the most prominent symptoms and signs. Diffuse and symmetric lymphadenopathy is also quite common, occurring in 75% of cases. In retrospect, patients often remember this illness as a severe case of flu. Its complex of symptoms most closely resembles acute mononucleosis. In fact, the appearance of either mononucleosis- or influenza-like symptoms should prompt the physician to consider the possibility of acute HIV infection and to initiate appropriate assessment of potential HIV transmission risk behaviors.

The laboratory markers of the acute HIV syndrome are, for the most part, nonspecific and incompletely characterized, but a burst of viremia occurs within the first several weeks of infection, detectable by transient HIVp24 antigenemia.[63,65] Laboratory evidence of subclinical hepatitis may be seen in the subsequent disease course.

Although most of the signs and symptoms of the acute retroviral syndrome are nonspecific and self-limited and abate within 2 weeks, others can persist into the prolonged asymptomatic phase of HIV disease. Most prominent among these is diffuse reactive lymphadenopathy, which persists in as many as one third of patients following the acute retroviral syndrome. Although recognized very early in the HIV epidemic and initially considered part of the AIDS-related complex, it is now apparent from prospective epidemiologic cohort studies that lymphadenopathy in and of itself does not affect the patient's clinical prognosis, and it is now considered to be compatible with asymptomatic HIV disease.

Headache is another clinical component of the acute retroviral syndrome.[66,67] This symptom, thought to be caused by HIV infection of the meninges, can persist beyond the acute syndrome, resulting in chronic or recurring headache in some patients. This clinical process is poorly characterized but seems to be relatively independent of immune deficiency and not necessarily a harbinger of more serious encephalopathic manifestations of HIV disease. Nevertheless, it can be a chronically debilitating problem.

The therapeutic implications of the diagnosis of acute retroviral syndrome remain uncertain. What is certain is that physicians, especially those caring for patients likely to be engaging in behaviors associated with a risk for HIV transmission, must recognize this syndrome in order to initiate further diagnostic and monitoring procedures. Some have postulated that antiretroviral therapy in the acute syndrome phase may be beneficial, but no controlled studies of benefit have been conducted. For the patient who is diagnosed with the acute retroviral syndrome, it is important that the physician initiate appropriate diagnostic tests and immediately begin counseling the patient to prevent further HIV transmission and to optimize ongoing medical monitoring and care.

Asymptomatic (Early) HIV Disease

No other area in the clinical spectrum of HIV disease has seen so rapid an increase in our understanding and at the same time so much controversy as has the asymptomatic phase of HIV disease. This phase begins with initial HIV infection or after the resolution of the acute retroviral syndrome. The diagnosis of asymptomatic HIV disease demands vigilance on the part of the physician and optimum communication between the physician and patient. Ideally, every physician at least considers the possibility of HIV infection in each of his or her patients. A nonobtrusive, confidential, and nonjudgmental assessment of each patient's risk of exposure to HIV should be made and followed by the recommendation for HIV testing if the patient is estimated to have any elevated probability of HIV exposure or if the patient expresses any concern about being infected.

HIV testing must increasingly be seen and used as a routine medical diagnostic test.[41,68] The stigma surrounding the use of this key procedure has contributed to a reluctance to recommend or accept early diagnosis. This reluctance, while understandable from a social and at times legal standpoint, results in underuse of the test, and runs counter to the current belief that the early diagnosis of HIV disease allows the patient access to medical care that is tailored to his or her specific medical condition and that can, with increasing success, lower the probability of further disease progression. Con-

cerned physicians must support efforts to limit the social liability of testing to increase the early diagnosis of HIV disease.

In contrast to the difficulties previously experienced in the definition of ARC, the definition of the asymptomatic phase of HIV disease is relatively straightforward. Other than diffuse reactive lymphadenopathy or headache, no chronic signs or symptoms potentially attributable to HIV infection should be present. Specifically, patients considered to be asymptomatic are those who *do not* experience unexplained fevers, diarrhea, unintentional weight loss, night sweats, or other symptoms suggestive of chronic viral infection. It is more difficult to be dogmatic about the presence of such complaints as depression, anxiety, or fatigue, as these states may follow the patient's knowledge of his or her infection, rather than resulting from physiologic changes due to HIV infection.

Although the clinical description of asymptomatic HIV disease is straightforward, there is a wide array of associated laboratory abnormalities. Some of these may indicate the presence of other diseases; others may be relatively nonspecific and are useful primarily because they lead to the diagnosis of HIV infection. These and other laboratory values can also serve as prognostic markers to assess the stage of the patient's HIV disease. The types of laboratory abnormalities seen in asymptomatic HIV disease are, in fact, typical of those that characterize the more advanced stages of the disease. In the hemogram, for example, any one combination of anemia, neutropenia, and thrombocytopenia can be seen. Neither anemia nor neutropenia is typically severe in these patients. The neutropenia that is seen often reflects a relative decrease in both neutrophils and lymphocytes. Thrombocytopenia can be more severe and, in fact, can occur without a close relationship to the underlying stage of HIV disease. The mechanisms for thrombocytopenia in HIV disease are incompletely understood but may reflect infection of progenitor cells as well as accelerated destruction of platelets.

Abnormalities in chemistry panels in patients with asymptomatic HIV disease are common but usually not severe. Usual abnormalities include a relative increase in total serum globulin levels and, especially as the disease progresses, a decrease in albumin and cholesterol levels. Transaminase levels may be elevated, owing either to chronic hepatitis, which is common among homosexual men and IV drug users, or to reactivation of previously quiescent viral hepatitis infections as the immune deficiency caused by HIV progresses.

More specific abnormalities in the asymptomatic phase of HIV disease are seen in studies of the immune system and in diagnostic tests for HIV infection itself. As the asymptomatic period progresses, laboratory evidence of immune deficiency correspondingly increases, which can be followed by monitoring the absolute circulating CD4+ T-lymphocyte count.[69,70] There is as much as a 15% variation in these results even in the best laboratories,[71] and some of this variation may be decreased by following, instead or in addition, the relative percentage of these peripheral CD4+ lymphocytes.[72] Most laboratories provide this information in routine CD4+ result forms. Regardless, the CD4+ cell count is an important marker, and is typically normal (750–1,000/mm³) in the earliest stages of asymptomatic HIV disease. As the asymptomatic phase continues, CD4+ cell count decreases by about 40 to 80 cells/mm³ per year, although this rate of decline varies widely among individuals.[73] In fact, each individual appears to have his or her own ''track'' of CD4+ cell decline which may be secondarily changed by antiretroviral therapy. As the probability of the development of various opportunistic diseases and the potential benefit of antiretroviral therapy can be predicted from the CD4+ cell count, these values are crucial for establishing a management plan to guide intervals between patient visits, the initiation of therapy directly against HIV infection itself, and the initiation of therapy to prevent complicating opportunistic infections.

A variety of other laboratory tests may be used to follow the course of asymptomatic HIV disease.[74] Among the most important of these are assays of serum levels of β_2-microglobulin[75,76] or neopterin,[77,78] and quantitative assays for HIV p24 antigen.[79,80] Each of these markers has independent predictive value in estimating the eventual probability of disease progression. The use of the CD4+ cell count has been favored because this cell is central to the pathogenesis of HIV disease. HIV p24 antigen is a more direct marker of HIV infection than serum β_2-microglobulin and neopterin, as the latter reflect the immune response to HIV infection rather than the ''quantity'' of the infection itself. HIV p24 antigen has major limitations, however, particularly in the clinical monitoring of individual patients with asymptomatic HIV disease, as it is only found in approximately 10% of such subjects whose risk of disease progression is not necessarily elevated. Also, the HIV p24 antigen level has not proved useful in predicting response to antiviral therapy.[81] Serum β_2-microglobulin and neopterin levels, while relatively nonspecific for HIV disease, are reproducibly measurable in all patients, irrespective of disease stage. Some studies have evaluated the usefulness of combinations of markers for predicting the probability of disease progression. Here, for example, abnormalities of both CD4+ cell count and serum β_2-microglobulin levels have been shown to be much more predictive of degree progression than abnormalities in either test alone.[75,82] While of interest, it is not yet certain if this type of prognostic panel will be of as much value in monitoring response to therapy as it seems to be in predicting the probability of progression of untreated HIV disease.

A variety of other laboratory abnormalities may be seen in patients with asymptomatic HIV disease. These abnormalities are of uncertain value in predicting prognosis but nevertheless may be useful in some patients, especially in estimating subsequent probabilities of specific opportunistic infections. The erythrocyte sedimentation rate, for example, may be so nonspecific as to be of limited value as a prognostic test unless a rapid increase is detected, which may be the harbinger of near-term clinical deterioration. Other tests are useful in subsequent medical care of the HIV-infected patient in that they predict complicating infections. For example, tests for *Toxoplasma gondii,* hepatitis B virus, syphilis, and tuberculosis are recommended early in a patient's care.

The expected duration of asymptomatic HIV disease becomes predictable with increasing certainty.[80] A variety of prospective studies have demonstrated that most patients remain asymptomatic for very prolonged periods of time after initial infection, regardless of the route of initial HIV infection. In the largest prospective cohort, comprising homosexual men, the median time from estimated initial infection to the development of signs and symptoms of advanced HIV disease (AIDS) was 10.8 years.[83] Similar estimates of 10- to 11-year asymptomatic periods have been made for HIV-infected blood transfusion recipients, IV drug users, and adult hemophiliacs.[84-87]

Considerable attention has been directed toward the differences in the appearance of HIV disease in various populations (see section on Variations in HIV Disease, below). Although the spectrum of opportunistic diseases may vary quite widely, the basic rate of progression of HIV infection appears to be similar across broad racial, ethnic, gender, and geographic groupings. Of course, the pace of this disease process is quite variable in individual patients. In some patients the disease progresses much more rapidly than in others. Cases have been reported, for example, in which advanced HIV disease was diagnosed within 12 months of documented primary infection. Conversely, in many individuals the disease progresses more slowly, and these patients remain asymptomatic well beyond the median.

In 1987, after the benefit of zidovudine was established in patients with advanced HIV disease, a clinical trial was designed by the AIDS Clinical Trials Group of the National Institutes of Allergy and Infectious Disease (NIAID) to compare zidovudine treatment with placebo in patients with asymptomatic HIV infection.[88] In this trial, which accrued more than 3,200 patients over the following 2 years, two daily dosages of zidovudine were compared, 500 mg and 1,500 mg, each administered in five divided daily oral doses. Patients were stratified by entry CD4+ cell count into two groups: those with greater than or equal to 500 cells/mm³ and those with less than 500 cells/mm³. The group with fewer than 500 CD4+ cells/mm³ was further subdivided at entry into patients with 200 to 500 cells/mm³ and those with fewer than 200 cells/mm³, to ensure subsequent comparability in these three treatment arms. All patients were followed closely for progression to symptomatic disease that met the CDC criteria for advanced ARC or AIDS. Laboratory end points, including CD4+ cell counts and HIV p24 antigen level changes, were considered secondary but nevertheless important in this trial.

In August 1989, the continuation of the placebo arm of the trial in the subgroup of patients with fewer than 500 CD4+ cells/mm^3 at entry was stopped by an independent data and safety monitoring board because of a higher clinical progression rate in the placebo recipients than in the zidovudine recipients. When adjusted for slightly differing median durations of therapy between the treatment groups, zidovudine was shown to decrease the rate of progression to AIDS by a factor of approximately 3, with a high degree of statistical significance. Furthermore, the development of serious adverse events, especially in the lower total daily dosage group, was less than reported with this drug when used in the treatment of more advanced HIV disease. Overall compliance in this study was very good, and the vast majority of patients were able to continue to receive zidovudine without interruptions in therapy and without a reduction in dosage. In addition to a demonstrated clinical effect, zidovudine also had significant beneficial effects on CD4+ cell counts and HIV p24 antigen levels.

Because of the comparable clinical benefits between the two zidovudine dosage groups, but with significantly less toxicity in the lower dosage group, this regimen— 500 mg/day given in five divided doses—was subsequently approved by the Food and Drug Administration (FDA) for use in asymptomatic HIV-infected patients with fewer than 500 CD4+ cells/mm^3. This recommendation was reinforced by a panel of the NIAID that similarly recommended this treatment for patients who were known to be HIV infected and in whom CD4 cell counts had dropped below 500 cells/mm^3 (Table 9–2).

Although the benefit of treatment of asymptomatic infection in the setting of a CD4+ cell count above 500 cells/mm^3 has been established, several issues have been the subject of debate,[89,90] and subsequent analyses have been made to shed more light on this clinical trial experience. Preliminary results of a study conducted by the Veterans Administration suggested that there might be differences in the clinical benefit of zidovudine between white and nonwhite participants with symptomatic disease. In contrast, an analysis of the asymptomatic patients in the AIDS Clinical Trials Group study showed no such differences. Also, subsequent analyses of this clinical trial showed a very low rate of development of resistance to zidovudine in patients who were asymptomatic when they began the antiretroviral treatment. In one analysis of patients who remained asymptomatic, very low levels of resistance (median ID$_{50}$ = 0.07 μmoles/L) were detected, even after more than 2 years of continuous zidovudine treatment. A second, similar study showed virtually no cases of high-level zidovudine resistance in asymptomatic patients, even after 2 years of treatment.[91]

The optimum time at which zidovudine treatment should be initiated in asymptomatic, HIV-infected individuals remains uncertain. The preliminary results of the Veterans Administration study mentioned above indicated that zidovudine, when initiated immediately in a group of symptomatic HIV-infected patients with 200 to 500 CD4+ cells/mm^3, was more likely to decrease progression to AIDS than when this therapy was withheld until the CD4+ cell count declined to below 200 cells/mm^3. The AIDS Clinical Trials Group controlled study is still continuing for asymptomatic patients with greater than 500 CD4+ cells/mm^3. It is not yet known whether clinical or laboratory benefit will be demonstrated for this less advanced HIV disease or whether these findings would warrant changes in the current recommendations for the initiation of zidovudine therapy.

There are various excellent reviews providing guidelines for the essential baseline evaluation and follow-up clinical care of asymptomatic HIV-infected patients. The essence of these guidelines is that HIV infection must be considered in each patient contact, with testing used to make the diagnosis as early as possible. Early diagnosis can facilitate appropriate counseling and medical monitoring and, when indicated, therapeutic intervention. Once HIV infection has been diagnosed, patients should be evaluated for other coincident non-HIV-related medical problems that are commonly associated with the risk-related behaviors by which they acquired HIV infection. For example, patients who acquired HIV infection by a sexual route should be evaluated for other sexually transmitted diseases. Testing for those non-HIV problems might include tests for exposure to tuberculosis, hepatitis B, and syphilis. Finally, the initial evaluation should consider the subsequent probability that certain HIV-specific diseases will develop, and should include appropriate serologic tests, including that for prior exposure to *Toxoplasma gondii*.

These guidelines also recommend the frequency and type of continuing assessment of the HIV-infected person, and the frequency of follow-up of laboratory markers of disease stage. Briefly, the guidelines call for

Table 9–2.   Treatment Guidelines for Early HIV Disease

Treatment	*Comments*
ANTIRETROVIRAL THERAPY	
e.g., zidovudine	CD4+ < 500/mm^3
	Severe toxicity uncommon
	Duration of benefit > 2 yr
	High-level drug resistance rare
PNEUMOCYSTIC PROPHYLAXIS	
e.g., trimethoprim/sulfamethoxazole, dapsone, aerosolized pentamidine	CD4+ < 200/mm^3 or <20%
MONITORING RECOMMENDATIONS	
Examine patient more frequently as CD4+ cell count declines:	
Every 6–12 months if >500/mm^3	
Every 3 months if <500/mm^3	

a diminishing interval between medical assessments as the disease progresses. For example, whereas asymptomatic patients with essentially normal CD4+ cell counts might be reassessed every 6 to 12 months, this interval becomes as short as 3 months as the patient's CD4+ cell count approaches the count at which zidovudine therapy is considered indicated. The follow-up interval may become even shorter as the disease progresses and the need for additional active medical intervention, such as prophylaxis against specific opportunistic infections, becomes apparent.

The main concerns in the management of asymptomatic HIV disease center on increasing the effectiveness of antiretroviral therapy and on preventing or delaying the onset of opportunistic infections and malignancies. New drugs and drug combinations are currently being investigated for the treatment of HIV disease, as are new agents for the prevention of opportunistic infection. Together these approaches can be expected to substantially prolong the period in which the asymptomatic patient remains free of clinical disease.[92-94]

Early Symptomatic HIV Disease

As the duration of HIV infection increases and as more CD4+ cells are lost, patients pass from the asymptomatic to the symptomatic phase of HIV disease. The existence of a symptomatic state, independent of AIDS *per se,* was appreciated very early in the epidemic. Large numbers of patients in the same geographic and risk-behavior groups as patients with AIDS were known to have significant and chronic medical problems, but those problems did not meet the Centers for Disease Control (CDC) case definition of AIDS.[95,96] Disease in such patients usually later progressed to meet the CDC's AIDS criteria. Thus, it was expected that whatever the etiology of AIDS, it probably had a prolonged natural history, perhaps including an asymptomatic phase but certainly including a "pre-AIDS" phase. Although clinicians could reasonably agree on a good working definition for AIDS itself, there remained substantial uncertainty as to the diagnostic criteria for symptomatic patients who potentially had pre-AIDS. Thus, in 1983, well after the term AIDS was accepted, a working group convened by the CDC attempted to define what they called the AIDS-related complex.[95] They proposed a definition that combined several signs, symptoms, and laboratory abnormalities that had been reported in patients before AIDS developed. With the widespread use of CD4+ cell testing after 1983, many physicians also required that patients have a specified decline in CD4+ cell count, typically to less than 200 cells/mm³, to be considered to have ARC.

There were many problems with using a single definition to encompass the large and varied constellation of clinical problems associated with HIV infection. For this reason, the concept of ARC currently is much less widely favored. Instead, clinicians more frequently use the term *symptomatic HIV disease,* and rely on the relative type and degree of signs and symptoms as well as laboratory markers of immune states (*i.e.,* CD4+ cell count) to assess the stage of HIV infection in an individual patient. This approach—assessing the stage of disease along the spectrum of disease caused by HIV—is commensurate with current levels of knowledge. Further, as therapies more effective in lowering the probabilities of progression to symptomatic HIV disease and development of certain opportunistic diseases become available, staging by symptomatic status and immune dysfunction is likely to remain relevant. In fact, with advances in medical management, much of the phase of HIV disease previously called AIDS may be further divided into two separate stages, each with specific and unique prognostic and therapeutic implications.

The array of symptoms experienced by patients with HIV disease is impressive, ranging from relatively minor problems to potentially life-threatening ones. Nearly every organ system in the body can be affected, and the symptoms may range in duration and frequency from brief and nonrecurrent to persistent and chronic. Similarly, symptom response to therapy ranges from excellent to minimal, and the effect of symptoms on the patient ranges from minimal to devastating. Some of the signs and symptoms of HIV infection have an obvious etiology; others are much less well understood. Frequently, but not always, there is a relationship between medical understanding of the cause of a particular problem and the ability to treat it effectively. Also, there tends to be a relationship between the severity of symptoms and the degree of underlying immune deficiency. A complete review of each of the signs and symptoms of HIV infection and their management is beyond the scope of this chapter. However, several of the more frequent and important problems are described below. As the complexity and severity of complicating medical problems increase with CD4+ cell counts below 200 cells/mm³, patients in this phase of disease are considered to have late symptomatic HIV disease and are discussed separately. It should be emphasized, however, that the specific symptoms of the early symptomatic phase can and usually do continue throughout the patient's subsequent course.

Fever Fever is a common feature of the acute retroviral syndrome. Seemingly coinciding with a temporarily effective host control of HIV replication, the fever abates and does not recur during the asymptomatic period. HIV-infected patients in the asymptomatic phase can of course experience common, minor viral infections that may cause febrile episodes. In addition, fever is a feature common to an array of specific opportunistic infections and malignancies, including, but not limited to, *Pneumocystis carinii* pneumonia, cryptococcal meningitis, and HIV-related non-Hodgkin's lymphomas.

Patients with HIV infection, however, are often febrile in the absence of any specific opportunistic disease.

A common clinical question is the degree to which a fever can be accepted as a symptom of HIV, rather than as a symptom of a treatable bacterial infection, for example, thus not requiring further clinical or laboratory evaluation. The management of fever in patients with symptomatic HIV disease often relies on the intermittent or long-term use of nonsteroidal anti-inflammatory drugs. No single agent seems consistently more effective for all patients, and the optimum drug and regimen are often achieved only after a period of trial and error.

Night Sweats Another common and nonspecific symptom of HIV disease is the presence of recurrent, drenching night sweats. As with fevers, the pathogenesis of this symptom is poorly understood, but it is presumed to be due to circulating factors, either produced by or in reaction to HIV infection itself. According to the most widely used definition, night sweats are those that are drenching in severity and occur repeatedly over at least a 2-week period. Because night sweats are often associated with fever, the management of fever with long-term, regular administration of antipyretic agents may help control the sweats as well.

Chronic Diarrhea Chronic diarrhea is often associated with specific opportunistic GI pathogens later in the course of HIV disease.[97] Early in the disease course, however, diarrhea can occur without an identified association with specific pathogens. This diarrhea may be induced by HIV infection of the cells of the GI tract itself, or there may be opportunistic infections present for which currently available diagnostic procedures are inadequately sensitive. Whatever its origin, diarrhea can be uncomfortable and in severe cases can be associated with cachexia, dehydration, and general debilitation. The presence of severe or chronic diarrhea in a patient with HIV infection should prompt an aggressive search for an infectious etiology. While diagnostic evaluations are underway, and in the event that no specific offending pathogen is identified, symptomatic treatment can be offered.[98] No specific contraindications exist in HIV-infected patients to this symptomatic treatment, and drugs such as loperamide (Imodium) and diphenoxylate HCl/atropine sulfate (Lomotil) are often quite effective. Some success has also been reported with somatostatin analogues.

Fatigue Fatigue, in contrast to other signs such as fever or weight loss, is extremely hard to quantitate. Some quantitation would seem important, as the severity of impairment from this symptom ranges from mild limitations in a usually active life-style to severe debilitation, leaving patients nearly bedridden and unable to perform even the most routine daily activities. Fatigue is typically progressive: it may be noticed first only in the later part of the day, but progressively becomes more noticeable earlier in the day. The complaint of fatigue should prompt an evaluation for thyroid or adrenal insufficiencies; the latter are especially common in HIV infection.

In the absence of endocrine deficits and of any evidence of neuropathy or myopathy, management again becomes symptomatic. Of course, a patient complaining of fatigue should be evaluated for depression, as this symptom, which is commonly associated with somatic complaints, is quite treatable.

Minor Oral Infections Early in the epidemic, a high incidence of apparent oral *Candida albicans* infection was observed in people who did not yet meet the criteria for AIDS.[99] It was soon appreciated that some cases of apparent candidiasis were in fact due to oral hairy leukoplakia, an Epstein-Barr virus-related lesion first recognized in patients with HIV infection.[100,101] As with the other signs and symptoms of symptomatic HIV disease, the oral lesions may develop across a broad range of CD4+ cell counts. There is the sense, however, that patients with oral candidiasis in particular might be in a somewhat more advanced stage of disease and at higher risk for the near-term development of life-threatening opportunistic diseases. Treatment of oral *Candida* infection is straightforward[102] and a variety of topical and oral agents are successful, although there is a high rate of recurrence. Oral hairy leukoplakia is less often symptomatic and is often left untreated. For particularly unsightly leukoplakia lesions, however, treatment with high doses of oral acyclovir appears successful in most cases. Finally, periodontal disease is frequently seen in HIV disease and may be extremely aggressive, leading to tooth loss and bone destruction. Referral to specialists in oral medicine is strongly advised for such cases, and treatment with chlorhexidene is effective in controlling this problem in many patients.

Headache As is the case with other signs and symptoms of HIV infection, headache can be associated with specific opportunistic infections or cancers. In the absence of these, headache can be an important symptom of HIV disease. Some patients experience a recurring pattern of headache that can persist, in extreme cases, for years. In this regard, headache can be a symptom of ''asymptomatic'' HIV disease. Headaches are often described as severe and bifrontal or occipital. Diagnostic evaluation, including imaging, is indicated for the HIV-infected patient with headaches. In many patients with recurring headaches, no specific pathogen is identified and the cerebrospinal fluid is rather unremarkable, with lymphocyte-predominant pleocytosis and mild protein elevations seen in approximately 50% of cases.[103,104] Treatment is symptomatic, and nonsteroidal anti-inflammatory agents are preferred over narcotics, owing to the chronicity of this complaint.

CLINICAL MANAGEMENT OF SYMPTOMATIC HIV DISEASE

Patients in the earlier stages of symptomatic HIV disease do not have immediately life-threatening opportunistic infections or malignancies. Therefore, management consists of treatment of the underlying HIV infection itself and symptomatic therapy for the many non-life-threatening illnesses they may experience. The frequency of follow-up for patients with symptomatic HIV disease is generally dictated by the desire to initiate antiretroviral therapy at an appropriate time, if such therapy had not been initiated while the patient was asymptomatic, and to adequately monitor patients receiving such therapy to prevent the occurrence of severe toxicity. The frequency of follow-up is also related to the need for careful, objective evaluation of symptoms that may portend a serious opportunistic disease. These goals are largely met by determining CD4+ cell counts at approximately 3-month intervals, by monitoring specific laboratory values and symptoms associated with the development of drug-related toxicities, and by paying attention to new or worsening symptoms. It can be anticipated that the adverse effects of antiretroviral therapy will become more prominent as the underlying HIV disease progresses. Also, concerns of HIV resistance to antiretroviral therapy will be more important in patients who are symptomatic, as preliminary evidence suggests that there is a much higher rate of high-level resistance in symptomatic than in asymptomatic patients.[91,105] Although a complete review of antiretroviral therapy for such patients is beyond the scope of this chapter, combinations of antiretroviral agents may prove beneficial for patients with symptomatic HIV infection.[106,107]

Late Symptomatic HIV Disease

As the CD4+ count declines below 200 cells/mm³ in the symptomatic HIV-infected patient, the rate of serious opportunistic diseases increases. Along with the continuing treatment of HIV and of symptomatic complaints, the clinician must address the important question of primary prophylaxis against opportunistic infections common in patients with HIV disease. Such prophylaxis should be considered when convenient, inexpensive, and nontoxic antibiotics that are effective against the specific opportunistic infection are available, and when the probability of the near-term development of this opportunistic infection is predictable and high. Such prophylactic therapy should be offered when the subsequent risk of disease is sufficiently high, to minimize unnecessary exposure to these antibiotics; almost all antibiotics used prophylactically in this setting have side-effects and may induce drug resistance in some cases.

Pneumocystis carinii pneumonia is the opportunistic infection that is most commonly and successfully treated prophylactically, because of the relative accuracy with which this infection can be predicted and because of the availability of effective and safe oral antibiotic regimens.[108–111] Ongoing cohort studies of HIV-infected persons have shown that there is a low 6-month risk of *Pneumocystis carinii* pneumonia (<0.5%) until the CD4+ cell count drops below 200 cells/mm³ or the total lymphocyte population declines to below 20%. After

such a drop, the 6-month risk rises to 8.4% and even higher if chronic symptoms of HIV infection are also present. Effective orally administered regimens include trimethoprim-sulfamethoxazole,[112] trimethoprimdapsone, and dapsone alone,[113] and newer experimental agents are being evaluated. Also, pentamidine given as an inhaled aerosol has activity and is approved for prophylaxis against *Pneumocystis carinii* pneumonia.

Prophylaxis against opportunistic infections other than *Pneumocystis carinii* pneumonia are currently under investigation, including orally administered fluconazole for cryptococcal meningitis and oral agents for CNS toxoplasmosis, *Mycobacterium avium-intracellulare,* and CMV retinitis. In these areas clinical trials are ongoing.

The frequency of follow-up for patients with late symptomatic HIV disease is driven more by the symptom complex and the rate of disease progression than by any simple algorithm. Obviously, as the stage of disease advances and as the immune dysfunction worsens, more frequent monitoring will be necessary. Also, more frequent diagnostic testing may be necessary to evaluate the symptoms of HIV infection as they appear, in order to provide the earliest possible diagnosis of specific life-threatening opportunistic infections and cancers.

Advanced HIV Disease

Patients with symptomatic disease pass from the stage of moderate symptomatology and immune deterioration to one of more life-threatening manifestations and more severe immune dysfunction. With the increasing use of antiretroviral drug therapy and primary prophylactic regimens, the term "AIDS" has seemed inadequate and restricted. It is now possible to prevent or delay certain AIDS-defining opportunistic diseases without a concomitant reduction in the severity of the HIV-induced immune deficiency. For this reason, many physicians rely more heavily on the laboratory staging of HIV disease, especially with CD4+ cell counts. Nevertheless, it is understood that the tempo of the disease may accelerate, and the psychological impact of its progression is qualitatively different in patients who have experienced a life-threatening manifestation of HIV infection than in those who have not. Thus, there is still some ambiguity in our terminology, which may lessen as our knowledge of this process increases. In this review, *advanced HIV disease* is used for those patients with an increasingly significant risk of mortality, which separate studies have seen when CD4+ cell counts drop below 50 cells/mm³. This staging thus avoids the term "AIDS" altogether and is helpful, insofar as the development of specific "AIDS-defining" opportunistic diseases can be delayed, to some degree, without improving the underlying immune dysfunction. Evidence from a carefully followed cohort of patients at the National Cancer Institute showed that there is a low probability of death until CD4+ cell counts drop below 50 cells/mm³. Below this level, however, this hazard increases greatly. Nevertheless, opportunistic diseases are central to the problem of advanced HIV disease and remain the cause of much of our concern because of their high morbidity and mortality rates. Other laboratory features of advanced HIV disease, in addition to those specific to each of the opportunistic diseases, deserve mention: low serum albumin and cholesterol levels, high levels of serum globulins, and features reflecting functional limitations of bone marrow. In patients with advanced disease, anemia and neutropenia may occur independent of the use of myelosuppressive medication.

CLINICAL MANAGEMENT OF ADVANCED HIV DISEASE

The management of patients with advanced HIV disease is even less driven by fixed algorithms than the management of patients with earlier stage HIV disease. The patient with advanced disease requires much more intensive and more frequent clinical examination because of the potentially short period to the development of life-threatening diseases or complications of therapy. Many patients are seen every 1 to 4 weeks, for example, and even more frequent examinations may be necessary. The management of advanced HIV disease is likely to change substantially with the availability of additional antiretroviral agents, some of which are just now entering clinical testing. As agents prove effective and become available, their use in combination with zidovudine or with each other may prove to be beneficial, particularly in patients in whom total viral burden, viral replication rate, and immune deficits appear to combine to make the rapid development of resistance to zidovudine quite common.

Ideally, especially for patients with advanced disease, laboratory markers that allow us to determine whether a given patient is responding to antiretroviral therapy, and to identify patients in whom previously beneficial therapy is no longer effective, will become available. Such markers would make rational treatment planning and followup possible; currently, however, this management is highly empirical.

The identification of surrogate markers of antiretroviral therapy is only now becoming possible as prospective epidemiologic cohorts are maturing and providing insight into the factors that predict disease progression. From the preliminary data, there is some optimism about the use of serial CD4+ cell counts in this setting; preliminary evidence suggests that patients in whom CD4+ cell counts increase after the initiation of zidovudine therapy have a better outcome.[75,81,82,114,115]

The duration of the advanced stage of HIV stage is variable but appears to be improving. Access to expert medical care is paramount for these patients, who will, by definition, die rapidly if prophylaxis against opportunistic infection, early diagnosis and treatment of opportunistic diseases, and continuous effective antiviral therapy are not made available. On the other hand, with good supportive care, survival for 2 or more years can

be expected. The key to continued progress appears to lie in broadening the success of opportunistic infection prophylaxis and in the availability of more effective agents or combinations of agents to more completely control the replication of HIV over a longer period of time. Ultimately, antiretroviral therapy alone or combined with immune-based therapy might restore some degree of immune function even in patients with established advanced HIV disease.

VARIATIONS IN HIV DISEASE

Because HIV infection is characterized by variability, it at first seems difficult to define specific types of variation in the disease process. Nevertheless, some of the interindividual or interpopulation differences in the course of HIV disease are instructive and suggest insights into the nature of the etiologic agent, the host, or the interaction between the two.

Perhaps the most evident patterns of variation in HIV disease are seen in specific subpopulations. For example, the manifestations of HIV disease, especially in advanced stages of disease, vary substantially in different geographic areas, in different racial and ethnic populations, between men and women, and between younger and older patients.

Geographic Variations in HIV Disease

Insofar as HIV disease involves a dynamic interaction between the virus, the host, and the environment, it is not surprising that substantial variations exist in the disease process in different parts of the world. Based on the nature of these variations, one might speculate that geographic or genetic differences exist in the locally dominant strain of HIV. It is also possible that regional manifestations of severe immunodeficiency might vary according to the prevalence of regional endemic diseases. Yet other factors, more difficult to quantify, might be involved. For example, access to skilled medical care may vary from region to region, as might the relative nutritional status of an affected population. Each of these factors, especially the specific endemic diseases, probably has some role in the geographic variations seen in HIV disease.

Geographic variability in the manifestations of HIV disease is present in the United States. For example, histoplasmosis is a common opportunistic infection in the Ohio River Valley and other parts of the United States where it is a common endemic disease.[116] Outside of these regions, histoplasmosis, even in patients with severe HIV-associated immunodeficiency, is quite rare. Conversely, tuberculosis as a complication of HIV disease is more common on the eastern seaboard, where, related to the excess uses of alcohol and illicit drugs in the urban underclass, tuberculosis is already much more common than in other parts of the United States.[117,118]

Geographic variation is also evident in the case of toxoplasmosis. In the United States, toxoplasmosis accounts for less than 2% of all primary diagnoses of severe HIV disease, while in France this figure is approximately 25%.[119,120] This difference is thought to reflect the baseline endemicity of this organism. In France, most likely owing to dietary habits that include the consumption of uncooked or undercooked meat, approximately 80% of the general population have serologic evidence of exposure to *Toxoplasma gondii*. In contrast, only 17% of HIV-infected individuals in San Francisco are serologically reactive for this organism. As about 30% of patients with endogenous *Toxoplasma gondii* infection develop *Toxoplasma* encephalitis during the course of their HIV disease, it can be expected that CNS toxoplasmosis should be more common in France than in the United States. Numerous other examples of geographic variations in the distribution of HIV-associated opportunistic infections can be cited: *Mycobacterium avium-intracellulare* complex infections are more common in the United States than in Europe,[121] and are very uncommon in Africa, and cryptococcal meningitis is more common in Africa than in other parts of the world.[122,123]

Race and Ethnicity

A third form of variation in the spectrum of HIV diseases is associated with the race and ethnicity of the patient. For reasons that may be partially genetic, HIV infection has spread less rapidly among Asian- and Pacific Island–origin Americans. Also, although more likely due to differences in the route of HIV acquisition, Kaposi's sarcoma is less common in African-Americans than in white Americans.[124] Recently, the preliminary results of the Veterans Administration placebo-controlled trial of zidovudine in patients with moderately symptomatic HIV disease became available. In this study, more than 350 patients were randomized either to begin zidovudine immediately or to wait until CD4+ cell counts declined. In the patient population overall, the preliminary results confirmed those of several other groups with regard to the benefit of this therapy. However, the Veterans Administration investigators observed that these benefits did not seem to accrue in the subgroup of African-American and Latino subjects in their study. In this subset of patients, there was no measurable effect of zidovudine therapy on CD4+ cell count, nor was there any apparent survival advantage to early as opposed to later initiation of treatment. Although these preliminary observations have been disputed, it is at least conceivable that differences do exist in the metabolism or efficacy of a drug such as zidovudine in certain groups of patients, and that these differences may ultimately limit the drug's effectiveness.

Sex-Based Differences

The sex of the HIV-infected individual as a variable in the disease process has become a center of much con-troversy.[47,125–127] While it stands to reason that some types of infections common in non-HIV-infected persons, such as vaginal candidiasis, may be increased in frequency and in severity in the setting of immune dysfunction associated with HIV infection, published evidence for such differences remains limited. One study does suggest that HIV-infected women have a higher rate of aggressive vaginal candidiasis, and other studies have indicated an apparent increase in the rate of clinical HIV disease progression in women. These conclusions are still tentative, however, and are expected to be the subject of future epidemiologic and clinical trials. Resolving these issues related to the clinical course of HIV disease in women is important to ensure that adequate diagnosis, reporting, management, and compensation for medical care are afforded these patients. For this reason, many investigators and laypeople have called for careful prospective studies of the natural history of HIV disease in women and for the more systematic inclusion of careful serial examinations of women participating in clinical trials, including more frequent and regular examinations for cervical dysplasia in women infected with HIV.

Age-Related Differences

The age of the HIV-infected individual is another potential source of variability in the manifestations of the disease process. It is clear that the rate of HIV progression can be very rapid in infants; and HIV-infected hemophiliacs older than 30 years appear to have a worse prognosis. However, advancing age between the periods of later childhood and about 30 years of age appears to have only a relatively small effect on the rate of disease progression. The reasons for these differences are unclear. Moreover, advocates for the care of adolescent HIV-infected individuals point to the nearly complete absence of information on the spectrum of disease and the rate of HIV disease progression in this important intermediate age group.

Chronologic Variations in the Spectrum of HIV Disease

In addition to obvious differences in the spectrum of HIV disease and the incidence of specific opportunistic infections and malignancies in different populations, there has been a clear change in the disease spectrum over time even within a given population. For example, the rate of occurrence of Kaposi's sarcoma in homosexual men, while much higher than in nonhomosexual HIV-infected populations, is decreasing over time. Initially accounting for nearly 50% of all reported cases of AIDs, Kaposi's sarcoma accounted for only approximately 18% of initial cases reported in 1989. This change does not simply reflect an increase in nonhomosexual cases (*e.g.,* IV drug users) of HIV disease, as similar, although in absolute terms smaller, changes were seen in all subpopulations infected with HIV. Of additional interest is the observation that although the relative incidence of Kaposi's sarcoma in homosexual men appears to be decreasing, the clinical course of this malignancy currently appears to be more aggressive.

The reasons for chronologic variation in the spectrum of HIV disease remain conjectural. One intriguing possibility is that the rates of HIV disease progression reflect some type of statistical distribution. Because the disease process requires an interaction between the host and the etiologic agent, in this case HIV, it has been speculated that individuals who become ill within a relatively short time after HIV exposure are qualitatively and quantitatively different from patients who become ill more than a decade after exposure.[128] In other epidemics, the initial case fatality rate has been high and has declined with continued progression of the epidemic, even in the absence of specific treatments. Although this pattern may or may not be observed with HIV disease, it is an important area to study, as knowledge may change and further information may improve our ability to predict the future course and spread of this epidemic disease.

Changing Epidemiology due to the Availability of Treatment

An obvious potential source of variation in the clinical spectrum of HIV disease over time relates to therapeutic advances. Certainly, the effects of antiretroviral therapy, the primary and secondary prophylaxis of opportunistic diseases, and a more effective diagnosis and management of opportunistic diseases are apparent to all. It would in fact be surprising if the more widespread use of these and other therapeutic and diagnostic approaches had not resulted in a change in the epidemiology and clinical spectrum of reported HIV disease. Evidence to support this change is already available. In the San Francisco men's health study, a prospective epidemiologic cohort of homosexual men, the projected incidence of AIDS decreased coincident with the introduction and widespread use of zidovudine.[129,130] Also, in the largest study of aerosolized pentamidine for prophylaxis of *Pneumocystis carinii* pneumonia, the risk of disease progression was much lower in those also reported to be taking zidovudine therapy. Lastly, a retrospective analysis of HIV mortality in the state of Maryland estimated an increase in duration of survival from 190 to 770 days coincident with the introduction of zidovudine therapy.[131] While encouraging, these reports and the absence of similar findings in poorer populations within the United States or in developing countries should give us pause. Clearly these advances are not possible unless the individual has access to competent medical care and appropriate diagnostic and therapeutic maneuvers. This access is far from widely available in many parts of the world, including India, Africa, and the American underclass, where HIV infection is still spreading rapidly.

A final aspect of the changing epidemiology coincident with therapy regards our basic terminology. As described, I favor the conceptualization of HIV infection with its subsequent disease process as one of continuous and progressive immune deterioration, which can be staged by the symptomatic state of the patient and by the use of laboratory markers such as CD4+ cell counts. As additional therapeutic agents become increasingly successful in preventing the specific manifestations of HIV disease without reversing the underlying immune deficit, it will be more important to avoid terms such as AIDS and ARC, which are limited in their definitions to the specific symptoms and opportunistic diseases that the individual patient is currently experiencing. Because these diseases and symptoms may be affected by ongoing therapy, it seems best to avoid these terms and adopt the approach of staging based primarily on symptoms and on measured immune competence.

SUMMARY

This chapter has reviewed the epidemiologic and clinical spectrum of HIV disease and of its associated sequelae. I have argued that HIV disease should be considered to be a progressive process, and that monitoring the spectrum of manifestations, combined with appropriate assessment of immune competence using serial CD4+ cell counts, permits the clinician and the patient to follow the tempo of the HIV disease and to initiate antiretroviral therapy, to initiate appropriate prophylaxis for specific opportunistic infections, and to be alert for the development of disease manifestations at the optimal times. As we observe the epidemic for longer periods of time, it is clear that we will find more relationships between those opportunistic diseases already reported in HIV disease and others yet to be reported to the overall disease process. By studying the variations in the spectrum of disease, we may better understand the dominant direction of disease progression within the affected population, and thus be able to deliver appropriate effective care.

REFERENCES

1. Greene WC: The molecular biology of human immunodeficiency virus type 1 infection. N Engl J Med 324:308, 1991
2. Brodsky MH, Warton M, Myers RM, Littman DR: Analysis of the site in CD4 that binds to the HIV envelope glycoprotein. J Immunol 144:3078, 1990
3. Dalgleish AG, Beverley PCL, Clapham PR et al: The CD4 (T4) antigen is an essential component of the receptor for the AIDS retrovirus. Nature 312:763, 1984
4. Deen KC, McDougal JS, Inacker R et al: A soluble form of CD4 (T4) protein inhibits AIDS virus infection. Nature 331:82, 1988

5. Klatzmann D, Champagne E, Chamaret S et al: T-lympho-cyte T4 molecule behaves as the receptor for human ret-rovirus LAV. Nature 312:767, 1984

6. Homsy J, Meyer M, Tateno M et al: The Fc and not CD4 receptor mediates antibody enhancement of HIV infection in human cells. Science 244:1357, 1989

7. Fauci AS, Schnittman SM, Poli G et al: Immunopathogenic mechanisms in human immunodeficiency virus (HIV) in-fection. Ann Intern Med 114:678, 1991

8. Lifson JD, Reyes GR, McGrath MS et al: AIDS retrovirus induced cytopathology: Giant cell formation and involve-ment of CD4 antigen. Science 232:1123, 1986

9. Schnittman SM, Greenhouse JJ, Psallidopoulos MC et al: Increasing viral burden in CD4+ T cells from patients with human immunodeficiency virus (HIV) infection re-flects rapidly progressive immunosuppression and clinical disease. Ann Intern Med 113:438, 1990

10. Levy JA, Shimabukuro J, McHugh T et al: AIDS-associated retroviruses (ARV) can productively infect other cells be-sides human T helper cells. Virology 147:441, 1985

11. Levy JA: Human immunodeficiency viruses and the pathogenesis of AIDS. JAMA 261:2997, 1989

12. Hammer SM, Gillis JM, Pinkston P, Rose RM: Effect of zidovudine and granulocyte-macrophage colony-stimu-lating factor on human immunodeficiency virus replication in alveolar macrophages. Blood 75:1215, 1990

13. Gartner S, Markovits P, Markovitz DM et al: The role of mononuclear phagocytes in HTLV-III/LAV infection. Sci-ence 233:215, 1986

14. Ho DD, Rota TR, Hirsch MS: Infection of monocyte/mac-rophages by human T lymphotropic virus Type III. JCI 77:1712, 1985

15. Perno C-F, Yarchoan R, Cooney DA et al: Replication of human immunodeficiency virus in monocytes. J Exp Med 169:933, 1989

16. Watkins BA, Dorn HH, Kelly WB et al: Specific tropism of HIV-1 for microglial cells in primary human brain cul-tures. Science 249:549, 1990

17. Nelson JA, Reynolds-Kohler C, Margaretten W et al: Hu-man immunodeficiency virus detected in bowel epithe-lium from patients with gastrointestinal symptoms. Lancet 1:259, 1988

18. Membreno L, Irony I, Dere W et al: Adrenocortical func-tion in acquired immunodeficiency syndrome. J Clin En-docrinol Metab 65:482, 1987

19. Acierno LJ: Cardiac complications in acquired immuno-deficiency syndrome (AIDS): A review. J Am Coll Cardiol 13:1144, 1989

20. Anderson RM: The role of mathematical models in the study of HIV transmission and the epidemiology of AIDS. J AIDS 1:241, 1988

21. Aronow HA, Brew BJ, Price RW: The management of the neurological complications of HIV infection and AIDS. AIDS 2:S151, 1988

22. Jacobson MA, Mills J: Serious cytomegalovirus disease in the acquired immunodeficiency syndrome (AIDS). Ann Intern Med 108:585, 1988

23. Lane HC, Masur H, Gelmann EP et al: Correlation between immunologic function and clinical subpopulations of pa-tients with the acquired immune deficiency syndrome. Am J Med 78:417, 1985

24. Krown SE, Metroka C, Wernz JC, AIDS Clinical Trials Group Oncology Committee: Kaposi's sarcoma in the ac-quired immune deficiency syndrome: A proposal for uni-form evaluation, response, and staging criteria. J Clin On-col 7:1201, 1989

25. Masur H, Ognibene FP, Yarchoan R et al: CD4 counts as predictors of opportunistic pneumonias in human im-munodeficiency virus (HIV) infection. Ann Intern Med 111:223, 1989

26. Stites DP, Moss AR, Bacchetti P et al: Lymphocyte subset analysis to predict progression to AIDS in a cohort of ho-mosexual men in San Francisco. Clin Immunol Immu-nopathol 52:96, 1989

27. Lang W, Perkins H, Anderson RE et al: Patterns of T lym-phocyte changes with human immunodeficiency virus in-fection: From seroconversion to the development of AIDS. J AIDS 2:63, 1989

28. Phair J, Munoz A, Detels R, Multicenter AIDS Cohort Study Group: The risk of *Pneumocystis carinii* pneumonia among men infected with human immunodeficiency virus type 1. N Engl J Med 322:161, 1990

29. Kaslow RA, Phair JP, Friedman HB et al: Infection with the human immunodeficiency virus: Clinical manifesta-tions and their relationship to immune deficiency. Ann Intern Med 107:474, 1987

30. Berry CD, Hooton TM, Collier AC, Lukehart SA: Neuro-logic relapse after benzathine penicillin therapy for sec-ondary syphilis in a patient with HIV infection. N Engl J Med 316:1587, 1987

31. Jones DR, Tierney M, Felsenstein D: Alteration in the nat-ural history of neurosyphilis by concurrent infection with the human immunodeficiency virus. N Engl J Med 316:1569, 1987

32. Pelstring RJ, Zellmer RB, Sulak LE et al: Hodgkin's disease in association with human immunodeficiency virus infec-tion. Cancer 67:1865, 1991

33. Baer DM, Anderson ET, Wilkinson LS: Acquired immune deficiency syndrome in homosexual men with Hodgkin's disease. Am J Med 80:738, 1986

34. Schoeppel SL, Hoppe RT, Dorfman RF et al: Hodgkin's disease in homosexual men with generalized lymphade-nopathy. Ann Intern Med 102:68, 1985

35. Volberding PA: Treatment of malignant disease in AIDS patients. AIDS 2:S169, 1988

36. Folks TM: Human immunodeficiency virus in bone mar-row: Still more questions than answers. Blood 77:1625, 1991

37. Folks T, Kessler SW, Orenstein JM et al: Infection and replication of HIV-1 in purified progenitor cells of normal human bone marrow. Science 242:919, 1988

38. Stahl RE, Friedman-Kien A, Dubin R et al: Immunologic abnormalities in homosexual men. Am J Med 73:171, 1982

39. Ammamm AJ, Abrams DI, Conant M et al: Acquired im-mune dysfunction in homosexual men: Immunologic profiles. Clin Immunol Immunopathol 27:315, 1983

40. Volberding PA: HIV infection as a disease: The medical indications for early diagnosis. J AIDS 2:421, 1989

41. Rhame FS, Maki DG: The case for wider use of testing for HIV infection. N Engl J Med 320:1248, 1989

42. Francis DP, Chin J: The prevention of acquired immu-nodeficiency syndrome in the United States. JAMA 257:1357, 1987

43. Gershon RRM, Vlahov D, Nelson KE: The risk of trans-mission of HIV-1 through non-percutaneous, non-sexual modes: A review. AIDS 4:645, 1990

44. Donegan E, Lenes BA, Tomasulo PA, Transfusion Safety Study Group: Transmission of HIV-1 by component type

and duration of shelf storage before transfusion. Transfusion 30:851, 1990

45. Donegan E, Stuart M, Niland JC, Transfusion Safety Group: Infection with human immunodeficiency virus type 1 (HIV-1) among recipients of antibody-positive blood donations. Ann Intern Med 113:733, 1990

46. Padian NS, Shiboski SC, Jewell NP: The effect of number of exposures on the risk of heterosexual HIV transmission. J Infect Dis 161:883, 1990

47. Haverkos HW, Edelman R: The epidemiology of acquired immunodeficiency syndrome among heterosexuals. JAMA 260:1922, 1988

48. Henderson DK, Fahey BJ, Willy M et al: Risk for occupational transmission of human immunodeficiency virus Type 1 (HIV-1) associated with clinical exposures. Ann Intern Med 113:740, 1990

49. Hagen MD, Meyer KB, Kopelman RI, Pauker SG: Human immunodeficiency virus infection in health care workers: A method for estimating individual occupational risk. Arch Intern Med 149:1541, 1989

50. Asjo B, Albert J, Karlsson A et al: Replication capacity of human immunodeficiency virus from patients with varying severity of HIV infection. Lancet 2:660, 1986

51. de Wolf F, Roos M, Lange JMA et al: Decline in CD4+ cell numbers reflects increase in HIV-1 replication. AIDS Res Hum Retroviruses 4:433, 1988

52. Burke DS, Fowler AK, Redfield RR, Walter Reed Retroviral Research Group: Isolation of HIV-1 from the blood of seropositive adults: Patient stage of illness and sample inoculum size are major determinants of a positive culture. J AIDS 3:1159, 1990

53. Weiss SH, Goedert JJ, Gartner S et al: Risk of human immunodeficiency virus (HIV-1) infection among laboratory workers. Science 239:68, 1988

54. Falloon J, Eddy J, Wiener L, Pizzo PA: Human immunodeficiency virus infection in children. J Pediatr 114:1, 1989

55. Goedert JJ, Drummond JE, Minkoff HL et al: Mother-to-infant transmission of human immunodeficiency virus type 1: Association with prematurity or low anti-gp120. Lancet 2:1351, 1989

56. Cowan MJ, Walker C, Culver K et al: Maternally transmitted HIV infection in children. AIDS 2:437, 1988

57. European Collaborative Study: Children born to women with HIV-1 infection: Natural history and risk of transmission. Lancet 337:253, 1991

58. Ziegler JB, Johnson RO, Cooper DA, Gold JWM: Postnatal transmission of AIDS-associated retrovirus from mother to infant. Lancet 1:896, 1985

59. Stiehm ER, Vink P: Transmission of human immunodeficiency virus infection by breast-feeding. J Pediatr 118:410, 1991

60. Cooper DA, Maclean P, Finlayson R et al: Acute AIDS retrovirus infection. Lancet 1:537, 1985

61. Wallace MR, Harrison WO: HIV seroconversion with progressive disease in health care worker after needlestick injury. Lancet 1:1454, 1988

62. Gaines H, von Sydow M, Pehrson PO, Lundbergh P: Clinical picture of primary HIV infection presenting as a glandular-fever-like illness. Br Med J 297:1363, 1988

63. Tindall B, Cooper DA, Donovan B et al: Primary human immunodeficiency virus infection: Clinical and serologic aspects. Infect Dis Clin North Am 2:329, 1988

64. Tindall B, Barker S, Donovan B, Sydney AIDS Study Group: Characterization of the acute clinical illness associated with human immunodeficiency virus infection. Arch Intern Med 148:945, 1988

65. Fox R, Eldred LJ, Fuchs EJ et al: Clinical manifestations of acute infection with human immunodeficiency virus in a cohort of gay men. AIDS 1:35, 1987

66. Grant I, Atkinson JH, Hesselink JR et al: Evidence for early central nervous system involvement in the acquired immunodeficiency syndrome (AIDS) and other human immunodeficiency virus (HIV) infections. Ann Intern Med 107:828, 1987

67. Carne CA, Smith A, Elkington SG et al: Acute encephalopathy coincident with seroconversion for anti-HTLV-III. Lancet 2:1206, 1985

68. Lo B, Steinbrook RL, Cooke M et al: Voluntary screening for human immunodeficiency virus (HIV) infection. Ann Intern Med 110:727, 1989

69. Burcham J, Marmor M, Dubin N et al: CD4% is the best predictor of development of AIDS in a cohort of HIV-infected homosexual men. AIDS 5:365, 1991

70. Phillips AN, Lee CA, Elford J et al: Serial CD4 lymphocyte counts and development of AIDS. Lancet 337:389, 1991

71. Malone JL, Simms TE, Gray GC et al: Sources of variability in repeated T-helper lymphocyte counts from human immunodeficiency virus type 1-infected patients: Total lymphocyte count fluctuations and diurnal cycle are important. J AIDS 3:144, 1990

72. Taylor JMG, Fahey JL, Detels R, Giorgi JV: CD4 percentage, CD4 number, and CD4:CD8 ratio in HIV infection. Which to choose and how to use. J AIDS 2:114, 1989

73. Munoz A, Carey V, Saah AJ et al: Predictors of decline in CD4 lymphocytes in a cohort of homosexual men infected with human immunodeficiency virus. J AIDS 1:396, 1988

74. Moss AR: Predicting who will progress to AIDS: At least four laboratory predictors available. Br Med J 2:1067, 1988

75. Anderson RE, Lang W, Shiboski S et al: Use of beta2-microglobulin level and CD4 lymphocyte count to predict development of acquired immunodeficiency syndrome in persons with human immunodeficiency virus infection. Arch Intern Med 150:73, 1990

76. Hofmann B, Wang Y, Cumberland WG et al: Serum beta2-microglobulin level increase in HIV infection: Relation to seroconversion, CD4 T-cell fall and prognosis. AIDS 4:207, 1990

77. Kramer A, Wiktor S, Fuchs D et al: Neopterin: A predictive marker of acquired immune deficiency syndrome in human immunodeficiency virus infection. J AIDS 2:291, 1989

78. Melmed RN, Taylor JMG, Detels R et al: Serum neopterin changes in HIV-infected subjects: Indicator of significant pathology, CD4 T cell changes, and the development of AIDS. J AIDS 2:70, 1989

79. Eyster ME, Ballard JO, Gail MH et al: Predictive markers for the acquired immunodeficiency syndrome (AIDS) in hemophiliacs: Persistence of p24 antigen and low T4 cell count. Ann Intern Med 110:963, 1989

80. Rinaldo C, Kingsley L, Neumann J et al: Association of human immunodeficiency virus (HIV) p24 antigenemia with decrease in CD4+ lymphocytes and onset of acquired immunodeficiency syndrome during the early phase of HIV infection. J Clin Microbiol 27:880, 1989

81. Machado SG, Gail MH, Ellenberg SS: On the use of laboratory markers as surrogates for clinical endpoints in the evaluation of treatment for HIV infection. J AIDS 3:1065, 1990

82. Moss AR: Laboratory markers as potential surrogates for clinical outcomes in AIDS trial. J AIDS 3:S69, 1990

83. Lemp GF, Payne SF, Rutherford GW et al: Projections of AIDS morbidity and mortality in San Francisco. JAMA 263:1497, 1990

84. Moss AR, Bacchetti P: Editorial review: Natural history of HIV infection. AIDS 3:55, 1989

85. Ward JW, Bush TJ, Perkins HA et al: The natural history of transfusion-associated infection with human immunodeficiency virus. N Engl J Med 321:947, 1989

86. Eyster ME, Gail MH, Ballard JO et al: Natural history of human immunodeficiency virus infections in hemophiliacs: Effects of T-cell subsets, platelet counts, and age. Ann Intern Med 107:1, 1987

87. Schoenbaum EE, Hartel D, Friedland G: HIV infection and intravenous drug use. Curr Opinion Infect Dis 3:80, 1990

88. Volberding PA, Lagakos SW, Koch MA, AIDS Clinical Trials Group of the National Institute of Allergy and Infectious Diseases: Zidovudine in asymptomatic human immunodeficiency virus infection. N Engl J Med 322:941, 1990

89. Cotton P: Controversy continues as experts ponder zidovudine's role in early HIV infection. JAMA 263:1605, 1990

90. Hamilton JD, Simberkoff MS, Hartigan P et al: Zidovudine in asymptomatic HIV infection (letter). N Engl J Med 323:754, 1990

91. Richman DD, Grimes JM, Lagakos SW: Effect of stage of disease and drug dose on zidovudine susceptibilities of isolates of human immunodeficiency virus. J AIDS 3:743, 1990

92. Arno PS, Shenson D, Siegel NF et al: Economic and policy implications of early intervention in HIV disease. JAMA 262:1493, 1989

93. Makadon HJ, Seage GR, Thorpe KE, Fineberg HV: Paying the medical cost of the HIV epidemic: A review of policy options. J AIDS 3:123, 1990

94. Friedland GH: Early treatment for HIV: The time has come. N Engl J Med 322:1000, 1990

95. Haverkos HW, Gottlieb MS, Killen JY, Edelman R: Classification of HTLV-III/LAV-related diseases. J Infect Dis 152:1095, 1985

96. Centers for Disease Control: The Centers for Disease Control's surveillance definition of AIDS. MMWR 35:334, 1986

97. Greenson JK, Belitsos PC, Yardley JH, Bartlett JG: AIDS enteropathy: Occult enteric infections and duodenal mucosal alterations in chronic diarrhea. Ann Intern Med 114:366, 1991

98. Johanson JF, Sonnenberg A: Efficient management of diarrhea in the acquired immunodeficiency syndrome (AIDS). Ann Intern Med 112:942, 1990

99. Klein RS, Harris CA, Small CB et al: Oral candidiasis in high-risk patients as the initial manifestation of the acquired immunodeficiency syndrome. N Engl J Med 311:354, 1984

100. Greenspan JS, Greenspan D, Lennette ET et al: Replication of Epstein-Barr virus within the epithelial cells of oral "hairy" leukoplakia, an AIDS-associated lesion. N Engl J Med 313:1564, 1985

101. Greenspan D, Conant M, Silverman S et al: Oral "hairy" leucoplakia in male homosexuals: Evidence of association with both papillomavirus and a herpes-group virus. Lancet 2:831, 1984

102. Greenspan JS, Greenspan D, Winkler JR: Diagnosis and management of the oral manifestations of HIV infection and AIDS. Infect Dis Clin North Am 2:373, 1988

103. Hollander H, Stringari S: Human immunodeficiency virus-associated meningitis. Am J Med 83:813, 1987

104. Hollander H: Cerebrospinal fluid normalities and abnormalities in individuals infected with human immunodeficiency virus. J Infect Dis 158:855, 1988

105. Larder BA, Kellam P, Kemp SD: Zidovudine resistance predicted by direct detection of mutations in DNA from HIV-infected lymphocytes. AIDS 5:137, 1991

106. Hirsch MS: Chemotherapy of human immunodeficiency virus infections: Current practice and future prospects. J Infect Dis 161:845, 1990

107. Yarchoan R, Mitsuya H, Broder S: Strategies for the combination therapy of HIV infection. J AIDS 3:99, 1990

108. Freedberg KA, Tosteson ANA, Cohen CJ, Cotton DJ: Primary prophylaxis for *Pneumocystis carinii* pneumonia in HIV-infected people with CD4 counts below 200/mm^3: A cost-effectiveness analysis. J AIDS 4:521, 1991

109. Hirschel B, Lazzarin A, Chopard P, Swiss Group for Clinical Studies on AIDS: A controlled study of inhaled pentamidine for primary prevention of *Pneumocystis carinii* pneumonia. N Engl J Med 324:1079, 1991

110. Ruskin J, LaRiviere M: Low-dose co-trimoxazole for prevention of *Pneumocystis carinii* pneumonia in human immunodeficiency virus disease. Lancet 337:468, 1991

111. Fischl MA: Treatment and prophylaxis of *Pneumocystis carinii* pneumonia. AIDS 2:s143, 1988

112. Shafer RW, Seitzman PA, Tapper ML: Successful prophylaxis of *Pneumocystis carinii* pneumonia with trimethoprim-sulfamethoxazole in AIDS patients with previous allergic reactions. J AIDS 2:389, 1989

113. Kemper CA, Tucker RM, Lang OS et al: Low-dose dapsone prophylaxis of *Pneumocystis carinii* pneumonia in AIDS and AIDS-related complex. AIDS 4:1145, 1990

114. Fahey JL, Taylor JMG, Detels R et al: The prognostic value of cellular and serologic markers in infection with human immunodeficiency virus type 1. N Engl J Med 322:166, 1990

115. de Wolf F, Lange JMA, Houweling JTM et al: Appearance of predictors of disease progression in relation to the development of AIDS. AIDS 3:563, 1989

116. Bonner JR, Alexander WJ, Dismukes WE et al: Disseminated histoplasmosis in patients with the acquired immune deficiency syndrome. Arch Intern Med 144:2178, 1984

117. Small PM, Schecter GF, Goodman PC et al: Treatment of tuberculosis in patients with advanced human immunodeficiency virus infection. N Engl J Med 324:289, 1991

118. Sunderam G, McDonald RJ, Maniatis T et al: Tuberculosis as a manifestation of the acquired immunodeficiency syndrome (AIDS). JAMA 256:362, 1986

119. Israelski DM: Toxoplasmic encephalitis in patients with AIDS. Infect Dis Clin North Am 2:429, 1988

120. Luft BJ, Brooks RG, Conley FK et al: Toxoplasmic encephalitis in patients with acquired immune deficiency syndrome. JAMA 252:913, 1984

121. Hawkins CC, Gold JWM, Whimby E et al: *Mycobacterium avium* complex infections in patients with the acquired immunodeficiency syndrome. Ann Intern Med 105:184, 1986

122. Chuck SL, Sande MA: Infections with *Cryptococcus neoformans* in the acquired immunodeficiency syndrome. N Engl J Med 321:794, 1989

123. Zuger A, Louie E, Holzman RS et al: Cryptococcal disease in patients with the acquired immunodeficiency syndrome. Ann Intern Med 104:234, 1986

124. Haverkos HW, Drotman DP, Morgan M, Amsel Z: Kaposi's sarcoma in homosexual men with AIDS, by race. Lancet 2:1075, 1988

125. Anastos K, Palleja SM: Caring for women at risk of HIV infection. J Gen Intern Med 6:S40, 1991

126. Kim HC, Raska K, Clemow L et al: Human immunodeficiency virus infection in sexually active wives of infected hemophilic men. Am J Med 85:472, 1988

127. Padian NS: Editorial review: Prostitute women and AIDS: Epidemiology. AIDS 2:413, 1988

128. Lang W: Frailty selection and HIV. Lancet 1:1397, 1989

129. Gail MH, Rosenberg PS, Goedert JJ: Therapy may explain recent deficits in AIDS incidence. J AIDS 3:296, 1990

130. Rosenberg PS, Gail MH, Schrager LK et al: National AIDS incidence trends and the extent of zidovudine therapy in selected demographic and transmission group. J AIDS 4:392, 1991

131. Moore RD, Hidalgo J, Sugland BW, Chaisson RE: Zidovudine and the natural history of the acquired immunodeficiency syndrome. N Engl J Med 324:1412, 1991

10

Serologic Tests for Human Immunodeficiency Virus Infection

Richard T. Davey, Jr.   *M. B. Vasudevachari*   *H. Clifford Lane*

With official recognition of the existence of a new clinical syndrome in 1981,[1,2] initial diagnoses of the acquired immunodeficiency syndrome (AIDS) were presumptive and were usually made on the basis of a distinct set of clinical illnesses occurring in the absence of other known causes of immunosuppression. These illnesses were primarily opportunistic infections and unusual malignancies that were diagnosed in association with laboratory evidence of defective immune function. Within this framework a comprehensive case definition was constructed that attempted to group presumptive cases of AIDS on the basis of common clinical and immunologic parameters even prior to the identification of a defined infectious etiology.[3,4] However, with isolation and identification of human immunodeficiency virus type 1 (HIV-1) as the causative agent in 1983–1984,[5,6] considerable emphasis was placed on the development and testing of accurate serologic methods by which to measure infection with the virus in patients even before they developed symptoms compatible with the clinical case definition.

Within a short period of time solid-phase assays were developed that, when used properly according to established guidelines, proved to be both highly sensitive and specific. Commercial production of these assays in relatively inexpensive kit form soon allowed them to be adopted for widescale use. In the past few years, more sophisticated virologic and immunologic techniques have also been developed that have further enhanced our ability to diagnose HIV-1 infection early and accurately and have also contributed to the longitudinal follow-up of patients with known infection.

However, the potential value of these newer techniques notwithstanding, various modifications of the original solid-phase serologic methods have remained the standard means by which the vast majority of infections with HIV-1 continue to be diagnosed in the United States and many developed nations. This chapter will review some of these standard serologic methods as they pertain to the laboratory diagnosis of HIV-1 infection.

HIV-1 ENZYME IMMUNOASSAYS

In the mid-1980s, much of the impetus for the development of rapid serologic screening methods for HIV-1 arose from the dual need to have available (1) a rapid, reliable, and inexpensive means of screening the nation's blood supply for occult infection, and (2) a sensitive method of screening patients for HIV-1 infection even in the absence of overt clinical disease. Prior to the development and commercial production of solid-phase screening methods, for example, the safety of donated blood or other transfusion products could only be assured by means of a system of voluntary self-deferral by members of groups believed to be at high risk for transmission of the virus. While clearly important in reducing the rate of transmission of virus from transfused blood products, such self-deferral methods were unreliable because of their strict dependence on the altruism of the donor population.

In March 1985 the routine testing of donated blood by a rapid solid-phase approach became available through the development, testing, and licensure of the first enzyme-linked immunoassay (ELISA) kit. Thereafter, it soon became evident that separate access to a system of testing at-risk individuals for infection with HIV-1 would assume equal importance if deliberate blood donation as a ready means of determining HIV-1 serostatus were to be avoided. Because of the relative ease with which standardized microtiter assays could be manufactured, by 1987 a total of at least eight different commercial preparations had been licensed by the Food and Drug Administration.[7,8] It was in this milieu that the HIV-1 ELISA was rapidly established as a primary diagnostic screening tool.[9,10] So-called "alternate test sites" that were established nationwide in government-sponsored clinics to allow the confidential or anonymous testing of at-risk individuals were soon supplemented by the widescale availability of these generally inexpensive assays through other means, such as through separate hospital-based or commercial laboratories.

An important principle underlying the successful development of the early serologic assays for HIV-1 infection was the observation that the overwhelming majority of infected individuals appeared to mount a detectable antibody response to various protein components of the virus within a brief period of time after exposure.[11,12] Whereas exceptional individuals or cohorts have been described in which a significant lag period (up to 3 years or more) has been documented between the time of presumed viral infection and the development of a measurable antibody response,[13,14] it is generally believed that such individuals are quite uncommon.[15] Rather, most exposed individuals will develop antibody against the virus within a few months, and some as early as a few weeks after viral infection. Widescale serologic testing of infected individuals has also revealed that the major antigens against which antibody is produced are also fairly consistent within the population, although the exact timing of appearance and the relative intensity of individual antibody specificities may vary from person to person. Although the genome of HIV-1 (Fig. 10–1) is known to code for a number of structural and regulatory proteins as well as for proteins whose function is as yet poorly understood, three major protein groups of HIV-1 account for the highest intensity of circulating antibody directed against the virus[16]: (1) the envelope (*env*) proteins: the precursor membrane glycoprotein gp160 and its two major subunits, gp120 and gp41; (2) the polymerase (*pol*) proteins: the reverse

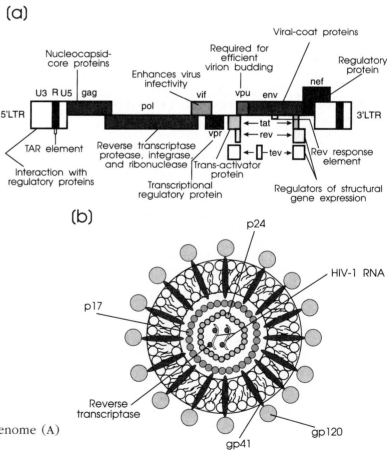

Figure 10–1.   Diagram of the HIV-1 viral genome (A) and the HIV-1 virion structure (B).

transcriptase p66 and the endonuclease p31; and (3) the core (*gag*) proteins: the precursor protein p55 and its components p24, p18, and p15.

Within a few weeks (4–8 weeks most commonly, although a duration as short as 8 days has been described) after exposure to the virus, infected individuals often experience a brief period of constitutional illness (fever, fatigue, myalgias, rash, gastrointestinal complaints, and, rarely, neurologic symptoms) that has been likened to an influenza-like viral illness.[12] This period lasts anywhere from a few days to a few weeks and is accompanied by a burst of active viral replication in the host, as documented by high levels of circulating virus in plasma as well as measurable p24 antigen expression. With subsidence of the acute symptomatology, increasing levels of virus-specific antibody begin to appear and can be quantified by a variety of serologic detection methods. Antibodies against p24 and against the viral envelope proteins (gp160 and gp41 in particular) are among the first detectable HIV-1–specific immunoglobulins produced during this period of acute seroconversion. Of note, conventional immunoassays appear to be especially sensitive to the early detection of anti-p24 antibody under these circumstances, whereas certain other tests, such as the radioimmunoprecipitation assay (RIPA) may show reactivity earlier with antibody directed against the higher molecular weight antigens such as gp160.[11]

The ELISA Method

The first generation of enzyme immunoassays that were licensed as diagnostic kits were based on the use of viral lysates derived from strains of HIV-1 propagated in infected cells, particularly those employing either the lymphoid leukemia cell line H9 (used in the kits produced by Abbott, Du Pont, Electronucleonics, Organon Teknika, Cellular Products, and Ortho, for example) or the CEM cell line (used in the kit produced by Genetic Systems).[7] The basis for a majority of these assay kits is an indirect antibody-binding system linked to a solid phase (use of microtiter plate wells is most common, although polystyrene or latex beads are also used) (Fig. 10–2). According to the method employed by most commercial manufacturers, viral lysate is prepared from common laboratory strains of virus (*e.g.,* lymphadenopathy virus, LAV) that have been passaged in tissue culture and then bound to the solid phase of the particular assay system. The relative amounts of each of the major structural and expressed proteins of HIV-1 may differ significantly between the various commercial preparations, although usually both the external envelope glycoproteins (*i.e.,* gp120 and its precursor, gp160) and the *gag*-derived products (p24 and p17 antigen in particular) are well represented in the bound material.

As with most conventional ELISA kits, patients' sera (often tested in duplicates or triplicates to reduce error) are allowed to react with antigens bound on the solid

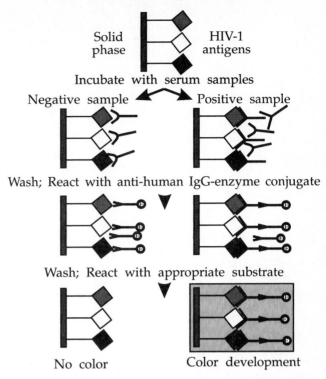

Figure 10–2. The standard commercial HIV-1 ELISA technique.

phase for a specified period of time, after which time unbound antibody is washed away in a rinse step. With some kits care must be taken to minimize the use of heat-inactivated sera, as a higher rate of false positivity has been reported when sera are treated in this fashion prior to testing.[17] If a patient's serum contains either specific anti-HIV-1 antibody or some nonspecific form of cross-reacting immunoglobulin, it will remain adherent to the viral preparation linked to the solid phase. Enzymatically labeled anti-human Ig is then added to the solid phase and allowed to incubate for a set period of time, and then the reaction mixture is washed as before. Most assays employ either alkaline phosphatase or horseradish peroxidase as the tagged enzyme. Finally, substrate material that is capable of undergoing a colorimetric reaction in the presence of the bound enzyme is added to the reaction well. The speed and intensity of the colorimetric reaction that follows are directly dependent on the amount of bound enzyme, which in turn is dependent on the quantity of anti-HIV-1 antibody bound to viral lysate on the solid phase. The intensity (recorded as the optical density, or O.D., of the reaction mixture) of this reaction is easily quantitated by means of a spectrophotometer calibrated to read at the optimal wavelength of the substrate material. A specific O.D. can then be assigned to each test well in a panel; in a typical microtiter plate assay, up to 96 wells can be read from a single plate. With the use of series of known positive and negative samples as controls, a standard curve for the colorimetric reaction is generated against which the O.D. of test samples can be compared. A "cutoff" value for the lowest O.D. still regarded as consistent with a positive determination can be calculated based on a statistical comparison of the intensity of a panel of positive control samples relative to known negative sera. Whereas test sera with O.D. values well above the cutoff point can be recorded as unequivocally positive, the scoring of samples with O.D. readings skirting the cutoff range can be more problematic. The propensity of test results to fall close to the cutoff range may vary from one manufacturer's kit to another. Thus, kits that produce positive readings closer to the cutoff range may exhibit slightly greater sensitivity than those requiring higher O.D. readings for a positive determination, but they may also be more prone to false-negative and false-positive findings as a consequence of this narrow margin.

In accord with its planned role as an initial screening device, it should not be surprising that the HIV-1 ELISA was designed to optimize sensitivity at the expense of specificity. Because of the availability of backup or confirmatory assays to validate positive findings as well as the potentially serious consequences of undiagnosed infections, a reduction in the number of false negatives even at the expense of a slightly higher rate of false positives was judged to be a reasonable trade-off. In this regard, most of the commercially marketed ELISA preparations have been shown to have a sensitivity of at least 99.5% and a specificity of greater than 99.8% in large-scale testing of individuals with high-risk behavior for HIV-1 acquisition.[16,18] However, the positive predictive value of the standard HIV-1 ELISA may fluctuate widely depending on the population being screened.[19] For example, the false-positive rate in low-risk populations is substantially higher than in high-risk populations, an observation that must be taken into account in the interpretation of preliminary test results. In a large study of volunteer blood donors (generally regarded as a low-risk pool) by the American Red Cross, only 13% of those individuals with a repeatedly reactive HIV-1 ELISA were determined to be HIV-1 infected on the basis of a confirmatory Western blot.[10] Such data have obvious implications for widescale screening of donated blood products, for which the majority of positive ELISA reactions may be expected to be false-positive readings on samples from uninfected donors. In contrast, the rate of false-negative results with conventional ELISA assays is believed to be quite small, currently no more than one in every 40,000 samples.[20] As advances in solid-phase technology lead to development of even more sensitive probes, this rate should continue to drop even further.

As with any assay capable of processing large numbers of test sera at one time, ELISA methodology is subject to a number of technical drawbacks that may diminish the significance of any single positive result. These range from frank procedural errors in the handling of samples, such as mislabeling of specimens, to deficiencies in the manual or automated performance of sample processing, such as well-to-well carry-over during pipetting and resultant contamination of neighboring wells. Apart from these purely technical considerations, the causes of false-positive ELISA results may be both varied and obscure. In some cases, however, certain common elements have been identified that may explain these findings. Chief among these is the presence of cross-reactive antibodies against certain common HLA antigens (HLA-DR and other class II antigens in particular) that may be present in some patients' sera. These antibodies presumably recognize and bind to cellular contaminants within the viral lysates used in these kits. The use of the CEM cell line (rather than H9 cells) to propagate virus in tissue culture has been reported to eliminate this particular cause of cross-reactivity.[21]

Other causes of false-positive ELISA readings that have been identified include the presence of autoreactive antibodies (*e.g.,* antinuclear or antimitochondrial antibodies), heat inactivation of sera prior to testing, repeated freeze-thaw cycles of test sera, severe hepatic disease, passive immunoglobulin administration (isolated cases of transient "seroconversion" have been reported in patients receiving passive IgG injections), and certain malignancies. Cross-reactivity of sera from patients with certain retroviral infections sharing antigenic similarity with HIV-1 (*e.g.,* HIV-2, whose *gag*-encoded proteins are closely related to those found in HIV-1) has also been reported; with other retroviral infections lacking these common epitopes (*e.g.,* HTLV-I), in contrast, cross-reactivity with HIV-1 on ELISA generally does not occur. The causes of false-negative ELISA findings are also varied and, in addition to improper handling of reagents in individual test kits, include performance of the assay too early in the period after HIV-1 exposure (*i.e.,* prior to seroconversion) as well as conditions that cause B-cell dysfunction and defective antibody synthesis, such as severe hypogammaglobulinemia.

A significant advance in the efforts to improve the sensitivity and specificity of existing solid-phase immunoassays came through the introduction of viral antigens produced through recombinant DNA technology to replace the crude mixtures of proteins derived from lysates. Not only can recombinant proteins be produced with considerably more purity and in higher amounts than protein derived from lysates, they can also be bound to solid-phase surfaces with much tighter control over protein ratios and concentrations. A potential drawback of such recombinant proteins is that they may afford a more limited repertoire of antigenic sites, and they may also differ somewhat from native proteins by virtue of altered patterns of glycosylation; nonetheless, the avidity between these antigens and anti-HIV-1 antibodies appears quite high. In addition to diagnostic utility in the screening of individuals and blood products, these newer generation immunoassays may prove especially valuable in the research setting. Immunoassays enriched in external envelope antigen such as gp160, for example, have already been utilized in the detection of anti-*env* antibody responses in individuals immunized with candidate anti-HIV-1 vaccines, particularly those employing either recombinant gp160 or gp120 protein as immunogen.[22,23] These assays have provided significantly enhanced sensitivity to early antibody responses over that afforded by a more conventional ELISA.

Most ELISA kits utilize enzyme-tagged anti-human IgG as the probe to detect the presence of bound HIV-1–specific antibody within a test well. Another refinement that may improve the sensitivity of existing immunoassays, as well as possibly lead to earlier detection of seroconversion, entails either the addition or substitution of enzyme-labeled anti-human IgM for anti-human Ig at this stage of the assay.

INTERPRETION OF ELISA RESULTS

Sera from an individual infected with HIV-1 should routinely test positive by commercial HIV-1 ELISA within a few months of exposure. Because these assays are variously enriched both in *gag*-derived proteins and envelope glycoproteins, antigens against which the humoral response in the host is characteristically brisk, the ELISA is usually quite sensitive in the early detection of seroconversion. Because of the uniformly high sensitivity of most commercial preparations, a negative ELISA reading at an appropriate interval following exposure strongly militates against the likelihood of infection. In general, barring procedural errors in the performance of the assay, there is usually no reason to require that a negative screening ELISA be immediately repeated in these circumstances. A common exception to this guideline would be if, as is often the case, the interval between testing and presumed exposure is unknown and there is the possibility that the original test was performed relatively early in the period after possible infection. In this situation it may be reasonable to repeat the test on a new sample within a few months of the initial assay. Negative findings on repeat testing undertaken in this manner may help rule out the possibility of a prolonged latency period between infection and seroconversion in any given individual. Alternatively, any of a number of newer, more sensitive methods (*e.g.,* polymerase chain reaction techniques, or PCR) of detecting the presence of the virus directly may be substituted for the standard serologic assays in these circumstances.[24–29]

Another circumstance in which repeat ELISA testing may be warranted is if the initial results showed borderline reactivity according to the internal O.D. standards generated within each test kit. O.D. readings falling slightly under (*e.g.,* less than 1 SD below) the cutoff value may simply reflect high negative signals from true seronegative sera or, alternatively, could represent the initial stages of reactivity in sera from an individual undergoing incipient seroconversion. Because the immunoassay is not capable of differentiating these two possibilities, either repeating the test on a fresh specimen, repeating the test with the same sera but using a different commercial assay, or a combination of these two approaches may be used to attempt to resolve this diagnostic uncertainty. If borderline reactivity persists despite repeated testing, a minimal recommendation is to repeat the ELISA within a few months' time. Failure of the O.D. to rise substantially over time, while not definitive evidence by itself, is suggestive of the likelihood that this low level of reactivity does not represent true infection. Again, the use of standard confirmatory procedures such as the Western blot or the use of newer direct-detection techniques may be quite helpful in these circumstances.

The HIV-1 Western Blot

Essential to the diagnosis of a true serologic response to HIV-1 infection is the requirement that a repeatedly positive result by ELISA or other rapid screening method be confirmed by specific delineation of the antibody profile associated with this finding. Because a positive ELISA result may be due to a number of causes, many of them unrelated to true HIV-1 infection, all ELISA readings in which the O.D. falls within the positive range must be verified by repeated testing prior to more detailed evaluation (Fig. 10–3). Although this algorithm should be followed on samples from all individuals, it is particularly applicable to individuals without risk factors for HIV-1 exposure, in whom the majority of positive ELISA test results will be false positives. Only samples that are repeatedly reactive on two or more separate ELISA runs merit further diagnostic evaluation with a confirmatory assay. In the United States and elsewhere, this confirmatory role most frequently involves the use of an HIV-1–specific Western blot, of which numerous commercial preparations have been marketed.[30] A positive Western blot not only confirms the presence of antibodies reactive with HIV-1 in the infected individual but also permits identification of the specific viral components to which that individual has raised a detectable humoral response. By serial application it can also be used to grade the intensity of the individual components of that response qualitatively and, in some cases, quantitatively during interval follow-up.

COMMERCIAL WESTERN BLOT PREPARATIONS

A conventional HIV-1 Western blot is an immunoblot preparation consisting of a crude lysate of HIV-1 cultivated in a continuous cell line, partially purified by differential centrifugation after cell lysis, separated by molecular weight into individual viral proteins *via* gel electrophoresis, and then electrophoretically transferred onto nitrocellulose paper (Fig. 10–4). The nitrocellulose paper is cut into narrow strips, which are then packaged in kit form along with an incubation tray and a set of developing reagents. Provision of seropositive and seronegative sera as controls is usually the responsibility of the individual laboratory performing the assay, and

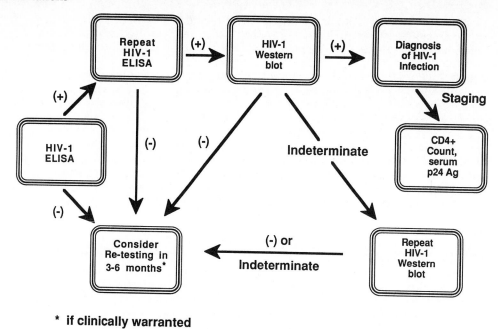

Figure 10–3.   Algorithm for the correct use and sequence of serologic testing in the diagnosis of HIV-1 infection.

such controls should be included in each separate run as an essential quality control measure. The standard assay is performed according to a modified method of Towbin *et al.*[31] Test sera are allowed to react with the individual viral components on the nitrocellulose paper, which serves as the solid support for the detection of antibodies in a manner analogous to the antigen-coated microtiter well in a standard ELISA. After washing and removal of unbound antibodies, recognition of various viral proteins by antibodies present within sera can be detected through addition of a second antibody directed against human immunoglobulin. The latter reagent is usually chemically tagged either with a radioactive probe that can be detected by autoradiographic means or, as

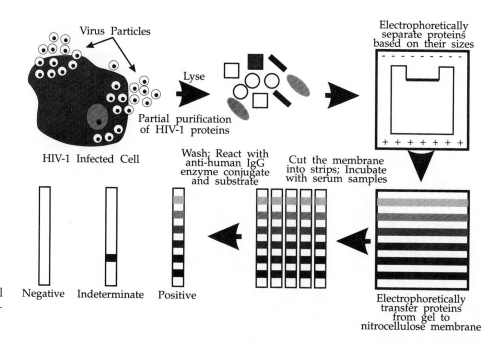

Figure 10–4. Commercial HIV-1 Western blot technique.

is more common in commercial preparations, with an enzyme capable of generating a colorimetric reaction in the presence of substrate added during a subsequent development step. Performance of many commercially available Western blot kits requires a minimal amount of sample handling and can now be completed within a few hours. By comparison with control sera as well as internal reference standards usually provided with each kit, results can be scored visually in terms of the pattern and number of antibody bands present. Alternatively, recently developed densitometry techniques now allow antibody banding to be evaluated quantitatively as well; in the research setting, for example, this may have particular value for following serologic reactivity to specific HIV-1 antigens over time. It has also been used to evaluate the humoral response to candidate AIDS vaccines in noninfected seronegative recipients following both primary and booster immunizations.[22]

When used to confirm seroreactivity in a patient with presumed HIV-1 infection, the Western blot will generally reveal variable degrees of antibody reactivity with the three major structural and/or enzymatic protein groups expressed by the virus: *env, gag,* and *pol* gene products (Fig. 10–5). The specific pattern of banding may vary from individual to individual, and the intensity

may fluctuate both according to the relative amounts of specific anti-HIV-1 antibody circulating at any given time and with the particular commercial preparation being used. Most commercial Western blot preparations are especially sensitive to the detection of anti-p24 antibody, and its appearance on immunoblotting may occur relatively early in the period after exposure, occasionally serving to herald the process of seroconversion. The appearance of detectable levels of antibody against *pol* and *env* gene products may be delayed until somewhat later, although this lag period is usually sufficiently brief that its impact on serodiagnosis is minor. Antibodies against other gene products of HIV-1, such as *nef* or other regulatory elements, are generally not detected by a conventional Western blot.

SCORING OF WESTERN BLOT RESULTS

Even predating official FDA licensure of the first commercial Western blot preparation (a kit manufactured by Biotech/Du Pont, Wilmington, DE) in April 1987, and further intensified by the introduction of several nonlicensed kits by different manufacturers, the correct interpretation or scoring of a Western blot result has been an area of considerable controversy in the medical literature. Even today not all laboratories have agreed on a common algorithm for the grading of test results. Occasionally this has led to some confusion in the reporting of test results, particularly when separate laboratories using different criteria have been asked to perform confirmatory assays on the same specimens.

Depending on the rigor of the definition applied, it is generally agreed that a negative Western blot is one in which either (1) no bands are present at any location or (2) at least no bands corresponding to the molecular weights of known viral proteins can be detected. The presence of bands at locations not corresponding to known viral antigens is a fairly common finding and is presumed to reflect contaminants within the preparation against which some degree of cross-reactive antibody recognition occurs. The molecular weights of these so-called aberrant bands may vary from manufacturer to manufacturer and even occasionally from lot to lot in kits produced by the same manufacturer.

The definition of what should constitute a positive Western blot result has been considerably more difficult to codify, particularly as there has been disagreement among investigators as to whether appropriate stringency of the definition should require the presence of antibody against any two *versus* all three of the major viral gene products. Antibody against a protein (or proteins) from all three groups has always been accepted as unequivocal evidence of a positive finding, and the Biotech/Du Pont kit was licensed with the manufacturer's recommendation that reactivity with all three gene products be present in order for a positive determination to be made.[32] This was also the position adopted by the American Red Cross at that time. More recently, however, there has been convincing evidence that antibody

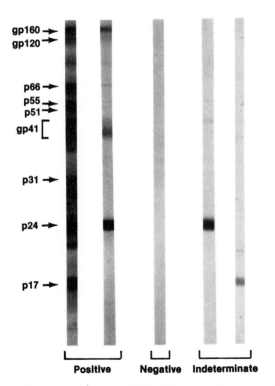

Figure 10–5. A positive HIV-1 Western blot, showing antibody banding at the major viral proteins that can be identified using this technique. For comparison, both a negative Western blot and an indeterminate Western blot are also shown.

against only two of the three major groups may also be equally diagnostic of true seroreactivity to HIV-1.[21,30] In 1988, the Consortium for Retrovirology Serology Standardization recommended that scoring of a positive Western blot could be made on the basis of the following pattern: anti-p24 or anti-p31 occurring in the presence of either anti-gp41 or anti-gp160/gp120.[33] Other groups, in contrast, have suggested that the presence or absence of antibody against *pol* gene products such as p31 should not be required within this definition.

While this controversy still continues to a lesser degree today, currently the most widely accepted criteria are those adopted by the Centers for Disease Control in 1989,[30] which were based on the standards established by the Association of State and Territorial Public Health Laboratory Directors the previous year.[34] According to these criteria, a Western blot can be considered reactive if it contains at least two of the three bands thought by the Association to be of diagnostic significance: namely, anti-p24, anti-gp41, and anti-gp160/gp120.

By definition, Western blot results that cannot be classified as either negative or positive are grouped into the category of "indeterminate" findings. Bands present may correspond to the molecular weights of known HIV-1 proteins[35] as well as to other proteins on the nitrocellulose paper of unknown (but presumably not viral) origin. Either isolated or joint reactivity at the p24 and/or p55 bands is particularly common in Western blots falling into the indeterminate category, regardless of whether one is surveying patients whose histories might classify them as being at high risk[36] or low risk[37-43] for HIV-1 infection. However, the vast majority of indeterminate Western blot results will occur in patients with no other evidence of HIV-1 infection, and it is presumed that this limited antibody recognition represents cross-reactivity by antibodies of low specificity with various contaminants of the immunoblot preparation. For example, cross-reactivity with class I and II HLA antigens present as cellular contaminants within the viral lysate appears to account for a significant percentage of false-positive banding. It is likely that newer immunoblot assays utilizing recombinantly derived viral antigens rather than viral lysates will reduce the incidence of indeterminate reactivity, although this remains to be established in large-scale testing.[44,45]

If clinically warranted (*e.g.,* in the setting of a recent history of possible HIV-1 exposure), the finding of an indeterminate Western blot pattern in the context of a positive HIV-1 ELISA result should prompt repetition of the Western blot on either the same or, if available, a fresh serum specimen. If the repeat assay is still indeterminate, the clinician should then consider retesting the patient within a few months time, inasmuch as it is possible that the patient was first tested early in the process of seroconverting and that, on serial examination, follow-up studies may reveal the full pattern of antibody reactivity. As several studies have confirmed, however, the likelihood that an indeterminate Western blot represents performance of the assay in the window of time between partial and complete seroconversion is low for most patients. Rather, on serial testing the vast majority of indeterminate findings will remain either indeterminate (with either identical or different patterns of banding), will revert to full seronegativity, or will vacillate between the two categories. Thus, failure of the Western blot to evolve from an indeterminate to a positive test within a few months strongly militates against the possibility that the patient is HIV-1 infected. Nonetheless, plagued by the anxiety generated during this period of diagnostic uncertainty, many physicians and patients understandably will want to undertake more definitive diagnostic procedures in an attempt to rule out more conclusively the possibility of occult infection.

It is particularly important to realize that the Western blot is comparatively poor as an initial screening test for HIV-1 infection. Among homosexual or bisexual men testing negative for HIV-1 by both ELISA and PCR techniques, 20% to 30% may still show one or more bands on Western blot.[22,36] Moreover, during evaluations performed every 1 to 3 months over the course of 1 year or more, 70% of an HIV-1–ELISA negative, PCR-negative cohort of homosexual men with an initial indeterminate Western blot continued to have one or more bands on serial immunoblots.[36] Other studies on low-risk populations have noted similar findings.[37] Because of this high frequency of indeterminate reactivity—the overwhelming preponderance of which will be nonspecific binding—the Western blot is not appropriate for use as a primary screening tool in the population at large. Rather, its strength is as a confirmatory assay in the setting of a positive HIV-1 ELISA or other initial screening test.

Although estimates for the sensitivity and specificity of the HIV-1 Western blot vary somewhat depending on the manufacturer, comparative surveys have shown that most preparations have a sensitivity of at least 96%.[21,33] When the Western blot is used properly as a confirmatory test in sequence with an initial positive screening assay, the combination of the two tests should have a positive predictive value greater than 99% in both low-risk and high-risk populations. The sensitivity of the newer generation of immunoblot preparations utilizing recombinant antigens also appears to be quite high.[45]

Indirect Immunofluorescence Assay

Although the performance standards of currently marketed Western blot kits are generally quite high and the processing time of some versions has been reduced to as short as a few hours, some laboratories prefer to use an indirect immunofluorescence assay (IFA) for screening or to substitute it for the conventional immunoblot as a confirmatory assay.[46-50] A potential advantage of the IFA is that it is rapid, relatively simple to perform, and requires a minimum of technical skill. It does, however, require the use of a fluorescent microscope, so that equipment and training expenses may be elevated accordingly. In this technique, slides containing fixed monolayers of HIV-1–infected cell lines (H9 or CEM lines are the principal cell lines used) are coated with various dilutions of test sera for a defined period of time (Fig. 10–6). During this incubation step, anti-HIV-1 antibodies present in the sera will bind to antigens contained in the monolayer. After washing, the slide preparation is allowed to react with anti-human IgG antibody tagged with an ultraviolet light–activated dye such as fluorescein isothiocyanate (FITC). The slide is again washed, dried, and scored by microscopic examination with a fluorescent microscope. With proper technique, background staining should be minimal and fluorescent cells can be scored for both number and intensity as well as for the character of the staining pattern. As a negative control, it is critical to measure immunofluorescence against a noninfected cell monolayer in order to reduce the possibility of nonspecific (false-positive) reactivity. Similarly, as with any of the standard antibody detection methods, proper quality control requires that sera from a known seropositive individual also be included as a positive control.

In addition to the relative ease with which it can be performed, the IFA has the advantage of generally turning positive earlier in the course of infection than either a conventional ELISA or Western blot. The time to development of a positive IFA after acute seroconversion to HIV-1 can be further reduced by substituting FITC-labeled anti-human IgM as the developing antiserum. Cooper *et al* studied eight individuals who presented with an acute mononucleosis-like illness consistent with primary infection with HIV-1.[12] In their experience, the IFA performed using FITC-conjugated anti-IgM turned positive a mean of 5 days after the onset of acute symptoms, as compared to a mean of 11 days when a more conventional anti-IgG antiserum was used. In contrast, reactivity on what they regarded as their most sensitive HIV-1 ELISA did not develop until a mean of 31 days after the beginning of the illness. Most authors agree that, in clinical use, the sensitivity and specificity of the IFA can match or exceed that of the Western blot, although occasionally there may be some variability in appropriate scoring of samples owing to inexperience with the technique. Its major limitation in the research setting is that, unlike the Western blot, it does not permit precise delineation of specific patterns of antibody reactivity.

Radioimmunoprecipitation Assay

The RIPA is another test that is sometimes favored for use as a confirmatory immunoassay, although its use is largely restricted to laboratories that have the facilities and expertise to propagate HIV-1 in continuous cell culture.[51] To perform this test (Fig. 10–7), infected lymphocytic cells (H9 cells are used predominantly) are

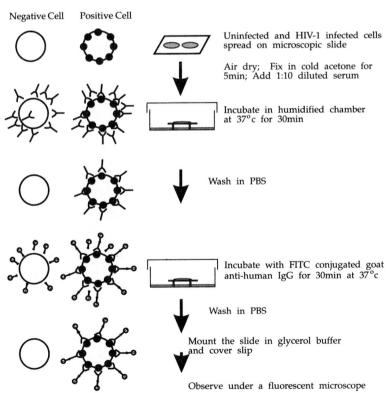

Negative Cell　　Positive Cell

Uninfected and HIV-1 infected cells spread on microscopic slide

Air dry; Fix in cold acetone for 5min; Add 1:10 diluted serum

Incubate in humidified chamber at 37°c for 30min

Wash in PBS

Incubate with FITC conjugated goat anti-human IgG for 30min at 37°c

Wash in PBS

Mount the slide in glycerol buffer and cover slip

Observe under a fluorescent microscope

No Fluorescence　　Fluorescence

Figure 10–6. A standard indirect immunofluorescent assay (IFA) for HIV-1 detection.

RADIOIMMUNOPRECIPITATION
(flow chart)

1. Preparation of labeled viral lysates:

Infect CD4 expressing cells with HIV-1
When the virus induced cytopathic effect is maximum, metabolically label cells with ^{35}S-methionine and ^{35}S-cysteine for 6 to 12 hours
Wash and lyse cells in buffer containing detergents
Clarify cell lysates by centrifugation
Collect the supernatant and preadsorb with protein-A sepharose beads
(Alternatively HIV-1 proteins can also be labeled with radioiodine-^{125}I)

2. Immunoprecipitation

Add serum sample to an aliquot of the labeled viral lysate
(Run a positive and a negative control serum simultaneously)
Incubate overnight at 4°C
Add protein-A sepharose beads of protein-A expressing *Staphylococcus* bacteria
Incubate overnight at 4°C
Wash the beads and elute the immunoprecipitated proteins by adding buffer-containing SDS/β-mercaptoethanol and heating the sample in boiling water bath
Centrifuge the sample and collect the supernatant

3. Gel electrophoresis and autoradiography

Load the samples, positive and negative controls along with protein molecular-weight markers, on a SDS-polyacrylamide (10–12.5%) gel and electrophorese at a constant current of 25 mA
Fix the proteins in the gel in methanol/acetic acid/water mixture
Impregnate the gel in radioactive-enhancing flours
Dry the gel and expose to an X-ray film
After a length of time develop the film and identify HIV-1 specific protein bands

Figure 10–7.   Flow diagram of a HIV-1 radioimmunoprecipitation assay (RIPA).

grown in the presence of radiolabeled amino acids such as [^{35}S]-methionine and [^{35}S]-cysteine to permit incorporation of radiolabel into HIV-1 proteins. Alternatively, surface labeling of HIV-1 with [^{125}-I] after purification of virus from a host cell line is utilized by some laboratories.[52] With metabolic radiolabeling, a cell lysate is then prepared by homogenization of cells in the presence of buffered detergent. Serum samples to be tested are reacted with the radiolabeled cell lysate, resulting in the generation of antigen-antibody complexes if anti-HIV-1 antibodies are present. The reaction mixture is next incubated with protein A–coated sepharose beads that will bind to the heavy chain (Fc region) of available IgG molecules. Radiolabel-containing immune complexes that are present will thus become attached to a solid phase (sepharose) *via* this protein–binding mechanism. Following binding, beads are removed from the lysate *via* centrifugation, the antibody-antigen complexes are eluted from the beads by heating and solubilization in detergent, and the resulting immunoprecipitates are separated electrophoretically according to molecular weight. Autoradiography of the separated proteins yields an immunoblot pattern similar to that produced by Western blotting, although resolution of the higher molecular weight envelope proteins is generally better.

Several aspects of the RIPA have made widescale adoption of this technology by clinical laboratories somewhat difficult. The need to maintain viral stocks and active cell culture lines, the requirement for storing and handling of radioactive tracer materials, the time and technical expertise required to perform the assay properly, and the overall expense of this test have all contributed to making the RIPA substantially less attractive than the Western blot for routine use. For this reason most assays of this type are performed in research laboratories where the skills and materials required are more readily accessible. Nonetheless, there are circumstances in which the clinician may find the RIPA particularly helpful, such as in the detection of low levels of antibody positivity or aiding in the evaluation of individuals with indeterminate Western blot patterns. The sensitivity and specificity of the RIPA usually exceed those of the Western blot under most circumstances, and the RIPA has provided insight into the nature of the antibody response to the higher molecular weight (gp160, gp120) envelope proteins early in the process of seroconversion.[53] However, early in the course of infection it may be relatively less sensitive than conventional immunoblotting as a means of monitoring the initial antibody response to other viral antigens, such as p24 or gp41.

Rapid Latex Agglutination Assay

The technical complexity and expense associated with some of the more conventional anti-HIV-1 antibody detection methods have led to a search for simplified, less costly methods of serologic screening,[54-56] particularly those that could be more suitable for use under field conditions such as might be found in central Africa or other medically disadvantaged regions with a high incidence of HIV-1 infection. These newer tests may also offer some practical advantages in developed nations as well. One such test that has been developed is the rapid latex agglutination assay, a procedure that can be performed within a matter of minutes and that requires a minimum of reagents and technical skill.[57,58] This assay, a modification of a standard latex agglutination assay, is based on the use of recombinant proteins derived from a highly conserved region of the HIV-1 genome that are chemically linked to polystyrene beads. The beads are incubated with various dilutions of test and control sera at room temperature and are observed for the appearance of a characteristic agglutination reaction. HIV-1 envelope proteins are usually used for this purpose, both because anti-*env* antibodies generally arise early in the process of seroconversion and because they exhibit limited cross-reactivity with, for example, HIV-2 or other human retroviruses that may be endemic in a particular region. One nonglycosylated envelope preparation marketed by Cambridge BioScience Corp, for example, consists of the carboxy terminal third of gp120 linked with the amino terminal half of gp41, minus 23 amino acids normally present at their junction. The rapid latex agglutination procedure is generally easy to perform but does require at least modest skill and experience in the proper interpretation of results. As with all of the serologic assays, it should always be conducted with both positive and negative controls. In using the latex agglutination assay to screen large panels of sera from several regions where HIV-1 infection is endemic, one group has reported estimates of sensitivity as high as 99.3% and specificity as high as 100% in comparison to Western blotting.[58] It should be cautioned, however, that because such estimates were derived from populations where the incidence of infection was as high as 18%, the applicability of this test as a screening tool in comparatively low-risk populations remains uncertain.

Dot-Blot Immunobinding and Other Assays

Another rapid screening test that appears to hold promise as a cost-effective alternative to conventional ELISA and Western blot testing is the dot-blot immunoassay. In this assay, a lysate of viral antigens is prepared from HIV-1 harvested from cell culture and is dotted onto a gridwork of absorbent nitrocellulose paper.[59,60] Alternatively, recombinantly produced HIV-1 envelope or other proteins have also be used for this purpose.[54] Ap-propriate dilutions of test sera (with a panel of positive and negative controls) are spotted onto the areas containing bound viral antigens and allowed to react. After incubation, the nitrocellulose is washed to remove unbound antibody, and then enzyme-linked goat anti-human IgG antibody is added to the paper. The dots are developed by the addition of an appropriate substrate for the bound enzyme, resulting in a colorimetric reaction whose intensity directly correlates with the amount of bound HIV-1–specific antibody. Using this method to screen sera from high-risk patients, one group reported a 93% concordance between results obtained by dot-blot immunoassay and ELISA.[60] Similarly, another group reported a 98.2% concordance of dot-blot immunoassay results with conventional Western blotting in evaluating sera from patients with and without risk factors for exposure.[54]

A number of other rapid and simple immunoassays have been proposed or developed for use in the detection of a serologic response to HIV-1, such as the passive hemagglutination assay.[61,62] One of the most elegant examples is the autologous red cell agglutination assay, described by Kemp and colleagues.[63] In this technique, a nonagglutinating mouse monoclonal antibody reactive with human red blood cells is chemically cross-linked to a synthetic peptide antigen derived from gp41 envelope protein (other immunogenic proteins of HIV-1 could also be adapted for this technique). Addition of this antigen-antibody complex to microliter quantities of whole blood obtained from a patient will cause that patient's red cells to become coated with the complex. Anti-HIV-1 antibodies present in the blood sample should bind to the cell-bound antigen and cause agglutination of red cells into a visible mass. This assay can be completed within a matter of minutes and has the advantage of using the patient's own blood. It also offers the potential for quantitative assessment in that it may be possible to titer the amount of specific anti-HIV-1 antibody in a patient's blood by performing competitive inhibition of the agglutination reaction with added peptide antigen. A false-positive rate as low as 0.1% (compared with 0.2% using a commercial ELISA) for this assay has been described in seronegative blood donors. The false-negative rate appears to be approximately 1%.

p24 Antigen Capture Assay

Once the diagnosis of HIV-1 infection has been established by serologic methods, a number of surrogate markers of HIV-1 activity may be of use in guiding clinical decision-making.[64-66] One serologic assay that has been shown to be of utility in the prognostic staging and management of the infected individual is the serum p24 antigen capture assay.[67] This assay, also known as the HIV-1 antigen capture assay, is a solid-phase technique designed to provide a quantitative measure of the level of viral p24 antigen present within serum or other body fluids. Viral p24 protein circulates in the bloodstream either as free antigen or bound to anti-p24 antibody in the form of immune complexes; the conventional p24 antigen capture assay detects only the unbound fraction.

Although the levels of serum p24 antigen may vary from individual to individual, in many patients this antigen can be detected relatively early in the period after exposure to HIV-1, often preceding the process of seroconversion by several weeks.[68] This rise in measurable p24 antigen levels presumably correlates with the burst in viral replication, detectable by other methods such as plasma viremia,[69,70] that occurs shortly after primary infection. However, because the timing of this p24 elevation and its rate of rise are generally not predictable, the p24 antigen capture assay is generally not useful as a primary screening tool in establishing independently an early diagnosis of HIV-1 infection. In any case, the p24 antigen level usually drops below the threshold of detection by conventional methods as anti-p24 antibody is formed during seroconversion, and it may remain in that state during the subsequent years of asymptomatic infection. Thereafter, depending on an individual's immune status as reflected in the dynamic equilibrium with levels of anti-p24 antibody, it may again become detectable as the infection enters more advanced stages.

Because only 20% to 30% of individuals with asymptomatic HIV-1 infection will have detectable levels of serum p24 antigen by standard methodology, this assay compares unfavorably with the conventional ELISA as a diagnostic tool for HIV-1 infection. Two large-scale studies of the utility of the serum p24 antigen capture assay in screening volunteer blood donors have shown that it provides no additional benefit over conventional screening for HIV-1 antibody in the detection of infected units of blood.[71,72] Its primary role lies in monitoring the levels of viral activity within the known infected host, such as in response to the initiation of antiretroviral chemotherapy, and in serving as an independent prognostic marker of disease activity over time. With regard to its role as an indicator of viral replication, for example, it is well established that conventional antiretroviral therapy with an agent such as zidovudine can at least temporarily reduce the level of serum p24 antigen in antigenemic patients, presumably reflecting an overall inhibition of the level of viral activity in the treated patient.[73] Based on these data, the p24 antigen test has been widely adopted for use as an important surrogate marker of antiviral efficacy in a number of clinical drug trials of putative antiretroviral agents.[74,75] Whether there exists a strict correlation between a declining level of serum p24 antigen on therapy and an improved clinical status for any given infected individual remains an area of considerable controversy, however.

With respect to its role in prognostic stratification, it has been shown that patients with detectable serum p24 antigen as a group may progress more rapidly to the development of AIDS-defining illnesses than a similar group of patients lacking this serum marker.[68,76–89] In a 1988 study of a cohort from San Francisco, for example, it was found that over a 3-year period, serum p24-antigenemic patients developed AIDS-defining conditions at a rate more than three times higher than within a similar cohort of p24 antigen–negative individuals.[90]

The serum p24 antigen capture assay is a solid-phase immunoassay that has been available since 1986. It is commercially marketed for research purposes in kit form by several manufacturers, including Abbott, Coulter, and Du Pont Laboratories. Although specific reagents differ between various manufacturers, the assay is generally performed as follows (Fig. 10–8): test sera and control sera are allowed to react with monoclonal or polyclonal anti-HIV-1 antibody (reactive to p24 antigen) bound either to the bottom of a microtiter well or coated on polystyrene beads. After appropriate incubation and washing, the well or beads are incubated with goat or rabbit anti-HIV-1 antibody, which in turn will bind in proportionate amounts to any p24 antigen captured on the solid phase. After washing, an enzyme-tagged anti-goat (or anti-rabbit) immunoglobulin is added that, in the presence of an appropriate substrate, will produce a colorimetric reaction whose intensity can be measured spectrophotometrically. With the use of dilutions of a serum with a known concentration of p24 antigen as a positive control, a standard curve of O.D. *versus* concentration can be generated against which the absor-

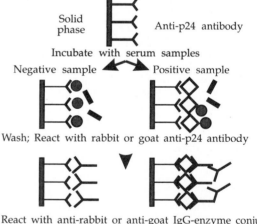

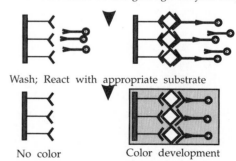

Figure 10–8. A conventional commercially available p24 antigen capture assay.

bance values of test sera can be compared quantitatively. Most commercially available kits define their lower limits of p24 antigen detection as being in the range of 50 pg/ml, although the actual linear portion of the standard curve will often permit reliable measurements as low as 10 to 20 pg/ml. To confirm the specificity of the assay, positive test serum should also be retested in the presence of human sera containing a known high concentration of anti-HIV-1 antibody. With most kits a reduction in the test serum's O.D. of 50% or greater by this "neutralization" procedure confirms the specificity of the p24 measurement.

A major limitation to the overall utility of the conventional p24 antigen capture assay is that it is only capable of detecting free p24 antigen and not antigen complexed with anti-p24 antibody. Recently, a significant improvement in the sensitivity of this test has been achieved through efforts to disrupt immune complexes prior to assay. In particular, alteration of the pH of samples through simple chemical pretreatment will markedly increase the level of detectable p24 antigen in sera from both asymptomatic patients and those with advanced HIV infection. One method that has been developed involves the addition of dilute hydrochloric acid to samples and subsequent neutralization with alkali.[91] A newer method involving acidification with a mild organic acid such as glycine (pH 2.2) has also been studied and offers the potential advantage of being less likely to denature epitopes on p24 antigen prior to measurement (M. B. Vasudevachari *et al*, unpubl. observ.).[92]

REFERENCES

1. Gottlieb MS, Schroff R, Schanker HM et al: *Pneumocystis carinii* pneumonia and mucosal candidiasis in previously healthy homosexual men: Evidence of a new acquired cellular immunodeficiency. N Engl J Med 305:1425, 1981
2. Masur H, Michelis MA, Greene JB et al: An outbreak of community-acquired *Pneumocystis carinii* pneumonia: Initial manifestation of cellular immune dysfunction. N Engl J med 305:1431, 1981
3. Centers for Disease Control: Revision of the case definition of acquired immunodeficiency syndrome for national reporting—United States. MMWR 34:373, 1985
4. Centers for Disease Control: Revision of the CDC surveillance case definition for acquired immunodeficiency syndrome. Council of State and Territorial Epidemiologists; AIDS Program, Center for Infectious Diseases. MMWR 36(suppl 1):1S, 1987
5. Barré-Sinoussi F, Cherman JC, Rey F et al: Isolation of a T-lymphotropic retrovirus from a patient at risk for acquired immune deficiency syndrome (AIDS). Science 220:868, 1983
6. Popovic M, Sarngadharan MG, Read E, Gallo RC: Detection, isolation, and continuous production of cytopathic retroviruses (HTLV-III) from patients with AIDS and pre-AIDS. Science 224:497, 1984
7. Schleupner CJ: Diagnostic tests for HIV-1 infection. In Mandell G, Douglas R, Bennett J (eds): Principles and Practice of Infectious Diseases, p S3. New York, Churchill Livingstone, 1989
8. Sandler SG, Dodd RY, Fang CT: Diagnostic tests for HIV infection: Serology. In DeVita VT, Hellman S, Rosenberg SA (eds): AIDS: Etiology, Treatment, and Prevention, 2nd ed, p 121. Philadelphia, JB Lippincott, 1988
9. Levinson SS, Denys GA: Strengths and weaknesses in methods for identifying the causative agent(s) of acquired immunodeficiency syndrome (AIDS). CRC Crit Rev Clin Lab Sci 26:277, 1988
10. Houn HY, Pappas AA, Walker EM Jr: Status of current clinical tests for human immunodeficiency virus (HIV): Applications and limitations. Ann Clin Lab Sci 17:279, 1987
11. Gaines H, Sydow MV, Sönnerborg A et al: Antibody response in primary human immunodeficiency virus infection. Lancet 1:1249, 1987
12. Cooper DA, Imrie AA, Penny R: Antibody response to human immunodeficiency virus after primary infection. J Infect Dis 155:1113, 1987
13. Ranki A, Valle SL, Krohn M et al: Long latency precedes overt seroconversion in sexually transmitted human-immunodeficiency-virus infection. Lancet 2:589, 1987
14. Imagawa DT, Lee MH, Wolinsky SM et al: Human immunodeficiency virus type 1 infection in homosexual men who remain seronegative for prolonged periods. N Engl J Med 320:1458, 1989
15. Horsburgh Jr CR, Ou CY, Jason et al: Duration of human immunodeficiency virus infection before detection of antibody. Lancet 2:637, 1989
16. Centers for Disease Control: Update: Serologic testing for antibody to human immunodeficiency virus. MMWR 36:833, 1988
17. Centers for Disease Control: Problems created by heat-inactivation of serum specimens before HIV-1 antibody testing. MMWR 38:407, 1989
18. Evans RP, Shanson DC, Mortimer PP: Clinical evaluation of Abbott and Wellcome enzyme linked immunosorbent assays for detection of serum antibodies to human immunodeficiency virus (HIV). J Clin Pathol 40:552, 1987
19. Carlson JR, Bryant ML, Hinrichs SH et al: AIDS serology testing in low and high risk groups. JAMA 253:3405, 1985
20 Ward JW, Holmberg SD, Allen JR et al: Transmission of human immunodeficiency virus (HIV) by blood transfusions screened as negative for HIV antibody. N Engl J Med 318:473, 1988
21. Schwartz JS, Dans PE, Kinosian BP: Human immunodeficiency virus test: Evaluation, performance, and use. JAMA 259:2574, 1988
22. Kovacs JA, Megil ME, Deyton L et al: Phase 1 trial of a recombinant gp160 candidate aids vaccine (abstr), Book II, p 289. In: Proceedings of the Fourth International Conference on AIDS, Stockholm, June 12–16, 1988
23. Redfield RR, Birx DL, Ketter N et al: A phase I evaluation of the safety and immunogenicity of vaccination with recombinant gp160 in patients with early human immunodeficiency virus infection. N Engl J Med 324:1677, 1991
24. Coombs RW, Collier AC, Allain JP et al: Plasma viremia in human immunodeficiency virus infection. N Engl J Med 321:1626, 1989
25. Ho DH, Moudgil T, Alam M: Quantitation of human immunodeficiency virus type 1 in the blood of infected persons. N Engl J Med 321:1621, 1989
26. Saiki RK, Gelfand DH, Stoffel S et al: Primer-directed enzymatic amplification of DNA with a thermostable DNA polymerase. Science 239:487, 1988
27. Lifson AR, Stanley M, Pane J et al: Detection of human immunodeficiency virus DNA using the polymerase chain

reaction in a well-characterized group of homosexual and bisexual men. J Infect Dis 161:436, 1990

28. Phair JP, Wolinsky S: Diagnosis of infection with the human immunodeficiency virus. J Infect Dis 159:320, 1989

29. Busch MP, Eble BE, Khayam-Bashi H et al: Evaluation of screened blood donations for human immunodeficiency virus type 1 infection by culture and DNA amplification of pooled cells. N Engl J Med 325:1, 1991

30. Centers for Disease Control: Interpretation and use of the Western blot assay for serodiagnosis of human immunodeficiency virus type 1 infections. MMWR 38:1, 1989

31. Towbin H, Staehelin T, Gordon J: Electrophoretic transfer of proteins from polyacrylamide gels to nitrocellulose sheets: Procedure and some applications. Proc Natl Acad Sci USA 76:4350, 1979

32. Du Pont Diagnostics: Human immunodeficiency virus (HIV): Biotech/Du Pont HIV Western blot kit for detection of antibodies to HIV. Wilmington, Delaware, Du Pont Diagnostics, 1987

33. Consortium for Retrovirus Serology Standardization: Serologic diagnosis of human immunodeficiency virus infection by Western blot testing. JAMA 260:674, 1988

34. Hausler WJ Jr: Report of the Third Consensus Conference on HIV Testing sponsored by the Association of State and Territorial Public Health Laboratory Directors. Infect Control Hosp Epidemiol 9:345, 1988

35. Povolotsky J, Gold JWM, Chein N et al: Differences in human immunodeficiency virus type 1 (HIV-1) anti-p24 reactivities in serum of HIV-1 infected and uninfected subjects: Analysis of indeterminate Western blot reactions. J Infect Dis 163:247, 1991

36. Davey R, Metcalf J, Easter M et al: Western Blot and PCR reactivity patterns in individuals at high risk for HIV exposure (abstr Th.B.P. 179). Presented at the V International Conference on AIDS, Montreal, June 1989

37. Midthun K, Garrison L, Clements ML et al, for the NIAID AIDS Vaccine Clinical Trials Network: Frequency of indeterminate Western blot tests in healthy adults at low risk for human immunodeficiency virus infection. J Infect Dis 162:1379, 1990

38. Dock NL, Lamberson HV, O'Brien TA et al: Evaluation of atypical human immunodeficiency virus immunoblot reactivity in blood donors. Transfusion 28:412, 1988

39. Kleinman SH, Niland JC, Azen SP et al: Prevalence of antibodies to human immunodeficiency virus type 1 among blood donors prior to screening. Transfusion 29:572, 1989

40. Leitman SF, Klein HG, Melpolder JJ et al: Clinical implications of positive tests for antibodies to human immunodeficiency virus type 1 in asymptomatic blood donors. N Engl J Med 321:917, 1989

41. Nusbacher J, Naiman R: Longitudinal follow-up of blood donors found to be reactive for antibody to human immunodeficiency virus (anti-HIV) by enzyme-linked immunoassay (EIA+) but negative by western blot (WB−). Transfusion 29:365, 1989

42. Jackson JB, MacDonald KL, Cadwell J et al: Absence of HIV infection in blood donors with indeterminate Western blot tests for antibody to HIV-1. N Engl J Med 322:217, 1990

43. Genesca J, Shih JW, Jett B et al: What do Western blot indeterminate patterns for human immunodeficiency virus mean in EIA-negative blood donors? Lancet 2:1023, 1989

44. Hofbauer JM, Schulz TF, Hengster P et al: Comparison of Western blot (immunoblot) based on recombinant-derived p41 with conventional tests for serodiagnosis of human immunodeficiency virus infections. J Clin Microbiol 26:116, 1988

45. Busch MP, el Amad Z, McHugh TM et al: Reliable confirmation and quantitation of human immunodeficiency virus type 1 antibody using a recombinant-antigen immunoblot assay. Transfusion 31:129, 1990

46. Lennette ET, Karpatkin S, Levy JA: Indirect immunofluorescence assay for antibodies to human immunodeficiency virus. J Clin Microbiol 25:199, 1987

47. Hedenskog M, Dewhurst S, Ludvigsen C et al: Testing for antibodies to AIDS-associated retrovirus (HLTV-III/LAV) by indirect fixed cell immunofluorescence: Specificity, sensitivity, and applications. J Med Virol 19:325, 1986

48. Gallo D, Diggs JL, Shell GR et al: Comparison of detection of antibody to the acquired immune deficiency syndrome virus by enzyme immunoassay, immunofluorescence, and Western blot methods. J Clin Microbiol 23:1049, 1986

49. Carlson JR, Yee J, Hinrichs SH et al: Comparison of indirect immunofluorescence and Western blot for detection of anti-human immunodeficiency virus antibodies. J Clin Microbiol 25:494, 1987

50. McHugh TM, Stites DP, Casavant CH et al: Evaluation of the indirect immunofluorescence as a confirmatory test for detecting antibodies to the human immunodeficiency virus. Diagn Immunol 4:233, 1986

51. Chiodi F, Bredberg-Raden U, Biberfeld G et al: Radioimmunoprecipitation and Western blotting with sera of human immunodeficiency virus infected patients: A comparative study. AIDS Res Hum Retroviruses 3:165, 1987

52. Tersmette M, Lelie PN, van der Poel CL et al: Confirmation of HIV seropositivity: Comparison of a novel radioimmunoprecipitation assay to immunoblotting and virus culture. J Med Virol 24:109, 1988

53. Saah AJ, Farzadegan H, Fox R et al: Detection of early antibodies in human immunodeficiency virus infection by enzyme-linked immunosorbent assay, Western blot, and radioimmunoprecipitation. J Clin Microbiol 25:1605, 1987

54. Carlson JR, Yee JL, Watson-Williams EJ et al: Rapid, easy, and economical screening tests for antibodies to human immunodeficiency virus. Lancet 1:361, 1987

55. Van de Perre P, Nzaramba D, Allen S et al: Comparison of six serological assays for human immunodeficiency virus antibody detection in developing countries. J Clin Microbiol 26:552, 1988

56. Heyward WL, Curran JW: Rapid screening tests for HIV infection. JAMA 260:542, 1988

57. Riggin CH, Beltz GA, Hung CH et al: Detection of antibodies to human immunodeficiency virus by latex agglutination with recombinant antigen. J Clin Microbiol 25:1772, 1987

58. Quinn TC, Riggin CH, Kline RL et al: Rapid latex agglutination assay using recombinant envelope polypeptide for the detection of antibody to the HIV. JAMA 260:510, 1988

59. Heberling RL, Kalter SS: Rapid dot-immunobinding assay on nitrocellulose for viral antibodies. J Clin Microbiol 23:109, 1986

60. Heberling RL, Kalter SS, Marx PA et al: Dot immunobinding assay compared with enzyme-linked immunosorbent assay for rapid and specific detection of retrovirus antibody induced by human or simian acquired immunodeficiency syndrome. J Clin Microbiol 26:765, 1988

61. Vasudevachari MB, Uffelman KU, Mast TC et al: Passive hemagglutination test for detection of antibodies to human

immunodeficiency virus type 1 and comparison of the test with enzyme-linked immunosorbent assay and Western blot (immunoblot) analysis. J Clin Microbiol 27:179, 1989

62. Scheffel JW, Wiesner D, Kapsalis A et al: Retrocell HIV-1 passive hemagglutination assay for HIV-1 antibody screening. J AIDS 3:540, 1990

63. Kemp BE, Rylatt DB, Bundesen PG et al: Autologous red cell agglutination assay for HIV-1 antibodies: Simplified test with whole blood. Science 241:1352, 1988

64. Cooper EH, Lacey CJN: Laboratory indices of prognosis in HIV infection. Biomed Pharmacother 42:539, 1988

65. Fahey JL, Taylor JMG, Detels R et al: The prognostic value of cellular and serologic markers in infection with human immunodeficiency virus type 1. N Engl J Med 322:166, 1990

66. Muñoz A, Carey V, Saah AJ et al: Predictors of decline in CD4 lymphocytes in a cohort of homosexual men infected with human immunodeficiency virus. J AIDS 1:396, 1988

67. Moss AR, Bacchetti P: Natural history of HIV infection. AIDS 3:55, 1989

68. Goudsmit J, Lange JM, Krone WJ et al: Pathogenesis of HIV and its implications for serodiagnosis and monitoring of antiviral therapy. J Virol Methods 17:19, 1987

69. Clark SJ, Saag MS, Decker WD et al: High titers of cytopathic virus in plasma of patients with symptomatic primary HIV-1 infection. N Engl J Med 324:954, 1991

70. Daar ES, Moudgil T, Meyer RD, Ho DD: Transient high levels of viremia in patients with primary human immunodeficiency virus type 1 infection. N Engl J Med 324:961, 1991

71. Busch MP, Taylor PE, Lenes BA et al, for the Transfusion Safety Study Group: Screening of selected male blood donors for p24 antigen of human immunodeficiency virus type 1. N Engl J Med 323:1308, 1990

72. Alter HJ, Epstein JS, Swensen SG et al, for the HIV-Antigen Study Group: Prevalence of human immunodeficiency virus type 1 p24 antigen in U.S. blood donors: An assessment of the efficacy of testing in donor screening. N Engl J Med 323:1312, 1990

73. Jackson GG, Paul DA, Falk LA et al: Human immunodeficiency virus (HIV) antigenemia (p24) in the acquired immunodeficiency syndrome (AIDS) and the effect of treatment with zidovudine (AZT). Ann Intern Med 108:175, 1988

74. Lane HC, Kovacs JA, Feinberg J et al: Anti-retroviral effects of interferon-alpha in AIDS-associated Kaposi's sarcoma. Lancet 2:1218, 1988

75. Yarchoan R, Pluda JM, Thomas RV et al: Long-term toxicity/activity profile of 2′,3′-dideoxyinosine in AIDS or AIDS-related complex. Lancet ii:526, 1990

76. Allain JP, Laurian Y, Paul DA et al: Long-term evaluation of HIV antigen and antibodies to p24 and gp41 in patients with hemophilia. N Engl J Med 317:1114, 1987

77. Raška K Jr, Kim HC, Raška K 3rd et al: Human immunodeficiency virus (HIV) infection in haemophiliacs: Long-term prognostic significance of the HIV serologic pattern. Clin Exp Immunol 77:1, 1989

78. Eyster ME, Ballard JO, Gail MH et al: Predictive markers for the acquired immunodeficiency syndrome (AIDS) in hemophiliacs: Persistence of p24 antigen and low T4 cell count. Ann Intern Med 110:963, 1989

79. Hofmann B, Bygbjerg I, Dickmeiss E et al: Prognostic value of immunologic abnormalities and HIV antigenemia in asymptomatic HIV-infected individuals: Proposal of immunologic staging. Scand J Infect Dis 21:633, 1989

80. Lindhardt BO, Ulrich K, Kusk P, Hofmann B: Serological response in patients with chronic asymptomatic human immunodeficiency virus infection. Eur J Clin Microbiol Infect Dis 7:394, 1988

81. Lindhardt BO, Gerstoft J, Hofmann B et al: Antibodies against the major core protein p24 of human immunodeficiency virus: Relation to immunological, clinical and prognostic findings. Eur J Clin Microbiol Infect Dis 8:614, 1989

82. Portera M, Vitale F, La Licata R et al: Free and antibody-complexed antigen and antibody profile in apparently healthy HIV seropositive individuals and in AIDS patients. J Med Virol 30:30, 1990

83. Kamani N, Krilov LR, Wittek AE, Hendry RM: Characterization of the serologic profile of children with human immunodeficiency virus infection: Correlation with clinical status. Clin Immunol Immunopathol 53:233, 1989

84. Sei Y, Tsang PH, Chu FN et al: Inverse relationship between HIV-1 p24 antigenemia, anti-p24 antibody and neutralizing antibody responses in all stages of HIV-1 infection. Immunol Lett 20:223, 1989

85. Weber JN, Clapham PR, Weiss RA et al: Human immunodeficiency virus infection in two cohorts of homosexual men: Neutralizing sera and association of anti-gag antibody with prognosis. Lancet 1:119, 1987

86. Forster SM, Osborne LM, Cheingsong-Popov R et al: Decline of anti-p24 antibody precedes antigenaemia as correlate of prognosis in HIV-1 infection. AIDS 1:235, 1987

87. Andrieu JM, Eme D, Venet A et al: Serum HIV antigen and anti-p24-antibodies in 200 HIV seropositive patients: Correlation with CD4 and CD8 lymphocyte subsets. Clin Exp Immunol 73:1, 1988

88. Lange JM, Paul DA, Huisman HG et al: Persistent HIV antigenaemia and decline of HIV core antibodies associated with transition to AIDS. Br Med J 293:1459, 1986

89. Murray HW, Godbold JH, Jurica KB, Roberts RB: Progression to AIDS in patients with lymphadenopathy or AIDS-related complex: Reappraisal of risk and predictive factors. Am J Med 86:533, 1989

90. Moss AR, Bacchetti P, Osmond D et al: Seropositivity for HIV and the development of AIDS or AIDS related condition: Three year follow up of the San Francisco General Hospital cohort. Br Med J 296:745, 1988

91. Nishanian P, Huskins KR, Stehn S et al: A simple method for improved assay demonstrates that HIV p24 antigen is present as immune complexes in most sera from HIV-infected individuals. J Infect Dis 162:21, 1990

92. Kestens L, Hoofd G, Gigase PL et al: HIV antigen detection in circulating immune complexes. J Virol Methods 31:67, 1991

Infectious Complications of HIV

Pneumocystis carinii and Other Protozoa

11A

Judith Falloon   Henry Masur

PNEUMOCYSTIS CARINII

Pulmonary disease caused by *Pneumocystis carinii* was rarely documented prior to the emergence of the acquired immunodeficiency syndrome (AIDS) in the early 1980s. Now, in areas where infection with the human immunodeficiency virus (HIV) is prevalent, it is one of the most commonly observed "community-acquired" pneumonias. Despite the widespread use of effective prophylaxis, infection with *P. carinii* remains an important cause of morbidity and mortality in patients infected with HIV.

On the basis of morphological appearance and antibiotic susceptibilities, *P. carinii* has traditionally been classified as a protozoon, but recent data suggest that the organism is phylogenetically more closely linked to the fungi.[1] The study of *Pneumocystis* has been hampered by an inability to propagate it in culture, so that research on human *Pneumocystis* depends on the harvest of *P. carinii* cysts and trophozoites from bronchoalveolar lavage (BAL) fluid or autopsy in patients with *Pneumocystis* pneumonia. Because of the limited quantities of organisms available for study, much of the pathogenesis of the disease remains an enigma. The most widely used animal model, the corticosteroid-treated rat, has been useful for harvesting rat *P. carinii* and for studying therapeutic and prophylactic agents.

Infection with *P. carinii* is thought to be transmitted by the respiratory route. It is presumed, but not proven, that infection occurs early in life and remains latent unless immunodeficiency permits the development of disease.[1] Direct person-to-person spread is not known to occur, and Centers for Disease Control recommended procedures do not now include the respiratory isolation of patients with acute *Pneumocystis* pneumonia. Clustering of cases has been documented in several episodes, however, and some authorities recommend that a susceptible patient not be exposed to a patient with active, untreated *Pneumocystis* pneumonia.

Although *Pneumocystis* pneumonia is the most common opportunistic infection in patients with AIDS, occurring at some time during the course of their illness in over 80% of patients not receiving anti-*Pneumocystis* prophylaxis, not all patients with HIV infection are at great risk of developing this disease. The identification of a subset of patients at particular risk for *Pneumocystis* pneumonia occurred after retrospective review of data, in which it was noted that patients with *Pneumocystis* pneumonia almost always had circulating CD4+ T-cell counts of 200 cells/mm³ or less.[2] Subsequently, these data were confirmed prospectively in a large cohort study in which the risk of *Pneumocystis* pneumonia over time was related to CD4+ T-cell counts at baseline.[3] In these patients, who were not receiving prophylaxis against *Pneumocystis* pneumonia, the risk of developing *Pneumocystis* pneumonia was less than 0.5% over the next 6 months in patients with CD4+ T-cell counts above 200 cells/mm³, but it was over 8% at 6 months and 18% at 12 months if the baseline CD4 count was less than 200 cells/mm³. In addition, patients with thrush or fever were more likely to develop *Pneumocystis* pneumonia than were those without these symptoms.[3]

The patients at greatest risk of developing *Pneumocystis* pneumonia, however, are those who have previously had an episode of *Pneumocystis* pneumonia.[4] In observations made in a cohort of patients with a history of *Pneumocystis* pneumonia who were randomized to receive one of two dosages of zidovudine, the risk of a recurrence of *Pneumocystis* pneumonia was 31% over the next 6 months and 66% during the next 12 months.[4] Thus, patients with prior *Pneumocystis* pneumonia and those with CD4 counts less than 200 cells/mm^3 are the prime targets for efforts to prevent *Pneumocystis* pneumonia.

Manifestations of Disease

Pneumocystis carinii disease in patients with HIV infection involves solely the lung in the majority of patients. *Pneumocystis* pneumonia in a patient with HIV infection generally manifests with fever and respiratory symptoms such as cough, which is usually nonproductive; chest pain, tightness, or discomfort, especially on inspiration; and dyspnea or exercise intolerance. Fatigue and weight loss are common. Patients who have previously had *Pneumocystis* pneumonia can sometimes recognize the return of symptoms while the disease is quite mild. When compared with patients without HIV infection, patients with AIDS tend to have a more indolent course, with a longer duration of symptoms and less hypoxemia at the time of diagnosis.[5] Physical examination is often unrevealing, although rales may be present on auscultation of the chest. The chest radiograph typically shows diffuse, bilateral, interstitial infiltrates, but many other patterns can be seen, including a normal chest radiograph, localized infiltrates, cavities and blebs, alveolar infiltrates, asymmetry, and predominantly upper lobe disease, which is associated with the use of aerosolized pentamidine for prophylaxis.[6,7] Both the chest radiograph and blood gas values can be normal in a patient with early *Pneumocystis* pneumonia, and the presenting manifestations may be limited to fever or subjective respiratory symptoms. The degree of disease evident on the chest radiograph correlates with the ultimate prognosis, as does the degree of hypoxemia at presentation.[8,9] The clinical presentation of *Pneumocystis* pneumonia, while often characteristic, is not specific, and cannot be distinguished from that of other pulmonary processes such as common viral or *Mycoplasma* infections, nonspecific pneumonitis, fungal pneumonia, cytomegalovirus pneumonia, or pulmonary Kaposi's sarcoma.

In addition to localized pulmonary disease, disseminated *P. carinii* disease occurs.[10,11] Although cases of disseminated disease were reported prior to the widespread use of aerosolized pentamidine, the frequency with which they are now recognized appears to be higher. Aerosolized pentamidine seems to predispose to extrapulmonary *Pneumocystis* infection, perhaps because diagnosis and therapy are delayed until after dissemination has occurred, and the few organisms that invade blood vessels or lymphatics are not treated by a regimen that results in useful concentrations only in the lungs. The manifestations of disseminated pneumocystosis are protean and depend on which organs are involved; thus, there is no characteristic presentation.

Diagnosis of *Pneumocystis* Disease

The diagnosis of *P. carinii* disease depends on demonstration of the cyst or trophozoite form of the organism within human tissues or body fluids. Human *Pneumocystis* cannot be cultured from clinical material, and serology currently has no role in diagnosis.[1] The diagnosis of *P. carinii* pneumonia is now generally made by BAL.[12-14] The presence of *Pneumocystis* in a BAL specimen indicates current or recent disease and therefore almost always merits active therapy. An exception to the requirement for treatment would be a patient who has recently been adequately treated for an episode of *Pneumocystis* pneumonia with good clinical response, because persistence of organisms in lavage specimens for many weeks after the termination of successful therapy has been documented.[15-17] The sensitivity of BAL alone in the diagnosis of *Pneumocystis* pneumonia is 86% to 97% in patients who have not received aerosolized pentamidine prophylaxis. In some centers, the diagnostic yield of BAL is reduced to 60% to 80% if the patient has received aerosolized pentamidine prophylaxis, and in this case, follow-up procedures, including transbronchial biopsies, may be necessary if the initial BAL does not reveal a causative process in a patient who is not improving clinically.[6] When transbronchial biopsy is used in addition to BAL, the sensitivity of bronchoscopy for the diagnosis of *Pneumocystis* pneumonia is well over 90%.[18,19] Although open lung biopsy is a time-honored way of making the diagnosis, such an invasive procedure is now rarely warranted for the diagnosis of *Pneumocystis* pneumonia.

A recent major advance in the diagnosis of *Pneumocystis* pneumonia is the development of the examination of noninvasively obtained expectorated sputum to provide a diagnosis. The simplicity of the procedure promotes early diagnosis, and early diagnosis (before the development of serious respiratory compromise) results in improved survival.[8] Because the test is very specific, if it reveals *Pneumocystis,* no bronchoscopy is needed unless there is reason to seek other diseases. The sensitivity varies considerably between institutions but reaches 80% to 92% in some centers in patients not receiving aerosolized pentamidine.[7,20] At our institution, the diagnostic yield of the induced sputum examination was 64% in patients receiving aerosolized pentamidine, compared to 92% in patients not receiving prophylaxis.[7] In a patient in whom *P. carinii* pneumonia is strongly suspected, bronchoscopy should follow a negative induced sputum examination because of the risk of a missed diagnosis.

The sensitivity and specificity of the induced sputum examination for the diagnosis of *Pneumocystis* pneumonia depend on the method of obtaining and processing the specimen, the stains used to examine it, and the experience of the laboratory personnel responsible for interpreting the resultant smear.[20,21] The best results have been observed when the patient gargles vigorously to remove debris prior to the nebulization, when high-flow ultrasonic nebulization with hypertonic saline is used to stimulate a cough for the production of a specimen, when sputum liquefaction and concentration steps are included in the preparation of the material, and when indirect immunofluorescence techniques using antibodies to *P. carinii* are used to examine the smear.[20] These techniques minimize the confusion that can result from the presence in the specimen of yeast from the oral cavity. Yeast will stain with such commonly used cyst-wall stains as toluidine blue O and Gomori's methenamine silver nitrate, and inexperienced readers may have difficult distinguishing yeast from the cysts of *Pneumocystis*.[22] The Giemsa and Diff-Quik stains, while useful in very experienced hands, can make distinguishing the trophozoites of *Pneumocystis* from cellular debris quite difficult.[1]

Although some centers have used radiographic, nuclear medicine, pulmonary function, or serum chemistry parameters to help in selecting those patients in whom invasive procedures are used to seek a diagnosis of *Pneumocystis* pneumonia, the low specificity and high cost of tests such as gallium citrate radioisotope scanning and pulmonary function testing make them cost-ineffective and thus not generally recommended.[23] Their use can delay making a definitive diagnosis and instituting specific therapy.

The diagnosis of disseminated pneumocystosis is generally made by the observation of organisms in tissues obtained at biopsy or autopsy. *Pneumocystis* has been observed histologically in almost every organ. When an eye examination reveals rounded, yellow-white choroidal lesions consistent with what has been described previously as *Pneumocystis* choroiditis, the diagnosis is suggested although not established.[24] In addition, certain radiographic observations are suggestive—but not diagnostic—of disseminated pneumocystosis: multiple lesions in visceral organs such as liver, spleen, or kidney with progressive calcification that may be best visualized by ultrasound.[25,26]

Treatment

Two antibiotic regimens are well-established as being effective for the treatment of disease caused by *P. carinii*: trimethoprim with sulfamethoxazole (oral or intravenous [IV]) and pentamidine isethionate (IV) (Table 11A–1). These agents appear to have comparable efficacy, so that the choice of therapy is based on toxicity and convenience.[16,27] Patients with HIV infection who are treated with trimethoprim-sulfamethoxazole (TMP-SMX) commonly develop side-effects such as rash, fever, leukopenia, anemia, thrombocytopenia, nausea, vomiting, increases in hepatic transaminase levels, and renal impairment.[16,27-29] The cause of these frequent serious side-effects remains to be explained. The severity of these drug reactions should not be overestimated, however. Some patients can continue to receive TMP-SMX despite the occurrence of maculopapular rash, nausea, or moderately severe laboratory abnormalities. In one study, reducing the dose (from the standard 20 mg/kg of trimethoprim component per day to 12–15 mg/kg/day by following drug levels in blood) and tolerating some adverse reactions permitted all of 36 patients to complete therapy with TMP-SMX.[27] In this study, 33 of 34 patients completed therapy with IV pentamidine at a dosage of 4 mg/kg/day, with a 30% to 50% dosage reduction if the serum creatinine level rose by more than 1 mg/dl. Most clinicians prefer to use TMP-SMX rather than pentamidine because the toxicity of TMP-SMX is less severe, and it can be administered orally, thus simplifying what is generally a 21-day course of therapy. Many physicians will withhold zidovudine or reduce the dose during the acute treatment of *Pneumocystis* pneumonia with TMP-SMX or pentamidine in order to diminish the likelihood that bone marrow suppression will limit anti-*Pneumocystis* therapy.

Pentamidine isethionate therapy can result in azotemia, pancreatitis, leukopenia, thrombocytopenia, nausea, vomiting, hypotension, cardiac arrhythmias, hy-

Table 11A–1. Drug Regimens for the Treatment of *Pneumocystis* Pneumonia

Drug	Dose	Comments
Trimethoprim + sulfamethoxazole	15–20 mg/kg/day IV or PO 75–100 mg/kg/day IV or PO	Fixed combination; recommended not to exceed 960 mg of trimethoprim/day administer in 3 divided doses
Pentamidine	4 mg/kg/day IV	Infuse over 1–2 hr to prevent hypotension
Dapsone + trimethoprim	100 mg/day PO 15–20 mg/kg/day PO	Investigational but readily available probably less toxic than trimethoprim-sulfamethoxazole
Primaquine + clindamycin	15–30 mg base PO 600 mg q6h to 900 mg q8h IV, or 300–450 mg q6h PO	Investigational but readily available
Trimetrexate + leucovorin	45 mg/m² /day IV 20 mg/m² PO or IV qid	Investigational, available under Treatment IND
Aerosolized pentamidine	600 mg/day via Respirgard nebulizer	Avoid using as sole therapy
566C80	750 mg tid	Investigational

perkalemia, a bitter taste that can diminish appetite, and dysregulation of glucose metabolism, including hyperglycemia or hypoglycemia that can be sudden in onset and fatal.[27,30] Pancreatic dysfunction and hyperglycemia may be permanent and severe. When pentamidine is administered intramuscularly, pain and sterile abscesses at the injection site can result, so that it is preferable to administer pentamidine by slow (1-hour) IV drip.[30] Some clinicians prefer to use lower doses of pentamidine (3 mg/kg), especially if the creatinine level has risen during therapy, or to treat for courses shorter than 21 days because the risk of hypoglycemia and pancreatitis appears to increase with the cumulative dose of pentamidine. There is evidence that a dosage of 3 mg/kg has efficacy, but it is not known if the efficacy is equal to that seen at 4 mg/kg.[31]

The optimal duration of therapy for an episode of *Pneumocystis* pneumonia has never been determined. A 21-day course is recommended, but it is reasonable to consider a 14-day course adequate in a patient who has responded and in whom continuing therapy involves significant toxicity or discomfort. In patients with mild to moderately severe pneumonia, most or all of this therapy can often safely be administered on an outpatient basis.

Some patients with a history of intolerance of conventional therapies can be safely rechallenged, so a patient labeled "allergic" to these therapies should have the intolerance defined before such therapy is abandoned. Rechallenge with TMP-SMX rarely results in life-threatening complications, although fatal Stevens-Johnson syndrome can occur. There are, however, patients who cannot tolerate either TMP-SMX or parenteral pentamidine. For patients with mild to moderate disease who are candidates for oral therapy, two investigational but readily available oral regimens can be used: dapsone plus trimethoprim and primaquine plus clindamycin (see Table 11A–1).[32,33] Small clinical trials have suggested that both regimens are effective and well tolerated, although side-effects are common. One small study suggests that trimethoprim-dapsone is less toxic but as effective as TMP-SMX, and some physicians use trimethoprim-dapsone as first-line therapy.[32] In that study, side-effects were frequent in dapsone-trimethoprim–treated patients but were not often dose limiting; they consisted of neutropenia, rash, nausea, hyperkalemia, methemoglobinemia, increases in hepatic transaminase levels, and anemia. Patients should be tested for glucose-6-phosphate dehydrogenase deficiency prior to receiving dapsone because this deficiency predisposes to severe dapsone-related hemolysis.

In an open trial of oral primaquine plus clindamycin for the treatment of *Pneumocystis* pneumonia, treatment was effective in all but two of 28 episodes; 20 of the patients had received initial therapy with other agents, however.[33] Rash occurred in half of the patients. It is likely that primaquine plus clindamycin will prove to be a useful alternative in patients with mild to moderate *Pneumocystis* pneumonia and intolerance of TMP-SMX.

A new drug, an investigational hydroxynaphthoquinone compound called 566C80, appears to have efficacy and minimal toxicity based on a small open trial; a large comparative trial is in progress.[34,35] Some investigators have reported therapeutic successes when using pentamidine delivered locally to the lung by aerosolization for the treatment of acute *P. carinii* pneumonia.[31,36] Because of reports of delayed responses, early relapses, and failures in patients with *Pneumocystis* infection outside of the lung, it is imprudent to use aerosolized pentamidine as sole therapy. Its potential for use in combination with other therapies remains to be defined. For the patient who requires IV therapy, trimetrexate, a folate antagonist administered with concomitant leucovorin, is available under Treatment IND.[17,37] Eflornithine (DFMO) has been given to a small number of patients; it has potential efficacy but substantial toxicity.[38,39]

The most recent advance in the treatment of *P. carinii* pneumonia involves the use of corticosteroids in conjunction with specific antimicrobial therapy.[9] After anecdotal reports suggested benefit when corticosteroids were administered to patients with *Pneumocystis* pneumonia, a number of clinical trials were undertaken to investigate this possibility.[40-42] The largest of these, a randomized, unblinded trial, enrolled 251 patients within 36 hours of initiating anti-*Pneumocystis* therapy and convincingly demonstrated that, in patients with more than mild disease at entry, the use of concomitant corticosteroids led to a decrease by approximately half in the risk of oxygenation failure, mechanical ventilation, and death.[40] In those patients with the most severe disease, death occurred in 42% of patients who did not receive corticosteroids and in 20% of those who did. There were few end points of death or respiratory failure in patients with mild disease, and efficacy was not demonstrated in this subset of patients, although it is possible that a larger study would have demonstrated benefit. Data from four other studies support the conclusion that corticosteroids are of benefit for the treatment of *Pneumocystis* pneumonia.[9]

In the large study of corticosteroids for *Pneumocystis* pneumonia, the regimen used was prednisone, 40 mg twice daily for 5 days, followed by 40 mg/day for 5 days and then 20 mg/day for the duration of anti-*Pneumocystis* therapy (Table 11A–2).[40] While other regimens have been either suggested or used, this regimen remains the one for which the greatest body of supporting data exist and is the one recommended by a consensus panel convened to examine the data and formulate recommendations for the use of corticosteroids in patients with HIV infection and acute *P. carinii* pneumonia.[9] This panel has recommended that patients with an entry PaO_2 of less than 70 mm Hg on room air or an alveolar-arterial gradient greater than 35 mm Hg receive this regimen of corticosteroids in addition to specific anti-*Pneumocystis* therapy. Corticosteroids should be begun as soon as possible and within 72 hours of beginning anti-*Pneumocystis* therapy. Although

Table 11A–2.   Recommendations for the Use of Corticosteroids in the Treatment of Acute *Pneumocystis* Pneumonia

Target population:	Patients with acute *Pneumocystis* pneumonia and Pao$_2$ < 70 mm Hg on room air or A-a gradient > 35 mm Hg at time therapy is initiated
Dosage:	Prednisone, 40 mg orally twice daily for 5 days, 20 mg twice daily for 5 days, then 20 mg/day until the end of antimicrobial therapy
Timing:	Begin during first 72 hours of anti-*Pneumocystis* therapy

theoretical risks from this use of corticosteroids exist, only an increase in thrush and mild herpesviral infections have been reported.[40] It is likely, however, that corticosteroid-associated side-effects will be observed in some patients, and that diseases such as tuberculosis, cryptococcosis, and histoplasmosis will be exacerbated at times. The beneficial effects of corticosteroids in all patients with more than mild *Pneumocystis* pneumonia, however, argue strongly in favor of their use in conjunction with close monitoring of the patient.

The mechanism by which corticosteroids produce benefit remains unexplained, but it appears to involve an amelioration of a treatment-induced deterioration in lung function that often occurs during the first week of therapy. Approximately 40% of patients will have worsening of their oxygenation (defined as a 10% drop in oxygen saturation) during the first week of treatment for *Pneumocystis* pneumonia.[42] In one study, this deterioration occurred in only 6% of corticosteroid-treated patients.[42] Although a host response to antigens released as organisms are killed by antimicrobial therapy has been postulated, the pathogenesis behind both the deterioration and its amelioration by corticosteroids remains unexplained. Because the deterioration is an early phenomenon, the early institution of corticosteroids is likely to be the most beneficial, and delaying their institution until after serious deterioration has occurred may limit or abolish their beneficial effect. In one clinical trial in which corticosteroids were administered after respiratory deterioration, no benefit was observed.[9]

The armamentarium for the treatment of patients who fail therapy is less satisfactory than that available for initial treatment. These patients have a poor prognosis despite a change in therapy.[18] Before primary therapy is abandoned, patients should have received at least 5 to 10 days of therapy at appropriate doses, and other pulmonary processes should have been considered as potential causes of part or all of the pulmonary dysfunction (bronchoscopy with transbronchial biopsies may be helpful). In such patients, a general recommendation is to switch from TMP-SMX to parenteral pentamidine or *vice versa;* the addition of one to the

other increases the risk of toxicity without known added benefit. The addition of corticosteroids in this situation as salvage therapy may be helpful, although the one existing study suggests that it may not.[9]

The reported mortality in some series of patients with AIDS, *Pneumocystis* pneumonia, and respiratory failure has been 80% to 100%, but more recent series have demonstrated improving survival. Thus, intubation should be considered where needed.[43-45] It is important to determine the wishes of a patient who is failing therapy regarding intubation, resuscitation, and admission to the intensive care unit.

There are no data that specifically address the treatment of patients with disseminated pneumocystosis. One reasonable approach would be to treat with conventional systemic agents for at least 21 days, with the duration of therapy dependent on the clinical response. In the absence of data, most clinicians would use oral systemic prophylaxis after the completion of acute therapy in a patient who has been successfully treated for disseminated pneumocystosis.

Prevention of *Pneumocystis* Pneumonia

Effective strategies to prevent the development of *P. carinii* pneumonia represent a major advance in the management of patients at risk for *Pneumocystis* disease. Recommended regimens for anti-*Pneumocystis* prophylaxis include oral TMP-SMX and inhaled, aerosolized pentamidine (Table 11A–3).[4] Although large comparative trials are in progress, there are currently no data to support a preference for one *versus* the other of these modalities of prophylaxis.

Aerosolized pentamidine is the prophylaxis of choice for some clinicians. In a large dose-comparative trial of aerosolized pentamidine, recurrences of *Pneumocystis* pneumonia were significantly fewer in patients receiving 300 mg of pentamidine by aerosol every 4 weeks than in patients receiving 30 mg every 2 weeks.[46] The aerosol was well tolerated, with side-effects consisting of cough or bronchospasm that could in most cases be ameliorated or prevented by pretreatment with an inhaled bronchodilator. In a European trial, aerosolized pentamidine was also effective for preventing primary episodes of *Pneumocystis* pneumonia.[47] In these studies, the Respirgard II nebulizer was used. More efficient, more convenient, and potentially more economical aerosol delivery systems are being studied, but their role is currently uncertain.[48]

Many clinicians use TMP-SMX as their prophylaxis regimen of choice. One small randomized trial of TMP-SMX (160 mg trimethoprim and 800 mg sulfamethoxazole twice daily) *versus* no prophylaxis has been completed in patients with Kaposi's sarcoma and no prior *Pneumocystis* pneumonia.[49] In this study, *Pneumocystis* pneumonia occurred in none of 30 TMP-SMX–treated patients and in 16 (53%) of 30 untreated patients. Side-effects occurred in half of the treated patients, but drug was discontinued in only 17% of patients. An effect on

Table 11A–3. Recommendations for the Prevention of *Pneumocystis* Pneumonia

Target populations:	a) Patients with prior *Pneumocystis* disease (secondary prophylaxis) b) Patients with CD4+ T cells < 200/mm³ or <20% of lymphocytes (primary prophylaxis)
Regimens of choice:	Aerosolized pentamidine (300 mg by Respirgard II nebulizer every 4 weeks; other nebulizer systems may be effective and may require lower doses) *or* Trimethoprim-sulfamethoxazole (one double-strength tablet orally twice daily, 2, 3, or 7 days per week)
Investigational alternatives:	Dapsone, 100 mg/day or several times per week; dapsone, 200 mg, plus pyrimethamine, 75 mg weekly

mortality was also noted, with a mean survival of 23 months in treated patients compared with 13 months in untreated patients. Other doses and schedules of administration for prophylactic TMP-SMX have been proposed.[50,51] In a retrospective analysis of the efficacy of low-dose, intermittent TMP-SMX prophylaxis (160 mg trimethoprim and 800 mg sulfamethoxazole three times per week), none of the 71 patients receiving secondary prophylaxis for a mean of 18.5 months and none of the 45 patients receiving primary prophylaxis for a mean of 24.2 months developed *Pneumocystis* pneumonia. Side-effects occurred in 28%, but only 13% discontinued TMP-SMX, suggesting that this lower dose regimen is better tolerated than the twice daily regimen. More rigorous trials are needed to confirm the desirability of such intermittent, low-dose approaches.

In addition to aerosolized pentamidine and oral TMP-SMX, dapsone alone or dapsone plus pyrimethamine have been used to prevent *Pneumocystis* pneumonia. Conceivably, either of these regimens could be effective even if given as infrequently as once weekly.[52] Controlled trials supporting the efficacy and safety of dapsone-containing regimens are not yet completed. It is also possible that investigational regimens such as 566C80 or clindamycin-primaquine may have a role in the prevention of *Pneumocystis* pneumonia.

Any regimen for the prevention of *Pneumocystis* pneumonia needs to be assessed on the basis of efficacy, safety, and cost. No regimen is completely effective and completely safe. The breakthrough rate for aerosolized pentamidine in patients with prior *Pneumocystis* pneumonia may be over 20% per year.[46] Oral TMP-SMX is probably much more effective, but it is not tolerated by 10% to 40% of patients, whereas almost all patients tolerate aerosolized pentamidine. Aerosolized pentami-

dine is significantly more costly than TMP-SMX and will remain so even after it no longer has orphan drug status. Thus, many clinicians prefer TMP-SMX for patients who can tolerate this regimen. A valid assessment of the comparative safety and efficacy of aerosolized pentamidine and oral TMP-SMX prophylaxis awaits the completion and analysis of randomized comparative trials.

Prophylaxis can alter the presentation of *Pneumocystis* infection and the ease of diagnosis, as well. In patients receiving aerosolized pentamidine prophylaxis, recurrences present more commonly in the upper lobes of the lung, presumably because of poorer distribution of the aerosol in these areas, and extrapulmonary pneumocystosis seems to be more common.[6,7,10,11] A number of cases of cystic or bullous lung disease and pneumothorax have occurred in patients who have been receiving aerosolized pentamidine.[53] Pneumothorax is associated with active *Pneumocystis* pneumonia, prior *Pneumocystis* pneumonia, and prior use of aerosolized pentamidine for prophylaxis; it may also correlate with extrapulmonary disease.[53,54] The diagnosis of *Pneumocystis* pneumonia by examination of induced sputum specimens and BAL fluid is inhibited by the use of aerosolized pentamidine because the cysts in respiratory specimens may be fewer and more often single, making interpretation of the smear more difficult, and the yield on BAL of the upper lobes may be higher than that of the traditionally performed lower lobe lavage.[6,7] At our institution, where indirect immunofluorescence with anti-*Pneumocystis* antibodies is routinely used to evaluate specimens, and where site-directed BAL is performed in the area of greatest radiographic abnormality, the diagnostic yield of BAL has continued to be close to 100% despite the use of aerosolized pentamidine.

In light of these factors, many clinicians prefer to use an oral systemic agent for prophylaxis unless the patient cannot tolerate such therapy or requires concomitant therapy that makes the use of one of these agents impractical. Aerosolized pentamidine remains a useful alternative for patients intolerant of TMP-SMX. In addition to the use of specific anti-*Pneumocystis* prophylaxis, the use of an effective antiretroviral agent such as zidovudine decreases (but does not eliminate) the risk of *Pneumocystis* pneumonia; thus, antiretroviral therapy is an important strategy in the prevention of *Pneumocystis* pneumonia and other opportunistic infections.[55]

TOXOPLASMA GONDII

Toxoplasmosis is caused by infection with *Toxoplasma gondii*, an obligate intracellular protozoon whose definitive host is the cat. Man usually acquires infection by ingesting oocysts excreted in cat feces or cysts present in inadequately cooked meat. Clinical disease in patients with AIDS is thought to represent reactivation of previously dormant cysts from a prior infection in most cases.[56]

Manifestations and Diagnosis of Toxoplasmosis

In patients with HIV infection, toxoplasmosis is most often confined to the brain, although chorioretinitis, pneumonia, and disseminated disease have also been documented.[57,58] Toxoplasmosis almost always occurs in patients with preexisting antibody to toxoplasma, and it occurs in patients with CD4+ T-cell counts below 100 cells/mm[3].[59] Cerebral toxoplasmosis generally presents with fever, headaches, seizures, altered consciousness, or focal neurologic abnormalities that reflect the intracerebral location and size of the foci of toxoplasmosis.[57,60-62] As visualized by computed tomography (CT) or magnetic resonance imaging (MRI), lesions are typically multiple but may be single. There is usually associated cerebral edema.[62] On CT scan, the lesions are often round and hypodense, with ring enhancement after the administration of contrast material.[57] A double-dose delayed contrast CT scan sometimes reveals lesions not apparent on conventional scanning. MRI is more sensitive than CT, with lesions not visible on CT scan often demonstrable by MRI.[57]

The definitive diagnosis of cerebral toxoplasmosis requires brain biopsy with confirmation of the presence of *T. gondii* by routine histopathologic examination, immunoperoxidase stain, or culture (which is generally unavailable).[59,62,63] The organisms are usually seen in the periphery of a lesion, not in the central area of necrosis. Since biopsy specimens typically are small, sampling error can result in missed diagnoses. When organisms are not found, the inflammatory cell infiltrate can be confused with lymphoma by less experienced pathologists. Because of the risks and insensitivity of biopsy and the rapid response of most patients to conventional therapy, patients are now typically given an empirical trial of therapy. A clinical response confirmed by improvement on imaging of the brain within 2 to 4 weeks of initiating therapy strongly suggests a diagnosis of toxoplasmosis. This approach can result in a delay in the diagnosis and treatment of central nervous system lymphoma, tuberculoma, or cryptococcoma. Brain biopsy should be performed in cases with atypical radiographic findings or in patients who fail to definitively improve after 2 to 4 weeks of empirical therapy.

The specific diagnosis of acute toxoplasmosis in patients with HIV infection relies primarily on the histologic demonstration of organisms (or, at research centers, on the culture of organisms) in specimens from any body site, including tissue, cerebrospinal fluid, blood, or BAL fluid. Serologic studies for IgG antibody to *T. gondii* cannot distinguish latent from active infection and are not diagnostically useful, although the absence of IgG antibody suggests another diagnosis.[59,62,63] IgM antibodies are generally absent. Lumbar puncture cannot unequivocally establish a specific diagnosis of toxoplasmosis (unless organisms are seen on smear), although evaluations of local antibody production have been published.[64,65]

Treatment and Prevention of Toxoplasmosis

Toxoplasmosis responds well to pyrimethamine in combination with sulfadiazine (Table 11A–4).[60] Leucovorin should be used concurrently to ameliorate bone marrow suppression, and patients should be well hydrated to avoid crystalluria and renal failure.[66] Corticosteroids are reserved for patients with substantial cerebral edema. Substantial or complete response is seen in almost 90% of treated patients during the first 2 months of therapy; however, 45% to 70% of patients develop side-effects from one or more of the components of therapy, with manifestations such as neutropenia, fever, rash, renal dysfunction, and thrombocytopenia.[60-62] Sulfadiazine must be discontinued in approximately one third of patients. Therapy of some type must be continued for the lifetime of the patient; cessation of therapy will be associated with relapses in most patients.[60,61] Relapses are usually in the site of prior disease, suggesting that therapy is not curative. It is possible that long-term suppression can be achieved with drug dosages substantially lower than those necessary to achieve an acute response.

Because conventional therapy is so effective, patients with toxoplasmosis who have a history of non-life-threatening sulfonamide toxicity should usually be rechallenged with pyrimethamine-sulfadiazine. In addition, patients who develop minor or transient toxicities such as a morbilliform rash (but not Stevens-Johnson syndrome or toxic epidermal necrolysis) should attempt to continue to receive conventional therapies.

For those who are truly intolerant or who have failed conventional therapy, alternative therapies are now being explored. In open, uncontrolled trials, pyrimethamine in combination with IV or oral clindamycin has shown efficacy.[67,68] A trial comparing this regimen with

Table 11–4. Treatment of Cerebral Toxoplasmosis

Regimen of choice:	Pyrimethamine (25–100 mg/day) + sulfadiazine (4–8 g/day in 4 divided doses) + leucovorin (5–25 mg/day)
Alternative regimens:	Pyrimethamine (25–100 mg/day) + clindamycin (1,200–2,400 mg/day IV in divided doses, then 300–900 mg PO q 6–8 hr)
	Pyrimethamine (25–100 mg/day) + dapsone (100 mg/day)
	566C80 (investigational hydroxy-napthoquinone)
	Azithromycin (investigational macrolide)
	Clarithromycin (investigational macrolide)

the standard pyrimethamine-sulfadiazine regimen has not yet been completed, but preliminary reports suggest that the overall outcome is similar in the two groups, although clindamycin may be less effective but less toxic.[69] Other agents currently in clinical trials that appear promising include 566C80, azithromycin, clarithromycin, dapsone, and high-dose pyrimethamine, as well as agents in combination with γ-interferon.[70,71]

No data exist on the utility and safety of drug regimens for the prevention of acute toxoplasmosis. Some regimens likely to be useful for the prevention of pneumocystosis, such as dapsone-pyrimethamine, could prove to be useful for reducing the frequency of toxoplasmosis. A prudent recommendation for patients with HIV infection would be to avoid cat feces and to eat only well-cooked meat.

CRYPTOSPORIDIOSIS, MICROSPORIDIOSIS, AND ISOSPORIASIS

Cryptosporidiosis

Cryptosporidium is a coccidian protozoon that can cause severe, protracted diarrhea in patients with HIV infection.[72] Sources of infection include exposure to infected persons, animals, and contaminated food or water. Fecal-oral transmission is the presumed mode. Nosocomial transmission occurs. Cryptosporidiosis in a patient with HIV infection and a depleted CD4+ T-cell count usually is characterized by persistent, voluminous watery diarrhea, weight loss, nausea, vomiting, and abdominal pain. Manifestations may be mild, however, and cryptosporidiosis occasionally remits spontaneously, especially in patients with relatively preserved immune function.[72,73] Fever is not a prominent finding. Lactose intolerance and malabsorption may occur. In some patients, cryptosporidiosis is life-threatening, and IV hydration and alimentation are required to sustain life.

Cryptosporidium can infect most of the gastrointestinal tract, including the gallbladder and bile ducts, in patients with AIDS, but the bowel is the major target organ.[74] Organisms have been observed in pulmonary specimens, but whether this generally represents contamination from gastrointestinal fluids is unclear. In enteritis, *Cryptosporidium* typically infects the microvillous border of intestinal cells. It can sporulate *in situ* and reinfect the same host.

The diagnosis of cryptosporidiosis can be made by the demonstration of oocysts in feces by one of several techniques. A modified acid-fast stain is rapid, easily interpreted, and convenient.[72,75] If few oocysts are present, concentration techniques such as the sucrose flotation method can facilitate diagnosis, as can obtaining multiple specimens.[73] Light and electron microscopic examination of gastrointestinal biopsy specimens can also provide a diagnosis.[76] In gallbladder disease, radiographic procedures may demonstrate thickening of the gallbladder, bile duct dilation and stricture, and lumenal irregularities.[75]

There is no specific therapy that has been shown to be effective for cryptosporidiosis. Spiramycin, diclazuril, hyperimmune bovine colostrum or globulin, eflornithine, erythromycin, oral bovine dialyzable leucocyte extract, azithromycin, and paramomycin have all been tried, with isolated reports of success.[72,73,75,77] No therapy has been convincingly demonstrated to be effective in a controlled or open clinical trial, however. Thus, the management of affected patients should emphasize fluid and electrolyte balance and nutrition. Antidiarrheal agents, including octreotide acetate (sandostatin), should be tried. Hyperalimentation may be required. Severe biliary obstruction may require endoscopic papillotomy, cholecystectomy, or T-tube placement.

Microsporidiosis

Microsporidia are spore-forming, obligate intracellular protozoa that have been recognized as a cause of illness in patients with HIV infection and low CD4+ T-cell counts.[78,79] Enteric microsporidial infections have been reported with increasing frequency in HIV-infected patients with chronic diarrhea and weight loss. Ocular, muscular, and hepatic infections have also been reported.[80-82] Because of difficulties in diagnosis, it is likely that microsporidial infections are a greater problem in patients with HIV infection than is currently realized.[76] Reliable serologic tests are not available, and the diagnosis requires biopsy of infected tissue. Routine histopathologic studies can provide identification, but microsporidia are often overlooked because they are small, stain poorly, and can evoke little tissue response.[78,83] Diagnostic confirmation requires electron microscopic visualization of the organism's characteristic ultrastructure. For enteric infection, upper endoscopy and biopsy with electron microscopy appears to be the most reliable way to make the diagnosis. There are no accepted techniques for the detection of microsporidia in human body fluids or excreta, although such techniques are currently being investigated.

There is no known effective antimicrobial therapy for microsporidiosis. Metronidazole has been reported to have some efficacy in a small number of patients.[79]

Isosporiasis

Isospora belli is a coccidian that causes an enteric infection that is uncommon in North American patients but common in Haitian or African patients with AIDS.[75,84] The resultant diarrhea, weight loss, nausea, and crampy abdominal pain can be chronic and debilitating. The syndrome is clinically indistinguishable from that of cryptosporidiosis. The diagnosis is made by detection of the organism in stools, either by use of the modified acid-fast method that is used to identify *Cryptosporidium* or by wet mounts. Concentration techniques may be useful. The oocysts of *Isospora* can be easily distinguished from those of *Cryptosporidium* by their characteristic size, shape, and number of sporocysts.

Isosporiasis can be effectively treated with 10 days

of TMP-SMX, with rapid resolution of symptoms and clearing of oocysts from the stool.[84,85] Because relapses (some of which may represent reinfection) have occurred in half of treated patients after the completion of therapy, patients are usually treated with three times weekly TMP-SMX for continued suppression. Pyrimethamine, metronidazole, or quinacrine may be alternatives for sulfonamide-intolerant patients.[75,86]

CONCLUSION

Infections with protozoa can cause severe and life-threatening disease in patients with HIV infection. While therapy exists for some of these infections, some remain without effective therapy. Toxicity from treatment often complicates the therapy of treatable protozoal infections, and relapse after the discontinuation of therapy is the rule. The development of safe, tolerable, effective, and inexpensive new antiprotozoal therapies and chemoprophylaxis is an important goal of ongoing research.

REFERENCES

1. Masur H, Lane HC, Kovacs JA et al: Pneumocystis pneumonia: From bench to clinic. Ann Intern Med 111:813, 1989
2. Masur H, Ognibene FP, Yarchoan R et al: CD4 counts as predictors of opportunistic pneumonias in human immunodeficiency virus (HIV) infection. Ann Intern Med 111:223, 1989
3. Phair J, Munoz A, Detels R et al: The risk of *Pneumocystis carinii* pneumonia among men infected with human immunodeficiency virus type 1. N Engl J Med 322:161, 1990
4. Centers for Disease Control: Guidelines for prophylaxis against *Pneumocystis carinii* pneumonia for persons infected with human immunodeficiency virus. MMWR 38(S5):1, 1989
5. Kovacs JA, Hiemenz JW, Macher AM et al: *Pneumocystis carinii* pneumonia: A comparison between patients with the acquired immunodeficiency syndrome and patients with other immunodeficiencies. Ann Intern Med 100:663, 1984
6. Jules-Elysee K, Stover D, Zaman M, White D: Aerosol pentamidine prophylaxis: Effect on yield of bronchoscopy for PCP. Am Rev Respir Dis 139:238, 1989
7. Levine SJ, Masur H, Gill VJ et al: The effect of aerosolized pentamidine prophylaxis on the diagnosis of *Pneumocystis carinii* pneumonia by induced sputum examination in patients infected with the human immunodeficiency virus. Am Rev Respir Dis, in press
8. Brenner M, Ognibene FP, Lack EE et al: Prognostic factors and life expectancy of patients with acquired immune deficiency syndrome and *Pneumocystis carinii* pneumonia. Am Rev Respir Dis 136:1199, 1987
9. The National Institutes of Health–University of California Expert Panel for Corticosteroids as Adjunctive Therapy for Pneumocystis Pneumonia: Consensus statement on the use of corticosteroids as adjunctive therapy for pneumocystis pneumonia in the acquired immunodeficiency syndrome: N Engl J Med 323:1500, 1990
10. Raviglione MC: Extrapulmonary pneumocystosis: The first 50 cases. Rev Infect Dis 12:1227, 1990
11. Telzac EE, Cote RJ, Gold JWM et al: Extrapulmonary *Pneumocystis carinii* infections. Rev Infect Dis 12:380, 1990
12. Hopewell PC: Diagnosis of *Pneumocystis carinii* pneumonia. Infect Dis Clin North Am 2:409, 1988
13. Golden JA, Hollander H, Stulbarg MS, Gamsu G: Bronchoalveolar lavage as the exclusive diagnostic modality for *Pneumocystis carinii* pneumonia: A prospective study among patients with acquired immunodeficiency syndrome. Chest 90:18, 1986
14. Weldon-Linne CM, Rhone DP, Bourassa R: Bronchoscopy specimens in adults with AIDS: Comparative yields of cytology, histology and culture for diagnosis of infectious agents. Chest 98:24, 1990
15. Shelhamer JH, Ognibene FP, Macher AM et al: Persistence of *Pneumocystis carinii* in lung tissue of acquired immunodeficiency syndrome patients treated for pneumocystis pneumonia. Am Rev Respir Dis 130:1161, 1984
16. Wharton JM, Coleman DL, Wofsy CB et al: Trimethoprim-sulfamethoxazole or pentamidine for *Pneumocystis carinii* pneumonia in the acquired immunodeficiency syndrome: A prospective randomized trial. Ann Intern Med 105:37, 1986
17. Allegra CJ, Chabner BA, Tuazon CU et al: Trimetrexate for the treatment of *Pneumocystis carinii* pneumonia in patients with the acquired immunodeficiency syndrome. N Engl J Med 317:978, 1987
18. Murray JF, Felton CP, Garay SM et al: Pulmonary complications of the acquired immunodeficiency syndrome. N Engl J Med 310:1682, 1984
19. Broaddus C, Dake MD, Stulbarg MS et al: Bronchoalveolar lavage and transbronchial biopsy for the diagnosis of pulmonary infections in the acquired immunodeficiency syndrome. Ann Intern Med 102:747, 1985
20. Kovacs JA, Ng V, Masur H et al: Diagnosis of *Pneumocystis carinii* pneumonia: Improved detection in sputum using monoclonal antibodies. N Engl J Med 318:589, 1987
21. Zaman MK, Wooten OJ, Suprahmanya B et al: Rapid non-invasive diagnosis of *Pneumocystis carinii* from induced liquified sputum. Ann Intern Med 109:7, 1988
22. Pintozzi RL, Blecka LJ, Nanos S: The morphologic identification of *Pneumocystis carinii*. Acta Cytol 23:35, 1979
23. Tuazon CV, Delaney MD, Simon GL et al: Utility of gallium-67 scintigraphy and bronchial washings in patients with the acquired immunodeficiency syndrome. Am Rev Respir Dis 132:1087, 1985
24. Rao NA, Zimmerman PL, Boyer D et al: A clinical, histopathologic, and electron microscopic study of *Pneumocystis carinii* choroiditis. Am J Ophthalmol 107:218, 1989
25. Radin DR, Baker EL, Klatt EC et al: Visceral and nodal calcification in patients with AIDS-related *Pneumocystis carinii* infection. AJR 154:27, 1990
26. Lubat E, Megibow AJ, Balthazar EJ et al: Extrapulmonary *Pneumocystis carinii* infection in AIDS: CT findings. Radiology 174:157, 1990
27. Sattler FR, Cowan R, Nielsen DM, Ruskin J: Trimethoprim-sulfamethoxazole compared with pentamidine for treatment of *Pneumocystis carinii* pneumonia in the acquired immunodeficiency syndrome: A prospective, noncrossover study. Ann Intern Med 109:280, 1988
28. Gordin FM, Simon GL, Wofsy CB, Mills J: Adverse reactions to trimethoprim-sulfamethoxazole in patients with the acquired immunodeficiency syndrome. Ann Intern Med 100:495, 1984
29. Wofsy CB: Use of trimethoprim-sulfamethoxazole in the treatment of *Pneumocystis carinii* pneumonitis in patients

with acquired immunodeficiency syndrome. Rev Infect Dis 9:S184, 1987

30. Pearson RD, Hewlett EL: Pentamidine for the treatment of *Pneumocystis carinii* pneumonia and other protozoal diseases. Ann Intern Med 103:782, 1985

31. Conte JE, Jr, Chernoff D, Feigal DW Jr et al: Intravenous or inhaled pentamidine for treating *Pneumocystis carinii* pneumonia in AIDS: A randomized trial. Ann Intern Med 113:203, 1990

32. Medina I, Mills J, Leoung G et al: Oral therapy for *Pneumocystis carinii* pneumonia in the acquired immunodeficiency syndrome: A controlled trial of trimethoprim-sulfamethoxazole versus trimethoprim-dapsone. N Engl J Med 323:776, 1990

33. Toma E, Fournier S, Poisson M et al: Clindamycin with primaquine for *Pneumocystis carinii* pneumonia. Lancet 1:1046, 1989

34. Hughes WT, Gray VL, Gutteridge WE et al: Efficacy of a hydroxynaphthoquinone, 566C80, in experimental *Pneumocystis carinii* pneumonitis. Antimicrob Agents Chemother 34:225, 1990

35. Hughes WT, Kennedy W, Shenep JL et al: Safety and pharmacokinetics of 566C80, a hydroxynaphthoquinone with anti-*Pneumocystis carinii* activity: A phase I study in human immunodeficiency virus (HIV)-infected men. J Infect Dis 163:843, 1991

36. Soo Hoo GW, Mohsenifar Z, Meyer RD: Inhaled or intravenous pentamidine therapy for *Pneumocystis carinii* pneumonia in AIDS: A randomized trial. Ann Intern Med 113:195, 1990

37. Sattler FR, Allegra CJ, Verdegem TD et al: Trimetrexate-leucovorin dosage evaluation study for treatment of *Pneumocystis carinii* pneumonia. J Infect Dis 161:91, 1990

38. Golden JA, Sjoerdsma A, Santi DV: *Pneumocystis carinii* pneumonia treated with α-difluoromethylornithine. West J Med 141:613, 1984

39. Sahai J, Berry AJ: Eflornithine for the treatment of *Pneumocystis carinii* pneumonia in patients with the acquired immunodeficiency syndrome: A preliminary review. Pharmacotherapy 9:29, 1989

40. Bozzette SA, Sattler FR, Chiu J et al: A controlled trial of early adjunctive treatment with corticosteroids for *Pneumocystis carinii* pneumonia in the acquired immunodeficiency syndrome. N Engl J Med 323:1451, 1991

41. Gagnon S, Boota AM, Fischl MA et al: Corticosteroids as adjunctive therapy for severe *Pneumocystis carinii* pneumonia in the acquired immunodeficiency syndrome: A double-blind, placebo-controlled trial. N Engl J Med 323:1444, 1990

42. Montaner JSG, Lawson LM, Levitt N et al: Corticosteroids prevent early deterioration in patients with moderately severe *Pneumocystis carinii* pneumonia and the acquired immunodeficiency syndrome (AIDS). Ann Intern Med 113:14, 1990

43. El-Sadr W, Simberkoff MS: Survival and prognostic factors in severe *Pneumocystis carinii* pneumonia requiring mechanical ventilation. Am Rev Respir Dis 137:1264, 1988

44. Friedman Y, Franklin C, Rackow EC, Weil MH: Improved survival in patients with AIDS, *Pneumocystis carinii* pneumonia, and severe respiratory failure. Chest 96:862, 1989

45. Wachter RM, Russi MB, Bloch DA et al: *Pneumocystis carinii* pneumonia and respiratory failure in AIDS: Improved outcomes and increased use of intensive care units. Am Rev Respir Dis 143:251, 1991

46. Leoung GS, Feigal DW Jr, Montgomery AB et al: Aerosolized pentamidine for prophylaxis against *Pneumocystis carinii* pneumonia: The San Francisco Community Prophylaxis Trial. N Engl J Med 323:769, 1990

47. Hirschel B, Lazzarin A, Chopard P et al: A controlled study of inhaled pentamidine for primary prevention of *Pneumocystis carinii* pneumonia. N Engl J Med 324:1079, 1991

48. Murphy RL, Lavelle JP, Allan JD et al: Aerosol pentamidine prophylaxis following *Pneumocystis carinii* pneumonia in AIDS patients: Results of a blinded dose comparison study using an ultrasonic nebulizer. Am J Med 1991; 90:418

49. Fischl MA, Dickinson GM, La Voie L: Safety and efficacy of sulfamethoxazole and trimethoprim chemoprophylaxis for *Pneumocystis carinii* pneumonia in AIDS. JAMA 259:1185, 1988

50. Hughes WT, Rivera GK, Schell MJ et al: Successful intermittent chemoprophylaxis for *Pneumocystis carinii* pneumonitis. N Engl J Med 316:1627, 1987

51. Ruskin J, LaRiviere M: Low-dose co-trimoxazole for prevention of *Pneumocystis carinii* pneumonia in human immunodeficiency virus disease. Lancet 337:468, 1991

52. Hughes WT: Comparison of dosages, intervals, and drugs in the prevention of *Pneumocystis carinii* pneumonia. Antimicrob Agents Chemother 32:623, 1988

53. Newsome GS, Ward DJ, Pierce PF: Spontaneous pneumothorax in patients with acquired immunodeficiency syndrome treated with prophylactic aerosolized pentamidine. Arch Intern Med 150:2167, 1990

54. Sepkowitz KA, Telzak EE, Gold JWM et al: Pneumothorax in AIDS. Ann Intern Med 114:455, 1991

55. Fischl MA, Richman DD, Grieco MH et al: The efficacy of azidothymidine (AZT) in the treatment of patients with AIDS and AIDS-related complex: A double-blind, placebo-controlled trial. N Engl J Med 317:185, 1987

56. Luft BJ, Remington JS: Toxoplasmic encephalitis. J Infect Dis 157:1, 1988

57. Navia BA, Petito CK, Gold JWM et al: Cerebral toxoplasmosis complicating the acquired immune deficiency syndrome: Clinical and neuropathological findings in 27 patients. Ann Neurol 19:224, 1986

58. Oksenhendler E, Cadranel J, Sarfati C et al: *Toxoplasma gondii* pneumonia in patients with the acquired immunodeficiency syndrome. Am J Med 88:5N, 1990

59. Luft BJ, Brooks RG, Conley FK et al: Toxoplasmic encephalitis in patients with acquired immune deficiency syndrome. JAMA 252:913, 1984

60. Leport C, Raffi F, Matheron S et al: Treatment of central nervous system toxoplasmosis with pyrimethamine/sulfadiazine combination in 35 patients with the acquired immunodeficiency syndrome: Efficacy of long-term continuous therapy. Am J Med 84:94, 1988

61. Haverkos HW, TE Study Group: Assessment of therapy for toxoplasma encephalitis. Am J Med 82:907, 1987

62. Wanke C, Tuazon CU, Kovacs A et al: *Toxoplasma* encephalitis in patients with acquired immune deficiency syndrome: Diagnosis and response to therapy. Am J Trop Med Hyg 36:509, 1987

63. Israelski DM, Remington JS: Toxoplasmic encephalitis in patients with AIDS. Infect Dis Clin North Am 2:429, 1988

64. Threlkeld MG, Graves AH, Cobbs CG: Cerebrospinal fluid staining for the diagnosis of toxoplasmosis in patients with the acquired immune deficiency syndrome. Am J Med 83:599, 1987

65. Potasman I, Resnick L, Luft BJ, Remington JS: Intrathecal production of antibodies against *Toxoplasma gondii* in

patients with toxoplasmic encephalitis and the acquired immunodeficiency syndrome (AIDS). Ann Intern Med 108:49, 1988

66. Oster S, Hutchison F, McCabe R: Resolution of acute renal failure in toxoplasmic encephalitis despite continuance of sulfadiazine. Rev Infect Dis 12:618, 1990

67. Dannemann BR, Israelski DM, Remington JS: Treatment of toxoplasmic encephalitis with intravenous clindamycin. Arch Intern Med 148:2477, 1988

68. Leport C, Bastuji-Garin S, Peronne C et al: An open study of the pyrimethamine-clindamycin combination in AIDS patients with brain toxoplasmosis. J Infect Dis 160:557, 1989

69. Katlama C, De Wit S, Guichard A et al: Pyrimethamine-clindamycin versus pyrimethamine-sulfadiazine in toxoplasma encephalitis in AIDS: A randomized prospective multicentric european study (abstr W.B.30). Presented at the VII International Conference on AIDS, Florence, Italy, June 16–21, 1991

70. Araujo FG, Huskinson J, Remington JS: Remarkable in vitro and in vivo activities of the hydroxynaphthoquinone 566C80 against tachyzoites and tissue cysts of *Toxoplasma gondii*. Antimicrob Agents Chemother 35:293, 1991

71. Suzuki Y, Orellana MA, Schreiber RD, Remington JS: Interferon-γ: The major mediator of resistance against *Toxoplasma gondii*. Science 240:516, 1988

72. Soave R, Armstrong D: *Cryptosporidium* and cryptosporidiosis. Rev Infect Dis 8:1012, 1986

73. Connolly GM, Dryden MS, Shanson DC, Gazzard BG: Cryptosporidial diarrhea in AIDS and its treatment. Gut 29:593, 1988

74. Schneiderman DJ, Cello JP, Laing FC: Papillary stenosis and sclerosing cholangitis in the acquired immunodeficiency syndrome. Ann Intern Med 106:546, 1987

75. Soave R, Johnson WD Jr: *Cryptosporidium* and *Isospora belli* infections. J Infect Dis 157:225, 1988

76. Kotler DP, Francisco A, Clayton F et al: Small intestinal injury and parasitic diseases in AIDS. Ann Intern Med 113:444, 1990

77. Rehg JE: Activity of azithromycin against cryptosporidia in immunosuppressed rats. J Infect Dis 163:1293, 1991

78. Shadduck JA: Human microsporidiosis and AIDS. Rev Infect Dis 11:203, 1989

79. Schattenkerk JKME, van Gool T, Van Ketel RJ et al: Clinical significance of small-intestinal microsporidiosis in HIV-1-infected individuals. Lancet 337:895, 1991

80. Orenstein JM, Chiang J, Steinberg W et al: Intestinal microsporidiosis as a cause of diarrhea in human immunodeficiency virus-infected patients: A report of 20 cases. Hum Pathol 21:475, 1990

81. Terada S, Reddy KR, Jeffers LJ et al: Microsporidan hepatitis in the acquired immunodeficiency syndrome. Ann Intern Med 107:61, 1987

82. Centers for Disease Control: Microsporidian keratoconjunctivitis in patients with AIDS. MMWR 39:188, 1990

83. Rijpstra AC, Canning EU, Van Ketel RJ et al: Use of light microscopy to diagnose small-intestinal microsporidiosis in patients with AIDS. J Infect Dis 157:817, 1988

84. DeHovitz JA, Pape JW, Boncy M et al: Clinical manifestations and therapy of *Isospora belli* infection in patients with the acquired immunodeficiency syndrome. N Engl J Med 315:87, 1986

85. Pape JW, Verdier R-I, Johnson WD Jr: Treatment and prophylaxis of *Isospora belli* infection in patients with the acquired immunodeficiency syndrome. N Engl J Med 320:1044, 1989

86. Weiss LM, Perlman DC, Sherman J, et al: *Isospora belli* infection: Treatment with pyrimethamine. Ann Intern Med 109:474, 1988

Fungal Infections in Patients with the Acquired Immunodeficiency Syndrome

11B

Michael A. Polis   *Joseph A. Kovacs*

Fungal infections are common complications of the immunosuppression of human immunodeficiency virus (HIV) infection. Such infections can result in life-threatening meningitis or in discomforting but not debilitating oral thrush. This chapter reviews the clinical presentation and management of fungal infections in patients with the acquired immunodeficiency syndrome (AIDS).

CRYPTOCOCCUS NEOFORMANS

Cryptococcus neoformans is the major cause of meningitis in AIDS patients. In addition to meningitis, *C. neoformans* can also cause local organ dysfunction as well as disseminated disease.

Organism Description

C. neoformans is a yeastlike fungus that reproduces by budding.[1] It produces no known toxins but does have a large polysaccharide capsule that appears to play a role in protecting the organism from host defense mechanisms. There are four serotypes of *C. neoformans*: A and D are classified as *C. neoformans* var. *neoformans*, and B and C are classified as *C. neoformans* var. *gatti*. The classification is based on several characteristics, including mating abilities.[1] Whereas in non-AIDS patients B and C serotypes occasionally cause disease, in AIDS patients, both in the United States and in Africa, cryptococcosis is caused almost exclusively by serotypes A and D.[2–4] Organisms isolated from AIDS patients have been reported to differ from those isolated from non-AIDS patients.[5] In primary culture, isolates from AIDS patients grew as nonmucoid, pasty colonies in one study, in contrast to the mucoid colonies of non-AIDS isolates. Further, the capsule in AIDS isolates has been reported to be significantly smaller than that in non-AIDS isolates.[5]

Epidemiology and Pathogenesis

C. neoformans is a ubiquitous fungus that can be isolated from a variety of environmental sites, including soil, and is found in especially high concentrations in pigeon feces.[1] Initial infection occurs *via* the respiratory route through inhalation of aerosolized organisms following exposure to environmental sources. There is no evidence that *C. neoformans* can be contracted directly from humans or animals, and thus isolation of patients with active infection is not necessary. In patients with intact immune systems the infection is controlled in the lung, usually without causing serious complications. In immunocompromised patients, however, especially patients with AIDS, the organism is inadequately controlled and may cause life-threatening extrapulmonary disease, primarily meningitis. Because there are no reliable serologic markers for prior exposure, at present it cannot be determined if disease in immunosuppressed hosts results from primary infection or, as is the case with many other opportunistic infections, such as toxoplasmosis, from reactivation of latent, previously controlled infection.

The incidence of cryptococcosis in AIDS patients in the United States has been reported in larger studies to range from approximately 6% to 12%.[6-9] Among 160,000 AIDS patients reported to the CDC, cryptococcosis was identified, usually as the AIDS-defining diagnosis, in 1.5%. This is clearly an underestimate of the incidence of cryptococcosis in this population, since in many patients cryptococcosis develops subsequent to other AIDS-defining opportunistic infections, such as *Pneumocystis carinii* pneumonia. Cryptococcosis has been reported to occur in 3.7% of AIDS patients in Great Britain and is a very common opportunistic infection in Africa, occurring in 13% to 17% of patients in one report.[10,11]

Cryptococcosis can present as either the initial AIDS-defining opportunistic process in HIV-infected patients (42% to 75% of cases) or as a later process. When cryptococcosis is the initial manifestation, other opportunistic processes, such as *P. carinii* pneumonia, are often identified simultaneously.[6-8,12] As for other infections such as *P. carinii* pneumonia, patients with low CD4 counts are at greatest risk for the development of cryptococcosis. In one report, 30 of 31 patients had CD4 counts below 100 cells/mm³ at the time of diagnosis.[13] In another report, all six patients in whom *C. neoformans* was cultured from bronchoscopy specimens had CD4 counts below 100 cells/mm³.[14] In a prospective study, among symptomatic HIV-infected patients with CD4 counts below 200 cells/mm³, the annual incidence of cryptococcal disease was greater than 3%.[15]

Clinical Manifestations

The most common site of infection with *C. neoformans* in both AIDS and non-AIDS patients is the central nervous system (CNS).[6-8,12] *C. neoformans* usually infects both the brain and the meninges diffusely, and thus produces both meningitis and encephalitis. Occasionally, cryptococcomas, which are large focal lesions, develop. In four published series, meningitis, alone or together with extrameningeal disease, was reported to occur in 67% to 85% of AIDS patients with cryptococcosis.[6-8,12] Cryptococcal meningitis in AIDS patients frequently presents in a subtle manner: headache and fever are the most common manifestations, occurring in 60% to 100% of patients, and may be the only presenting symptoms (Table 11B-1).[6-8,12] Nausea or vomiting has been reported in about 40%. Meningeal signs and an altered mental status are seen in about one fourth of patients, and seizures or focal neurologic abnormalities are seen infrequently. Symptoms are usually present for 2 to 4 weeks prior to diagnosis, although occasionally they may be present for up to 4 months.[12]

Abnormal computed tomography (CT) scans of the head have been reported in 20% to 30% of patients with meningitis, although the abnormalities were not always related to cryptococcosis. Abnormalities attributable to cryptococcosis have included multiple ring enhancing lesions in patients with cryptococcomas, nonenhancing focal lesions, and meningeal enhancement.[7,8,12]

Examination of the cerebrospinal fluid (CSF) in AIDS patients with cryptococcal meningitis usually reveals a large organism burden but often a minimal inflammatory response. From 10% to 35% of patients will have a CSF white blood cell count over 20 cells/mm³, 35% to 70% have elevated CSF protein levels, and 17%

Table 11B-1. Incidence of Symptoms, Signs, and Laboratory Values in Patients with Cryptococcal Meningitis

Characteristic	*Incidence (%)*
Heachache	67–100
Fever	62–95
Altered mental status	18–28
Meningeal signs	25–30
Seizures	4–9
Focal neurologic abnormality	6–17
Positive serum cryptococcal antigen test	94–100
Positive CSF cryptococcal antigen	91–100
Positive CSF India ink	64–88
Positive CSF culture	95–100
Abnormal CSF glucose	17–64
Abnormal CSF protein	35–69
Abnormal CSF WBC count	13–35

Data summarized from Kovacs et al,[6] Clark et al,[7] Chuck and Sande,[8] and Zuger et al.[12]

to 64% have low glucose levels.[6–8,12] In one study all three parameters were normal in 15% of patients[6]; in another, only 41% had at least one abnormality.[7] Despite the minimal CSF abnormalities, India ink preparations are positive in 64% to 88% of patients, and often many organisms are seen. CSF cryptococcal antigen is present in over 90% of patients with meningitis, and titers are often very elevated; titers were greater than 1:1,024 in 39% to 48% of patients in two reports.[7,8] Patients with cryptococcomas may have a negative CSF cryptococcal antigen test.[12] Serum cryptococcal antigen is present in an even higher proportion of patients with meningitis, being detectable in 94% to 100% of patients.[6–8,12] CSF culture for *C. neoformans* is positive in virtually 100% of patients with meningitis. Patients with cryptococcomas may have negative CSF cultures but positive biopsy cultures.[12]

Disease exclusively outside the CNS has been reported in 10% to 33% of AIDS patients with cryptococcosis. Pneumonia and fungemia are the most common extraneural presentations. Some 4% to 10% of patients with cryptococcosis have presented with pneumonia without meningitis; up to 40% of all patients with cryptococcosis will have evidence of pulmonary infection. Patients with pneumonia may present with fever, productive cough, dyspnea, and occasionally hemoptysis. On chest radiography a variety of abnormalities have been seen, including lobar consolidation, nodules that may cavitate, diffuse interstitial infiltrates, bilateral miliary infiltrates, pleural effusions, and hilar adenopathy. Chest radiographs may also be normal. Histopathologically, cryptococci are most often located in the interstitium of alveoli, but occasionally they are found within capillaries and lymphatics (Fig. 11B–1) (see Color Fig. 1).[16] There is often little or no inflammatory response despite the presence of large numbers of organisms.

Fungemia as the sole manifestation of *C. neoformans* infection has been noted in 4% to 8% of patients.[6,8] Positive blood cultures have also been reported in 33% to 68% of patients with meningitis.[6,7,12] Fungemia may be associated with minimal complaints: fever, malaise, and fatigue are often the only symptoms suggesting a systemic infection. Disseminated disease may also be demonstrated by bone marrow biopsy.[17] In occasional patients all cultures are negative but serum cryptococcal antigen assays are positive.[6,8]

Other sites of infection are also occasionally seen. Eye involvement, including retinitis, is seen in patients with meningitis. Mucocutaneous manifestations of cryptococcal infection in AIDS patients have included skin and oral lesions. Oral manifestations have included palatal and tongue ulcers, which are indurated and tender on palpation.[18,19] Skin lesions can manifest in a variety of forms: papules, plaques, nodules, and ulcerated lesions have all been reported.[19–24] Frequently the lesions have characteristics resembling other processes

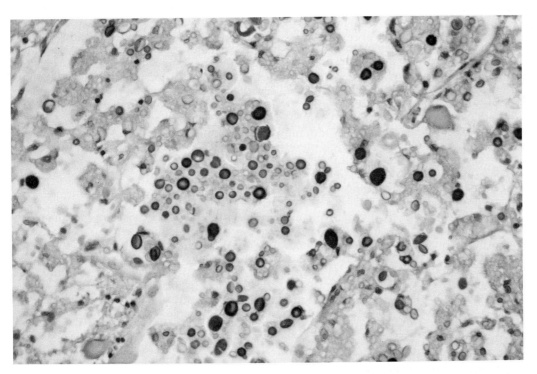

Figure 11B–1.   Mucicarmine stain of cryptococcus in the lung showing massive disruption of the pulmonary architecture in a patient with AIDS and cryptococcal pneumonia.

commonly seen in AIDS patients, such as Kaposi's sarcoma, herpes simplex or zoster, and molluscum contagiosum. Cryptococcal arthritis is a rare complication of infection.[25] Gastrointestinal (GI) involvement, including infection of the stomach, duodenum, colon, pancreas, and liver, has also been reported.[26] Omental involvement presented as an incarcerated hernia in one case, and massive abdominal adenopathy was initially thought due to a lymphoma in another.[6,27] Cryptococcal myocarditis manifesting with or without heart failure has also been seen.[28] Rarely, asymptomatic patients have positive urine, blood, or bone marrow cultures for *C. neoformans* without evidence of clinically significant disease attributable to cryptococcal infection.[12] The prostate may also be a site of asymptomatic infection, especially in patients who have completed a course of antifungal therapy.[29]

Diagnosis

The diagnosis of cryptococcosis in AIDS patients relies on culturing the organism or detecting cryptococcal antigen in a clinical specimen. Histopathologic diagnosis without culture confirmation is also utilized; however, other fungal pathogens with similar morphology should then be considered and the diagnosis of cryptococcosis confirmed by staining with mucicarmine. Although the diagnosis can usually be established quickly and easily when it is considered, a high index of suspicion is necessary to ensure that appropriate specimens are obtained and cultured. Because of the subtle manifestations of *C. neoformans* infection in AIDS patients, it is easy for both physicians and patients to dismiss seemingly minor complaints such as headache or fever, insofar as such symptoms are common and most often not due to cryptococcosis. Patients at highest risk for developing cryptococcosis, including those with CD4 counts below 200/mm[3], and especially those with counts below 100 cells/mm[3], should be diligently evaluated. Patients with other life-threatening opportunistic infections will inevitably have low CD4 counts and thus should also be considered at high risk.

The simplest and most rapid method for diagnosing cryptococcosis at any site is the serum cryptococcal antigen test. This test can be performed in a few hours and is positive in over 90% of patients with meningitis, as well as in most patients without meningitis.[6–8,12] Although occasional false positive results occur, the use of appropriate controls will minimize these. The serum cryptococcal antigen test is thus an appropriate screening test in patients with or without headache, and is especially useful in patients with a fever but no localizing signs or symptoms. In such patients blood should also be submitted for fungal culture, although such cultures will not become positive for at least a few days.

All patients suspected of having cryptococcal meningitis should undergo a lumbar puncture. The diagnosis is confirmed by detecting cryptococcal antigen in CSF, by visualizing organisms in CSF using India ink, and by culturing the organism from CSF. Because CSF protein and glucose levels and cell counts are frequently normal in AIDS patients, all CSF samples should be cultured and assayed for antigen, regardless of the characteristics of the fluid. Patients with detectable antigen should be started on therapy immediately while culture results are pending. Although the India ink test is positive in the majority of patients with meningitis, it is less sensitive than antigen detection and requires greater experience for correct interpretation; thus, some laboratories will perform only the antigen test.[6–8,12]

The diagnosis of extraneural cryptococcosis depends on culturing the organism or detecting it histopathologically in biopsy or other clinical specimens. For patients with pneumonitis, bronchoscopy appears to be very useful in making the diagnosis. Transbronchial biopsy was positive in six (75%) of eight patients in one series.[16] Cryptococci were also identified in five (63%) of eight bronchial brush specimens, five (83%) of six bronchoalveolar lavage (BAL) specimens, and seven (100%) of seven cell blocks prepared from BAL fluid. Bronchoscopy specimens may also be positive without radiographic or histopathologic evidence of pneumonitis.[14]

Isolation of *C. neoformans* from any site should be considered significant and an indication for further evaluation and therapy. Although the organism may be detected in the urine or BAL fluid of patients with no evidence of disease, such patients should receive antifungal therapy because of the risk of life-threatening dissemination or meningitis. As previously noted, some patients will have fungemia without localized infection, and the diagnosis thus relies on positive blood cultures exclusively. Lysis-centrifugation techniques as well as radiometric techniques appear to increase the sensitivity of cultures, although occasionally cultures will be false negative if the radiometric technique alone is used.[30] In rare patients positive serum cryptococcal antigen is the exclusive evidence of cryptococcal infection.[8,12] Although the site of infection in such patients may not be identified, it is prudent to treat such patients to prevent life-threatening complications.

Differential Diagnosis

In AIDS patients meningitis is caused predominantly by *C. neoformans.* Other organisms such as *Listeria,* other fungi, and mycobacteria can occasionally cause meningitis. Headaches may be due to cryptococcal meningitis as well as to focal mass lesions, including those due to toxoplasmosis, lymphoma, and tuberculosis. Sinusitis also is commonly seen in HIV-infected patients, although it will frequently coexist with another, more life-threatening process.

Therapy

Prior to the AIDS epidemic, *C. neoformans* infections were treated with amphotericin B alone or combined with flucytosine. In a randomized study of non-AIDS patients with cryptococcal meningitis, the combination of amphotericin B (0.3 mg/kg/day) and flucytosine (150 mg/kg/day) administered for 6 weeks was as effective as amphotericin B alone (0.4 mg/kg/day) administered for 10 weeks, and combination therapy was associated with more rapid sterilization of the CSF.[31] Based on these data, 6 weeks of combination therapy became the standard treatment regimen for non-AIDS patients.

For patients with AIDS and cryptococcal infection, it became clear early in the epidemic that treatment with standard courses of amphotericin B alone or combined with flucytosine was successful in many patients but was associated with a high relapse rate once therapy was discontinued. In two series, a combined response rate of 54% (28/52) was seen, but the relapse rate in the absence of suppressive therapy was 56% (10/18) among patients who had initially responded to therapy.[6,12] From these early retrospective studies it was not clear if combination therapy was more beneficial than therapy with amphotericin B alone. Moreover, toxicity with the combination therapy was greater than with amphotericin B alone, and flucytosine was frequently discontinued because of this toxicity.

Based on these early data, patients were routinely treated with a total of 1 to 2 g of amphotericin B; flucytosine was often added if the patient was not receiving other marrow suppressive agents, and was discontinued if toxicity developed. Following completion of amphotericin B therapy, patients were placed on a suppressive antifungal regimen in an attempt to prevent relapse. Amphotericin B administered in a dosage of 1 mg/kg once weekly was commonly used, although more frequent dosing of amphotericin B or the use of an oral agent such as ketoconazole was also common.[32]

In a recently published retrospective study of 89 patients with cryptococcal meningitis, the experience at San Francisco General Hospital in the first 6 years of the epidemic was reviewed.[8] In that study no difference in survival was found between patients receiving amphotericin B alone and those receiving amphotericin B plus flucytosine. However, median survival was significantly increased in patients receiving suppressive therapy after the initial treatment regimen compared to those not receiving suppression. Interestingly, no difference was seen between those receiving amphotericin B and those receiving ketoconazole for suppression, even though ketoconazole does not penetrate into the CNS. Although the reason for the benefit of ketoconazole is uncertain, one possible explanation is that disease may reactivate from an extrameningeal site, and that ketoconazole was effective in preventing this extrameningeal relapse. In one report, cultures of prostatic secretions were positive in 22% of patients who had no evidence of active disease elsewhere, and the authors postulated that the prostate thus served as a nidus for recurrent dissemination.[29]

Recently important new advances in the management of cryptococcal meningitis have been made. These advances have been based on the availability of a new oral antifungal agent, fluconazole, and its evaluation in well-designed randomized studies. Fluconazole is a triazole with good activity against *C. neoformans;* it crosses the blood-brain barrier efficiently, achieving levels in the CSF that are 25% to 88% of serum levels.[33] Preliminary uncontrolled studies suggested that fluconazole was effective in the treatment of cryptococcal meningitis in AIDS patients.[33,34] However, in a small randomized study, therapy failed in eight of 14 patients receiving fluconazole, compared to none of six patients receiving amphotericin B plus flucytosine, and four of the patients receiving fluconazole died, whereas no patient in the amphotericin B group died.[35] More recently, a randomized blinded study of 194 patients, conducted by the NIAID Mycoses Study Group, that compared fluconazole (200 mg/day) to amphotericin B (mean, 0.5 mg/kg/day) with or without flucytosine found no significant difference in outcome between the two groups. However, the time to sterilization of the CSF was more rapid in the amphotericin B group (2 weeks *vs.* 4 weeks), and a higher proportion of the patients receiving fluconazole died during the first 2 weeks of therapy (M. Saag, pers. commun.). The NIAID Mycoses Study Group has undertaken a subsequent study to evaluate 2 weeks of amphotericin B followed by long-term fluconazole therapy.

Although the use of fluconazole as initial therapy is controversial, the role of fluconazole as a suppressive agent has recently been validated in two randomized trials. In a placebo-controlled trial conducted by the California Collaborative Treatment Group, fluconazole proved significantly more effective than placebo in preventing relapse at any site in patients with cryptococcal meningitis who had previously responded to standard therapy.[36] Ten (37%) of 27 placebo recipients *versus* only one (3%) of 34 patients receiving fluconazole (100 or 200 mg/day) experienced recurrence during a median follow-up of 4 to 5 months. In another study conducted by the NIAID Mycoses Study Group that compared the efficacy of amphotericin B (1 mg/kg/wk) to fluconazole (200 mg/day) as suppressive regimens following successful treatment with amphotericin B, a significantly higher proportion of patients receiving amphotericin B relapsed (14 [18%] of 78, *vs.* 3 [3%] of 111 for the fluconazole group) during a median 1 year of follow-up (M. Saag, pers. commun.).[37]

Based on the above data, the initial therapy of cryptococcal meningitis should be with amphotericin B alone or together with flucytosine. After a total of 1 to 2 g of amphotericin B has been administered, suppressive therapy with fluconazole (200 mg/day) should be started and continued for the life of the patient. Further studies are needed to determine if shorter courses of amphotericin B followed by fluconazole are as effective as this regimen. Although treatment of extrameningeal disease has not been as thoroughly evaluated, the above regimen should be used for such patients as well.

Alternative regimens are also being evaluated for the treatment of cryptococcal disease in AIDS patients. Itraconazole is another triazole that has poor penetration into the CSF but has been found effective in animal models of cryptococcal meningitis. In an open, uncontrolled study, 13 of 20 assessable patients had a complete response (negative cultures with clinical resolution), although two of these experienced relapses at 6 and 10 weeks while continuing therapy.[38] Itraconazole may also play a role as a suppressive agent in patients with no active meningeal disease.[39] Sch-39304, a new triazole that was in clinical trials, is no longer being developed.[40]

Although intrathecal amphotericin B has been advocated for the treatment of cryptococcal meningitis, there is currently no evidence that such therapy is beneficial or necessary in AIDS patients.[41]

Prognostic Factors

In non-AIDS patients a number of factors, such as low CSF glucose or leukocyte levels and positive India ink smear, have been associated with a poor prognosis.[42] In AIDS patients, however, such factors appear less important in prognosis. In the largest retrospective study published to date, only a low sodium level at presentation and positive cultures of specimens from extrameningeal sites were associated with shorter survival.[8] In other studies, abnormal CT scans, altered mental status at presentation, or high mean serum and CSF cryptococcal antigen levels were associated with a poor prognosis.[7,12]

Prophylaxis

Although primary prophylaxis with fluconazole to prevent cryptococcal meningitis is being used by some physicians, the benefits of such an approach in patients with no history of cryptococcosis have not been investigated. Because at present no factors other than low CD4 count are useful in identifying an at-risk population, and because the incidence of cryptococcosis is relatively low, the potential side-effects, the risk that resistant organisms may develop, and the high cost of such an approach may outweigh the benefit. Well-controlled clinical trials are clearly needed to address these issues. Avoidance of exposure to possible environmental sources of *C. neoformans* should help minimize the risk of developing infection.

CANDIDA SPECIES

Organism Description

Candida species are yeasts that exist predominantly in unicellular forms. They are 2.5 to 6 μm ovoid cells that reproduce by budding. More than 150 species exist and at least ten are pathogenic in humans.

Epidemiology and Pathogenesis

Candida organisms are ubiquitous; they have been recovered from soil, hospital environments, and food.

Clinical Manifestations

Candida species are the most common causative agents of fungal infections in HIV-infected persons. Fortunately, these infections are seldom invasive, can usually be easily treated, and, with appropriate management, can often be prevented. It was established early in the course of the HIV epidemic that oral candidiasis is a marker of an impaired immune system and a prognostic marker for the subsequent development of opportunistic infections.[43] Candidal infections of the esophagus, trachea, bronchi, or lungs are recognized as indicator diseases for AIDS.[44] Whereas oropharyngeal candidal infections (and candidal vaginosis in women) regularly occur in HIV-infected persons with CD4 counts above 200 cells/mm³, esophageal candidiasis is indicative of more advanced immunodeficiency and seldom occurs with CD4 counts above 100 cells/mm³.[45] Oropharyngeal and vaginal candidiasis may recur frequently.[45,46] *Candida* species seldom cause disseminated infections in patients with AIDS unless there are associated factors such as the presence of chronic indwelling catheters or neutropenia.

Diagnosis

Oropharyngeal candidiasis (thrush) is generally diagnosed from the characteristic appearance of white plaques on the tongue, buccal mucosa, or palate. Microscopic examination of a scraping of the plaque, using Gram stain or potassium hydroxide, will reveal sheets of hyphae, pseudohyphae, and yeast forms.

The diagnosis of *Candida* esophagitis is frequently made on the basis of the characteristic clinical presentations of odynophagia, dysphagia, a feeling of obstruction, and/or substernal chest pain, often accompanied by oropharyngeal candidiasis.[47] Radiographically, an esophageal contrast study may reveal discrete, widely separated plaques on a normal background mucosa, diffuse plaque formation without ulcers, or a grossly irregular esophagus as a result of multiple plaques and ulcers (Fig. 11B–2).[48] In one study, with radiologists experienced in the diagnosis of esophageal disease in persons with AIDS, *Candida* esophagitis was distinguished from esophagitis due to herpes or cytomegalovirus (CMV) without the need for endoscopy.[48] Blind brushing of the esophagus *via* nasogastric tube is highly sensitive and specific in the diagnosis of *Candida* esophagitis.[49] Most often, however, the diagnosis of *Candida* esophagitis is made from its characteristic clinical presentation without the need for endoscopy or radiologic intervention.[50] Esophagoscopy or radiographic contrast procedures may be reserved for persons not responding to empirical therapy.

Differential Diagnosis

Oropharyngeal candidiasis may often be mistaken for oral hairy leukoplakia. Although esophagitis due to

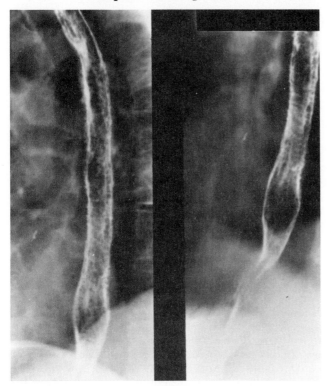

Figure 11B–2. Esophagogram of esophageal candidiasis showing a markedly irregular esophagus due to multiple plaques in a patient with AIDS and severe odynophagia.

Candida is the most common cause of esophagitis in patients with HIV infection, CMV and herpes simplex virus (HSV) may also produce a similar constellation of radiographic and clinical findings.[48,51] Other causes of esophageal lesions in these patients include Kaposi's sarcoma, mycobacteria, and lymphoma.

Therapy

Oropharyngeal candidiasis usually responds readily to topical agents such as nystatin or clotrimazole troches, and these agents should be the initial treatment of choice because of their ease of administration and relatively low cost. Prior to the introduction of the azoles, there were no oral antifungal agents available that could effectively treat esophageal candidiasis. Presently ketoconazole, an imidazole, administered orally in a dosage of 200 mg/day, is well tolerated and can successfully treat esophageal as well as oropharyngeal candidiasis. Ketoconazole requires an acidic pH for dissolution, however, and may not be well absorbed in patients with hypochlorhydria or in those taking H_2-blocking agents or antacids.[52] Some patients have had persistent *Candida* esophagitis despite prolonged therapy with ketoconazole.[53] Fluconazole, a triazole, given at a dosage of 50

mg/day, may be better tolerated and more effective than ketoconazole for oropharyngeal candidiasis,[54,55] but its higher cost will likely prohibit its routine use as primary therapy. Fluconazole may be successful in treating some cases of refractory oral candidiasis.[56] For severe cases of esophageal candidiasis not responding to the azoles, amphotericin B, 0.6 mg/kg given intravenously (IV) for 7 to 10 days, may still be necessary.

Prophylaxis

Oropharyngeal candidiasis frequently recurs when treatment is stopped. Lifelong therapy with the least expensive effective agent is recommended for patients with frequent recurrences.

HISTOPLASMA CAPSULATUM

Organism Description

Histoplasma capsulatum exists in the soil in the mycelial phase, but converts to the yeast form at the body temperature of mammals. The mycelial form has septate, branching hyphae (1 to 2.5 μm across) with lateral and terminal spores. The yeast form is ovoid, 1.5 to 2.0 by 3.0 to 3.5 μm, and reproduces by budding.

Epidemiology and Pathogenesis

The major endemic focus of histoplasmosis is in the central United States. Examination of soil specimens has shown the organism is present in large numbers in areas frequented by birds or bats. An estimated 500,000 new cases occur in the United States per year, but most cases are either asymptomatic or acute self-limited illnesses. Because of the endemicity of histoplasmosis in the central United States, and the initial presentation and propagation of the HIV epidemic on the coasts of the United States, histoplasmosis has been reported in less than 0.5% of patients with AIDS.[57] As the AIDS epidemic spreads through the central United States, however, the numbers of cases of histoplasmosis will correspondingly increase. Whereas in immunocompetent patients, *H. capsulatum* rarely disseminates,[58] disseminated disease is the primary presentation in patients with AIDS.[59-62] Disseminated histoplasmosis (at a site other than the lungs or cervical or hilar lymph nodes), diagnosed definitively, with laboratory evidence of HIV infection, is included in the CDC surveillance case definition for AIDS.[44]

Clinical Manifestations

The most common presentation of disseminated histoplasmosis is that of fever and weight loss. Respiratory complaints are common, but chest radiographs may be normal in more than 40% of cases. Hepatomegaly, splenomegaly, and lymphadenopathy each occur in about one fourth of the cases.[59,60,62,63] CNS involvement is common, manifesting as a meningitis or as a space-occupying lesion. It occurs in about 15% of patients.[59,61,64] Hematologic abnormalities, including thrombocytopenia, neutropenia, and anemia, are found in more than 20% of patients at presentation.[62,64] A syndrome resembling bacterial septicemia has been reported in about 10% of cases.[59,63,65] Disseminated histoplasmosis not uncommonly manifests with various types of cutaneous lesions, including maculopapular rashes,[66] tender pustules,[67,68] papules, skin or oral ulcers,[67,69] and ulcerated palatal nodules.[70] GI masses,[71,72] chorioretinitis,[73] and pleural effusion[74] have also been reported in association with disseminated histoplasmosis. CD4 counts in one series of patients in whom counts were obtained within 60 days of diagnosis of disseminated histoplasmosis showed a median count of 33 cells/mm^3; only two of 17 patients had counts above 250 cells/mm^3.[75]

Diagnosis

The definitive diagnosis of disseminated histoplasmosis rests on biopsy and culture of the organism from tissue. Positive cultures are often obtained from bone marrow, blood, lung biopsy or lavage, sputum, lymph nodes, skin, or CSF.[59,60,62,75] Diff-Quik, Wright-Giemsa, or methenamine silver stains, among others, can be used on tissue, sputum, or BAL specimens for a rapid diagnosis (Fig. 11B–3) (see Color Fig. 2). Immunodiffusion or complement fixation anti-*H. capsulatum* antibody tests are frequently negative, but may be helpful when positive.[59] Demonstration by radioimmunoassay of *H. capsulatum* polysaccharide antigen in blood and urine specimens has been reported to correlate well both with response to therapy and with relapse. This technique may prove useful in diagnosing and managing patients with disseminated histoplasmosis and AIDS.[76] The assay is not routinely available, but samples can be sent to Dr. L. Joseph Wheat at the Indiana University Medical Center, Indianapolis.

Differential Diagnosis

The presentation of histoplasmosis in the patient with AIDS is similar to that of tuberculosis or *P. carinii* pneumonia. Less commonly, pulmonary cryptococcosis, coccidioidomycosis, nocardiosis, CMV, or Kaposi's sarcoma may be seen. Because the infection may endogenously reactivate, patients may not have a recent history of travel to endemic areas.

Therapy

Amphotericin B, 0.6 mg/kg/day IV, is the standard treatment and is highly effective.[76] Nearly all patients, however, experience relapses within 1 year, even after receiving more than 35 mg/kg, an observation that supports the use of maintenance therapy to prevent recurrence. Weekly or biweekly doses of amphotericin B, 1 mg/kg, appears to be better in preventing relapses than ketoconazole.[59,77] Anecdotal data on the results of treatment with fluconazole are equivocal; patients have relapsed on maintenance doses of 50 to 100 mg/day, but higher doses may be effective.[57] Itraconazole maintenance therapy has produced prolonged remissions for more than 12 months.[57] Preliminary results of a larger open trial suggest similar results. None of the azole compounds has been shown to be effective in the initial treatment of disseminated histoplasmosis in patients with AIDS.

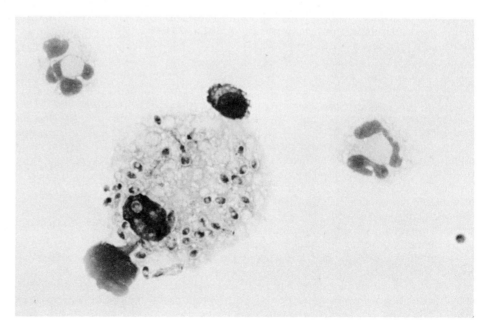

Figure 11B–3. Diff-Quik stain of a cytopathologic specimen from a bronchoalveolar lavage showing multiple *Histoplasma capsulatum* organisms within a macrophage in a patient with AIDS and pulmonary histoplasmosis.

Prophylaxis

The efficacy of prophylaxis for a disease of low incidence is difficult to ascertain. Only in areas highly endemic for histoplasmosis would it be reasonable to consider prophylaxis. Ketoconazole has not been effective for maintenance therapy and would not be a likely candidate.

COCCIDIOIDES IMMITIS

Organism Description

Coccidioides immitis is a fungus that lives in the soil as a mold. Arthroconidia, produced from the hyphae of the mycelial phase, infect the host when they are released into the air and inhaled. In tissues, the fungus grows as spherules, large structures containing hundreds of endospores.[78]

Epidemiology and Pathogenesis

Coccidioidomycosis is endemic in certain areas in North, Central, and South America, including the deserts of the southwestern United States. Most cases are concentrated in these regions, and in susceptible, non-AIDS persons the annual rate of infection has been estimated to be about 3%.[78] Early in the course of the AIDS epidemic, coccidioidomycosis was only rarely seen as a complication of AIDS.[79-81] Whereas in immunocompetent patients, disseminated coccidioidomycosis occurs in only 1.2% of patients with coccidioidomycosis who require hospitalization, dissemination is more common in patients with AIDS.[82] Presently, disseminated coccidioidomycosis (involving sites other than the lungs or cervical or hilar lymph nodes), diagnosed definitively, with laboratory evidence of HIV infection, is included in the CDC surveillance definition of AIDS.[44]

It has not been established whether coccidioidomycosis in patients with AIDS represents reactivation of latent infection or primary infection. In the largest reported series, positive serologies were reported for complement-fixing (CF) antibodies, indicative of an IgG response, and were generally negative for tube precipitin (TP) serologies, which would indicate an IgM response.[83] This suggests that much of the disease results from reactivation rather than primary infection. A smaller study calculated an annual rate of coccidioidal infection in some AIDS patients in Tucson to be 27%, much higher than the annual rate of less than 4% in non-AIDS patients in Tucson. This suggests that either the disease reactivates or that susceptibility to infection is enhanced in patients with AIDS.[82]

Clinical Manifestations

Because the route of infection of *C. immitis* is via inhalation of arthroconidia, coccidioidomycosis most fre-quently involves the lungs. The most common presentation is that of fever, weight loss, and cough. Diffuse reticulonodular infiltrates on chest radiographs are characteristic of its presentation in patients with AIDS (Fig. 11B–4).[82-84] In contrast to the presentation in patients with AIDS, a review of 300 non-AIDS patients hospitalized with coccidioidomycosis identified only 13 patients with the same extent of disease.[82]

In the largest reported series of AIDS patients with coccidioidomycosis, 77 patients were grouped into six clinical categories according to disease manifestation: focal pulmonary disease, diffuse pulmonary disease, cutaneous disease, meningitis, lymph node or liver involvement, and positive serologies only.[83] Focal pulmonary disease occurred in 20 patients (26%), most commonly as a focal alveolar infiltrate, but also as discrete nodules, pulmonary cavities, hilar adenopathy, and bilateral pleural effusions. Thirty-one patients (40%) had diffuse reticulonodular infiltrates. Four patients (5%) presented with cutaneous disease; three of these patients also had pulmonary involvement. Nine patients (12%) presented with coccidioidal meningitis. The CSF generally showed an elevated white blood cell count (range, 2 to 772 cells/mm^3), decreased glucose levels, increased protein levels, and a positive CF antibody titer to *C. immitis*. *C. immitis* was cultured from the CSF in five of nine patients. Seven patients (9%) presented with localized extrathoracic lymph node or liver involvement. An additional six patients (8%) were positive only by coccidioidal serology.[83] Of the patients in whom CD4 counts were determined at the time of diagnosis, 84%

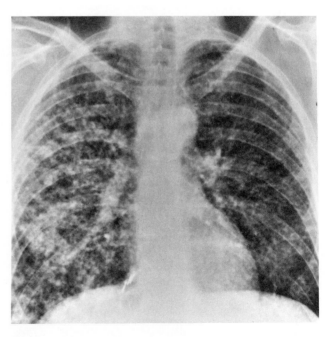

Figure 11B–4.   Chest radiograph of a patient with AIDS and pulmonary coccidioidomycosis showing a characteristic diffuse, reticulonodular pattern.

had counts below 250 cells/mm³. Those patients with diffuse pulmonary disease had a lower median CD4 count of only 44 cells/mm³. Isolated cases of peritonitis[85] and fungemia[86] due to *C. immitis* have also been reported.

Diagnosis

The diagnosis of coccidioidomycosis is easily made because the fungus can readily be cultured in most media. Visualization of the distinctive spherule in tissues is also diagnostic of invasive disease (Fig. 11B–5) (see Color Fig. 3). Coccidioidal serologies may be helpful in the diagnosis of the disease, but both CF antibody assays and TP serologies may be negative in as many as 25% of patients.[83,86] A high index of suspicion must be maintained for the diagnosis of coccidioidomycosis in the patient with AIDS and negative coccidioidal serologies who has traveled through an endemic area.[87]

Differential Diagnosis

The pulmonary manifestations of coccidioidomycosis may mimic the more common presentations of pulmonary disease in patients with AIDS, particularly *P. carinii* pneumonia, tuberculosis, and histoplasmosis. The reticulonodular pattern may be similar to that seen with pulmonary Kaposi's sarcoma. The presentation

of meningitis may be similar to that of cryptococcal meningitis.

Therapy

Standard treatment for disseminated or diffuse pulmonary coccidioidomycosis remains amphotericin B, 1 to 1.5 mg/kg/day IV, up to a total of at least 1 to 2.5 g before maintenance therapy with oral agents is considered.[88] The optimal treatment of patients with AIDS and limited disease due to coccidioidomycosis is unknown. Ketoconazole has been used in doses of 400 mg/day orally. However, three patients who were taking ketoconazole for other reasons developed active coccidioidomycosis.[83] The experience with the triazoles, itraconazole (200 mg twice daily orally) and fluconazole (400 mg/day orally), has been limited but encouraging.[83,88] Itraconazole for coccidioidal meningitis has shown some anecdotal success in non-HIV-infected patients.[89]

Prognostic Factors

Patients with diffuse pulmonary disease appear to have a worse prognosis than do those patients with more limited disease; median survival was only 1 month from the date of diagnosis in the former group, though survival ranged up to 17 months. Correspondingly, a high mortality was seen in patients with low CD4 counts.[83]

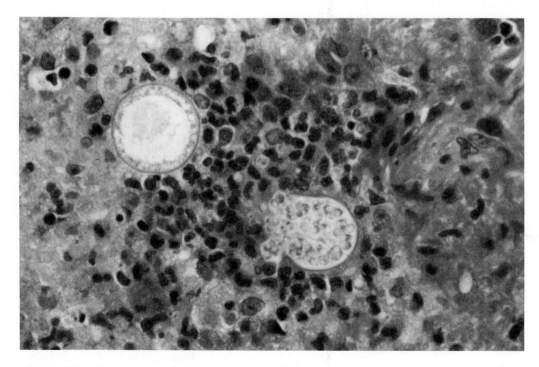

Figure 11B–5. Hematoxylin-eosin stain of a lung biopsy from the patient in Figure 11B–4 showing a rupturing endosporulating spherule and an empty spherule.

Color Figures

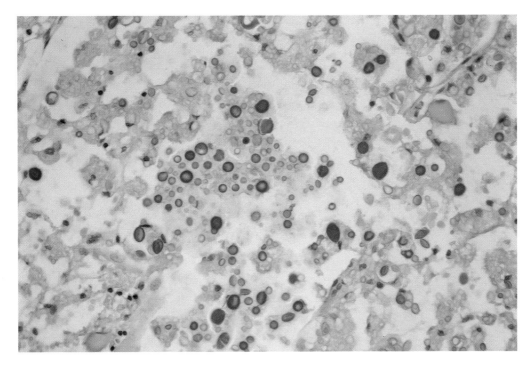

Color Figure 1.

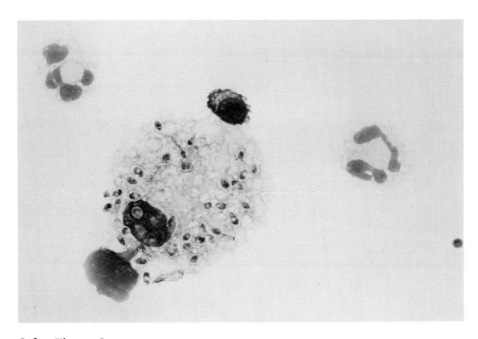

Color Figure 2.

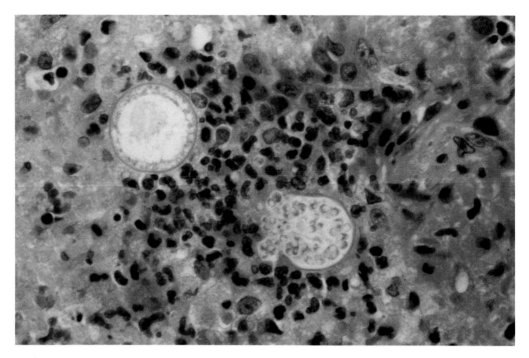

Color Figure 3.

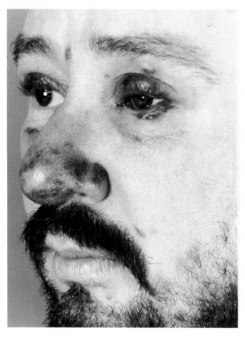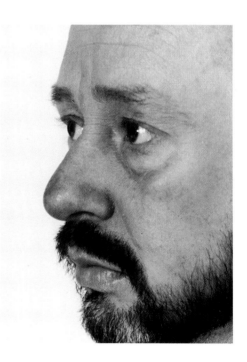

Color Figure 4.

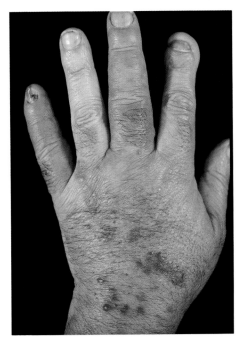

Color Figure 5. Classic KS. Plaque and nodular lesion.

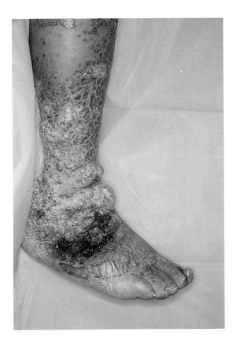

Color Figure 6. Classic KS. Extensive infiltration, tumor, and secondary lymphedema.

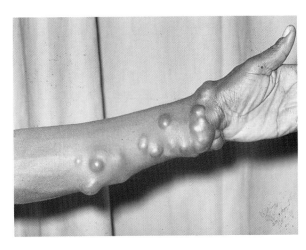

Color Figure 7. Endemic KS. Nodular form.

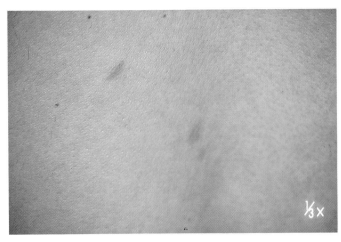

Color Figure 8. AIDS-KS. Early patch lesion.

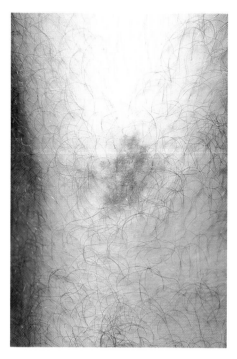

Color Figure 9. AIDS-KS. More advanced patch lesion.

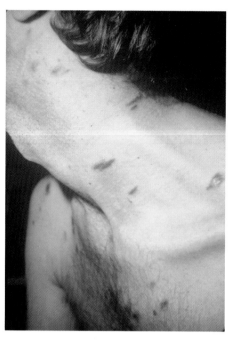

Color Figure 10. AIDS-KS. Patch lesions distributed symmetrically along Langer's (skin cleavage) lines.

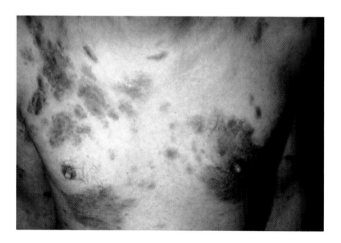

Color Figure 11. AIDS-KS. Hemorrhagic presentation.

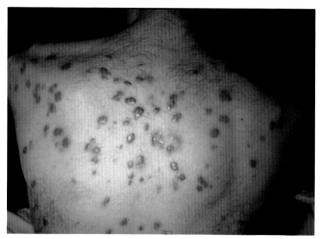

Color Figure 12. AIDS-KS. Extensive symmetric distribution of plaque and tumor lesions.

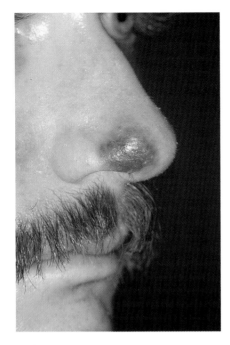

Color Figure 13. AIDS-KS. Large patch lesion of the nose (a common site for AIDS-KS).

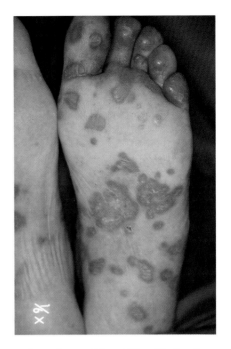

Color Figure 14. AIDS-KS. Patches, plaques, and nodules on the sole.

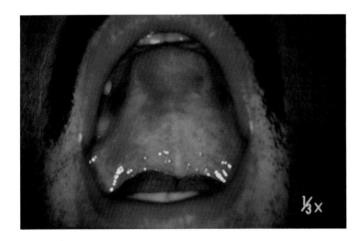

Color Figure 15. AIDS-KS. Involvement of the hard and soft palate.

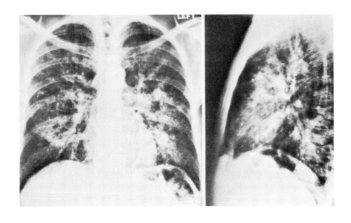

Figure 12–16. AIDS-KS. Chest X-ray showing extensive central infiltrate.

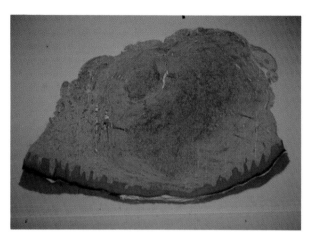

Color Figure 17. Gross microscopic view showing the hemorrhagic and cellular nature of KS.

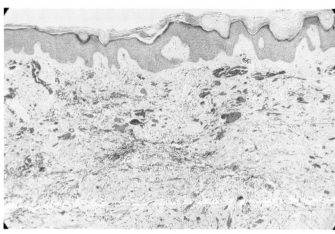

Color Figure 18. Low-power view of a patch lesion showing slitlike vascular spaces and inflammatory cell infiltrate of the dermis.

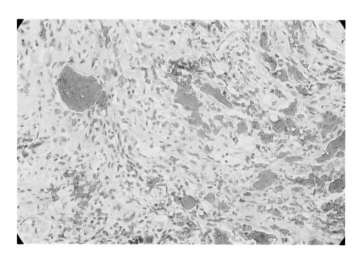

Color Figure 19. High-power view showing irregularly shaped vascular channels, extravasated erythrocytes, and spindle cells.

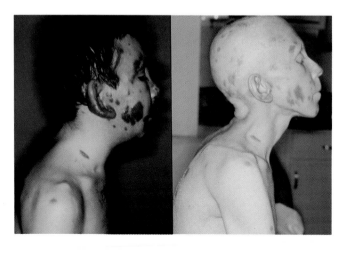

Color Figure 20. AIDS-KS. Extensive facial tumors, pre- and postradiation therapy.

ASPERGILLUS SPECIES

Organism Description

Aspergillus is a common mold found in soil that frequently causes invasive pulmonary and obstructing bronchial disease in immunocompromised patients. Pulmonary aspergillosis, however, has been a rare complication of AIDS, occurring as a late manifestation of the disease.[90] Spores (conidia) of *Aspergillus* are approximately 3 μm in size and their hyphae, which are 2 to 5 μm wide, are often septate and exhibit Y-shaped branching. The hyphae cannot be easily distinguished from those of other pathogenic molds. *A. fumigatus* and *A. flavus* are the most common causes of aspergillosis.

Clinical Manifestations

Both invasive pulmonary and obstructing bronchial aspergillosis have been described in patients with AIDS.[90] In one report, the most common clinical presentation entailed the insidious development of cough and fever in a profoundly immunocompromised patient with neutropenia.[90] Four of 13 patients were reported to have received corticosteroids previously, and four patients were users of marijuana. Radiographically, cavitary lung disease or diffuse infiltrates were the most common findings. Ten of the 13 patients died a median of 3 months after diagnosis.

Other organs, including the heart,[91,92] the pancreas,[93] and the brain and spinal cord,[94] may rarely be infected by *Aspergillus* in patients with AIDS.

Diagnosis

Isolation of *Aspergillus* from biopsy cultures together with microscopic identification in tissue assures the diagnosis of aspergillosis. Isolation of *Aspergillus* from sputum or the appearance of hyphae in a smear or a biopsy specimen can be suggestive but not diagnostic of aspergillosis.

Differential Diagnosis

Because pulmonary aspergillosis is seen only infrequently in patients with AIDS, the diagnosis of invasive pulmonary aspergillosis in an AIDS patient must be made with caution. More common etiologies of pulmonary disease, such as *P. carinii*, nonspecific interstitial pneumonitis, tuberculosis, histoplasmosis, CMV, and Kaposi's sarcoma, must be ruled out.

Therapy

Response to treatment has been poor. IV amphotericin B and oral itraconazole have been used, with some response.[90] Owing to the paucity of data, the treatment of invasive pulmonary aspergillosis in a patient with AIDS should be the same as in other immunocompromised patients, with IV amphotericin B, 0.5 to 0.6 mg/kg/day. Early treatment may be beneficial.[95] Itraconazole, 200 to 400 mg/day given for extended periods, has shown promise in the treatment of aspergillosis in other immunocompromised patients.[96–98] Its utility in the treatment of aspergillosis in patients with AIDS remains to be shown.[90]

BLASTOMYCES DERMATITIDIS

Blastomyces dermatitidis is an 8 to 15 μm yeast cell with daughter cells forming a bud with a broad base. Pulmonary or miliary blastomycosis has only rarely been reported in persons with AIDS.[99,100] Immunocompromised persons traveling through the endemic areas of the Ohio and Mississippi river basins may be at risk for developing disease with *Blastomyces*.

REFERENCES

1. Diamond RD: *Cryptococcus neoformans.* In Mandell GL, Douglas RG Jr, Bennett JE (eds): Principles and Practice of Infectious Diseases, 3rd ed, p 1980. New York, Churchill Livingstone, 1990
2. Bottone EJ, Salkin IF, Hurd NJ, Wormser GP: Serogroup distribution of *Cryptococcus neoformans* in patients with AIDS. J Infect Dis 156:242, 1987
3. Swinne D, Nkurikiyinfura JB, Muyembe TL: Clinical isolates of *Cryptococcus neoformans* from Zaire. Eur J Clin Microbiol 5:50, 1986
4. Rinaldi MG, Drutz DJ, Howell A et al. Serotypes of *Cryptococcus neoformans* in patients with AIDS (letter). J Infect Dis 153:642, 1986
5. Bottone EJ, Toma M, Johansson BE, Wormser GP: Poorly encapsulated *Cryptococcus neoformans* from patients with AIDS: I. Preliminary observations. AIDS Res 2:211, 1986
6. Kovacs JA, Kovacs AA, Polis M et al: Cryptococcosis in the acquired immunodeficiency syndrome. Ann Intern Med 103:533, 1985
7. Clark RA, Greer D, Atkinson W et al: Spectrum of *Cryptococcus neoformans* infection in 68 patients infected with human immunodeficiency virus. Rev Infect Dis 12:768, 1990
8. Chuck SL, Sande MA: Infections with *Cryptococcus neoformans* in the acquired immunodeficiency syndrome. N Engl J Med 321:794, 1989
9. Dismukes WE: Cryptococcal meningitis in patients with AIDS. J Infect Dis 157:624, 1988
10. Mackenzie DW: Cryptococcosis in the AIDS era. Epidemiol Infect 102:361, 1989
11. Clumeck N, Carael N, Van de Perre P: The African AIDS experience in contrast with the rest of the world. In Leoung G, Mills J (eds): Opportunistic Infections in Patients with the Acquired Immunodeficiency Syndrome, p 43. New York, Marcel Dekker, 1989
12. Zuger A, Louie E, Holzman RS et al: Cryptococcal disease in patients with the acquired immunodeficiency syndrome: Diagnostic features and outcome of treatment. Ann Intern Med 104:234, 1986
13. Lecomte I, Meyohas MC, De Sa M: Relation between decreasing serial CD4 lymphocytes count and outcome of cryptococcosis in AIDS patients: A basis for new diagnosis

strategy (abstr), p 235. In: Proceedings of the VI International Conference on AIDS, San Francisco, CA 1990

14. Masur H, Ognibene FP, Yarchoan R et al: CD4 counts as predictors of opportunistic pneumonias in human immunodeficiency virus (HIV) infection. Ann Intern Med 111:223, 1989

15. Bozzette SA, Waskin HA: Cryptococcal disease in AIDS. In Volberding P, Jacobson M (eds): AIDS Clinical Review 1990, p 149. New York, Marcel Dekker, 1990

16. Gal AA, Koss MN, Hawkins J et al: The pathology of pulmonary cryptococcal infections in the acquired immunodeficiency syndrome. Arch Pathol Lab Med 110:502, 1986

17. Witt D, McKay D, Schwam L et al: Acquired immune deficiency syndrome presenting as bone marrow and mediastinal cryptococcosis. Am J Med 82:149, 1987

18. Glick M, Cohen SG, Cheney RT et al: Oral manifestations of disseminated *Cryptococcus neoformans* in a patient with acquired immunodeficiency syndrome. Oral Surg Oral Med Oral Pathol 64:454, 1987

19. Lynch DP, Naftolin LZ: Oral *Cryptococcus neoformans* infection in AIDS. Oral Surg Oral Med Oral Pathol 64: 449, 1987

20. Hernandez AD: Cutaneous cryptococcosis. Dermatol Clin 7:269, 1986

21. Jones C, Orengo I, Rosen T, Ellner K: Cutaneous cryptococcosis simulating Kaposi's sarcoma in the acquired immunodeficiency syndrome. Cutis 45:163, 1990

22. Borton LK, Wintroub BU: Disseminated cryptococcosis presenting as herpetiform lesions in a homosexual man with acquired immunodeficiency syndrome. J Am Acad Dermatol 10:387, 1984

23. Rico MJ, Penneys NS: Cutaneous cryptococcosis resembling molluscum contagiosum in a patient with AIDS. Arch Dermatol 121:901, 1985

24. Concus AP, Helfand RF, Imber MJ et al: Cutaneous cryptococcosis mimicking molluscum contagiosum in a patient with AIDS. J Infect Dis 158:897, 1988

25. Ricciardi DD, Sepkowitz DV, Berkowitz LB et al: Cryptococcal arthritis in a patient with acquired immune deficiency syndrome: Case report and review of the literature. J Rheumatol 13:455, 1986

26. Bonacini M, Nussbaum J, Ahluwalia C: Gastrointestinal, hepatic, and pancreatic involvement with *Cryptococcus neoformans* in AIDS. J Clin Gastroenterol 12:295, 1990

27. Scalfano FP, Prichard JG, Lamki N et al: Abdominal cryptococcoma in AIDS: A case report. J Comput Tomogr 12: 237, 1988

28. Lewis W, Lipsick J, Cammarosano C: Cryptococcal myocarditis in acquired immune deficiency syndrome. Am J Cardiol 55:1240, 1985

29. Larsen RA, Bozzette S, McCutchan JA et al: Persistent *Cryptococcus neoformans* infection of the prostate after successful treatment of meningitis. California Collaborative Treatment Group. Ann Intern Med 111:125, 1989

30. Robinson PG, Sulita MJ, Matthews EK, Warren JR: Failure of the Bactec 460 radiometer to detect *Cryptococcus neoformans* fungemia in an AIDS patient. Am J Clin Pathol 87:783, 1987

31. Bennett JE, Dismukes WE, Duma RJ et al: A comparison of amphotericin B alone and combined with flucytosine in the treatment of cryptococcal meningitis. N Engl J Med 301:126, 1979

32. Zuger A, Schuster M, Simberkoff MS et al: Maintenance

amphotericin B for cryptococcal meningitis in the acquired immunodeficiency syndrome (AIDS). Ann Intern Med 109:592, 1988

33. Stern JJ, Hartman BJ, Sharkey P et al: Oral fluconazole therapy for patients with acquired immunodeficiency syndrome and cryptococcosis: Experience with 22 patients. Am J Med 85:477, 1988

34. Sugar AM, Saunders C: Oral fluconazole as suppressive therapy of disseminated cryptococcosis in patients with acquired immunodeficiency syndrome. Am J Med 85:481, 1988

35. Larsen RA, Leal MA, Chan LS: Fluconazole compared with amphotericin B plus flucytosine for cryptococcal meningitis in AIDS: A randomized trial. Ann Intern Med 113: 183, 1990

36. Bozzette SA, Larsen RA, Chiu J et al: A placebo-controlled trial of maintenance therapy with fluconazole after treatment of cryptococcal meningitis in the acquired immunodeficiency syndrome. N Engl J Med 324:580, 1991

37. Powderly W, Saag M, Cloud G et al: Fluconazole vs. amphotericin B as maintenance therapy for prevention of relapse in AIDS-associated cryptococcal meningitis (abstr 1162). In: Abstracts of the 1990 Intersciences Conference on Antimicrobial Agents and Chemotherapy. Washington, DC, American Society of Microbiology, Washington, DC 1990

38. Denning DW, Tucker RM, Hanson LH et al: Itraconazole therapy for cryptococcal meningitis and cryptococcosis. Arch Intern Med 149:2301, 1989

39. Larsen RA: Azoles and AIDS. J Infect Dis 162:727, 1991

40. Walsh TJ, Lester-McCully C, Rinaldi MG et al: Penetration of SCH-39304, a new antifungal triazole, into cerebral spinal fluid of primates. Antimicrob Agents Chemother 34: 1281, 1990

41. Polsky B, Depman MR, Gold JWM et al: Intraventricular therapy of cryptococcal meningitis via a subcutaneous reservoir. Am J Med 81:24, 1986

42. Diamond RD, Bennett JE: Prognostic factors in cryptococcal meningitis: A study in 111 cases. Ann Intern Med 80:176, 1974

43. Klein RS, Harris CA, Small CB et al: Oral candidiasis in high-risk patients as the initial manifestation of the acquired immunodeficiency syndrome. N Engl J Med 311: 354, 1984

44. Centers for Disease Control: Revision of the CDC surveillance case definition for acquired immunodeficiency syndrome. MMWR 36:1S, 1987

45. Imam N, Carpenter CCJ, Mayer KH et al: Hierarchical pattern of mucosal candida infections in HIV-seropositive women. Am J Med 89:142, 1990

46. Carpenter CCJ, Mayer KH, Fisher A et al: Natural history of acquired immunodeficiency syndrome in women in Rhode Island. Am J Med 86:771, 1989

47. Tavitian A, Raufman JP, Rosenthal LE: Oral candidiasis as a marker for esophageal candidiasis in the acquired immunodeficiency syndrome. Ann Intern Med 104:54, 1986

48. Levine MS, Woldenberg R, Herlinger H, Laufer I: Opportunistic esophagitis in AIDS: Radiographic diagnosis. Radiology 165:815, 1987

49. Bonacini M, Laine L, Gal AA et al: Prospective evaluation of blind brushing of the esophagus for *Candida* esophagitis in patients with human immunodeficiency virus infection. Am J Gastroenterol 85:385, 1990

50. Porro GB, Parente F, Cernushi M: The diagnosis of esoph-

ageal candidiasis in patients with acquired immune deficiency syndrome: Is endoscopy always necessary? Am J Gastroenterol 84:143, 1989

51. Gould E, Kory WP, Raskin JB et al: Esophageal biopsy findings in the acquired immunodeficiency syndrome (AIDS): Clinicopathologic correlation in 20 patients. South Med J 81:1392, 1988

52. Lake-Bakaar G, Tom W, Lake-Bakaar D et al: Gastropathy and ketoconazole malabsorption in the acquired immunodeficiency syndrome (AIDS). Ann Intern Med 109:471, 1988

53. Tavitian A, Raufman JP, Rosenthal LE et al: Ketoconazole-resistant *Candida* esophagitis in patients with acquired immunodeficiency syndrome. Gastroenterology 90:443, 1991

54. Dupont B, Drouhet E: Fluconazole in the management of oropharyngeal candidosis in a predominantly HIV antibody-positive group of patients. J Med Vet Mycol 26:67, 1988

55. DeWit S, Weerts D, Goossens H et al: Comparison of fluconazole and ketoconazole for oropharyngeal candidiasis in AIDS. Lancet 1:746, 1989

56. Lucatorto FM, Franker C, Hardy WD, Chafey S: Treatment of refractory oral candidiasis with fluconazole: A case report. Oral Surg Oral Med Oral Pathol 71:42, 1991

57. Graybill JR: AIDS commentary: Histoplasmosis and AIDS. J Infect Dis 158:623, 1988

58. Sathapatayavongs B, Batteiger BE, Wheat J et al: Clinical and laboratory features of disseminated histoplasmosis during two large urban outbreaks. Medicine 62:263, 1983

59. Wheat LJ, Connolly-Stringfield PA, Baker RL et al: Disseminated histoplasmosis in the acquired immune deficiency syndrome: Clinical findings, diagnosis and treatment, and review of the literature. Medicine 69:361, 1990

60. Johnson PC, Hamill RJ, Sarosi GA: Clinical review: Progressive disseminated histoplasmosis in the AIDS patient. Semin Respir Infect 4:139, 1989

61. Anaissie E, Fainstein V, Samo T et al: Central nervous system histoplasmosis: An unappreciated complication of the acquired immunodeficiency syndrome. Am J Med 84:215, 1988

62. Johnson PC, Khardori N, Najjar AF et al: Progressive disseminated histoplasmosis in patients with acquired immunodeficiency syndrome. Am J Med 85:152, 1988

63. Ankobiah WA, Vaidya K, Powell S et al: Disseminated histoplasmosis in AIDS: Clinicopathologic features in seven patients from a non-endemic area. NY State J Med 90:234, 1990

64. Wheat LJ, Batteiger BE, Sathapatayavongs B: *Histoplasma capsulatum* infections of the central nervous system. Medicine 69:244, 1990

65. Huang CT, McGarry T, Cooper S et al: Disseminated histoplasmosis in the acquired immunodeficiency syndrome: Report of five cases from a nonendemic area. Arch Intern Med 147:1181, 1987

66. Barton EN, Roberts L, Ince WE et al: Cutaneous histoplasmosis in the acquired immune deficiency syndrome: A report of three cases from Trinidad. Trop Geogr Med 40:153, 1988

67. Cohen PR, Bank DE, Silvers DN, Grossman ME: Cutaneous lesions of disseminated histoplasmosis in human immunodeficiency virus–infected patients. J Am Acad Dermatol 23:422, 1990

68. Ibanez HE, Ibanez MA: Case report: A new presentation of disseminated histoplasmosis in a homosexual man with AIDS. Am J Med Sci 298:407, 1989

69. Eisig S, Boguslaw B, Cooperband B, Phelan J: Oral manifestations of disseminated histoplasmosis in acquired immunodeficiency syndrome: Report of two cases and review of the literature. J Oral Maxillofac Surg 49:310, 1991

70. Oda D, McDougal L, Fritsche T, Worthington P: Oral histoplasmosis as a presenting disease in acquired immunodeficiency syndrome. Oral Surg Oral Med Oral Pathol 70:631, 1990

71. Graham BD, McKinsey DS, Driks MR, Smith DL: Colonic histoplasmosis in acquired immunodeficiency syndrome: Report of two cases. Dis Colon Rectum 34:185, 1991

72. Haggerty CM, Britton MC, Dorman JM, Marzoni JFA: Gastrointestinal histoplasmosis in suspected acquired immunodeficiency syndrome. West J Med 143:244, 1985

73. Macher A, Rodrigues MM, Kaplan W et al: Disseminated bilateral chorioretinitis due to *Histoplasma capsulatum* in a patient with the acquired immunodeficiency syndrome. Ophthalmology 92:1159, 1985

74. Marshall BC, Cox JK, Carroll KC, Morrison RE: Case report: Histoplasmosis as a cause of pleural effusion in the acquired immunodeficiency syndrome. Am J Med Sci 300:98, 1990

75. Nightingale SD, Parks JM, Pounders SM et al: Disseminated histoplasmosis in patients with AIDS. South Med J 83:624, 1990

76. Wheat LJ, Connolly-Stringfield P, Kohler RB et al: *Histoplasma capsulatum* polysaccharide antigen detection in diagnosis and management of disseminated histoplasmosis in patients with acquired immunodeficiency syndrome. Am J Med 87:396, 1989

77. McKinsey DS, Gupta MR, Riddler SA et al: Long-term amphotericin B therapy for disseminated histoplasmosis in patients with the acquired immunodeficiency syndrome (AIDS). Ann Intern Med 111:655, 1989

78. Knoper SR, Galgiani JN: Coccidioidomycosis. Infect Dis Clin North Am 2:861, 1988

79. Abrams DI, Robia M, Blumenfeld W et al: Disseminated coccidioidomycosis in AIDS (letter). N Engl J Med 310:986, 1984

80. Roberts CJ: Coccidioidomycosis in acquired immune deficiency syndrome: Depressed humoral as well as cellular immunity. Am J Med 76:734, 1984

81. Kovacs A, Forthal DN, Kovacs JA, Overturf GD: Disseminated coccidioidomycosis in a patient with acquired immune deficiency syndrome. West J Med 140:447, 1984

82. Bronnimann DA, Adam RD, Galgiani JN et al: Coccidioidomycosis in the acquired immunodeficiency syndrome. Ann Intern Med 106:372, 1987

83. Fish DG, Ampel NM, Galgiani JN et al: Coccidioidomycosis during human immunodeficiency virus infection: A review of 77 patients. Medicine 69:384, 1990

84. Galgiani JN, Ampel NM: *Coccidioides immitis* in patients with human immunodeficiency virus infections. Semin Respir Infect 5:151, 1990

85. Byrne WR, Dietrich RA: Disseminated coccidioidomycosis with peritonitis in a patient with acquired immunodeficiency syndrome: Prolonged survival associated with positive skin test reactivity to coccidioidin. Arch Intern Med 149:947, 1989

86. Ampel NM, Ryan KR, Carry PJ et al: Fungemia due to *Coccidioides immitis*: An analysis of 16 episodes in 15 patients and a review of the literature. Medicine 65:312, 1986

87. Antoniskis D, Larsen RA, Akil B et al: Seronegative disseminated coccidioidomycosis in patients with HIV infection. AIDS 4:691, 1990
88. Galgiani JN, Ampel NM: AIDS commentary: Coccidioidomycosis in human immunodeficiency virus–infected patients. J Infect Dis 162:1165, 1990
89. Tucker RM, Denning DW, Dupont B, Stevens DA: Itraconazole therapy for chronic coccidioidal meningitis. Ann Intern Med 112:108, 1990
90. Denning DW, Follansbee SE, Scolaro M et al: Pulmonary aspergillosis in the acquired immunodeficiency syndrome. N Engl J Med 324:654, 1991
91. Cox JN, diDio F, Pizzolato GP et al: *Aspergillus* endocarditis and myocarditis in a patient with the acquired immunodeficiency syndrome (AIDS): A review of the literature. Virchows Archiv [A] Pathol Anat 417:255, 1991
92. Henochowicz S, Mustafa M, Lawrinson WE et al: Cardiac aspergillosis in acquired immune deficiency syndrome. Am J Cardiol 55:1239, 1985
93. Bhatt B, Cappell MS: A perihepatic abscess containing *Aspergillus* in a patient with the acquired immune deficiency syndrome. Am J Gastroenterol 85:1200, 1990
94. Woods GL, Goldsmith JC: *Aspergillus* infection of the central nervous system in patients with acquired immunodeficiency syndrome. Arch Neurol 47:181, 1990
95. Aisner J, Schimpff SC, Wiernik PH: Treatment of invasive aspergillosis: Relation of early diagnosis and treatment to response. Ann Intern Med 86:539, 1977
96. Denning DW, Tucker RM, Hanson LH, Stevens DA: Itraconazole in opportunistic mycoses: Cryptococcosis and aspergillosis. J Am Acad Dermatol 23:602, 1990
97. Dupont B: Itraconazole therapy in aspergillosis: Study in 49 patients. J Am Acad Dermatol 23:607, 1990
98. Viviani MA, Tortorano AM, Langer M et al: Experience with itraconazole in cryptococcosis and aspergillosis. J Infect 18:151, 1989
99. Kitchen LW, Clark RA, Hoadley DJ et al: Concurrent pulmonary *Blastomyces dermatitidis* and *Mycobacterium tuberculosis* infection in an HIV-1 seropositive man. J Infect Dis 160:911, 1991
100. Herd AM, Greenfield SB, Thompson WS, Brunham RC: Miliary blastomycosis and HIV infection. Can Med Assoc J 143:1329, 1990

Tuberculosis and Other Bacterial Infections

11C

Gerald Friedland   *Robert Klein*

Unusual opportunistic infections caused by parasites, fungi, and viruses signaled the onset of and remain most prominently associated with the human immunodeficiency virus (HIV) epidemic. More recently, mycobacterial and other bacterial infections have been appreciated as frequent and important causes of morbidity and mortality in people with HIV infection.

The most prominent immunologic abnormality in HIV infection and AIDS, depletion of the CD4 or T-helper/inducer cells,[1] leads to the characteristic increased susceptibility to opportunistic infection with nonbacterial pathogens and bacteria for which an intact cell-mediated immune response is necessary, such as tuberculosis. However, polyclonal activation and dysfunction of B cells, including impaired responses to T-cell–independent antigens such as bacterial polysaccharides, impaired monocyte function, and impaired neutrophil function, also occur with HIV infection.[2-15] These abnormalities probably explain, in large part, an increased susceptibility of individuals with HIV infection to community-acquired bacterial infections. In addition, the frequent need for intravenous (IV) lines and other invasive procedures places symptomatic patients at risk for a wide array of nosocomial bacterial infections.

This chapter discusses the characteristics and significance of mycobacterial and other bacterial infections associated with HIV disease.

TUBERCULOSIS

The worldwide epidemic of HIV infection has resulted in a major secondary epidemic of tuberculosis. The recent epidemiologic patterns of the two diseases can be superimposed temporally and demographically. As the case rate of acquired immunodeficiency syndrome (AIDS) has increased, the 20-year decline in tuberculosis cases in the United States ended and was reversed in 1986.[16] This increasing rate resulted in a cumulative excess of 9,226 cases of tuberculosis in the United States through 1987, 23,495 excess cases by 1989, and an expected further 6% increase through 1990.[17] The 25- to 44-year-old age group in which most HIV infection occurs also experienced the most substantial increase in tuberculosis cases.[16] In addition, the increase in tuberculosis cases has been greatest in geographic areas with high rates of prevalence of HIV infection.[18-24] The increase in New York City has been greater than in any other locality in the United States and has been striking among 30- to 39-year-old blacks and Hispanics, the age group accounting for 80% of all AIDS cases in New York City.[16]

Tuberculosis and AIDS case matches have revealed substantial overlap of the two diseases and similar demographic patterns. Recent available data on tuberculosis patients in Africa and other Third World countries reveal high rates of HIV co-infection. Serosurveys in Kinshasa, Zaire, have shown an HIV seroprevalence of 17% to 38% in tuberculosis patients, as compared to 4% to 9% in the general adult population.[18] In Cite Soleil, Haiti, where the prevalence of HIV infection is 10% in pregnant women, 39% of adult patients with tuberculosis were infected with HIV in 1989.[17]

Pathogenesis

Most of the cases of active tuberculosis among persons infected with HIV represent reactivation of latent tuberculosis infection rather than progression of recently acquired infection. The strongest evidence supporting this hypothesis comes from a prospective study of IV drug users enrolled in a methadone program in the Bronx, New York.[25] Over a 2-year period, eight cases of active tuberculosis occurred among 215 HIV-positive subjects and none among 298 HIV-negative subjects. Of the eight cases, seven occurred among the 49 methadone program enrollees who were previously known to have had a positive result on the purified protein derivative (PPD) test (case rate, 7.9/100 person-years). Only one case occurred in a patient who was HIV positive and without a previously known positive PPD test (OR = 25). No cases occurred among 62 enrollees who were PPD-positive but HIV-negative (p = 0.0025) (Table 11C–1). The potential magnitude of the secondary tuberculosis epidemic in New York City can be estimated from these findings. It is believed that there are approximately 200,000 IV drug users in New York City. Approximately 20% may be PPD positive and 55% HIV infected; resulting in populations of 40,000 and 110,000, respectively, and 22,000 (11%) who are co-infected.

With an expected 15% tuberculosis reactivation rate in 2 years, an excess of 3,300 new cases of tuberculosis might be expected in HIV-infected IV drug users in New York alone.[26] There are an estimated 10 million persons with latent tuberculosis infection in the United States and as many as 1 million persons with HIV infection[17] (Table 11C–2). The extent to which these two infected populations overlap will be a significant factor in the substantial number of tuberculosis cases that may be expected to develop over the next decade in the United States. Worldwide, approximately 1 billion people are infected with *M. tuberculosis*[27] and an estimated 5 to 10 million are infected with HIV. In geographic areas such as central Africa, where both infections coexist, enormous numbers of new cases of tuberculosis in young adults must be anticipated and with them, the potential for overwhelming of existing control programs.[27–29]

Clinical Features

Several clinical features of tuberculosis associated with HIV infection are worthy of note. First, the diagnosis of tuberculosis usually coincides with or precedes the diagnosis of AIDS.[21–25] In a Florida series comprising patients with both diagnoses, tuberculosis was diagnosed more than 1 month before AIDS in 50%, and within 1 month after the diagnosis of AIDS in another 30%.[30] It appears that a lesser degree of immunosuppression may be required for *M. tuberculosis* reactivation than for other opportunistic infections characterizing the AIDS diagnosis. For example, in San Francisco, among HIV-positive patients with tuberculosis, the median CD4 cell count was 326 cells/mm³ (range, 23 to 742/mm³),[24] whereas *Pneumocystis carinii* pneumonia usually oc-

Table 11C–1. Incidence of Active Tuberculosis During the Study Period, According to HIV Status and Prior Status of PPD Tuberculin Skin Test

Group	HIV Positive	HIV Negative	p value
All study subjects*			
New cases of active TB, n/n (%)	8/215 (4)	0/298 (0)	<0.002
Cases/100 person-years	2.1	0	<0.001†
Prior positive PPD test			
New cases of active TB, n/n (%)	7/49 (14)	0/62 (0)	<0.005
Cases/100 person-years	7.9‡	0	<0.005§
No prior positive PPD test			
New cases of active TB, n/n (%)	1/166 (0.6)	0/236 (0)	NS
Cases/100 person-years	0.3‡	0	NS

Abbreviations: TB = tuberculosis; NS = not significant, PPD = purified protein derivative.
* Two HIV-positive and five HIV-negative subjects with a history of active tuberculosis treated before entry into the study have been excluded.
† Total person-years for HIV-positive subjects, 389.8; for HIV-negative subjects, 582.2.
‡ Rate ratio, 24.0; p <0.00001.
§ Total person-years for HIV-positive subjects, 88.1; for HIV-negative subjects, 119.6.
Reproduced with permission from Selwyn PA, Hartel D, Lewis VA *et al:* A prospective study of the risk of tuberculosis among intravenous drug users with human immunodeficiency virus infection. N Engl J Med 320:545, 1990, and Schoenbaum EE, Hartel D, Friedland G: HIV infection and intravenous drug use. Curr Opin Infect Dis 3:80, 1990.

Table 11C–2. Characteristics of Mycobacterial Infection in Association With HIV Disease

Characteristic	M. tuberculosis	Disseminated M. avium Complex
Time of onset in HIV disease	Early to late (CD4+ $\leq$ 350 cells/mm³)	Late (CD4+ < 100 cells/mm³)
Site	Pulmonary, extrapulmonary	Extrapulmonary (GI and reticuloendothelial system)
Demography	IV drug users, poor socioeconomic status, Third World	Equally distributed by risk, confined to industrialized countries
Disease mechanism	Reactivation of dormant foci	Recent acquisition
Therapy	Isoniazid, rifampin, pyrazinamide, $\pm$ ethambutol	Clofazamine, ciprofloxacin, ethambutol, rifampin, $\pm$ amikacin
Response	Excellent	Variable

curs when the CD4 cell count falls below 200/mm³.[31] The earlier appearance of tuberculosis is likely a measure of the relative virulence of *M. tuberculosis* compared with other opportunistic pathogens. Tuberculosis may also appear later in the course of HIV disease, after the initial AIDS diagnosis, and may be found at autopsy, unrecognized clinically in substantial numbers of patients.[23]

In most series, the clinical presentation of active tuberculosis among HIV-infected individuals differs from that seen in persons with normal immunity. The degree of difference is related to the degree of immunosuppression resulting from HIV disease.[17] Early in HIV infection, tuberculosis usually presents in a typical clinical form, whereas late in HIV disease, after AIDS has already been diagnosed, subtle and atypical presentations are more common. Although pulmonary disease still predominates,[24] extrapulmonary disease, often lymphatic or hematogenously disseminated, with or without coexisting pulmonary tuberculosis may appear in 40% to 75% of patients with both diagnoses.[32-36] The proportion of extrapulmonary cases increases as HIV disease progresses. In San Francisco, 60% of patients with AIDS and tuberculosis had at least one extrapulmonary site of disease, compared to 28% of non-AIDS patients with tuberculosis (p < 0.001).[33] In a series from Barcelona, Spain,[32] pulmonary tuberculosis occurred in 96% of HIV-negative tuberculosis cases and in only 39% of HIV-positive cases. In 1988, extrapulmonary tuberculosis in persons known to be HIV-positive represented 21% of national extrapulmonary tuberculosis morbidity.[36] Of note, extrapulmonary tuberculosis was substantially more common in AIDS patients who were black and whose risk factors included IV drug use or heterosexual contact. Many unusual clinical presentations have been recorded, including disease in bone, brain, and visceral abscesses.[37,38] Although the rate of occurrence is not precisely known, tuberculosis mycobacteremia appears to be more frequent in HIV-infected persons.[17,39] Patients with extrapulmonary disease may have lower CD4 counts and a poorer prognosis than those with pulmonary disease.[33] Among those presenting with pulmonary disease, cavitation and/or upper lobe apical disease appears to be less common than in other pop-

ulations with reactivation disease.[24,25,34,35] Further, symptoms may be subtle and may not point to a specific organ system location.

Diagnosis

The diagnosis of active tuberculosis should be considered in persons with known or possible HIV infection and pulmonary disease, focal disease at extrapulmonary sites, and generalized symptoms and signs of wasting and fever. Chest radiographs should be obtained in all patients with HIV infection and respiratory or constitutional symptoms. The radiologic appearance of tuberculosis may vary with the degree of patient's immunosuppression. Focal disease is more likely early in HIV infection and hematogenous, diffuse infiltrates are more likely as immunosuppression advances.[24] In late stages of HIV infection the presence of peripheral or intrathoracic lymphadenopathy (hilar, cervical, mediastinal, paratracheal) should raise the suspicion of tuberculosis. Peripheral adenopathy usually regresses as immunosuppression increases in HIV disease, so that newly enlarged nodes may herald the presence of extrapulmonary tuberculosis. Intrathoracic lymphadenopathy is not seen with the more common bacterial or *P. carinii* pneumonias.

Mycobacterial stains and cultures should be performed on all well-collected respiratory specimens, including sputum, lavage, and biopsy specimens. Acid-fast smears of sputum are positive in 31% to 82% of patients with pulmonary tuberculosis and HIV infection.[17] When tuberculosis is potentially in the differential diagnosis of persons with known or suspected HIV infection and undiagnosed pulmonary disease, appropriate respiratory precautions should be followed. Recent instances of transmission of tuberculosis, including multidrug-resistant organisms, to unsuspecting health care workers and others have occurred in association with aerosol pentamidine administration[40] in a substance abuse treatment facility[41] and in a hospital setting.[42] Particular attention should be directed toward sputum induction or diagnostic or treatment procedures that induce excessive coughing. Under such circumstances, if airborne exposure of patients or staff may occur, procedures should be performed in negative pressure rooms or in booths in which air is exhausted to the outside environment.[43]

Because of the strong association of active tuberculosis with HIV infection, the Centers for Disease Control (CDC) recommends that all patients with tuberculosis should be offered counseling and HIV antibody testing,[44] especially individuals with extrapulmonary disease and persons in the demographic and risk groups in which the overlap of tuberculosis and HIV infection is known to occur. Tuberculin skin testing with 5 tuberculin units of PPD placed intradermally should be performed on all HIV-positive individuals. Anergy may be present in over half of patients with advanced HIV disease, but a substantial percentage may still demonstrate a 5-mm or greater induration reaction. In patients with HIV infection, a reaction of this size is considered indicative of *M. tuberculosis* infection.[44] One half to three quarters of HIV-seropositive patients without advanced disease who have active tuberculosis may still have a tuberculin reaction of this size,[44] although higher rates of skin test anergy among HIV-infected individuals have been reported.[45] If the skin test is reactive, a chest radiograph should be obtained and the patient examined for extrapulmonary tuberculosis.

Preventive Therapy for Tuberculous Infection

All persons, regardless of age, with HIV and *M. tuberculosis* co-infection (≥5 mm induration) are at substantial risk for the reactivation of latent tuberculosis and should be considered for isoniazid preventive therapy (300 mg/day) unless it is medically contraindicated.[44] HIV-infected individuals with a positive PPD test who are anergic and those in close contact with persons with active pulmonary disease should receive prophylaxis as well. Because of the high rates of HIV positivity among IV drug users, the CDC recommends isoniazid preventive therapy for all IV drug users with a tuberculin reaction of 10 mm or more induration, regardless of age.[44] In one published uncontrolled series comprising IV-drug using methadone recipients in the Bronx, none of 13 dually infected patients who received isoniazed developed tuberculosis, whereas seven (19%) of 36 who did not receive isoniazid developed tuberculosis within a 2-year period of observation.[25] A recently reported but unpublished randomized controlled study of isoniazid *versus* placebo in over 500 HIV-infected patients in Zambia showed a reduction in tuberculosis incidence in the treated group (8.3% *vs.* 0) in 1 year of observation.[46] Primary care sites as well as drug treatment programs represent ideal settings for administration of tuberculosis preventive treatment in a supervised fashion, with excellent potential for compliance.[47] The recommended duration of preventive therapy is 12 months, although some authorities favor continued isoniazid preventive therapy in the face of declining immune status as HIV disease progresses. Because of the emergence of isoniazid-resistant organisms in the United States and developing countries and the possibility of adverse reactions to isoniazid, alternative regimens for prophylaxis are clearly needed. A promising regimen of rifampin and pyrazinamide administered for 2 to 3 months is currently undergoing controlled clinical trials.

Antituberculosis Therapy

Multiple studies have demonstrated that standard antituberculosis drug regimens are equally as effective in HIV-infected individuals as in noninfected individuals in clearing sputum cultures and producing a clinical response.[22,33,48] Tuberculosis treatment appears to be highly effective for both pulmonary and extrapulmonary disease in individuals with HIV disease. Most isolates of *M. tuberculosis* in AIDS patients remain susceptible to first-line antituberculosis drugs. The recommended initial regimen in adults is isoniazid (300 mg/day), rifampin (600 mg/day), and pyrazinamide (20–30 mg/kg/day). Ethambutol (15–25 mg/kg/day) is added if isoniazid drug resistance is suspected. This four-drug regimen is usually continued for 2 months, and if the isolate is isoniazid sensitive, isoniazid and rifampin are continued for a total of 6 to 12 months for both pulmonary and extrapulmonary tuberculosis. Both the CDC and the American Thoracic Society also recommend maintenance of therapy for at least 6 months beyond the conversion of sputum cultures to negative in patients with HIV disease and pulmonary tuberculosis.[44] A recent retrospective study from San Francisco of 132 patients with known tuberculosis and AIDS from 1981 to 1988 seems to support the adequacy of the short-course conventional regimen.[48] In this study, 50 (38%) patients had only pulmonary tuberculosis, 40 (30%) had only extrapulmonary tuberculosis, and 42 (32%) had both pulmonary and extrapulmonary disease. In 59%, tuberculosis preceded the diagnosis of AIDS, in 14% AIDS and tuberculosis were concordant, and in 27% tuberculosis was diagnosed after AIDS. Several treatment regimens were used but all for an intended 6- to 9-month duration. Sputum samples were sterilized at a median of 10 weeks of therapy, and chest radiographs at 3 months were stable or improved for all pulmonary cases. Only one treatment failure occurred, in a noncompliant patient with multiple drug-resistant organisms. The median survival for all treated patients was 16 months from the diagnosis of tuberculosis and the median duration of follow-up for patients after completion of therapy was 9.6 months (range, 1–85 months). Disease relapsed in only three patients (5%). The relapses occurred in a total of 823 patient-years of follow-up (3.6 relapses per 100 patient-years). These rates of treatment failure (<1%) and relapses (<5%) are within the ranges previously reported for patients with treated tuberculosis without HIV infection in San Francisco. Nevertheless, the results should be interpreted with some caution.

The retrospective assessment of patients might not have uncovered some patients who died of tuberculosis. Further, the demographic characteristics of the patients in this study reflected the HIV-infected population in San Francisco, which is substantially different from that in New York, New Jersey, Florida, or Third World countries. White homosexual men predominated in the San Francisco study, whereas persons of minority race and ethnic background and IV drug using risk predominate in the eastern United States. Finally, recent advances in therapy for HIV infection have resulted in prolongation of life and the potential for an increased time in which relapses might occur.

A similar study conducted in Zaire showed good response to therapy among patients dually infected with tuberculosis and HIV, but death from other AIDS-related causes occurred so soon after the tuberculosis diagnosis was made that the relapse rate could not be adequately assessed.[49] Finally, a surprisingly high rate of adverse drug reactions of sufficient severity to cause a change in therapy was noted in the San Francisco study.[48] Adverse reactions occurred in 18% of patients and were particularly common with rifampin, consisting mostly of rash and hepatitis. Despite excellent clinical results in patient series with this and other standard regimens in the United States,[48] Europe,[32] and Africa,[49] isolated reports of treatment failures[50,51] and the preliminary nature of current available data have led many authorities to continue to advocate a more cautious and conservative approach[17,52,53] in which isoniazid therapy is continued indefinitely after the conclusion of short-course therapy with multiple drugs.

Several drug interactions are important to note in the increasingly common treatment of IV drug users for tuberculosis. Rifampin will induce hepatic enzymes, which rapidly metabolize methadone. The combination of rifampin and methadone may result in rapid, unpleasant opiate withdrawal symptoms. An increase in the methadone dosage of 10 mg/day, to a total increase of 25% to 50% of the initial dosage, is often routinely required. The commonly used antifungal agents ketoconazole and fluconazole interact with isoniazid and rifampin, with resultant reduced serum levels and ineffective antifungal therapy in some patients.[17] Finally, rifampin absorption may be inhibited by ketoconazole, with resultant failure of treatment for tuberculosis.[54]

NONTUBERCULOUS MYCOBACTERIAL INFECTION

Nontuberculous mycobacteria have long been known to cause serious localized infections in nonimmunocompromised patients and, rarely, disseminated disease in immunocompromised patients. During the past decade, however, an epidemic of nontuberculous mycobacterial infection has occurred concurrent with the AIDS epidemic. Disseminated nontuberculous myco-

bacterial disease is now the most common reported bacterial infection in patients with AIDS. AIDS case surveillance by the CDC disclosed disseminated nontuberculous mycobacterial disease in 5.5% of patients with AIDS from 1981 to 1987.[55] Over 95% of these infections were due to *Mycobacterium avium* complex. More recently the proportion of patients with AIDS and disseminated *M. avium* complex has increased further, with a cumulative incidence of 7.6%. Through December 31, 1990, 12,202 cases had been reported among 161,073 patients with AIDS.[56] This substantial number of reported cases likely represents only a small percentage of actual cases, insofar as CDC AIDS case reporting is weighted toward the initial AIDS indicator diagnosis. Several hospital-based studies have noted that between 76% and 90% of disseminated *M. avium* complex infections occur after the AIDS diagnoses.[56-58] Cumulative incidence studies of disseminated *M. avium* complex infection indicate occurrence rates of 15% to 35% in AIDS patients.[56] It can be estimated, therefore, that disseminated *M. avium* complex infections had occurred in 24,000 to 39,000 of the 161,073 patients with AIDS whose cases had been reported through December 1990.[55]

The late development of disseminated *M. avium* complex infection is believed to result from the requirement for more severe immunosuppression with this relatively virulent organism than with other more virulent opportunistic pathogens such as *M. tuberculosis* and *P. carinii*. Disseminated *M. avium* complex infection rarely occurs in patients until the absolute CD4+ count falls below 100 cells/mm^3.[56] The mean number of CD4+ cells at its occurrence is less than 60 cells/mm^3.[56-58]

In contrast to *M. tuberculosis* infection, disseminated *M. avium* complex infection does not differ in occurrence by risk behavior or race and ethnicity, and may be evenly distributed throughout the United States.[55] In addition, this opportunistic infection appears to be rare in Africa among patients with AIDS. In one recent study, *M. avium* complex could not be identified by blood culture in 50 consecutive patients with AIDS in Uganda.[59] Further, whereas *M. tuberculosis* disease in patients with AIDS or HIV infection is most likely the result of reactivation of dormant foci, most evidence suggests that disseminated *M. avium* complex infection is the result of recent acquisition from environmental sources[55,60] such as water, food, and soil, the recognized habitats of these organisms.[61] The GI tract rather than the respiratory tract is believed to be the usual site of entry.[56]

The most commonly described clinical manifestations of disseminated *M. avium* complex infection are fever, weight loss, profound anemia, abdominal pain, and diarrhea. Patients may often present late in HIV disease without organ system localization, and only with fever and inanition. Pulmonary symptoms and radiographic abnormalities are unusual. In contrast, disseminated *M. kansasii* infection in patients with AIDS, a far less common entity, frequently presents with pulmonary disease, including upper lobe cavitation.[62]

The diagnosis of disseminated infection is established by culture of *M. avium* complex from normally sterile sites. Because the infection is widely disseminated, involving the blood, bone marrow, liver, spleen, and lymph nodes, many opportunities for diagnosis are available. The preferred test is culture of the blood. A high-grade continuous bacteremia is almost always seen,[63] with colony counts ranging from 350 to 28,000 cfu/ml.[63,64] Two successive blood cultures are positive in 95% of cases.[65] More rapid preliminary diagnoses may be obtained by acid-fast stain of fecal specimens[64] and/or histologic examination of bone marrow, lymph node, or liver tissue.[66] Poorly formed granulomas are usually seen, with large numbers of organisms present on acid-fast stains.

Patients presenting with disseminated *M. avium* complex infection as the AIDS indicator diagnosis have a shorter survival than those presenting with *P. carinii* pneumonia or Kaposi's sarcoma.[55,56,67] The estimated median survival of patients with AIDS and disseminated *M. avium* complex infection was 4.5 months in a series of patients in the Bronx[67] and 4.1 months in patients reported to the CDC with this diagnosis, compared to 11.1 months in patients without disseminated *M. avium* complex infection.[56] The severe degree of immunosuppression at the time of development of disseminated *M. avium* complex infection may account for the shortened survival. Alternatively, disseminated *M. avium* complex infection itself may hasten mortality. The exact contribution of *M. avium* infection to mortality in patients with AIDS remains debatable.[68] Certainly significant morbidity is associated with this infection, and attempts to develop successful treatment have been made over the past decade. Initial experience with multiple-drug regimens was disappointing.[60,69] More recently, four- and five-drug regimens have been shown to reduce or eliminate mycobacteremia and to alleviate symptoms of fever, diarrhea, and abdominal pain.[57,58] These regimens have consisted of prolonged therapy with combinations of ethambutol, clofazamine, ciprofloxacin, rifampin, or riftabutin, with or without amikacin. Controlled clinical trials of several potentially efficacious regimens are currently underway through the AIDS Clinical Trials Group. Treatment regimens are associated with substantial adverse reactions and may be difficult to administer, requiring a case-by-case assessment of risk and benefit.

PNEUMONIA

Pneumonia due to causes other than *P. carinii* is a major cause of morbidity and mortality among individuals infected with HIV.[70] Bacterial pneumonia occurs with increased frequency in patients with HIV infection and AIDS.[71–73] The majority of cases are due to either *Strep-*

tococcus pneumoniae or *Hemophilus influenzae.*[72,74,75] However, a large number of pathogenic or opportunistic bacteria may cause pneumonia in these patients. Gram-negative bacilli, especially in nosocomial infections,[76,77] *Staphylococcus aureus,*[75–77] *Nocardia asteroides,*[78,79] *Legionella* species,[71,72,76,80,81] *Branhamella catarrhalis, Rhodococcus equi,*[82–85] and group B streptococci[74,76] have all been described as pulmonary pathogens in this setting.

The actual incidence of bacterial pneumonia in HIV-infected individuals is unclear, for a variety of reasons. Many individuals may develop pneumonia before their HIV status is known; patients with known HIV infection who present with respiratory complaints have often been taking as prophylaxis or are often given therapeutically trimethoprim-sulfamethoxazole for presumed or proven *P. carinii* pneumonia, rendering a specific diagnosis of bacterial pneumonia difficult; variations in frequency of occurrence may exist, depending on HIV risk or other behaviors (*e.g.,* smoking, alcoholism); and limited prospective cohort studies are available. One prospective study of IV drug users reported a cumulative yearly incidence of bacterial pneumonia of 97 per 1,000 among HIV seropositive patients who had not yet developed AIDS, as compared with 21 per 1,000 for seronegative patients (p < 0.001).[72]

The clinical manifestations of bacterial pneumonia in these patients generally are similar to those in immunocompetent hosts, with fever, productive cough with purulent sputum, and consolidation on physical examination and chest radiographs.[72–75,86–89] In contrast to pyogenic bacteria, *Nocardia* infection may commonly manifest as subacute disease with reticulonodular infiltrates or solitary masses with or without cavitation, as well as with lobar or multilobar consolidation.[90] *Rhodococcus equi* also frequently causes cavitation.[84,85] A large proportion of patients with pneumonia due to pyogenic bacteria develop bacteremia, and the course of the illness may be more severe and prolonged than in immunocompetent hosts.[72,73,75,77,91] Recurrent episodes, not necessarily due to the same pathogen, may occur.[75,77]

Appropriate management of the patient with pneumonia should include an attempt to make a specific diagnosis. Sputum Gram stain and sputum and blood cultures will often lead to a diagnosis. Antimicrobial therapy should be chosen based on the infecting organism. In community-acquired infections treated prior to identification of the causative organism, therapy should include agents active against *S. pneumoniae* and *H. influenzae.* In nosocomial infections, effective therapy against gram-negative bacilli and *S. aureus* is advisable.[73] Although severely immunodeficient persons with HIV infection have poor responses to pneumococcal vaccine,[92,93] individuals earlier in the course of HIV infection may have adequate antibody responses.[94,95] It is recommended that all HIV-infected individuals receive pneumococcal vaccine,[96] although the clinical utility of this is not yet proven.

ENTERIC INFECTIONS

The GI tract is frequently affected in AIDS. In addition to direct effects of HIV and infections due to protozoan organisms, bacterial infections of the GI tract are common. Thorough evaluation may often lead to a specific diagnosis, so that appropriate therapy can be given.[97] Prior to and early in the AIDS epidemic, it was recognized that sexually active homosexual men were at risk for GI infections due to *Shigella*,[98–102] *Campylobacter*,[98,103,104] and possibly, to a lesser extent, *Salmonella*.[105,106] However, in the presence of immunodeficiency due to HIV infection, bacterial GI infections are frequently more severe, commonly are accompanied by bacteremia, and often relapse after antimicrobial therapy is discontinued.[97,106–110] In addition, *Salmonella* infection occurs much more frequently than in the absence of HIV infection.[111] These enteric infections are not limited to homosexual men with HIV infection; other individuals, including heterosexual white, Haitian, and African patients, IV drug users, and blood transfusion recipients, have been reported.[107,112–123] In all cases, supportive treatment should accompany any specific antimicrobial therapy given.

Salmonella

Salmonellosis may occur in the HIV-infected individual prior to, concomitant with, or following an AIDS-defining opportunistic infection.[107,108,112,124–126] *S. typhimurium* is most commonly involved, but other species of nontyphoidal *Salmonella* have been reported.[106,111,114–116] A recent report from Peru suggests that in areas where *S. typhi* is prevalent, the risk of infection with this pathogen is similarly increased in HIV-infected persons, and with severe immunodeficiency severe gastroenteritis can occur.[124]

The HIV-infected patient with salmonellosis typically presents with nonspecific symptoms and diarrhea, although diarrhea may be absent.[125] The nonspecific symptoms may include fever, anorexia, cachexia, fatigue, malaise, and weight loss. Symptoms may be subacute and may be present for weeks before the patient seeks medical attention. Rigors suggest bacteremia, which is clearly more common in the HIV-infected patient with salmonellosis than in an immunocompetent host. The diagnosis is made by culturing the organism from blood or stool; in some patients, bacteremia may be present without positive stool cultures.[106,107] With bacteremia, infection may involve other organs.

In immunocompetent individuals, *Salmonella* gastroenteritis is generally a self-limited disease and antimicrobial therapy is not recommended. The high rate of bacteremia and the severity of disease in the presence of HIV infection suggest that even gastroenteritis should be treated in these individuals. Most isolates are susceptible to the antibiotics commonly used to treat *Salmonella* infections, and therapy should be guided by *in vitro* susceptibility testing. It appears that 2 to 3 weeks of parenteral therapy will be effective in the majority of patients. Oral quinolones have been reported to be effective in the treatment of salmonellosis, including bacteremia,[127,128] but further evidence is needed before they can be considered effective first-line therapy. After discontinuation of therapy, relapse is frequent, so that chronic suppressive therapy with an oral agent that is effective *in vitro* and well tolerated should be considered.[108,113]

Campylobacter

Campylobacter infections are increased in frequency among patients with AIDS.[129] Infections are typically associated with diarrhea and abdominal cramping. The diarrhea is commonly bloody, and fever is usually present.[125] *Campylobacter jejuni* and *Campylobacter fetus* infections occur in HIV-infected persons[97,123,130–132] as well as in immunocompetent hosts. However, with underlying HIV infection, *Campylobacter* infections may be atypical, severe, persistent or recurrent, associated with bacteremia, and require prolonged therapy.[123,129,132] In addition, newer species, such as *C. cinaedi, C. fennelliae,* and *C. hyointestinalis,* have also been recognized as pathogens in individuals with or at risk for HIV infection.[103,118,133–136] Examination of the stool generally reveals fecal leukocytes.[125] The diagnosis is confirmed by isolation of the organism in culture. In immunocompetent individuals ill enough to require treatment, erythromycin has been the antimicrobial of choice.[137] Information on the response to antimicrobial therapy in patients with HIV infection is limited. Antimicrobial therapy probably should be prolonged to prevent relapse. However, there are already reports of *C. jejuni* isolates resistant to erythromycin in patients with HIV infection,[117,123] so that optimal therapy remains to be determined.

Shigella

Like *Campylobacter, Shigella* causes infections that may be associated with severe diarrhea or dysentery with fever.[125] In patients with HIV infection, shigellosis has been described as particularly severe, persistent, or both.[110,119,120,122] *S. flexneri* is the most common species involved.[97,119–122] Bacteremia, which occurs uncommonly in shigellosis and is rare in immunocompetent adults,[119,137] has been present in approximately one half of reported cases in individuals with HIV infection in whom the results of blood cultures were noted.[119,120] Although this likely reflects, in part, a bias due to reporting of the most severe cases, it seems likely that the rate of bacteremia due to *Shigella* is higher in the setting of HIV infection, as appears to be true for other enteric pathogens. Therapy with an antimicrobial to which the organism is susceptible *in vitro* should be used, with careful follow-up evaluation for relapse after discontinuation of treatment.

BACTEREMIA

Most cases of community-acquired bacteremia in individuals with HIV infection are due to organisms that cause pneumonia or enteric infections,[75,138] including those noted above. Symptoms or physical findings suggesting the lung or GI tract as the primary site of infection may be minimal or absent altogether. Isolation from blood cultures may be the first clue as to the infecting organism.

As with any other patient, an individual with HIV infection may be at risk for nosocomial local infection or bacteremia from an indwelling IV catheter. An indwelling catheter is the most important risk factor for *S. aureus* bacteremia in non-drug-using patients with HIV infection.[139] Strict adherence to recommended infection control precautions should minimize this risk. Often, because of the need for long-term venous access for administration of ganciclovir, foscarnet, or other IV medications for treatment or suppression of infections, or because peripheral access may be difficult, as is true for many IV drug users, central venous catheterization is required. The risk of central catheter–associated infections is increased in the presence of HIV infection.[140,141] Patients with indwelling lines maintained in the ambulatory setting are also at risk. The infecting microorganisms are similar to those seen in catheterized patients without HIV infection and include *Staphylococcus aureus, Staphylococcus epidermidis, Candida albicans,* and gram-negative bacilli, including *Pseudomonas aeruginosa.*[7,140–142] There are no data available to suggest that these infections should be managed differently in the HIV-infected patient.

SYPHILIS

An understanding of the natural history, diagnosis, and optimal therapy of syphilis in HIV-infected individuals has been limited by a paucity of prospective studies of large cohorts of co-infected individuals and controlled clinical trials. In addition, the frequent occurrence of cerebrospinal fluid abnormalities due to HIV infection or other HIV-associated conditions in the individual being evaluated for neurosyphilis, and uncertainty about the expected serologic response when patients are treated for syphilis, have made diagnosis and management particularly confusing.

However, anecdotal reports, small series of cases, and reviews of syphilis in HIV-infected individuals show that syphilis in the presence of HIV infection may manifest as early neurosyphilis,[143–147] may fail to respond to conventional therapy,[143–149] and may relapse after treatment.[145–147,150] Furthermore, although anecdotal reports of the delayed development of positive results on serologic tests for syphilis in the HIV-infected individual have appeared,[146,151] the majority of individuals appear to have appropriately reactive serologies despite HIV infection.[146,147] It has also been reported that specific treponemal tests, ordinarily expected to persist lifelong, may disappear in HIV-infected patients with a history of syphilis,[152,153] but recently this has been recognized in immunocompetent individuals as well.[154] Neurosyphilis should be considered in the differential diagnosis of unexplained neurologic, psychiatric, or ophthalmologic illness in HIV-infected patients.[149] Evaluation for syphilis should be routine in all persons who have acquired HIV infection *via* sexual contact, and HIV testing should be recommended for all patients with syphilis.[155]

The CDC recommends standard treatment (2.4 million units of benzathine penicillin) for the treatment of primary or secondary syphilis, even in HIV-infected persons.[155] However, others have suggested that regimens effective against neurosyphilis should be the minimal accepted regimen for primary or secondary syphilis in the setting of concomitant HIV infection.[146,156] All patients treated for syphilis should undergo careful prolonged follow-up to determine the long-term response to therapy and for evaluation for possible relapse.[145–147,155,157]

LISTERIOSIS

Cell-mediated immunity, including normal functioning of T lymphocytes and macrophages, is important in resistance to infection with *Listeria monocytogenes;* more than one half of cases in reported large series occur in immunosuppressed hosts.[158] Therefore, it is surprising that *Listeria* infection appears to be uncommon in individuals with HIV infection. It has been suggested that in AIDS patients elevated levels of tumor necrosis factor, important in the inhibition of *Listeria in vivo,* may explain the infrequency of this infection.[159] However, at least 17 patients with listeriosis and known HIV infection have been reported.[159–161] Meningitis or meningoencephalitis and bacteremia, clinical syndromes that are similar to listeriosis in patients without HIV infection, are common.[160] Response to therapy with ampicillin, with or without an aminoglycoside, is generally good, although some cases have been fatal.[159–161] Relapse after therapy has not yet been reported to be a major problem.

NOCARDIOSIS

Infection due to *Nocardia* is apparently uncommon in the setting of HIV infection. As is true with *Listeria,* this is somewhat surprising in view of the frequent association of immune deficiencies with *Nocardia* infection.[162] There have been at least 14 cases of *Nocardia* infection in patients with AIDS.[163] The occurrence of six cases (0.28%) among 2,167 patients with AIDS at one medical center[163] suggests that this infection is rare, but as the number of AIDS cases increases it will be seen with increasing frequency. Of note, one half of reported cases have involved multiple sites, and the majority of cases involved viscera or bone. The lung was the site most commonly involved, with seven (50%) of patients having lung infection. Antimicrobial therapy with a sulfonamide and a tetracycline was successful in four of six patients. Early diagnosis appeared to carry a more favorable prognosis. In three cases the disease was diagnosed only post mortem.

BACILLARY ANGIOMATOSIS

Bacillary angiomatosis is a vascular proliferative disease that affects the skin and lymph nodes of patients with HIV infection[164-166]; disseminated visceral or bone involvement may also occur.[167-171] The patient usually presents with cutaneous erythematous papules and nodules; the lesions may be confused clinically and histologically with Kaposi's sarcoma.[171,172] A history of recent cat scratches can sometimes be elicited.[167-170,173] Peliosis hepatis, a rare condition in which hepatic parenchyma contains cystic, blood-filled spaces, causing hepatomegaly and abdominal pain, has also been reported in patients with HIV infection[174,175] and recently was associated with bacillary angiomatosis in two patients with HIV infection.[172] The presence in the lesions of bacillary angiomatosis of bacilli that stain similarly to those found in cat-scratch disease has led to the use of the term "disseminated cat-scratch disease" in some patients. However, it is not clear whether the etiology of bacillary angiomatosis is identical to that of cat-scratch disease. The presence of these organisms and of certain histologic characteristics allows the distinction from Kaposi's sarcoma to be made.[171,172,176] Recent studies using molecular techniques have identified the likely causative organism as *Rickettsia*-like, most closely related to *Rochalimaea quintana,* the cause of trench fever.[170] Another recent report has described isolation of a newly recognized fastidious gram-negative curved bacillus from the blood of symptomatic HIV-infected and other immunosuppressed patients with persistent fever.[177] Although the fatty acid composition of these isolates was similar to that of *R. quintana,* they apparently differed from this organism more than the agent identified in bacillary angiomatosis. The relationship of these two syndromes, if any, remains to be determined.

Bacillary angiomatosis is potentially fatal if not treated.[166] Successful treatment has been accomplished with erythromycin or tetracyclines.[164,165,167,171-173,176,178]

MISCELLANEOUS BACTERIAL INFECTIONS

Clinicians have noted recurrent episodes of sinusitis in patients with HIV infection.[179-181] The relative contributions of infection and allergy in the pathogenesis of this disorder, the optimal diagnostic methods to be used, and the therapy of choice remain to be clarified. Most patients respond to a combination of decongestants and antibiotics; chronic suppressive therapy may be required if recurrences are frequent, and surgical drainage may be necessary in some cases.

A variety of skin and soft-tissue infections have been reported in patients with HIV infection or AIDS, including subcutaneous and perirectal abscesses, furunculosis, folliculitis, ecthyma, erysipelas, otitis externa, impetigo, and pyomyositis.[76,142,181-183] *S. aureus* is a common pathogen. Until additional information becomes available, therapy should be the same as for individuals without HIV infection.

Periodontal disease, including gingivitis and periodontitis, is common and may be rapidly progressive in patients with HIV infection.[184,185] Although information about the exact causes of periodontal diseases remains incomplete, data suggest that a variety of oral bacteria may play a causal role in periodontitis.[186]

All parenteral drug users are at risk for infective endocarditis. Preliminary evidence suggests that HIV-infected drug users with bacterial endocarditis have disease similar to that seen in HIV-seronegative parenteral drug users. However, patients with advanced symptomatic HIV disease have a higher mortality.[187]

REFERENCES

1. Ho DD, Pomerantz RJ, Kaplan JC: Pathogenesis of infection with human immunodeficiency virus. N Engl J Med 317:278, 1987
2. Ellis M, Gupta S, Galant S et al: Impaired neutrophil function in patients with AIDS or AIDS-related complex: A comprehensive evaluation. J Infect Dis 158:1268, 1988
3. Lane HC, Masur H, Edgar LC et al: Abnormalities of B-cell activation and immunoregulation in patients with the acquired immunodeficiency syndrome. N Engl J Med 309:453, 1983
4. Amman AS, Schiffman G, Abrams D et al: B-cell deficiency in acquired immune deficiency syndrome. JAMA 251:1447, 1984
5. Pahwa SG, Quilop MTJ, Lange M et al: Defective B-lymphocyte function in homosexual men in relation to the acquired immunodeficiency syndrome. Ann Intern Med 101:757, 1984
6. Janoff EN, Douglas JM Jr, Gabriel M et al: Class-specific antibody response to pneumococcal capsular polysaccharides in men infected with human immunodeficiency virus type 1. J Infect Dis 158:983, 1988
7. Ballet JJ, Sulcebe G, Courderc LJ et al: Impaired antipneumococcal antibody response in patients with AIDS-related persistent generalized lymphadenopathy. Clin Exp Immunol 68:479, 1987
8. Bernstein LJ, Ochs HD, Wedgwood RJ, Rubinstein A: Defective humoral immunity in pediatric immune deficiency syndrome. J Pediatr 107:352, 1985
9. Bernstein LJ, Krieger BZ, Novick B et al: Bacterial infection in the acquired immune deficiency syndrome of children. Pediatr Infect Dis 4:472, 1985
10. Oleske J, Minnefor A, Cooper R Jr et al: Immune deficiency syndrome in children. JAMA 249:2345, 1983
11. Smith PD, Ohura K, Masur H et al: Monocyte function in the acquired immune deficiency syndrome: Defective chemotaxis. J Clin Invest 74:2121, 1984
12. Poli G, Bottazzi B, Acero R et al: Monocyte function in intravenous drug abusers with lymphadenopathy syndrome and in patients with acquired immunodeficiency

syndrome: Selective impairment of chemotaxis. Clin Exp Immunol 62:136, 1985

13. Ras GJ, Aftychis HA, Anderson R, van der Walt I: Mononuclear and polymorphonuclear leukocyte dysfunction in male homosexuals with acquired immunodeficiency syndrome (AIDS). S Afr Med J 66:806, 1984

14. Lazzarin A, Foppa CU, Galli M et al: Impairment of polymorphonuclear leucocyte function in patients with acquired immunodeficiency syndrome and with lymphadenopathy syndrome. Clin Exp Immunol 65:105, 1986

15. Bowen DL, Lane HC, Fauci AS: Immunopathogenesis of the acquired immunodeficiency syndrome. Ann Intern Med 103:704, 1985

16. Reider HL, Cauthen GM, Kelly GD et al: Tuberculosis in the United States. JAMA 262:385, 1989

17. Barnes PF, Bloch AB, Davidson DT, Snider DE: Tuberculosis in patients with human immunodeficiency virus infection. N Engl J Med 324:1644, 1991

18. Colebunders RL, Ryder RW, Nzilambi N et al: HIV infection in patients with tuberculosis in Kinshasa, Zaire. Am Rev Respir Dis 139:1082, 1989

19. Centers for Disease Control: Tuberculosis in acquired immunodeficiency syndrome—Florida. MMWR 35:587, 1986

20. Centers for Disease Control: Tuberculosis and AIDS—New York City. MMWR 36:785, 1987

21. Centers for Disease Control: Tuberculosis and AIDS—Connecticut. MMWR 36:133, 1987

22. Pitchenik AE, Cole C, Russell BW et al: Tuberculosis, atypical mycobacteriosis in the acquired immunodeficiency syndrome among Haitian and non-Haitian patients in South Africa. Ann Intern Med 101:641, 1984

23. Sunderm A, McDonald RJ, Maniatis T et al: Tuberculosis as a manifestation of the acquired immunodeficiency syndrome (AIDS). JAMA 256:363, 1986

24. Theuer CP, Hopewell PC, Elias D et al: Human immunodeficiency virus infection in tuberculosis patients. J Infect Dis 162:8, 1990

25. Selwyn PA, Hartel D, Lewis VA et al: A prospective study of the risk of tuberculosis among intravenous drug users with human immunodeficiency virus infection. N Engl J Med 320:545, 1989

26. Schoenbaum EE, Hartel D, Friedland GH: Intravenous drug use and HIV infection. Curr Opin Infect Dis 3:80, 1990

27. Centers for Disease Control: Tuberculosis in developing countries. MMWR 3:561, 1990

28. Pitchenik AE: Tuberculosis control and the AIDS epidemic in developing countries. Ann Intern Med 113:39, 1990

29. Styblo K: The potential impact of AIDS in the tuberculosis situation in developed and developing countries. Bull Int Union Tuberc Lung Dis 63(2):25, 1988

30. Reider HL, Canthen GM, Bloch AB et al: Tuberculosis and acquired immunodeficiency syndrome—Florida. Arch Intern Med 149:1268, 1989

31. Phair J, Munoz A, Detels R et al: The risk of *Pneumocystis carinii* pneumonia among men infected with human immunodeficiency virus type 1. N Engl J Med 322:161, 1990

32. Soriano L, Mallolas J, Gatell J et al: Characteristics of tuberculosis in HIV-infected patients: A case-control study. AIDS 2:429, 1988

33. Chaisson RE, Schecter GF, Theuer CP et al: Tuberculosis in patients with the acquired immunodeficiency syndrome: Clinical features, response to therapy and survival. Am Rev Respir Dis 136:570, 1987

34. Handwerger S, Mildvan D, Senie R, McKinley FU: Tuberculosis and the acquired immunodeficiency syndrome at a NYC hospital 1978–1985. Chest 91:176, 1987

35. Louie E, Ricel B, Holzman RS: Tuberculosis in non-Haitian patients with AIDS. Chest 90:542, 1986

36. Braun MM, Byers RH, Heyward WL et al: Acquired immunodeficiency syndrome and extrapulmonary tuberculosis in the United States. Arch Intern Med 150:1913, 1990

37. Bishburg E, Sunderm G, Reichman LB, Kapila R: Central nervous system tuberculosis with the acquired immunodeficiency syndrome and its related complex. Ann Intern Med 105:210, 1986

38. Moreno S, Pacho E, Lopez-Hence JA et al: Mycobacteria tuberculosis visceral abscesses in the acquired immunodeficiency syndrome (AIDS). Ann Intern Med 109:437, 1988

39. Saltzman BR, Motyl MR, Friedland GH et al: *Mycobacterium tuberculosis* bacteremia in the acquired immunodeficiency syndrome. JAMA 256:390, 1986

40. Centers for Disease Control: *Mycobacterium tuberculosis* transmission in a health clinic—Florida, 1988. MMWR 38(No. 15):256, 1989

41. Centers for Disease Control: Transmission of multidrug-resistant tuberculosis from an HIV-positive client in a residential substance-abuse treatment facility—Michigan. MMWR 40:129, 1991

42. Centers for Disease Control: Nosocomial transmission of multidrug-resistant tuberculosis to health-care workers and HIV-infected patients in an urban hospital—Florida. MMWR 39(No. 40):718, 1990

43. Centers for Disease Control: Guidelines for preventing the transmission of tuberculosis in health-care settings, with special focus on HIV-related issues. MMWR 39(No. RR-17), 1990

44. Tuberculosis and human immunodeficiency virus infection: Recommendations of the Advisory Committee for the Elimination of Tuberculosis. MMWR 38:236, 1989

45. Robert CF, Hirschel B, Rochat T et al: Tuberculin skin reactivity in HIV-1 seropositive intravenous drug addicts (letter). N Engl J Med 321:1268, 1989

46. Wadhawan D, Hira S, Mwansa N et al: Isoniazid prophylaxis among patients with HIV-1 infection (abstr Th.B.510). Presented at the VI International Conference on AIDS, San Francisco, June 1990

47. Selwyn P, Feingold AR, Iezza A et al: Primary care for patients with HIV infection in a methadone maintenance treatment program. Ann Intern Med 111:761, 1989

48. Small PM, Schechter GF, Goodman PC et al: Treatment of tuberculosis in patients with advanced human immunodeficiency virus infection. N Engl J Med 325:289, 1991

49. Mukadi Y, Perriens J, Willame JC et al: Short course antituberculous therapy for pulmonary tuberculosis: A prospective controlled study (abstr Th.B.507). Presented at the VI International Conference on AIDS, San Francisco, June 1990

50. Sunderm G, Mangura BT, Lombardo JM, Reichman LB: Failure of ''optimal'' four-drug short-course tuberculosis chemotherapy in a compliant patient with human immunodeficiency virus. Am Rev Respir Dis 136:1475, 1987

51. Dylewski J, Thilbert L: Failure of tuberculosis chemotherapy in a human immunodeficiency virus–infected patient. J Infect Dis 162:S778, 1990

52. Iseman MD: Is standard chemotherapy adequate in tuberculosis patients infected with the HIV? Am Rev Respir Dis 136:1326, 1987

53. Davidson P: Treating tuberculosis: What drugs, for how long? Ann Intern Med 112:393, 1990

54. Enselhard D, Stutman HR, Marks MI: Interaction of ketoconazole with rifampin and isoniazid. N Engl J Med 311:1681, 1984

55. Horsburgh CR Jr, Selik RM: The epidemiology of disseminated non-tuberculous mycobacterial infection in the acquired immunodeficiency syndrome (AIDS). Am Rev Respir Dis 139:4, 1989

56. Horsburgh CR Jr: *Mycobacterium avium* complex infection in the acquired immunodeficiency syndrome. N Engl J Med 324:1332, 1991

57. Chiu J, Nussbaum J, Bozzette S et al: Treatment of disseminated *Mycobacterium avium* complex infection in AIDS with amikacin, ethambutol, rifampin, and ciprofloxacin. Ann Intern Med 113:358, 1990

58. Hoy J, Mijch A, Sandland M et al: Quadruple-drug therapy for *Mycobacterium avium-intracellulare* bacteremia in AIDS patients. J Infect Dis 161:801, 1990

59. Okello DO, Sewankambo N, Goodgame R et al: Absence of bacteremia with *Mycobacterium avium-intracelluare* in Ugandan patients with AIDS. J Infect Dis 162:208, 1990

60. Hawkins CC, Gold JWM, Whimby E et al: *Mycobacterium avium* complex infections in patients with the acquired immunodeficiency syndrome. Ann Intern Med 105:184, 1986

61. Wolinsky E: Non-tuberculous mycobacterium and associated diseases. Am Rev Respir Dis 119:107, 1979

62. Levine B, Chaisson RE: *Mycobacterium kansasii:* A cause of treatable pulmonary disease associated with advanced human immunodeficiency virus (HIV) infection. Ann Intern Med 114:861, 1991

63. Wong B, Edwards FF, Kiehn TE et al: Continuous high-grade *Mycobacterium avium-intracellulare* bacteremia in patients with the acquired immunodeficiency syndrome. Am J Med 75:38, 1985

64. Keihn TE, Edwards FF, Brannon EP et al: Infections caused by *Mycobacterium avium* complex in immunocompromised patients: Diagnoses by blood culture and fecal examination, antimicrobial susceptibility tests, and morphological and seroagglutination characteristics. J Clin Microbiol 21:168, 1985

65. Barnes PF, Arevado C: Blood culture positivity patterns in bacteremia due to *Mycobacterium avium-intracellulare.* South Med J 81:1059, 1988

66. Kahn SA, Saltzman BR, Klein RS et al: Hepatic disorder in acquired immunodeficiency syndrome: A clinical and pathological study. Am J Gastroenterol 81:1145, 1986

67. Friedland GH, Saltzman B, Vileno J et al: Survival differences in patients with the acquired immunodeficiency syndrome. J AIDS 4:144, 1991

68. Chaisson RE, Hopewell PC: Mycobacteria and AIDS mortality. Am Rev Respir Dis 139:1, 1989

69. Young LS, Inderlied CB, Berlin OG, Gottlieb MS: Mycobacterial infections in AIDS patients, with an emphasis on the *Mycobacterium avium* complex. Rev Infect Dis 8:1024, 1986

70. Centers for Disease Control: Increase in pneumonia mortality among young adults and the HIV epidemic—New York City, United States. MMWR 37:593, 1988

71. Murray JF, Felton CP, Garay SM et al: Pulmonary complications of the acquired immunodeficiency syndrome. N Engl J Med 310:1682, 1984

72. Selwyn PA, Feingold AR, Hartel D et al: Increased risk of bacterial pneumonia in HIV-infected intravenous drug users without AIDS. AIDS 2:267, 1988

73. Chaisson RE: Bacterial pneumonia in patients with human immunodeficiency virus infection. Semin Respir Infect 4:133, 1989

74. Polsky B, Gold JWM, Whimbey E et al: Bacterial pneumonia in patients with the acquired immunodeficiency syndrome. Ann Intern Med 104:38, 1986

75. Whimbey E, Gold JWM, Polsky B et al: Bacteremia and fungemia in patients with the acquired immunodeficiency syndrome. Ann Intern Med 104:511, 1986

76. Witt DJ, Craven DE, McCabe WR: Bacterial infections in adult patients with the acquired immune deficiency syndrome (AIDS) and AIDS-related complex. Am J Med 82:900, 1987

77. Levine SJ, White DA, Stover DE, Fels AOS: The incidence and significance of *Staphylococcus aureus* in respiratory cultures from HIV+ patients (abstr). Am Rev Respir Dis 137:355, 1988

78. Holtz HA, Lavery DP, Kapila R: Actinomycetales infection in the acquired immunodeficiency syndrome. Ann Intern Med 102:203, 1985

79. Rodriguez JL, Barrio JL, Pitchenik AE: Pulmonary nocardiosis in the acquired immunodeficiency syndrome: Diagnosis with bronchoalveolar lavage and treatment with non-sulphur containing drugs. Chest 90:912, 1986

80. Armstrong D, Gold JWM, Dryjanski J et al: Treatment of infections in patients with the acquired immunodeficiency syndrome. Ann Intern Med 103:738, 1985

81. Niedt GW, Schinella RA: Acquired immunodeficiency syndrome: Clinicopathologic study of 56 autopsies. Arch Pathol Lab Med 109:727, 1985

82. Samies JH, Hathaway BN, Echols RM et al: Lung abscess due to *Corynebacterium equi.* Am J Med 80:685, 1986

83. Sane DC, Durack DT: Infection with *Rhodococcus equi* in AIDS. N Engl J Med 314:56, 1986

84. Harvey RL, Sunstrom JC: *Rhodococcus equi* infection in patients with and without human immunodeficiency virus infection. Rev Infect Dis 13:139, 1991

85. Emmons W, Reichwein B, Winslow DL: *Rhodococcus equi* infection in the patient with AIDS: Literature review and report of an unusual case. Rev Infect Dis 13:91, 1991

86. Stover DA, White DE, Romano PA et al: Spectrum of pulmonary diseases associated with the acquired immune deficiency syndrome. Am J Med 78:429, 1985

87. Heron CW, Hine AL, Pozniak AL et al: Radiographic features in patients with pulmonary manifestations of the acquired immune deficiency syndrome. Clin Radiol 36:583, 1985

88. Schlamm HT, Yancovitz SR: *Haemophilus influenzae* pneumonia in young adults with AIDS, ARC, or risk of AIDS. Am J Med 86:11, 1989

89. Amorosa JK, Nahass RG, Nosher JL, Gocke DJ: Radiologic distinction of pyogenic pulmonary infection from *Pneumocystis carinii* pneumonia in AIDS patients. Radiology 175:721, 1990

90. Kramer MR, Uttamchandani RB: The radiographic appearance of pulmonary nocardiosis associated with AIDS. Chest 98:382, 1990

91. Murata GH, Ault MJ, Meyer RD: Community-acquired bacterial pneumonias in homosexual men: Presumptive evidence for a defect in host resistance. AIDS Res 1:379, 1984–85

92. Ammann AJ, Schiffman G, Abrams D et al: B-cell immu-

nodeficiency in acquired immune deficiency syndrome. JAMA 251:1447, 1984

93. Simberkoff MS, Sadr WE, Schiffman G, Rahal JJ: *Streptococcus pneumoniae* infection and bacteremia in patients with acquired immunodeficiency syndrome, with report of a pneumococcal vaccine failure. Am Rev Respir Dis 130:1174, 1984

94. Klein RS, Selwyn PA, Maude D et al: Response to pneumococcal vaccine among asymptomatic heterosexual partners of persons with AIDS and intravenous drug users infected with human immunodeficiency virus. J Infect Dis 160:826, 1989

95. Huang KL, Ruben FL, Rinaldo CR Jr et al: Antibody responses after influenza and pneumococcal immunization in HIV-infected homosexual men. JAMA 257:2047, 1987

96. Centers for Disease Control: Recommendations of the Immunization Practices Advisory Committee. Pneumococcal polysaccharide vaccine. MMWR 38:64, 1989

97. Smith PD, Lane HC, Gill VJ: Intestinal infections in patients with the acquired immunodeficiency syndrome (AIDS): Etiology and response to therapy. Ann Intern Med 108:328, 1988

98. Quinn TC, Stamm WE, Goodell SE et al: The polymicrobial origin of intestinal infections in homosexual men. N Engl J Med 309:576, 1983

99. Dritz SK, Back AF: *Shigella* enteritis venereally transmitted. N Engl J Med 291:1194, 1974

100. Bader M, Pedersen AH, Williams R et al: Venereal transmission of shigellosis in Seattle–King county. Sex Trans Dis 4:89, 1977

101. Sohn N, Robilotti JG: The gay bowel syndrome: A review of colonic and rectal conditions in 200 male homosexuals. Am J Gastroenterol 67:478, 1977

102. Drusin LM, Genvert G, Topf-Olstein B, Levy-Zombeck E: Shigellosis: Another sexually transmitted disease? Br J Vener Dis 52:348, 1976

103. Quinn TC, Goodell SE, Fennel C et al: Infections with *Campylobacter jejuni* and *Campylobacter*-like organisms in homosexual men. Ann Intern Med 101:187, 1984

104. Felman YM, Nikitas JA: Sexually transmitted disease in the male homosexual community. Cutis 30:706, 1982

105. Dritz SK, Braff EH: Sexually transmitted typhoid fever. N Engl J Med 296:1359, 1977

106. Nadelman RB, Mathur-Wagh U, Yankovitz SR, Mildvan D: *Salmonella* bacteremia associated with the acquired immunodeficiency syndrome (AIDS). Arch Intern Med 145:1968, 1985

107. Glaser JB, Morton-Kute L, Berger SR et al: Recurrent *Salmonella typhimurium* bacteremia associated with the acquired immunodeficiency syndrome. Ann Intern Med 102:189, 1985

108. Jacobs JL, Gold JWM, Murray HW et al: *Salmonella* infections in patients with the acquired immunodeficiency syndrome. Ann Intern Med 102:186, 1985

109. Baskin DH, Lax JD, Barenberg D: *Shigella* bacteremia in patients with the acquired immunodeficiency syndrome. Am J Gastroenterol 82:338, 1987

110. Glupczynski Y, Hansen W, Jonas C, Deltenre M: *Shigella flexneri* bacteraemia in a patient with acquired immunodeficiency syndrome. Acta Clin Belg 40:388, 1985

111. Celum CL, Chaisson RE, Rutherford GW et al: Incidence of salmonellosis in patients with AIDS. J Infect Dis 156:998, 1987

112. Smith PD, Macher AM, Bookman MA et al: *Salmonella typhimurium* enteritis and bacteremia in the acquired immunodeficiency syndrome. Ann Intern Med 102:207, 1985

113. De Wit S, Taelman H, Van de Perre P et al: *Salmonella* bacteremia in African patients with human immunodeficiency virus infection. Eur J Clin Microbiol Infect Dis 7:45, 1988

114. Profeta S, Forrester C, Eng RHK et al: *Salmonella* infections in patients with acquired immunodeficiency syndrome. Arch Intern Med 145:670, 1985

115. Fischl MA, Dickinson GM, Sinave C et al: *Salmonella* bacteremia as manifestation of acquired immunodeficiency syndrome. Arch Intern Med 146:113, 1986

116. Sperber SJ, Schleupner CJ: Salmonellosis during infection with human immunodeficiency virus. Rev Infect Dis 9:925, 1986

117. Dworkin B, Wormser GP, Abdoo RA et al: Persistence of multiply antibiotic-resistant *Campylobacter jejuni* in a patient with acquired immune deficiency syndrome. Am J Med 80:965, 1986

118. Ng VL, Hadley WK, Fennell CL et al: Successive bacteremias with "*Campylobacter cinaedi*" and "*Campylobacter fennelliae*" in a bisexual male. J Clin Microbiol 25:2008, 1987

119. Baskin DH, Lax JD, Barenberg D: *Shigella* bacteremia in patients with the acquired immune deficiency syndrome. Am J Gastroenterol 82:338, 1987

120. Boers M, Peeters AJ, van Berkel M et al: Shigellosis and AIDS. Neth J Med 34:93, 1989

121. Blaser MJ, Hale TL, Formal SB: Recurrent shigellosis complicating human immunodeficiency virus infection: Failure of pre-existing antibodies to confer protection. Am J Med 86:105, 1989

122. Simor AE, Poon R, Borczyk A: Chronic *Shigella flexneri* infection preceding development of acquired immunodeficiency syndrome. J Clin Microbiol 27:353, 1989

123. Perlman DM, Ampel NM, Schiffman RB et al: Persistent *Campylobacter jejuni* infections in persons infected with human immunodeficiency virus (HIV). Ann Intern Med 108:540, 1988

124. Gotuzzo E, Frisancho O, Sanchez J et al: Association between the acquired immunodeficiency syndrome and infection with *Salmonella typhi* or *Salmonella paratyphi* in an endemic typhoid area. Arch Intern Med 151:381, 1991

125. Chaisson RE: Infections due to encapsulated bacteria, salmonella, shigella, and campylobacter. Infect Dis Clin North Am 2:475, 1988

126. Bottone EJ, Wormser GP, Duncanson FP: Nontyphoidal salmonella bacteremia as an early infection in the acquired immunodeficiency syndrome. Diagn Microbiol Infect Dis 2:247, 1984

127. Heseltine PNR, Causey DM, Appleman M et al: Norfloxacin in the eradication of enteric infections in AIDS patients. Eur J Cancer Clin Oncol 24(suppl 1):S25, 1988

128. Jacobson MA, Hahn SM, Gerberding JL et al: Ciprofloxacin for salmonella bacteremia in the acquired immunodeficiency syndrome (AIDS). Ann Intern Med 110:1027, 1989

129. Sorvillo FJ, Lieb LE, Waterman SH: Incidence of campylobacteriosis among patients with AIDS in Los Angeles County. J AIDS 4:598, 1991

130. Rolston KVI, Rodriguez S, Hernandez M, Bodey GP: Diarrhea in patients infected with the human immunodeficiency virus. Am J Med 86:137, 1989

131. Miro JM, Mallolas J, Moreno A et al: Infectious gastroen-

teritis with the acquired immunodeficiency syndrome (AIDS). Ann Intern Med 109:342, 1988

132. Wheeler AP, Gregg CR: *Campylobacter* bacteremia, cholecystitis, and the acquired immunodeficiency syndrome. Ann Intern Med 105:804, 1986

133. Cimolai N, Gill MJ, Jones A et al: "*Campylobacter cinaedi*" bacteremia: Case report and laboratory findings. J Clin Microbiol 25:942, 1987

134. Edmonds P, Patton CM, Griffin PM et al: *Campylobacter hyointestinalis* associated with human gastrointestinal disease in the United States. J Clin Microbiol 25:685, 1987

135. Pasternack J, Bolivar R, Hopfer RL et al: Bacteremia caused by *Campylobacter*-like organisms in two male homosexuals. Ann Intern Med 101:339, 1984

136. Totten PA, Fennell CL, Tenover FC et al: *Campylobacter cinaedi* (sp. nov.) and *Campylobacter fennelliae* (sp. nov.): Two new *Campylobacter* species associated with enteric disease in homosexual men. J Infect Dis 151:131, 1985

137. Streulens MJ, Patte D, Kabir I et al: *Shigella* septicemia: Prevalence, presentation, risk factors and outcome. J Infect Dis 152:784, 1985

138. Gilks CF, Brindle RJ, Otieno LS et al: Life-threatening bacteraemia in HIV-1 seropositive adults admitted to hospital in Nairobi, Kenya. Lancet 2:545, 1990

139. Skoutelis AT, Murphy RL, MacDonell KB et al: Indwelling central venous catheter infections in patients with acquired immune deficiency syndrome. J AIDS 3:335, 1990

140. Jacobson MA, Gellerman H, Chambers H: *Staphylococcus aureus* bacteremia and recurrent staphylococcal infection in patients with acquired immunodeficiency syndrome and AIDS-related complex. Am J Med 85:172, 1988

141. Raviglione MC, Battan R, Pablos-Mendez A et al: Infections associated with Hickman catheters in patients with acquired immunodeficiency syndrome. Am J Med 86:780, 1989

142. Krumholz HM, Sande ME, Lo B: Community-acquired bacteremia in patients with acquired immunodeficiency syndrome: Clinical presentation, bacteriology and outcome. Am J Med 86:776, 1989

143. Johns DR, Tierney M, Felsenstein D: Alteration in the natural history of neurosyphilis by concurrent infection with the human immunodeficiency virus. N Engl J Med 316:1569, 1987

144. Spence MR, Abrutyn E: Syphilis and infection with the human immunodeficiency virus. Ann Intern Med 107:587, 1987

145. Hook EW III: Syphilis and HIV infection. J Infect Dis 160:530, 1989

146. Musher DM, Hamill RJ, Baughn RE: Effect of human immunodeficiency virus (HIV) infection on the course of syphilis and on the response to treatment. Ann Intern Med 113:872, 1990

147. Musher D: Syphilis, neurosyphilis, penicillin, and AIDS. J Infect Dis 163:1201, 1991

148. Lukehart SA, Hook EW III, Baker-Zander SA et al: Invasion of the central nervous system by *Treponema pallidum*: Implications for diagnosis and treatment. Ann Intern Med 109:855, 1988

149. Katz DA, Berger JR: Neurosyphilis in acquired immunodeficiency syndrome. Arch Neurol 46:895, 1989

150. Berry CD, Hooton TM, Collier AC, Lukehart SA: Neurologic relapse after benzathine penicillin therapy for secondary syphilis in a patient with HIV infection. N Engl J Med 316:187, 1987

151. Hicks CB, Benson PM, Lupton GP, Tramont EC: Seronegative secondary syphilis in a patient infected with the human immunodeficiency virus (HIV) with Kaposi sarcoma. Ann Intern Med 107:492, 1987

152. Haas JS, Bolan G, Larsen SA et al: Sensitivity of treponemal tests for detecting prior treated syphilis during human immunodeficiency virus infection. J Infect Dis 162:862, 1990

153. Johnson PDR, Graves SR, Stewart L et al: Specific syphilis serological tests may become negative in HIV infection. AIDS 5:419, 1991

154. Romanowski B, Sutherland R, Fick GH et al: Serologic response to treatment of infectious syphilis. Ann Intern Med 114:100, 1991

155. Centers for Disease Control: Recommendations for diagnosing and treating syphilis in HIV-infected patients. MMWR 37:600, 1988

156. Tramont EC: Syphilis in the AIDS era. N Engl J Med 316:1600, 1987

157. Lukehart SA: Serologic testing after therapy for syphilis: Is there a test for cure? Ann Intern Med 114:107, 1991

158. Armstrong DA: *Listeria monocytogenes.* In Mandell GL, Douglas RG Jr, Bennett JE (eds): Principles and Practice of Infectious Diseases, 3rd ed, p 1587. New York, Churchill Livingstone, 1990

159. Decker CF, Simon GL, DiGiola RA, Tuazon CU: *Listeria monocytogenes* infections in patients with AIDS: Report of five cases and review. Rev Infect Dis 13:413, 1991

160. Kales CP, Holzman RS: Listeriosis in patients with HIV infection: Clinical manifestations and response to therapy. J AIDS 3:139, 1990

161. Berenguer J, Sloera J, Diaz MD et al: Listeriosis in patients infected with human immunodeficiency virus. Rev Infect Dis 13:115, 1991

162. Lerner PI: *Nocardia* species. In Mandell GL, Douglas RG Jr, Bennett JE (eds): Principles and Practice of Infectious Diseases, 3rd ed, p 1926. New York, Churchill Livingstone, 1990

163. Kim Jungmee K, Minamoto GY, Grieco MH: Nocardial infection as a complication of AIDS: Report of six cases and review. Rev Infect Dis 13:624, 1991

164. Stoler MH, Bonfiglio TA, Steigbigel RT, Pereira M: An atypical subcutaneous infection associated with acquired immune deficiency syndrome. Am J Clin Pathol 80:714, 1983

165. Cockerell CJ, LeBoit PE: Bacillary angiomatosis: A newly characterized, pseudoneoplastic, infectious, cutaneous vascular disorder. J Am Acad Dermatol 22:501, 1990

166. Cockerell CJ, Whitlow MA, Webster GF, Friedman-Kien AE: Epithelioid angiomatosis: A distinct vascular disorder in patients with the acquired immunodeficiency syndrome or AIDS-related complex. Lancet 2:654, 1987

167. Koehler JE, LeBoit PE, Egbert BM, Berger TG: Cutaneous vascular lesions and disseminated cat-scratch disease in patients with the acquired immunodeficiency syndrome (AIDS) and AIDS-related complex. Ann Intern Med 109:449, 1988

168. Milam MW, Balerdi MJ, Toney JF et al: Epithelioid angiomatosis secondary to disseminated cat-scratch disease involving the bone marrow and skin in a patient with acquired immune deficiency syndrome: A case report. Am J Med 88:180, 1990

169. Kemper CA, Lombard CM, Deresinski SC, Tomkins LS: Visceral bacillary epithelioid angiomatosis: Possible manifestations of disseminated cat scratch disease in the

immunosuppressed host. A report of two cases. Am J Med 89:216, 1990

170. Relman DA, Loutit JS, Schmidt TM et al: The agent of bacillary angiomatosis: An approach to the identification of uncultured pathogens. N Engl J Med 323:1573, 1990

171. LeBoit PE, Berger TG, Egbert BM et al: Bacillary angiomatosis: The histopathology and differential diagnosis of a pseudoneoplastic infection in patients with human immunodeficiency virus disease. Am J Surg Pathol 13:909, 1989

172. Perkocha LA, Geaghan SM, Yen TSB et al: Clinical and pathological features of bacillary peliosis hepatis in association with human immunodeficiency virus infection. N Engl J Med 323:1581, 1990

173. Pilon VA, Echols RM: Cat-scratch disease in a patient with AIDS. Am J Clin Pathol 92:236, 1989

174. Czapar CA, Weldon-Linne M, Moore DM, Rhone DP: Peliosis hepatis in the acquired immunodeficiency syndrome. Arch Pathol Lab Med 110:611, 1986

175. Scoazec J-Y, Marche C, Giradr P-M et al: Peliosis hepatis and sinusoidal dilatation during infection by the human immunodeficiency virus (HIV): An ultrastructural study. Am J Pathol 131:38, 1988

176. Walford N, van der Wouw PA, Das PK, ten Velden JJAM: Epithelioid angiomatosis in the acquired immunodeficiency syndrome: Morphology and differential diagnosis. Histopathology 16:83, 1990

177. Slater LN, Welch DF, Hensel D, Coody DW: A newly recognized fastidious gram-negative pathogen as a cause of fever and bacteremia. N Engl J Med 323:1587, 1990

178. Rudikoff D, Phelps RG, Gordon RE, Bottone EJ: Acquired immunodeficiency syndrome-related bacillary vascular proliferation (epithelioid angiomatosis): Rapid response to erythromycin therapy. Arch Dermatol 125:706, 1989

179. Rubin JS, Honigberg R: Sinusitis in patients with the acquired immunodeficiency syndrome. Ear Nose Throat J 69:460, 1990

180. Slavit DH, Yocum MW, Kern EB: Chronic sinusitis and dyspnea: Could this be AIDS? Otolaryngol Head Neck Surg 103:650, 1990

181. Schrager LK: Bacterial infections in AIDS patients. AIDS 2(suppl 1):S183, 1988

182. Follansbee SE: Other infections associated with AIDS. In Levy JA (ed): AIDS: Pathogenesis and Treatment, p 467. New York, Marcel Dekker, 1989

183. Blumberg HM, Stephens DS: Pyomyositis and human immunodeficiency virus infection. South Med J 83:1092, 1990

184. Winkler JR, Murray PA: Periodontal disease: A potential intraoral expression of AIDS may be rapidly progressive periodontitis. Can Dent Assoc J 1:20, 1987

185. Klein RS, Quart AM, Small CB: Periodontal disease in heterosexuals with acquired immunodeficiency syndrome. J Periodontol 62:535, 1991

186. Williams RC: Periodontal disease. N Engl J Med 322:373, 1990

187. Nahass RG, Weinstein MP, Bartels J, Gocke DJ: Infective endocarditis in intravenous drug users: A comparison of human immunodeficiency virus type 1-negative and -positive patients. J Infect Dis 162:967, 1990

Herpesvirus Infection in Individuals With HIV Infection

Chapter 11D

Robert T. Schooley

Herpesvirus infections account for more morbidity and mortality in individuals with advanced human immunodeficiency virus (HIV) infection than any other group of viral pathogens. Herpes simplex or herpes zoster infection may be the heralding clinical manifestation of HIV-related immune dysfunction.[1,2] Cytomegalovirus (CMV) is, in contrast, a pathogen that is likely to be present in HIV-infected individuals throughout the course of HIV infection, but it rarely causes disease until HIV-associated immunologic abnormalities are well advanced.[3] It has been speculated that Epstein-Barr virus (EBV) might play a role in the pathogenesis of lymphoid interstitial pneumonitis[4] and in the induction of non-Hodgkin's lymphoma in this patient population, especially lymphomas confined to the central nervous system (CNS).[5] Human herpesvirus type 6 (HHV-6) has not been demonstrated to directly cause morbidity in individuals with HIV infection, but it has been proposed as a potential cofactor that enhances replication of HIV in infected individuals.

In addition to their roles as pathogens in the setting of HIV infection, it has been suggested that the herpesviruses might play important roles in facilitating progression of HIV infection. Herpesviruses are potent immunomodulating agents, both in the context of primary infection[6,7] and in association with reactivation following immunosuppression.[8] Finally, molecular biologic studies have indicated that herpes group virus enhancing elements may promote HIV replication through effects on the *tat* gene product, and that HIV replication may promote replication of herpes group viruses.[9–12]

Thus, herpesviruses play important direct roles in induction of morbidity and mortality in HIV-infected individuals, and may in addition contribute to the progression of the underlying disease process. Although effective chemotherapy of herpesvirus infection in the setting of HIV infection may greatly reduce morbidity and mortality, significant unique problems with antiviral chemotherapy are present in this patient population. The first problem relates to the additional toxicity of antiviral chemotherapy in this setting because of the underlying degree of HIV-associated bone marrow dysfunction. This problem is further compounded by the fact that antiretroviral chemotherapeutic agents may also be myelosuppressive. Second, the prolonged immune dysfunction associated with HIV infection requires that antiherpesvirus therapy be continued for prolonged periods, thus enhancing problems associated with the emergence of herpesviruses with reduced susceptibility to chemotherapeutic agents.[13-15] Thus, effective management of herpesvirus infections poses significant challenges in the setting of HIV infection; nonetheless, successful recognition and management of these infections may play a major role in reducing morbidity and, possibly, may retard progression of the underlying HIV-associated immune dysfunction.

CYTOMEGALOVIRUS INFECTION

CMV infection is ubiquitous in the adult population. Several studies have demonstrated an extremely high seroprevalence rate among most HIV-infected populations.[16-18] Rates of isolation of CMV from urine and blood increase with progressive evidence of HIV-related immune dysfunction.[19,20] The increasing burden of CMV presumably reflects progressive depletion of CMV-specific cell-mediated immune responses.[21-24] Despite evidence of increasing CMV replication with progressive HIV-related immune dysfunction, morbidity directly due to CMV infection rarely is demonstrable until immune dysfunction is profound. Clinical manifestations of CMV infection in HIV-infected individuals most frequently involve the eye, but the gastrointestinal (GI) tract, the lungs, and the adrenal glands are also frequently affected.[25]

Clinical Syndromes Associated With CMV Infection

CMV RETINITIS

Retinitis due to CMV may be the presenting manifestation of HIV infection.[26,27] Usually, however, CMV retinitis does not occur until CD4 cell counts in the peripheral blood have declined to less than 50 cells/mm^3. CMV retinitis usually presents initially as a painless progressive loss of vision in individuals with advanced HIV infection. Depending on the location of the lesion and the frequency and vigor of routine ophthalmoscopic examination, the first manifestation of CMV retinitis may be the characteristic funduscopic abnormalities on physical examination. The funduscopic findings of CMV retinitis are usually quite distinctive[28-30] and include a localized yellowish lesion or lesions that initially favor the vascular arcades. As the lesion expands, a characteristic accompanying deep and superficial hemorrhagic retinitis develops.

In the setting of advanced HIV infection, unless treated with affective antiviral chemotherapeutic agents,

lesions of CMV retinitis expand in all directions and gradually coalesce to result in complete loss of vision in the affected eye.[29,30] The rate at which vision is lost depends on the tempo of the process and the degree to which the macula is involved by the process. Although CMV retinitis usually begins as a unilateral process, CMV infection is a systemic disease, and involvement of the contralateral retina almost always appears eventually if the process is not treated.

The microinfarctions of the retinal nerve fiber layer that appear funduscopically as cotton wool spots are a major differential diagnostic possibility in this setting. Such lesions are detected rather frequently in HIV infection and may represent direct involvement of the retina by HIV.[31] Although early CMV retinitis may be morphologically indistinguishable from cotton wool spots, the lesions of CMV retinitis progress and become hemorrhagic with ongoing observation. Cotton wool spots tend to be scattered and vary in number and distribution over time in HIV-infected individuals.

Although ocular *Toxoplasma* infection may occasionally mimic CMV retinitis,[32] the typical *Toxoplasma* lesion is more elevated because of choroidal involvement and the more intense vitritis and uveitis associated with *Toxoplasma gondii* infection.[29] Acute retinal necrosis[33-35] is a syndrome that may be seen in immunocompetent or immunocompromised individuals. This process is usually sudden in onset and rapidly progressive. The process is usually unilateral at presentation, but progresses to involve both eyes in roughly one third of cases.[34] Unlike most cases of CMV retinitis, patients with acute retinal necrosis frequently note mild to moderate pain, which is sometimes exacerbated by eye movement because of myositis or optic neuritis.[34] In contrast to CMV retinitis, individuals with acute retinal necrosis usually exhibit extraretinal ocular involvement with conjunctivitis, episcleritis, and keratic precipitates. The distribution and ophthalmoscopic appearance of retinal lesions are often useful in distinguishing CMV retinitis from acute retinal necrosis in that CMV retinitis often initially follows arcade vessels or involves the optic nerve, while acute retinal necrosis may initially be more peripheral in distribution. Acute retinal necrosis frequently includes a more prominent vitreous reaction and is more frequently associated with retinal detachment.[34] Evidence is emerging that herpes simplex virus (HSV) and varicella-zoster virus (VZV) are the most frequent etiologic agents for acute retinal necrosis.[35-41] Thus, the diagnostic distinction between CMV retinitis and acute retinal necrosis is quite important, because the initial antiviral chemotherapy preferred for acute retinal necrosis is high-dose intravenous (IV) acyclovir, rather than ganciclovir, and because more attention to the management of retinal detachment is required in acute retinal necrosis.

The diagnostic evaluation of individuals with HIV infection with possible CMV retinitis is relatively straightforward: the clinical setting, the tempo of the process, and the ophthalmoscopic findings are usually sufficient to make a firm diagnosis. Serologic studies for antibodies to CMV, *T. gondii,* HSV, or VZV are not helpful because of the frequency with which these agents occur in the adult population, and because seropositivity provides little insight into intraocular pathogenesis. In that CMV retinitis is a late-stage manifestation of HIV infection, isolation of CMV from urine or buffy coat cells would be expected in many individuals at risk for CMV retinitis, with or without ocular disease.[17,20] Thus, in most cases of CMV retinitis, the diagnosis hinges primarily on clinical rather than laboratory features. Although lesions of CMV retinitis are usually recognizable to experienced clinicians without ophthalmologic consultation, involvement of an ophthalmologist in the management of such cases is usually quite helpful from several standpoints. First, CMV retinitis is merely an ocular manifestation of a systemic process. In some cases the initial involvement may affect primarily peripheral areas of the retina, and thus may be most demonstrable with indirect ophthalmoscopy. In individuals with advanced HIV infection and unexplained weight loss and fever, ophthalmologic consultation for early evidence of CMV retinitis is often quite helpful. Ophthalmologic consultation is mandatory in cases in which the presentation is atypical, and in which other differential diagnostic possibilities are more important. Perhaps the most important aspect of ophthalmologic consultation is the role an ophthalmologist can play in documenting the extent of retinal involvement for assessment of response to therapy. The initial and subsequent ophthalmologic evaluation should include detailed mapping of the extent of the process, including the distribution of hemorrhage. Funduscopic photography is often a useful adjunct in the management of patients with CMV retinitis. The utility of routine prospective ophthalmologic consultation in individuals with HIV infection is controversial. Although some clinicians advocate ophthalmologic evaluations as frequently as every 6 months, the cost-effectiveness of this approach is debatable. It is more prudent to perform a baseline evaluation at the time of diagnosis of HIV infection and to reserve subsequent evaluations for HIV-infected individuals with ocular symptoms or with late-stage disease, who are thus at greatly increased risk of CMV infection.

The natural history of untreated CMV retinitis involves progressive enlargement of individual lesions and the appearance of scattered new lesions. Lesions gradually coalesce to lead to blindness. Although involvement may initially be unilateral, eventual bilateral involvement is the rule rather than the exception. Thus, patients with CMV retinitis should receive antiviral chemotherapy from the time of initial diagnosis.

GASTROINTESTINAL INVOLVEMENT WITH CMV

The GI manifestations of CMV infection may include any portion of the GI tract from the mouth to the anus.[25] As in the case of retinitis, GI tract involvement usually is not encountered until late in the HIV-related disease process. GI tract involvement by CMV infection may be isolated manifestation of the disease, but it is also seen in individuals with CMV retinitis.

CMV Stomatitis   Oral ulceration is frequently encountered in HIV infection. Although the most frequent cause of oral ulceration is aphthous stomatitis, the process may be associated with HIV chemotherapy[42] or with a number of pathogens, including HSV[1] and CMV.[43] Aphthous stomatitis is usually diagnosed on the basis of the clinical appearance of the lesions. In aphthous stomatitis the lesions are painful and appear as scattered shallow ulcerations that appear intermittently. These lesions may be difficult to distinguish from the stomatitis associated with dideoxycytidine therapy.[42] Evaluation of persistent or progressive ulcerating oral lesions should include cultures for HSV and biopsies for evidence of CMV infection or malignancy.

CMV Esophagitis   Esophagitis is a frequent GI manifestation of CMV infection.[44,45] The process is indistinguishable clinically from that attributable to *Candida albicans* or HSV. The presence of extensive oral candidiasis may suggest esophageal candidal involvement in individuals with esophageal symptoms; however, candidal esophagitis may be present without oral involvement, particularly in individuals using topical oral prophylaxis with nystatin or clotrimazole. In addition, the pathogenesis of esophagitis may be multifactorial, involving both CMV and topical fungal colonization. An esophagogram that demonstrates discrete ulcerative lesions against a background of normal esophageal mucosa is suggestive of herpetic or CMV esophagitis,[44] but the definitive diagnosis usually requires direct endoscopic visualization, cultures, and biopsies. Because CMV is frequently found in the salivary secretions of healthy people, the isolation of CMV from cultures of material obtained endoscopically must be interpreted with caution.

CMV Gastritis   CMV gastritis may manifest with abdominal pain or with antral involvement and obstruction.[46–48] CMV gastritis is often accompanied by esophagitis. Thus, such patients will often also complain of dysphagia, odynophagia, and epigastric pain. The major differential diagnostic possibilities are peptic ulcer disease or involvement by *C. albicans* or HSV. Establishing a firm diagnosis of CMV gastritis requires endoscopy with a biopsy that demonstrates histologic evidence of CMV infection.

CMV Colitis   The colon is the most frequently symptomatic target of CMV replication in the GI tract. Patients with CMV colitis present with diarrhea and abdominal pain that may initially be intermittent, and the diarrhea usually is not bloody.[49–52] The initial clinical evaluation should include an investigation for other enteric pathogens, including *Mycobacterium avium-intracellulare, Salmonella* spp., *Shigella* spp., *Campylobacter jejuni,*

Yersinia enterocolitica, Entamoeba histolytica, Cryptosporidium, and *Giardia lamblia.* In that many individuals at risk for CMV colitis may also be receiving courses of antimicrobial therapy, *Clostridium difficile*–induced colitis must also be ruled out. If fecal examinations fail to demonstrate the presence of any of these pathogens, a barium enema examination and colonscopy are indicated. Barium enema examination may reveal mucosal granularity, thickened folds, superficial erosions, and spasticity.[53,54] Involvement may be focal or diffuse.[53] A normal barium enema examination does not rule out CMV colitis. Colonoscopy characteristically reveals a hemorrhagic colitis that may be diffuse or segmental. The diagnosis rests on the demonstration of typical intranuclear inclusions in rectal or colonic mucosal tissue. Neutrophilic infiltration and CMV inclusions in endothelial cells are also often observed. Viral cultures may be obtained from GI mucosal biopsies, but cultures of stool for CMV are not helpful.

If untreated, CMV colitis is associated with ongoing diarrhea, inanition, and wasting. Ulcerative lesions may progress to colonic perforation.[55-58] Thus, all patients with proven CMV colitis are candidates for antiviral chemotherapy.

CMV HEPATITIS AND CHOLECYSTITIS

CMV may also affect the biliary tract.[59-62] Although CMV inclusions in the liver are not infrequently seen at autopsy,[63] CMV-induced hepatitis *per se* is extremely unusual in individuals with HIV infection.[3] Biliary tract involvement may manifest as right upper quadrant pain associated with elevated serum alkaline phosphatase levels and mildly elevated hepatic transaminase levels. Such individuals may develop papillary stenosis with secondary bacterial cholangitis,[61] acalculous cholecystitis,[62] and dual infection with *Cryptosporidium.*[59] The treatment of patients with biliary disease due to CMV includes attention to mechanical issues associated with obstruction[61] and antiviral chemotherapy, although there have been no controlled trials of antiviral therapy in this setting.

CMV INVOLVEMENT OF THE CNS

Histologic changes in the CNS compatible with CMV infection have been noted in several clinical series.[64-67] CMV has also been reported in association with ascending myelitis[68] and subacute polyneuropathy[69] in patients with AIDS. Despite the histologic findings at autopsy suggestive of CMV infection, it is highly likely that many of the earlier reports of CNS morbidity due to CMV in HIV-infected individuals failed to take into account the direct role of HIV as an etiologic agent for encephalitis in this clinical setting.[70-73] Thus, a diagnosis of CMV encephalitis in the setting of HIV infection must be viewed with skepticism. Evidence of a role for CMV in radicular neuropathy is more compelling,[69] and certainly warrants a trial of antiviral chemotherapy.

CMV PNEUMONITIS

CMV is frequently isolated from materials recovered from pulmonary sources in HIV-infected individuals.[74,75] The high frequency with which the organism occurs in HIV-infected individuals undergoing pulmonary diagnostic procedures renders interpretation of isolation of CMV difficult.[76] Although demonstration of both CMV and *P. carinii* is associated with a worse prognosis than when only *P. carinii* is demonstrated,[77] it is difficult to determine whether such findings should be interpreted as an indication of a dual contribution to pathology, or whether CMV isolation is simply a surrogate marker for a more severely immunocompromised state. In other series it has not been demonstrated that isolation of CMV from bronchoalveolar lavage (BAL) fluid represents a worse prognosis in patients with *P. carinii* pneumonia.[78] One rather extensive autopsy series demonstrated that CMV inclusions were frequently found in pulmonary tissues of those dying of HIV infection; however, CMV as an isolated cause of pneumonia was extremely infrequent.[79] Thus, as in the case of the CNS, determining whether isolation of CMV from pulmonary sources indicates pathology or colonization is difficult. Therapeutic decisions about the importance of CMV isolated from BAL fluid must often be made in patients who have undergone bronchoscopy for presumed *P. carinii* pneumonia and who have not responded to anti-*Pneumocystis* therapy. The recent demonstration that early corticosteroid therapy improves the prognosis of those with moderate to severe CMV pneumonitis suggests that much of the morbidity that in the past had been attributed to CMV might reflect unrelated inflammatory processes initiated by anti-*Pneumocystis* therapy.[80,81] Thus, CMV pneumonia is a rare entity in the setting of HIV infection. Definitive diagnosis requires the demonstration of typical intranuclear inclusions in pulmonary tissue, and should not rest solely on isolation of CMV from BAL fluid. Once the diagnosis of CMV pneumonia is established, antiviral therapy is indicated.

CMV ADRENALITIS

Reports of adrenal insufficiency associated with CMV infection have also appeared.[82,83] The diagnosis should be suspected in individuals with symptoms or signs of adrenal insufficiency in the setting of advanced HIV disease, particularly if disease attributable to CMV has been demonstrated in other organs. The diagnosis is made by a cosyntropin stimulation test.

CMV INVOLVEMENT OF OTHER TISSUES

CMV inclusions have been demonstrated in a wide variety of other organs at autopsy.[77] It is difficult to discern how frequently such demonstrations indicate a role for CMV in the induction of pathology. Nonetheless, cases of epididymitis,[84] cervicitis,[85] and pancreatitis[86-88] attributable to CMV have been reported in the setting of HIV infection, suggesting that, on occasion, the presence of CMV in such sites may be indicative of CMV-associated morbidity.

Treatment of CMV Infection in the Setting of HIV Infection

Antiviral chemotherapy for CMV infection has evolved rapidly in the past 5 years. With the initial descriptions of the efficacy of ganciclovir for CMV retinitis,[89,90] it became apparent both that therapy for CMV infection was plausible and that HIV infection was an excellent setting for the evaluation of antiviral agents with putative activity against CMV.

GANCICLOVIR

Ganciclovir (9-[1,3-dihydroxy-2-propoxy)methyl]-guanine) is a nucleoside analogue with substantial activity against CMV, HSV, VZV, and EBV.[91,92] The drug is metabolized to its triphosphate derivative (ganciclovir-TP) by a process that involves cellular kinases.[93,94] The drug is administered by IV infusion and has a terminal serum half-life of 3 to 4 hours.[95] The half-life of intracellular ganciclovir-TP is in excess of 12 hours; thus, dosing regimens with 12-hour dosing intervals are quite feasible. In that excretion is almost exclusively renal, ganciclovir clearance correlates directly with the creatinine clearance. Ganciclovir is removed by hemodialysis. Serum levels following a 4-hour hemodialysis are roughly half predialysis levels.[95] Oral absorption of ganciclovir is limited,[96] although several studies of oral administration are underway.

The toxicity of ganciclovir is primarily hematologic. In the initial clinical trials of ganciclovir in patients with HIV infection, neutropenia was encountered in 25% to 35% of the study subjects.[97,98] Thrombocytopenia has also been reported with ganciclovir therapy,[97] as have thrombophlebitis,[99] nausea, and transient disorientation.[97] The hematologic toxicity of ganciclovir is further exacerbated by co-administration of zidovudine.[100,101] Because most HIV-infected patients with CMV-induced morbidity have advanced HIV infection, almost all will be candidates for concomitant antiretroviral chemotherapy.

Although there have been case reports of individuals with HIV infection who presented with CMV retinitis not previously treated with zidovudine and in whom the CMV retinitis transiently remitted with zidovudine therapy,[102] most HIV-infected patients with CMV-induced morbidity either will be taking or will have previously received antiretroviral therapy. It is clear that, once established in HIV-infected patients, CMV infection is progressive, particularly in the case of CMV colitis[56-58] and retinitis.[103] Thus, observation for evidence of progression of CMV disease is rarely warranted.

Therapy with ganciclovir is usually initiated at 5 mg/kg twice daily and maintained for 14 days. Initial response rates in the range of 80% to 90% are to be expected for CMV retinitis and colitis.[97,98,104,105] Response rates for other CMV syndromes are less well delineated, as few organized clinical trials restricted to other syndromes have been undertaken.

In the setting of CMV infection, relapse is virtually certain if maintenance therapy is not employed after the initial induction phase.[97] Maintenance therapy with ganciclovir is recommended at a daily dosage of 5 mg/kg IV. This should be continued indefinitely in almost all patients with HIV infection and CMV-induced morbidity.

Concomitant administration of zidovudine and ganciclovir is possible, although management of dual therapy requires close attention to hematologic toxicity.[101,106] In individuals who are already receiving zidovudine and who present with CMV-associated morbidity, temporary discontinuation of antiretroviral therapy during the period of induction therapy with ganciclovir is prudent. After patients are stable on maintenance ganciclovir therapy, reintroduction of zidovudine is warranted. If patients are unable to tolerate both drugs, the use of agents such as granulocyte colony-stimulating factor[107] or granulocyte-macrophage colony-stimulating factor[108,109] may be indicated. Substitution of dideoxyinosine[110] or dideoxycytidine[111] for zidovudine is also an acceptable approach.

Prolonged ganciclovir therapy for CMV infection is associated with the emergence of resistant isolates of CMV.[112] This observation was first made in two patients with AIDS and in another with leukemia. In each patient, emergence of ganciclovir-resistant isolates of CMV was noted after 2 to 5 months of therapy. The mechanism by which resistance develops is not clear, but it is clear that the HIV-infected patient treated with prolonged ganciclovir therapy is at great risk for the development of resistance.

FOSCARNET

In the setting of resistant virus, or in individuals with CMV infection requiring therapy but who are unable to tolerate ganciclovir therapy, foscarnet is an acceptable alternative agent. Foscarnet is active against all five herpes group viruses, including CMV, and HIV.[113,114] The drug is poorly absorbed after oral administration.[115] The pharmacokinetics following IV administration are complex and influenced by the competing uptake of foscarnet by bone and elimination by the kidneys.[115] After intermittent bolus dosing the serum half-life in man is in the range of 3 to 4 hours.[116]

In the case of CMV retinitis, foscarnet has been used primarily for individuals who are intolerant of ganciclovir or in whom disease progresses despite ganciclovir therapy. A recently completed randomized study of foscarnet and ganciclovir as initial therapy for CMV retinitis revealed that, although ophthalmologic response rates were similar, mortality rates were substantially higher in those randomized to initial ganciclovir therapy.[119a]

The reason for the decreased mortality rate among foscarnet recipients could not be determined, but it might be a reflection of the increased antiretroviral therapy received by foscarnet recipients and/or the synergistic antiretroviral activity exhibited by zidovudine and foscarnet.[119b] As a result of this study, the role of foscarnet as an alternative agent to ganciclovir is currently under reassessment. In these settings foscarnet has the advantage of exhibiting no bone marrow toxicity and of maintaining antiviral activity against ganciclovir-resistant strains of CMV.[112] In the case of newly diagnosed CMV retinitis, response rates to foscarnet are similar to those for ganciclovir.[117–119] The major toxic effect associated with foscarnet is renal dysfunction, which is exacerbated in individuals who have not been fully hydrated.[118,110] Anemia and tremors have also been observed. Acute overdosing with foscarnet results in decreases in serum ionized calcium levels owing to the calcium chelating properties of the drug. Although the nephrotoxicity associated with foscarnet is easily monitored, most clinicians prefer to initiate therapy with ganciclovir and to reserve foscarnet for individuals with ganciclovir intolerance or in whom disease progresses despite ganciclovir therapy. *In vitro* susceptibility testing of CMV isolates from individuals with progressive disease who are receiving ganciclovir therapy correlates well with the clinical response to therapy; thus, routine susceptibility testing of CMV isolates is rarely required for clinical decision-making.

FUTURE DEVELOPMENTS

Several future developments in the treatment of CMV infection are to be expected. Several groups have investigated the use of intravitreal ganciclovir as maintenance therapy for individuals with CMV retinitis and HIV infection who do not tolerate IV therapy.[120–122] It has been demonstrated in bone marrow allograft recipients with CMV pneumonia that combination therapy with ganciclovir and CMV immune globulin is superior to treatment with either component alone.[123–126] Similar approaches are currently under investigation in the setting of HIV infection. The demonstration of synergistic antiviral activity *in vitro*[127,128] with combined ganciclovir and foscarnet has led to early pilot trials of combination chemotherapy with these two agents. Finally, several additional compounds, such as the phosphonylmethoxyalkylpurines and pyrimidines, have demonstrated substantial antiviral activity *in vitro*[129,130] and are currently entering clinical trials. Thus, over the next several years, it is to be expected that the introduction of novel agents and the application of combination chemotherapy will further improve CMV therapy in patients with HIV infection.

HERPES SIMPLEX VIRUS

Progressive oral and perianal HSV infection was one of the initial clinical manifestations that brought AIDS to medical attention.[1] In the past decade it became apparent that HSV may cause major morbidity in individuals with HIV infection, and that, as in the case of CMV infection, such individuals need prolonged therapy and are at risk for the emergence of resistant viruses. As in the case of CMV infections, HSV infection in individuals with HIV infection may cause substantial direct morbidity.[1,131] In addition, destruction of mucosal and cutaneous barriers by progressive HSV infection may increase the risk of infection with bacterial or fungal agents. It has been demonstrated that HSV-2 seropositivity is an independent risk factor for HIV seroconversion.[132] Although HSV seropositivity could be a surrogate marker for sexual activity, it is also quite possible that cutaneous and mucosal disruption caused by HSV infection could enhance the transmissibility of HIV infection.

Clinical Syndromes due to HSV Infection

As in the nonimmunocompromised patient population, oral and genital sites account for the majority of morbidity due to HSV in individuals with HIV infection. In either site, the process is usually due to reactivation of latent virus rather than to primary infection. Many individuals note progressively more frequent or more severe bouts of oral or genital herpes simplex infection as HIV-induced immune dysfunction progresses. In the case of homosexual men, perianal herpes simplex lesions may also become more frequent or severe.[1,131] In most cases the diagnosis is relatively straightforward and does not require confirmation by culture, biopsy, or Tsanck preparation. Nonetheless, particularly in the setting of more advanced disease, perianal and genital lesions may have an atypical appearance because of maceration or superinfection with other organisms. Under these circumstances, clinicians should maintain a low threshold for obtaining viral cultures, even when lesion morphology might make HSV infection seem unlikely.

HSV is also a common cause of esophagitis in advanced HIV infection.[44] Although many patients with HSV esophagitis exhibit concurrent oral lesions due to HSV, such lesions may be absent or atypical. Furthermore, the presence of orolabial HSV infection does not ensure that esophageal disease is due to HSV. Radiographic studies may help distinguish lesions from *Candida* esophagitis but cannot distinguish between CMV- and HSV-induced esophagitis.[44] The definitive diagnosis rests with esophagoscopy and biopsy, although many clinicians advocate a therapeutic trial of acyclovir therapy before subjecting patients to endoscopy. As in the case of CMV, however, isolation of virus from esophageal washings must be interpreted with caution because of the high prevalence of HSV excretion in oral secretions in the general population.

Cutaneous herpesvirus infections, particularly those involving the digits (herpetic whitlow), may also cause substantial morbidity in HIV-infected individuals.[133–136] As in the case of oral or genital lesions, herpetic whitlow may initially appear intermittently and become progressive and persistent as the HIV-associated immunodeficiency becomes more severe. The major differential diagnostic problem with herpetic whitlow stems from the fact that if the diagnosis is not considered, bacterial pathogens may receive the major attention in the initial evaluation.

HSV may also cause aseptic meningitis in patients with or without immune dysfunction.[137] In most cases, these individuals will exhibit concurrent genital or perianal lesions. Virus may be isolated from the cerebrospinal fluid if a lumbar puncture is performed during an acute exacerbation. One case of central diabetes insipidus in association with aseptic meningitis has been reported.[138] Despite the occurrence of HSV-induced aseptic meningitis in the setting of HIV infection, encephalitis due to HSV is extremely uncommon.

Treatment of HSV Infection in the Setting of HIV

Acyclovir is the drug of choice for the initial management of HSV infection in HIV-infected patients. The drug is available in IV, oral, and topical formulations and is well tolerated by most individuals with HIV infection. Acyclovir is active *in vitro* against HSV-1, HSV-2, VZV, and EBV in concentrations that are easily achievable after oral or IV administration.[134-143] The major toxic effect associated with the drug is reversible nephrotoxicity, which is most easily demonstrable when acyclovir administered by rapid bolus to individuals who are not well hydrated.

The renal dysfunction is related to the serum level achieved following bolus administration of acyclovir.[144,145] In that oral administration is not associated with high peak serum levels, renal dysfunction is not a feature of oral administration. Occasional patients have been reported with confusion, seizures, or altered mental status associated with acyclovir therapy.[146-148] An early report that acyclovir and zidovudine exhibited synergistic antiretroviral activity has not been confirmed by other investigators.[149] Thus, acyclovir should be reserved for the treatment or suppression of HSV-associated morbidity.

In HIV-infected individuals with mild recurrent oral, genital, or perianal HSV infection, the same general approach used in the nonimmunocompromised patient population is warranted. Although topical therapy has been shown to be useful in primary herpes simplex genitalis infection,[150] it has not demonstrated utility in recurrent oral[151] or genital disease.[152] Despite the demonstration that topical acyclovir may decrease mucocutaneous disease in immunocompromised patients,[153] topical therapy has little role in this patient population.

Oral therapy may be used for individuals with mild recurrent disease, either for acute bouts of infection[154-156] or for chronic suppression in individuals with frequently recurrent disease.[157-159] In these settings initiation of therapy at a dosage of 200 mg five times daily is appropriate. If the suppressive strategy is adopted,

the daily maintenance dose needed to prevent recurrence may vary between 600 and 1,000 mg. In the case of primary disease, or if the disease is extensive, or if compliance or GI absorption is in question, initiation of therapy with IV acyclovir is warranted.[160,161] As in the case of CMV infection, in patients with HIV infection and severe mucocutaneous disease due to HSV, particularly those with extensive orolabial, perianal, genital, or esophageal disease, maintenance therapy is usually necessary. Under most circumstances successful suppression can be maintained for prolonged periods with oral therapy.

Resistance of HSV to acyclovir was well described prior to the widespread use of the agent in the setting of HIV infection.[162-165] This problem is being recognized increasingly frequently in the setting of HIV infection, because these individuals often present with extensive lesions (and thus with a large viral burden) and require prolonged or repeated treatment with acyclovir.[166-171] Isolates are usually resistant to acyclovir on the basis of altered thymidine kinase activity and thus are cross-resistant to ganciclovir. Thymidine kinase activity is not required for induction of antiviral activity of either vidarabine (ara-A) or foscarnet; thus, most acyclovir-resistant isolates remain susceptible to vidarabine and foscarnet. Although both foscarnet[169,172-174] and vidarabine have been used in the treatment of acyclovir-resistant HSV infections, a randomized controlled trial has demonstrated that foscarnet is superior to vidarabine in this setting because of its antiviral activity and lower toxicity.[175]

VARICELLA-ZOSTER VIRUS

Primary VZV infection manifests clinically as chickenpox. Following primary infection the virus remains in latent form within dorsal nerve root ganglia. Reactivation of VZV replication, which is observed more frequently with aging or in the setting of immunosuppression, manifests clinically as herpes zoster. In that most individuals with HIV infection are adults, the major morbidity associated with VZV in HIV-infected individuals results from reactivation of infection rather than from primary infection. Indeed, because herpes zoster is relatively uncommon in individuals less than 50 years old, the occurrence of herpes zoster in younger individuals should raise the question of underlying HIV infection.[2,176,177]

Chickenpox

Primary VZV infection in the setting of HIV infection is observed relatively infrequently in the United States. Because varicella tends to be more severe in adults[178] and in immunocompromised individuals,[179] the occurrence of chickenpox in an adult known to be HIV seropositive should usually be treated with antiviral therapy. If an HIV-infected adult with chickenpox is known to have a relatively intact cell-mediated immune response by virtue of a recent CD4 cell determination, and if there is no evidence of pulmonary or CNS involvement,[180–182] oral therapy with acyclovir at a dosage of 800 mg five times daily is warranted.[183] If the individual is known to be significantly immunocompromised or if there is evidence of visceral involvement, IV acyclovir therapy is required.[184] Oral acyclovir has also been shown to be beneficial in the treatment of chickenpox in nonimmunocompromised children.[185] In HIV-infected children with any significant degree of immune dysfunction, however, IV acyclovir therapy should be used, as in the case of other immunocompromised children.[186] The long-term effects of chickenpox in individuals with HIV infection have not been delineated, although it is quite possible that such individuals will suffer from herpes zoster relatively soon after the bout of chickenpox because of the decreased ability to mount vigorous immune response.[177]

Herpes Zoster

Herpes zoster infection may be the initial clinical manifestation of HIV infection,[2,176,177] although it is important to emphasize that herpes zoster occurs without demonstrable underlying immunodeficiency in middle-aged individuals.[187–189] Herpes zoster is usually self-limiting, even in individuals with relatively advanced HIV infection, although such individuals are at risk of developing chronic progressive cutaneous[190–195] or CNS[196] infection following herpes zoster infection. It is the impression (not proved) of many clinicians that herpes zoster is both more severe and more prolonged in individuals with advanced HIV infection, and that such individuals are more likely to develop chronic scarring or postherpetic neuralgia than are individuals with intact immune responses.

The management of HIV-infected individuals with herpes zoster has not yet been subjected to randomized controlled trials. By analogy with the approach outlined earlier for chickenpox, it seems prudent to treat HIV-infected individuals know to be relatively immunocompetent with high-dose oral acyclovir, and to use IV acyclovir in individuals with advanced immune dysfunction or with extensive dermatomal involvement, severe pain, or evidence of cutaneous or visceral dissemination. Although insight into the recently recognized syndrome of chronic varicella is rapidly emerging, acyclovir-resistant isolates of VZV have already been recognized in this setting.[193–194] Foscarnet has been used in the treatment of chronic VZV infection resistant to acyclovir, but the results in one small series of patients were equivocal at best.[195]

EPSTEIN-BARR VIRUS

EBV is very common in individuals with or at risk for HIV infection.[17,197] EBV expression, as quantitated by oropharyngeal isolation,[198,199] the number of EBV-infected B cells in the peripheral blood,[200] or EBV DNA in oropharyngeal secretions,[201] is elevated in individuals with HIV infection. In that EBV replication is controlled primarily by cell-mediated immune responses,[202,203] and in that EBV-specific cytotoxic T-cell responses decline in parallel with increasing HIV-associated immune dysfunction,[204,205] the increased rates of viral expression[198–201] and the compensatory increases in EBV-specific humoral immune responses[205–208] would be expected from knowledge of the immunobiology of herpes group and retroviral infections. EBV is a potent immunomodulatory agent in the setting of either primary infection[6] or reactivation.[8] The role of EBV as an immunomodulator, coupled with the transactivating capabilities of herpes group and retroviral regulatory elements,[9,10] has led to speculation that EBV might serve as a cofactor that could stimulate progression of HIV-associated immune dysfunction. Despite these biologic interactions, no sero-epidemiologic support for this hypothesis has yet been obtained.[209]

AIDS-Associated Lymphoma

Non-Hodgkin's lymphoma was recognized early in the AIDS epidemic as one of the major AIDS-associated malignancies.[210,211] The presence of EBV nucleic acid in all cases of African Burkitt's lymphoma, the demonstration of decreased EBV-specific cell-mediated immune responses, and the increased replicative rate of EBV in HIV infection have led to speculation that EBV might play a contributory or etiologic role in the pathogenesis of HIV-associated lymphoma. EBV sequences are detectable in a relatively large fraction of B-cell lymphomas in the setting of HIV infection,[5,212–218] particularly CNS lymphomas.[5,219–222] As more sophisticated histologic, immunocytochemical, and molecular biologic analyses have been applied to AIDS-associated lymphomas, it has become apparent that these malignancies are a heterogeneous group of disorders.[5,214,215] It is clear that EBV sequences are detectable in virtually all CNS lymphomas in the setting of HIV infection.[5,219–222] These tumors are usually not associated with B-cell malignancy outside the CNS. On the other hand, investigations of extracranial tumors has revealed the presence of EBV sequences in a variable portion of tumors. The histologic heterogeneity and the varying clinical courses seen in these peripheral lymphomas suggest that multiple factors may play a role in their pathogenesis. Despite the presence of EBV DNA in many AIDS-associated lymphomas, the precise role of EBV in the pathogenesis of AIDS-associated malignancy has not been fully delineated.

Hairy Leukoplakia

Oral hairy leukoplakia is characterized by white, frond-like lesions that are adherent to the tongue, particularly to its lateral aspects.[223] These lesions are noted in individuals with HIV infection and may be confused with oral candiasis. In contrast to oral candidiasis, the lesions associated with hairy leukoplakia are difficult to scrape from the tongue and are usually not painful. *In situ* hybridization studies have demonstrated the presence of EBV sequences within these lesions.[223–225] Although one study has suggested that hairy leukoplakia is a prognostic feature associated with progression of HIV infection,[226] the association is much less strong than with immunologic markers such as CD4 cell enumeration. Even though hairy leukoplakia will often regress with high-dose oral acyclovir therapy,[227] the lesions are rarely painful enough to warrant therapy and are most important as an oral indication that HIV infection should be considered when such lesions are noted. EBV DNA has also been detected in biopsy specimens obtained from esophageal ulcers, suggesting that EBV may also contribute to esophageal morbidity in individuals with HIV infection.[228]

Lymphoid Interstitial Pneumonitis

Several investigators have detected EBV DNA in pulmonary tissue obtained from children with HIV-associated lymphoid interstitial pneumonitis (LIP).[4,229–230] As in the case of AIDS-associated lymphoma, the role of EBV in the pathogenesis of HIV-associated LIP remains unclear.

HUMAN HERPESVIRUS TYPE 6

HHV-6 was initially isolated from the peripheral blood of six individuals with lymphoproliferative disorders.[231] Two of these individuals had AIDS. The virus is a gamma herpesvirus that has since been isolated from the peripheral blood and saliva of both healthy and immunocompromised individuals.[232–235] It has been demonstrated that most individuals acquire antibodies to HHV-6 during the first year of life,[236] and that the virus is the etiologic agent for exanthem subitum.[237] HHV-6 has been postulated to be a cofactor in the progression of HIV disease in that it, too, can upregulate the HIV long terminal repeat segment,[238] and it has been shown to enhance HIV expression in one tissue culture system.[239] Epidemiologic investigations suggest that HHV-6 infection does not play a significant role in acceleration of HIV infection *in vivo*.[240–242] Thus, it is clear that HHV-6 is a common agent that shares many epidemiologic features with other herpes group viruses. At this point a role for HHV-6 in the pathogenesis of HIV infection has not been convincingly demonstrated.

REFERENCES

1. Siegal FP, Lopez C, Hammer GS et al: Severe acquired immunodeficiency in male homosexuals manifested by chronic perianal ulcerative herpes simplex lesions. N Engl J Med 305:1439, 1981
2. Friedman-Kein AE, Lafleur FL, Gendler E et al: Herpes zoster: A possible early clinical sign for development of acquired immunodeficiency syndrome in high-risk individuals. J Am Acad Dermatol 14:1023, 1986
3. Jacobson MA, Mills J: Serious cytomegalovirus disease in the acquired immunodeficiency syndrome (AIDS). Ann Intern Med 108:585, 1988
4. Andiman WA, Gradoville L, Heston R et al: Use of cloned probes to detect Epstein Barr viral DNA in tissues of patients with neoplastic and lymphoproliferative diseases. J Infect Dis 148:967, 1983
5. McGrath MS, Shiramizu B, Meeker TC et al: Aids-associated polyclonal lymphoma: Identification of a new HIV-associated disease process. J AIDS 4:408, 1991
6. Reinherz EL, O'Brien C, Rosenthal P, Schlossman SF: The cellular basis for viral-induced immunodeficiency: Analysis by monoclonal antibodies. J Immunol 125:1269, 1980
7. Carney WP, Rubin RH, Hoffman RA et al: Analysis of T lymphocyte subsets in cytomegalovirus mononucleosis. J Immunol 126:2114, 1981
8. Schooley RT, Hirsch MS, Colvin RB et al: Association of herpesvirus infections with T-lymphocyte-subset alterations, glomerulopathy, and opportunistic infections after renal transplantation. N Engl J Med 308:307, 1983
9. Gendelman HE, Phelps W, Feigenbaum L et al: *Trans*-activation of the human immunodeficiency virus long terminal repeat sequence by DNA viruses. Proc Natl Acad Sci USA 83:9759, 1986
10. Mosca JD, Bednarik DP, Raj NBK et al: Herpes simplex virus type-1 can reactivate transcription of latent human immunodeficiency virus. Nature 325:67, 1987
11. Skolnik PR, Kosloff BR, Hirsch MS: Bidirectional interactions between human immunodeficiency virus type 1 and cytomegalovirus. J Infect Dis 157:508, 1988
12. Montagnier L, Gruest J, Chamaret S et al: Adaptation of lymphadenopathy associated virus (LAV) to replication in EBV-transformed B lymphoblastoid cell lines. Science 225:63, 1984
13. Hirsch MS, Schooley RT: Resistance to antiviral drugs: The end of innocence (editorial). N Engl J Med 320:313, 1989
14. Drew WL: Clinical use of ganciclovir for cytomegalovirus infection and the development of drug resistance. J AIDS 4:542, 1991
15. Erlich KS, Mills J, Chatis P et al: Acyclovir-resistant herpes simplex virus infections in patients with the acquired immunodeficiency syndrome. N Engl J Med 320:293, 1989
16. Drew WL, Mintz L, Miner RC, Sands M et al: Prevalence of cytomegalovirus infection in homosexual men. J Infect Dis 143:188, 1981
17. Quinnan GV, Masur H, Rook AH et al: Herpesvirus infections in the acquired immune deficiency syndrome. JAMA 252:72, 1984
18. Quinn TC, Piot P, McCormick JB et al: Serologic and immunologic studies in patients with AIDS in North America and Africa: The potential role of infectious agents as cofactors in human immunodeficiency virus infection. JAMA 257:2617, 1987
19. Lange M, Klein EB, Kornfield H et al: Cytomegalovirus isolation from healthy homosexual men. JAMA 252:1908, 1984
20. Collier AC, Meyers JD, Corey L et al: Cytomegalovirus infection in homosexual men: Relationship to sexual practices, antibody to human immunodeficiency virus, and cell-mediated immunity. Am J Med 82:593, 1987
21. Quinnan GV, Siegel JP, Epstein JS et al: Mechanisms of

T-cell functional deficiency in the acquired immunodeficiency syndrome. Ann Intern Med 103:710, 1985

22. Rook AH, Manischewitz JF, Frederick WR et al: Deficient, HLA-restricted, cytomegalovirus-specific cytotoxic T cells and natural killer cells in patients with the acquired immunodeficiency syndrome. J Infect Dis 152:627, 1985

23. Epstein JS, Frederick WR, Rook AH et al: Selective defects in cytomegalovirus- and mitogen-induced lymphocyte proliferation and interferon release in patients with acquired immunodeficiency syndrome. J Infect Dis 152:727, 1985

24. Rook AH, Masur H, Lane HC et al: Interleukin-2 enhances the depressed natural killer and cytomegalovirus-specific cytotoxic activities of lymphocytes from patients with the acquired immune deficiency syndrome. J Clin Invest 72:398, 1983

25. Schooley RT: Cytomegalovirus infection in the setting of infection with human immunodeficiency virus. Rev Infect Dis 17:S811, 1990

26. Henderly DE, Freeman WR, Smith RE et al: Cytomegalovirus retinitis as the initial manifestation of the acquired immune deficiency syndrome. Am J Ophthalmol 103:316, 1987

27. Jabs DA, Enger C, Bartlett JG: Cytomegalovirus retinitis and acquired immunodeficiency syndrome. Arch Ophthalmol 107:75, 1989

28. Hennis HL, Scott AA, Apple DJ: Cytomegalovirus retinitis. Surv Ophthalmol 34:193, 1989

29. Henderly DE, Jampol LM: Diagnosis and treatment of cytomegalovirus retinitis. J AIDS 4:S6, 1991

30. Palestine AG: Clinical aspects of cytomegalovirus retinitis. Rev Infect Dis 10:S515, 1988

31. Pomerantz RJ, Kuritzkes DR, de la Monte SM et al: Infection of the retina by human immunodeficiency virus type 1 (HIV-1). N Engl J Med 317:1643, 1987

32. Holland GN, Engstrom RE, Glasgow BJ et al: Ocular toxoplasmosis in patients with the acquired immunodeficiency syndrome. Am J Ophthalmol 106:653, 1988

33. Willerson D Jr, Aaberg TM, Reeser FH et al: Necrotizing vaso-occlusive retinitis. Am J Ophthalmol 84:209, 1977

34. Duker JS, Blumenkranz MS: Surv Ophthalmol 35:327, 1991

35. Grutzmacher RD, Henderson D, McDonald PJ, Coster DJ: Herpes simplex chorioretinitis in a healthy adult. Am J Ophthalmol 96:788, 1983

36. Ludwig IH, Zegerra H, Zakov ZN: The acute retinal necrosis syndrome: Possible herpes simplex retinitis. Ophthalmology 91:1659, 1984

37. Imura N, Imura R, Oku H et al: Rise of antibody titer for varicella zoster virus in the aqueous and vitreous in two cases with Kirasawa uveitis. Jpn J Clin Ophthalmol 39:101, 1985

38. Yeo JH, Pepose JS, Stewart JA et al: Acute retinal necrosis syndrome following herpes zoster dermatitis. Ophthalmology 93:1418, 1986

39. Culbertson WW, Blumenkranz MS, Pepose JS et al: Varicella zoster is a cause of the acute retinal necrosis syndrome. Ophthalmology 93:559, 1986

40. Forster DJ, Dugal PU, Frangeih GT et al: Rapidly progressive outer retinal necrosis in the acquired immune deficiency syndrome. Am J Ophthalmol 110:431, 1990

41. Jabs DA, Schachat AP, Liss R et al: Presumed varicella zoster retinitis in immunocompromised patients. Retina 7:9, 1987

42. Yarchoan R, Perno CF, Thomas RV et al: Phase 1 studies of 2′,3′-dideoxycytidine in severe human immunodeficiency viral infection as a single agent and alternating with zidovudine. Lancet 1:76, 1988

43. Kanas RJ, Jensen HL, Abrams AM, Wuerker RB: Oral mucosal cytomegalovirus as a manifestation of the acquired immune deficiency syndrome. Oral Surg Oral Med Pathol 64:183, 1987

44. Levine MS, Woldenberg R, Herlinger H, Laufer I: Opportunistic esophagitis in AIDS: Radiographic diagnosis. Radiology 165:815, 1987

45. Villar LA, Massanari RM, Mitros FA: Cytomegalovirus infection with acute erosive esophagitis. Am J Med 76:924, 1984

46. Elta G, Turnage R, Eckhasuer FE et al: A submucosal antral mass caused by cytomegalovirus infection in a patient with acquired immunodeficiency syndrome. Am J Gastroenterol 81:714, 1986

47. Victoria MS, Nagia BS, Jindrak K: Cytomegalovirus pyloric obstruction in a child with acquired immunodeficiency syndrome. Pediatr Infect Dis 550, 1985

48. Balthazar EJ, Megibou AJ, Hulnick DH: Cytomegalovirus esophagitis and gastritis in AIDS. AJR 144:1201, 1985

49. Knapp AB, Horst DA, Eliopoulos G et al: Widespread cytomegalovirus gastroenterocolitis in a patient with acquired immunodeficiency syndrome. Gastroenterology 85:399, 1983

50. Gertler SL, Pressman J, Price P et al: Gastrointestinal cytomegalovirus infection in a homosexual man with severe acquired immunodeficiency syndrome. Gastroenterology 85:1403, 1983

51. Meiselman MS, Cello JS, Margaretten W: Cytomegalovirus colitis: Report of the clinical endoscopic and pathologic findings in two patients with acquired immunodeficiency syndrome. Gastroenterology. 88:171, 1985

52. Dieterich DT, Rahmin M: Cytomegalovirus colitis in AIDS: Presentation in 44 patients and a review of the literature. J AIDS 4:S29, 1991

53. Frager HH, Frager JD, Wolf EL et al: Cytomegalovirus colitis in acquired immune deficiency syndrome: Radiologic spectrum. Gastrointest Radiol 11:241, 1986

54. Balthazar EJ, Megibow AJ, Fazzini E et al: Cytomegalovirus colitis in AIDS: Radiographic findings in 11 patients. Radiology 155:585, 1985

55. Fernandes B, Brunton J, Koven I: Ileal perforation due to cytomegaloviral enteritis. Can J Surg 29:453, 1986

56. Frank D, Ratent RF: Intestinal perforation associated with cytomegalovirus infection in patients with acquired immunodeficiency syndrome. Am J Gastroenterol 79:201, 1984

57. Freedman PG, Weiner BC, Balthazar EJ: Cytomegalovirus esophagogastritis in a patient with acquired immunodeficiency syndrome. Am J Gastroenterol 79:201, 1984

58. Burke G, Nichols L, Balogh K et al: Perforation of the terminal ileum with cytomegalovirus vasculitis and Kaposi's sarcoma in a patient with acquired immunodeficiency syndrome. Surgery 102:540, 1987

59. Blumberg RS, Kelsey P, Perrone T et al: Cytomegalovirus and cryptosporidium-associated acalculous gangrenous cholecystis. Am J Med 76:1118, 1984

60. Agha FP, Nostrant TT, Abrams GD et al: Cytomegalovirus cholangitis in a homosexual man with acquired immune deficiency syndrome. Am J Gastroenterol 81:1068, 1986

61. Schneiderman DJ, Cello JP, Laing FC: Papillary stenosis and sclerosing cholangitis in the acquired immunodeficiency syndrome. Ann Intern Med 106:546, 1987

62. Aaron JS, Wynter CD, Kirton OC, Simko V: Cytomegalo-

virus associated with acalculous cholecystitis in a patient with acquired immune deficiency syndrome. Am J Gastroenterol 83:879, 1988

63. Guarda LA, Luna MA, Smith JL Jr et al: Acquired immune deficiency syndrome: Postmortem findings. Am J Clin Pathol 81:549, 1984

64. Reichert CM, O'Leary TJ, Levens DL et al: Autopsy pathology in the acquired immune deficiency syndrome. Am J Pathol 112:357, 1983

65. Hawley DA, Schaffer JF, Schulz DM, Muller J: Cytomegalovirus encephalitis in acquired immunodeficiency syndrome. Am J Clin Pathol 80:874, 1983

66. Morgello S, Cho ES, Nielson S et al: Cytomegalovirus encephalitis in patients with acquired immunodeficiency syndrome: An autopsy study of 30 cases and a review of the literature. Hum Pathol 18:289, 1987

67. Masdeu JC, Small CB, Weiss L et al: Multifocal cytomegalovirus encephalitis in AIDS. Ann Neurol 23:97, 1988

68. Tucker T, Dix RD, Katzen C et al: Cytomegalovirus and herpes simplex virus ascending myelitis in a patient with acquired immune deficiency syndrome. Ann Neurol 18:74, 1985

69. Jeantils V, Lemaitre MO, Robert J et al: Subacute polyneuropathy with encephalopathy in AIDS with human cytomegalovirus pathogenicity. Lancet 1:1039, 1986

70. Shaw GM, Harper ME, Han BH et al: HTLV-III infection in brains of children and adults with AIDS encephalopathy. Science 227:177, 1985

71. Ho DD, Rota TR, Schooley RT et al: Isolation of HTLV-III from cerebrospinal fluid and neural tissues of patients with neurologic syndromes related to the acquired immunodeficiency syndrome. N Engl J Med 313:1493, 1985

72. Koenig S, Gendelman HE, Orenstein JM et al: Detection of AIDS virus in macrophages in brain tissue from AIDS patients with encephalophathy. Science 233:1089, 1986

73. Gabuzda DH, Ho DD, de la Monte SM et al: Immunohistochemical identification of HTLV-III antigen in brains of patients with AIDS. Ann Neurol 20:289, 1986

74. Murray JF, Felton CP, Garay SM et al: Pulmonary complications of the acquired immunodeficiency syndrome: Report of a National Heart, Lung and Blood Institute Workshop. N Engl J Med 310:1682, 1984

75. Broaddus C, Dake MD, Stulbarg MS et al: Bronchoalveolar lavage and transbronchial biopsy for the diagnosis of pulmonary infections in the acquired immunodeficiency syndrome. Ann Intern Med 102:747, 1985

76. Abdallah PS, Mark JB, Merigan TC: Diagnosis of cytomegalovirus pneumonia in compromised hosts. Am J Med 61:326, 1976

77. Pass HI, Potter DA, Macher AM et al: Thoracic manifestations of the acquired immunodeficiency syndrome. J Thorac Cardiovasc Surg 88:654, 1984

78. Brodie HR, Broaddus C, Blumenfield W et al: Is cytomegalovirus a cause of lung disease in patients with AIDS? (abstr). Clin Res 33:396A, 1985

79. Wallace JM, Hannah J: Cytomegalovirus pneumonia in patients with AIDS. Chest 92:198, 1987

80. Bozzette SA, Sattler FR, Chiu J et al: A controlled trial of early adjunctive treatment with corticosteroids for pneumocystis carinii pneumonia in the acquired immunodeficiency syndrome. California Collaborative Treatment Group. N Engl J Med 323:1451, 1990

81. Consensus statement on the use of corticosteroids as adjunctive therapy for pneumocystis pneumonia in the acquired immunodeficiency syndrome. The National Institutes of Health—University of California Expert Panel for Corticosteroids as Adjunctive Therapy for Pneumocystis Pneumonia. N Engl J Med 323:1500, 1990

82. Tapper MI, Rotterdam HZ, Lerner CW et al: Adrenal necrosis in the acquired immunodeficiency syndrome. Ann Intern Med 100:239, 1984

83. Greene LW, Cole W, Greene JB et al: Adrenal insufficiency as a complication of the acquired immunodeficiency syndrome. Ann Intern Med 101:497, 1984

84. Randazzo RF, Hulette CM, Gottlieb MS, Rajfer J: Cytomegaloviral epididymitis in a patient with the acquired immune deficiency syndrome. J Urol 136:1095, 1986

85. Brown S, Senekkian EK, Montag AG: Cytomegalovirus infection of the uterine cervix in a patient with acquired immunodeficiency syndrome. Obstet Gynecol 71:489, 1988

86. Bigio EH, Haque AK: Disseminated cytomegalovirus infection presenting with acalculous cholecystitis and acute pancreatitis. Arch Pathol Lab Med 1131:1287, 1989

87. Wilcox CM, Forsmark CE, Grendell JH et al: Cytomegalovirus-associated acute pancreatic disease in patients with acquired immunodeficiency syndrome: Report of two patients. Gastroenterology 99:263, 1990

88. Joe L, Ansher AF, Gordin FM: Severe pancreatitis in an AIDS patient in association with cytomegalovirus infection. South Med J 82:1444, 1989

89. Felsenstein D, D'Amico DJ, Hirsch MS et al: Treatment of cytomegalovirus retinitis with 9-[2-hydroxy-1(hydroxymethyl)-ethoxymethyl]guanine. Ann Intern Med 103:377, 1985

90. Bach MC, Bagwell SP, Knapp NP et al: 9-(1,3-dihydroxy-2-propoxymethyl) guanine for cytomegalovirus infections in patients with the acquired immunodeficiency syndrome. Ann Intern Med 103:381, 1985

91. Field AK, Davies ME, Dewitt C et al: 9-([2-hydroxyl-1-(hydroxymethyl)ethoxyl]methyl) guanine: A selective inhibitor of herpes group virus replication. Proc Natl Acad Sci USA 80:4139, 1983

92. Cheng Y-C, Huang E-S, Lin J-C et al: Unique spectrum of activity of 9-[(1,3-dihydroxy-2-propoxy)methyl]guanine against herpes viruses in vitro and its mode of action against herpes simplex virus type 1. Proc Natl Acad Sci USA 80:2767, 1983

93. Boehme RE: Phosphorylation of the antiviral precursor 9-(1,3-dihydroxy-2-propoxymethyl)guanine monophosphate by guanylate kinase isoenzymes. J Biol Chem 259:12346, 1984

94. Biron KK, Stanat SC, Sorrell JB et al: Metabolic activation of the nucleoside analog 9-([2-hydroxy-1-(hydroxymethyl)ethoxy]methyl) guanine in human diploid fibroblasts infected with human cytomegalovirus. Proc Natl Acad Sci USA 82:2473, 1985

95. Somadossi J-P, Bevan R, Ling T: Clinical pharmacokinetics of ganciclovir in patients with normal and impaired renal function. Rev Infect Dis 105:507, 1988

96. Jacobson MA, de Miranda P, Cederberg DM et al: Human pharmacokinetics and tolerance of oral ganciclovir. Antimicrob Agents Chemother 31:1251, 1987

97. Collaborative DHPG Treatment Study Group: Treatment of serious cytomegalovirus infections with 9-(1,3-dihydroxy-2-propoxymethyl)guanine in patients with AIDS and other immunodeficiencies. N Engl J Med 314:801, 1986

98. Masur H, Lane HC, Palestine A et al: Effect of 9-(1,3-dihydroxy-2-propoxy-methyl)guanine on serious cyto-

megalovirus disease in eight immunosuppressed homosexual men. Ann Intern Med 104:41, 1986

99. Peterson P, Stahl-Bayuss CM: Cytomegalovirus thrombophlebitis after successful DHPG therapy (letter). Ann Intern Med 106:632, 1987

100. Jacobson MA, de Miranda P, Gordon SM et al: Prolonged pancytopenia due to combined ganciclovir and zidovudine therapy. J Infect Dis 158:489, 1988

101. Hochster H, Dietrich D, Bozzette S et al: Toxicity of combined ganciclovir and zidovudine for cytomegalovirus disease associated with AIDS: An AIDS Clinical Trials Group study. Ann Intern Med 113:111, 1990

102. D'Amico DJ, Skolnik PR, Kosloff BR et al: Resolution of cytomegalovirus retinitis with zidovudine therapy. Arch Ophthalmol 106:1168, 1988

103. Guyer DR, Jabs DA, Brant AM et al: Regression of cytomegalovirus retinitis with zidovudine: A clinicopathologic correlation. Arch Ophthalmol 107:868, 1989

104. Laskin OL, Cederberg DM, Mills J et al, for the Ganciclovir Study Group: Ganciclovir for the treatment and suppression of serious infections caused by cytomegalovirus. Am J Med 83:201, 1987

105. Chachoua A, Dieterich D, Krasinski K et al: 9-(1,3-dihydroxy-2-propoxymethyl)guanine (ganciclovir) in the treatment of cytomegalovirus gastrointestinal disease with the acquired immunodeficiency syndrome. Ann Intern Med 107:133, 1987

106. Causey P: Concomitant ganciclovir and zidovudine treatment for cytomegalovirus retinitis in patients with HIV infection: An approach to treatment. J AIDS 4:S16, 1991

107. Miles SA, Mitsuyasu RT, Moreno J et al: Combined therapy with recombinant granulocyte colony-stimulating factor and erythropoietin decreases hematologic toxicity from zidovudine. Blood 77:2109, 1991

108. Pluda JM, Yarchoan R, Smith PD et al: Subcutaneous recombinant granulocyte-macrophage colony-stimulating factor used as a single agent and in an alternating regimen with azidothymidine in leukopenic patients with severe human immunodeficiency virus infection. Blood 76:463, 1990

109. Israel RJ, Levine JD: Granulocyte-macrophage colony-stimulating factor and azidothymidine in patients with acquired immunodeficiency syndrome. Blood 77:2085, 1991

110. Lambert JS, Seidlin M, Reichman RC et al: 2',3'-dideoxyinosine (ddI) in patients with the acquired immunodeficiency syndrome or AIDS-related complex: A phase I trial. N Engl J Med 322:1333, 1990

111. Merigan TC, Skowron G, Bozzette SA et al: Circulating p24 antigen levels and response to dideoxycytidine in human immunodeficiency virus (HIV) infections: A phase I and II study. Ann Intern Med 110:189, 1989

112. Erice A, Chou S, Biron K et al: Progressive disease due to ganciclovir resistant cytomegalovirus in immune compromised patients. N Engl J Med 320:289, 1989

113. Oberg B: Antiviral effects of phosphonoformate (PFA, foscarnet sodium). Pharmacol Ther 19:387, 1983

114. Sandstrom EG, Kaplan JC, Byington RE, Hirsch MS: Inhibition of human T cell lymphotropic virus type III in vitro by phosphonoformate. Lancet 1:1480, 1985

115. Sjovall J, Karlsson A, Ogenstad S et al: Pharmacokinetics and absorption of foscarnet after intravenous and oral administration to patients with human immunodeficiency virus. Clin Pharmacol Ther 44:65, 1988

116. Aweeka F, Gambertoglio J, Mills J, Jacobson MA: Pharmacokinetics of intermittently administered intravenous foscarnet in the treatment of acquired immunodeficiency syndrome patients with serious cytomegalovirus retinitis. Antimicrob Agents Chemother 33:742, 1989

117. Singer DRJ, Fallon TJ, Schulenburg WE et al: Foscarnet for cytomegalovirus retinitis (letter). Ann Intern Med 103:962, 1985

118. Walmsley SL, Chew E, Read SE et al: Treatment of cytomegalovirus retinitis with trisodium phosphonoformate hexahydrate (foscarnet). J Infect Dis 157:569, 1988

119. Jacobson MA, O'Donnell JJ, Mills J: Foscarnet treatment of cytomegalovirus retinitis in patients with the acquired immunodeficiency syndrome. Antimicrob Agents Chemother 33:736, 1989

119a. Studies of the Ocular Complications of AIDS Research Group: Foscarnet–ganciclovir cytomegalovirus retinitis trial: 2. Mortality. N Engl J Med 326, 1992 (in press)

119b. Jacobson MA, Van der Horst C, Causey DM et al: In vivo additive antiretroviral effect of combined zidovudine and foscarnet therapy for human immunodeficiency virus infection. J Infect Dis 163:1219, 1991

120. Ussery FM, Gibson SR, Conklin RH et al: Intravitreal ganciclovir in the treatment of AIDS-associated cytomegalovirus retinitis. Ophthalmology 95:640, 1988

121. Cantrill HL, Henry K, Melrose NH et al: Treatment of cytomegalovirus retinitis with intravitreal ganciclovir: Long-term results. Ophthalmology 96:367, 1989

122. Heinemann MH: Long-term intravitreal ganciclovir therapy for cytomegalovirus retinopathy. Arch Ophthalmol 107:1767, 1989

123. Reed E, Bowden R, Dandiker T et al: Efficacy of cytomegalovirus immunoglobulin in marrow transplant recipients with cytomegalovirus pneumonia. J Infect Dis 156:641, 1986

124. Reed EC, Dandiker PS, Meyers JD: Treatment of cytomegalovirus pneumonia with 9-[2-hydroxy-1-(hydroxymethyl)ethoxymethyl]guanine and high-dose corticosteroids. Ann Intern Med 105:214, 1986

125. Reed EC, Bowden RA, Dandiker PS et al: Treatment of cytomegalovirus pneumonia with ganciclovir and intravenous cytomegalovirus immunoglobulin in patients with bone marrow transplants. Ann Intern Med 109:783, 1988

126. Emanuel D, Cunningham I, Jules-Elysee K et al: Cytomegalovirus pneumonia after bone marrow transplantation successfully treated with the combination of ganciclovir and high-dose intravenous immune globulin. Ann Intern Med 109:777, 1988

127. Manischewitz JF, Quinnan GV Jr, Lane HC et al: Synergistic effect of ganciclovir and foscarnet on cytomegalovirus replication in vitro. Antimicrob Agents Chemother 34:373, 1990

128. Freitas VR, Fraser-Smith EB, Matthews TR: Increased efficacy of ganciclovir in combination with foscarnet against cytomegalovirus and herpes simplex virus type 2 in vitro and in vivo. Antiviral Res 12:205, 1989

129. Deray G, Martinez F, Katlama C et al: Foscarnet nephrotoxicity: Mechanism, incidence and prevention. Am J Nephrol 9:316, 1989

130. DeClercq E, Holy A, Rosenberg I et al: A novel selective broad-spectrum anti-DNA virus agent. Nature (London) 323:464, 1986

131. Goodell SE, Quinn TC, Mkrtichian E et al: Herpes simplex virus proctitis in homosexual men: Clinical, sigmoidoscopic, and histopathologic features. N Engl J Med 308:868, 1983

132. Holmberg SD, Stewart JA, Gerber AR et al: Prior herpes

simplex virus type 2 infection as a risk factor for HIV infection. JAMA 259:1048, 1988

133. Silverman S Jr, Wara D: Oral manifestations of pediatric AIDS. Pediatrician 16:185, 1989

134. Coldiron BM, Orcutt VL, Barbaro DJ: Resolution of resistant chronic herpetic lesions with zidovudine in a patient with the acquired immunodeficiency syndrome (letter). Arch Dermatol 124:1571, 1988

135. Lee JY, Peel R: Concurrent cytomegalovirus and herpes simplex virus infections in skin biopsy specimens from two AIDS patients with fatal CMV infection. Am J Dermatopathol 11(2):136, 1989

136. Baden LA, Bigby M, Kwan T: Persistent necrotic digits in a patient with the acquired immunodeficiency syndrome: Herpes simplex virus infection. Arch Dermatol 127:113, 1991

137. Dahan P, Haettich B, Le Parc JM, Paolaggi JB: Meningoradiculitis due to herpes simplex virus disclosing HIV infection (letter). Ann Rheum Dis 47:440, 1988

138. Madhoun ZT, DuBois DB, Rosenthal J et al: Central diabetes insipidus: A complication of herpes simplex type 2 encephalitis in a patient with AIDS (letter). Am J Med 90:658, 1991

139. Elion GB, Furman PA, Fyfe JA et al: Selectivity of action of an antiherpetic agent, 9-(2-hydroxyethoxymethyl)-guanine. Proc Natl Acad Sci USA 74:5716, 1977

140. Biron KK, Elion GB: In vitro susceptibility of varicella-zoster to acyclovir. Antimicrob Agents Chemother 18:443, 1980

141. Datta AR, Colby BM, Shaw JE, Pagano JS: Acyclovir inhibition of Epstein-Barr virus replication. Proc Natl Acad Sci USA 77:5163, 1980

142. Laskin OL, Longstreth JA, Saral R et al: Pharmacokinetics and tolerance of acyclovir, a new antiherpesvirus agent, in humans. Antimicrob Agents Chemother 21:393, 1982

143. Van Dyke RB, Conner JD, Wyborny C et al: Pharmacokinetics of orally administered acyclovir in patients with herpes progenitalis. Am J Med 73A:172, 1982

144. Peterslund NA, Black FT, Tauris P: Impaired renal function after bolus injections of acyclovir (letter). Lancet 1:243, 1983

145. Bean B, Aeppli D: Adverse effects of high-dose intravenous acyclovir in ambulatory patients with acute herpes zoster. J Infect Dis 151:362, 1985

146. Bataille P, Devos P, Noel JL et al: Psychiatric side-effects with acyclovir (letter). Lancet 2:724, 1985

147. Cohen SMZ, Minkove JA, Zebley JW III et al: Severe but reversible neurotoxicity from acyclovir. Ann Intern Med 100:920, 1984

148. Wade JC, Meyers JD: Neurologic symptoms associated with parenteral acyclovir treatment after marrow transplantation. Ann Intern Med 98:921, 1983

149. Mitsuya H, Broder S: Strategies for antiviral therapy in AIDS. Nature 325:773, 1987

150. Thin RN, Mabarro JM, Parker JD, Fiddian AP: Topical acyclovir in the treatment of initial genital herpes. Br J Vener Dis 59:116, 1983

151. Spruance SL, Schnipper LE, Overall JC Jr et al: Treatment of herpes simplex labialis with topical acyclovir in polyethylene glycol. J Infect Dis 146:85, 1982

152. Reichman RC, Badger GJ, Guinan ME et al: Topically administered acyclovir in the treatment of recurrent herpes simplex genitalis: A controlled trial. J Infect Dis 147:336, 1983

153. Whitley RJ, Levin M, Barton N et al: Infections caused by herpes simplex virus in the immunocompromised host: Natural history and topical acyclovir therapy. J Infect Dis 1150:323, 1984

154. Salo OP, Lassus A, Hovi T: Double-blind placebo-controlled trial of oral acyclovir in recurrent genital herpes. Eur J Sex Transm Dis 1:95, 1983

155. Reichman RC, Badger GJ, Mertz GJ et al: Treatment of recurrent genital herpes simplex infections with oral acyclovir: A controlled trial. JAMA 251:2103, 1984

156. Shepp DH, Newton BA, Dandliker PS et al: Oral acyclovir therapy for mucocutaneous herpes simplex virus infections in immunocompromised marrow transplant recipients. Ann Intern Med 102:703, 1985

157. Douglas JM, Critchlow C, Benedetti J et al: A double-blind study of oral acyclovir for suppression of recurrences of genital herpes simplex virus infection. N Engl J Med 310:1551, 1984

158. Mindel A, Weller IV, Faherty A et al: Prophylactic oral acyclovir in recurrent genital herpes. Lancet 2:57, 1984

159. Straus SE, Siedlin M, Takiff H et al: Oral acyclovir to suppress recurring herpes simplex virus infections in immunodeficient patients. Ann Intern Med 100:522, 1984

160. Corey L, Fife KH, Benedetti JK et al: Intravenous acyclovir for the treatment of primary genital herpes. Ann Intern Med 98:914, 1983

161. Mindel A, Adler MW, Sutherland S, Fiddian AP: Intravenous acyclovir treatment for primary genital herpes. Lancet 1:697, 1982

162. Schnipper LE, Crumpacker CS: Resistance of herpes simplex virus to acycloguanosine: Role of viral thymidine kinase and DNA polymerase loci. Proc Natl Acad Sci USA 77:2270, 1980

163. Coen DM, Schaffer PA: Two distinct loci confer resistance to acycloguanosine in herpes simplex type 1. Proc Natl Acad Sci USA 77:2265, 1983

164. Crumpacker CS, Schnipper LE, Marlowe SI et al: Resistance to antiviral drugs of herpes simplex virus isolated from a patient treated with acyclovir. N Engl J Med 306:343, 1982

165. Norris SA, Kessler HA, Fife KH: Severe, progressive herpetic whitlow caused by an acyclovir-resistant virus in a patient with AIDS. J Infect Dis 157:209, 1988

166. Youle MM, Hawkins DA, Collins P et al: Acyclovir-resistant herpes in AIDS treated with foscarnet. Lancet 2:341, 1988

167. Erlich KS, Mills J, Chatis P et al: Acyclovir-resistant herpes simplex virus infections in patients with the acquired immunodeficiency syndrome. N Engl J Med 320:293, 1989

168. Marks GL, Nolan PE, Erlich KS et al: Mucocutaneous dissemination of acyclovir-resistant herpes simplex virus in a patient with AIDS. Rev Infect Dis 11:474, 1989

169. Chatis PA, Miller CH, Schrager LE et al: Successful treatment with foscarnet of an acyclovir-resistant mucocutaneous infection with herpes simplex virus in a patient with acquired immunodeficiency. N Engl J Med 320:297, 1989

170. Gateley A, Gander RM, Johnson PC et al: Herpes simplex type 2 meningoencephalitis resistant to acyclovir in a patient with AIDS. J Infect Dis 161:711, 1990

171. Birch CJ, Tachedjian G, Doherty RR et al: Altered sensitivity to antiviral drugs of herpes simplex virus isolates from a patient with the acquired immunodeficiency syndrome. J Infect Dis 162:731, 1990

172. Erlich KS, Jacobson MA, Koehler JE et al: Foscarnet therapy of severe acyclovir-resistant herpes simplex virus type-2

infections in patients with the acquired immunodeficiency syndrome (AIDS). Ann Intern Med 110:710, 1989

173. MacPhail LA, Greenspan D, Schiodt M et al: Acyclovir-resistant, foscarnet-sensitive oral herpes simplex type-2 lesion in a patient with AIDS. Oral Surg Oral Med Oral Pathol 67:427, 1989

174. Safrin S, Assaykeen T, Follansbee S et al: Foscarnet therapy for acyclovir-resistant mucocutaneous herpes simplex virus infection in 26 AIDS patients: Preliminary data. J Infect Dis 161:1078, 1990

175. Safrin S, Crumpacker C, Chatis P et al: A controlled trial comparing foscarnet with vidarabine for acyclovir-resistant mucocutaneous herpes simplex in the acquired immunodeficiency syndrome. N Engl J Med 8:551, 1991

176. Colebunders R, Mann JM, Francis H et al: Herpes zoster in African patients: A clinical predictor of human immunodeficiency viral infection. J Infect Dis 157:314, 1988

177. Patterson LE, Butler KM, Edwards MS: Clinical herpes zoster shortly following primary varicella in two HIV-infected children. Clin Pediatr (Phila) 28:354, 1989

178. Whitley RJ, Mandell GM, Douglas RA, Bennett JE: Varicella zoster virus. In (eds): Principles and Practice of Infectious Diseases, 3rd ed, p 1153. New York, Churchill Livingstone, 1990

179. Feldman S, Hughes WT, Daniel CB: Varicella in children with cancer: Seventy-seven cases. Pediatrics 56:388, 1975

180. Preblud SR: Varicella: Complications and costs. Pediatrics 78:728, 1986

181. Johnson R, Milbourn PE: Central nervous system manifestations of chickenpox. Can Med J 102:831, 1970

182. Triebwasser JH, Harrie RE, Bryant RE et al: Varicella pneumonia in adults: Report of seven cases and a review of literature. Medicine (Baltimore) 46:409, 1967

183. Feder HM Jr: Treatment of adult chickenpox with oral acyclovir. Arch Intern Med 150:2061, 1990

184. Haake DA, Zakowski PC, Haake DL et al: Early treatment with acyclovir for varicella pneumonia in otherwise healthy adults: Retrospective controlled study and review. Rev Infect Dis 12:788, 1990

185. Balfour HH Jr, Kelly JM, Suarez CS et al: Acyclovir treatment of varicella in otherwise healthy children. J Pediatr 116:633, 1990

186. Prober CG, Kirk LE, Keeney RE: Acyclovir therapy of chickenpox in immunosuppressed children: A collaborative study. J Pediatr 101:622, 1982

187. Ragozzino MW, Melton LJ III, Kurland LT et al: Population-based study of herpes zoster and its sequelae. Medicine (Baltimore) 51:310, 1982

188. Hope-Simpson RE: The nature of herpes zoster: A long-term study and a new hypothesis. Proc R Soc Med 58:9, 1965

189. McGregor RM: Herpes zoster, chickenpox, and cancer in general practice. Br Med J 1:84, 1957

190. Acheson DW, Leen CL, Tariq WU et al: Severe and recurrent varicella-zoster virus infection in a patient with the acquired immune deficiency syndrome. J Infect 16:193, 1988

191. Whitley RJ: Varicella-zoster virus infections: Chronic disease in the immunocompromised host. Evidence for persistent excretion of virus. Pediatr Infect Dis J 8:584, 1989

192. Hoppenjans WB, Bibler MR, Orme RL et al: Prolonged cutaneous herpes zoster in acquired immunodeficiency syndrome. Arch Dermatol 126:1048, 1990

193. Linneman CC Jr, Biron KK, Hoppenjans WB et al: Emer-gence of acyclovir-resistant varicella zoster virus in an AIDS patient on prolonged acyclovir therapy. AIDS 4:577, 1990

194. Jacobson MA, Berger TG, Fikrig S et al: Acyclovir-resistant varicella zoster virus infection after chronic oral acyclovir therapy in patients with the acquired immunodeficiency syndrome (AIDS). Ann Intern Med 112:187, 1990

195. Safrin S, Berger TG, Gilson I et al: Foscarnet therapy in five patients with AIDS and acyclovir-resistant varicella-zoster virus infections. Ann Intern Med 115:19, 1991

196. Gilden DH, Murray RS, Wellish M et al: Chronic progressive varicella-zoster virus encephalitis in an AIDS patient. Neurology 38:1150, 1988

197. Cheeseman SH, Sullivan JL, Brettler DB et al: Analysis of cytomegalovirus and Epstein-Barr virus antibody responses in treated hemophiliacs: Implications for the study of acquired immune deficiency syndrome. JAMA 252:83, 1984

198. Crawford DH, Weller I, Iliescu V et al: Epstein-Barr (EB) virus infection in homosexual men in London. Br J Vener Dis 60:258, 1984

199. Chang RS, Thompson H, Pomerantz S et al: Epstein-Barr virus infections in homosexual men with chronic, persistent generalized lymphadenopathy. J Infect Dis 151:459, 1985

200. Yarchoan R, Redfield RR, Broder S: Mechanisms of B cell activation in patients with acquired immunodeficiency syndrome and related disorders. J Clin Invest 78:439, 1986

201. Alsip GR, Ench Y, Sumaya CV et al: Increased Epstein-Barr virus DNA in oropharyngeal secretions from patients with AIDS, AIDS-related complex, or asymptomatic human immunodeficiency virus infections. J Infect Dis 157: 1072, 1988

202. Moss DJ, Rickinson AB, Pope JH: Long-term T-cell mediated immunity to Epstein-Barr virus in man: III. Activation of cytotoxic T cells in virus-infected leukocyte cultures. Int J Cancer 23:618, 1979

203. Schooley RT, Hanyes BF, Grouse J et al: Development of suppressor T lymphocytes for Epstein-Barr virus-induced B-lymphocyte outgrowth during acute infectious mononucleosis: Assessment by two quantitative systems. Blood 57:510, 1981

204. Birx DL, Redfield RR, Tosato G: Defective regulation of Epstein-Barr virus infection in patients with acquired immunodeficiency syndrome (AIDS) or AIDS-related disorders. N Engl J Med 314:874, 1986

205. Blumberg RS, Paradis T, Byington R et al: Effects of human immunodeficiency virus on the cellular immune response to Epstein-Barr virus in homosexual men: Characterization of the cytotoxic response and lymphokine production. J Infect Dis 155:877, 1987

206. Rinaldo CR Jr, Kingsley LA, Lyter DW et al: Association of HTLV-III with Epstein-Barr virus infection and abnormalities of T lymphocytes in homosexual men. J Infect Dis 154:556, 1986

207. Sumaya CV, Boswell RN, Ench Y et al: Enhanced serological and virological findings of Epstein-Barr virus in patients with AIDS and AIDS-related complex. J Infect Dis 154:864, 1986

208. Rahman MA, Kingsley LA, Breinig MK et al: Enhanced antibody responses to Epstein-Barr virus in HIV-infected homosexual men. J Infect Dis 159:472, 1989

209. Lang DJ, Kovacs AA, Zaia JA et al: Seroepidemiologic studies of cytomegalovirus and Epstein-Barr virus infec-

tions in relation to human immunodeficiency virus type 1 infection in selected recipient populations. Transfusion Safety Study Group. J AIDS 2:540, 1989

210. Ziegler JL, Beckstead JA, Volberding PA et al: Non-Hodgkin's lymphomas in 90 homosexual men: Relation to generalized lymphadenopathy and the acquired immunodeficiency syndrome. N Engl J Med 311:565, 1984

211. Beckhardt RN, Farady N, May M et al: Increased incidence of malignant lymphoma in AIDS: A comparison of risk groups and possible etiologic factors. Mt Sinai J Med 55:383, 1988

212. Lind SE, Gross PL, Andiman WA et al: Malignant lymphoma presenting as Kaposi's sarcoma in a homosexual man with the acquired immunodeficiency syndrome. Ann Intern Med 102:338, 1985

213. Bashir RM, Hochberg FH, Harris NL et al: Variable expression of Epstein-Barr virus genome as demonstrated by in situ hybridization in central nervous system lymphomas in immunocompromised patients. Mod Pathol 3:429, 1990

214. Borisch-Chappuis B, Nezelof C, Muller H et al: Different Epstein-Barr virus expression in lymphomas from immunocompromised and immunocompetent patients. Am J Pathol 136:5751, 1990

215. Hamilton-Dutoit SJ, Pallesen G, Franzman MB et al: AIDS-related lymphoma: Histopathology, immunophenotype, and association with Epstein-Barr virus as demonstrated by in situ nucleic acid hybridization. Am J Pathol 138:149, 1991

216. Voelkerding KV, Sandhaus LM, Kim HC et al: Plasma cell malignancy in the acquired immune deficiency syndrome: Association with Epstein-Barr virus. Am J Clin Pathol 92:222, 1989

217. Neri A, Barriga F, Inghirami G et al: Epstein-Barr virus infection precedes clonal expansion in Burkitt's and acquired immunodeficiency syndrome-associated lymphoma. Blood 77:1092, 1991

218. Subar M, Neri A, Inghirami G et al: Frequent c-myc oncogene activation and infrequent presence of Epstein-Barr virus genome in AIDS-associated lymphoma. Blood 72:667, 1988

219. Rosenberg NL, Hochberg FH, Miller G et al: Primary central nervous system lymphoma related to Epstein-Barr virus in a patient with acquired immune deficiency syndrome. Ann Neurol 20:98, 1986

220. Rosenblum ML, Levy RM, Bredesen DE et al: Primary central nervous system lymphomas in patients with AIDS. Ann Neurol 23:S13, 1988

221. Del Mistro A, Laverda A, Balabrese F et al: Primary lymphoma of the central nervous system in two children with acquired immune deficiency syndrome. Am J Clin Pathol 94:722, 1990

222. Bashir RM, Harris NL, Hichberg FH et al: Detection of Epstein-Barr virus in CNS lymphomas by in-situ hybridization. Neurology 39:813, 1989

223. Greenspan JS, Greenspan D, Lennette ET et al: Replication of Epstein-Barr virus within the epithelial cells of oral "hairy" leukoplakia, an AIDS-associated lesion. N Engl J Med 313:564, 1985

224. Eversole LR, Stone CE, Beckman AM: Detection of EBV and HPV DNA sequences in oral "hairy" leukoplakia by in situ hybridization. J Med Virol 26:271, 1988

225. De Souza YG, Greenspan D, Felton JR et al: Localization of Epstein-Barr virus DNA in the epithelial cells of oral "hairy" leukoplakia by in situ hybridization of tissue sections (letter). N Engl J Med 320:1599, 1989

226. Moniaci D, Greco D, Flecchia G et al: Epidemiology, clinical features and prognostic value of HIV-1 related oral lesions. J Oral Pathol Med 19:477, 1990

227. Resnick L, Herbst JS, Raab-Traub N: Oral "hairy" leukoplakia. J Am Acad Dermatol 22:1278, 1990

228. Kitchen VS, Helbert M, Francis ND et al: Epstein-Barr virus associated oesophageal ulcers in AIDS. Gut 31:1223, 1990

229. Andiman WA, Eastman R, Martin K et al: Opportunistic lymphoproliferations associated with Epstein-Barr viral DNA in infants and children with AIDS. Lancet 2:1390, 1985

230. Fackler JC, Nagel JE, Adler WH: Epstein-Barr virus infection in a child with acquired immunodeficiency syndrome. Am J Dis Child 139(10):1000, 1985

231. Salahuddin SZ, Ablashi DV, Markham PD et al: Isolation of a new virus, HBLV, in patients with lymphoproliferative disorders. Science 234:596, 1986

232. Downing RG, Sewankambo N, Serwadda D et al: Isolation of human lymphotropic herpes viruses from Uganda. Lancet 2:390, 1987

233. Okuno T, Higashi K, Shiraki K et al: Human herpes viruses 6 (HHV-6) infection in renal transplantation. Transplantation 49:519, 1990

234. Harnet GB, Farr TJ, Pietroboni GR et al: Frequent shedding of human herpes virus 6 in saliva. J Med Virol 30:128, 1990

235. Levy JA, Greenspan D, Ferro F et al: Frequent isolation of HHV-6 from saliva: High seroprevalence of the virus in the population. Lancet 1:1047, 1990

236. Okuno T, Takahashi K, Balachandra K et al: Seroepidemiology of human herpes virus 6 infection in normal children and adults. J Clin Microbiol 27:651, 1989

237. Yamanishi K, Okuno T, Shiraki K et al: Identification of human herpes virus-6 as a causal agent for exanthem subitum. Lancet 1:1065, 1988

238. Horvat RT, Wood C, Balachandran N: Transactivation of human immunodeficiency virus promoter by human herpes virus 6. J Virol 63:970, 1989

239. Lusso R, Ensoli B, Markham PD et al: Productive dual infection by human CD4+ T-lymphocytes by HIV-1 and HHV-6. Nature 337:370, 1989

240. Fox J, Briggs M, Tedder RS: Antibody to human herpes virus-6 in HIV-1 positive and negative homosexual men. Lancet 2:396, 1988

241. Brown NA, Kovacs A, Lui CR et al: Prevalence of antibody to human herpes virus-6 among blood donors infected with HIV. Lancet 2:1146, 1988

242. Spira TJ, Bozeman LH, Sanderlin KC et al: Lack of correlation between human herpes virus-6 infection and the course of human immunodeficiency virus infection. J Infect Dis 161:567, 1990

12

Kaposi's Sarcoma and the Acquired Immunodeficiency Syndrome

Bijan Safai   *Joseph J. Schwartz*

In early 1981, the acquired immunodeficiency syndrome (AIDS) was initially recognized from the outbreak of Kaposi's sarcoma and *Pneumocystis carinii* pneumonia among young, previously healthy homosexual men.[1,2] Kaposi's sarcoma was among the first AIDS-defining conditions, and it has remained one of the major diseases associated with human immunodeficiency virus type 1 (HIV-1) infection. With the increased incidence of Kaposi's sarcoma, much interest has been focused on what was considered a rare and relatively indolent tumor. Many challenging questions, such as the association of Kaposi's sarcoma with HIV-1, the pathogenic mechanisms of Kaposi's sarcoma, and methods of treatment, have undergone reexamination. Considerable new and interesting information has accumulated, and previously held views are being challenged. This review summarizes the recent developments in Kaposi's sarcoma and proposes a coherent model for its pathogenesis.

HISTORICAL INFORMATION

In 1872 the Hungarian physician Moriz Kaposi first described this disease as "multiple idiopathic pigmented hemangiosarcoma."[3] He described the condition as localized, nodular, brown-red to blue-red tumors that appeared first on the soles and then the hands. He recognized the disease as a rare, chronic cutaneous disorder affecting men more than 40 years old. He was also aware of the multifocal nature of the disease, the occurrence of visceral involvement, and the vascular nature of the tumor. This form of Kaposi's sarcoma, known as classic Kaposi's sarcoma, occurs most commonly in Eastern Europe and North America among men of Italian or Jewish ancestry.[4] In the 1950s and 1960s, endemic Kaposi's sarcoma, a more aggressive form of the disease that occurred in younger individuals, was described in central Africa, accounting for 9% of all cancers in Uganda.[5-7] During the 1970s, Kaposi's sarcoma was reported among a new group of patients receiving immunosuppressive therapy for renal transplantation and other medical conditions.[8-11] Individuals infected with HIV, especially homosexual or bisexual men,[2,12] are currently the group with the highest incidence of an aggressive form of Kaposi's sarcoma, known as epidemic or AIDS-associated Kaposi's sarcoma.

EPIDEMIOLOGY

Prior to the AIDS epidemic, Kaposi's sarcoma was considered to be a rare disease appearing in patients originating from Eastern Europe, Italy, or Russia.[4] Before the AIDS epidemic, the annual incidence of Kaposi's sarcoma in the United States was 0.021 to 0.061 per 100,000 population.[13,14] Although classic Kaposi's sarcoma is mostly seen in persons of European descent, it has been seen in other groups, including three people of pure Eskimo inheritance.[15]

Since the onset of the AIDS epidemic, more than 24,000 cases of AIDS-associated Kaposi's sarcoma have been reported to the Centers for Disease Control (CDC). AIDS-associated Kaposi's sarcoma occurs in patients of all ages, with a mean age of 38 years. It has been seen and reported among all risk groups for HIV infection[16]; however, in the United States, it is most common in

HIV-infected homosexual or bisexual men. Approximately 96% of all reported cases of AIDS-associated Kaposi's sarcoma in the United States have been diagnosed in homosexual or bisexual men, representing 26% of all homosexual men with AIDS.[17] In comparison to other groups with AIDS, Kaposi's sarcoma is seen in 9% of Haitians, 3% of heterosexual intravenous (IV) drug abusers, 3% of transfusion recipients, 3% of women with AIDS, 3% of children with AIDS, and 1% of hemophiliacs.[16]

The incidence of AIDS-associated Kaposi's sarcoma has decreased steadily since the mid-1980s. Initially it accounted for 35% to 40% of all reported AIDS cases; however, presently it is seen in approximately 14% of all AIDS cases reported to the CDC.[18,19] This trend has been the subject of several reviews and discussions.[20–26] One explanation may be the decreased use of unlabeled amyl nitrate, an inhalant recreational drug and a possible mutagen.[20–23] Other epidemiologic studies suggest that changes in certain sexual practices may account for the decreasing incidence of Kaposi's sarcoma. Sexual activities such as anal lingus, anal intercourse, and anal fisting, which may increase the chance of developing Kaposi's sarcoma,[24,25] have been identified as high-risk behaviors for contracting HIV and have decreased. Another theory, one that suggests co-transmission of a second Kaposi's sarcoma–causing agent with the HIV-1 virus,[26] would also expect a decreased incidence of Kaposi's sarcoma with safer sexual practices.

In Africa, AIDS-associated Kaposi's sarcoma appears to be transmitted by heterosexual contact and has an approximately equal incidence among men and women.[27] This is in contrast to the male predominance observed in all other populations, and a male-female ratio of approximately 8:1 for AIDS-associated Kaposi's sarcoma in the United States.[16]

The infrequency of the disease in members of the same family, even in the endemic areas, is of special interest.[5,28,29] To date fewer than ten families with multiple cases of Kaposi's sarcoma have been reported.

CLINICAL FEATURES

Currently there exist four categories of Kaposi's sarcoma: classic, endemic African, iatrogenic, and AIDS-associated. Classic Kaposi's sarcoma usually manifests with blue to reddish purple macules, plaques, or nodules. Untreated lesions may coalesce to form large plaques and tumors that may produce fungating masses with ulceration. Lesions are frequently located on the extremities, most often on the feet and lower leg, but may appear anywhere on the skin or mucous membranes. Edema of the lower extremities, often painful, may precede or follow tumor invasion into the superficial and deep lymphatics. Lymph nodes and internal organs are rarely involved (see Color Figs. 5 and 6).[30]

In Africa, clinical forms of Kaposi's sarcoma have been described[31] as nodular, florid, infiltrative, and lymphadenopathic (Table 12–1, see Color Fig. 7). This classification is based on the clinical presentation and the clinical behavior of the disease. The lymphadenopathic form is usually seen in African children and young adults. It manifests mainly with involvement of the lymph nodes, and the disease is often rapidly fatal.[32,33]

In transplant recipients, Kaposi's sarcoma is the second most common tumor after lymphoma to arise. It has been reported to occur more often (10% *vs.* 3% of all transplant-associated neoplasms) in patients who receive cyclosporin as part of their immunosuppressive regimen.[34] The mean duration of therapy before the development of Kaposi's sarcoma is 23 months.[34,35] In iatrogenic Kaposi's sarcoma cutaneous involvement is most common; however, lymphatic and visceral dissemination can occur.

The clinical features of AIDS-associated Kaposi's sarcoma are markedly different from those seen in the other forms (see Color Figs. 8–15). The disease is characterized by a multifocal, widespread distribution that may involve any location on the skin or mucous membranes, as well as the lymph nodes, gastrointestinal (GI) tract, and visceral organs.[36,37] There is considerable variability in the timing of the initial development of Kaposi's sarcoma in HIV-infected individuals. We have seen patients with AIDS-associated Kaposi's sarcoma who lacked evidence of immune impairment.[36] Kaposi's sarcoma may be the first sign of HIV infection, especially in populations where HIV testing is not routinely performed. It can also arise in the later stages of HIV infection, when patients are suffering from various degrees of immune deficiency and opportunistic infections,[39] or even during the last months or weeks of life.

Table 12–1. Taylor Classification of Kaposi's Sarcoma

Clinical Type	Behavior	Age (yr)	Bone Involvement	Lymph Node Involvement	Predominant Skin Tumor
Nodular plaques	Indolent	>25	Rare	Rare	Nodules
Florid (exophytic)	Locally aggressive	>25	Often	Rare	Fungating
Infiltrative	Locally aggressive	>25	Always	Rare	Diffuse
Lymphadenopathic	Disseminated aggressive	<25	Rare	Always	Nodules

Reproduced with permission from Taylor JF, Templeton AC, Vogel CL *et al*: Kaposi's sarcoma in Uganda: A clinicopathologic study. Int J Cancer 8:122, 1971.

The natural course of the disease and the rate of the progression of Kaposi's sarcoma vary greatly with the clinical form of the disease. In classic Kaposi's sarcoma the majority of cases follow a slow and indolent course. Endemic Kaposi's sarcoma follows a more aggressive course, especially in children with the lymphadenopathic form. In AIDS-associated Kaposi's sarcoma the majority of cases follow a rapidly progressive course. Skin lesions appear most often on the lower extremity, followed by upper extremity, trunk, and, less commonly, the face, oral mucosa, and genitalia.[38] The initial few localized lesions frequently progress to widespread skin and mucosal involvement and, in some cases, involvement of lymph nodes, solid visceral organs, and most commonly the GI tract. Although AIDS-associated Kaposi's sarcoma is an aggressive form of the disease, patients usually succumb to opportunistic infections rather than to the sarcoma itself. In a report on 112 patients followed for a minimum of 15 months, 65 died within this time period. All but ten of the deaths were attributed to opportunistic infections. Two of the ten patients died of non-Hodgkin's lymphoma, and the other eight apparently of AIDS-associated Kaposi's sarcoma.[40,41] Many of the fatal cases of Kaposi's sarcoma are due to pulmonary involvement, and, although infrequent, pulmonary involvement carries a poor prognosis (see Figs. 12–16, Color insert).[42,43] At the other extreme are a few cases of indolent disease that show minimal progression over several years (B. Safai, unpubl. observ.).[36,44]

Patients with AIDS-associated Kaposi's sarcoma who do not develop opportunistic infections are estimated to have an 80% survival rate at 28 months from diagnosis, compared to a less than 20% survival rate in those with opportunistic infections.[45] We have observed a small group of patients with AIDS-associated Kaposi's sarcoma who lived at least 36 months from the time of biopsy diagnosis of Kaposi's sarcoma without developing opportunistic infections. These patients have survived from 36 to 124 months (average, 69 months) (B. Safai, unpubl. observ.).

Spontaneous regression has been reported in both classic and AIDS-associated Kaposi's sarcoma. The regression normally occurs early in the disease and affects only some of the lesions. By contrast, in iatrogenic Kaposi's sarcoma, discontinuation of immunosuppressive therapies has been reported to result in complete regression of the disease.[46,47]

STAGING

A successful staging classification system should yield prognostic information, be a useful guide to therapeutic interventions, and simplify analysis of different clinical trials. As a multicentric neoplasm, Kaposi's sarcoma does not lend itself to a TNM classification as do other solid tumors. There are, however, certain clinical features that can identify different presentations of Kaposi's sarcoma and, in general, the overall clinical course.

The most widely used staging system for Kaposi's sarcoma prior to the AIDS epidemic[31] was based on the experience from equatorial Africa (see Table 12–1). With the emergence of epidemic Kaposi's sarcoma and its aggressive features, it became apparent that a new staging system was needed to identify the distinctive features of this new group of patients. The initial classification[40] took into account the clinical presentation of Kaposi's sarcoma and subtypes A (without) and B (with) systemic "B" symptoms (Table 12–2).[48]

A more recent classification system, developed specifically for AIDS-associated Kaposi's sarcoma, takes into account both clinical and laboratory factors and recognizes the importance of the T-helper cell counts, as did the earlier Walter Reed staging system for HIV disease.[49,50] A multivariate analysis of nine variables in 212 patients showed three variables to be significant: a T4 cell count below 300 cells/mm³, B symptoms, and prior or coexisting opportunistic infection. A staging system based on these three variables that identifies four distinct prognostic groups has been proposed (Table 12–3). The variables found not to be significant on multivariate analysis were age, T4/T8 ratio, β_2-microglobulin, acid-labile interferon-α (IFN-α) skin and/or lymph node disease only, and GI/palatal lesions. Only on univariate analysis was extent of disease, defined as limited *versus* extensive skin involvement, and skin and/or lymph node *versus* GI tract and/or palatal involvement, found to be significant.

Another staging classification, recommended by the AIDS Clinical Trials Group (ACTG), uses three parameters (extent of tumor, immune status, and severity of systemic illness) to divide patients into good- and poor-risk groups (Table 12–4).[51] Only with use in prospective trials can the value of these much-needed staging systems in predicting treatment outcome and survival be realized.

Table 12–2. Staging Classification for Kaposi's Sarcoma*

Stage	Clinical Manifestations
I	Cutaneous, locally indolent
II	Cutaneous, locally aggressive, with or without lymph node involvement
III	Generalized mucocutaneous and/or lymph node involvement
IV	Visceral
Subtype	
A	No systemic signs or symptoms
B	Systemic signs: weight loss (10%) or fever (>100° F orally, unrelated to an identifiable source of infection lasting > 2 weeks.

Reproduced with permission from Krigel RL, Laubenstein LJ, Muggia FM: Kaposi's sarcoma: A new staging classification. Cancer Treat Rep 67:531, 1983.
* The first staging classification for AIDS-associated Kaposi's Sarcoma. Now superseded by classification by Chachoua *et al*[50] and Krown *et al*.[51]

Table 12–3. Staging Classification of AIDS-Associated Kaposi's Sarcoma Based on Multivariate Analysis of Nine Clinical and Laboratory Variables in 212 Patients

Stage	Variable
I	No opportunistic infection, no B symptoms, T4 > 300
II	No opportunistic infection, no B symptoms, T4 < 300
III	No opportunistic infection, B symptoms
IV	Opportunistic infection

Reproduced with permission from Chachoua A, Krigel R, Lafleur F *et al:* Prognostic factors and staging classification of patients with epidemic Kaposi's sarcoma. J Clin Oncol 7:774, 1989.

HISTOPATHOLOGIC FEATURES

The histopathologic process is believed to start in the mid-dermis and extend upward toward the epidermis. A fully developed lesion has a characteristic histopathologic picture consisting of interwoven bands of spindle cells and vascular structures embedded in a network of reticular and collagen fibers. Spindle cells may exhibit a wide range of nuclear pleomorphism. The vascular component may appear as slitlike spaces between the spindle cells or as very early, delicate capillaries. Extravasated erythrocytes and hemosiderin-laden macrophages are also present. Mononuclear cell infiltrates are seen, especially in younger lesions. Based on the quantity of the vascular component, the presence of nuclear pleomorphism, the number of spindle cells, and the amount of fibrosis in the tumor, three histopathologic patterns have been identified: (1) a mixed cellular pattern containing equal proportions of vascular slits, well-formed vascular channels, and spindle cells, (2) a mononuclear pattern consisting of proliferation of one cell type, usually spindle cells, and (3) an anaplastic pattern characterized by cellular pleomorphism and frequent mitosis. The mixed cellular pattern is seen in all clinical forms of Kaposi's sarcoma, but the anaplastic pattern has only been reported in the florid type associated with AIDS.[52]

The increase in the number of patients with AIDS-associated Kaposi's sarcoma in the past few years has made it possible to study the histopathologic changes of Kaposi's sarcoma in relation to clinical progression. As the clinical tumor develops from a prepatch stage to patch, plaque, nodular, and tumor stages, the histopathologic features progress to the more characteristic features described above. In the early clinical patch stage, histologic features include a slight increase in the number of bizarrely shaped endothelial-lined vascular spaces, and a sparse mononuclear cell infiltrate, composed of lymphocytes and plasma cells, which is seen in perivascular areas.[53,54] As the disease progresses to the plaque stage, the number of irregularly shaped vessels and the inflammatory cell infiltrate increase, and grouped spindle-shaped cells appear between collagen bundles. During the nodular stage, the histologic appearance consists of few thin endothelial-lined vascular channels in a matrix of dense, interweaving bundles of spindle-shaped cells. The mononuclear infiltrate is absent or sparse, but extravasated erythrocytes and hemosiderin-laden macrophages are present. Nuclear and cytologic atypia and a few mitotic cells are seen. The histopathology of Kaposi's sarcoma in lymph nodes and in viscera is similar to that seen in skin. Foci of tumors located in the sinusoid and capsular areas of the lymph nodes and a generalized lymphoid hyperplasia are characteristic of Kaposi's sarcoma in lymph nodes (see Color Figs. 13–15).[52,54]

Table 12–4. Staging Classification for Kaposi's Sarcoma

	Good Risk (0)	Poor Risk (1)
Tumor (T)	Confined to skin and/or lymph nodes and/or minimal oral disease*	Tumor-associated edema, or ulceration Extensive oral KS Gastrointestinal KS KS in other nonnodal viscera
Immune system (I)	CD4 cells > 200/μl	CD4 cell count < 200/μl
Systemic illness (S)	No history of opportunistic infection or thrush No B symptoms† Karnofky performance status > 70	History of opportunistic infection and/or thrush B symptoms present Performance status < 70 Other HIV-related illnesses (*e.g.,* lymphoma, neurologic disease)

* Minimal oral disease is nonnodular Kaposi's sarcoma confined to the palate.
† B symptoms are unexplained fever, night sweats, greater than 10% involuntary weight loss, or diarrhea persisting more than 2 weeks.
Reproduced with permission from Krown SE, Metroka C, Wernz JC *et al:* Kaposi's sarcoma in the acquired immune deficiency syndrome: A proposal for a uniform evaluation, response, and staging criteria. J Clin Oncol 7:1201, 1989.

CURRENT CONCEPTS ON THE DEVELOPMENT OF AIDS-ASSOCIATED KAPOSI'S SARCOMA

In recent years, advances in biotechnology have made available new methods to investigate the cellular and molecular events leading to the development and progression of Kaposi's sarcoma. This has resulted in a wealth of new knowledge about the pathogenesis of Kaposi's sarcoma.

Cell of Origin

The cell of origin of Kaposi's sarcoma has remained in question for many decades. Several different cell types have been suggested; however, histochemical staining, culture studies, and ultrastructural examinations have all yielded controversial results (Table 12–5).[55–67]

A major recent breakthrough in the study of the cellular nature of Kaposi's sarcoma came with the establishment of a long-term culture of AIDS-associated Kaposi's sarcoma–derived spindle cells. Cell growth is supported by conditioned media obtained from CD4+ T cells infected with HTLV-II.[69] Conditioned media from HTLV-I– or HIV-I–infected CD4+ T cells similarly maintained the growth of Kaposi's sarcoma cells, but to a lesser degree. These cells and some other long-term cultured cells have been characterized by phenotypic markers and cytochemical studies, and it has been demonstrated that the Kaposi's sarcoma spindle cells have features of vascular channel and endothelial cell lineage.[64] The same cells have some features of vascular smooth muscle when grown on a three-dimensional matrix.[66] A recent study shows that Kaposi's sarcoma spindle cells share morphology with vascular smooth muscle cells, and stain for and express the gene for smooth muscle a-actin.[67] The conclusion drawn from these studies suggests that the spindle cells originate from a mesenchymal precursor cell, possibly for smooth muscle. Despite the abundance of new information and technology, the identity of the cell of origin in Kaposi's sarcoma remains contested to this day.

None of the currently reported Kaposi's sarcoma cell lines show evidence of viral infection or chromosomal abnormalities[64]; however, a recently developed but as yet unpublished Kaposi's sarcoma cell line is said to show chromosomal aberration (R. C. Gallo, unpubl. observ.).

Cytokine Cascade

Detailed studies[64,69] of long-term Kaposi's sarcoma cell lines demonstrate that these cells express a variety of potent biologic activities, including (1) growth-promoting activities for Kaposi's sarcoma spindle cells, normal endothelial cells, fibroblasts, and some other mesenchymal cell types; (2) neoangiogenic activity; (3) induction of a tumor histologically similar to Kaposi's sarcoma, but of mouse origin, when the cells are inoculated subcutaneously into nude mice; (4) chemotactic and chemoinvasive activities for Kaposi's sarcoma spindle cells, normal endothelial cells, and fibroblasts[66]; and (5) interleukin-1 (IL-1) and granulocyte-macrophage colony-stimulating factor (GM-CSF)–like activities.[69] In addition, mRNA extracted from long-term Kaposi's sarcoma cell cultures and probed for a number of cytokines showed the cell to express high levels of mRNA for IL-1β and basic fibroplast growth factor (bFGF), and moderate levels of mRNA for GM-CSF and TGF-β.[69] Messenger RNA for platelet-derived growth factor-α (PDGF-α) and IL-6 has also been shown in significant quantities.[70] These results have been further confirmed by determining the rate of production and release of these cytokines in conditioned media using ELISA and radioimmunoprecipitation assays. The sequence analysis of several cDNA clones, Southern blot analysis, and quantitative slot blot analysis further confirmed high levels of expression of bFGF and IL-1β by Kaposi's sarcoma cells (G. Barillari *et al,* unpubl. observ.).

Table 12–5.   Cell of Origin of Kaposi's Sarcoma

Reference, Year	Putative Cell of Origin	Method of Analysis
Pepler, 1959[55]	Neural origin	Histochemistry
Pepler and Theron, 1962[56]	Schwann cell	Electron microscopy
Hashimoto *et al,* 1964[57]	Endothelial, perithelial	Histochemistry, electron microscopy
Dayan AD and Lewis, 1967[58]	Reticuloendothelial	Silver staining
Harrison and Kahn LB, 1978[59]	Pluripotential mesenchymal cell	Electron microscopy
Nadji *et al,* 1981[60]	Endothelial cell	Immunohistochemistry
Beckstead *et al,* 1985[61]	Lymphatic endothelium	Enzyme-, immuno-, lectin histochemistry
Rutgers *et al,* 1986[62]	Vascular endothelium	Immunohistochemistry
Russel Jones *et al,* 1986[63]	Lymphatic endothelium	Immuno-, lectin histochemistry
Salahuddin *et al,* 1988[64]	Lymphatic endothelium	Cytochemical, immuno-, enzyme histochemistry
Nickoloff and Christopher, 1989[65]	Dermal dendrocyte (reticuloendothelial)	Immunohistochemistry
Thompson *et al,* 1991[66]	Smooth muscle	Cell culture, Matrigel culture
Weich *et al,* 1991[67]	Vascular smooth muscle precursor	Northern blot, immunohistochemistry

Both bFGF and IL-1β, which are found in high levels along with other cytokines expressed by Kaposi's sarcoma cell cultures, have been demonstrated to exert significant effects on Kaposi's sarcoma cells, mesenchymal cells, and immune cells.[71,72] It has also been demonstrated that Kaposi's sarcoma cells proliferate in response to the mitogenic effects of recombinant IL-1α, IL-1β, PDGF, and TNF-α,β (G. Barillari et al, unpubl. observ.), whereas smooth muscle cells respond to acidic and basic FGF, IL-1, and PDGF.[72] These observations indicate that Kaposi's sarcoma cells produce cytokines that support their own growth (autocrine) as well as the growth of other cells (paracrine), and that these cytokines may play a major role in the pathogenesis of AIDS-associated Kaposi's sarcoma.[71,72]

Of special interest is the isolation of a vascular permeability factor from the conditioned media that is believed to be responsible for the development of the tissue edema that sometimes precedes development of the lesions of Kaposi's sarcoma (S. Sakurada, unpubl. observ.). Further analysis of the Kaposi's sarcoma spindle cell line–conditioned media led to the isolation of a 30-kilodalton protein. Preliminary studies indicate that this protein is responsible for most of the activities of the conditioned media resulting in the growth and maintenance of Kaposi's sarcoma cells (R. C. Gallo, Florence, Italy).

HIV-1 Transactivating Gene

Recent investigations have implicated the HIV-1 transactivating (tat) gene and its product, the Tat protein, as important in the pathogenesis of Kaposi's sarcoma.[73,74] An experimental model has been developed by inserting the tat gene into the genome of nude mice. These "transgenic mice" were found to express tat gene mRNA only in skin, and most male mice went on to develop skin lesions histologically suggestive of early Kaposi's sarcoma. Interestingly, Kaposi's sarcoma-like lesions developed only in male mice, which suggested once again a possible hormonal influence in the development of this tumor. Also of interest is that tat gene mRNA was not found in tumor cells. This implies that the tat gene product (Tat protein), released by nearby or perhaps distant cells, is able to affect the growth of the Kaposi's sarcoma-like tumor. Further investigations using long-term culture of cells derived from AIDS-associated Kaposi's sarcoma have shown that supernatant containing Tat protein stimulates the growth of these cells but not of normal mesenchymal cells. This growth-promoting effect was inhibited by anti-Tat antibodies.[74] Recent studies have demonstrated Tat protein uptake in tissue culture and localization of Tat protein to the nucleus.[75] This is the first example of a human retrovirus regulatory gene product that is released biologically active and acts as a growth factor for tumor cells.[74] Thus, tat may produce the primary growth stimulus for the development of Kaposi's sarcoma cells in HIV-1–infected individuals.

Immune Activation

Neither the data concerning the cytokine cascade nor the data describing the contribution of Tat protein explain the predominance of Kaposi's sarcoma among certain high-risk groups such as homosexual or bisexual men; thus, other factors must play a role in the development of AIDS-associated Kaposi's sarcoma. Previously described clinical, epidemiologic, and laboratory data suggest that activation of the immune system may play a role in the pathogenesis of AIDS-associated Kaposi's sarcoma.[39,76–80] This may also prove to be true in the cases of classic, endemic, and iatrogenic Kaposi's sarcoma. Patients with classic Kaposi's sarcoma have high levels of anti-cytomegalovirus (CMV) antibodies[81] which suggests that persistent infection with this virus could provide the necessary stimulus for immune activation. In endemic Kaposi's sarcoma seen in Africa, parasitic and other infections could be the source of continuous antigenic stimulation. In the case of iatrogenic Kaposi's sarcoma, because of the host's lowered resistance, a variety of infections with agents such as CMV, Epstein-Barr virus (EBV), and herpes simplex virus (HSV) occur.[11] In addition, there is immune stimulation from the alloantigens from the transplanted tissue. Furthermore, it has been shown that corticosteroids have a direct stimulatory growth effect on AIDS-associated Kaposi's sarcoma cells (S. Nakamura et al, unpubl. observ.), and drugs such as cyclosporin can reduce T-suppressor cell activity.[82] Removal of these suppressor cells might result in disregulation and activation of the immune system. In AIDS-associated Kaposi's sarcoma, the life-style of homosexual or bisexual men exposes them to chronic antigenic stimuli in the form of multiple viral, bacterial, and parasitic infections, and sperm alloantigens.[80,83] Homosexual men with AIDS-associated Kaposi's sarcoma, when compared with a group of "healthy" homosexual controls, had a much higher rate of passive (receptive) anal-genital intercourse associated with rectal deposition of the sexual partner's semen as well as traumatic sexual practices such as fisting, which would allow entry of infections and exposure to sperm alloantigens.[25] Further support for this hypothesis comes from the observation that in early AIDS-associated Kaposi's sarcoma, patients often show no evidence of immunosuppression, but rather show signs of immune activation[36,78–80]; and as mentioned earlier, patients with AIDS who present with Kaposi's sarcoma live much longer than those presenting with opportunistic infections.[45] Finally, there are recent reports of Kaposi's sarcoma in individuals doubly infected with HTLV-II/HIV-1 in whom HTLV-II may act as the source of antigenic stimulation. It is unclear why the doubly infected IV drug abusers are not developing Kaposi's sarcoma at a greater rate.[84]

A series of new laboratory studies support the role of immune activation in the pathogenesis of Kaposi's sarcoma: (1) HTLV-II–conditioned media, which support the long-term culture of AIDS-associated Kaposi's sarcoma cells, contain several cytokines normally produced by activated immune cells. (2) TNF-α enhanced the progression of Kaposi's sarcoma lesions and augmented HIV-1 replication in AIDS-associated Kaposi's sarcoma cases.[85–88] (3) Conditioned media from phytohemagglutinin-stimulated peripheral blood mononuclear cells, enriched T cells, and HTLV-I–infected CD4+ cells have been shown to contain cytokines (IL-1α, 1β, IL-6, TNF-α, -β, GM-CSF, IL-2) with additive and/or synergistic mitogenic effects on the AIDS-associated Kaposi's sarcoma cells, human umbilical vein endothelial cells (hUVE) and adult aortic smooth muscle cells (aa-SMC) (Barillari *et al,* unpubl. observ.). (4) Increased levels of intracellular and extracellular cytokines may interrupt HIV-1 latency and increase *tat* gene expression.[89–91] (5) Using the above mentioned conditioned media and recombinant Tat, it has been demonstrated that hUVE cells, and aa-SMC cells, could become re-

sponsive to the mitogenic effects of Tat (similar to AIDS-associated Kaposi's sarcoma–derived cells) following exposure to these conditioned media (G. Barillari *et al,* unpubl. observ.). Thus, under the appropriate conditions, some cells of mesenchymal origin could be made responsive to Tat protein by the conditioned media from activated lymphocytes (G. Barillari *et al,* unpubl. observ.).

A recently proposed hypothetical model for the pathogenesis of AIDS-associated Kaposi's sarcoma (Fig. 12–1) brings together much of the current knowledge of this disease.[72] In this model, excessive T-cell activation in an HIV-1–infected individual leads to the release of cytokines at levels sufficient to (1) stimulate proliferation of the AIDS-associated Kaposi's sarcoma cells and normal mesenchymal cells; (2) induce Tat responsiveness in SMC and endothelial cells; and (3) activate HIV-1 replication and *tat* gene expression. In ad-

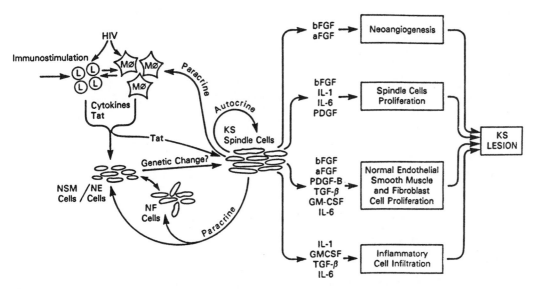

Figure 12–1. Model for the pathogenesis of the KS lesion in AIDS patients, showing normal endothelial cells (NE), normal smooth muscle cells (NSM), normal fibroblasts (NF), lymphocytes (L), and monocyte–macrophages (M). HIV-infected and activated cells (L and M) release TAT or other viral and cellular factor(s) capable of stimulating activation and proliferation of a particular cell type of mesenchymal origin. These cells (smooth muscle cells, endothelial cells?) then acquire the peculiar spindle-shaped morphology characteristic of KS cells. The KS cells, in turn, begin to produce and release several cytokines that maintain and amplify the cellular response via autocrine and paracrine pathways. Paracrine activation of normal cells (NE, NSM, NF, L, and M) leads to endothelial, smooth-muscle cell and fibroblast proliferation, neoangiogenesis, and inflammatory cell infiltrates. These phenomena, together with the spindle-cell proliferation, could underlie the typical histologic changes observed in early KS lesions. Later, interactions between cells of the immune system and mesenchymal cells could amplify cell activation and cytokine production. If the initial stimulus persists, a vicious cycle could be established that, under certain circumstances (*e.g.,* specific genetic changes) would lead to tumor transformation. (From Ensoli B, Salahuddin SZ, Gallo RC: Pathogenesis of AIDS-associated Kaposi's sarcoma. Hematol/Oncol Clin NA 5(2), April 1991)

dition, the extracellular Tat protein that is released transiently may (1) stimulate proliferation of AIDS-associated Kaposi's sarcoma cells and preactivated mesenchymal cells, (2) induce transactivation of the HIV-1 long terminal repeat and further amplify HIV-1 gene expression and replication, and (3) increase the effect of T-cell activation products on both cell growth and HIV-1 transactivation. Furthermore, the proliferation of AIDS-associated Kaposi's sarcoma cells leads to a release of cytokines owing to autocrine and paracrine activity, which induces neoangiogenesis and proliferation of mesenchymal cell types.[72]

In summary, HIV-1 infection and immunostimulation, through the effects of their extracellular products, might act together to initiate pathologic cellular and molecular events leading to the proliferation of spindle and mesenchymal cells observed in Kaposi's sarcoma lesions.[72] The recent experimental observations clearly delineate some of the mechanisms that explain the increased appearance of Kaposi's sarcoma among HIV-1–infected homosexual and bisexual men. Nevertheless, other factors such as hormonal influences,[73] sexual practices,[25] genetics,[92] environment,[22] and other infectious agents[26] might play roles in the initiation and development of Kaposi's sarcoma.

Immune Deficiency and Kaposi's Sarcoma

It has been generally believed that immune deficiency is one of the prerequisites for the development of Kaposi's sarcoma. This notion stemmed from the observation that some renal transplant recipients who were taking immunosuppressive drugs to prevent organ rejection developed Kaposi's sarcoma, and when the immunosuppressive drugs (such as prednisone, cyclophosphamide, azathioprine, or cyclosporin) were discontinued, the Kaposi's sarcoma lesions regressed.[46,48] The appearance of Kaposi's sarcoma as one of the first manifestations of the AIDS epidemic gave further support to the possible role of immune deficiency in the development of this disease. However, only a few years into the epidemic of AIDS, a small population of HIV-1–infected patients who developed Kaposi's sarcoma without any clinical or laboratory evidence of impaired immunity was recognized (B. Safai, unpubl. observ.). It became apparent that the mechanism by which HIV-1 causes Kaposi's sarcoma is different from the mechanism causing immune deficiency. Furthermore, studies of classic and endemic Kaposi's sarcoma did not show any true evidence of immune deficiency.[93] Based on this information and the recent studies implicating immune activation in the development of Kaposi's sarcoma, it no longer appears that immune deficiency is necessary for the development of Kaposi's sarcoma. More likely, chronic antigenic stimulation and disregulation of the immune system are important in the development of AIDS-associated Kaposi's sarcoma as well as the other forms of the disease.

Genetics

The appearance of Kaposi's sarcoma in elderly Italian and Jewish men, the endemic form of Kaposi's sarcoma seen in localized areas of Africa, and the occurrence of AIDS-associated Kaposi's sarcoma among a subpopulation of HIV-infected individuals all suggest a possible genetic susceptibility to the development of the disease. The number of reported cases of Kaposi's sarcoma among members of the same family is very small and speaks against involvement of a mendelian recessive or dominant inheritance.[28,29] An increased frequency of HLA-DR5 in Italian and Jewish patients with Kaposi's sarcoma and of HLA-DR2 among patients of other European descent with the disease, had been reported and confirmed during the early years of the AIDS epidemic.[94] However, HLA typing in a larger population with AIDS-associated Kaposi's sarcoma no longer shows an increased frequency of any HLA antigen (B. Safai, unpubl. observ.). It is difficult to explain the discrepancies seen in HLA typing. One possible reason may be that in the group of HIV-1–infected persons, Kaposi's sarcoma developed first among those most susceptible, perhaps with an association with HLA-DR5. This would result in the currently observed smaller percentage of HIV-1–infected persons with Kaposi's sarcoma who have no recognized genetic marker.

The absence of familial cases, and the lack of increased frequency of one or more HLA subtype, do not rule out the possibility of a genetic susceptibility factor in Kaposi's sarcoma. Further investigation in the area using more recently developed molecular genetic techniques may be beneficial.

Viral Etiology

The new model of pathogenesis of AIDS-associated Kaposi's sarcoma that has been proposed, based on recent studies, fails to answer many perplexing questions about the disease, such as why Kaposi's sarcoma occurs more frequently in homosexual men than in IV drug abusers and hemophiliacs, who are exposed to many blood-borne pathogens. Some recently described epidemiologic observations support the theory of a possible sexually transmitted co-agent involved in AIDS-associated Kaposi's sarcoma: (1) The recent reduction in the number of cases of AIDS-associated Kaposi's sarcoma as compared to rates in earlier years of the AIDS epidemic is attributed by some investigators to the current "safe" sexual practices of homosexual and bisexual men. (2) Only 1% of hemophiliacs are reported to have AIDS-associated Kaposi's sarcoma, *versus* 21% of homosexuals. (3) Homosexual men with AIDS who live in New York City or San Francisco have a greater risk of developing Kaposi's sarcoma than men from the central states. (4) AIDS-associated Kaposi's sarcoma is reported to be four times more common in women who had sex with bisexual men than with other HIV-1 seropositive men.[26]

(5) Women from Great Britain who developed AIDS-associated Kaposi's sarcoma were more likely to have contracted HIV-1 infection through sexual contact with persons from the United States. (6) Homosexual men who engaged in oral-anal contact and those who were the receptive partners had higher incidence of AIDS-associated Kaposi's sarcoma.[25] (7) The epidemiology of Kaposi's sarcoma in Sweden prior to the AIDS epidemic points to a causative infectious agent other than HIV. It was found by retrospective study of 529 cases that the incidence of Kaposi's sarcoma began to rise significantly two decades prior to the AIDS epidemic in Sweden.[95]

Another observation that suggests a transmissible agent other than HIV-1 comes from the study of a small group of HIV-seronegative patients with Kaposi's sarcoma. These individuals belong to the high-risk population (homosexual/bisexual) who have developed biopsy-proven Kaposi's sarcoma. They have normal immune status and the course of their disease is generally indolent. They have remained negative for HIV-1 by all tests, including polymerase chain reaction (PCR). They are younger than patients with classic Kaposi's sarcoma but slightly older than patients with the AIDS-associated form.[96–98]

The search for a putative agent of Kaposi's sarcoma has been on for many years. Early in the epidemic, much attention was given to the role of CMV and EBV in Kaposi's sarcoma.[99] Although these viruses are frequently found in AIDS-associated Kaposi's sarcoma cases, neither serologic nor molecular genetic studies have been able to identify them as etiologic agents.[100,101] Recently other viruses, possibly retroviruses, have come under suspicion. In the study of a cluster of cases from the Greek Peloponnesus Peninsula, retrovirus-like particles were found in close association with Kaposi's sarcoma cells in five of 12 specimens tested by ultrastructural studies.[102] All patients had antibodies to herpesvirus but were negative for HIV-1 and HTLV-I.

Although the data cited above support the hypothesis that a sexually transmissible agent other than HIV is involved in Kaposi's sarcoma, this appears unlikely, for a number of reasons: (1) no single causative agent has been consistently isolated in the tissue of Kaposi's sarcoma; (2) it does not explain the male predominance in African AIDS-associated Kaposi's sarcoma, where HIV-1 is transmitted through heterosexual contact; and (3) it does not explain the development of classic disease or transplantation-associated disease, in which there is no evidence of sexual transmission.

Alternatively, rather than a second novel agent, a different subtype of HIV or a defective form of HIV-1 may be involved and potentiate the development of Kaposi's sarcoma but by itself may not lead to immunodeficiency. In support of this, a recent case of Kaposi's sarcoma with normal immune test results, seronegative for HIV-1 by all routine tests, was found by sensitive assays to have antibodies against gp41 and *nef*. This antibody response to HIV-1 constituents may represent reactivity to such an agent.[103]

TREATMENT

Systemic Chemotherapy

The treatment of Kaposi's sarcoma has been a challenge since the onset of the AIDS epidemic. Unlike other HIV-associated neoplasms, such as non-Hodgkin's lymphoma, there was relatively little experience with systemic chemotherapy, since the classic form of the disease is usually indolent and responds well to local therapy. The aggressive nature of AIDS-associated Kaposi's sarcoma, which often presents with widespread disease and frequent lymph node and visceral involvement, makes the earlier experience with chemotherapy for the classic form of the disease not readily applicable. Furthermore, the anemia, multiple infections with opportunistic organisms, and immune deficiency often associated with AIDS-associated Kaposi's sarcoma were additional obstacles to aggressive chemotherapeutic regimens. Nevertheless, a number of trials of chemotherapy for Kaposi's sarcoma were undertaken, and some reported successful results. The initial trials for AIDS-associated Kaposi's sarcoma followed the recommendations of the National Cancer Institute,[104] with single-drug therapy used for minimal disease and combination chemotherapy for advanced disease. Partial response rates have ranged from 26% to 76%, with tolerable side-effects in the more current regimens in which low-dose therapy has been employed (Table 12–6).[104–116] The most successful regimen, with an overall response rate of 88%, has been low-dose ABV (adriamycin, bleomycin, and vincristine).[113] The frequency of opportunistic infections in this group was 25%, compared to 61% in patients treated with the same regimen with a standard dose.[105] Another promising treatment is reported to be the use of oral etoposide (VP-16), which may be more effective than parenteral vinblastine monotherapy and has the additional advantage of ease of administration.[116]

There are many difficulties in comparing different chemotherapeutic trials in patients with AIDS-associated Kaposi's sarcoma. No uniform staging system has been used to group patients in many of the clinical trials. Therefore, it must be kept in mind that the high partial remission rates seen in some trials employing a single drug may reflect patients who are in a better prognostic group or have limited disease. Some of the more aggressive regimens with multiple drugs have been employed only after single-drug treatment failure, or in patients with aggressive, widespread disease.

Variables that have been found to predict a poor therapeutic response have been low T4 counts, anemia, an increased erythrocyte sedimentation rate, and systemic B symptoms. Some of these variables correlate with those used in the prognostic staging classification recently proposed.[50] Although the more current treatment regimens have fewer immunosuppressive effects, it is difficult to determine whether they lead to a decreased survival owing to death from opportunistic infections, because none of the clinical trials enrolled pa-

Table 12–6. Chemotherapy Trials in AIDS-Associated Kaposi's Sarcoma

Regimen*	No. of Pts.	No. of Complete Responses	No. of Partial Reponses	Overall Response No. (%)	Reference
VP-16	41	12	19	31 (76)	105
ABV	31	7	19	26 (84)	105
Vb	38	1	9	10 (26)	106
ABV/AdVcD	27	8	12	20 (74)	107
Vc	18	0	11	11 (61)	108
VcVb	21	1	8	9 (42)	109
BVel	31	0	24	(62)	110
B	9	7		(78)	110
Vel/MTX	9	3	4	7 (77)	111
BVc	18	2	11	13 (72)	112
ABV	24	9	12	21 (88)	113
A	29	1	13	14 (48)	113

* A = Adriamycin, B = bleomycin, Vc = vincristine, Vb = vinblastine, Vel = velbane, MTX = methotrexate, Ad = actinomycin D, D = dacarbazine.

tient controls matched for disease stage. In addition, although some of the regimens have shown favorable response rates, none of the responses have been durable, with a mean duration of less than 8 months. Clearly, much work needs to be done to find the optimal regimen for each individual patient. The recent use of hematopoietic growth factors such as GM-CSF concomitantly with chemotherapy and antiviral therapy may lead to further protection against opportunistic infections and prolong survival.

Immune Response Modifiers

IFN-α has emerged as the only immune modulating agent to play a role in the treatment of AIDS-associated Kaposi's sarcoma, and it has been approved for this use by the FDA. Besides its antiproliferative effects, IFN-α has antiviral and immune stimulatory properties, which make it theoretically advantageous over cytotoxic, immunosuppressive regimens. Although the exact mechanism of action of IFN-α in Kaposi's sarcoma is not known, it is most likely due to its antiproliferative properties, because no improvement in immunologic parameters has been reported in patients who received the drug.[117–123]

Clinical trials using high-dose (20 MU or greater) IFN-α have shown response rates in the range of 20% to 50% (Table 12–7).[118–124] The rate of response and the time to response have been found to be dose related, although a complete remission has been reported with low-dose therapy (1 MU/day).[120] In one large study, the median disease-free interval and the median response duration were reported to be 13 and 18 months respectively, an improvement over the results achieved with chemotherapy.[118] Recent studies have shown that IFN-α can be used safely as long-term therapy for AIDS-associated Kaposi's sarcoma. In one study of five patients

treated for 24 to 30 months with medium-dose therapy, there was one sustained remission, and regression and stabilization occurred in two other patients.[125] None of the patients developed opportunistic infections or protocol-interrupting side-effects. This result demonstrates that early and sustained treatment with IFN-α may lead to prolonged disease control and increased survival.

The clinical trials have led to recognition of certain features predictive of a positive or negative response to IFN-α. Clinical features associated with a poor response include opportunistic infections, systemic B symptoms, and anemia. The most important laboratory factor is the number of CD4+ lymphocytes. Patients with CD4+ counts above 600 cells/mm³ have response rates greater than 80%. Patients with CD4+ counts below 200 cells/mm³ are unlikely to have a response.[121,126]

The subjective toxic effects associated with IFN-α are frequent and can be severe. Frequent symptomatic complaints include flulike symptoms, which occur in almost all patients receiving high-dose IFN-α. Other adverse effects include somnolence, headache, dizziness, and GI disturbances. Fortunately, tolerance increases as treatment progresses. Hematologic and hepatic toxicity are infrequent and usually mild, and rarely necessitate a dose reduction.

The combination of IFN-α and zidovudine has been shown to result in synergistic suppression of HIV replication *in vitro,* and studies have been conducted to evaluate these drugs in AIDS-associated Kaposi's sarcoma. In two preliminary reports,[126,127] the maximum tolerated dose combinations were 18 MU of IFN-α daily and 100 mg of zidovudine every 4 hours. The dose-limiting toxic effects were anemia and neutropenia for zidovudine and hepatotoxicity for IFN-α. Tumor response rates were higher than expected given the relatively low dose of IFN-α used, suggesting antitumor synergy. However, one study showed no treatment ad-

Table 12–7. Interferon Trials for AIDS-Associated Kaposi's Sarcoma

IFN Regimen	No. of Pts.	No. of Complete Responses	No. of Partial Responses	Total Responses No. (%)	Reference
INTERFERON-α_{2a}					
3 mu/day IM	36	0	1	1 (3)	118
3–36 mu/day IM	30	3	2	5 (17)	118
36 mu/day IM	34	8	5	13 (38)	118
36 mu/day IM + VBL	20	1	5	6 (30)	119
INTERFERON-α_{2b}					
1 mu/mm² 5 d/wk SC q.o.w.	10	1	1	2 (20)	120
1–50 mu/mm² 5 d/wk Sc-IV q.o.w.	4	1	1	2 (50)	120
50 mu/mm² 5 d/wk IV q.o.w.	1	0	4	4 (40)	120
1 mu/mm² 5 d/wk SC q.o.w.	9	2	1	3 (33)	121
30 mu/mm² 3 d/wk SC	65	5	13	18 (28)	121
50 mu/mm² 5 d/wk IV q.o.w.	33	4	11	15 (45)	121
INTERFERON-α-N1 (LYMPHOBLASTOID)					
6–15 mu/mm²/day × 28 d IM	27	3	1	4 (15)	122
20 mu/mm²/day × 2 mo IM	12	4	4	8 (67)	123
20 mu/mm²/day × 8 wk IV	20	3	9	12 (60)	124
20 mu/mm²/day × 8 wk + VBL	12	1	7	8 (67)	124
INTERFERON + ZIDOVUDINE					
4.5, 9, 18 mu/day IM + zidovudine, 100–200 mg q.4h.	37	1	16	17 (46)	125
9, 18, 27 mu/day IM + zidovudine, 100–200 mg q.4h.	43	16	4	20 (47)	126
9–18 mu/day SC + zidovudine, 300 mg b.i.d.	20	0	1	1 (5)	126

VBL = vinblastine, q.o.w. = every other week.

vantage with the addition of zidovudine.[128] As in studies of IFN-α alone, tumor response was associated with a CD4 count greater than 200 cells/mm³.

Studies have also been done using IFN-α in combination with vinblastine and etoposide.[115,124] There was no positive synergistic effect found in either study, and the hematologic and subjective toxic effects were more severe. Although the antitumor mechanisms for both cytotoxic chemotherapy and IFN-α are unknown, tumor response and perhaps survival benefits can only be expected in earlier stages of immune deficiency as measured by CD4+ cell counts above 200 to 300 cells/mm³.

Local Treatment of Kaposi's Sarcoma

The local treatment of Kaposi's sarcoma is important for the control of pain, edema, improvement of function, and the improvement of cosmetic appearance. There are numerous relatively safe therapeutic modalities for the control of local lesions. Small isolated lesions can be treated by excision, or by electrodesiccation and curettage. Another common treatment entails cryotherapy, although there is often residual brown pigmentation and, in darker skinned individuals, cosmetically unacceptable hypo- and hyperpigmentation. Radiotherapy, which has been frequently employed in the treatment

of classic Kaposi's sarcoma has become the most important therapeutic modality in the local treatment of AIDS-associated Kaposi's sarcoma.[129] Radiotherapy can be especially useful for the treatment of lesions in difficult anatomic areas such as the oral mucosa, conjunctiva, the face, and the sole (see Color Figs. 14 & 15). In a review of 226 lesions in 129 patients, there was a complete regression in 68% of the lesions. In only 9% of the lesions was there local regrowth within the radiation field.[130] Drawbacks to this mode of treatment are that it requires a specialized treatment facility, it is time-consuming (treatments are typically delivered in ten fractions over a 2-week period), and expensive.

Local treatment employing intralesional vinblastine in 190 lesions resulted in a complete response in 13% and a partial response in 78%.[131] The side-effects were mainly local pain (100%) and skin irritation (90%). Future trials of intralesional chemotherapy and biologic response modifiers may add safer and more effective treatment for mucocutaneous Kaposi's sarcoma.

Future Prospects

With the advent of new knowledge about the pathogenic mechanisms involved in Kaposi's sarcoma, it is foreseeable that safer and more effective therapeutic approaches will be developed. The availability of *in vitro* Kaposi's sarcoma cell culture allows for the screening of a large number of potentially therapeutic drugs. For example, a recent study indicated that a naturally occurring bacterial wall component (a polysaccharide peptido-glycan product) known as SP-PG is effective in tissue culture in controlling growth of Kaposi's sarcoma cells and inhibiting angiogenesis in an animal model of this disease. This compound will most likely be in clinical trials within the next 12 months (S. Nakamura *et al,* unpubl. observ.). (See color insert for Color Figs. 17–20.)

REFERENCES

1. Centers for Disease Control: *Pneumocystis* pneumonia—Los Angeles. MMWR 30:250, 1981
2. Centers for Disease Control (Friedman-Kien A et al): Kaposi's sarcoma and *Pneumocystis* pneumonia among homosexual men—New York and California. MMWR 30:305, 1981
3. Kaposi M: Idiopathic multiple pigmented sarcoma of the skin. Cancer 31:3, 1982
4. Digiovanna JJ, Safai B: Kaposi's sarcoma: Retrospective study of 90 cases with particular emphasis on the familial occurrence, ethnic background and prevalence of other diseases. Am J Med 71:779, 1981
5. Loethe R: Kaposi's sarcoma in Ugandan Africans. Acta Pathol Microbiol Scand 161:1, 1963
6. Dutz W, Stout AP: Kaposi's sarcoma in infants and children. Cancer 13:684, 1960
7. Davies JNP, Loethe R: Kaposi's sarcoma in African children. Acta Unio Int Contra Cancrum 18:394, 1962
8. Myers BD, Kessler E, Levi J et al: Kaposi's sarcoma in kidney transplant recipients. Arch Intern Med 133:307, 1974
9. Gange RW, Wilson JE: Kaposi's sarcoma and immunosuppressive therapy: An appraisal. Clin Exp Dermatol 3:135, 1978
10. Penn I: Kaposi's sarcoma in organ transplant recipients. Transplantation 27:8, 1979
11. Shmueli D, Shapira Z, Yussim A et al: The incidence of Kaposi's sarcoma in renal transplant patients and its relation to immunosuppression. Transplant Proc 21:3209, 1989
12. Haverkos HW, Curran JW: The current outbreak of Kaposi's sarcoma and opportunistic infections. CA 32:330, 1982
13. Oettle AG: Geographical and racial differences in the frequencies of Kaposi's sarcoma as evidence of environmental or genetic causes. Acta Unio Int Contra Cancrum 18:330, 1962
14. Rothman S: Remarks on sex, age, and racial distribution of Kaposi's sarcoma and on possible pathogenetic factors. Acta Unio Int Contra Cancrum 18:326, 1962
15. Mikkelsen F, Nielsen N, Hansen JP: Kaposi's sarcoma in polar Eskimos. Acta Derm Venereol (Stockh) 57:539, 1977
16. Haverkos HW, Friedman-Kien AE, Drotman P et al: The changing incidence of Kaposi's sarcoma among patients with AIDS. J Am Acad Dermatol 22:1250, 1990
17. Lifson AR, Darrow WW, Hessol NA et al: Kaposi's sarcoma in a cohort of homosexual and bisexual men. Am J Epidemiol 131:221, 1990
18. Centers for Disease Control Task Force on Kaposi's Sarcoma and Opportunistic Infections: Epidemiologic aspects of the current outbreak of Kaposi's sarcoma and opportunistic infections. N Engl J Med 306:248, 1982
19. Centers for Disease Control: HIV/AIDS Surveillance Report. Atlanta, CDC, January 1990
20. Selik RM, Starcher ET, Curran JW: Opportunistic diseases reported in AIDS patients: Frequencies, associations, and trends. AIDS 1:175, 1987
21. Goedert JJ, Wallen WC, Mann DL et al: Amyl nitrite may alter T lymphocytes in homosexual men. Lancet 11:412, 1982
22. Haverkos HW, Pinsky PF, Dortman DP, Bergman DJ: Disease manifestation among homosexual with acquired immunodeficiency syndrome: A possible role of nitrites in Kaposi's sarcoma. Sex Transm Dis 12:203, 1985
23. Dunkel VC, Rogers-Back AM, Lawlor TE et al: Mutagenicity of some alkyl nitrites used as recreational drugs. Environ Mol Mut 14:115, 1989
24. Jaffe HW, Choi K, Thomas PA et al: National case-control study of Kaposi's sarcoma and *Pneumocystis carinii* pneumonia in homosexual men: Part I. Epidemiologic results. Ann Intern Med 99:145, 1983
25. Darrow WW, Jaffe HW, Curran JW: Passive and intercourse as a risk factor for AIDS in homosexual men. Lancet 2:160, 1983
26. Beral V, Peterman TA, Berkelman RL et al: Kaposi's sarcoma among persons with AIDS: A sexually transmitted infection? Lancet 2:123, 1990
27. Bayley AC, Downing RG, Cheingsong-Popov R et al: HTLV-III serology distinguishes atypical and endemic Kaposi's sarcoma in Africa. Lancet 1:359, 1985
28. Epstein E: Kaposi's sarcoma and parapsoriasis en plaque in brothers (letter). JAMA 219:1477, 1972
29. Brownstein MH, Shapiro L, Skolnik P: Kaposi's sarcoma in community practice (letter). Arch Dermatol 107:137, 1973
30. Rothman S: Some clinical aspects of Kaposi's sarcoma in the European and North American populations. Acta Unio Int Contra Cancrum 18:364, 1962
31. Taylor JF, Templeton AC, Vogel CL et al: Kaposi's sarcoma in Uganda: A clinicopathological study. Int J Cancer 8:122, 1971
32. Slavin G, Cameron HM, Forbes C et al: Kaposi's sarcoma in East African children: A report of 51 cases. J Pathol 100:187, 1970
33. Dutz W, Stout AP: Kaposi's sarcoma in infants and children. Cancer 12:289, 1959
34. Civati G, Busnach G, Brando B et al: Occurrence of Kaposi's sarcoma in renal transplant recipients treated with cyclosporine. Transplant Proc 20(suppl 3):924, 1988
35. Harwood AR, Osoba SD, Hofstadler SL et al: Kaposi's sarcoma in recipients of renal transplants. Am J Med 67:759, 1979
36. Safai B, Johnson KG, Myskowski PL et al: The natural history of Kaposi's sarcoma in the acquired immunodeficiency syndrome. Ann Intern Med 103:744, 1985
37. Niedt GW, Schinella RA: Acquired immunodeficiency syndrome: A clinicopathologic study of 56 autopsies. Arch Pathol Lab Med 109:727, 1985
38. Myskowski PL, Niedzwiecki D, Shurgot BA et al: AIDS-associated Kaposi's sarcoma: Variables associated with survival. J Am Acad Dermatol 18:1299, 1988
39. Safai B, Sarngadharan MG, Koziner B et al: Spectrum of Kaposi's sarcoma in the epidemic of AIDS. Cancer Res 45:4646s, 1985

40. Krigel RL: The treatment and nature history of Kaposi's sarcoma. Proc NY Acad Sci 437:447, 1984

41. Krigel R: Prognostic factors in Kaposi's sarcoma. In Friedman-Kien AE, Laubenstein LJ (eds): Epidemic Kaposi's Sarcoma and Opportunistic Infections in Homosexual Men. New York, Masson, 1984

42. Meduri GU, Stover DE, Lee M et al: Pulmonary Kaposi's sarcoma in the acquired immunodeficiency syndrome. Am J Med 81:11, 1986

43. Hamm PG, Judson MA, Aranda CP: Diagnosis of pulmonary Kaposi's sarcoma with fiberoptic bronchoscopy and endobronchial biopsy. Cancer 59:807, 1987

44. Hardy AM: Characterization of long term survivors of acquired immunodeficiency syndrome. J AIDS 4:386, 1991

45. Rothenberg R, Woelfel M, Stoneburner R et al: Survival with the acquired immunodeficiency syndrome: Experience with 5,833 cases in New York City. N Engl J Med 317:1297, 1987

46. Pilgrim M: Spontaneous manifestation of regression of a Kaposi's sarcoma under cyclosporin A. Hautarzt 39:368, 1988

47. Wijnveen AC, Persson H, Bjorck S et al: Disseminated Kaposi's sarcoma: Full regression after withdrawal of immunosuppressive therapy of a case. Transplant Proc 19: 3735, 1987

48. Krigel RL, Laubenstein LJ, Muggia FM: Kaposi's sarcoma: A new staging classification. Cancer Treat Rep 67:531, 1983

49. Redfield RR, Wright DC, Tramont EC: The Walter Reed staging classification for HTLV-III/LAV infection. N Engl J Med 314:131, 1986

50. Chachoua A, Krigel R, Lafleur F et al: Prognostic factors and staging classification of patients with epidemic Kaposi's sarcoma. J Clin Oncol 7:774, 1989

51. Krown SE, Metroka C, Wernz JC et al: Kaposi's sarcoma in the acquired immune deficiency syndrome: A proposal for a uniform evaluation, response, and staging criteria. J Clin Oncol 7:1201, 1989

52. Gottleib GJ, Ackerman AB (eds): Kaposi's Sarcoma: A Text and Atlas. Baltimore, Lea & Febiger, 1988

53. McNutt NS, Fletcher V, Conant MA: Early lesions of Kaposi's sarcoma in homosexual men: An ultrastructural comparison with other vascular proliferations in skin. Am J Pathol 11:62, 1983

54. Gottleib GJ, Ackerman AB: Kaposi's sarcoma: An extensive disseminated form in young homosexual men. Hum Pathol 13:882, 1982

55. Pepler WJ: The origin of Kaposi's haemangiosarcoma: A histochemical study. J Pathol Bacteriol 78:553, 1959

56. Pepler WJ, Theron JJ: An electron microscopic study of Kaposi's haemangiosarcoma. J Pathol Bacteriol 83:521, 1962

57. Hashimoto K, Lever WF: Kaposi's sarcoma: Histochemical and electron microscopic studies. J Invest Dermatol 43: 539, 1964

58. Dayan AD, Lewis PD: Origin of Kaposi's sarcoma from the reticulo-endothelial system. Nature 2:889, 1967

59. Harrison AC, Kahn LB: Myogenic cells in Kaposi's sarcoma: An ultrastructural study. J Pathol 124:157, 1978

60. Nadji M, Morales AR, Ziegles-Weissman J, Penneys NS: Kaposi's sarcoma: Immunohistologic evidence for an endothelial origin. Arch Pathol Lab Med 105:274, 1981

61. Beckstead JH, Wood GS, Fletcher V: Evidence for the origin of Kaposi's sarcoma from lymphatic endothelium. Am J Pathol 119:294, 1985

62. Rutgers JL, Wieczorek R, Bonetti F et al: The expression of endothelial cell surface antigens by AIDS-associated Kaposi's sarcoma: Evidence for a vascular endothelial cell origin. Am J Pathol 122:493, 1986

63. Jones RR, Spaull J, Spry C, Jones EW: Histogenesis of Kaposi's Sarcoma in patients without acquired immune deficiency syndrome (AIDS). J Clin Pathol 39: 742, 1986

64. Salahuddin SZ, Nakamura S, Biberfeld P et al: Angiogenic properties of Kaposi's sarcoma-derived cells after long-term culture in vitro. Science 242:430, 1988

65. Nickoloff BJ, Griffiths CEM: The spindle-shaped cells in cutaneous Kaposi's sarcoma. Am J Pathol 135:793, 1989

66. Thompson EW, Nakamura S, Shima TB et al: Supernatants of acquired immunodeficiency syndrome–related Kaposi's sarcoma cells induce endothelial cell chemotaxis and invasiveness. Cancer Res 51:2670, 1991

67. Weich HA, Salahuddin SZ, Nakamura S et al: AIDS-Kaposi's derived cells in long-term culture express and synthesize smooth muscle a-actin (in press)

68. Nakamura S, Salahuddin SZ, Biberfeld P et al: Kaposi's sarcoma cells: Long-term culture with growth factor from retrovirus-infected CD4+ T cells. Science 242:426, 1988

69. Ensoli B, Nakamura S, Salahuddin SZ et al: AIDS-Kaposi's sarcoma-derived cells express cytokines with autocrine and paracrine growth effects. Science 243:223, 1989

70. Miles SA, Rezai AR, Salazar-Gonzalez JF et al: AIDS Kaposi's sarcoma–derived cells produce and respond to interleukin 6. Proc Natl Acad Sci USA 87:4068, 1990

71. Ensoli B, Salahuddin SZ, Gallo RC: AIDS-associated Kaposi's sarcoma: A molecular model for its pathogenesis. Cancer Cells 1:93, 1989

72. Ensoli B, Barillari G, Gallo RC: Pathogenesis of AIDS-associated Kaposi's sarcoma. Hematol Oncol Clin North Am 5:2281, 1991

73. Vogel J, Hinrichs SH, Reynolds RK et al: The HIV *tat* gene induces dermal lesions resembling Kaposi's sarcoma in transgenic mice. Nature 335:606, 1988

74. Ensoli B, Barillari G, Salahuddin SZ et al: Tat protein of HIV-1 stimulates growth of cells derived from Kaposi's sarcoma lesions of AIDS patients. Nature 345:84, 1990

75. Frankel AD, Paba CO: Cellular uptake of the Tat protein from human immunodeficiency virus. Cell 55:1189, 1988

76. Rabkin CS, Goedert JJ, Biggar RJ et al: Kaposi's sarcoma in three HIV-1-infected cohorts. J AIDS 3(suppl 1):s38, 1990

77. Mitsuyasu RT, Taylor JMG, Glaspy J et al: Heterogeneity of epidemic Kaposi's sarcoma. Cancer 57:1657, 1986

78. Ballard HS: Dissemination of Kaposi's sarcoma without lymphocyte abnormalities. Arch Intern Med 145:547, 1985

79. Lane HC, Masur H, Gelman EP et al: Correlation between immunologic function and clinical subpopulations of patients with the acquired immunodeficiency syndrome. Am J Med 78:417, 1985

80. Jacobson LP, Munos A, Fox R et al: Incidence of Kaposi's sarcoma in a cohort of homosexual men with human immunodeficiency virus type 1. J AIDS 3(suppl 1):s24, 1990

81. Giraldo G, Beth E, Huang ES: Kaposi's sarcoma and its relationship to cytomegalovirus (CMV): III. CMV DNA and CMV early antigens in Kaposi's sarcoma. Int J Cancer 26:23, 1980

82. Cohen DJ, Loertscher R, Rubin MF et al: Cyclosporine: A new immunosuppressive agent for organ transplantation. Ann Intern Med 101:667, 1984

83. Mavligit GM, Talpaz M, Hsia FT et al: Chronic immune stimulation by sperm alloantigens. JAMA 251:237, 1984

84. Gorter RW, Osmond D, Gallo D et al: Coinfection of HIV-

I and HTLV-I/II in intravenous drug users in treatment programs in San Francisco. Presented at the VII International Conference on AIDS, Florence, Italy, June 1991

85. Aboulafia D, Miles SA, Saks SR, Mitsuyasu RT: Intravenous recombinant tumor necrosis factor in the treatment of AIDS-related Kaposi's sarcoma. J AIDS 2:54, 1989

86. Duh EJ, Maury WJ, Folks TM et al: Tumor necrosis factor α activates human immunodeficiency virus type 1 through induction of nuclear factor binding to the NF-κB sites in the long terminal repeat. Microbiology 86:5974, 1989

87. Poli G, Kinter A, Justement JS et al: Tumor necrosis factor α functions in an autocrine manner in the induction of human immunodeficiency virus expression. Immunology 87:782, 1990

88. Osborn L, Kunkel S, Nabel GJ: Tumor necrosis factor α and interleukin 1 stimulate the human immunodeficiency virus enhancer by activation of the nuclear factor kB. Proc Natl Acad Sci USA 86:2336, 1989

89. Folks T, Justement J, Kinter A et al: Cytokine-induced expression of HIV-1 in a chronically infected promonocyte cell line. Science 238:800, 1988

90. Koyanagi Y, O'Brien WA, Zhao JQ: Cytokines alter production of HIV-1 from primary mononuclear phagocytes. Science 241:1673, 1988

91. Latham PS, Lewis AM, Varesio L et al: Expression of human immunodeficiency virus long terminal repeat in the human promonocyte cell line U937: Effect of endotoxin and cytokines. Cell Immunol 129:513, 1990

92. Pomerantz RJ, Feinberg MB, Trono D et al: Lipopolysaccharide is a potent monocyte/macrophage-specific stimulator of human immunodeficiency virus type 1 expression. J Exp Med 172:253, 1990

93. Safai B, Mike V, Giraldo G et al: Association of Kaposi's sarcoma with second primary malignancies. Cancer 45:1472, 1980

94. Pollack MS, Safai B, DuPont B: HLA-DR5 and DR2 are susceptibility factors for acquired immunodeficiency syndrome with Kaposi's sarcoma in different ethnic subpopulations. Dis Markers 1:135, 1983

95. Dictor M, Attewell R: Epidemiology of Kaposi's sarcoma in Sweden prior to the acquired immunodeficiency syndrome. Int J Cancer 42:346, 1988

96. Friedman-Kien AE, Saltzman BR, Cao Y et al: Kaposi's sarcoma in HIV-negative homosexual men. Lancet 335:168, 1990

97. Garcia-Muret MP, Oujol RM, Pig L et al: Disseminated Kaposi's sarcoma not associated with HIV infection in a bisexual man. J Am Acad Dermatol 23:1038, 1990

98. Safai B, Peralta H, Menzies K et al: Kaposi's sarcoma among HIV-seronegative high risk population (abstr). Presented at the VII International Conference on AIDS, Florence, Italy, June 1991

99. Giraldo G, Buonaguro FM, Beth-Giraldo E: The role of viruses in Kaposi's sarcoma (KS) evolution. APMIS Suppl 8:62, 1989

100. Holmberg SD: Possible cofactors for the development of AIDS-related neoplasms. Cancer Detect Prevent 14:331, 1990

101. Jahan N, Razzaque A, Greenspan J et al: Analysis of human KS biopsies and cloned cell lines for cytomegalovirus, HIV-1, and other selected DNA virus sequences. AIDS Res Hum Retroviruses 5:225, 1989

102. Rappersberger K, Tschachler E, Zonzits E et al: Endemic Kaposi's sarcoma in human immunodeficiency virus type 1–seronegative persons: Demonstration of retrovirus-like particles in cutaneous lesions. J Invest Dermatol 95:371, 1990

103. Bowden F, McFee D, Sonza S et al: Antibodies to GP41 and *nef* in a male homosexual with Kaposi's sarcoma who is seronegative for HIV by conventional testing (abstr). Presented at the VII International Conference on AIDS, Florence, Italy, June 1991

104. DeWys WD, Curran J, Henle W, Johnson G: Workshop on Kaposi's Sarcoma: Meeting report. Cancer Treat Rep 66:1387, 1982

105. Laubenstein LJ, Krigel RL, Odajnyk CM et al: Treatment of epidemic Kaposi's sarcoma with etoposide or a combination of doxorubicin, bleomycin, and vincristine. J Clin Oncol 2:1115, 1984

106. Volberding PA, Abrams DI, Conant M et al: Vinblastine therapy for Kaposi's sarcoma in the acquired immunodeficiency syndrome. Ann Intern Med 103:335, 1985

107. Gelmann E, Longo D, Lane H et al: Combination chemotherapy of disseminated Kaposi's sarcoma in patients with the acquired immune deficiency syndrome. Am J Med 82:456, 1987

108. Minzter D, Real F, Jovino F et al: Treatment of Kaposi's sarcoma and thrombocytopenia with vincristine in patients with the acquired immunodeficiency syndrome. Ann Intern Med 102:200, 1985

109. Kaplan L, Abrams D, Volberding P: Treatment of Kaposi's sarcoma in acquired immunodeficiency syndrome with an alternating vincristine-vinblastine regimen. Cancer Treat Rep 70:1121, 1986

110. Wernz J, Laubenstein L, Hymes K et al: Chemotherapy and assessment of response in epidemic Kaposi's sarcoma (EKS) with bleomycin and velbane (abstr). Proc Am Soc Clin Oncol 5:4, 1986

111. Minor R, Brayes T: Velban and methotrexate combination chemotherapy for epidemic Kaposi's sarcoma (abstr). Proc Am Soc Clin Oncol 5:1, 1986

112. Gill P, Rarick M, Bernstein-Singer M: Treatment of advanced Kaposi's sarcoma using a combination of bleomycin and vincristine. Am J Oncol 13:315, 1990

113. Gill PS, Rarick M, McCutchan LA et al: Systemic treatment of AIDS-related Kaposi's sarcoma: Results of a randomized trial. Am J Med 90:427, 1991

114. Glaspy J, Miles S, McCarthy S et al: Treatment of advanced stage Kaposi's sarcoma with vincristine and bleomycin (abstr). Proc Am Soc Clin Oncol 5:3, 1986

115. Krigel RL, Slywotzky VW, Lonberg M et al: Treatment of epidemic Kaposi's sarcoma with a combination of interferon-alpha 2b and etoposide. J Biol Response Mod 7:359, 1988

116. Brambilla L, Fossati S, Boneschi V, Clerici M: Oral etoposide versus parenteral vinblastine in chemotherapy for Kaposi's sarcoma (abstr). Presented at the Fourth European Conference on Clinical Oncology and Cancer Nursing, November 1–4, 1987

117. Krown SE, Real FX, Cunningham-Rundles S et al: Preliminary observations on the effect of recombinant leukocyte A interferon in homosexual men with Kaposi's sarcoma. N Engl J Med 308:1071, 1983

118. Real FX, Oettgen HF, Krown SE: Kaposi's sarcoma and the acquired immunodeficiency syndrome: Treatment with high and low doses of recombinant leukocyte A interferon. J Clin Oncol 4:544, 1986

119. Krown SE, Gold JWM, Real FX et al: Interferon alpha-2a ± vinblastine (VLB) in AIDS-associated Kaposi's sarcoma (KS/AIDS): Therapeutic activity, toxicity and effects on HTLV-III/LAV viremia (abstr). J Interferon Res 6:3, 1986

120. Groopman JE, Gottleib MS, Goodman J et al: Recombinant alpha-2 interferon therapy for Kaposi's sarcoma associated with acquired immunodeficiency syndrome. Ann Intern Med 100:671, 1984

121. Volberding PA, Mitsuyasu RT, Golando JP, Spiegel RJ: Treatment of Kaposi's sarcoma with interferon alpha-2b (Intron A). Cancer 59:620, 1987

122. Gelmann EP, Preble OT, Steis R et al: Human lymphoblastoid interferon treatment of Kaposi's sarcoma in the acquired immune deficiency syndrome: Clinical response and prognostic parameters. Am J Med 78:737, 1985

123. Rios A, Mansell PWA, Newell GA et al: Treatment of acquired immunodeficiency syndrome–related Kaposi's sarcoma with lymphoblastoid interferon. J Clin Oncol 3:506, 1985

124. Fischl M, Lucas S, Gorowski E et al: Interferon alpha-N1 Welferon (WFN) in Kaposi's sarcoma: Single agent or combination with vinblastine (VBL) (abstr). J Interferon Res 6(suppl 1):4, 1986

125. Schaart FM, Bratzke B, Ruszczak Z et al: Long-term therapy of HIV-associated Kaposi's sarcoma with recombinant interferon α-2a. Br J Dermatol 124:62, 1991

126. Krown SE, Gold JWM, Niedzwiecki D et al: Interferon-α with zidovudine: Safety, tolerance, and clinical and virologic effects in patients with Kaposi's sarcoma associated with the acquired immunodeficiency syndrome (AIDS). Ann Intern Med 112:812, 1990

127. De Wit R, Danner SA, Bakker JM et al: Combined zidovudine and interferon-alpha treatment in patients with AIDS-associated Kaposi's sarcoma. J Intern Med 229:35, 1991

128. Fischl MA, Uttamchandani RB, Resnick L et al: A phase I study of recombinant human interferon-α_{2a} or human lymphoblastoid interferon-α_{n1} and concomitant zidovudine in patients with AIDS-related Kaposi's sarcoma. J AIDS 4:1, 1991

129. Nisce L, Safai B: Radiation therapy of Kaposi's sarcoma in AIDS. Front Radiat Ther Oncol 19:126, 1985

130. Cooper JS, Steinfeld AD, Lerch I: Intentions and outcomes in the radiotherapeutic management of epidemic Kaposi's sarcoma. Int J Radiat Oncol Biol Phys 20:422, 1991

131. Newman SB: Treatment of epidemic Kaposi's sarcoma (KS) with intralesional vinblastine injection (IL-VBL). Proc Annu Meet Am Soc Clin Oncol 7:A19, 1988

13

Lymphoma and Other Miscellaneous Cancers

Alexandra M. Levine

CANCER OCCURRING IN VARIOUS STATES OF ABNORMAL IMMUNE FUNCTION

The development of certain cancers in various states of abnormal immune function had been described well before the onset of the acquired immunodeficiency syndrome (AIDS) epidemic. An understanding of these conditions may serve to place the AIDS-related malignancies in proper perspective.

Congenital Immune Deficiency States

Over 70 different congenital immune deficiency states have now been defined, representing abnormalities of one or multiple components of the immune system. Although these disorders may be quite distinct from one another, they share the propensity for development of malignant disease; in general, the risk of cancer in these settings is approximately 100 times greater than would be expected in the general population.[1] Although the specific frequencies of different cancers vary among the diverse congenital immune deficiency states, the cancer most frequently encountered is malignant lymphoma. This cancer accounts for approximately 49% of all cancers seen in this setting, while leukemias account for 13% and miscellaneous solid cancers account for the remainder. Interestingly, full immune reconstitution by means of bone marrow transplantation has prolonged survival in these individuals by preventing the development of serious opportunistic infections and inhibiting the development of malignant disease. For example, Kersey *et al* noted no case of lymphoma in 48 patients with severe combined immunodeficiency syndrome who were followed up for a median of 4.8 years

after transplantation, or in 15 patients with Wiskott-Aldrich syndrome who were followed for 3.7 years.[2]

Organ Transplantation: Iatrogenic Immunosuppression

Patients undergoing organ transplantation have routinely received long-term immunosuppressive regimens designed to prevent graft rejection. The drugs used most commonly in this setting have included prednisone and azathioprine. In recent years, more extensive immunosuppression has been achieved by use of cyclosporin, with or without monoclonal antibody therapy to depress the T-cell count. In the setting of iatrogenic immunosuppression in the course of transplantation, extraordinary increases in several unusual cancers have been described.[3] The transplantation model provides insight into the malignancies seen in patients infected by the human immunodeficiency virus (HIV), not only in terms of the specific cancers that occur, but also in terms of the time course or latent period of these cancers.

The first cancer that occurs in organ transplant recipients is Kaposi's sarcoma. This entity occurs at a median of 20 months after transplantation and at a frequency of approximately 500 times greater than expected.[1-5] Interestingly, spontaneous remission of Kaposi's sarcoma has been reported in approximately 30% of posttransplantation patients after simple discontinuation of or reduction in the immunosuppressive therapy.[5]

The second malignancy seen in the setting of organ transplantation is malignant lymphoma, which occurs 28 to 49 times more frequently than expected, with a latent period of approximately 33 months.[5] The clinical and pathologic characteristics of posttransplantation

225

malignant lymphoma are very similar to those described in the setting of HIV infection, with widespread extranodal disease at presentation and a predominance of high-grade, B-cell types;[6,7] lymphoma primary to the brain has been reported in 28% of these individuals. Of interest, in approximately 18% of transplant recipients the lymphoma has developed in the allograft tissue.[5] With the use of newer, more effective immunosuppressive regimens, lymphoma now accounts for a greater percentage of all cancers than before, and the latent period between transplantation and the diagnosis of lymphoma has decreased. For example, Swinnen *et al* reported a ninefold increase in lymphoma prevalence in 154 cardiac transplant recipients who received OKT3 monoclonal antibody, compared with patients who received less immunosuppressive regimens; the risk of lymphoma also increased with the higher total dose of OKT3 employed.[8] The incidence of lymphoma is also higher in individuals receiving nonrenal organ transplants, presumably because the degree of immunosuppression is higher in these settings, in which the physician does not have the option of reverting to dialysis in the event of graft rejection.[5] Thus, as reported by the Cincinnati Transplant Tumor Registry, lymphoma now accounts for 13% of cancers in renal transplant recipients but 38% of cancers in heart transplant recipients, 60% of cancers in liver transplant recipients, and 83% of cancers in bone marrow transplant recipients. As with transplantation-associated Kaposi's sarcoma, in approximately 20% of transplant recipients with lymphoma the lymphoma has regressed spontaneously on discontinuation of the immunosuppressive agents. It is clear that increasing degrees of immunosuppression, even in the iatrogenic setting, may be associated with the development of malignant lymphoma.

The third cancer that occurs in the setting of organ transplantation is squamous cell cancer of the lips and skin, accounting for 38% of the cancers recorded in the Cincinnati Transplant Tumor Registry.[5] The incidence of these cancers is 18 to 29 times higher than expected and increases over time. Thus, in a review of 3,846 renal transplants, the incidence of squamous cell carcinoma was 11% at 5 years, 29% at 10 years, and 43% at 14 years after transplantation.[9] Although squamous cell carcinoma usually remains localized for many years, this is not universally the case in the transplantation setting, in which distant metastases and death due to squamous cell carcinoma have been noted.

The final cancers consistently noted in organ transplant recipients include cancers of the anogenital region.[10] These cancers, which may be associated with prior infection with the human papillomavirus (HPV), are seen quite late after transplantation, at a median of 107 months.[5,11] Rather aggressive disease may be seen.

Acquired Autoimmune Disease

The spectrum of cancers occurring with increased frequency in association with autoimmune disease is similar to that seen in the transplantation model, although the incidence is far lower, presumably because the degree of immunosuppression is not as significant or prolonged. In a long-term retrospective study of patients with rheumatoid arthritis, those who received cyclosphosphamide had a greater rate of lymphoma, skin cancers, and bladder cancer than those who did not receive cyclosphosphamide.[12] Lymphoma has also been described with increased frequency in patients with Sjögren's syndrome, Hashimoto's thyroiditis, celiac disease, and other diseases; the lymphoma may develop specifically in the sites of prior immune disease, even in the absence of immunosuppressive therapy.[13-15]

It is thus apparent that states of abnormal immunity, whether congenital, acquired, or iatrogenic, may be associated with an increased prevalence of certain rather unusual cancers. Further, the degree of immunosuppression seems to predict the development of one type of malignancy in preference to another, as does the time required for development of that particular malignancy.

The first cancer associated with underlying HIV infection, Kaposi's sarcoma, was also the cancer seen first in the transplantation model.[1,16] Similarly, lymphoma, which was not statistically related to the AIDS epidemic until 4 years after its onset, is the second cancer to develop in organ transplant recipients.[1,17] Although there are no epidemiologic data to suggest that squamous cell carcinoma or cancers of the anogenital region are statistically increased in the HIV-infected population, individual cases have been reported, and an increased incidence of anal intraepithelial neoplasia has been noted in homosexual men with symptomatic HIV infection.[18,19] It is possible that these entities will become significantly more prevalent in HIV-infected patients in the future, as effective antiretroviral therapy extends the lifetime of such patients.

ETIOLOGY AND PATHOGENESIS OF AIDS-RELATED LYMPHOMA

Although HIV is capable of infecting Epstein-Barr virus (EBV)–infected B lymphocytes and of allowing direct polyclonal activation of human B lymphocytes,[20-23] there is no evidence to suggest that this retrovirus is the direct cause of the lymphomas seen in HIV-infected individuals. Nonetheless, HIV likely plays some critical role in this regard, and may provide the underlying requisite immunosuppression.

The role of EBV in the pathogenesis of AIDS-related lymphomas has been discussed for some time, based on observations made in various animal systems and in diverse settings of immunosuppression. EBV has been linked to the development of lymphoma in cotton-top marmosets[1]; and after exposure to EBV, boys with the X-linked lymphoproliferative syndrome may develop fatal or chronic infectious mononucleosis or high-grade B-cell lymphoma.[24-27] EBV-induced lymphomas have also been described in the organ transplantation model.[28-30] A role for EBV in the pathogenesis of AIDS-related lymphomas has also been suggested, based on data on African Burkitt's lymphoma: the EBV genome has been found within tumor cell DNA in 97% of cases.[31] Although a direct relationship between EBV and endemic Burkitt's lymphoma has never been demonstrated, the presence of high-titer antibody to EBV prior to the development of Burkitt's lymphoma,[32] and the possibility of underlying immunosuppression induced by chronic malarial infection, have made this hypothesis an attractive one.

A possible role for EBV in the lymphomas associated with HIV was given credence by the findings of Birx *et al*,[20] who described defective regulation of EBV infection in patients with AIDS; in this setting, EBV immune T cells, which normally suppress EBV-induced B-cell activation, instead enhanced B-cell activation. Ernberg *et al*[33] subsequently described the presence of EBV genome within lymphoma cell DNA in a patient with underlying HIV infection. Additional data were collected in a review of 29 tumors; EBV antigens and/or genome were found in 58%. Hamilton-Dutoit *et al,* using *in situ* hybridization techniques, detected EBV genome in eight of 16 lymphomas.[34] Further, Shibata *et al* demonstrated an increased likelihood of progression to lymphoma in a group of HIV-infected men in whom B cells derived from enlarged reactive lymph nodes were found to contain EBV DNA by the polymerase chain reaction. The presence of EBV genome within lymphoma DNA was also demonstrated in approximately 40% of patients with AIDS-related lymphoma.[35]

Although the data are intriguing, the fact that less than half of HIV lymphomas exhibit integration of EBV genome indicates that EBV cannot be the sole cause of these tumors. In fact, Subar *et al* in 1988 reported finding EBV genome in only six of 16 cases.[36]

Chromosomal abnormalities have been well described in patients with AIDS-associated lymphoma. The abnormalities are most commonly t(8;14) or t(8;22), as had previously been described in endemic and sporadic Burkitt's lymphoma.[37-40] Rearrangement of the *c-myc* oncogene has also been described with frequency, occurring in 12 of 16 cases reported by Subar *et al.*[36] Interestingly, in one well-studied case, immunoglobulin gene rearrangement without *c-myc* rearrangement was present; sequencing of the translocation junction disclosed that the breakpoint was situated seven base pairs from the chromosome 14 site involved in a previously studied case of endemic Burkitt's lymphoma, which was far from the *myc* locus on chromosome 8. The molecular biology of this case suggests that common molecular mechanisms may be operating in both endemic Burkitt's lymphoma and the AIDS-associated tumors.[41]

Although lymphoma is expected to be genotypically monoclonal, with specific immunoglobulin gene rearrangement, this has not been uniformly demonstrated in patients with AIDS-associated lymphoma, in whom multiple clonal expansions may be seen. The evolution of this clonal ambiguity was described in two patients by Lippman *et al*,[42] while Pelicci *et al*[43] described multiple monoclonal B-cell expansions in a group of patients with AIDS-related lymphoproliferative disorders. Similar findings have been described in the setting of organ transplantation,[6] although genetic monoclonality has also been well described in a group of cardiac transplant recipients studied by Cleary *et al.*[7]

It is probable that the full pathogenesis of lymphoma in the setting of HIV infection may involve multiple steps. With underlying immunosuppression, current or prior EBV infection may be activated, with resultant ongoing B-cell proliferation. Even in the absence of EBV-driven lymphoproliferation, however, HIV may itself allow ongoing B-cell activation and proliferation, either directly or *via* production of certain cytokines such as interleukin-6 from HIV-infected cells, resulting in a state of ongoing B-cell replication.[44] In this setting, a chance chromosomal abnormality could occur, leading to immunoglobulin gene rearrangements and the selection of several clones with the potential of growth advantage. With further chromosomal aberrations leading to *c-myc* translocation, a single clone may subsequently be selected, leading to a monoclonal B-cell malignancy.

EPIDEMIOLOGIC ASPECTS

Malignant lymphoma is a relatively late manifestation of infection by HIV. Thus, true epidemic of lymphoma was not evident until 1985, 4 years after the initial recognition of AIDS.[16,17] Recent data from the National Cancer Institute appear to confirm this hypothesis.[45] Of a group of 55 patients with symptomatic HIV infection enrolled in various antiretroviral trials from 1985 to 1987, eight developed high-grade B-cell lymphoma a median of 23.8 months (range, 13 to 35 months) after entry into the study. The actuarial risk of lymphoma development at 36 months was predicted to be in the range of 46%. Although this precise figure may be falsely high, owing to the small number of individuals involved, the point may still be made that ever-increasing numbers of patients with AIDS-related lymphoma may be expected as patients live longer with effective antiretroviral intervention.

AIDS-related lymphoma has now been described in all populations at risk for HIV infection, and the precise clinical or pathologic aspects of disease appear quite similar, as do response to therapy and survival.[46-48]

PATHOLOGIC ASPECTS OF LYMPHOMATOUS DISEASE

Approximately 90% of the lymphomas described in AIDS have been of high-grade, B-cell types, including B immunoblastic lymphoma and small non-cleaved cell lymphoma, which may be of the Burkitt or non-Burkitt variants.[46,49-53] Older terminologies for the former subtype include "diffuse histiocytic lymphoma," while the latter tumor was called "undifferentiated lymphoma."[54,55]

Although these tumor types are common in the setting of congenital immune deficiency disease, autoimmune disorders, and organ transplantation, they are distinctly unusual in routine settings, accounting for only about 10% of newly diagnosed cases.[55,56]

Diffuse large cell lymphoma has also been described in association with AIDS; these intermediate-grade lymphomas may simply represent diverse pathologic classification in a field that is known to be complex and problematic.[57]

No prospective therapeutic trial has yet established any difference in outcome between patients with intermediate-grade large cell lymphoma and those with high-grade B-cell disease. However, in a retrospective series reported by Knowles *et al,* the median survival of patients with immunoblastic lymphoma was only 2 months, *versus* 5.5 months for those with small non-cleaved cell disease and 7.5 months for those with large non-cleaved cell lymphoma.[51] These figures may be biased in that multivariate analyses were not performed, and it is certainly possible that other factors were operative to explain the survival differences.

Although low-grade lymphomas, including small cleaved cell lymphomas, chronic lymphocytic leukemia, and multiple myeloma, have been described in a small number of HIV-infected patients, there is no evidence that the prevalence of these subtypes has increased in the epidemic.[17,49,58-60] Furthermore, the response to treatment—whether the treatment includes "watchful waiting" or the use of single alkylating agents—and the natural history of disease, including prolonged survival in patients with known lymphomatous disease, are very similar to what is seen in patients without HIV infection.

Although T-cell lymphomas have been described in several HIV-infected patients, they are actually quite unusual, with fewer than 15 reported to date. The entities have included T8 lymphocytosis,[51,60,61] precurser (lymphoblastic) T-cell lymphoma,[62,63] peripheral T-cell lymphoma,[64,65] lymphomatoid granulomatosis,[66,67] and pseudo-Sézary syndrome.[68] Interestingly, several cases of HTLV-I–associated adult T-cell lymphoma/leukemia have been reported in patients dually infected with HIV and HTLV-I.[69-71]

CLINICAL ASPECTS OF LYMPHOMATOUS DISEASE

Presenting Symptoms and Signs

Approximately 75% of patients with AIDS-related lymphoma present with systemic "B" symptoms, consisting of fever, drenching night sweats, and/or weight loss.[46,49-53,60,72,73] Although such symptoms are common in lymphoma, it is imperative to exclude other potential causes, such as occult opportunistic infection.

Aside from systemic symptoms, the patient with AIDS-associated lymphoma may present with any conceivable symptom, depending on the extent and sites of the lymphomatous disease. It is also possible to encounter patients who seemingly have no significant symptoms but seek medical attention because of an infected tooth, for example, which on biopsy is found to represent lymphomatous involvement of the maxilla; or very subtle changes in personality or behavior, which may be the only early symptom of primary central nervous system (CNS) lymphoma.[74]

Sites of Lymphomatous Involvement

One of the distinguishing features of AIDS-related lymphoma is the widespread extent of disease at presentation, with extranodal involvement recorded in 80% to 90% of all patients.[46,49-53,60,72,73] Such extranodal disease (stage IV, or IE) would be expected in approximately 40% of non-AIDS-related cases.[75]

The most common sites of involvement are the CNS (32%), the gastrointestinal tract (26%), bone marrow (25%), and liver (12%).[49,50,76] However, virtually any site of the body may be involved. A multi-institutional report on 90 patients noted that lymphoma was found in the earlobe, maxilla, gallbladder, popliteal fossa, orbit, skin, adrenal, kidney, pancreas, and other unusual sites.[50] Additional case reports have described primary lymphoma of the bile duct,[77] presentation as a perianal abscess,[78] and pulmonary involvement, including an isolated coin lesion in the lung, as well as interstitial or alveolar infiltrates, nodules, and/or pleural effusions.[79]

Prognostic Factors for Survival

Multivariate analyses have recently defined those factors that affect the survival of patients with HIV-associated lymphoma. As demonstrated by Levine *et al* in a series of 49 patients with systemic lymphoma, Karnofsky performance status less than 70%, the development of AIDS prior to the lymphoma, and bone marrow involvement were each associated with a significant decrease in survival.[80] Lower CD4 counts, as a continuous variable, was also associated with a poor prognosis. The median survival of patients who presented with one or more of these factors was 4 months, while individuals who lacked all of the factors survived a median of 11 months. In the series published by Kaplan *et al,* a CD4 level of 100 cells/dl or less was the most significant factor in predicting shortened survival. Other significant factors included low Karnofsky performance status, the development of AIDS prior to the lymphoma, and presence of stage IV disease.[52]

In considering the survival of patients with primary CNS (P-CNS) *versus* systemic lymphoma, Levine *et al* noted that patients with P-CNS lymphoma had the shortest median survival. Of interest, patients with P-CNS lymphoma were distinct in regard to the severity of HIV-related immunosuppression. Thus, the median

CD4 count in patients with P-CNS lymphoma was 37 cells/dl, versus 189 cells/dl in those with systemic disease. Further, 73% of patients with P-CNS lymphoma had a history of AIDS before the lymphoma developed, *versus* 37% of patients with systemic disease.[80] The poor prognosis in patients with P-CNS lymphoma, then, is related to severe immune depression, with the onset of multiple AIDS-defining pathologic processes.

It is important to note that leptomeningeal disease does not indicate a poor outcome, and attention to this site has become mandatory.[80] The incidence of asymptomatic leptomeningeal lymphoma is approximately 17%, and lumbar puncture should routinely be performed as part of the staging evaluation and for the purpose of CNS prophylaxis.[81]

Treatment Options in AIDS-Associated Lymphoma

In the 1970s and 1980s, treatment regimens for patients with intermediate- or high-grade lymphoma became progressively more intensive,[82-85] based in part on the Goldie-Coldman hypothesis, which predicted that spontaneous resistance to multiple agents would occur after exposure to one or two.[86] When additional data became available indicating the importance of relative dose intensity,[85,87] it was logical to assume that the same relationships might be valid in patients with HIV infection, in whom the lymphoma was frequently extensive and bulky.

Accordingly, Gill *et al* devised a very intensive novel regimen that consisted of high-dose cytosine arabinoside, methotrexate, and cyclophosphamide, interspersed with other, routine agents.[88] In a pilot study in nine patients placed on this regimen, complete remission occurred in only 33%, and relapse or progression of CNS disease occurred in 67%. Furthermore, 78% of patients developed opportunistic infections, of which they died. These results caused an early termination of the trial and led to the hypothesis that perhaps less intensive therapy might be indicated.

Other investigators also employed dose-intensive regimens with similar results. Thus, Dugan *et al* used the ProMACE-MOPP regimen and noted a complete remission rate of only 20%, with extensive delays and dose reductions necessary in subsequent cycles.[89] Odajnyk *et al* noted that the COMP regimen, used in 25 patients with small non-cleaved cell lymphoma, produced complete remission in only 28%, and the median survival time was 3 months.[90] In a trial consisting of high-dose cytosine arabinoside, methotrexate, cyclophosphamide, and other agents, Kaplan *et al* reported a median survival time of only 5.2 months, which compared unfavorably with the median survival time of 11.3 months in patients who received less intensive regimens ($p < 0.05$).[52] Furthermore, a median survival time of 4.6 months was seen in patients who received 1 g/m^2 or more of cyclophosphamide, compared to 12.2 months in those who received less than 1 g/m^2 ($p < 0.05$).[52]

Only two trials have demonstrated efficacy of a very dose intensive regimen. Bermudez *et al* employed the MACOP-B regimen in 11 patients and reported complete remission in seven.[91] By contrast, complete remission was achieved in only two (17%) of 12 patients who received less intensive therapy, usually consisting of CHOP.[82] Of note, however, essentially all complete responders in the MACOP-B trial had a Karnofsky performance status of 100%, and none had a history of AIDS prior to lymphoma. Gisselbrecht *et al* employed the LNH-84 regimen in 60 patients with "good-prognosis" AIDS-associated lymphoma and reported a complete remission rate of 72% and long-term (15-month) disease-free survival in 40% of all patients treated.[92] It is possible, then, that good-prognosis patients with HIV-associated lymphoma may fare well with intensive multi-agent chemotherapy. The majority of affected patients, however, do not fall into this category and would be expected to do poorly after such dose-intensive therapy.

In an attempt to evaluate the concept that "less may be better" in the lymphomas associated with HIV infection, Levine *et al*[81] used a low-dose modification of the M-BACOD regimen[83] in a prospective multi-institutional trial sponsored by the AIDS Clinical Trials Group of the National Institute of Allergy and Infectious Disease (Table 13-1). A complete remission rate of 46% was achieved in 35 evaluable patients. Partial responses were seen in 5%, with an overall response rate of 51%. Responses were seen in patients with and without poor prognostic indicators and were durable in the majority, although additional HIV-related illnesses continued to occur, with 20% of patients developing opportunistic infections while on therapy. The median survival of complete responders was 15 months. With the use of intrathecal cytosine arabinoside, no case of isolated CNS relapse was observed. Thus, less intensive regimens of combination chemotherapy with early CNS prophylaxis may indeed be fully equivalent to more intensive regimens, which have been associated with higher rates of opportunistic infection.

In an attempt to ascertain the safety of the combined use of hematopoietic growth factors (rGM-CSF) plus chemotherapy in patients with AIDS-associated lymphoma, Kaplan *et al* reported on a Phase I trial that used differing doses and schedules of rGM-CSF along with the CHOP regimen.[93] No increase in p24 antigenemia was found in patients treated with CHOP plus rGM-CSF, compared with patients who received CHOP alone.

Walsh *et al* have recently completed another Phase I trial of rGM-CSF, used with the low-dose M-BACOD regimen discussed above, in 17 patients within the AIDS Clinical Trials Group. Doses of M-BACOD were escalated to achieve the full dose regimen. A complete remission rate of 51% was achieved, and no patient developed dose-limiting hematologic toxicity. Opportunistic infections were not obviated, occurring in 17% of subjects.[94]

The AIDS Clinical Trials Group has now embarked on a Phase III trial in which patients are stratified by

Table 13–1. Low-Dose Regimen for AIDS-Related Lymphoma[81]

Treatment	Current Regimen	M-BACOD Regimen[83]
Bleomycin	4 mg/m² IV, day 1	4 mg/m² IV, day 1
Doxorubicin	25 mg/m² IV, day 1	45 mg/m² IV, day 1
Cyclophosphamide	300 mg/m² IV, day 1	600 mg/m² IV, day 1
Vincristine	1.4 mg/m² IV, day 1 (not to exceed 2 mg)	1.0 mg/m² IV, day 1
Dexamethasone	3 mg/m² PO, days 1–5	6 mg/m² PO, days 1–5
Methotrexate	500 mg/m² IV on day 15, with folinic acid rescue, 25 mg PO q6h × 4, beginning 6 hr after completion of methotrexate	3,000 mg/m² IV on day 14, with folinic acid rescue, 10 mg/m² IV or PO q 6 h for 72 hr, beginning 24 hr after completion of methotrexate
Cytosine arabinoside	50 mg intrathecally on days 1, 8, 21, 28	None
Helmet field radiotherapy	2,400 cGy with marrow involvement; 4,000 cGy with known CNS involvement	None
Azidothymidine	200 mg every 4 hr for 1 year, starting after chemotherapy	None
Total treatment	4–6 cycles at 28-day intervals	10 cycles at 21-day intervals

*(From Levine A: JAMA 266:84, 1991)

prognostic indicators and randomly assigned to receive either the low-dose M-BACOD regimen or standard-dose M-BACOD with rGM-CSF. The goal is to ascertain the precise role of dose intensity in this setting, provided that the chemotherapy may be safely administered by the concomitant use of the hematopoietic growth factor.

Aside from the use of chemotherapy with hematopoietic growth factors, recent trials have studied the use of multi-agent chemotherapy with concomitant antiretroviral therapy, as reported by Levine *et al,* who used the low-dose M-BACOD regimen with dideoxycytidine.[95] The results of these trials are awaited.

PRIMARY CNS LYMPHOMA

Lymphoma primary to the brain is not unusual in patients with congenital immune deficiency diseases, in organ transplant recipients, and in patients infected with HIV.[1] In fact, P-CNS lymphoma was considered a criterion for the diagnosis of AIDS from the outset of the epidemic.[16]

The prognosis of patients with P-CNS lymphoma is the poorest of any subgroup with AIDS-related lymphoma, with a median survival time of only 2 to 3 months despite therapy.[80]

Presenting symptoms include focal neurologic deficits, headache, seizure, or cranial neuropathies. Subtle abnormalities may also occur, such as changes in personality.[74,96]

Findings on brain computed axial tomography are not pathognomonic for P-CNS lymphoma, although certain features are expected. Lesions tend to be relatively few in number, with one to three mass lesions found in the majority of cases. The individual lesions are relatively large, usually between 3 and 5 cm. With the use of con-

trast material, ring enhancement may be seen, similar to what has been described in toxoplasmosis.[96,97]

Essentially any site in the brain may be involved, including the basal ganglia, the parietal, frontal or frontoparietal lobes, and the cerebellum and pons.[74,96–98]

The treatment of affected individuals is quite problematic, owing to the presence of multiple other AIDS-defining illnesses. Although radiation therapy may be associated with complete remission in approximately half of treated patients, these remissions tend to be short, and the median survival time is less than 6 months.[99] Death may be secondary to recurrent lymphoma, to other pathologic processes within the brain, or to other AIDS-defining illnesses.

The optimal therapeutic intervention in these patients is unknown at present, although it is apparent that radiation therapy alone will be inadequate, and that intensive chemotherapeutic intervention simply is not tolerated by these frail, severely immunocompromised individuals.

HODGKIN'S DISEASE IN THE HIV-INFECTED INDIVIDUAL

Epidemiologic data from San Francisco, Los Angeles, and New York indicate that there has been no increase in Hodgkin's disease since the onset of the AIDS epidemic.[72,100,101] This would be fully consistent with other settings of immunocompromise, in which Hodgkin's disease has not been reported as increased.

Nonetheless, historically, the clinical and pathologic characteristics of Hodgkin's disease have been well appreciated within the context of the host's underlying immune status, and the overall prognosis may reflect the balance between the malignancy and the host's defense against it. Thus, the worldwide epidemiologic pattern of Hodgkin's disease varies, with poor prognostic pathologic types such as lymphocyte depletion or mixed cellularity types and extensive, symptomatic disease reported from various developing areas of the world, where malnutrition and chronic infection by malaria or other pathogens may serve to immunosuppress. In contrast, reports from centers that serve patients of middle or upper socioeconomic status note a preponderance of nodular sclerosis or lymphocyte-predominant disease, with the majority of patients presenting with limited stage disease and no systemic B symptoms.[102,103]

The characteristics of Hodgkin's disease that have been described in HIV-infected patients are fully consistent with these concepts. With underlying immunodeficiency, it is logical to assume that affected individuals would present with widespread symptomatic disease, and that poor-prognosis pathologic subtypes would predominate. This is exactly the case. Thus, while there has been no statistical increase in or epidemic of Hodgkin's disease in association with AIDS, the chance occurrence of Hodgkin's disease in the HIV-infected patient has influenced the nature of the malignancy, such that extensive symptomatic disease of the mixed cellularity type or lymphocyte depletion type is expected.[104,105]

Although a typical, non-AIDS-related case of Hodgkin's disease in the United States may be curable with radiation therapy or multi-agent chemotherapy, cure is much less likely for HIV-infected patients, in whom the median survival time has been in the range of 12 to 15 months despite therapy.[72,104,105] The optimal therapeutic intervention is currently undefined, although the use of combination chemotherapy, such as the ABVD regimen, together with hematopoietic growth factors (rG-CSF) is currently under investigation by the AIDS Clinical Trials Group.

MISCELLANEOUS CANCERS IN THE HIV-INFECTED PATIENT

There is no evidence at present that any particular cancer, other than Kaposi's sarcoma and lymphoma, is statistically increased in the same pattern as has been described in AIDS.[100,101] However, using the model of organ transplantation, it may be reasonable to postulate that certain cancers, such as squamous cell carcinomas of the skin or cancers of the anogenital tract, will be seen in increasing numbers as the epidemic proceeds. In recent years, numerous case reports have described squamous cell carcinomas of the skin in HIV-infected individuals. Furthermore, an interesting relationship between HIV infection, HPV infection, and anal intraepithelial neoplasia has been reported. It will be imperative to follow these cases carefully in an attempt to understand the full natural history of neoplasia occurring in the setting of HIV-induced immunosuppression.

Anal Intraepithelial Neoplasia

The incidence of anal carcinoma began to increase statistically in the late 1970s. An abrupt increase first emerged in 1978 in single men from New York City, in whom a 10-fold increase was noted.[101,106,107] Since that time, there has been no further increase. These cancers have been associated with a history of receptive anal intercourse, which has been strongly correlated (relative risk = 33) with a homosexual or bisexual life-style.[106,107] In addition, a correlation has also been demonstrated between prior HPV infection and the subsequent development of anal carcinoma.[108] The HPV types most commonly associated with anal cancer have included types 16, 18, 31, 33, and 35, while HPV types 6 and 11 have been associated with genital warts.[109]

Palefsky et al recently reported an interesting relationship between HIV infection and the development of anal intraepithelial neoplasia.[18] A group of 97 homosexual males with symptomatic HIV infection and without anal symptoms were studied by anal cytology; techniques included the Papanicolaou smear and the DNA/RNA dot blot technique for the presence of HPV DNA. Abnormal anal cytologic findings were detected in 39% and consisted of anal intraepithelial neoplasia in 15%, atypical cytology in 20%, and condyloma in 4%. A subset of patients underwent anal biopsy, with results consistent with the findings on the anal Papanicolaou smear. Of importance, neither the cytologic findings nor the anal biopsy results correlated with the detection of external anal disease or with symptoms related to this site.

HPV DNA was found in 54% of Palefsky's subjects. Of these, infection by HPV types 16/18 or 31/33/35 was present in 75%, and 12% had been infected by multiple subtypes. The presence of two or more types of HPV infection correlated with a 39-fold increased risk of abnormal cytologic findings.

Similar data were reported by Frazer et al, who studied 61 homosexual men by means of anal Papanicolaou smear and HPV analysis.[19] Cytologic dysplasia with concomitant HPV infection was found in 40%, while another 40% had evidence of HPV infection without dysplasia. A subgroup of these men were studied serially, and 66% were found to have persistent dysplasia, lasting over 1 year. The presence of long-standing dysplastic changes in the anorectal epithelium would be most worrisome in regard to eventual evolution to frank invasive carcinoma.

The long-term consequences of anal dysplastic changes, and even intraepithelial neoplasia, remain unknown. However, the model of HPV infection, long-term cervical dysplasia, cervical intraepithelial neoplasia (CIN), and the subsequent development of invasive cancer may serve as an appropriate model.[110–112] In the setting of chronic HPV infection, increasing degrees of cytologic atypia and CIN are eventually followed by the development of invasive cervical cancer. Thus, Campion et al[110] reported that 85% of women infected by HPV type 16 progressed from CIN grade I to CIN grade III within a 5-year period. Furthermore, McIndoe *et al* noted that 22% of patients with persistent CIN III progressed to invasive cervical cancer within a follow-up interval of 28 years.[111] Thus, if the course of anal intraepithelial neoplasia is similar to that of CIN, it is probable that HIV-infected patients, as they live longer, may be at ever increasing risk for the development of this tumor.

Cervical Intraepithelial Neoplasia

Women with HIV infection must be followed for the possibility of cervical dysplasia, CIN, and cervical carcinoma. Routine Papanicolaou smears should be done and HPV status determined. These evaluations become even more pertinent, because the risk of developing cervical or vulvar cancer in association with HPV is greatly increased in the setting of immunosuppression, as noted by Penn in organ transplant recipients.[10] It is probable, then, that the full malignant potential of underlying HPV infection in women with HIV-induced immunosuppression has not yet been fully realized, and it will be extremely important to follow these women very carefully in the years ahead.

Miscellaneous Cancers

Numerous small series and single case reports have described the development of miscellaneous diverse cancers in HIV-infected patients. Common to most reports is the relatively young age of the individuals and a more aggressive course of disease than is usually expected.[113]

Both squamous cell carcinomas of the skin and melanoma have been reported in HIV-infected patients, and, as demonstrated by Tindall *et al,* the course of disease in three cases of melanoma was directly related to the degree of HIV-induced immunosuppression.[114]

The development of germinal testicular tumors has also been described in HIV-infected patients; in fact, the largest group in the series of solid cancers published by Monfardini *et al* consisted of pure seminomas in six patients, pure embryonal tumors in two, and embryonal mixed tumors in four. The course of illness did not seem particularly aggressive in these patients.[115]

HIV-infected patients with gastric adenocarcinomas, pancreatic carcinoma, thymoma, thyroid carcinoma, glioblastoma, and medulloblastoma have been reported, as have patients with various types of lung cancer.[113] Once again, although there is no evidence to suggest that these cancers have increased in incidence, it would seem wise to follow such patients closely in time, in an attempt to ascertain the true malignant potential of the severe immunosuppression induced by HIV.

REFERENCES

1. Penn I: Principles of tumor immunity: Immunocompromised patients. AIDS Updates 3:1, 1990
2. Kersey JH, Shapiro RS, Heinitz KJ et al: Lymphoid malignancy in naturally occurring and post bone marrow transplantation immunodeficiency diseases. In Good RA, Lindenlaub E (eds): The Nature, Cellular and Biochemical Basis and Management of Immunodeficiencies. Symposia Medica Hoechst, vol 21, p 289. Stuttgart, FK Shattauer Verlag, 1987
3. Fraumeni JF Jr, Hoover R: Immunosurveillance and cancer: Epidemiologic observations. Natl Cancer Inst Monogr 47:121, 1977
4. Penn I: Kaposi's sarcoma in organ transplant recipients: Report of 20 cases. Transplantation 27:8, 1979
5. Penn I: Cancers complicating organ transplantation. N Engl J Med 323:1767, 1990
6. Ferry JA, Jacobson JO, Conti D et al: Lymphoproliferative disorders and hematologic malignancies following organ transplantation. Mod Pathol 2:583, 1989
7. Cleary ML, Warnke R, Sklar J: Monoclonality of lymphoproliferative lesions in cardiac-transplant recipients: Clonal analysis based on immunoglobulin-gene rearrangements. N Engl J Med 310:477, 1984
8. Swinnen LJ, Costanzo-Nordin MR, Fisher SG et al: Increased incidence of lymphoproliferative disorder after immunosuppression with the monoclonal antibody OKT3 in cardiac transplant recipients. N Engl J Med 323:1723, 1990
9. Schiel AGR, Flavel S, Disney APS et al: Cancer development in patients progressing to dialysis and renal transplantation. Transplant Proc 7:685, 1985
10. Penn I: Cancers of the anogenital region in renal transplant recipients: Analysis of 65 cases. Cancer 58:611, 1986
11. zur Hausen H: Human papillomaviruses and their possible role in squamous cell carcinomas. Curr Top Microbiol Immunol 78:1, 1977
12. Baker JL, Kahl LE, Zee BC et al: Malignancy following treatment of rheumatoid arthritis with cyclophosphamide: Long term case-control follow-up study. Am J Med 83:1, 1987
13. Zulman J, Jaffe R, Talal N: Evidence that the malignant lymphoma of Sjögren's syndrome is a monoclonal B-cell neoplasm. N Engl J Med 299:1215, 1978
14. Good AE, Russo RH, Schnitzer B et al: Intracranial histiocytic lymphoma with rheumatoid arthritis. J Rheumatol 5:75, 1978
15. Levine AM, Taylor CR, Schneider DR et al: Immunoblastic sarcoma of T-cell versus B-cell origin: I. Clinical features. Blood 58:52, 1981
16. Centers for Disease Control: Diffuse, undifferentiated non-Hodgkin's lymphoma in homosexual males—United States. MMWR 31:277, 1982
17. Centers for Disease Control: Revision of the case definition of acquired immunodeficiency syndrome for national reporting—United States. Ann Intern Med 103:402, 1985
18. Palefsky JM, Gonzales J, Greenblatt RM et al: Anal intraepithelial neoplasia and anal papillomavirus infection among homosexual males with group IV HIV disease. JAMA 263:2911, 1990
19. Frazer IH, Crapper RM, Medley G et al: Association between anorectal dysplasia, human papillomavirus, and human immunodeficiency virus infection in homosexual men. Lancet 2:657, 1986
20. Birx DL, Redfield RR, Tosato G: Defective regulation of Epstein-Barr infection in patients with acquired immunodeficiency syndrome (AIDS) or AIDS-related disorders. N Engl J Med 314:874, 1986
21. Lane HC, Masur H, Edgar LC et al: Abnormalities of B-

cell activation and immunoregulation in patients with the acquired immunodeficiency syndrome. N Engl J Med 309: 453, 1983

22. Yarchoan R, Redfield RR, Broder S: Mechanisms of B cell activation in patients with acquired immunodeficiency syndrome and related disorders. J Clin Invest 78:439, 1986

23. Schittman SM, Lane HC, Higgins SE et al: Direct polyclonal activation of human B-lymphocytes by the AIDS virus. Science 233:1084, 1986

24. Ziegler JL, Magrath IT, Gerber P et al: Epstein-Barr virus and human malignancy. Ann Intern Med 86:323, 1977

25. Grierson H, Purtilo OT: Epstein-Barr virus infections in males with the X-linked lymphoproliferative syndrome. Ann Intern Med 106:538, 1987

26. Purtilo DT: Immune deficiency predisposing to Epstein-Barr virus induced lymphoproliferative diseases: The X-linked lymphoproliferative syndrome as a model. Adv Cancer Res 34:279, 1981

27. Purtilo DT: Epstein-Barr virus induced oncogenesis in immune deficient individuals. Lancet 1:300, 1980

28. Dummer JS, Bound LM, Singh G et al: Epstein-Barr virus induced lymphoma in a cardiac transplant recipient. Am J Med 77:179, 1984

29. Krammer P: Persistent Epstein-Barr infection and a histiocytic sarcoma in a renal transplant recipient. Cancer 55:503, 1985

30. Sullivan JL, Medveczky P, Forman SJ et al: Epstein-Barr virus induced lymphoproliferation: Implications for antiviral chemotherapy. N Engl J Med 311:1163, 1984

31. Purtilo DT: Malignant lymphoproliferative diseases induced by Epstein-Barr virus in immunodeficient patients, including X-linked, cytogenetic and familial syndromes. Cancer Genet Cytogenet 4:251, 1981

32. de The G, Geser A, Day NE et al: Epidemiological evidence for causal relationship between Epstein-Barr virus and Burkitt's lymphoma from Ugandan prospective study. Nature 274:756, 1978

33. Ernberg I, Bjorkholm M, Zech L et al: An Epstein-Barr virus genome carrying pre-B leukemia in a homosexual man with characteristic karyotype and impaired EBV specific immunity. J Clin Oncol 4:1481, 1986

34. Hamilton-Dutoit S, Pallensen G, Karkov J et al: Identification of EBV-DNA in tumor cells of AIDS-related lymphomas by in situ hybridization (letter). Lancet 1:554, 1989

35. Shibata D, Weiss LM, Nathwani BN et al: Epstein-Barr virus in benign lymph node biopsies from individuals infected with the human immunodeficiency virus is associated with the concurrent or subsequent development of non-Hodgkin's lymphoma. Blood, 77:1527, 1991

36. Subar M, Neri A, Inghirami G et al: Frequent c-myc oncogene activation and infrequent presence of Epstein-Barr virus genome in AIDS-associated lymphoma. Blood 72:667, 1988

37. Peterson JM, Tubbs RR, Savage RA et al: Small noncleaved B-cell Burkitt-like lymphoma with chromosome t(8;14) translocation and Epstein-Barr virus nuclear-associated antigen in a homosexual man with acquired immune deficiency syndrome. Am J Med 78:141, 1985

38. Wang PG, Lee EC, Sieverts H et al: Burkitt's lymphoma in AIDS: Cytogenetic study. Blood 63:190, 1984

39. Chaganti RSK, Jhanwar SC, Koziner B et al: Specific translocations characterize Burkitt's-like lymphoma of homosexual men with the acquired immunodeficiency syndrome. Blood 61:1265, 1983

40. Magrath I, Erikson J, Whang-Peng J et al: Synthesis of kappa light chains by cell lines containing an 8;22 chromosomal translocation derived from a male homosexual with Burkitt's lymphoma. Science 222:1094, 1983

41. Haluska F, Russo G, Kant J et al: Molecular resemblance of an AIDS associated lymphoma and endemic Burkitt lymphomas: Implications for their pathogenesis. Proc Natl Acad Sci USA 86:8907, 1989

42. Lippman SM, Volk JR, Spier CM, Grogen TM: Clonal ambiguity of human immunodeficiency virus associated lymphoma: Similarity to post transplant lymphomas. Arch Pathol Lab Med 112:128, 1988

43. Pelicci P, Knowles DM, Arlin ZA et al: Multiple monoclonal B cell expansions and c-myc oncogene rearrangements in acquired immune deficiency syndrome-related lymphoproliferative disorders: Implications for lymphomagenesis. J Exp Med 164:2049, 1986

44. Nakajima K, Martinez-Maza O, Hirano T et al: Induction of IL-6 (B-cell stimulatory factor-2/IFN-beta 2) production by human immunodeficiency virus. J Immunol 142:531, 1989

45. Pluda JM, Yarchoan R, Jaffe ES et al: Development of lymphoma in a cohort of patients with severe human immunodeficiency virus (HIV) infection on long term antiretroviral therapy. Ann Intern Med 113:276, 1990

46. Levine AM, Meyer PR, Begandy MK et al: Development of B-cell lymphoma in homosexual men: Clinical and immunologic findings. Ann Intern Med 100:7, 1984

47. Ragni M, Kingsley L, Duzyk A, Obrams I: HIV associated malignancy in hemophiliacs: Preliminary report from the Hemophilia Malignancy Study (HMS). Blood 74:38a, 1988

48. Monfardini S, Vaccher E, Tirelli U: AIDS associated non-Hodgkin's lymphoma in Italy: Intravenous drug users versus homosexual men. Ann Oncol 1:208, 1990

49. Levine AM, Gill PS, Meyer PR et al: Retrovirus and malignant lymphoma in homosexual men. JAMA 254:1921, 1985

50. Ziegler JL, Beckstead JA, Volberding PA et al: Non-Hodgkin's lymphoma in 90 homosexual men: Relation to generalized lymphadenopathy and the acquired immunodeficiency syndrome. N Engl J Med 311:565, 1984

51. Knowles DM, Chamulak GA, Subar M et al: Lymphoid neoplasia associated with the acquired immunodeficiency syndrome (AIDS): The New York University experience. Ann Intern Med 108:744, 1988

52. Kaplan LD, Abrams DI, Feigal E et al: AIDS-associated non-Hodgkin's lymphoma in San Francisco. JAMA 261:719, 1989

53. Lowenthal DA, Straus DJ, Campbell SW et al: AIDS-related lymphoid neoplasia: The Memorial Hospital Experience. Cancer 61:2325, 1988

54. Lukes RJ, Collins RD: Immunologic characterization of human malignant lymphomas. Cancer 34:1488, 1974

55. Non-Hodgkin's Lymphoma Pathologic Classification Project: National Cancer Institute sponsored study of classifications of non-Hodgkin's lymphomas: Summary and description of a working formulation for clinical usage. Cancer 49:2112, 1982

56. Lukes RJ, Parker JW, Taylor CR et al: Immunologic approach to non-Hodgkin's lymphomas and related leukemias. Analysis of the results of multiparameter studies of 425 cases. Semin Hematol 15:322, 1978

57. National Cancer Institute, Non-Hodgkin's Lymphoma Classification Project Writing Committee: Classification of non-Hodgkin's lymphomas: Reproducibility of major classification systems. Cancer 55:91, 1985

58. Ross RK, Dworsky RL, Paganini-Hill A et al: Non-Hodgkin's lymphomas in never married men in Los Angeles. Br J Cancer 52:785, 1985

59. Vandermolen LA, Fehir KM, Rice L: Multiple myeloma in a homosexual man with chronic lymphadenopathy. Arch Intern Med 145:91, 1985

60. Kaplan MH, Susin M, Pahwa SG et al: Neoplastic complications of HTLV-III infection: Lymphomas and solid tumors. Am J Med 82:389, 1987

61. Itescu S, Brancato LJ, Buxbaum J et al: A diffuse infiltrative CD8 lymphocytosis syndrome in human immunodeficiency virus infection: Host immune response associated with HLA-DR5. Ann Intern Med 112:3, 1990

62. Ruff P, Bagg A, Papadopoulos K: Precurser T cell lymphoma associated with human immunodeficiency virus type 1: First reported case. Cancer 64:39, 1989

63. Presant CA, Gala K, Wiseman C et al: HIV-associated T cell lymphoblastic lymphoma in AIDS. Cancer 60:1459, 1987

64. Nasr SA, Brynes RK, Garrison CP, Chan WC: Peripheral T cell lymphoma in a patient with acquired immune deficiency syndrome. Cancer 61:947, 1988

65. Sternlieb J, Mintzer D, Kwa D, Bluckman S: Peripheral T cell lymphoma in a patient with the acquired immunodeficiency syndrome. Am J Med 85:445, 1988

66. Anders KH, Latta H, Chang BS et al: Lymphomatoid granulomatosis and malignant lymphoma of the central nervous system in the acquired immunodeficiency syndrome. Hum Pathol 20:326, 1989

67. Colby TV: Central nervous system lymphomatoid granulomatosis in AIDS? Hum Pathol 20:301, 1989

68. Janier M, Katlama C, Flageul B et al: The pseudo-Sézary syndrome with CD8 phenotype in a patient with the acquired immunodeficiency syndrome. Ann Intern Med 110:738, 1989

69. Kobayashi M, Yoshimoto S, Figishita M et al: HTLV-1 positive cell lymphoma/leukemia in and AIDS patient. Lancet 1:1360, 1984

70. Baurmann H, Miclea JM, Ferchal F et al: Adult T cell leukemia associated with HTLV-I and simultaneous infection by HIV type 2 and human herpesvirus 6 in an African woman: A clinical, virologic and familial serologic study. Am J Med 85:853, 1988

71. Shibata D, Brynes R, Rabinowitz A et al: HTLV-I associated adult T cell leukemia lymphoma in a patient infected with HIV-1. Ann Intern Med 111:871, 1989

72. Kaplan LD: AIDS associated lymphoma. Bailliere Clin Haematol 3:139, 1990

73. Kalter SP, Riggs SA, Cabanillas F et al: Aggressive non-Hodgkin's lymphomas in immunocompromised homosexual males. Blood 66:655, 1985

74. Gill PS, Levine AM, Meyer PR et al: Primary central nervous system lymphoma in homosexual men: Clinical, immunologic and pathologic features. Am J Med 78:742, 1985

75. Jones SE, Fuks Z, Bullm M et al: Non-Hodgkin's lymphomas: IV. Clinicopathologic correlation of 405 cases. Cancer 31:806, 1973

76. Levine AM: Reactive and neoplastic lymphoproliferative disorders and other miscellaneous cancers associated with HIV infection. In DeVita VT Jr, Hellman S, Rosenberg SA (eds): AIDS: Etiology, Diagnosis, Treatment and Prevention, 2nd ed, p 263. Philadelphia, JB Lippincott, 1988

77. Kaplan LD, Kahn J, Jacobson J et al: Primary bile duct lymphoma in the acquired immunodeficiency syndrome. Ann Intern Med 110:161, 1989

78. Mehta S, Pawel BR: Human immunodeficiency virus associated large cell immunoblastic lymphoma presenting as a peri-anal abscess. Arch Pathol Lab Med 113:531, 1989

79. Sider L, Weiss AJ, Smith MD et al: Varied appearance of AIDS related lymphoma in the chest. Radiology 171:629, 1989

80. Levine AM, Sullivan-Halley J, Pike MC et al: HIV-related lymphoma: Prognostic factors predictive of survival. Cancer 68:2466, 1991

81. Levine AM, Wernz JC, Kaplan L et al: Low dose chemotherapy with CNS prophylaxis and zidovudine maintenance for AIDS-related lymphoma: A prospective multi-institutional trial. JAMA 266:84, 1991

82. McKelvey EM, Gottlieb JA, Wilson HE et al: Hydroxyldaunomycin (Adriamycin) combination chemotherapy in malignant lymphoma. Cancer 38:1484, 1976

83. Skarin AT, Canellos GP, Rosenthal DS et al: Improved prognosis of diffuse histiocytic and undifferentiated lymphoma by use of high dose methotrexate alternating with standard agents (M-BACOD). J Clin Oncol 1:91, 1983

84. Klimo P, Connors JM: MACOP-B chemotherapy for the treatment of diffuse large cell lymphoma. Ann Intern Med 102:596, 1985

85. Frei E III, Canellos GP: Dose: A critical factor in cancer chemotherapy. Am J Med 69:585, 1980

86. Goldie JH, Coldman AJ, Gudauskas GA: Rationale for the use of alternating non-cross resistant chemotherapy. Cancer Treat Rep 66:439, 1982

87. Kwak LW, Halpern J, Olshen RA, Horning SJ: Prognostic significance of actual dose intensity in diffuse large cell lymphoma: Results of a tree-structured survival analysis. J Clin Oncol 8:963, 1990

88. Gill PS, Levine AM, Krailo M et al: AIDS-related malignant lymphoma: Results of prospective treatment trials. J Clin Oncol 5:1322, 1987

89. Dugan M, Subar M, Odajnyk C et al: Intensive multiagent chemotherapy for AIDS related diffuse large cell lymphoma. Blood 68:124a, 1986

90. Odajnyk C, Subar M, Digan M et al: Clinical features and correlates with immunopathology and molecular biology of a large group of patients with AIDS associated small non-cleaved cell lymphoma. Proc Am Soc Hematol 68:131a, 1986

91. Bermudez MA, Grant KM, Rodvien R, Mendes F: Non-Hodgkin's lymphoma in a population with or at risk for acquired immunodeficiency syndrome: Indications for intensive chemotherapy. Am J Med 86:71, 1989

92. Gisselbrecht C, Tirelli U, Oksenhendler E et al: Non-Hodgkin's lymphoma associated with HIV: Intensive treatment by LNH 84 regimen (abstr 1324). Presented at the VI International Conference on AIDS, San Francisco, June 20–24, 1990

93. Kaplan L, Kahn J, Crowe J et al: A randomized trial of chemotherapy with or without recombinant granulocyte-monocyte colony-stimulating factor in HIV associated non-Hodgkin's lymphoma: Effect of treatment on serum p24 antigen levels (abstr 4546). Presented at the VI International Conference on AIDS, San Francisco, June 20–24, 1990

94. Walsh C, Wernz J, Levine A et al: Phase I trial of m-BACOD and granulocyte macrophage colony stimulating factor (GM-CSF) in HIV associated non-Hodgkin's lymphoma. Unpublished manuscript

95. Levine AM, Rarick MU, Willson E, et al: Combined use of chemotherapy (low dose modification of M-BACOD regimen) with dideoxycytidine (ddC) in patients with HIV related systemic lymphoma: Preliminary results. Presented at the VII International Conference on AIDS, Florence, 1991

96. So YT, Beckstead JH, Davis RL: Primary central nervous system lymphoma in acquired immune deficiency syndrome: A clinical and pathological study. Ann Neurol 20: 566, 1986

97. Gill PS, Graham RA, Boswell W et al: A comparison of imaging, clinical and pathologic aspects of space occupying lesions within the brain in patients with acquired immune deficiency syndrome. Am J Physiol Imag 1:134, 1986

98. Shibata S: Sites of origin of primary intracerebral malignant lymphoma. Neurosurg 25:14, 1989

99. Formenti SC, Gill PS, Lean E et al: Primary central nervous system lymphoma in AIDS: Results of radiation therapy. Cancer 63:1101, 1989

100. Bernstein L, Levin D, Menck H, Ross R: AIDS related secular trends in cancer in Los Angeles County men: A comparison by marital status. Cancer Res 49:466, 1989

101. Biggar RJ, Burnett W, Mikl J, Nasca P: Cancer among New York men at risk of acquired immunodeficiency syndrome. Int J Cancer 43:979, 1989

102. MacMahon B: Epidemiology of Hodgkin's disease. Cancer Res 26:1189, 1966

103. Lukes RJ, Butler JJ, Hicks ED: Natural history of Hodgkin's disease as related to HD pathologic picture. Cancer 19: 317, 1966

104. Schoppel SL, Hoppe RT, Dorfman RF et al: Hodgkin's disease in homosexual men with generalized lymphadenopathy. Ann Intern Med 102:68, 1985

105. Tirelli U, Vaccher E, Rezza G et al: Hodgkin's disease in association with AIDS: A report on 36 patients. Acta Oncol 28:637, 1989

106. Daling JR, Weiss NS, Klopfenstein LL et al: Correlates of homosexual behavior and the incidence of anal cancer. JAMA 247:1988, 1982

107. Daling JR, Weiss NS, Hislop TG et al: Sexual practices, sexually transmitted diseases, and the incidence of anal cancer. N Engl J Med 317:973, 1987

108. Beckmann AM, Daling JR, Sherman KJ et al: Human papilloma virus infection and anal cancer. Int J Cancer 43: 1042, 1989

109. Reid R, Greenberg M, Jenson AB et al: Sexually transmitted papilloma viral infection: I. The anatomic distribution and pathologic grade of neoplastic lesions associated with different viral types. Am J Obstet Gynecol 156:212, 1987

110. Campion MJ, McCance DJ, Cuzick J, Singer A: Progressive potential of mild cervical atypia: Prospective cytological, culposcopic, and virological study. Lancet 2:237, 1986

111. McIndoe WA, McLean MR, Jones RW, Mullins PR: The invasive potential of carcinoma in situ of the cervix. Obstet Gynecol 64:451, 1984

112. Scholefield JH, Talbot IC, Whatrup C et al: Anal and cervical intraepithelial neoplasia: Possible parallel. Lancet 2: 765, 1989

113. Levine AM: Miscellaneous cancers associated with HIV infection. Curr Opin Oncol 2:1171, 1990

114. Tindall B, Finlayson R, Mutimer K et al: Malignant melanoma associated with human immunodeficiency virus infection in three homosexual men. J Am Acad Dermatol 20:587, 1989

115. Monfardini S, Vaccher E, Pizzocaro KG et al: Unusual malignant tumors in 49 patients with HIV infection. AIDS 3: 449, 1989

14

Central and Peripheral Nervous System Complications of HIV-1 Infection and AIDS

Richard W. Price   *Bruce J. Brew*   *Marian Roke*

The neurologic complications of HIV-1 infection are both common and varied, and contribute importantly to patient morbidity and mortality. Disorders of both the central nervous system (CNS) and peripheral nervous system (PNS) may complicate all stages of systemic HIV-1 infection, from the period following initial infection through the end-stage of severe immunosuppression. These neurologic complications may be classified in a number of ways: according to their neuroanatomic localization, in relation to the stage of systemic HIV-1 infection in which they occur, and in relation to the underlying pathophysiology of the particular disease process. Table 14–1 presents a neuroanatomic classification, dividing conditions according to the major pattern of symptom and sign localization; this classification provides a framework for the initial approach to diagnosis pursued by the neurologist.[1]

This chapter is organized principally according to a pathophysiologic classification and is subdivided into sections that address, in turn, disorders known or suspected to relate to effects of HIV-1 itself on the CNS, with an emphasis on the AIDS dementia complex; CNS opportunistic infections; CNS opportunistic neoplasms; other CNS disorders that relate to systemic illness; and PNS and skeletal muscle disorders. Because discussion of some of the conditions overlaps with a more extensive treatment presented in other chapters, the present discussion emphasizes the neurologic aspects of these disorders, the conditions caused by HIV-1 itself, and approaches to diagnosis. A final section summarizes the principles of diagnosis and management.

The diagnosis of neurologic complications of HIV-1 infection and AIDS is far from an academic exercise. Rather, a precise diagnosis is critical to the practical management of patients and frequently leads to specific therapy, with a consequent reduction in morbidity and preservation of meaningful function and quality of life. It is our impression that all too often, AIDS clinicians faced with neurologic complications "give up" on the patient when further diagnostic and therapeutic avenues remain open and capable of preserving worthwhile life.

CNS CONDITIONS KNOWN OR PRESUMED TO RELATE TO AN EFFECT OF HIV-1

Although it is clear that HIV-1 can directly infect the CNS, understanding is still limited regarding the nature of this infection, including its frequency, timing, pathobiology, and relation to clinical manifestations.[2-7] Accumulating clinical and laboratory observations are beginning to clarify these issues and have allowed at least a partial definition of what may be considered overlapping phases of infection and clinical sequelae. These include (1) CNS disorders occurring in the context of acute HIV-1 infection and seroconversion, (2) asymptomatic infection, (3) aseptic meningitis and headache, and (4) the AIDS dementia complex. These different manifestations appear to relate to the varying interactions of the virus and immune reactions.

CNS Disorders Complicating Primary HIV-1 Infection

Although a variety of CNS disorders have been noted in the context of initial HIV-1 infection and seroconversion, reports of these have involved principally individual

Table 14–1. Major Neurologic Complications in HIV-1–Infected Patients, Classified by Neuroanatomic Localization

BRAIN

PREDOMINANTLY NONFOCAL

Common
  AIDS dementia complex
  Metabolic encephalopathies (alone or as exacerbating influence)
  Cytomegalovirus (CMV) encephalitis (clinical impact uncertain)
  Toxoplasmosis (encephalitic form)

Rare
  Herpes encephalitis
  Aspergillosis

PREDOMINANTLY FOCAL

Common
  Cerebral toxoplasmosis
  Primary CNS lymphoma
  Progressive multifocal leukoencephalopathy (PML)

Uncommon/Rare
  Tuberculous brain abscess/tuberculoma
  Cryptococcoma
  Varicella-zoster virus (VZV) encephalitis
  Vascular disorders

SPINAL CORD

Common
  Vacuolar myelopathy (part of AIDS dementia complex)

Uncommon
  VZV myelitis (complicating herpes zoster)
  Spinal epidural or intradural lymphoma
  HTLV-I–associated myelopathy

MENINGES

Common
  Cryptococcal meningitis
  Aseptic meningitis (HIV-1?)

Uncommon
  Lymphomatous meningitis (metastatic)
    Tuberculous meningitis (*M. tuberculosis*)
    Syphilitic meningitis

Rare
  Listeria monocytogenes meningitis

PERIPHERAL NERVE AND ROOT

Very Common
  Distal sensory polyneuropathy

Common
  Autonomic neuropathy
  Herpes zoster
  Acute and chronic demyelinating neuropathies
  Nucleoside toxic neuropathies (ddI, ddC)

Uncommon
  Mononeuritis multiplex
    Early limited form
    Late malignant form
  CMV polyradiculopathy
  Mononeuropathy associated with aseptic meningitis
  Mononeuropathy secondary to lymphomatous meningitis

MUSCLE
  Polymyositis
  Noninflammatory myopathies
  Zidovudine toxic myopathy

cases.[8–16] Hence, a general picture of their incidence and natural history is unavailable, and indeed, the full spectrum of neurologic involvement has yet to be clearly defined.

Headaches and photophobia may be frequent in the acute phase of the seroconversion-related mononucleosis-like syndrome associated with HIV-1 infection.[8] Such symptoms may indicate a subclinical meningitis, and usually are mild and resolve spontaneously. From available reports, the more severe neurologic deficits usually appear clinically after the mononucleosis-like illness begins to subside; they may take the form of encephalitis, meningitis, ataxia, or myelopathy, either alone or together with PNS abnormalities that have included brachial plexopathy or neuropathy.[9–16] The course of these neurologic disorders is monophasic, and most patients have recovered within a number of weeks. The cerebrospinal fluid (CSF) in some cases has shown a minor lymphocyte-predominant pleocytosis with a modest rise in protein levels. Brain computed tomography (CT) has generally been reported as normal, although we are aware of one case in which changes similar to those reported in acute disseminated allergic encephalomyelitis were identified. The electroencephalogram (EEG) may show focal or diffuse slow waves.

Although these early syndromes are apparently uncommon, their incidence may be underappreciated. Clinically they are indistinguishable from other acute viral or postinfectious encephalitides, most of which never achieve specific diagnosis. Additionally, there may be no background systemic illness to engender suspicion of HIV-1 infection, and, even when present, the acute systemic manifestations of HIV-1 may be overshadowed by the prominent neurologic symptoms and signs. If the patient is not identified as a member of a high-risk group or if serologic testing is not done, there may be no clue to the etiologic diagnosis. Moreover, in those serotested in the acute phase, anti-HIV-1 antibodies may not be detected. Immunologic assessment will likewise usually be unrewarding since T-lymphocyte subsets are often normal or include only transient elevations of the CD8+ subset, but usually without depression of the CD4+ subset. Consequently, acute and convalescent (extended to 6 to 12 weeks or longer) serologic data in these encephalitides are needed, and in some patients virus isolation, p24 antigen detection, or the polymerase chain reaction (PCR) may be needed for diagnosis. The effect of zidovudine or other therapy on these conditions has not been assessed.

HIV-1 Infection of the CNS During the Asymptomatic Phase

Evidence is now accumulating that early in the course of asymptomatic HIV-1 infection, involvement of the CNS, or at least of the leptomeninges, is common and may, in fact, be the rule. This early nervous system infection has been demonstrated principally in studies of CSF from asymptomatic seropositive subjects, which have shown (1) abnormalities on "routine" studies, including cell count, protein, and immunoglobulin, (2) local, "intra-blood-brain barrier" synthesis of anti-HIV-1 antibodies, and (3) isolation of virus.[17-23] These observations have both biologic and practical clinical implications. They reveal that both CNS exposure and host reactions to HIV-1 occur early in infection and continue through the asymptomatic period, yet are without apparent immediate clinical sequelae. Additionally, these background abnormalities must be taken into account in the interpretation of CSF results obtained for other diagnostic purposes.

During this asymptomatic phase, the biology of CNS infection appears to diverge from that of symptomatic disease. Thus, abnormal CSF has not yet been shown to confer an adverse prognosis *vis-à-vis* the AIDS dementia complex or other CNS involvement. Although early controversy centered on the isolated development of the AIDS dementia complex in the absence of systemic disease, from a broad population perspective this seems to be rare. Particularly compelling in this regard are the results of the Multicenter AIDS Cohort Study (MACS), which has shown preservation of neurologic function in infected subjects who were otherwise asymptomatic.[24-26]

In the face of these and other laboratory abnormalities, it may still be fair to ask whether there are subclinical CNS abnormalities in these patients. From a pathologic perspective there may be important indolent infection and inflammatory events within the CNS. Yet from a practical clinical standpoint, the risk of isolated cognitive decline in asymptomatic individuals is sufficiently small that there is clearly no basis for disability assignment or disqualification of individuals from work based simply on HIV-1 seropositive status.

Recently a multiple sclerosis-like illness was reported in HIV-1–infected patients in the asymptomatic phase of infection.[27,28] The presentation included remissions and exacerbations, with corticosteroid responsiveness in the setting of preserved CD4+ cell counts. Although it is possible that these cases may represent the concurrence of two diseases, it is more likely that an autoimmune disease indistinguishable from multiple sclerosis is triggered by HIV-1 infection. This illness may involve pathogenetic processes similar to those that underlie immune thrombocytopenic purpura or demyelinating polyneuropathy (see below) in this same group of patients.

Aseptic Meningitis and Headache

Although the seroconversion-related illness may be accompanied by headache and aseptic meningitis, these clinical problems are more common and more important later in the course of HIV-1 infection, apparently occurring most frequently in patients in whom HIV-1 infection is progressing, with falling CD4+ T-lymphocyte counts and clinical manifestations of the AIDS-related complex.[29,30]

Hollander and Stringari have segregated aseptic meningitis into two clinical types, an acute form and a chronic form.[30] Both are accompanied by meningeal symptoms, including headache, whereas meningeal signs are largely confined to the acute group. Cranial nerve palsies may also complicate the course, most often affecting cranial nerves V, VII, or VIII, with Bell's palsy sometimes recurring. The CSF shows a mononuclear pleocytosis, usually with a normal glucose and slightly elevated protein levels. The syndrome itself is benign, although affected patients may have an overall poor prognosis with respect to progression to AIDS-defining complications. There is nothing to suggest that these patients are more or less likely to develop the AIDS dementia complex than patients without headache, but there is little population-based data on the issue.

It is presumed that these aseptic meningitis syndromes relate to HIV-1 itself, because this retrovirus can be isolated from the CSF of some of these patients.[29] However, it is also possible that another infection might actually cause the meningeal inflammation and secondarily induce the entry and proliferation of HIV-1–infected cells in the meninges.

Isolated headache is a common symptom and occurs in the same clinical setting as aseptic meningitis[31,32]; indeed, it may be difficult to segregate true aseptic meningitis, in which local inflammation causes symptoms, from this headache when the headache is accompanied by incidental mild pleocytosis. The cause of this type of headache is uncertain, but the headache may be severe and intractable. In some patients it appears to relate to development of systemic disease (*e.g., Pneumocystis carinii* pneumonia) and hence may be caused by systemic production of vasoactive cytokines. In other patients a relation to systemic inflammation is not clear. We have observed that low doses of amitriptyline appear effective in controlling the headaches in some patients, but controlled study of this issue is needed.

AIDS Dementia Complex

The AIDS dementia complex, characterized by cognitive, motor, and behavioral dysfunction, usually develops later in the course of HIV-1 infection and is in fact one of the commonest CNS complications of late, untreated HIV-1 infection.[4,33-35] Characteristically this syndrome manifests after patients have developed major opportunistic infections or neoplasms that define systemic AIDS, although a small number of patients present before these major systemic complications have developed, at a time when they do not yet fulfill formal criteria for the diagnosis of AIDS on the basis of systemic disease.[36] Recognition of this early presentation has resulted in the addition of the AIDS dementia complex to the diagnostic criteria for AIDS.[37] Usually, however, such patients have already evinced minor complications of HIV-1 infection such as lymphadenopathy, malaise, weight loss, or oral candidiasis. It is only a very small number of patients who develop major dementia when they are otherwise medically well and systemically asymptomatic, and even these patients characteristically meet laboratory criteria of immunosuppression.

CLASSIFICATION AND TERMINOLOGY

The term *AIDS dementia complex* was introduced to describe a clinical syndrome—a cohesive constellation of symptoms and signs—rather than a clearly established disease entity of uniform etiopathogenesis.[4,33,35] It remains useful both to adhere to this original intent and to continue to segregate the concept of the AIDS dementia complex from that of HIV-1 brain infection. As discussed below, HIV-1 clearly infects the CNS and likely accounts for at least one of the pathologic subtypes of the AIDS dementia complex, and thus the syndrome overlaps with HIV-1 brain infection, but infection and disease are not synonymous.

The distinct character of the cognitive changes associated with AIDS dementia complex, which include prominent mental slowing and inattention, along with concomitant affliction of motor performance (described below) underlies the classification of this syndrome among the *subcortical dementias.* Thus, it is placed into a group of conditions that also includes the cognitive impairment found in Parkinson's disease, Huntington's disease, hydrocephalus, and progressive supranuclear palsy.[38] This presentation is in contradistinction to the cortical dementias, such as Alzheimer's disease, in which memory impairment predominates, or Creutzfeldt-Jakob disease, which variously manifests with aphasia, apraxia, or other focal features. Although the anatomic justification for this designation remains to be fully demonstrated, it is a clinically useful distinction and emphasizes the inappropriateness of applying to AIDS patients the definitions and measurement tools that were originally developed for Alzheimer's disease.

Each of the three terms in "AIDS dementia complex" was chosen for a reason. *AIDS* was included because the morbidity of the condition may be comparable to that of other AIDS-defining complications of HIV-1 infection. *Dementia* was included because acquired and persistent cognitive decline is characteristically unaccompanied by alterations in the level of alertness, and it is this cognitive impairment which is generally the most disabling manifestation. The third component, *complex,* was added because the syndrome also importantly includes impaired motor performance and, at times, behavioral change, and therefore the syndrome is not simply an isolated dementia. Myelopathy, *but not peripheral neuropathy,* and organic psychosis, *but not reactive anxiety or depression,* were included within this term because they may coexist with or be difficult to separate from the "core" cognitive and motor abnormalities.

Once the diagnosis of the AIDS dementia complex is made, it is useful to apply a staging scheme based on functional severity in the cognitive and motor spheres (Table 14–2).[26,35] This staging relies on relatively simple functional evaluation and provides a common vocabulary for practical clinical use and for comparing patients assessed by different physicians. It also provides a simple framework for correlations with various laboratory studies.

Recently the World Health Organization (WHO) introduced a new terminology with certain useful features that had been omitted from previous classifications.[39] The WHO classification can be roughly translated

Table 14–2. Staging Scheme for the AIDS Dementia Complex*

Stage of AIDS Dementia Complex	Characteristics
Stage 0: (Normal)	Normal mental and motor function.
Stage 0.5: (Equivocal/ subclinical)	Either minimal or equivocal *symptoms* of cognitive or motor dysfunction characteristic of AIDS dementia complex, or mild signs (snout response, slowed extremity movements), but without impairment of work or capacity to perform activities of daily living. Gait and strength are normal.
Stage 1: (Mild)	Unequivocal evidence (symptoms, signs, neuropsychological test performance) of functional intellectual or motor impairment characteristic of AIDS dementia complex, but patient is able to perform all but the more demanding aspects of work or activities of daily living. Can walk without assistance.
Stage 2: (Moderate)	Patient cannot work or maintain the more demanding aspects of daily life, but can perform basic activities of self-care. Ambulatory, but may require a single prop.
Stage 3: (Severe)	Major intellectual incapacity (patient cannot follow news or personal events, cannot sustain complex conversation; considerable slowing of all output) or motor disability (patient cannot walk unassisted, requiring walker or personal support, usually with slowing and clumsiness of arms as well).
Stage 4: (End stage)	Nearly vegetative. Intellectual and social comprehension and responses are at a rudimentary level. Nearly or absolutely mute. Paraparetic or paraplegic with double incontinence.

* Descriptions summarized from Sidtis and Price[26] and Price and Brew.[35]

into the AIDS dementia complex staging scheme. WHO introduced the term *HIV-1 associated cognitive/motor complex* to encompass the full constellation of the AIDS dementia complex, and added subcategories to refer to patients with predominantly cognitive (*HIV-1 associated dementia*) or myelopathic (*HIV-1 associated myelopathy*) presentations of sufficient severity to interfere with work or activities of daily living (hence severe enough to qualify as Stage 2 or greater in AIDS dementia complex staging). The term *HIV-1 associated minor cognitive/motor disorder* was introduced to designate patients with mild symptoms and signs and only minimal functional impairment of work or activities of daily living (Stage 1 AIDS dementia complex). In addition to the advantage of attempting to separate the patients with predominantly myelopathy from those with cognitive changes, this terminology restricts the term *dementia* to the level of cognitive impairment consistent with that used in other formal definitions. It might also simplify reporting this condition as an AIDS-defining disorder if one restricts this designation to a presentation with sufficient functional severity to be termed *HIV-1 associated dementia* or *HIV-1 associated myelopathy*. The requirement for this level of severity (equivalent to Stage 2 or greater in the AIDS dementia complex terminology) is probably both biologically and prognostically consistent with other AIDS-defining conditions. The WHO classification also does not make the implicit assumption that the disorder is a single disease entity differing only in severity, but allows for the possibility that milder and more severe disease may be discontinuous processes.

CLINICAL FEATURES

The clinical features of the AIDS dementia complex are briefly summarized in Table 14–3.[33] The earliest symptoms usually consist of difficulties with concentration and memory. Patients begin to lose track of their train of thought or conversation, and many complain of "slowness" in thinking. Complex tasks become more difficult and take longer to complete, while forgetfulness or difficulty in concentration lead to missed appointments and the need to keep lists. If patients need a high level of concentration or organization for their occupation or activities at home, the AIDS dementia complex may be recognized early from impaired performance. In other instances, a friend or family member may be the first to notice subtle cognitive and personality changes as the patient begins to withdraw socially and appears apathetic and unusually quiet or forgetful.

Although psychological depression is usually mild or absent in these patients, in mild cases it may be difficult to separate depression or fatigue from early AIDS dementia complex. In a minority, a more agitated organic psychosis may be the presenting or predominant aspect of the illness. Such patients are irritable, hyperactive, and may become overtly manic.

Although cognitive manifestations usually appear earlier than motor symptoms and continue to predom-

Table 14–3. Clinical Features of the AIDS Dementia Complex

EARLY MANIFESTATIONS
SYMPTOMS
  Cognition
    Impaired concentration
    Forgetfulness
    Mental slowing
  Motor
    Unsteady gait
    Leg weakness
    Loss of coordination, impaired handwriting
    Tremor
  Behavior
    Apathy, withdrawal, personality change
    Agitation, confusion, hallucinations
SIGNS
  Mental status
    Psychomotor slowing
    Impaired serial 7s or reversals
    Organic psychosis
  Neurologic examination
    Impaired rapid movements (limbs, eyes)
    Hyperreflexia
    Release reflexes (snout, glabellar, grasp)
    Gait ataxia (impaired tandem gait, rapid turns)
    Tremor (postural)
    Leg weakness

LATE MANIFESTATIONS
  Mental status
    Global dementia
    Psychomotor slowing: verbal responses delayed, near or absolute mutism, vacant stare
    Unawareness of illness, disinhibition
    Confusion, disorientation
    Organic psychosis
  Neurologic signs
    Weakness (legs ≫ arms)
    Ataxia
    Pyramidal tract signs: spasticity, hyperreflexia, extensor plantar responses
    Bladder and bowel incontinence
    Myoclonus

inate, in those with motor dysfunction early in the course of the disease, poor balance and incoordination are the most common complaints. Gait incoordination may result in more frequent tripping or falling, or a perceived need to exercise new care in walking. Patients may drop things more frequently, or may become slower and less precise with manual activities such as writing.

Early in the evolution of the illness, the patient may appear remarkably normal on formal bedside mental status testing, although responses are characteristically slow even when their content is accurate. As the disease progresses, patients perform poorly on tasks requiring concentration and attention such as word and digit reversals and serial 7s. With a further increase in severity, results of a larger array of mental status tests become abnormal. Slowing remains prominent, and afflicted individuals often appear apathetic, have poor insight, and are indifferent to their illness.

Even when not symptomatic, motor abnormalities can usually be detected on careful examination early in the course of the disease. Slowing of rapid successive and alternating movements of the fingers, wrists, or feet and impaired ocular motility with interruption of smooth pursuit and slowing or inaccuracy of saccade are common early findings. Also frequent is a generalized hyperreflexia, including the jaw jerk, followed later by the development of pathologic reflexes, including snout, glabellar, and, less commonly, grasp responses. As the disease evolves, ataxia, which at first affects only rapid turns or tandem gait, may become disabling, although usually as the syndrome worsens the leg weakness increases and paraparesis limits walking. Postural tremor is not unusual, and a few patients exhibit multifocal myoclonus as well. Bladder and bowel incontinence is common in the late stages of the disease. In the end stage patients become nearly vegetative, lying in bed with a vacant stare, unable to ambulate, and incontinent. However, with the exception of occasional hypersomnolence, the level of arousal is usually preserved in the absence of intercurrent illness. Characteristically, the course is notable for the absence of focal neurologic deficits (*e.g.,* aphasia, hemiparesis).

In children, the disorder has the same general features, although the course may vary somewhat and present in either a progressive or a static form.[40,41] The progressive form is characterized by the gradual loss of previously acquired motor skills in conjunction with the evolution of motor abnormalities ranging from spastic paraparesis to quadriplegia with pseudobulbar palsy and rigidity. Acquired microcephaly is the rule. The CDC surveillance criteria and classification for childhood AIDS now include neurologic disease with one or more of the following progressive findings: (1) loss of developmental milestones or intellectual ability, (2) impaired brain growth (acquired microcephaly and/or brain atrophy) demonstrated on CT or magnetic resonance imaging (MRI), or (3) symmetric motor deficits manifested by two or more of the following: paresis, abnormal tone, pathologic reflexes, ataxia, or gait disturbance.[42]

NEUROPSYCHOLOGICAL TEST PROFILE

Formal neuropsychological testing may be useful in assessing AIDS dementia complex patients, both in the context of clinical research studies on epidemiology and treatment and, in some cases, for practical patient diagnosis and management.[24–26,43,44] Appropriately chosen neuropsychological assessments address the same cardinal dysfunction sought by the AIDS-directed clinical examination and provide a formal, quantitative means of following patients serially. Assessments focus on alterations in motor speed, concentration, and mental manipulation. It is important to understand that the results of neuropsychological assessments should not be

used as the sole or even major criterion for diagnosis, and thus do not substitute for the clinical neurologic evaluation. The results are not disease specific and should always be interpreted in the clinical context. Thus, some patients with AIDS dementia complex will perform within the population norms, while others will do poorly on testing for other reasons. However, with proper interpretation, such studies may provide useful ancillary data by clarifying whether the magnitude and profile of the functional deficit are consistent with the history and hence with a diagnosis of the AIDS dementia complex and the clinical staging.

NEUROIMAGING STUDIES

Neuroimaging procedures are essential to the evaluation of AIDS patients with CNS dysfunction and are useful both in establishing the diagnosis of the AIDS dementia complex and, perhaps even more important, in excluding other neurologic conditions complicating AIDS. Neuroradiologic abnormalities in the AIDS dementia complex include the nearly universal finding of cerebral atrophy, detected by either CT or MRI.[33] In some affected patients MRI will additionally show abnormalities in the hemispheric white matter and, less commonly, in the basal ganglia or thalamus, with either patchy or diffusely increased signal intensity that is most apparent in T2-weighted images.[45–48] Children with AIDS-related dementia often have basal ganglia calcification in addition to atrophy.[49]

Metabolic imaging of patients with the AIDS dementia complex has also been reported, using both positron emission tomography (PET) and single photon emission computed tomography (SPECT), although the diagnostic utility of these modalities remains to be clearly delineated.[50–52] In the case of PET, improvement in the abnormalities of cerebral glucose metabolism have been used to corroborate the therapeutic effect of antiviral treatment.[53]

CEREBROSPINAL FLUID

A CSF examination, like neuroimaging, is used principally to exclude diagnoses other than the AIDS dementia complex. Routine examination of the CSF of these patients reveals the nonspecific findings of a mildly elevated protein level in approximately two thirds of patients and a mild mononuclear pleocytosis in nearly one fourth.[33] Additionally, HIV-1 can be directly isolated from the CSF of some.[23] However, as noted above, HIV-1 can also be isolated from the CSF of a variety of infected patients, including those who are asymptomatic or suffering from aseptic meningitis, as well as those with overt dementia. In some severely affected AIDS dementia-complex patients, HIV-1 p24 antigen in the CSF may be detected by immunoassay.[54] This study is usually of limited practical utility because the diagnosis is most often clinically quite evident in such patients.

Of perhaps greater potential value, certain surrogate

markers of immune cell activation have been noted to be increased in the CSF of AIDS dementia patients, with concentrations correlating, to some extent, with clinical severity. These markers include β_2-microglobulin (a noncovalently bound portion of the class 1 major histocompatibility complex) and neopterin (a product of pteridine metabolism that appears to be released by activated macrophages).[55-59] Quinolinic acid is similarly elevated[60]; this product of tryptophan metabolism can be induced by interferon-γ and perhaps other cytokines, and can act at the N-methyl-D-aspartate (NMDA) receptor as an endogenous excitotoxin. It has been speculated that quinolinic acid may contribute to the CNS injury in patients with the AIDS dementia complex. Whether or not quinolinic acid is a major factor in brain injury, elevation of these surrogate markers in the CSF indicates that, while AIDS patients are immunosuppressed, certain immune cell responses are upregulated as the disease progresses. In fact, this occurs in both the blood and CSF compartments and reflects parallel processes in systemic and CNS disease. Because these markers may be increased by the action of cytokines, these observations suggest that cytokine-related reactions might be involved in the production of CNS injury.[5,61,62]

CSF surrogate markers may also turn out to be clinically useful, although further study is needed to clearly delineate such utility. Certainly, elevated levels of β_2-microglobulin, neopterin, and quinolinic acid in the CSF are *not diagnostically specific;* these markers are also elevated in the CSF of patients with opportunistic CNS infections and CNS lymphoma.[55,56,60] However, in the absence of such conditions, increased concentrations of these markers may be helpful in assessing mild or equivocal cases of AIDS dementia complex. They may also prove useful in following the effects of therapy, as zidovudine treatment lowers the elevated CSF concentration of these markers.[37,38]

EPIDEMIOLOGY AND NATURAL HISTORY

The epidemiology of the AIDS dementia complex, including its prevalence at various stages of systemic HIV-1 infection, is not yet clearly defined.[5] Current understanding derives largely from clinical case observations rather than from prospective epidemiologic investigations. Several recent epidemiologic studies have, however, more clearly characterized some of the neurologic and neuropsychological aspects of asymptomatic HIV-1–seropositive subjects.[24,25] Additionally, the epidemiology of the AIDS dementia complex may be undergoing modification related to the widespread early use of antiviral therapy.[63]

Available information allows some approximations of the prevalence of the AIDS dementia complex at different phases of untreated systemic HIV-1 infection. Both its prevalence and severity increase as systemic disease progresses and helper (CD4+) T-lymphocyte counts fall. Our own impression is that this syndrome is a frequent and significant clinical problem in the late

stages of systemic HIV-1 infection, and prior to death the majority of AIDS patients exhibit its symptoms and signs, with perhaps one half showing functionally important (Stages 2 to 4) disability. Somewhat earlier in the evolution of systemic illness, when patients first present with AIDS-defining opportunistic infections (*e.g., P carinii* pneumonia), mild (Stage 1) AIDS dementia complex is detectable in perhaps 10% to 30% of patients, while more severe neurologic impairment (Stages 2 to 4) is present in perhaps another 5% to 15%. In the transitional phase of HIV-1 infection, when immunosuppression begins to manifest with constitutional symptoms and the AIDS-related complex, subclinical abnormalities (Stage 0.5) may be present in a third or more, although probably less than 10% exhibit features of Stage 1 or higher. In contrast, during the clinical latent period, when patients are constitutionally well, functionally significant abnormalities are rare.

The course of the AIDS dementia complex is also variable. Steadily progressive and severe disease (Stages 2 to 4) develops principally in individuals with advanced immunosuppression, whereas the course in those without systemic disease is more likely to be indolently progressive or even static (Stage 0.5 or 1). Exceptional patients may progress to Stages 2 to 4 without experiencing major systemic complications of HIV-1 infection, although characteristically laboratory evidence of severe immunosuppression is present and most have suffered constitutional, although not AIDS-defining, symptoms and signs before or concomitant with neurologic deterioration.[36] At the other extreme, some patients remain neurologically intact and continue to function at a high level despite recurrent, severe episodes of opportunistic infections. Thus, systemic immunosuppression appears to be a general prerequisite but not the sole determinant of severe, progressive AIDS dementia complex.

NEUROPATHOLOGY

Histologic abnormalities in patients with the AIDS dementia complex are most prominent in the subcortical structures: the central white matter, deep gray structures (including the basal ganglia and thalamus), the brain stem, and the spinal cord, with relative sparing of the cortex.[6,34,64] These abnormalities can be segregated into three overlapping major sets: (1) white matter pallor and gliosis, (2) multinucleated cell encephalitis, and (3) vacuolar myelopathy.[65] A less common additional finding is diffuse or focal spongiform change of the cerebral white matter.

The most common abnormality is diffuse white matter pallor accompanied by astrocytic reaction. This change involves particularly the central and periventricular white matter and diencephalic nuclei. When simple pallor is present without multinucleated cells, inflammation is characteristically scant.

Multinucleated cells are found in a subgroup of patients with more severe clinical disease. In these brains reactive infiltrates are more prominent and consist of perivascular and parenchymal foamy macrophages, microglia, and lymphocytes, along with the multinucleated cells. Because of the association of these findings with direct HIV-1 brain infection, as described below, this pathologic subset may be legitimately termed *HIV-1 encephalitis.*[66,67] The characteristic multinucleated cell and macrophage infiltrates are most often concentrated in the white matter and deep gray structures. In the white matter, they may be surrounded by focal rarefaction and, less commonly, by frank demyelination.

Vacuolar myelopathy pathologically resembles subacute combined degeneration caused by vitamin B12 deficiency,[65] but levels of this vitamin are usually normal in serum. Although there is a general correlation between the incidence of vacuolar myelopathy and the other pathologic abnormalities found in the brain, the myelopathy can occur in the absence of the multinucleated cell–associated changes, and *vice versa.* These discrepancies leave open the question of whether vacuolar myelopathy is an etiopathogenetically independent process. Patients with this pathology usually manifest hyperactive deep tendon reflexes, ataxia, spasticity, or paraplegia, depending on its severity.

ETIOLOGY AND PATHOGENESIS

Accumulating evidence from clinical observations, animal models, and direct demonstration of the virus in the brain supports the hypothesis that the AIDS dementia complex is due to an effect of HIV-1 itself on the nervous system, and that in a subset of patients this effect relates to direct brain infection. Infection of the CNS by HIV-1 has now been detected with a variety of techniques, beginning with studies using Southern blot analysis, which showed a high frequency of proviral DNA (comparable to that of lymphatic tissue) and high copy number in the brains of some patients with the AIDS dementia complex.[68] Both integrated and nonintegrated forms of the genome have been found. *In situ* studies have also detected the presence of viral DNA and RNA within these brains,[69,70] and HIV-1 has been cultured and even cloned directly from the brain.[29,71,72] In addition, HIV-1 antigens have been observed in brain by means of immunohistochemical techniques,[73–77] and HIV-1 virions have been identified by electron microscopy.[78,79]

With respect to the cell types involved in productive HIV-1 brain infection, an emerging consensus implicates macrophages and microglia, as well as multinucleated cells derived from these two cell forms, as the principal if not sole participants.[75,77,80,81] Although not an invariant finding in HIV-1–infected brains, the multinucleated cells are histologic markers of productive HIV-1 brain infection, and likely the multinucleation results from direct virus-induced cell fusion. Whether other cell types in the brain, including the native astrocytes, oligodendrocytes, or neurons, are also infected is less clear and requires further investigation. Cell culture studies have demonstrated low-level infection of glial cells and in glial and neuroblastoma cell lines.[82–85] Whether parallel infection of these cell types occurs *in vivo* has not yet clearly been demonstrated. Recent studies of ''neuropathic'' strains of HIV-1 suggest that the capacity of certain isolates to grow well in brain relates to macrophage tropism and that this is conferred by sequence changes in the viral genome coding for the V3 loop of gp120.[86–89]

Perhaps the central unresolved question of pathogenesis is this: How does HIV-1 infection confined to macrophages and microglia result in brain dysfunction? In the absence of direct cytopathic infection of neurons, oligodendrocytes, and other functional elements of the brain, speculation has now centered on *indirect* mechanisms whereby either (1) viral gene products released from infected cells or (2) cytokines, either released from infected cells or stimulated by the presence of infection, act as neurotoxins that in turn damage neighboring neurons, oligodendrocytes, or astrocytes.[3,4,61,62,90–92]

MANAGEMENT AND THERAPY OF CNS HIV-1 INFECTION AND THE AIDS DEMENTIA COMPLEX

Accumulating evidence indicates that the AIDS dementia complex can be treated and perhaps to some extent prevented with antiretroviral drug therapy. Initial anecdotal case reports[93] have been supplemented by controlled studies showing that in adult patients with HIV-1 infection, zidovudine has resulted in improved neuropsychological performance compared to placebo.[94,95] Likewise, a trial in children in which a constant infusion regimen of zidovudine was used showed striking improvement in neuropsychological performance in a group of children with and without overt neurodevelopmental abnormalities.[96,97] Pertinent to the issue of prevention, a study of the epidemiology of AIDS dementia complex in the Netherlands suggested that zidovudine reduced the incidence of new cases when it was first widely adopted in clinical practice.[63]

Unresolved issues with zidovudine include the question of optimal doses in both prophylactic and therapeutic situations. In the absence of precise dosage guidelines, a conventional dosage (500–600 mg/day) is recommended in both situations. In patients who exhibit neurologic deterioration on this dosage, the clinician may either attempt to increase the zidovodine dosage to 1,000 mg/day or more, thereby increasing the risk of toxicity, or may switch to another antiretroviral drug such as dideoxyinosine (ddI). Although there is some suggestion of activity,[98] the efficacy of ddI in the AIDS dementia complex has not yet been clearly shown in a controlled trial and is under further investigation.

The possible role of toxins in the genesis of the AIDS dementia complex has also given rise to proposals to attempt to block the effects of these putative intermediaries. For example, the calcium channel blocker nimodipine, which appeared to block the neuronal toxicity of HIV-1 gp120 in cell culture,[90] is now being considered for clinical trial.

Finally, less specific symptomatic management is also important in AIDS dementia complex patients. For example, in the subset of patients who present with mania, lithium or neuroleptics may be helpful. However, these patients may be unusually susceptible to the side-effects of neuroleptics and other psychotropic drugs, and thus treatment should be cautious and begin with low doses.

OPPORTUNISTIC CNS INFECTIONS

A variety of infections of the CNS complicate AIDS,[1,99,100] including, most importantly, *Toxoplasma gondii, Cryptococcus neoformans,* JC virus causing progressive multifocal leukoencephalitis (PML), and cytomegalovirus (CMV). The specific diagnosis of these and other CNS infections is important because several can be effectively treated.

Cerebral Toxoplasmosis

Cerebral toxoplasmosis is the most frequent of the CNS opportunistic infections that occur in the setting of AIDS and complicates the course in 5% to 15% or more of patients, with the incidence depending on geographic origin.[101-106] The varying incidence relates principally to the likelihood of earlier environmental exposure to the etiologic protozoan parasite, *Toxoplasma gondii.* Cerebral toxoplasmosis almost invariably results from recrudescence of previously acquired infection and relates to loss of the immune defenses that maintain *T. gondii* in an inactive encysted form. One study estimated that approximately one quarter of HIV-1–infected patients with antibodies against this parasite would eventually develop cerebral toxoplasmosis.[107]

The clinical presentation of cerebral toxoplasmosis is characteristically subacute, evolving over several days from initial symptoms to presentation with neurologic deficit.[101] Focal cerebral dysfunction usually predominates but is often combined with or occasionally overshadowed by nonfocal "encephalitic" symptoms and signs. Focal manifestations usually relate to hemispheric lesions and include hemiparesis, hemianesthesia, aphasia, apraxia, or seizures. Cerebellar ataxia and brain stem abnormalities are far less common. The encephalitic features include general confusion or altered consciousness with lethargy or even coma. Headache and fever are also relatively common. The typical patient thus appears ill and lethargic, and exhibits lateralizing neurologic symptoms or signs.

Pathologically, the disease is characterized by a variable number of cerebral abscesses.[101] In the acute encephalitic form of the disease, the brain may exhibit numerous small lesions with little in the way of cellular reaction. The more common, slowly developing lesions are often larger and surrounded by mononuclear cell reaction, edema, and at times vascular occlusion or an element of microscopic hemorrhage. Chronic healed lesions exhibit minor fibrotic changes. Untreated disease is characterized by the presence of free forms (tachyzoites) of *T. gondii,* whereas after treatment these forms are no longer seen, although encysted forms may persist.

The diagnosis of cerebral toxoplasmosis relies on ready clinical suspicion, the use of neuroimaging procedures, and therapeutic trial, with blood serology being of ancillary help.[101] In the approach to AIDS patients with suspected toxoplasmosis or other focal disorders, MRI or, less optimally, CT is critical, both to confirm the presence of macroscopic focal disease and to determine the nature of the abnormalities.[108] Multiple lesions involving the cortex or deep brain nuclei (thalamus, basal ganglia) surrounded by edema strongly favor cerebral toxoplasmosis. In most cases the abscesses of *T. gondii* infection exhibit ringlike contrast enhancement on either MRI or CT, but homogeneous contrast enhancement or nonenhancing hypodense lesions may be noted in some cases. It is now clear that MRI is generally superior to CT in demonstrating *Toxoplasma* abscesses and thus in revealing the location and multiplicity of lesions. If MRI is unavailable, there may be some advantage to using "double-dose" contrast-enhanced CT to detect these lesion. Table 14–4 com-

Table 14–4. Salient Aspects of the Differential Diagnosis of Four Common CNS Complications of AIDS

	Clinical		*Neuroimaging*		
Disorder	*Temporal Evaluation*	*Alertness*	*No. of Lesions*	*Type of Lesions*	*Location of Lesions*
Cerebral toxoplasmosis	Days	Reduced	Multiple	Spherical, enhancing, mass effect	Cortex, basal ganglia
Primary CNS lymphoma	Days to weeks	Variable	One or few	Diffuse enhancement, mass effect	Periventricular, white matter
Progressive multifocal leukoencephalitis	Weeks	Preserved	Multiple	Nonenhancing, no mass effect	White matter, adjacent to cortex
AIDS dementia complex	Weeks to months	Preserved	None, multiple or diffuse	Increased T2 signal, no enhancement or mass effect	White matter, basal ganglia

pares cerebral toxoplasmosis with two other common causes of focal brain disease in AIDS, primary CNS lymphoma and PML, and with the AIDS dementia complex. Cerebral lymphoma may produce a similar CT or MRI appearance, although the lesions of lymphoma commonly exhibit more diffuse or less clear-cut contrast enhancement on CT, tend to be radiologically less numerous, and are more often located in the white matter adjacent to the lateral ventricles. The lesions of PML are in the white matter, often at the cortical junction, and do not have mass effect.

Toxoplasma serology is of additional help if the results are appropriately interpreted. Because the disease is typically due to reactivation of the organism, patients with cerebral toxoplasmosis rarely have negative serum IgG antibody titers.[101,107] However, these titers may be low (occasionally an apparently negative titer will be positive when a more concentrated specimen, such as a 1:4 dilution, is tested) and frequently do not rise during the course of the disease. Thus, a positive titer indicates susceptibility and a negative titer casts doubt on the diagnosis.

The practical diagnosis of cerebral toxoplasmosis now relies principally on a therapeutic trial of antitoxoplasmosis treatment.[101,105] Brain biopsy is reserved for treatment failures or clinically atypical patients, such as those who are seronegative or have uncharacteristic MRI or CT findings. When treated promptly, toxoplasmosis responds with clear clinical and neuroimaging improvement within 1 to 2 weeks. In fact, many patients are clinically better within 24 to 48 hours. When brain biopsy is done, immunoperoxidase staining considerably increases the sensitivity in detecting *T. gondii.*

Pyrimethamine in combination with sulfadiazine is the standard therapy for cerebral toxoplasmosis, although there is some uncertainty regarding the appropriate dosage.[103,104] Some now suggest beginning with a loading dose of 100 to 200 mg of pyrimethamine, followed by a single oral daily dose of 50 to 75 mg thereafter, together with sulfadiazine, 6 to 8 g/day given in four divided doses. Patients also receive folinic acid, 10 mg/day, as a single oral dose. Once a therapeutic response is obtained, the dosage can be reduced somewhat to 25 to 50 mg/day of pyrimethamine and 2 g/day of sulfadiazine. Adverse reactions to sulfa, including allergy and bone marrow depression, are common and may necessitate substitution with clindamycin.[109,110] During the acute phase this may be given intravenously (IV) at doses of 1,200 mg every 6 hours, while later a chronic dose of 300 mg orally four times a day has been recommended by some. Treatment must be lifelong. Newer antitoxoplasmosis agents currently under trial include azithromycin, clarithromycin, and BW 566. From preliminary data these agents appear to be effective. BW 566 has the potential great advantage of being active against the cyst form of *Toxoplasma,* so that maintenance therapy might not be necessary.

In the treatment of cerebral toxoplasmosis, and indeed in all AIDS patients, corticosteroids should be avoided when possible. This is particularly important if a therapeutic trial is being considered to differentiate between toxoplasmosis and CNS lymphoma. Because the latter may respond symptomatically and radiologically to corticosteroids alone, clinical or neuroimaging improvement on combination antibiotic and steroid treatment is difficult to interpret. More generally, corticosteroids intensify the impairment of immune defenses in AIDS patients, potentially worsening not only toxoplasmosis but also other systemic opportunistic infections. Thus, we use corticosteroids only if mass effect is sufficient to threaten brain herniation. Once such patients improve, corticosteroids are then tapered rapidly.

Cryptococcal Meningitis

Cryptococcal meningitis is the commonest CNS fungal infection in AIDS patients,[111-115] most frequently presenting as a subacute meningitis with headache, nausea, vomiting, confusion, and lethargy, just as in non-AIDS patients. However, in some patients symptoms and signs are remarkably mild. Similarly, the CSF formula may be bland, with few or no cells and little or no perturbation in glucose or protein levels. Accordingly, one should routinely obtain India ink preparations, CSF cryptococcal antigen titers, and fungal cultures in all AIDS patients at lumbar puncture. The serum cryptococcal antigen assay is almost always positive,[114] so that it may serve as a screen in patients in whom the diagnostic suspicion is low, or if a spinal tap is refused or should be avoided (for example, in the presence of thrombocytopenia or other bleeding diathesis).

The optimal treatment of cryptococcal meningitis at present is still somewhat uncertain. It has recently been demonstrated that fluconazole is likely as effective as amphotericin B.[116-118] One recommendation is that amphotericin be used initially in more severely ill patients (*e.g.,* patients who are obtunded or who have a CSF antigen titer of greater than 1:256) and that fluconazole can be used in the remainder or after the severely affected patients improve and stabilize. Fluconazole appears to clear the CSF less quickly than amphotericin, whereas amphotericin is more often associated with organ toxicity, predominantly renal, and also must be administered *via* a central venous catheter, with the attendant complications of infection. The dose of fluconazole that is used is between 200 and 400 mg/day, while that for amphotericin B is 0.4 to 0.8 mg/kg/day. The efficacy of 5-flucytosine (5-FC) in this group of patients is now in doubt, and so it is not routinely administered.

Patients who do not respond to the regimens described above should undergo careful assessment to determine the precise reason for the failure. In broad terms, failure may result from continued active infection or from the residua of infection, including particularly hydrocephalus. Patients who develop hydrocephalus as the cause of persistent headache or other symptoms may require ventriculoperitoneal shunting or repeated spinal taps. Persistent cryptococcal infection may also result from poor oral absorption of fluconazole or from drug resistance. Although fluconazole levels are not generally determined, it has been our anecdotal experience that such determination been useful by demonstrating poor oral absorption, necessitating higher than usual doses. Drug resistance with respect to fluconazole at the moment does not appear to be common, but again, it has proved to be of some use in difficult cases.

Following successful induction therapy the relapse rate is still high, and virtually all patients require maintenance therapy. Usually this consists of a lower dose of the agent used for induction. For example, amphotericin may be given at a dosage of 1 mg/kg one to three times per week.

Primary prophylaxis against cryptococcal meningitis is unfortunately still under development. There is some evidence that ketoconazole may be useful, and one would anticipate that fluconazole will also prove useful. However, neither of these agents has been studied in a prospective trial, and the theoretical risk of the development of drug resistance as a consequence of long-term administration argues for caution at the present time.

Progressive Multifocal Leukoencephalitis

PML is an opportunistic infection caused by the human papovavirus, JC.[119-123] It may develop in about 4% of AIDS patients. The disease is characterized by selective demyelination. The pathologic lesions begin as small foci, most often in the subcortical white matter, which then coalesce to form larger lesions. Lesions of the hemispheres are most common, but the cerebellum and brain stem may also be affected. The microscopic appearance includes pathognomonic inclusion-bearing swollen oligodendrocyte nuclei and bizarre pleomorphic, hyperchromatic astrocytes. The oligodendrocyte inclusions relate to the presence of JC virus nucleocapsids, which can be identified by electron microscopy, and the demyelinating lesions are caused by the death of these cells, with secondary degeneration of their myelin-forming processes. Inflammation is inconspicuous in the majority of cases.

Like toxoplasmosis and primary CNS lymphoma, PML presents with focal neurologic deficit. However, in the case of PML the clinical evolution is usually more protracted, and altered consciousness or other "encephalitic" signs are usually not present (see Table 14–4). Rather, the picture is one of worsening focal deficits, such as hemiparesis, hemianopsia, aphasia, hemisensory deficit, ataxia, and the like. The hemispheres are more commonly involved than the posterior fossa structures. The diagnosis can often be suspected clinically, while neuroimaging usually helps to support the diagnosis and rule out confounding diseases.[124,125] Again, MRI is superior to CT and shows white matter lesions, often adjacent to the cortex and usually most evident on T2-weighted images. These abnormalities should correlate with clinical deficits, and one should not confuse the white matter changes associated with the AIDS dementia complex with those of PML. A useful aphorism is, "In PML the patient is worse than the scan, in the AIDS dementia complex the scan looks worse than the patient." This refers particularly to focal clinical deficits, which are characteristic of PML and absent in the AIDS dementia complex. Usually the PML abnormalities do not enhance and are not accompanied by mass effect. Neither serum nor CSF serologies are useful in the diagnosis since positive serum antibody titers against JC virus are found in the majority of the normal population and CSF titers are negative. The definitive diagnosis is made by brain biopsy or at autopsy. Light microscopy is usually adequate to establish the diagnosis, but occasionally either immunocytochemistry or *in situ* hybridization may be useful.

There is no proven effective therapy for the disease. Recent uncontrolled studies have raised the question of whether zidovudine, interferon-γ, or intrathecal cytosine arabinoside might be helpful in some cases, but this requires further study.[126,127] Spontaneous sustained remission of PML in two AIDS patients has recently been reported and provides hope for the development of new interventional strategies.[128]

Cytomegalovirus Infection

Systemic CMV infection is common in AIDS patients, and evidence of minor brain CMV infection, in the form of isolated inclusion-bearing cells within an occasional microglial nodule, can be found at autopsy in as many as one third.[34,66,129,130] The contribution of this level of CMV infection to neurologic symptoms and signs in AIDS patients is uncertain; likely it is generally minor and most often overshadowed by the AIDS dementia complex.[34] However, CMV may occasion cause clinically overt encephalitis, although its presentation has been poorly characterized. The illness generally seems to develop over days rather than weeks and includes fever, obtundation, and, often, seizures. MRI or CT may show ventricular ependymitis or small focal cortical lesions.

If CMV infection of the brain is highly suspected, specific antiviral therapy with ganciclovir should be considered, although its efficacy in CNS CMV infection other than retinopathy[131] has not yet been adequately tested.

Mycobacterial Infections

Although not strictly an opportunistic pathogen, *Mycobacterium tuberculosis* appears to produce an infection more common and perhaps more severe in certain groups of HIV-1–infected individuals. The development of *M. tuberculosis* infection is additionally influenced by socioeconomic factors, and predominantly affects IV drug abusers or others from lower socioeconomic groups rather than patients with homosexuality or transfusion as risk factors for AIDS.[132-134] However, even in AIDS patients with systemic tuberculosis, CNS involvement appears to be uncommon, although some have suggested that such infection, when present, may be more aggressive. Clinical presentations can include meningitis, acute abscess, and indolent, chronic tuberculoma. The diagnosis in some cases may be difficult to make and may require brain biopsy. Although systemic atypical mycobacteria, especially *M. avium-intracellulare,* commonly infect AIDS patients, they do not appear to cause clinical CNS disease. Thus, although organisms have been detected on occasion in the CSF or even brain, they have not been shown to infiltrate the brain parenchyma or to cause clinical symptoms and signs.

Varicella Zoster Virus and Herpes Simplex Virus Infections

Although unusual, VZV and, to a lesser extent, HSV-1 and HSV-2 have been reported to cause CNS disease in AIDS patients. VZV infections are of three types: (1) multifocal direct brain infection affecting principally the white matter and partially mimicking PML,[135-137] (2) cerebral vasculitis, which characteristically occurs in the setting of ophthalmic herpes zoster and causes contralateral hemiplegia,[138,139] and (3) myelopathy complicating herpes zoster.[140] Both HSV-1 and HSV-2 have been identified in the brains of some AIDS patients, but the clinical correlates of these infections in AIDS patients have not been wholly delineated.[141,142]

Syphilis

The influence of HIV-1 infection on the course, diagnosis, and treatment of syphilis in the setting of HIV-1 infection is presently somewhat controversial.[143-149] There is some evidence that syphilis may have a more aggressive course, with neurologic complications occurring at an earlier time, and that the complications may be atypical. Patients have been described who have presented with meningovascular syphilis after seemingly adequate treatment for primary syphilis. In addition to meningovascular syphilis, a polyradiculopathy has also been emphasized.[150] Despite these disturbing reports, it should be remembered that such treatment failures have been known for a considerable time and that unusually short times to progression have been recorded in the absence of HIV-1 infection. Of more importance is that both the diagnosis and the therapeutic monitoring of neurosyphilis in these patients may be problematic, because it may be difficult to know what process is responsible for the CSF abnormalities. Moreover, neurosyphilis may occur with a negative CSF VDRL and, on occasion, a negative FTA. From a practical viewpoint, clinical suspicion should be high in these patients, and if neurosyphilis is suspected, full-dose treatment (*e.g.,* 1–2 million units of IV penicillin for 10 days) should

be given and benzathine penicillin should not be relied on.

OPPORTUNISTIC CNS NEOPLASMS

The CNS of AIDS patients is subject to the development of opportunistic neoplasms, particularly lymphomas, that either arise in the brain itself or metastasize from extraneural sites. Although Kaposi's sarcoma involving the brain has been reported,[83] it is so exceedingly rare that it does not warrant general consideration in the differential diagnosis of brain disease.

Primary CNS Lymphoma

Primary CNS lymphomas of B-cell origin are opportunistic neoplasms that complicate the course of AIDS in approximately 5% of patients, although this estimate includes lymphomas noted incidentally at autopsy.[151-159] The incidence of primary CNS lymphoma in non-AIDS patients is increasing,[157,158] and our own recent experience suggests that this may also be the case in AIDS patients, perhaps related to their increased longevity and the efficacy of both prophylactic and therapeutic measures against various opportunistic infections. Primary brain lymphomas manifest with progressive focal or multifocal neurologic deficits similar to those seen in toxoplasmosis and PML, although the tempo of disease evolution is usually somewhere between the tempo of these two other diseases, with patients presenting after several days to a few weeks of progressive symptoms (see Table 14–4). These symptoms include changes in personality or behavior, hemiparesis, dysphasia, or other indications of hemispheral dysfunction. Headache is relatively common, but in the absence of systemic infection, fever and constitutional symptoms are also absent. Because of the deep location of the lymphoma in some patients, they may appear dull and apathetic, with gait disturbance but few lateralizing signs; in such cases the AIDS dementia complex may be a principal differential diagnosis.

Neuroradiologic studies are most important in the evaluation of AIDS patients with CNS lymphomas. Both MRI and CT usually can demonstrate symptomatic lesions, with MRI the more sensitive method. Characteristically, primary CNS lymphoma tumors are microscopically multicentric, but often only one or two lesions are disclosed on MRI or CT. Their location is characteristically deep in the brain, adjacent to the lateral ventricles, and often in the white matter rather than the gray matter. On CT they may enhance after contrast agent administration, but often the enhancement is weak, assuming a diffuse rather than ringlike pattern, or is absent. There is mass effect but there may be little surrounding edema. CSF cytology is unfortunately frequently negative or equivocal, and the definitive diagnosis therefore almost always relies on brain biopsy. Most often brain biopsy is undertaken when a trial of anti-*Toxoplasma* therapy fails to result in clinical improvement. However, the decision to proceed with biopsy can be accelerated when the lesions have the characteristic appearance and periventricular distribution of lymphoma and when blood toxoplasmosis serology is negative. Clinicians familiar with CNS lymphoma can often predict the correct diagnosis and accelerate the decision to proceed with biopsy. The use of stereotaxic biopsy techniques has increased the access to these tumors and reduced the morbidity of biopsy.

The current standard therapy for lymphoma in AIDS patients consists of whole brain irradiation and corticosteroids. When corticosteroids are used, the patient should also receive prophylaxis against *P carinii* pneumonia. At present there is no defined role for systemic chemotherapy. Because aggressive chemotherapy has become the treatment of choice for primary CNS lymphoma in non-AIDS patients,[158] it might be conjectured that the same will eventually prove true for these tumors in AIDS patients. However, primary CNS lymphomas characteristically occur late in the course of HIV-1 infection, when systemic disease is advanced and patients are more vulnerable to the toxic effects of cytoreductive drugs. Their bone marrow reserve is limited and their tolerance for chemotherapy is reduced by HIV-1 infection itself and often by the use of zidovudine. Chemotherapy might also preclude the continued chronic use of concurrent zidovudine. Moreover, these patients most often die of other HIV-1–related complications rather than of the lymphoma before sufficient time has passed for the recurrence that characterizes lymphoma in non-AIDS patients to develop.[151,154] Overall, primary CNS lymphomas in AIDS patients respond relatively well to radiation therapy, and many patients can remain "cured" for the remainder of their lives. For these reasons, the diagnosis should be pursued with vigor and treatment advocated. On the other hand, these patients are usually in a poor prognostic group with respect to systemic disease and their overall survival time is short. One can question whether corticosteroids or other therapeutic measures may even accelerate systemic disease in these patients, but this is difficult to judge.

Metastatic Lymphoma

Systemic lymphoma complicating HIV-1 infection may secondarily involve the CNS, with an incidence of CNS spread as high as 40%.[155,159] Unlike primary brain lymphomas, metastatic lymphomas most frequently involve the meninges or dura rather than the brain parenchyma and therefore manifest with cranial nerve palsies, headaches, spinal epidural cord compression, or increased intracranial pressure rather than with hemiparesis or other hemispheric signs. However, metastatic parenchymal brain disease or multifocal disease appearing simultaneously in both the brain and systemic organs may also occur, and in some cases the course may be fulminant. Otherwise the clinical and diagnostic features resemble those of non-AIDS-associated lymphomas. Because systemic lymphomas often occur early in HIV-

1 infection rather than late, as do the primary CNS lymphomas, some patients tolerate systemic and intrathecal chemotherapy along with whole brain irradiation. Aggressive chemotherapy may therefore be warranted in these patients, depending on the stage of HIV-1 infection and immunosuppression.

OTHER CNS DISORDERS

Cerebrovascular Complications

Some HIV-1–infected patients suffer transient neurologic deficits that are unrelated to an underlying opportunistic infection or neoplasm. In approximately half, no cause is found, although a vascular pathogenesis is suspected.[160,161] Preliminary clinical data suggest that such events are uncommon, although in one autopsy study as many as 20% of patients had evidence of small areas of infarction.[66,162] Despite the autopsy data, few patients with transient deficits appear to progress to a clinically significant stroke. The pathogenesis of these vascular disorders is completely unknown, but they may resemble the vascular complications noted in cancer patients and include nonbacterial thrombotic endocarditis. It is also possible that anticardiolipin antibodies, which have been demonstrated in HIV-1–infected patients,[163] may play a role. Another speculation is that changes may relate directly to HIV-1 infection of blood vessels.[164,165] Treatment is empirical and currently follows practices used in similarly affected, non-HIV-1–infected patients. Less common, but more severe, are agonal vascular events, including cerebral hemorrhage from thrombocytopenia and cerebral infarction from more aggressive nonbacterial thrombotic endocarditis and cerebral venous occlusion.

Metabolic and Nutritional Diseases

Patients with AIDS are subject to a constellation of metabolic brain disorders as a result of their complex systemic illnesses. These disorders include encephalopathies related to hypoxia and pulmonary disease, to sepsis and disseminated intravascular coagulation, and, less commonly, to renal failure. Likewise, toxic encephalopathies may relate to various medications with CNS side-effects. Such metabolic and toxic influences may exacerbate or unmask the AIDS dementia complex, leading to abrupt functional deterioration. Wernicke's disease and other nutritional disorders may occur in these patients and should be prevented or promptly treated with appropriate supplements. The diagnostic approach to and treatment of these disorders are similar in patients with and without AIDS.

Seizures

Seizures may occur in HIV-1 infection as a result of the various underlying opportunistic infections and neoplasms discussed above, and also perhaps in relation to the AIDS dementia complex or HIV-1 infection *per se.*[166,167] Seizures should lead to careful clinical and neuroimaging, preferably MRI, evaluation for focal disease. In the absence of a definable cause, these seizures should still probably be treated with chronic anticonvulsant therapy, even after a single seizure. Both phenytoin and carbamazepine are reasonable first-line drugs in these patients, although rashes are a common side-effect, particularly with phenytoin. Valproic acid is probably the next line of therapy for patients intolerant of phenytoin.

DISORDERS OF PERIPHERAL NERVOUS SYSTEM AND MUSCLE

Peripheral Neuropathies

Peripheral neuropathies are common and may complicate HIV-1 infection at each of its stages.[168–170] During the earliest stage, at or near the time of seroconversion, a variety of neuropathies have been described, although their incidence appears to be low. These have included brachial plexopathy, mononeuritides involving either peripheral or cranial nerves, and polyneuropathy.[9,13,14,16] Each appears to be self-limiting, with good general recovery. These likely have a postinfectious, autoimmune pathogenesis.

Apparently much more common is the development of demyelinating neuropathies during the asymptomatic or latent phase of HIV-1 infection.[171–173] These resemble Guillain-Barré syndrome, or more commonly, chronic inflammatory demyelinating polyneuropathy seen in other contexts, with the exception that the CSF often exhibits an uncharacteristic mild pleocytosis. Affected patients are usually otherwise well. It is probable that the pathophysiology of the neuropathy in HIV-1–infected patients parallels that of the disorder in other settings and has an autoimmune basis. Patients respond favorably to plasmapheresis or corticosteroids, and plasmapheresis is now recommended as the treatment of choice.[174] Intravenous immune globulin infusion may provide an alternative therapy.[175]

In the setting of ARC, and more commonly AIDS, several other neuropathies have been described. These include the infectious neuropathies caused by a varicella-zoster virus (*i.e.,* herpes zoster), and an ascending polyradiculopathy caused by CMV.[176–178] The latter deserves particular attention because it apparently can be arrested if recognized and treated promptly. The syndrome is clinically subacute and fulminating in onset and course, and involves painful ascending sensorimotor neuropathy with early bladder and bowel impairment. The CSF characteristically contains a high percentage of polymorphonuclear leukocytes, a finding that is otherwise rare in AIDS patients except in the setting of acute bacterial meningitis. Although CMV can be cultured from the CSF, this procedure often takes time, and ganciclovir should be started on the basis of clinical suspicion alone.[177] Often there is evidence of CMV infection elsewhere.

Cranial mononeuritides may also complicate the aseptic meningitis[179] that is presumably related to HIV-1 infection and metastatic lymphomatous meningitis, as described above. Mononeuritis multiplex has also been described in AIDS patients.[180,181] Recent studies suggest that mononeuritis multiplex in the setting of HIV-1 infection might be divided into two general forms.[181,182] The first is a more benign mononeuritis that occurs earlier in the disease course and possibly is related to a vasculitis. This condition is less aggressive and may be self-limiting; plasmapheresis may be helpful in affected patients. The second form is more aggressive, subacutely involving major nerves or roots and leading to progressive paralysis and death in some patients. There is some evidence that the later, aggressive form of mononeuritis multiplex may relate to CMV infection of peripheral nerves.[181] It may be worthwhile treating these patients with ganciclovir, but there is no clear evidence of ganciclovir's effects in this setting.

The most common neuropathy in AIDS patients is a distal, predominantly sensory axonal neuropathy.[168,172] It is usually a late complication of HIV-1 infection and occurs in the setting of AIDS. Characteristically, the sensory symptoms far exceed either sensory or motor dysfunction. The incidence is uncertain, but a mild form of the disease is likely common. A variant of this sensory axonal neuropathy is a less frequent but clinically important sensory polyneuropathy characterized by a severe "burning feet" sensation clinically reminiscent of severe alcoholic or diabetic neuropathy. Even in these patients sensory loss and motor weakness are usually relatively mild, but the painful paresthesias and burning sensation may preclude walking. The pathogenesis of this disorder is uncertain. It has been suggested that it may be related to direct HIV-1 infection of nerve or dorsal root ganglia, although this relationship has not been clearly demonstrated.[37,95] Treatment is symptomatic and entails tricyclic antidepressants or, if there is a ticklike component to the pain, carbamazepine or phenytoin. Narcotic analgesics may be helpful in some patients.

Several of the nucleoside antiretroviral agents, including ddI, dideoxycytosine (ddC), and d4T, have peripheral neurotoxicity as a major, dose-related side-effect.[183,184] The pathogenesis of the neurotoxicity is uncertain but may relate to an effect of these drugs on the mitochondrial DNA polymerase of dorsal root ganglia. Symptoms usually begin with pain in the feet that is described as aching, burning, or bruiselike. Such symptoms should provide warning to discontinue the drug. Although patients may continue to worsen for a few weeks—a phenomenon known as "coasting"—the condition is usually reversible if recognized early.

Autonomic neuropathy has also been reported in AIDS patients, often in conjunction with the more general sensory polyneuropathy.[184,185] The clinical features have ranged from postural hypotension to cardiovascular collapse in the setting of invasive procedures such as lung biopsy.

Myopathies

Myopathies of various types may also occur at several stages of HIV-1 infection, although they are less common and have not been so well characterized and classified as the neuropathies.[186,188] They may have a wide range of presentations, extending from asymptomatic creatine kinase (CK) elevation to progressive and severe proximal weakness. Some patients present with a typical polymyositis picture with proximal weakness and inflammatory changes on muscle biopsy. These patients may respond to corticosteroids or other immunomodulatory therapies. Less clear-cut are the myopathies without inflammatory changes. In some cases nemaline rods are found on biopsy. Simpson and Bender have reported that some affected patients may respond to corticosteroids.[186] Treatment with IV γ-globulin may provide an alternative avenue of therapy without further compromise of the immune system.

Confounding the diagnostic and therapeutic spectrum is the fact that zidovudine causes a toxic myopathy.[189-192] The myopathy occurs after prolonged exposure and may be less likely to occur with currently recommended doses, compared with the higher doses used earlier. It is thought to result from an effect of the drug on muscle mitochondrial DNA polymerase. Characteristically, the myopathy manifests as wasting of the buttock and thigh muscles associated with proximal leg weakness, although this may be mild. Serum CK levels are usually elevated. The diagnosis of zidovudine-related myopathy and its differentiation from the other myopathies occurring in HIV-1–infected patients may be difficult. Muscle biopsy may be helpful if it shows mitochondrial abnormalities, either ragged red fibers by light microscopy or abnormal mitochondrial morphology by electron microscopy. However, not all patients will exhibit these changes. If zidovudine is still thought to be responsible, it may be necessary to withdraw the drug and see if there is clinical and laboratory (CK) improvement.[191] The latter may take several weeks or even a few months to become evident. In the absence of clearer guidelines, we have generally evaluated these patients fully with muscle biopsy and, if a clear diagnosis cannot be established, switched patients to ddI or ddC (if not otherwise contraindicated) for at least 2 to 3 months.

GENERAL APPROACH TO DIAGNOSIS AND MANAGEMENT OF NERVOUS SYSTEM COMPLICATIONS

The approach to the diagnosis of CNS disease in patients with HIV-1 infection or AIDS follows that of neurologic diagnosis in general but takes into account the particular vulnerabilities of these patients. The steps involved are outlined in Table 14–5.

Table 14–5. Diagnosis of Neurologic Disease in HIV-1-Infected and AIDS Patients: Approach and Methods

DIAGNOSIS AND STAGING OF HIV-1 INFECTION
  Serostatus, virus identification (antigen, cultures, PCR)
  Systemic disease record, immune status, serum surrogate markers
NEUROLOGIC HISTORY
  Temporal profile of evolution
  Provisional anatomic localization
  Functional severity
NEUROLOGIC EXAMINATION
  Refined anatomic localization
NEUROIMAGING (MRI, CT; LESS COMMONLY MYELOGRAPHY, ANGIOGRAPHY)
  Refined anatomic localization
  Preliminary or presumptive etiologic diagnosis
CSF ANALYSIS
  Presence of host response (cells, protein, surrogate markers)
  Etiologic diagnosis (culture, cytology)
NEUROPSYCHOLOGICAL TESTING
  Quantitation and confirmation of deficit, staging the AIDS dementia complex
ELECTRODIAGNOSIS (EEG, EVOKED POTENTIALS, EMG, NERVE CONDUCTION)
  Physiologic diagnosis and localization
THERAPEUTIC TRIAL
  Focal brain lesions: targeted to toxoplasmosis
  Withdrawal of potential toxin (*e.g.,* zidovudine for myopathy)
TISSUE BIOPSY
  Diagnosis of focal brain lesions: lymphoma, PML
  Diagnosis of neuropathies, myopathies

It is, of course, critical to establish a diagnosis of systemic HIV-1 infection in order to confirm the arena of diagnosis. This becomes paramount in patients who first present with neurologic disease. In addition to serologic or virologic confirmation of HIV-1 infection, it also is important to establish the stage of HIV-1 infection in each patient, because the probabilities of the neurologic differential diagnosis vary with the changing immunologic and virologic status. The blood CD4+ T-lymphocyte count is probably the most useful laboratory index in this regard. Thus, in the early, "asymptomatic seropositive" phase of HIV-1 infection, when CD4+ cells are above 500/mm³, neurologic diseases related to autoimmunity (*e.g.,* demyelinating polyneuropathies) are more likely than those due to opportunistic infection. However, neurologic disorders are still relatively uncommon in these individuals, and the differential diagnosis must include diseases occurring in the general population or in the particular risk groups, such as endocarditis or intoxication in the case of drug abusers. However, in the late phase of HIV-1 infection, when severe immunosuppression ensues, AIDS-related complications are so common as to clearly predominate. Thus, the differential diagnosis shifts toward those conditions associated with AIDS. An additional consideration in the late phase of HIV-1 infection is that more than one neurologic disease may be present; usually they occur sequentially, and thus repeated evaluations may be needed as new symptoms or signs develop or old symptoms progress in the face of seemingly adequate therapy.

As in the non-AIDS patient, the approach to a specific neurologic diagnosis begins with a careful *neurologic history* to establish the background setting of the illness, its temporal profile, and an initial impression of its anatomic localization. The tempo of neurologic disease is a critical factor in the differential diagnosis, allowing acute events (vascular episodes or seizures) to be separated from those evolving more slowly, over days (toxoplasmosis) or weeks (AIDS dementia complex or PML). The *neurologic examination* serves to refine the anatomic localization and uncover additional asymptomatic abnormalities. The anatomic-physiologic diagnosis segregates diffuse brain disease with concomitant depressed alertness (*e.g.,* metabolic encephalopathies), diffuse brain disease with preserved alertness (*e.g.,* AIDS dementia complex), focal brain diseases (*e.g.,* cerebral toxoplasmosis, primary CNS lymphoma, PML), meningitides (*e.g.,* aseptic or cryptococcal meningitis), myelopathies, peripheral neuropathies, and myopathies (see Table 14–1).

Neuroimaging studies—MRI or CT, and much less commonly myelography or angiography—add further precision to anatomic localization and narrow the range of possible underlying pathologic processes. Thus, the AIDS dementia complex is typically marked by cerebral atrophy, at times accompanied by white matter abnormalities demonstrable with MRI, while the predominantly focal brain diseases show mass lesions (*e.g.,* toxoplasmosis or primary lymphoma) or demyelination (PML). Spinal MRI is usually negative in vacuolar myelopathy. *Electrodiagnosis* using EEG or evoked potentials may also be helpful in delineating and localizing physiologic dysfunction (*e.g.,* seizures, metabolic encephalopathies or myelopathies), and nerve conduction studies and electromyography can similarly refine the diagnosis of neuromuscular disorders, providing information regarding the anatomy (neuropathy *vs.* myopathy) or type (*e.g.,* demyelinating *vs.* axonal neuropathies) of disease.

Examination of the CSF provides a direct view of inflammatory reactions in the meninges and can precisely diagnose invading organisms (HIV-1, *Cryptococcus*) or neoplasms (lymphoma). Surrogate markers in the CSF may be helpful in confirming the presence of disease. In certain cases *tissue biopsy* may be needed. Brain biopsy may be necessary prior to therapy (*e.g.,* primary CNS lymphoma or tuberculosis) or may be done to establish the prognosis (PML). Nerve or muscle biopsy may be needed to further differentiate axonal from demyelinating neuropathy, or to distinguish polymyositis from zidovudine myopathy.

In some cases biopsy can be avoided with the use of a *therapeutic trial*. Thus, focal brain lesions with sur-

rounding edema and mass effect are usually managed with a trial of antitoxoplasmosis therapy and biopsy is performed only when such therapy fails, unless there is reason to consider *T. gondii* infection unlikely (negative serology, single or few lesions centered in the periventricular white matter). Similarly, toxic drug effects may be diagnosed from clinical improvement following their discontinuation.

In general, traditional *serologic studies* are of limited use, because most infections represent reactivated latent infection or are caused by ubiquitous organisms to which most HIV-1–infected patients have developed antibodies, whether or not they are suffering active CNS infection. Moreover, antibody titers do not reliably rise in association with active infection, and therefore a search for a fourfold increase is usually useless. However, the presence of antibodies can be used as an index of susceptibility, as in the case of *T. gondii* infection or CMV.

These clinical and laboratory evaluations, when pursued with a background understanding of the spectrum of neurologic disorders affecting HIV-1–infected patients, allows an exact neurologic diagnosis to be established in the majority of patients. As with other aspects of AIDS, this is an important and often fruitful exercise with gratifying relief of morbidity and prevention of death.

Acknowledgment: Our studies of the neurologic complications of AIDS were supported by Public Health Service grant NS-21703 from the National Institutes of Health.

REFERENCES

1. Price RW, Brew B: Management of the neurologic complications of HIV-1 infection and AIDS. In Sande MA, Volberding PA (eds): The Medical Management of AIDS. Philadelphia, WB Saunders, 1990
2. Price RW, Sidtis JJ, Rosenblum M: The AIDS dementia complex: Some current questions. Ann Neurol 23(suppl): 527, 1988
3. Wiley CA, Budka H: HIV-induced CNS lesions. Brain Pathol 1:153, 1991
4. Price RW, Sidtis JJ, Brew BJ: AIDS dementia complex and HIV-1 infection: A view from the clinic. Brain Pathol 1: 155, 1991
5. Price RW, Brew BJ, Sidtis J et al: The brain in AIDS: Central nervous system HIV-1 infection and AIDS dementia complex. Science 239:586, 1988
6. Budka H: Neuropathology of human immunodeficiency virus infection. Brain Pathol 1:163, 1991
7. Achim CL, Schrier RD, Wiley CA: Immunopathogenesis of HIV encephalitis. Brain Pathol 1:177, 1991
8. Tindall B, Cooper DA: Primary HIV infection: Host responses and intervention strategies. AIDS 5:1, 1991
9. Brew BJ, Perdices M, Darveniza P et al: The neurological features of early and 'latent' human immunodeficiency virus infection. Aust NZ J Med 19:700, 1989

10. Ho DD, Sarngadharan MG, Resnick L et al: Primary human T lymphotropic virus type III infection. Ann Intern Med 103:880, 1985

11. Denning DA, Anderson J, Rudge P et al: Acute myelopathy associated with primary infection with human immuno-deficiency virus. Br Med J 294:143, 1987

12. Piette AM, Tusseau F, Vignon D et al: Letter to the editor. Lancet 1:852, 1986

13. Wiselka MJ, Nicholson KG, Ward SC, Flower AJE: Acute infection with human immunodeficiency virus associated with facial nerve palsy and neuralgia. J Infect 15:189, 1987

14. Hagberg L, Malmvall BE, Svennerholm L et al: Guillain-Barré syndrome as an early manifestation of HIV central nervous system infection. Scand J Infect Dis 18:591, 1986

15. Carne CA, Smith A, Elkington SG et al: Acute encepha-lopathy coincident with seroconversion for anti HTLV-III. Lancet 2:1206, 1985

16. Calabrese LH, Proffitt MR, Levin KH et al: Acute infection with the human immunodeficiency virus (HIV) associated with acute brachial neuritis and exanthematous rash. Ann Intern Med 107:849, 1987

17. Resnick L, DiMarzo-Veronese F, Schupbach J et al: Intra-blood-brain barrier synthesis of HTLV-III specific IgG in patients with neurologic symptoms associated with AIDS or AIDS-related complex. N Engl J Med 313:1498, 1985

18. Goudsmit J, Wolters EC, Bakker M et al: Intrathecal syn-thesis of antibodies to HTLV-III in patients without AIDS or AIDS related complex. Br Med J 292:1231, 1986

19. Marshall DW, Brey RL, Cahill WT et al: Spectrum of ce-rebrospinal fluid findings in various stages of human im-munodeficiency virus infection. Arch Neurol 45:954, 1988

20. McArthur JC, Cohen BA, Farzadegan H et al: Cerebrospinal fluid abnormalities in homosexual men with and without neuropsychiatric findings. Ann Neurol 23(suppl):S34, 1988

21. Resnick L, Berger JR, Shapshak P, Tourtellotte WW: Early penetration of the blood-brain barrier by HIV. Neurology 38:9, 1988

22. Elovaara I, Iivanainen M, Sirkka-Liisa V et al: CSF protein and cellular profiles in various stages of HIV infection related to neurological manifestations. J Neurol Sci 78: 331, 1987

23. Ho DD, Rota TR, Schooley RT et al: Isolation of HTLV-III from cerebrospinal fluid and neural tissues of patients with neurologic syndromes related to the acquired im-munodeficiency syndrome. N Engl J Med 313:1493, 1984

24. Selnes OA, Miller E, McArthur J et al: No evidence of cognitive decline during the asymptomatic stages. Neu-rology 40:204, 1990

25. Miller EB, Selnes OA, McArthur JC et al: Neuropsycho-logical performance in HIV-1-infected homosexual men: The Multi center AIDS Cohort Study (MACS). Neurology 40:197, 1990

26. Sidtis JJ, Price RW: Early HIV infection and the AIDS de-mentia complex. Neurology 40:323, 1990

27. Berger JR, Sheremata WA, Resnick L et al: Multiple sclerosis-like leukoencephalopathy revealing human im-munodeficiency virus infection. Neurology 39:324, 1989

28. Gray F, Chimelli L, Mohr M et al: Fulminating multiple sclerosis-like leukoencephalopathy revealing human im-munodeficiency virus infection. Neurology 41:105, 1991

29. Levy JA, Shimabukuro J, Hollander H et al: Isolation of AIDS associated retroviruses from cerebrospinal fluid and brain of patients with neurological symptoms. Lancet 2: 586, 1985

30. Hollander H, Stringari S: Human immunodeficiency virus-associated meningitis: Clinical course and correlations. Am J Med 83:813, 1987

31. Goldstein J: Headache and acquired immunodeficiency syndrome. Neurol Clin 8:947, 1990

32. Brew BJ, Miller J: Human immunodeficiency virus related headache (abstr). Presented at the 7th International Con-ference on AIDS, Florence, Italy, 1991

33. Navia BA, Jordan BD, Price RW: The AIDS dementia com-plex: I. clinical features. Ann Neurol 19:517, 1986

34. Navia BA, Cho ES, Petito CK et al: The AIDS dementia complex: II. Neuropathology. Ann Neurol 19:525, 1986

35. Price RW, Brew BJ: The AIDS dementia complex. J Infect Dis 158:1079, 1988

36. Navia BA, Price RW: The acquired immunodeficiency syn-drome dementia complex as the presenting or sole man-ifestation of human immunodeficiency virus infection. Arch Neurol 44:65, 1987

37. Centers for Disease Control: Revision of the CDC sur-veillance case definition for acquired immunodeficiency syndrome. MMWR 36:1S, 1987

38. Cummings JL, Benson DF: Subcortical dementia: Review of an emerging concept. Arch Neurol 41:874, 1984

39. World Health Organization Consultation on the Neuro-psychiatric Aspects of HIV-1 Infection. Geneva, 11–13 January 1990. AIDS 4:935, 1990

40. Epstein LG, Sharer LR, Joshi V et al: Progressive enceph-alopathy in children with acquired immune deficiency syndrome. Ann Neurol 17:488, 1985

41. Belman AL, Ultmann MH, Horoupian D et al: Neurological complications in infants and children with acquired im-mune deficiency syndrome. Ann Neurol 18:560, 1985

42. Centers for Disease Control: Classification system for hu-man immunodeficiency virus (HIV) infection in children under 13 years of age. MMWR 36:225, 1987

43. Tross S, Price RW, Navia BA et al: Neuropsychological characterization of the AIDS dementia complex: A pre-liminary report. AIDS 2:81, 1988

44. Price RW, Sidtis JS: Evaluation of the AIDS dementia com-plex in clinical trials. J AIDS 3(suppl 2):S51, 1990

45. Post MJ, Tate LG, Quencer RM et al: CT, MR, and pathology in HIV encephalitis and meningitis. AJR 151:373, 1988

46. Jakobsen J, Gyldensted C, Brun B et al: Cerebral ventric-ular enlargement relates to neuropsychological measures in unselected AIDS patients. Acta Neurol Scand 79:59, 1989

47. Moeller AA, Backmund HC: Ventricle brain ratio in the clinical course of HIV infection. Acta Neurol Scand 81: 512, 1990

48. Jarvik JG, Hesselink JR, Kennedy C et al: Acquired im-munodeficiency syndrome: Magnetic resonance patterns of brain involvement with pathologic correlation. Arch Neurol 45:731, 1988

49. Belman AL, Lantos G, Horoupian D et al: Calcification of the basal ganglia in infants and children. Neurology 36: 1192, 1986

50. Rottenberg DA, Moeller JR, Strother SC et al: The meta-bolic pathology of the AIDS dementia complex. Ann Neu-rol 22:700, 1987

51. Kramer EL, Sanger JJ: Brain imaging in acquired immu-nodeficiency syndrome dementia complex. Semin Nucl Med 20:353, 1990

52. Pohl P, Vogl G, Fill H: Single photon emission computed tomography in AIDS dementia complex. J Nucl Med 29: 1382, 1988

53. Brunetti A, Berg G, DiChiro G et al: Reversal of brain metabolic abnormalities following treatment of AIDS dementia complex with 3'-azido-2',3'-dideoxythymidine (AZT, zidovudine): A PET-FDG study. J Nucl Med 30:581, 1989

54. Paul MO, Brew BJ, Khan A et al: Detection of HIV-1 in cerebrospinal fluid (CSF): Correlation with presence and severity of the AIDS dementia complex (abstr 238). Presented at the International Conference on AIDS, 1989

55. Brew BH, Bhalla RB, Fleisher M et al: Cerebrospinal fluid β_2 microglobulin in patients infected with human immunodeficiency virus. Neurology 39:830, 1989

56. Brew BJ, Bhalla RB, Paul M et al: Cerebrospinal fluid neopterin in human immunodeficiency virus type 1 infection. Ann Neurol 28:556, 1990

57. Griffin DE, McArthur JC, Cornblath DR: Neopterin and interferon-gamma in serum and cerebrospinal fluid of patients with HIV-associated neurologic disease. Neurology 41:69, 1991

58. Fuchs D, Chiodi F, Albert J et al: Neopterin concentrations in cerebrospinal fluid and serum of individuals infected with HIV-1. AIDS 3:285, 1989

59. Sonnerborg AB, von Stedingk L-V, Hansson L-O, Strannegard OO: Elevated neopterin and beta$_2$-microglobulin levels in blood and cerebrospinal fluid occur early in HIV-1 infection. AIDS 3:277, 1989

60. Heyes MP, Brew BJ, Martin A: Quinolinic acid in cerebrospinal fluid and serum in HIV-1 infection: Relationship to clinical and neurological status. Ann Neurol 29:202, 1991

61. Price RW, Brew BJ, Rosenblum M: The AIDS dementia complex and HIV-1 infection: A pathogenetic model of virus-immune interaction. In Waksman BH (ed): Immunologic Mechanisms in Neurologic and Psychiatric Disease, p. 269. New York, Raven Press, 1989

62. Merrill JE, Chen ISY: HIV-1, macrophages, glial cells, and cytokines in AIDS nervous system disease. FASEB J 5: 2391, 1991

63. Portegies P, de Gans J, Lange JM et al: Declining incidence of AIDS dementia complex after introduction of zidovudine treatment. Br Med J 299:819, 1989

64. Rosenblum MK: Infection of the central nervous system by the human immunodeficiency virus type 1: Morphology and relation to syndromes of progressive encephalopathy and myelopathy in patients with AIDS. Pathol Annu 25(Pt 1):117, 1990

65. Petito CK, Navia BA, Cho E-S: Vacuolar myelopathy pathologically resembling subacute combined degeneration in patients with acquired immunodeficiency syndrome (AIDS). N Engl J Med 312:874, 1985

66. Petito CK, Cho E-S, Lemann W et al: Neuropathology of acquired immunodeficiency syndrome (AIDS): An autopsy review. J Neuropathol Exp Neurol 45:635, 1986

67. Budka H, Wiley CA, Kleihues P et al: HIV-associated disease of the nervous system: Review of nomenclature and proposal for neuropathology-based terminology. Brain Pathol 1:143, 1991

68. Shaw GM, Harper ME, Hahn BH et al: HTLV-III infection in brains of children and adults with AIDS encephalopathy. Science 227:177, 1985

69. Koenig S, Gendelman HE, Orenstein JM et al: Detection of AIDS virus in macrophages in brain tissue from AIDS patients with encephalopathy. Science 233:1089, 1986

70. Stoler MH, Eskin TA, Benn S et al: Human T cell lymphotropic virus type III infection of the central nervous system: A preliminary in situ analysis. JAMA 256:2360, 1986

71. Gartner S, Markovits P, Markovits DM et al: Virus isolation from an identification of HTLV-III/LAV producing cells in brain tissue from a patient with AIDS. JAMA 256:2365, 1986

72. Li Y, Kappes JC, Conway JA, Price RW et al: Molecular characterization of human immunodeficiency virus type 1 cloned directly from uncultured human brain tissue: Identification of replication-competent and -defective viral genomes. J Virol 65:3973, 1991

73. Wiley CA, Schrier RD, Nelson JA et al: Cellular localization of human immunodeficiency virus infection within the brains of acquired immune deficiency syndrome patients. Proc Natl Acad Sci USA 83:7089, 1986

74. Gabuzda DH, Ho DD, De La Monte SM et al: Immunohistochemical identification of HTLV-III antigen in brains of patients with AIDS. Ann Neurol 20:289, 1986

75. Vazeux R, Brousse N, Jarry A et al: AIDS subacute encephalitis: Identification of HIV-infected cells. Am J Pathol 126:403, 1987

76. Pumarola-Sune T, Navia BA, Cordon-Cardo C et al: HIV antigen in the brains of patients with the AIDS dementia complex. Ann Neurol 21:490, 1987

77. Michaels J, Price RW, Rosenblum MK: Microglia in the human immunodeficiency virus encephalitis of acquired immune deficiency syndrome: Proliferation, infection and fusion. Acta Neuropathol 76:373, 1988

78. Epstein LG, Sharer LR, Cho ES et al: HTLV-III/LAV-like retrovirus particles in the brains of patients with AIDS encephalopathy. AIDS Res 1:447, 1985

79. Gyorkey F, Melnick JL, Gyorkey P: Human immunodeficiency virus in brain biopsies of patients with AIDS and progressive encephalopathy. J Infect Dis 155:870, 1987

80. Peudenier S, Hery C, Montagnier L, Tardieu M: Human microglial cells: Characterization in cerebral tissue and in primary culture, and study of their susceptibility to HIV-1 infection. Ann Neurol 29:152, 1991

81. Watkins B, Dorn HH, Kelly WB et al: Specific tropism of HIV-1 for microglial cells in primary human brain cultures. Science 249:549, 1990

82. Cheng-Mayer C, Rutka JT, Rosenblum ML et al: Human immunodeficiency virus can productively infect cultured human glial cells. Proc Natl Acad Sci USA 84:3526, 1987

83. Shapshak P, Sun NC, Resnick L et al: HIV-1 propagates in human neuroblastoma cells. J AIDS 4:228, 1991

84. Cheng-Mayer C, Weiss C, Seto D, Levy JA: Isolates of human immunodeficiency virus type 1 from the brain may constitute a special group of the AIDS virus. Proc Natl Acad Sci USA 86:8575, 1989

85. Keys B, Albert J, Kovamess J, Chiodi F: Brain-derived cells can be infected with HIV isolates derived from both blood and brain. Virology 183:834, 1991

86. Koyanagi Y, Miles S, Mitsuyasu RT et al: Dual infection of the central nervous system by AIDS viruses with distinct cellular tropisms. Science 236:819, 1987

87. O'Brien WA, Koyanagi Y, Namazie A: HIV-1 tropism for mononuclear phagocytes can be determined by regions of gp 120 outside the CD4-binding domain. Nature 348: 69, 1990

88. Shioda T, Levy JA, Cheng-Mayer C: Macrophage and T cell-line tropisms of HIV-1 are determined by specific regions of the envelope gp120 gene. Nature 349:167, 1991

89. Hwang SS, Boyle TJ, Lyerly HK, Cullen BR: Identification

of the envelope V3 Loop as the primary determinant of cell tropism in HIV-1. Science 253:71, 1991

90. Dreyer EV, Kaiser PK, Offermann JT, Lipton SA: HIV-1 coat protein neurotoxicity prevented by calcium channel antagonists. Science 248:364, 1990

91. Giulian D, Vaca K, Noonan CA: Secretion of neurotoxins by mononuclear phagocytes infected with HIV. Science 250:1593, 1990

92. Pulliam L, Herndier BG, Tang HM, McGrath MS: Human immunodeficiency virus-infected macrophages produce soluble factors that cause histological and neurochemical alterations in cultured human brains. J Clin Invest 87:503, 1991

93. Yarchoan R, Berg G, Brouwers P et al: Response of human immunodeficiency virus associated neurological disease to 3'-azido-3'-deoxythymidine. Lancet 1:132, 1987

94. Schmitt FA, Bigley JW, McKinnis R et al: Neuropsychological outcome of zidovudine (AZT) treatment of patients with AIDS and AIDS-related complex. N Engl J Med 319:1573, 1988

95. Sidtis JJ, Gatsonis C, Price RW et al: Zidovudine treatment of the AIDS dementia complex: Results of a placebo-controlled trial. (Unpublished manuscript)

96. Pizzo PA, Eddy J, Falloon J et al: Effect of continuous intravenous infusion of zidovudine (AZT) in children with symptomatic HIV infection. N Engl J Med 319:889, 1988

97. Brouwers P, Moss H, Wolters P et al: Effect of continuous-infusion zidovudine therapy on neuropsychologic functioning in children with symptomatic human immunodeficiency virus infection. J Pediatr 116:908, 1990

98. Yarchoan R, Mitsuya H, Thomas RV et al: In vivo activity against HIV and favorable toxicity profile of 2',3'-dideoxyinosine. Science 245:412, 1989

99. Snider WD, Simpson DM, Nielsen S et al: Neurological complications of acquired immune deficiency syndrome: Analysis of 50 patients. Ann Neurol 14:403, 1983

100. McArthur JC: Neurologic manifestations of AIDS. Medicine 66:407, 1987

101. Navia BA, Petito CK, Gold JWM et al: Cerebral toxoplasmosis complicating the acquired immune deficiency syndrome: Clinical and neuropathological findings in 27 patients. Ann Neurol 19:224, 1986

102. Haverkos H: Assessment of therapy for *Toxoplasma* encephalitis. Am J Med 82:907, 1987

103. Isrealski DM, Dannemann BR, Remington JS: Toxoplasmosis in patients with AIDS. In Sande MA, Volberding PA (eds): The Medical Management of AIDS. Philadelphia, WB Saunders, 1990

104. Leport C, Raffi F, Matheron S et al: Treatment of central nervous system toxoplasmosis with pyrimethamine/sulfadiazine combination in 35 patients with the acquired immunodeficiency syndrome: Efficacy of long-term continuous therapy. Am J Med 84:94, 1988

105. Cohn JA, McMeeking A, Cohen W et al: Evaluation of the policy of empiric treatment of suspected *Toxoplasma* encephalitis in patients with the acquired immunodeficiency syndrome. Am J Med 86:521, 1989

106. Gray F, Gherardi R, Wingate E et al: Diffuse "encephalitic" cerebral toxoplasmosis in AIDS: Report of four cases. J Neurol 236:273, 1989

107. Grant IH, Gold JWM, Rosenblum M et al: *Toxoplasma gondii* serology in HIV-infected patients: The development of central nervous system toxoplasmosis in AIDS. AIDS 4:519, 1990

108. Jarvik JG, Hasselink JR, Kennedy C et al: Acquired immunodeficiency syndrome: Magnetic resonance patterns of brain involvement with pathologic correlation. Arch Neurol 45:731, 1988

109. Dannemann BR, Israelski DM, Remington JS: Treatment of toxoplasmic encephalitis with intravenous clindamycin. Arch Intern Med 148:2477, 1988

110. Rolston KVI, Hoy J: Role of clindamycin in the treatment of central nervous system toxoplasmosis. Am J Med 83:551, 1987

111. Panther LA, Sande MA: Cryptococcal meningitis in AIDS. In Sande MA, Volberding PA (eds): The Medical Management of AIDS. Philadelphia, WB Saunders, 1990

112. Kovacs JA, Kovacs AA, Polis M et al: Cryptococcosis in the acquired immunodeficiency syndrome. Ann Intern Med 103:533, 1985

113. Zuger A, Louie E, Holzman RS et al: Cryptococcal disease in patients with the acquired immunodeficiency syndrome. Ann Intern Med 104:234, 1986

114. Chuck SL, Sande MA: Infections with *Cryptococcus neoformans* in the acquired immunodeficiency syndrome. N Engl J Med 321:794, 1989

115. Dismukes WE: Cryptococcal meningitis in patients with AIDS. J Infect Dis 157:624, 1988

116. Stern JJ, Hartman BJ, Sharkey P et al: Oral fluconazole therapy for patients with acquired immunodeficiency syndrome and cryptococcosis: Experience with 22 patients. Am J Med 85:477, 1988

117. Larsen RA, Leal MAE, Chan LS: Fluconazole compared with amphotericin B plus flucytosine for cryptococcal meningitis in AIDS: A randomized trial. Ann Intern Med 85:481, 1988

118. Sugar AM, Saunders C: Oral fluconazole as suppressive therapy of disseminated cryptococcosis in patients with the acquired immunodeficiency syndrome. Am J Med 85:481, 1988

119. Richardson EP: Progressive multifocal leukoencephalopathy. In Vinken PJ, Bruyn GW (eds): Handbook of Clinical Neurology, vol 34, p 307. Amsterdam, Elsevier, 1978

120. Padgett BL, Walker DL, Zu Rhein GM et al: JC papovavirus in progressive multifocal leukoencephalopathy. J Infect Dis 133:686, 1976

121. Houff SA, Major EO, Katz DA et al: Involvement of JC virus–infected mononuclear cells from the bone marrow and spleen in the pathogenesis of progressive multifocal leukoencephalopathy. N Engl J Med 318:301, 1988

122. Schmidbauer M, Budka H, Shah KV: Progressive multifocal leukoencephalopathy (PML) in AIDS and in the pre-AIDS era. Acta Neuropathol 80:375, 1990

123. Berger JR, Kaszovitz B, Donovan Post MJ, Dickinson G: Progressive multifocal leukoencephalopathy in association with human deficiency virus infection: A review of the literature with a report of sixteen cases. Ann Intern Med 107:78, 1987

124. Krupp LB, Lipton RB, Swerdlow ML et al: Progressive multifocal leukoencephalopathy: Clinical and radiographic features. Ann Neurol 17:344, 1985

125. Mark AS, Atlas SW: Progressive multifocal leukoencephalopathy in patients with AIDS: Appearance on MR images. Radiology 173:517, 1989

126. Conway B, Halliday WC, Brunham RC: Human immunodeficiency virus–associated progressive multifocal leukoencephalopathy: Apparent response to 3'-azido-3'-deoxythymidine. Rev Infect Dis 12:479, 1990

127. Portegies P, Algra PR, Hollak CEM et al: Response to cytarabine in progressive multifocal leukoencephalopathy in AIDS. Lancet 1:680, 1991

128. Berger JR, Mucke L: Prolonged survival and partial recovery in AIDS-associated progressive multifocal leukoencephalopathy. Neurology 38:1060, 1988

129. Morgello S, Cho ES, Nielsen S et al: Cytomegalovirus encephalitis in patients with acquired immunodeficiency syndrome. Hum Pathol 18:289, 1987

130. Vinters HV, Kwok MK, Ho HW et al: Cytomegalovirus in the nervous system of patients with the acquired immune deficiency syndrome. Brain 112:245, 1989

131. Mills J, Jacobson MA, O'Donnell JJ et al: Treatment of cytomegalovirus retinitis in patients with AIDS. Rev Infect Dis 10(suppl 3):S522, 1988

132. Sunderam G, McDonald RJ, Maniatis T et al: Tuberculosis as a manifestation of the acquired immunodeficiency syndrome (AIDS). JAMA 256:362, 1986

133. Guarner J, Del Rio C, Slade B: Tuberculosis as a manifestation of the acquired immunodeficiency syndrome. JAMA 256:3092, 1986

134. Bishburg E, Sunderam G, Reichman LB, Kapila R: Central nervous system tuberculosis with the acquired immunodeficiency syndrome and its related complex. Ann Intern Med 105:210, 1986

135. Horten B, Price RW, Jimenez D: Multifocal varicella-zoster virus leukoencephalitis temporally remote from herpes zoster. Ann Neurol 9:251, 1981

136. Ryder JW, Croen K, Kleinschmidt-De-Masters BK et al: Progressive encephalitis three months after resolution of cutaneous zoster in a patient with AIDS. Ann Neurol 19:182, 1986

137. Morgello S, Block GA, Price RW et al: Varicella-zoster virus leukoencephalitis and cerebral vasculopathy. Arch Pathol Lab Med 112:173, 1988

138. Hilt DC, Bucholz D, Krumholz A et al: Herpes zoster ophthalmicus and delayed contralateral hemiparesis caused by cerebral angiitis: Diagnosis and management approaches. Ann Neurol 14:543, 1983

139. Eidelberg D, Sotrel A, Horoupian DS et al: Thrombotic cerebral vasculopathy associated with herpes zoster. Ann Neurol 19:7, 1986

140. Devinsky O, Cho ES, Petito CK, Price RW: Herpes zoster myelitis. Brian 114:1181, 1991

141. Levy RL, Bredesen DE, Rosenblum ML: Neurological manifestations of the acquired immunodeficiency syndrome (AIDS): Experience at UCSF and review of the literature. J Neurosurg 62:475, 1985

142. Rhodes RH: Histopathology of the central nervous system in the acquired immunodeficiency syndrome. Hum Pathol 18:636, 1987

143. Berger JR: Neurosyphilis in human immunodeficiency virus type 1–seropositive individuals. Arch Neurol 48:700, 1991

144. Johns DR, Tierney M, Felsenstein D: Alteration in the natural history of neurosyphilis by concurrent infection with the human immunodeficiency virus. N Engl J Med 316:1569, 1987

145. Berry CD, Hooton TM, Collier AC, Lukehart SA: Neurologic relapse after benzathine penicillin therapy for secondary syphilis in a patient with HIV infection. N Engl J Med 316:1587, 1987

146. Katz DA, Berger JA: Neurosyphilis in acquired immunodeficiency syndrome. Arch Neurol 46:895, 1989

147. Simon RP: Neurosyphilis. Arch Neurol 42:606, 1985

148. Davis LE: Neurosyphilis in the patient infected with human immunodeficiency virus. Ann Neurol 27:211, 1990

149. Lukehart SA, Hook EW, Baker-Zander SA: Invasion of the central nervous system by *Treponema pallidum:* Implications for the diagnosis and treatment. Ann Intern Med 109:855, 1988

149a. Musher DM, Hamill RJ, Baughn RE: Effect of human immunodeficiency virus (HIV) infection on the course of syphilis and on the response to treatment. Ann Intern Med 113:872, 1990

150. Lanska M, Lanska DJ, Schmidley JW: Syphilitic polyradiculopathy in an HIV-positive man. Neurology 38:1297, 1988

151. So YT, Beckstead JH, Davis RL: Primary central nervous system lymphoma in acquired immune deficiency syndrome: A clinical and pathological study. Ann Neurol 20:566, 1986

152. Levine AM: Non-Hodgkin's lymphomas and other malignancies in the acquired immune deficiency syndrome. Semin Oncol [Suppl] 14:34, 1987

153. Meeker TC, Shiramizu B, Kaplan L: Evidence for molecular subtypes of HIV-associated lymphoma: Division into peripheral monoclonal, polyclonal and central nervous system lymphoma. AIDS 5:669, 1991

154. Baumgartner JE, Rachlin JR, Beckstead JH et al: Primary central nervous system lymphomas: Natural history and response to radiation therapy in 55 patients with acquired immunodeficiency syndrome (AIDS). J Neurosurg 73:206, 1990

155. Formenti SC, Gill PS, Lean E et al: Primary central nervous system lymphoma in AIDS: Results of radiation therapy. Cancer 63:1101, 1989

156. Remick SC, Diamond C, Migliozzi JA et al: Primary central nervous system lymphoma in patients with and without the acquired immune deficiency syndrome: A retrospective analysis and review of the literature. Medicine 69:345, 1990

157. DeAngelis LM: Primary CNS lymphoma: A new clinical challenge. Neurology 41:619, 1991

158. DeAngelis LM, Yaholom J, Heineman MH: Primary CNS lymphoma: Combined treatment with chemotherapy and radiotherapy. Neurology 40:80, 1990

159. Zeigler JL, Beckstead JA, Volberding PA et al: Non-Hodgkin's lymphoma in 90 homosexual men: Relation to generalized lymphadenopathy and the acquired immunodeficiency syndrome. N Engl J Med 311:565, 1984

160. Engstrom JW, Lowenstein DH, Bredesen DE: Cerebral infarctions and transient neurologic deficits associated with acquired immunodeficiency syndrome. Am J Med 86:528, 1989

161. Mizusawa H, Hirano J, Llena JR, Shintaku M: Cerebral lesions in acquired immune deficiency syndrome (AIDS). Acta Neuropathol 76:451, 1988

162. Maclean C, Flegg PJ, Kilpatrick DC: Anti-cardiolipin antibodies and HIV infection. Clin Exp Immunol 81:263, 1990

163. Yankner BA, Skolnik PR, Shoukimas GM et al: Cerebral granulomatous angiitis associated with isolation of human T lymphotropic virus type III from the central nervous system. Ann Neurol 20:362, 1986

164. Cho ES, Sharer LR, Peress NS et al: Intimal proliferation of leptomeningeal arteries and brain infarcts in subjects with AIDS. J Neuropathol Exp Neurol 46:385, 1987

165. Wong MC, Suite NA, Labar DR: Seizures in human immunodeficiency virus infection. Arch Neurol 47:640, 1990

166. Holtzman DM, Kaku DA, So YT: New onset seizures associated with human immunodeficiency virus infection: Causation and clinical features in 100 cases. Am J Med 87:173, 1989

167. So YT, Holtzman DM, Abrams DI, Olnery RK: Peripheral neuropathy associated with acquired immunodeficiency syndrome: Prevalence and clinical features from a population based survey. Arch Neurol 45:945, 1988

168. Miller RG, Parry G, Pfaeffl W et al: The spectrum of peripheral neuropathy associated with ARC and AIDS. Muscle Nerve 11:857, 1988

169. Leger JM, Bouche P, Bolger F, Chaunu MP et al: The spectrum of polyneuropathies in patients infected with HIV. J Neurol Neurosurg Psychiatry 52:1369, 1989

170. Cornblath DR, McArthur JC, Kennedy PGE et al: Inflammatory demyelinating peripheral neuropathies associated with human T-cell lymphotropic virus type III infection. Ann Neurol 21:32, 1986

171. Cornblath DR, McArthur JC: Predominantly sensory neuropathy in patients with AIDS and AIDS-related complex. Neurology 38:794, 1988

172. Lipkin WI, Parry G, Kiprov D et al: Inflammatory neuropathy in homosexual men with lymphadenopathy. Neurology 35:1479, 1985

173. Cornblath D: Treatment of the neuromuscular complications of human immunodeficiency virus infection. Ann Neurol 23(suppl):S88, 1988

174. Cornblath DR, Chaudhry V, Griffin JW: Treatment of chronic inflammatory demyelinating polyneuropathy with intravenous immunoglobulin. Ann Neurol 30:104, 1991

175. Eidelberg D, Sotrel A, Vogel H et al: Progressive polyradiculopathy in acquired immune deficiency syndrome. Neurology 36:912, 1986

176. Miller RG, Storey JR, Greco CM: Ganciclovir in the treatment of progressive AIDS-related polyradiculopathy. Neurology 40:569, 1990

177. Fuller GN, Gill SK, Guilloff RJ et al: Ganciclovir treatment of lumbosacral polyradiculopathy in AIDS. Lancet 335:48, 1990

178. Bredesen DE, Lipkin WI, Messing R: Prolonged, recurrent aseptic meningitis with prominent cranial nerve abnormalities: A new epidemic in gay men? (abstr). Neurology 33:85, 1984

179. Miller RG, Parry G, Lang W et al: AIDS-related inflammatory polyradiculoneuropathy: Successful treatment with plasma exchange (abstr). Neurology 36(suppl):206, 1986

180. Said G, Lacroix C, Chemouilli P et al: CMV neuropathy in AIDS: A clinical and pathological study. Ann Neurol 29:139, 1991

181. So YT, Olney RK: The natural history of mononeuropathy multiplex and simplex in patients with HIV infection (abstr). Neurology 41(suppl):374, 1991

182. Dubinsky RM, Yarchoan R, Dalakas M, Broder S: Reversible axonal neuropathy from the treatment of AIDS and related disorders with 2′,3′-dideoxyinosine (ddI). Muscle Nerve 12:856, 1989

183. Lambert JS, Seidlin M, Reichman RC: 2′,3′-dideoxyinosine (ddI) in patients with the acquired immunodeficiency syndrome or AIDS-related complex. N Engl J Med 322:1333, 1990

184. Lin-Greenberg A, Taneja-Uppal N: Dysautonomia and infection with the human immunodeficiency virus. Ann Intern Med 106:167, 1987

185. Craddock C, Pasvol G, Bull R et al: Cardiorespiratory arrest and autonomic neuropathy in AIDS. Lancet 2:16, 1987

186. Simpson CM, Bender AN: Human immunodeficiency virus-associated myopathy: Analysis of 11 patients. Ann Neurol 24:79, 1988

187. Bailey RO, Turok DI, Jaufmann BP et al: Myositis and acquired immunodeficiency syndrome. Hum Pathol 18:749, 1987

188. Illa I, Nath A, Dalakas M: Immunocytochemical and virological characteristics of HIV-associated inflammatory myopathies: Similarities with seronegative polymyositis. Ann Neurol 29:474, 1991

189. Mhiri C, Baudrimont M, Bonne G et al: Zidovudine myopathy: A distinctive disorder associated with mitochondrial dysfunction. Ann Neurol 29:606, 1991

190. Chalmers AC, Greco CM, Miller RG: Prognosis in AZT myopathy. Neurology 41:1181, 1991

191. Dalakas MC, Illa I, Pezeshkpour GH et al: Mitochondrial myopathy caused by long term zidovudine therapy. N Engl J Med 322:1098, 1990

192. Arnaudo E, Dalakas M, Shanske S et al: Depletion of muscle mitochondrial DNA in AIDS patients with zidovudine-induced myopathy. Lancet 1:508, 1991

15

Gastrointestinal Manifestations of HIV Infection and AIDS

Donald P. Kotler

Gastrointestinal (GI) symptoms are exceedingly common in patients with acquired immunodeficiency syndrome (AIDS) as they are in other immune deficiency states.[1-3] The GI tract, like other mucous membranes, is inherently vulnerable to pathogens, owing to the lack of a strong physical barrier. It is in intimate contact with the external (luminal) environment in order to perform its essential function of solute absorption. An elaborate defense has evolved to protect the GI tract, including a multicompartmental immune system. The immune defenses of the various mucous membranes are linked as a common mucosal immune system.[4]

Gastrointestinal involvement in human immunodeficiency virus (HIV) infection and AIDS may be significant on several levels. Epidemiologic studies imply that HIV infection is efficiently transmitted via rectal mucosa.[5] Bidirectional transmission is likely. Evidence from several laboratories indicates that cellular reservoirs for HIV exist in the intestines. Alterations in bowel habits, associated with "nonspecific" inflammation, are common in HIV-infected people without AIDS and are related to the expression of HIV protein antigens in tissue.[6] In addition, opportunistic GI infections producing malabsorption or progressive wasting cause considerable morbidity and contribute to debilitation and a terminal course.

This chapter discusses the effects of HIV infection and AIDS on the GI tract. The topic of mucosal immunity is reviewed and the results of studies localizing HIV to the intestine are discussed. Specific infectious and neoplastic complications are covered. The diagnosis and management of these complications, which have variable and overlapping clinical expressions, are grouped by the clinical syndromes that develop.

MUCOSAL IMMUNITY AND IMMUNE DEFICIENCY

Normal Mucosal Immunity

The systemic and mucosal immune systems function largely independently, although they share a common embryologic heritage. The mucosal immune system is composed of lymphoid aggregates in the tonsils, Peyer's patches, and mucosal lymphoid follicles, and diffuse collections of cells in the lamina propria.[7] The epithelium overlying mucosal lymphoid follicles and Peyer's patches contains specialized cells (M cells) that allow penetration of particulate antigens.[8]

Lymphoid follicles are the sites of luminal antigen uptake and presentation. Sensitized B- and T-cell precursors then migrate to mesenteric lymph nodes and distant sites, where they proliferate and differentiate. Both B cells and helper T cells return to the intestine, while suppressor T cells home to the spleen.[9] Several elegant studies have demonstrated the distinctive trafficking patterns of gut-associated lymphocytes.[10]

The intestinal mucosa contains a diversity of immunologically active cells. The proportion of mucosal helper T lymphocytes to suppressor T lymphocytes is approximately the same in mucosa and peripheral blood.[11] B lymphocytes comprise about 10% of the mononuclear cells in the lamina propria. Plasma cells also are an important constituent of the cell population. Macrophages are the major form of phagocytic cell in the lamina propria, though eosinophils as well as mast cells may be found in mucosal biopsy specimens from healthy individuals.[12] Extravascular neutrophils are not a normal inhabitant of the lamina propria.

Mononuclear cells also course through the epithelium. The phenotypic composition of the intraepithelial mononuclear cell population is different from the lamina propria. The major cell type found is the CD8+ T cell, and the normal helper to suppressor ratio is about 0.05.[13] Intraepithelial macrophages are another important cell type. Occasional mast cells or eosinophils may be seen in normal epithelium. On the other hand, the presence of neutrophils in the epithelium is indicative of a pathologic process.

The mucosa contains elements of both humoral (secretory) and cell-mediated immunity. The antibody system in the intestine produces mainly secretory IgA, though substantial quantities of B cells containing IgM are normally present.[14] Secretory IgA binds and excludes foreign luminal antigens from the body. Most of the IgA exists in dimeric form linked by a peptide (J piece). IgA is actively secreted from the epithelial cell after binding to a glycoprotein of epithelial cell origin (secretory component), which protects the antibody from degradation in the lumen. Hepatic bile also contains secretory IgA. Cell-mediated immune reactions in the GI tract are similar to reactions in other body compartments.

Mucosal immunity is highly coordinated. Despite its proximity to many potential pathogens, the mucosa is uninflamed. The system of immune suppression and immune activation (contrasuppression) is finely regulated and limits the intensity, extent, and duration of an immune reaction, thus protecting the integrity of the mucous membrane.[15]

Mucosal immune function also is integrated with systemic immunity in several ways. The most striking is the active suppression of systemic immune responses to previously encountered luminal antigens (tolerance).[16] Potential adverse responses to the inadvertent systemic introduction of foreign antigens, such as food antigens, are limited by tolerance.

Other, nonimmunologic factors promote the defense of the GI tract.[17] Gastric acid is antiseptic, while salivary, pancreatic, and biliary secretions contain specific anti-infective factors. Secreted mucus is a lubricant; a diffusion barrier for particulate materials but not soluble materials such as water, electrolytes, or nutrients; and a structure to which IgA, lysozyme, and other proteins attach.[18] Intestinal motility is an important factor in maintaining low intraluminal bacterial counts in the upper intestine; a stable colonic flora also contributes to homeostasis.[19] Bacteria serve physiologic functions, such as fermentation of unabsorbed carbohydrates and salvage of metabolizable carbons, as well as a defensive function, by suppressing the proliferation of potential pathogens. This property is illustrated by *Clostridium difficile,* a bacterium present in the intestines of many healthy people that causes colitis only when antibiotics are given.[20]

Mucosal Immunity in AIDS

Mucosal immunity in HIV-infected patients has received little study, and the available data are spotty. Clinical and experimental observations suggest that homologous defects are present in the mucosal and systemic immune systems. Studies of mucosal biopsy specimens conducted using immunohistochemical techniques have demonstrated equivalent decreases in the helper T-cell population in blood and intestinal mucosa.[21–23] In one study, peripheral blood helper cell numbers were decreased in *healthy* homosexual men while the number of mucosal helper cells was normal.[21] In the same study, the number of cells bearing surface antigens of a cytotoxic cell phenotype were normal in the mucosa. In another study, flow cytometric analysis of isolated mucosal lymphocytes disclosed increased expression of the killer cell markers Leu-7 and Leu-11a (CD16).[24] Although the functional activity of the killer cells was not assessed, deficient killer cell activity in peripheral blood lymphocytes has been demonstrated repeatedly.[25]

Electron microscopic studies have demonstrated evidence of activation of intraepithelial lymphocytes in AIDS patients.[26] Flow cytometric studies showed increased cell membrane expression of DR antigen in lamina propria and intraepithelial mononuclear cells from rectal mucosa, implying cell activation.[24] However, a decrease in the number of activated T cells was found to be associated with villous atrophy in duodenal biopsy specimens.[27]

Immunohistologic studies have demonstrated a depletion of plasma cells containing IgA in mucosal biopsy specimens from AIDS patients as well as a decrease in salivary IgA secretion.[28] IgM-containing plasma cell numbers were increased in several patients, implying a defect in T-lymphocyte–directed gene rearrangement in plasma cell precursors (switching). In contrast to evidence of decreased secretory immunity, serum IgA concentrations often are elevated in HIV-infected people. IgA also is commonly found in immune complexes,[29] and has been shown to possess rheumatoid factor-like activity.[30]

HIV AND THE GI TRACT

Several investigators have found evidence of HIV in the GI tract. Evidence of HIV DNA was found in mucosal homogenates with the aid of the polymerase chain reaction technique in 70% of patients.[31] *In situ* hybridization studies demonstrated HIV-1 RNA in lymphocytes and macrophages in intestinal lamina propria in a subset of AIDS patients.[32,33] Other studies have shown HIV DNA in intestinal cells, including the crypt epithelium and enterochromaffin cells.[34,35] HIV core antigen (p24) has been localized by immunohistologic techniques to various cell types in the GI tract.[31,36–38] Primary intestinal cell lines and colonic tumor epithelial cell lines can be productively infected with HIV.[39,40] *In vitro* studies demonstrated apparent endocytosis of HIV by an epithelial cell line.[41]

Animal studies indicate that intestinal cells are reservoirs for retroviruses. Infection of intestinal crypt epithelium by a feline retrovirus isolate produced an acquired immune deficiency associated with diarrhea and wasting.[42]

DISEASE COMPLICATIONS

Infections (Table 15–1)

VIRUSES

HIV The potential role of HIV as an enteric pathogen is undefined. A prospective study of HIV-infected subjects with GI or proctologic symptoms demonstrated significant correlations between altered bowel habits and histologic evidence of intestinal injury, which was independent of the presence of enteric pathogens.[6] Mucosal HIV p24 contents, determined by quantitative enzyme-linked immunosorbent assay (ELISA), were highest in non-AIDS patients in Walter Reed classes 3 and 4. The expression of p24 correlated both with altered bowel habits and with histologic alterations. Other

results included elevated tissue contents of the cytokines, tumor necrosis factor and interleukin-1, and lesser elevations of the inflammatory mediators, prostaglandin E_2 and leukotriene B_4, adding biochemical evidence in support of mucosal inflammation.

In a companion study, qualitative and quantitative histopathologic studies were performed on rectal biopsy specimens from HIV-infected patients and control subjects and correlated with disease stage.[43] Mucosal cellularity and the numbers of lymphocytes and degranulating eosinophils were maximal in Walter Reed class 3/4 patients. The rise in lymphoid cellularity occurred while CD4+ lymphocyte counts in peripheral blood were falling. Mucosal lymphoid cellularity correlated with mucosal p24 content. Although these studies provide no insight into the pathogenesis of the colonic inflammation, the results strongly suggest that inflammation and HIV expression in mucosa are related. An HIV-associated inflammatory bowel disease could be an important factor in the pathogenesis of the immune deficiency as well as a factor in disease transmission.

Cytomegalovirus Cytomegalovirus (CMV) infection is common in AIDS patients, and evidence of CMV infection is found in up to two thirds of autopsies.[44] Disseminated CMV infection is a progressive disease and frequently contributes to mortality. Serologic evidence of infection is extremely common worldwide and almost invariably present in patients from groups at high risk for the development of AIDS.[45] CMV infects many cell types, including epithelial cells in mucous membranes, so that CMV may be shed in secretions. Thus, it is likely that sexually promiscuous people are infected with multiple strains of the virus.

The primary viral infection is not a significant clinical illness in most cases, although a mononucleosis-like syndrome has been observed. The infection then enters a latent phase, which is lifelong in most immunocompetent people. In the HIV-infected patient with diminished T-cell function, repeated episodes of viral reactivation occur, as demonstrated by intermittent virus shedding and the reappearance of anti-CMV IgM antibodies in the serum.[46] Reactivations become more frequent and prolonged over time, until persistent reactivation and dissemination occur and lead to widespread tissue injury.

Several GI syndromes have been associated with CMV, including esophageal ulcers, esophagitis, gastritis, isolated intestinal ulcers, terminal ileitis, intestinal perforation, focal or diffuse colitis, hepatitis, pancreatitis, sclerosing cholangitis, and unexplained wasting. The clinical approach is based on the usual evaluation of presenting signs and symptoms, and the diagnosis is made by biopsy and histologic analysis.

The key histopathologic feature of CMV infection is the intracellular inclusion (Fig. 15–1). A large argyrophilic nuclear inclusion is seen, often surrounded by a clear halo. The cytoplasm is markedly enlarged and may

Table 15–1. Gastrointestinal Pathogens in AIDS Patients

Parasites
Cryptosporidium parvum
Enterocytozoon bieneusi
Isospora belli
Giardia lamblia
Entamoeba histolytica
*Blastocystis hominis**
Bacteria
Salmonella spp.
Shigella spp.
Campylobacter spp.
Helicobacter pylori
Mycobacterium tuberculosis
Mycobacterium avium-intracellulare
Clostridium difficile
Viruses
Cytomegalovirus
Herpes simplex
Human immunodeficiency virus
Adenovirus
Epstein-Barr virus
Human papilloma virus
Hepatitis B, C, D
Fungi
Candida albicans
Torulopsis glabrata
Histoplasma capsulatum
Coccidioides immitis
Cryptococcus neoformans

* Uncertain pathogenetic potential.

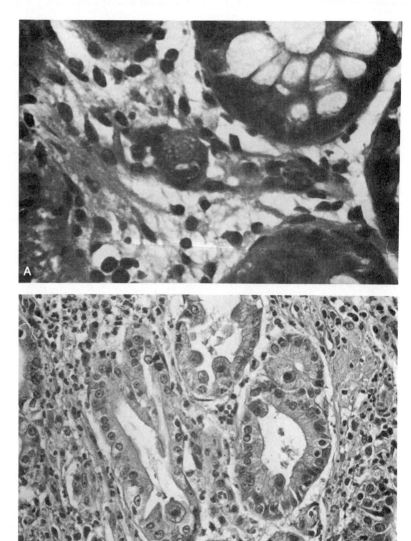

Figure 15–1. (**A**) Intranuclear and cytoplasmic inclusions of CMV in an endothelial cell in the lamina propria of the colon (H&E ×600). (**B**) CMV inclusion bodies in gastric epithelial cells (H&E ×250).

contain numerous small, granular, basophilic inclusions. Inclusions are seen most often in endothelial cells but occasionally are seen in crypt epithelial cells. CMV inclusions are found in multiple cell types in inflamed, ulcerated tissues. When inclusions are rare or atypical, immunohistologic or *in situ* hybridization techniques developed for clinical use may be helpful.[47,48] Other available diagnostic techniques generally are less useful. The presence of anti-CMV IgG is nonspecific, while some patients with disseminated infection lack serum IgM or even serum IgG anti-CMV. Viral culture is of little value, because asymptomatic individuals may intermittently shed CMV[49,50] while some patients with widespread disease have negative cultures.

Several agents capable of inhibiting CMV replication are available. The most widely studied is ganciclovir.[51] Clinical benefit from ganciclovir therapy in patients with serious CMV infection includes clinical stabilization, repletion of body mass, and prolonged survival.[52–54] Ganciclovir is administered intravenously (IV) using an induction regimen followed by maintenance therapy. The drug has hematologic toxicity, the most relevant of which is neutropenia. In most cases a chronic indwelling IV catheter must be placed. Despite the potential problems, patients receiving ganciclovir have been followed for as long as 4 years and have reported reasonable comfort and exhibited good functional performance. An oral form of ganciclovir is being developed.

Foscarnet is an antiviral agent with activity against CMV as well as HIV. Evidence of clinical benefit has been reported.[55] Like ganciclovir, foscarnet must be given by IV infusion. Further development of treatment regimens is expected. Other orally bioavailable antiviral agents with *in vitro* efficacy are being developed for clinical testing.

Immune globulins with high titer antibodies to CMV

are being evaluated for prophylaxis or adjunctive therapy,[56] but there are no data on possible favorable effects on GI disease. Interferon and other nucleoside analogues have not been found to be of value in the treatment of serious CMV infections.

Herpes Simplex Virus Herpes simplex virus infections are common in HIV-infected persons and may cause esophagitis or proctitis. However, the major clinical syndrome in AIDS is a slowly spreading, painful, shallow, clean-based perianal or perineal ulcer.[57] Herpesvirus is readily cultured from the ulcerated surface. These ulcers respond favorably to acyclovir.

Epstein-Barr Virus There has been surprisingly little study of Epstein-Barr virus (EBV) in the GI tract despite its prevalence in other epithelia.[58] Diverse GI symptoms are common in patients with sustained serologic evidence of EBV reactivation.[59] EBV has been found in lesions of oral hairy leukoplakia.[60] EBV genome also has been found in a small percentage of B-cell lymphomas.[61] It is possible that EBV plays a pathologic role in the GI tract.

Adenovirus Adenoviruses are occasionally isolated from rectal swabs or biopsy specimens from AIDS patients with diarrheal disorders, as well as from other sites.[62] The patients otherwise may be clinically stable and do not necessarily have progressive disease. A diarrheal syndrome attributed to adenovirus has been described, with cytoplasmic inclusion bodies seen in superficial epithelial cells identified as adenovirus on electron microscopy.[63]

PARASITES

Cryptosporidium parvum Cryptosporidium is the most widely recognized enteric pathogen in patients with AIDS. Cryptosporidiosis has a worldwide distribution and is responsible for 5% to 10% of cases of severe diarrhea in American AIDS patients. *Cryptosporidium* is a cause of "slim" disease, a wasting syndrome described in African AIDS patients.[64,65] The parasite may infect immunocompetent as well as immunodeficient people.[66] Prolonged shedding of cysts may occur after clinical resolution,[67] and evidence of latent infection in the GI tract has been reported.[68] Cryptosporidiosis has been implicated in traveler's diarrhea and in outbreaks of diarrheal disease in day care centers.[69] There is little host specificity,[70] and bidirectional infection of humans and animals has been reported.[71] Cases of chronic intestinal cryptosporidiosis have been reported in agammaglobulinemic patients without AIDS,[72] suggesting that secretory immune deficiency might promote chronicity, as has been shown in a murine model of giardiasis.[73]

After ingestion and excystation of the oocysts, the sporozoite invades the epithelial cell, possibly *via* specific receptor binding,[74] and occupies an extracytoplasmic site beneath the brush border.[75] Cycles of asexual division with autoinfection occur, as does sexual division with production and fecal excretion of thick-walled oocysts. Destruction of epithelial cells with villous atrophy and inflammation results from the infection.

Cryptosporidiosis usually is chronic and protracted in AIDS patients. Spontaneous remissions occur infrequently and may be related to a temporal rise in CD4+ lymphocyte counts,[76,77] sometimes associated with zidovudine therapy.[77]

There is considerable variation in disease localization, clinical severity, and the course of cryptosporidiosis in AIDS. A majority of patients have diffuse small intestinal disease without or with mild colonic involvement. A smaller percentage have a cryptosporidial colitis and ileitis with no clinical or laboratory evidence of jejunal disease.[78] Massive secretory diarrhea reminiscent of cholera occurs in some patients with AIDS. The most severe clinical form of the disease is biliary and pancreatic infection, associated with pancreatitis, sclerosing cholangitis, or (acalculous) cholecystitis.[79] Isolated cases of *Cryptosporidium* in gastric or respiratory epithelium or invading the lamina propria have been reported.[80,81]

Cryptosporidiosis can be diagnosed by special examination of stool specimens or intestinal aspirates. Several methods of concentration and staining of the oocysts have been described.[82] In addition, cryptosporidia are readily seen in intestinal biopsies (Fig. 15–2). The infection may be patchy, especially in the colon.

The therapeutic options for cryptosporidiosis are limited. Many antibiotics have been tried. Spiramycin, a macrolide antibiotic available in Europe and Canada (Rhone Poulenc), may improve symptoms and occasionally results in clearance of the parasite, but no objective benefit was demonstrated when spiramycin was given orally or parenterally in controlled trials. Immune bovine colostrum suppressed cryptosporidial infection in a child with congenital agammaglobulinemia and in a few AIDS patients.[83–85] Uncontrolled observations have demonstrated a positive clinical effect of paromomycin (Humatin) in some patients.[86]

The treatment of diarrhea due to cryptosporidiosis may be difficult. Diet modification may be helpful in patients with clinically mild disease. A lactose-free, low-fat diet with calorie-rich fluid supplements containing extra protein may be well tolerated. Standard formulas containing substantial quantities of long chain fats and high concentrations of sugar often cause bloating and worsened diarrhea. Hydrophilic bulking agents generally are unhelpful. Opiates such as diphenoxylate, paregoric, or tincture of opium may be effective, although the amount required sometimes causes excessive sedation, and escalating doses may be required.

A subset of patients with AIDS have severe secretory diarrhea with fluid losses of up to 15 L/day. Rapid volume depletion with azotemia and electrolyte abnormalities may occur. The disease resembles cholera clinically, though secretory enterotoxins have not been reported in cryptosporidiosis. Diminished diarrheal

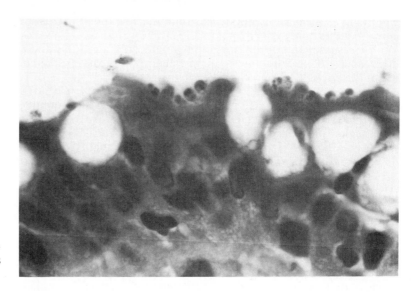

Figure 15–2. Localization of cryptosporidia along the luminal membrane of villus epithelial cells (H&E ×1000).

volume may occur during treatment with indomethacin or the phenothiazines, chlorpromazine (Thorazine) or trifluoperazine (Stelazine), which inhibit chloride secretion by crypt epithelial cells. Therapy with a somatostatin analogue may be successful,[87] though patients with severe disease may not respond. Despite these approaches, parenteral fluid administration often is necessary to maintain a normal state of hydration.

Enterocytozoon bieneusi Microsporidia are protozoa only recently recognized to infect man, although they are known to cause disease in other animals.[88] The first case of microsporidiosis reported was in 1985, and the illness has been seen worldwide.[88–89] The infecting species has been identified as *Enterocytozoon bieneusi*. The prevalence of microsporidiosis in AIDS is unknown. It likely is a common cause of unexplained small intestinal injury. Microsporidial spores have been identified in stool specimens and intestinal aspirates by electron microscopy but cannot be definitively distinguished by light microscopy.[90,91] Presently, the diagnosis on intestinal biopsy also requires electron microscopy for confirmation.

A recent electron microscopic study of small intestinal biopsy specimens from patients with AIDS and unexplained diarrhea revealed 20 cases of microsporidiosis.[92] In another study, microsporidiosis was found to be associated with partial jejunal villous atrophy, xylose malabsorption, and diminished specific activities of brush border disaccharidases, implying a pathogenic role for this organism.[93,94] Electron microscopic studies have limited the infection to the small intestine, with the jejunum more heavily infested than the duodenum,[95] though one report documented microsporidia in colonic epithelial cells.[96]

Clinically, infection with microsporidia resembles infection with cryptosporidia, other diffuse small intestinal diseases, or short bowel syndrome. Microscopically, partial villous atrophy and crypt hyperplasia are seen. The presence of prominent cytopathic changes in villous epithelial cells, especially in the upper villi, is a clue to the diagnosis (Fig. 15–3). The supranuclear regions contain globular inclusions (meronts and sporonts) which may deform the nucleus (see Fig. 15–3). The fully developed spores erupt through the luminal membrane, destroying the cell.

Little is known of the life cycle of *E. bieneusi* in nature or of the existence of other animal hosts. There is no known effective therapy. Patients later shown to have microsporidiosis have been treated with a variety of antibiotics. Symptoms may respond to treatment with trimethoprim-sulfa drugs or paromomycin, although evidence of microsporidiosis, intestinal injury, and malabsorption persists (pers. observ.). Nutritional therapy is based on diet modification to decrease the fat and lactose content. Elemental diets may be well tolerated. Parenteral nutrition has been utilized in some patients.

Microsporidiosis is an important and newly recognized pathogen. The organism may be a significant cause of enteric disease in patients with AIDS in the United States and elsewhere, and in infectious diarrhea in general. Further studies are needed to enhance the diagnostic and therapeutic armamentarium.

Isospora belli *Isospora belli* is a coccidium closely related to *Cryptosporidium*. It has been reported frequently in AIDS patients from Haiti and west Africa.[97,98] The symptoms of isosporiasis are similar to those of cryptosporidiosis. Oocysts may be scarce in stool specimens,[99,100] and the diagnosis is easily missed. On biopsy, *Isospora* is found in the apical cytoplasm of villous epithelial cells and produces partial villous atrophy and crypt hyperplasia (Fig. 15–4). A case of disseminated isosporiasis with extensive infection in the mesenteric

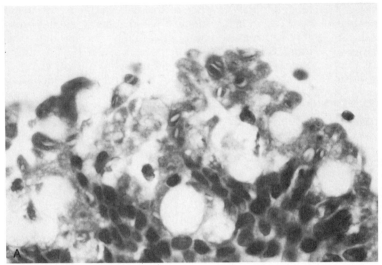

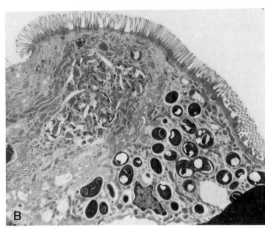

Figure 15–3. (**A**) Developing forms of microsporidia located in an area of cell necrosis and sluffing at the villus tip (H&E ×600). (**B**) Transmission electron micrograph demonstrating a developing sporont in the cell on the left and maturing spores in the cell on the right (H&E ×8000).

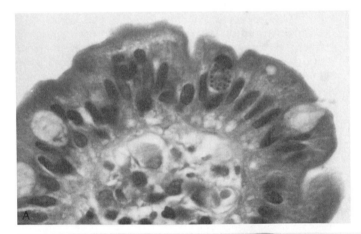

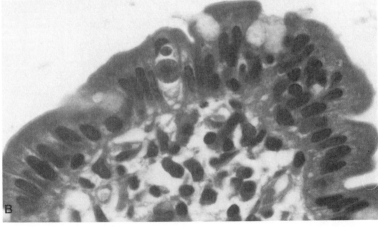

Figure 15–4. (**A**) Microgametocyte form of isospora. (**B**) Merozoite form of isospora (H&E ×600).

lymph nodes and other organs has been reported.[101] Successful disease suppression with improved intestinal function has been reported with trimethoprim-sulfa at various dosages[98,99] but does not occur in every patient. Diarrhea recurs on discontinuation of therapy, so that chronic therapy with trimethoprim-sulfa, trimethoprim alone, or pyrimethamine and folinic acid is necessary.

Giardia lamblia   Enteric infection with *Giardia lamblia* is an important problem in many parts of the world. Giardiasis was diagnosed commonly in sexually active homosexual men during the 1970s and early 1980s and was a frequent cause of the "gay bowel" syndrome.[102] The infection is acquired during ingestion of cysts in contaminated water or through sexual activity involving oral-anal contact. The organism elicits a strong immune response but the infection may not be eradicated completely, owing to temporal alterations in giardial antigens.[103]

Giardiasis is not a common cause of acute diarrhea in AIDS. Cysts are seen occasionally in stool specimens, or trophozoites may be identified in intestinal biopsies (Fig. 15–5). Mucosal structure may be normal since small intestinal injury in giardiasis is T cell mediated.[104] The serum antibody response to acute giardial infection was lower in HIV-seropositive people than in seronegatives.[105] In the absence of intestinal injury, *Giardia* might affect nutrient absorption by local effects on brush border proteins, bile salt deconjugation in the lumen, or other mechanisms. Drug therapy with quinacrine or metronidazole is indicated if cysts or trophozoites are found, though suspicion of other etiologies should be high.

Amebiasis   Intestinal infection with *Entamoeba histolytica* is another common infection in homosexual men[106] and a cause of gay bowel syndrome. Like giardiasis, amebiasis is not a common cause of severe illness in HIV-infected patients, despite frequent shedding in the stool. The virulence of strains of *E. histolytica* is related to the presence of specific zymogens, which are not present in all isolates,[107] so that many isolates probably represent commensal organisms. Although metronidazole therapy should be prescribed, the possibility of coexisting pathogens should be kept in mind.

Other parasites have been reported, including *Strongyloides stercoralis* (Fig. 15–6), which may produce a hyperinfection syndrome.[108] *Blastocystis hominis,* thought by some to be an enteric pathogen,[109] has been found in several HIV-seropositive people with diarrhea.

BACTERIA

Mycobacteria   Systemic infections with *Mycobacterium avium-intracellulare* (MAI) and *Mycobacterium tuberculosis* are common in AIDS patients.[110] Extrapulmonary tuberculosis often is an early complication of AIDS. The major GI manifestation is granulomatous hepatitis, though isolated ulcers of the intestine, especially of the ileum, have been noted.

MAI infections have been seen with increasing frequency in the setting of AIDS. The infection usually occurs late in the course of AIDS. MAI rarely causes infections in immunocompetent people as it is less virulent than *M. tuberculosis.* It is acquired orally or possibly by aerosol. Atypical mycobacteria may be cultured from the water supplies in urban areas.[111]

MAI produces a systemic infection with widespread tissue distribution that is usually most prominent in the liver, spleen, mesenteric lymph nodes, bone marrow, and intestinal mucosa (Fig. 15–7). Organomegaly is present. Intra-abdominal lymphadenopathy is prominent on ultrasound or computed tomography (CT), and MAI must be differentiated from other infections and neoplasms. On occasion, nodes undergo liquefaction necrosis and produce a mycobacterial peritonitis. It is important to diagnose this complication, as the clinical presentation may mimic an acute abdominal crisis.

The intestinal lesion of MAI is the result of mucosal and submucosal infiltration with macrophages contain-

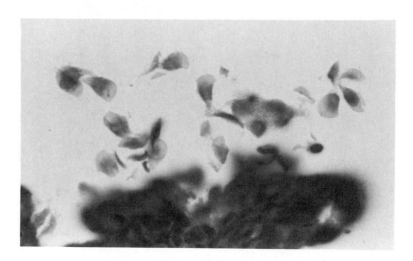

Figure 15–5.   Trophozoites of giardia adjacent to villus cells (H&E ×800).

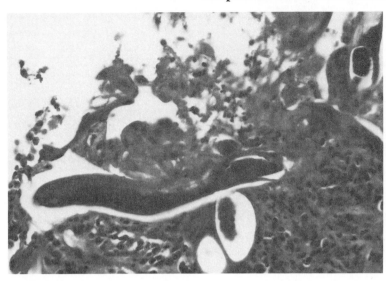

Figure 15–6. Larval forms of strongyloides in a patient with a hyperinfection syndrome (H&E ×400).

ing intracellular organisms that are not lysed, possibly owing to a local deficiency of interferon-γ.[112] The cellular infiltration blocks intramucosal lymphatic flow and produces fat malabsorption with exudative enteropathy. The infection, therefore, is a pathophysiologic counterpart to Whipple's disease.[113] In severe cases there is villous atrophy and impaired absorption of sugars and amino acids.

The major clinical syndrome in patients with disseminated MAI infection is characterized by fever, progressive wasting, and debilitation, with or without diarrhea.[110] The fever and constitutional symptoms may respond promptly to therapy with prostaglandin syn-

thesis inhibitors. Diagnosis is by culture or biopsy (Fig. 15–8). An enlarged left supraclavicular node (Virchow's node) may contain MAI (pers. observ.) and is a clue to intra-abdominal disease. Blood cultures may become positive before local symptoms develop, and bacteremia usually is sustained.[114] Histologic demonstration of acid-fast bacilli in intestinal or liver tissue is straightforward. Molecular hybridization techniques are being developed to allow species identification on tissue sections.

The treatment of *M. tuberculosis* in HIV-infected and non-HIV-infected patients generally is similar and includes multidrug regimens. The optimal length of treatment is not known. Some clinicians continue an-

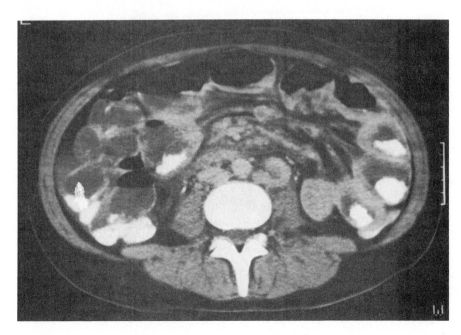

Figure 15–7. CT scan of the abdomen demonstrating mesenteric lymphadenopathy, tethering of the mesentery, and thickening of the bowel wall in a patient with MAI.

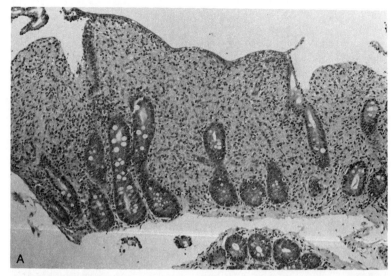

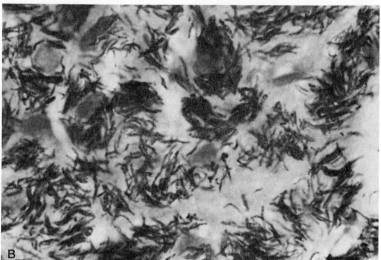

Figure 15–8. (**A**) Massive infiltration of the jejunum with MAI (H&E ×250). (**B**) Acid-fast stain demonstrating intracellular bacilli. The characteristic beaded appearance of the bacilli can be detected (Ziehl Nielson ×1000).

tituberculosis therapy indefinitely, whereas others have found that standard regimens are adequate for HIV-infected patients.

MAI is less responsive to therapy than *M. tuberculosis.* Early trials failed to show benefit of single-drug or two-drug regimens.[115] However, recent studies have demonstrated clinical benefit of four- and five-drug regimens, including parenteral amikacin therapy for 2 to 6 weeks.[116,117]

Other mycobacterial species have been found on occasion, with variable clinical consequences, based on their sensitivity to antibiotics.[118] A few patients have had an MAI-like intestinal lesion in which the foamy macrophages contained gram-positive bacilli rather than acid-fast organisms. Some of these cases could be due to infection with *Rhodococcus equus,* a complication previously reported in AIDS.[119] Interestingly, the foamy macrophages seen in Whipple's disease also contain gram-positive, non-acid-fast rods.

Bacterial Enteritides Bacterial enteritides in HIV-infected persons include salmonellosis, shigellosis, and *Campylobacter* infection.[120–122] The incidence of serious disease is higher than in the general population. One study found a high incidence of *Campylobacter*-like organisms, but their presence did not correlate with clinical symptoms.[123] Enhanced susceptibility could be related to achlorhydria, which is found in a proportion of AIDS patients.[124] Classic studies demonstrated the relationship between gastric acidity and the infective dose of various enteric pathogens.[125]

Bacterial enteritides in AIDS may have a chronic relapsing course, often with bacteremia. The presentation resembles that of enteric fever, with abdominal pain, distention, and a diarrheal syndrome varying from ileocolitis to proctocolitis. The diagnosis is straightforward with routine evaluation. Blood cultures should be part of the workup of suspected infectious diarrhea with fever in an HIV-infected patient. Patients respond to antibiotic therapy with parenteral agents.

An unusual feature of bacterial enteritides in AIDS is the tendency for clinical or microbiologic relapse. It is possible that disease recurrence is due to impaired intracellular killing in macrophages. The intracellular reservoir may protect the organisms against lysis. Quinolones such as ciprofloxacin are felt to be bactericidal to intracellular organisms,[126] though the drug was unable to eliminate the carrier state after *Salmonella* infections in a non-AIDS treatment group.[127] Further studies will be needed to determine if complete eradication of enteric bacterial pathogens in AIDS is possible, or if chronic therapy will continue to be needed.

Antibiotic-associated colitis, related to elaboration of *C. difficile* toxin, is common in AIDS patients who receive prolonged courses of broad-spectrum antibiotics. The clinical syndrome is similar in AIDS and non-AIDS patients. Suspicion should be raised by the clinical situation, and the diagnosis is confirmed with a stool toxin assay. Treatment with vancomycin or metronidazole is as effective in AIDS as in non-AIDS patients. Residual symptoms can be managed with oral cholestyramine (Questran), which binds the bacterial toxin. Surveillance for recurrent colitis may be necessary in patients who require chronic antibiotic therapy.

FUNGI

Candida albicans   Candidiasis is a very common opportunistic infection, occurring in over 80% of AIDS patients. Early clinical observations associated the occurrence of thrush, not related to antibiotic usage or other immune impairment, with an increased risk of progression to AIDS within 6 months.[128] The most common species is *C. albicans,* which is part of the normal enteric flora. However, infection by *Torulopsis glabrata* has been reported and may be a cause of treatment failure.[129] Candidiasis in AIDS is predominantly a mucosal disease, which differs from what is seen in other states of immune derangement such as uncontrolled diabetes mellitus or drug-induced leukopenia. In those circumstances, tissue invasion and septicemia is common. Systemic candidiasis in AIDS patients usually is associated with idiopathic or drug-induced neutropenia.

Other Fungi   The luminal GI tract, liver, spleen, and mesenteric lymph nodes may be involved by histoplasmosis, coccidiodomycosis, or other fungal infections.[130–131] Systemic fungal infections in AIDS usually are rapidly progressive diseases. Although the fungi are not primary enteric pathogens, visceral dissemination and involvement of the luminal GI tract may occur. Typically, there is a chronic febrile illness with constitutional symptoms. Suspicion should be aroused by a history of residence in an endemic area. The diagnosis is made by culture or examination of tissue samples with special stains (Fig. 15–9). Treatment with antifungal agents must be continued for months and perhaps indefinitely.

Neoplasms

KAPOSI'S SARCOMA

The diagnosis of Kaposi's sarcoma in young homosexual males in 1981 was one of the earliest observations indicating a new disorder of immune function.[132] The lesion is indistinguishable histopathologically from the classic Kaposi's sarcoma that occurs in elderly men, from endemic forms of Kaposi's sarcoma found in Africa, or from the form that occurs during immunosuppressive therapy. Kaposi's sarcoma in association with AIDS is demographically limited: it is more common in white homosexual men than in other people with AIDS,[133] which suggests the existence of a separate cofactor for this complication.

Visceral involvement in Kaposi's sarcoma is more common in AIDS patients than in patients with classic Kaposi's sarcoma.[134] GI tract lesions are common and often asymptomatic, but may cause a swallowing disorder, luminal obstruction, intussusception, disturbed motility from neural involvement, or lymphatic blockade with exudative enteropathy. Severe bleeding is uncommon and perforation is rare. Severe diarrhea is not a common finding in uncomplicated Kaposi's sarcoma, and patients with diarrhea should be evaluated for the presence of other pathogens.

The diagnosis of Kaposi's sarcoma can be made by visual inspection and confirmed by biopsy. Endoscopic biopsy may be false negative because of a submucosal location of the tumor.[135] Kaposi's sarcoma responds to chemotherapy[136] or radiation therapy, but no treatment is needed in asymptomatic cases. Obstructive lesions can be treated effectively by laser ablation.[137]

LYMPHOMA

An increased incidence of extranodal, high-grade, non-Hodgkin's B-cell lymphomas in young men was noticed in the early 1980s.[138] The development of lymphoma later was shown to be related to HIV infection. B-cell lymphomas have a special predilection for the central nervous system (CNS) and the GI tract. EBV genomes have been identified in some of these tumors,[61] suggesting a possible etiologic role. Lymphoproliferative disease involving T cells has been seen in some HIV-infected persons and appears to be related to coexisting infection with HTLV-I, a T-lymphotropic oncogenic retrovirus.[139]

GI lymphomas in AIDS are biologically aggressive, especially the Burkitt's lymphoma subtype. However, the lesions may respond to combination chemotherapy. There are few long-term survivors because of the underlying immune deficiency.

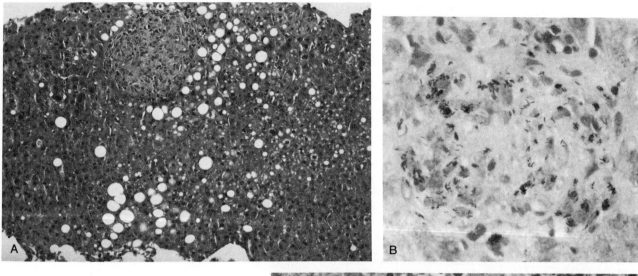

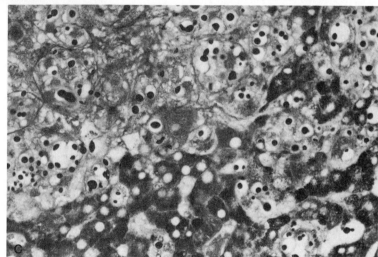

Figure 15–9. (**A**) Well-formed granuloma in the liver (H&E ×250). (**B**) Acid-fast bacilli located within a granuloma (Ziehl Nielson ×400). (**C**) Cryptococcal hepatitis (GMS ×600). (**D**) Histoplasmosis of the liver (GMS ×600). (**E**) Cocciodomycosis of the liver (H&E ×400).

OTHER CANCERS

Sporadic reports of carcinomas in the GI tract have been published, including carcinomas of the tongue, esophagus, stomach, colon, and anus. In some cases the tumors are biologically aggressive, with widespread hematogenous dissemination and short survival. The relationship of these tumors to AIDS is uncertain but might be related either to infection with a co-carcinogenic agent or to loss of immune surveillance against developing tumors.

CLINICAL SYMDROMES

Disorders of Food Intake

Oral candidiasis is the most commonly encountered complication in HIV-seropositive patients. Clinically, the infection presents as erosions or plaques on the gin-giva, palate, hypopharynx, and/or esophagus (Fig. 15–10). Isolated involvement of the oral cavity and the esophagus has been reported.[140] Bronchial, gastric, and intestinal mucosae are not involved grossly or microscopically. On radiologic examination, plaques with or without erosions are seen.

The most common complaints are sore throat and/or odynophagia, sometimes with choking or even aspiration, plus a mild to moderate substernal discomfort. Food intake is decreased, and increased sensitivity of the oral cavity to temperature and acidity may be noted.

In most cases the diagnosis can be made by inspection and confirmed by a response to treatment. Culture, biopsy, or brush cytology can be used to confirm the diagnosis. A cytology brush for the esophagus has been developed that avoids possible contamination by oral secretions.[141] Candidiasis can be successfully treated with topical or systemic agents. Topical therapies include nystatin and clotrimazole troches (Mycelex), ke-

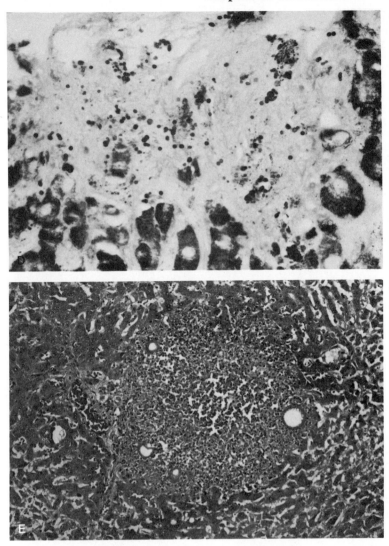

Figure 15–9. (*Continued*)

toconazole (Nizoral), and fluconazole (Diflucan). Ketoconazole and fluconazole occasionally are associated with abnormal liver function tests. A potential problem with treatment is decreased bioavailability; ketoconazole absorption is best at an acid pH, but many AIDS patients are achlorhydric.[124,142] Administration of an acidifying agent may improve effectiveness. The infection is resistant to oral therapy in a small percentage of cases and must be treated with IV amphotericin.

Oral hairy leukoplakia is a whitish, verrucous excrescence that occurs mainly along the sides of the tongue[143] and has been mistaken for candidiasis. EBV has been found in the lesions by molecular hybridization studies as well as by electron microscopy.[60] The diagnosis is made by inspection and confirmed, if necessary, by biopsy. Acyclovir or ganciclovir therapy causes resolution.[144]

Painful ulcers of the oral cavity, hypopharynx, or esophagus may cause significant impairment of food intake. The most common etiologies are viral and idiopathic, though ulcerating neoplasms and mycobacterial or fungal infections are seen rarely. Small aphthous ulcers in the oral cavity are common and may resolve spontaneously or after administration of topical steroids. Acute necrotizing ulcerative gingivitis is a focally destructive process of uncertain etiology that may extend to the bone.[145] The most common virus-associated ulcer is due to CMV, which occurs in the oral cavity or esophagus. The lesions usually appear as erosions or as shallow coalescing ulcerations with abundant intracellular viral inclusions. The lesion responds symptomatically and undergoes healing in response to ganciclovir therapy.[56]

Many esophageal ulcers are seen in which no etiologic agent can be identified. The ulcers are atypical in their large size and in the extensively undermining of the mucosa (Fig. 15–11). The ulcers typically are refractory to therapy against gastric acid secretion, and the

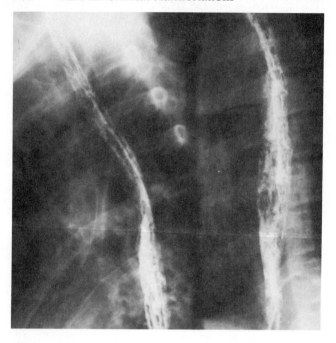

Figure 15–10. Two views of a barium swallow demonstrating mucosal plaques due to candidiasis.

pain may respond poorly to opiates. Progressive malnutrition is the usual result in untreated cases. Biopsies are recommended to rule out CMV esophagitis or ulcerated tumor and show inflamed granulation tissue, sometimes with rare CMV inclusions. Ganciclovir therapy does not bring symptomatic relief or healing, though viral inclusions disappear. The presence of HIV in esophageal ulcers has been shown by RNA *in situ* hybridization techniques and by the detection of an HIV core protein, p24, in cells in the ulcer.[146–147] Viral particles suggestive of HIV were seen in transient esophageal ulcers associated with primary HIV infection.[148] One study also found evidence of EBV-infected cells in esophageal ulcers.[149] Corticosteroid therapy has been shown to produce symptomatic relief, weight gain, and ulcer healing in a substantial proportion of patients.[147,150–151] Therapy has been administered by oral, parenteral, and intralesional routes. Despite the potential hazards of steroid therapy, clinical experience has demonstrated that the treatment can be administered with relative safety. Prophylaxis against tuberculosis, herpesviruses, fungi, or other pathogens should be considered.

Neoplasms such as Kaposi's sarcoma or lymphoma may affect food intake by interfering with mastication or swallowing. These lesions may respond to a variety of therapies.

In many cases, food intake is diminished in the absence of pathologic lesions. The causes are diverse but fall into several general categories. Organic neurologic diseases may interfere with the initiation or coordination of eating. More diffuse lesions such as HIV-associated encephalitis cause anorexia due either to alterations in consciousness, damage to neurons involved in appetite behavior, or the release of cytokines such as tumor necrosis factor that reversibly suppress food intake.[152] Secondary anorexia is a common feature of both systemic infections and malabsorptive illnesses, owing to the release of inhibitory factors acting at the level of the CNS.[153–154] Alterations in taste, anorexia, and nausea are common side-effects of medications. Psychosocial factors such as depression, isolation, and poverty, and debilitation itself may lead to inadequate intake. Such considerations are an important part of clinical therapeutics in AIDS.

Dyspepsia

Nausea and dyspepsia are very common symptoms in AIDS but rarely dominate the clinical picture. These symptoms may be due to a variety of pathologic processes. The stomach may be involved by disseminated infections such as CMV, MAI, or fungus, or by tumors such as Kaposi's sarcoma, lymphoma, or adenocarci-

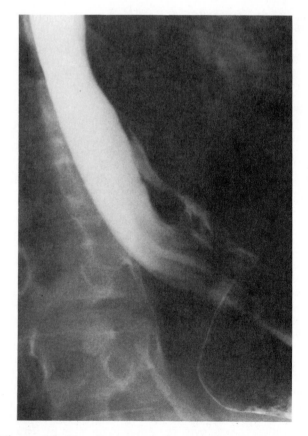

Figure 15–11. Barium esophagram demonstrating an idiopathic ulcer that is undermining the superior edge and tracking submucosally to the gastric cardia.

noma. Symptomatic gastritis due to *Helicobacter pylori* has been found but is not common, possibly because of frequent antibiotic usage in AIDS patients. Some medications, such as nonsteroidal anti-inflammatory agents, promote gastric ulceration and produce dyspepsia. On the other hand, symptomatic peptic ulcer disease is uncommon in AIDS patients, possibly because of the decreased gastric acid secretion.[124] Achlorhydria may alter drug absorption or lead to increased bacterial colony counts in the stomach and upper small intestine, with potential adverse affects on nutrient absorption. Dyspepsia is due to a low-grade pancreatitis in some patients and may precede the development of biliary tract disease.

The clinical symptoms are nonspecific. The presence of weight loss or fever implies a serious complication such as a systemic infection or ulcerating tumor.

The treatment of dyspeptic complications depends on their exact nature. Symptomatic *Helicobacter pylori* infection in an AIDS patient is treated in a similar manner as the infection in other symptomatic patients. The diagnosis of CMV or MAI infection is an indication for systemic anti-infective therapy. Widespread or ulcerating Kaposi's sarcoma is an indication for systemic chemotherapy, as is the presence of lymphoma.

Diarrhea and Wasting

Diarrhea and weight loss are very common problems in AIDS patients, occurring in up to 80% of cases in some series. Symptoms are associated either with small intestinal injury and malabsorption or with enterocolitis (Table 15–2). Although early studies reported large numbers of patients with unexplained diarrhea, an infectious agent can be found in most comprehensively evaluated AIDS patients.[93,155] In contrast, unexplained

Table 15–2. Causes of Diarrhea and Wasting

Malabsorptive diseases
   Cryptosporidiosis
   Isosporiasis
   Microsporidiosis
   Giardiasis
   M. avium-intracellulare
     group
   Bacterial overgrowth
Enterocolitis
   Cytomegalovirus
   M. avium-intracellulare
   M. tuberculosis
   Cryptosporidiosis
   Adenovirus
   Salmonella spp.
   Shigella spp.
   Campylobacter spp.
   Fungal infections
   HIV?
   Clostridium difficile toxin

diarrhea is common in HIV-infected patients without AIDS.

Nutrient malabsorption is an extremely common occurrence in AIDS. In many cases it is clinically occult and involves fat[156] or vitamin B_{12}.[33] A subset of AIDS patients have severe malabsorption associated with histologic evidence of small intestinal injury. Many cases are due to cryptosporidiosis, isosporiasis, or microsporidiosis.[93] The intestinal injury appears similar to tropical sprue and includes partial villous atrophy and crypt hyperplasia. Total villous atrophy such as occurs in celiac disease is rare. Malabsorption also may occur as a result of MAI infection. Severe malabsorption is not a feature of giardiasis. CMV produces a diffuse disease in the lamina propria but rarely causes severe injury to the villous epithelium. There is little evidence implicating bacterial overgrowth as a cause of intestinal injury, despite reports of alterations in the upper intestinal flora.[157] While intraluminal bacterial colony counts may be somewhat elevated as a result of hypochlorhydria or achlorhydria, unpublished series have shown most AIDS patients to have jejunal colony counts within the normal range (M. Kapembwa, D. P. Kotler, pers. observ.).

A proportion of patients have severe intestinal dysfunction, with an etiologic agent found after comprehensive evaluation.[34-35,90,156-157,159-162] It is possible that HIV or another unidentified pathogen is responsible for the damage. However, the report of clinical improvement in response to a gluten-free diet[163] suggests another possible pathogenesis related to luminal antigens and immune dysregulation.

There are several causes of enterocolitis in patients with AIDS. CMV colitis is diagnosed frequently and produces a progressive disease that may result in bowel infarction and perforation. MAI produces an infiltrative disease without specific findings in the colon. Disseminated *M. tuberculosis* also has been found in the GI tract and causes focal ulcerations, especially in the ileocecal region. Some patients with cryptosporidiosis have disease limited to the colon and present with symptoms of severe proctocolitis without significant malabsorption. Fungal infection may involve the bowel. Adenovirus also may cause a persistent colitis. Adenovirus infection is limited to epithelial cells, and the diagnosis can be made with certainty only by electron microscopy. Other causes of proctitis and colitis include bacteria such as *Salmonella*, *Shigella*, and *Campylobacter,* and antibiotic-associated colitis.

Clinical differentiation of malabsorptive from colitic disease is important to focus the diagnostic evaluation, though the possibility of multiple coexisting diseases may require a comprehensive workup (Table 15–3). An algorithmic approach may be used (Fig. 15–12).[164] Important information often can be obtained from the patient's history. The symptoms related to small intestinal infection are those of malabsorption and are similar to symptoms in patients with tropical sprue or short bowel syndrome.[93,164] Enterocolitic diseases produce typical symptoms of colitis, often associated with

Table 15–3. Clinical Differentiation of Malabsorptive and Colitic Diarrhea

Parameter Studied	Malabsorption	Colitis
Stool frequency (per 24 hr)	3–8	3–30
Stool volume (per 24 hr)	750–10,000 ml	250–1000 ml
Stool volume (per bowel movement)	Variable, often large	Small
Regularity of bowel movements	Variable	Regular
Formed stools	Rarely	Never
Occult blood in stools	No	Yes
Fecal leukocytes	No	Yes
Tenesmus	No	Sometimes
Fever	No	Yes
Debility	Yes	Yes
Appetite	Fair to good	Fair to poor

fever, anorexia, progressive weight loss, and extreme debilitation.

Optimal diagnostic techniques vary with the specific pathogen. The diagnosis of cryptosporidiosis is made readily by examination of the stool or tissue sections. Isosporiasis also can be diagnosed by stool examination or tissue biopsy. The diagnosis of microsporidiosis is more difficult as spores cannot by specifically identified in stool specimens except by electron microscopy. In some cases the presence of microsporidia in intestinal biopsies can be suggested by histopathologic features on light microscopy.[92,165]

The spectrum of endoscopic lesions in CMV colitis varies from essentially normal-appearing mucosa, to scattered groups of vesicles or erosions, to broad shallow ulcerations that may coalesce. CMV usually causes a pancolitis, though specific regions of the bowel may be affected earlier or more severely than others. CMV dissemination is not expressed at all sites simultaneously and can be more extensive in the right colon and cecum, so that the diagnosis may be missed if the evaluation is limited. Isolated deep ulcers due to CMV may also occur in the absence of diffuse disease. The diagnosis of CMV infection is made by histologic examination of tissue biopsy specimens (see Fig. 15–1).

Acid-fast bacilli can be seen on stool examination and their presence suggests possible intestinal involvement with MAI. Mucosal abnormalities on barium x-rays or thickening of the intestinal wall plus enlargement of mesenteric and retroperitoneal nodes on CT is characteristic of MAI. Diagnosis by biopsy (see Figs. 15–8 and 15–9) often can be made in 1 day, whereas mycobacterial cultures may take as long as 6 weeks to become positive.

Maintenance of nutritional status and fluid balance is an important clinical task, especially in patients with malabsorption. Oral rehydration solutions are hypocaloric and may promote wasting if used excessively. A low-fat, lactose-free diet supplemented with medium chain triglycerides[166] may be beneficial. Standard poly-meric formula diets generally are tolerated poorly, while elemental diets may lead to less diarrhea.[167] Palatability is a problem with elemental diets. In refractory cases, parenteral hydration or parenteral nutrition may be employed and has been shown to improve nutritional status.[168]

Nutritional support is less effective in patients with enterocolitis associated with systemic infections than in patients with malabsorptive diseases due to the associated metabolic derangements. In one study, total parenteral nutrition resulted in weight gain due entirely to an increase in body fat content, while the body cell mass progressively diminished.[168] Although nutritional support might slow the rate of protein depletion, the key to successful therapy is proper diagnosis and treatment of the specific disease complication. Ganciclovir treatment of CMV colitis was shown to lead to body mass repletion in the absence of formal nutritional support.[53]

Anorectal Diseases

The anorectal region may be affected by ulcers, masses, warts, infections, and hemorrhoids. Anorectal ulcers may arise from stratified squamous epithelium in the anal canal, perianal and perineal skin, or rectal mucosa. Herpes simplex virus type II is a common cause of anorectal ulceration. The primary lesion occurs at the pectinate line. Vesicles in the anal canal may be missed, as they rupture during defecation. Large, shallow, spreading perianal ulcers are recognized more commonly. A proctitis may occur, but is more common in non-HIV-infected subjects. Most cases respond to therapy with acyclovir or ganciclovir. Parenteral acyclovir therapy is required for extensive lesions. Herpes simplex virus resistant to acyclovir has been demonstrated in patients with refractory ulcerations. The use of foscarnet may bring resolution.[169] CMV also can cause anorectal ulcerations. The diagnosis is established by biopsy. Ganciclovir therapy may be associated with clinical resolution.

A variety of classic venereal diseases can produce anorectal ulcerations. Epidemiologic studies in Africa strongly suggest that genital ulceration promotes the transmission of HIV infection.[170] The diagnosis and therapy of *Neisseria gonorrhoeae* proctitis are similar in AIDS and non-AIDS patients. Syphilis may have an atypical presentation in HIV-infected subjects, and serologic diagnosis may be problematic.[171] Darkfield examination or flourescent antibody techniques disclose the *Treponema pallidum* spirochete. Prolonged IV antibiotic therapy is required.

Chlamydial infections are the most prevalent sexually transmitted diseases in sexually active groups, and the risk of infection rises with the level of sexual activity.[172] Definitive diagnosis is made by cell culture. Usual therapy is oral tetracycline or doxycycline. The frequency of chancroid, caused by *Hemophilus ducreyi,* in HIV-infected patients is unknown. The diagnosis usually is suggested on clinical grounds and confirmed

Diagnostic Algorithm for Diarrhea and Wasting in AIDS

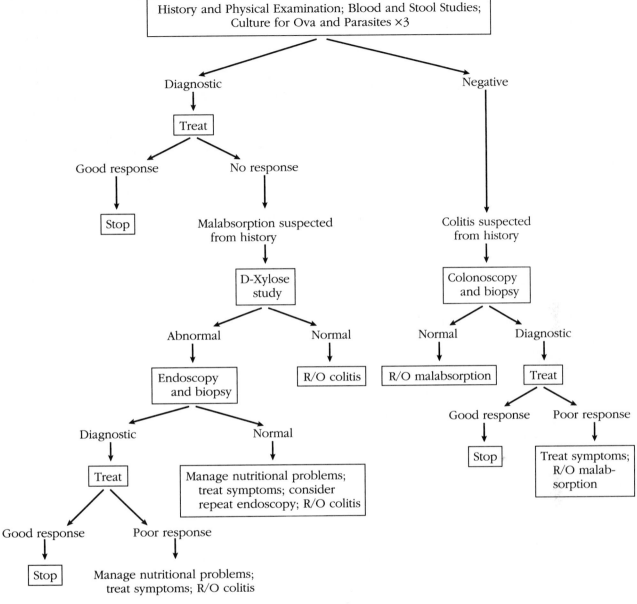

Figure 15–12.   Diagnostic algorithm for diarrhea and wasting in AIDS. (Adapted with permission from Hecker LM, Kotler DP: Gastrointestinal manifestations in AIDS. In Conn RB (ed): Current Diagnosis. Philadelphia, JB Lippincott, 1991.)

after infection with *T. pallidum* is excluded. Therapy with either trimethoprim-sulfamethoxasole or a sulfa drug alone may be successful.

Rectal spirochetosis has been recognized in homosexual men with or without HIV infections.[173] The infection usually is asymptomatic and an incidental finding on evaluation (Fig. 15–13).

Idiopathic ulcers of the anorectal region, similar to

those occurring in the esophagus, are seen in AIDS patients.[146] As with esophageal ulcers, they may contain detectable quantities of p24. CMV, HSV, HPV, acid-fast bacilli, fungi, and bacteria must be excluded by culture or histologic studies. The pathogenesis of the ulceration is unknown. Intralesional or systemic corticosteroids produce a prompt clinical response but have a variable effect on healing.

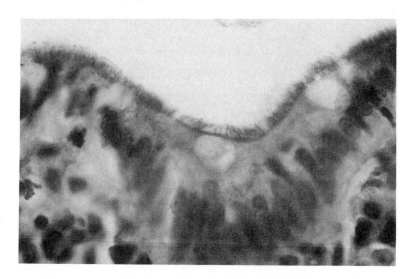

Figure 15–13. Spirochetes located along the luminal membrane of rectal crypt epithelial cells, giving it a shaggy appearance (H&E ×800).

The incidence of anogenital neoplasms is increased in AIDS patients as it is in immunosuppressed renal transplant recipients.[174] Kaposi's sarcoma and lymphoma are the most common neoplasms and present as mass lesions or as ulcers. Epidermoid cancers, including squamous cell and cloacagenic cancer, occur in anal skin and rectal glands, respectively. Although these cancers rarely metastasize in immunocompetent persons, they may do so in patients with AIDS. For these lesions, management after diagnostic biopsy includes excision, chemotherapy, or laser photocoagulation. Laser therapy of rectal Kaposi's sarcoma also is effective and may cause dramatic regression of bulky disease.[137]

The role of papillomavirus, the etiologic agent of condylomata acuminata (common venereal warts), in anorectal cancers is unclear. Specific serotypes of papillomaviruses are suspected as being cofactors in carcinogenesis in the anogenital region, particularly of squamous cell carcinomas of the cervix or anus.[175] Leukoplakia of the anal canal is thought to be an intermediate form of the lesion and is a common finding in HIV-infected homosexual men.[176] Of note, the prevalence of squamous cell carcinoma of the anus was known to be increased in homosexual men prior to the recognition of AIDS.[177]

Hemorrhoids are common in HIV-infected persons. Factors predisposing to hemorrhoids may have predated the HIV infection. Severe diarrhea or proctitis may promote thrombosis, ulceration, and secondary infection. Fleshy skin tags, resembling those seen in Crohn's disease, also are commonly seen and are related to underlying inflammation.

Other Syndromes

HEMORRHAGE

GI hemorrhage is not a common consequence of AIDS, but serious or life-threatening bleeding does occur.

Bleeding may result from the same conditions occurring in the non-HIV-infected patient as well as from the tumors and ulcers seen in AIDS. Episodes of massive arterial hemorrhage have been seen in patients with acute or chronic intestinal ulcers or with rapidly progressive Kaposi's sarcoma.

The clinical presentation of GI hemorrhage in an AIDS patient is the same as in a non-AIDS patient, and the basic concepts of diagnosis and treatment also are the same. Bleeding lesions may be visualized by endoscopy and bleeding controlled locally while diagnostic material is obtained. Angiographic localization of obscure lesions and pharmacologic control may be successful. If bleeding is related to a discrete ulcer, surgical excision may be indicated. Surgery is less appropriate for patients with widespread disease. Proper management of bleeding neoplasms involves effective local control followed by systemic chemotherapy.

Surgical Complications

Disease complications requiring consideration of emergency surgical intervention occur in patients with AIDS. Perforated viscus occurs in AIDS, but the cause may be a solitary ulcer, CMV infection,[178] or tumor[179] rather than peptic ulcer disease or diverticulitis. Malignant obstruction usually is due to Kaposi's sarcoma or lymphoma rather than to adenocarcinoma. Kaposi's sarcoma or lymphoma also may be the leading edge in an intussusception. Some patients with peritonitis have had only mild fibrinous exudate at laparotomy.[180]

The clinical appearance of appendicitis, cholecystitis, or generalized peritonitis is the same in AIDS and non-AIDS patients. Appendicitis typically responds well to surgery. In contrast, patients with acute acalculous cholecystitis associated with sclerosing cholangitis, CMV, or cryptosporidial infections, may respond less well to surgery.

Though the physical findings of an acute abdomen are not significantly affected by the presence of AIDS, the laboratory evaluation differs markedly from expected. Elevated leukocyte counts with early forms in the circulation may not be present, especially if there is preexisting leukopenia or prior treatment with myelosuppressive drugs. Isotopic imaging studies such as an indium-labeled white blood cell study or gallium scan may appear normal in the presence of severe leukopenia. Imaging studies such as CT with luminal contrast may be particularly valuable in detecting extraluminal collections of pus or fluid.

Although the indications for surgery are the same in AIDS patients and non-HIV-infected patients, the expected outcomes may differ. One can anticipate unusual pathogens, prolonged recovery times, and the possibility of impaired wound healing. The incidence of postoperative complications and mortality is high in several series,[181-183] but this is due, at least in part, to the seriousness of the underlying illness and other complications, so that the presence of the immune deficiency itself may not be an important independent risk factor. Complete recovery after major abdominal surgery is possible in AIDS patients and may be followed by prolonged survival.[184]

Hepatobiliary Diseases

Liver dysfunction in AIDS may be related to preexisting hepatic diseases, infectious or neoplastic disease complications, or drug toxicity. Three distinct clinical syndromes have been recognized: diffuse hepatocellular injury, granulomatous hepatitis, and sclerosing cholangitis (Fig. 15–14). However, many patients with ab-

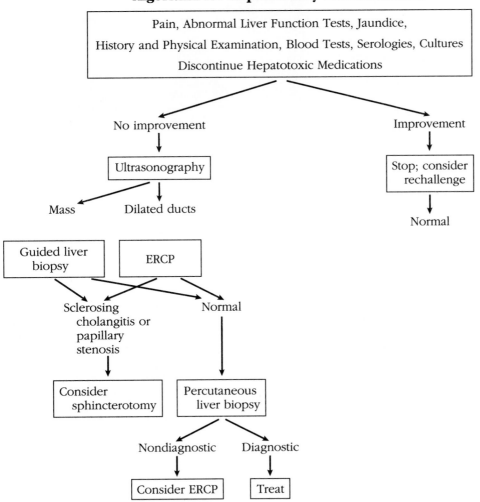

Algorithm for Hepatobiliary Disease in AIDS

Figure 15–14. Algorithm for diagnosing hepatobiliary disease in AIDS. (Adapted with permission from Hecker LM, Kotler DP: Gastrointestinal manifestations in AIDS. In Conn RB (ed): Current Diagnosis. Philadelphia, JB Lippincott, 1991.)

normal results on liver function tests are found to have macrovesicular or microvesicular fatty infiltration or other nonspecific changes.

Diffuse hepatitis is most commonly a result of drug toxicity or hepatitis C[185] or hepatitis D infection.[186] Acute hepatitis B infection is uncommon, owing to prior exposure in most patients, and may be clinically mild, because hepatocyte injury is produced by the immune reaction. Autoimmune chronic active hepatitis and chronic hepatitis B infections also are clinically mild syndromes in HIV-seropositive people.

Granulomatous hepatitis in AIDS is related to mycobacterial or fungal diseases or drug toxicity (see Fig. 15–9). *Pneumocystis carinii* may cause a hepatitis and other evidence of disseminated disease in patients receiving aerosol prophylaxis.[187] Isolated cases of cryptosporidiosis or microsporidiosis affecting the liver have been reported.[188] Fever and constitutional symptoms are prominent. Liver function tests demonstrate progressive elevations in the levels of alkaline phosphatase and γ-glutamyltranspeptidase, but bilirubin concentrations are less affected. Liver biopsy reveals granulomas, which may be poorly formed. Giant cells are seen only rarely. Special stains can presumptively identify the causative organisms, though mycobacterial and fungal cultures of liver tissue should be done routinely.

Peliosis hepatis has been described in AIDS patients.[189] As opposed to the syndrome in non-AIDS patients, the lesion in AIDS patients is due to infection by a *Rickettsia*-like organism related to the organism that causes cat scratch fever.

A syndrome of sclerosing cholangitis has been recognized in AIDS patients[78] and resembles the non-AIDS variety. The etiologies and pathogenetic mechanisms of sclerosing cholangitis in AIDS and the non-AIDS variety are unknown. Patients present with nonspecific abdominal complaints and progressive cholestasis. Retrograde endoscopy demonstrates single or multiple areas of narrowing and dilation of the intrahepatic or extrahepatic ducts, with mucosal ulceration in many cases (Fig. 15–15). Examination of bile and pancreatic juice may reveal bacterial overgrowth, viruses, or cryptosporidia; in some cases no identifiable pathogens are found. The short-term results of endoscopic therapy are variable and the long-term results are poor. Operative decompression may be helpful if there is an isolated stricture at the ampulla of Vater that is not adequately treated endoscopically. In long-term cases, progressive jaundice and liver failure may develop.

Pancreatic Diseases

Pancreatic diseases in AIDS have received little attention. The pancreas may be affected as part of a systemic complication such as CMV, MAI, fungal infection, Kaposi's sarcoma, or lymphoma.[190] Pancreatic involvement often is not recognized before death. Some AIDS patients have presented with an acute pancreatitis. The disease, which is clinically mild in most cases, is asso-

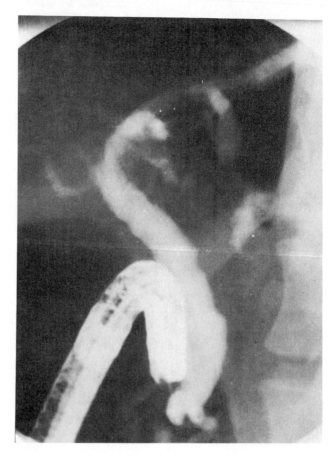

Figure 15–15.   Endoscopic retrograde cholangiogram demonstrating irregularity of the intrahepatic and extrahepatic bile ducts.

ciated with abdominal pain, nausea, vomiting, and elevations in serum amylase and lipase concentrations. In some cases a medication such as trimethoprim-sulfa can be implicated, while in others no etiologic agent can be found. IV pentamidine therapy for *Pneumocystis* pneumonia has been associated with hypoglycemia, owing to selective damage to beta cells in the islets of Langerhans.[191] A few patients have become insulin-requiring diabetics after pentamidine therapy. Hyperlipidemic pancreatitis has been observed in a few patients receiving IV lipids. There are no reports of chronic pancreatitis occurring as a specific complication of AIDS. Pancreatic insufficiency is an uncommon cause of fat malabsorption in AIDS patients.[192]

REFERENCES

1. Connolly GM, Shanson D, Hawkins DDA et al: Non-cryptosporidial diarrhoea in human immunodeficiency virus (HIV) infected patients. Gut 30:195, 1989
2. Rene E, Marche C, Requier B et al: Intestinal infections in patients with acquired immunodeficiency syndrome:

A prospective study in 132 patients. Dig Dis Sci 34:773, 1989

3. Horowitz S, Lorenzsonn VW, Olsen WA et al: Small intestinal disease in T cell deficiency. J Pediatr 85:457, 1974

4. Bienenstock J: The mucosal immunological network. Ann Allergy 53:535, 1984

5. Berkelman RB, Heyward WL, Stehr-Green JK, Curran JW: Epidemiology of human immunodeficiency virus infection and acquired immunodeficiency syndrome. Ann Intern Med 86:761, 1989

6. Kotler DP, Reka S: Intestinal mucosal inflammation associated with human immunodeficiency virus infection. Unpublished manuscript, 1991

7. Hodges JR, Wright R: Normal immune responses in the gut and liver. Clin Sci 63:339, 1982

8. Wolf JL, Bye WA: The membraneous epithelial (M) cell and the mucosal immune system. Annu Rev Med 35:95, 1984

9. Richman LK, Graeff AS, Yarchoan R, Strober W: Simultaneous induction of antigen-specific IgA helper T cells and IgG suppressor T cells in the murine Peyer's patch after protein feeding. J Immunol 126:2079, 1981

10. Guy-Grand D, Griscelli C, Vassalli P: The mouse gut lymphocyte, a novel type of T cell: Nature, origin and trafficking in normal and graft-vs-host conditions. J Exp Med 148:1661, 1978

11. Selby WS, Janossy G, Goldstein G, Jewell DP: T lymphocyte subsets in human intestinal mucosa: The distribution and relationship to MHC-derived antigens. Clin Exp Immunol 44:453, 1981

12. Marsh MN, Hinde J: Inflammatory component of celiac sprue mucosa: I. Mast cells, basophils and eosinophils. Gastroenterology 89:92, 1985

13. Selby WS, Janossy G, Bofill M, Jewell DP: Lymphocyte subpopulations in the human small intestine: The findings in normal mucosa and in the mucosa of patients with adult celiac disease. Clin Exp Immunol 52:219, 1983

14. Tomasi TB Jr, Tan EM, Solomon A, Prendergast RA: Characteristics of an immune system common to certain external secretions. J Exp Med 121:101, 1965

15. Green DR, Gold J, St Martin S, Gershon R, Gershon RK: Microenvironmental immunoregulation: Possible role of contrasuppressor cells in maintaining immune responses in gut-associated lymphoid tissues. Proc Natl Acad Sci USA 79:889, 1982

16. Kagnoff MF: Oral tolerance. Ann NY Acad Sci 392:248, 1982

17. Walker WA: Host defense mechanisms in the gastrointestinal tract. Pediatrics 57:901, 1976

18. Edwards PAW: Is mucus a selective barrier for macromolecules? Br Med Bull 34:55, 1971

19. Zubrzycki L, Spaulding EH: Studies on the stability of the normal fecal flora. J Bacteriol 83:968, 1962

20. Bartlett JG, Chang T, Taylor NS, Onderdonk AB: Colitis induced by *Clostridium difficile*. Rev Infect Dis 1:370, 1979

21. Rodgers VD, Fassett R, Kagnoff MF: Abnormalities in intestinal mucosal T cells in homosexual populations including those with the lymphadenopathy syndrome and acquired immunodeficiency syndrome. Gastroenterology 90:552, 1986

22. Ellakany S, Whiteside TL, Schade RR, van Thiel DH: Analysis of intestinal lymphocyte subpopulations in patients with acquired immunodeficiency syndrome (AIDS) and AIDS-related complex. Am J Clin Pathol 87:356, 1987

23. Budhraja M, Levandoglu H, Kocka F et al: Duodenal mucosal T cell subpopulation and bacterial cultures in acquired immune deficiency syndrome. Am J Gastroenterol 82:427, 1987

24. Kotler DP, Francisco A, Goldie P et al: Preservation of natural killer cell phenotypes in rectal mucosa in AIDS. Gastroenterology 88:1455A, 1985

25. Bekesi JG, Tsang P, Lew F et al: Functional integrity of T, B, and natural killer cells in homosexual subjects with prodromata and in patients with AIDS. Ann NY Acad Sci 437:28, 1984

26. Weber JR, Dobbins WO: The intestinal and rectal epithelial lymphocyte in AIDS. Am J Surg Pathol 10:627, 1986

27. Ulrich R, Zeitz M, Heise W et al: Mucosal atrophy is associated with loss of activated T cells in the duodenal mucosa of human immunodeficiency virus (HIV)-infected patients. Digestion 46:302, 1990

28. Kotler DP, Tierney AR, Scholes JV: Intestinal plasma cell alterations in the acquired immunodeficiency syndrome. Dig Dis Sci 32:129, 1987

29. Jackson S, Dawson LM, Kotler DP: IgA$_1$ is the major immunoglobulin component of immune complexes in the acquired immune deficiency syndrome. J Clin Immunol 8:64, 1988

30. Jackson S, Tarkowski A, Collins JE et al: Occurrence of polymeric immunoglobulin A1 rheumatoid factor in the acquired immune deficiency syndrome. J Clin Immunol 9:390, 1988

31. Kotler DP, Reka S, Borcich A, Cronin WJ: Detection, localization and quantitation of HIV-associated antigens in intestinal biopsies from HIV-infected patients. Am J Pathol 139:823, 1991

32. Fox CH, Kotler DP, Tierney AR et al: Detection of HIV-1 RNA in intestinal lamina propria of patients with AIDS and gastrointestinal disease. J Infect Dis 159:467, 1989

33. Harriman GR, Smith PD, McDonald KH et al: Vitamin B$_{12}$ malabsorption in patients with the acquired immunodeficiency syndrome. Arch Intern Med 149:2039, 1989

34. Nelson JA, Wiley CA, Reynolds-Kohler C et al: Human immunodeficiency virus detected in bowel epithelium from patients with gastrointestinal symptoms. Lancet 2:259, 1988

35. Mathijs JM, Hing M, Grierson J et al: HIV infection of rectal mucosa. Lancet 1:1111, 1988

36. Jarry A, Cortez A, Rene E et al: Infected cells and immune cells in the gastrointestinal tract of AIDS patients: An immunohistochemical study of 127 cases. Histopathology 16:133, 1990

37. Ullrich R, Zeitz M, Heise M et al: Small intestinal structure and function in patients infected with human immunodeficiency virus (HIV): Evidence for HIV-induced enteropathy. Ann Intern Med 111:15, 1989

38. Heise C, Dandekar S, Donovan R et al: HIV infection of jejunal mucosa in AIDS and ARC: Association with intestinal function. FASEB J 3:757A, 1989

39. Moyer MP, Huot RI, Ramirez A Jr et al: Infection of human gastrointestinal cells by HIV-1. AIDS Res Hum Retroviruses 66:1409, 1990

40. Adachi A, Koenig S, Gendelman HE et al: Productive, persistent infection of human colorectal cell lines with human immunodeficiency virus. J Virol 61:209, 1987

41. Bourinbaiar AS, Phillip DM: Transmission of human immunodeficiency virus from monocytes to epithelia. J AIDS 4:55, 1991

42. Hoover EA, Mullins JI, Quackenbush SL et al: Experi-

mental transmission and pathogenesis of immunodeficiency syndrome in cats. Blood 70:1880, 1987

43. Clayton F, Sigal S, Reka S, Kotler DP: Colonic mucosal injury and inflammation associated with human immunodeficiency virus type-1 (HIV) infection (abstr). Lab Invest 64:34A, 1991

44. Reichert CM, O'Leary TJ, Levens DL et al: Autopsy pathology in the acquired immune deficiency syndrome. Am J Pathol 112:357, 1983

45. Drew WL, Mintz L, Miner RC et al: Prevalence of cytomegalovirus infection in homosexual men. J Infect Dis 143:188, 1981

46. Lange M, Klein EB, Kornfield H et al: Cytomegalovirus isolation from healthy homosexual men. JAMA 252:1908, 1984

47. Rotterdam H: Tissue diagnosis of selected AIDS-related opportunistic infections. Am J Surg Pathol 11(suppl):3, 1987

48. Martin DC, Katzenstein DA, Yu GSM et al: Cytomegalovirus viremia detected by molecular hybridization and electron microscopy. Ann Intern Med 100:222, 1984

49. Culpepper-Morgan J, Kotler DP, Tierney AR, Scholes JV: Evaluation of diagnostic criteria for disseminated cytomegalovirus infection in the acquired immune deficiency syndrome. Am J Gastroenterol 82:1264, 1987

50. Clayton F, Klein EB, Kotler DP: Correlation of in situ hybridization with histology and viral culture in AIDS patients with cytomegalovirus colitis. Arch Pathol Lab Med 113:124, 1989

51. Koretz SH, Buhles WC, Brewin A et al: Treatment of serious cytomegalovirus infections using 9-(1,3-dihydroxy-2-propoxy-methyl) guanine in patients with AIDS and other immunodeficiencies. N Engl J Med 314:801, 1986

52. Kotler DP, Tierney AR, Altilio D et al: Body mass repletion during ganciclovir therapy of cytomegalovirus infections in patients with the acquired immunodeficiency syndrome. Arch Intern Med 149:901, 1989

53. Kotler DP, Culpepper-Morgan J, Tierney AR, Klein EB: Treatment of disseminated cytomegalovirus infection with 9-(1,3-dihydroxy-2-propoxymethyl)guanine: Evidence of prolonged survival in patients with the acquired immunodeficiency syndrome. AIDS Res 2:299, 1987

54. Dieterich DT, Chachoua A, Lafleur F, Worrell C: Ganciclovir treatment of gastrointestinal infections caused by cytomegalovirus in patients with AIDS. Rev Infect Dis 10(suppl):S532, 1988

55. Weber JN, Thom S, Barrison I et al: Cytomegalovirus colitis and esophageal ulceration in the context of AIDS: Clinical manifestations and preliminary report of treatment with foscarnet. Gut 28:482, 1987

56. Snydman DR, Werner BG, Heinze-Lacey B et al: Use of cytomegalovirus immune globulin to prevent cytomegalovirus disease in renal-transplant recipients. N Engl J Med 317:1049, 1987

57. Siegel FP, Lopez C, Hammer GS et al: Severe acquired immunodeficiency in male homosexuals manifested by chronic perianal ulcerative herpes simplex lesions. N Engl J Med 305:1439, 1981

58. Sixbey JW, Nedrud JG, Raab-Traub N et al: Epstein-Barr virus replication in oropharyngeal epithelial cells. N Engl J Med 310:1225, 1984

59. Lipscomb H, Tatsumi E, Harada S et al: Epstein-Barr virus and chronic lymphadenomegaly in male homosexuals with acquired immunodeficiency syndrome (AIDS). AIDS Res 1:59, 1983

60. Greenspan JS, Greenspan D, Lennette ET et al: Replication of Epstein-Barr virus within the epithelial cells of oral "hairy" leukoplakia, an AIDS-associated lesion. N Engl J Med 313:1564, 1985

61. Knowles DN, Inghirami G, Ubriaco A, Della-Favera R: Molecular genetic analysis of three AIDS-associated neoplasms of uncertain lineage demonstrates their B-cell derivation and the possible pathogenetic role of Epstein-Barr virus. Blood 73:792, 1989

62. Horowitz MS, Valdarrama G, Hatcher V et al: Characteristics of adenovirus isolates from AIDS patients. Ann NY Acad Sci 437:161, 1984

63. Janoff EN, Orenstein JM, Manischewitz JF, Smith PD: Adenovirus colitis in the acquired immunodeficiency syndrome. Gastroenterology 100:976, 1991

64. Sewankambo N, Mugerwa RD, Godgame RD et al: Enteropathic AIDS in Uganda: An endoscopic, histologic and microbiologic study. AIDS 1:9, 1987

65. Serwadda D, Mugerwa RD, Sewankambo NK et al: Slim disease: A new disease in Uganda and its association with HTLV-III infection. Lancet 2:849, 1985

66. Current WL, Reese NC, Ernst JV et al: Human cryptosporidiosis in immunocompetent and immunodeficient persons: Studies of an outbreak and experimental transmission. N Engl J Med 308:1252, 1985

67. Jokiph L, Jokiph AMM: Timing of symptoms and oocyst excretion in human crytosporidiosis. N Engl J Med 315:1643, 1986

68. Zar F, Geiseler PJ, Brown VA: Asymptomatic carriage of *Cryptosporidium* in the stool of a patient with acquired immunodeficiency syndrome. J Infect Dis 151:195, 1985

69. Alpert G, Bell LM, Kirkpatrick CE et al: Outbreak of cryptosporidiosis in a day-care center. Pediatrics 77:152, 1986

70. Tzipori S, Angus KW, Campbell I, Grey EW: *Cryptosporidium:* Evidence for a single-species genus. Infect Immun 30:884, 1980

71. Tzipori S, Angus KW, Campbell I et al: Experimental infection of lambs with cryptosporidium isolated from a human patient with diarrhoea. Gut 23:71, 1982

72. Sloper KS, Dourmashkin RR, Bird RB et al: Case report: Chronic malabsorption due to cryptosporidiosis in a child with immunoglobulin deficiency. Gut 23:80, 1982

73. Snider DP, Gordon J, McDermott MR, Underdown BJ: Chronic *Giardia muris* infection in anti-IgM-treated mice: I. Analysis of immunoglobulin and parasite-specific antibody in normal and immunoglobulin-deficient animals. J Immunol 134:4153, 1985

74. Thea DM, Pereira MEA, Sterling C, Keusch GT: Novel sporozoite surface lectin in *Cryptosporidium parvum.* (abstr 608A). In: Proceedings of the V International Conference on AIDS, Montreal, Canada 1989

75. Marcial MA, Madara JL: Cryptosporidium localization, structural analysis of absorptive cell-parasite membrane interactions in guinea pigs, and suggestion of protozoan transport by M cells. Gastroenterology 90:583, 1986

76. Flanigan TP, Soave R, Kotler D, Toerner J: Clearance of cryptosporidial infection in HIV positive men: A positive correlation with CD4 counts (abstr). In: Proceedings of the Sixth International Conference on AIDS, 1990, San Francisco, CA vol 1, p 251A

77. Greenberg R, Bank S, Siegal P: Resolution of intestinal cryptosporidiosis after treatment of AIDS with AZT. Gastroenterology 97:1327, 1989

78. Heller TD, Tierney AR, Kotler DP: Variable localization of intestinal cryptosporidiosis in AIDS (abstr). In: Pro-

ceedings of the V International Conference on AIDS, Montreal, Canada 1989, p 358A

79. Cello JP: Acquired immunodeficiency syndrome cholangiopathy: Spectrum of disease. Am J Med 86:539, 1989

80. Gross TL, Wheat J, Bartlett M, O'Connor KW: AIDS and multiple system involvement with cryptosporidium. Am J Gastroenterol 81:456, 1986

81. Ma P, Villanueva TG, Kaufman D et al: Respiratory cryptosporidiosis in acquired immune deficiency syndrome. JAMA 252:1298, 1984

82. Casemore DP, Armstrong M, Sands RL: Laboratory diagnosis of cryptosporidiosis. J Clin Pathol 38:1337, 1985

83. Tzipori S, Roberton D, Chapman C: Remission of diarrhoea due to cryptosporidiosis in an immunodeficient child treated with hyperimmune bovine colostrum. Br Med J 293:1276, 1986

84. Ungar BLP, Ward DJ, Fayer R, Quinn CA: Cessation of cryptosporidium-associated diarrhea in an acquired immunodeficiency syndrome patient after treatment with hyperimmune bovine colostrum. Gastroenterology 98:486, 1990

85. Nord J, Ma P, DiJohn D et al: Treatment with bovine hyperimmune colostrum of cryptosporidial diarrhea in AIDS patients. AIDS 4:581, 1990

86. Gathe J, Piot D, Hawkins K et al. Treatment of gastrointestinal cryptosporidiosis with paromomycin (abstr). In: Proceedings of the VI International Conference on AIDS, San Francisco, CA 1990, vol 1, p 384A

87. Cook DJ, Kelton JG, Stanisz AM, Collins SM: Somatostatin treatment for cryptosporidial diarrhea in a patient with the acquired immunodeficiency syndrome. Ann Intern Med 108:708, 1988

88. Canning EU, Lom J: The Microsporidia of Vertebrates. New York, Academic Press, 1986

89. Dobbins WO III, Weinstein WM: Electron microscopy of the intestine and rectum in acquired immunodeficiency syndrome. Gastroenterology 88:738, 1985

90. van Gool J, Hollister JS, Eeftinck Schattenkerk J et al: Diagnosis of *Enterocytozoon bieneusi* microsporidiosis in AIDS patients by recovery of spores from faeces. Lancet 336:697, 1991

91. Orenstein JM, Zierdt W, Zierdt C, Kotler DP: Identification of microsporidial spores in stool and duodenal fluid from AIDS patients. Lancet 336:1127, 1990

92. Orenstein JM, Chiang J, Steinberg W et al: Intestinal microsporidiosis as a cause of diarrhea in HIV-infected patients: A report of 20 cases. Hum Pathol 21:475, 1990

93. Kotler DP, Francisco A, Clayton F et al: Small intestinal injury and parasitic disease in the acquired immunodeficiency syndrome (AIDS). Ann Intern Med 113:444, 1990

94. Chow K, Reka S, Orenstein JM, Kotler DP: Structural and functional correlations of intestinal coccioides in AIDS (abstr). In: Proceedings of the Sixth International Conference on AIDS, 1990, San Francisco, CA vol 2, p 383A

95. Orenstein JM, Tenner M, Kotler DP: Localization of infection by microsporidia *Enterocytozoon bieneusi* in the gastrointestinal tracts of AIDS patients. Gastroenterology 98:467A, 1990

96. Gourley WK, Swedo JL: Intestinal infection by microsporidia *Enterocytozoon bieneusi* of patients with AIDS: An ultrastructural study of the use of human mitochondria by a protozoan. Lab Invest 58:35A, 1988

97. Malebranche R, Arnoux E, Guerin JM et al: Acquired immunodeficiency syndrome with severe gastrointestinal manifestations in Haiti. Lancet 1:873, 1983

98. Kobayashi LM, Kort MP, Berline OGW et al: Isospora infection in a homosexual man. Diagn Microbiol Infect Dis 3:363, 1985

99. DeHovitz JA, Pape JW, Boncy M, Johnson WD Jr: Clinical manifestation of *Isospora belli* infection in patients with the acquired immunodeficiency syndrome. N Engl J Med 315:87, 1986

100. Soave R, Johnson WD Jr: Cryptosporidium and *Isospora belli* infections. J Infect Dis 157:225, 1988

101. Restropo C, Macher AM, Radany EH: Disseminated extraintestinal isosporiasis in a patient with acquired immunodeficiency syndrome. Am J Clin Pathol 87:536, 1987

102. Kazal HL, Sohn N, Carasco JI et al: The gay bowel syndrome: Clinico-pathological correlations in 260 patients. Ann Clin Lab Sci 6:184, 1976

103. Nash TE, Agrawal A, Adam RD et al: Antigenic variation in *Giardia lamblia.* J Immunol 141:636, 1988

104. Stevens D, Frank D, Mahmoud AAF: Thymus dependency of host resistance to *Giardia muris* infection in nude mice. J Immunol 120:680, 1978

105. Janoff EN, Smith PD, Blaser MJ: Acute antibody responses to *Giardia lamblia* are depressed in patients with human immunodeficiency virus-1 infection. J Infect Dis 157:798, 1988

106. Schmerin MJ, Gelston A, Jones TC: Amebiasis: An increasing problem among homosexuals in New York City. JAMA 238:1386, 1977

107. Allason-Jones E, Mindel A, Sargeaunt P, Williams P: *Entameba histolytica* as a commensal parasite in homosexual men. N Engl J Med 315:353, 1986

108. Maayan S, Wormser GP, Widerhorn J et al: *Strongyloides stercoralis* hyperinfection in a patient with the acquired immunodeficiency syndrome. Am J Med 83:945, 1987

109. Russo AR, Stone SL, Taplin ME et al: Presumptive evidence for *Blastocystis hominis* as a cause of colitis. Arch Intern Med 148:1064, 1986

110. Young LS, Interlied CB, Berlin OG, Gottlieb MS: Mycobacterial infections in AIDS patients, with an emphasis on the *Mycobacterium avium* complex. Rev Infect Dis 8:1024, 1986

111. Goslee S, Wolinsky E: Water as a source of potentially pathogenic mycobacteria. Am Rev Respir Dis 113:287, 1976

112. Murray HW, Rubin BY, Masur H, Roberts RB: Impaired production of lymphokines and immune (gamma) interferon in the acquired immunodeficiency syndrome. N Engl J Med 310:883, 1984

113. Roth RI, Owen RL, Keren DF, Volberding PA: Intestinal infection with *Mycobacterium avium* in acquired immunodeficiency syndrome (AIDS): Histological and clinical comparison with Whipple's disease. Dig Dis Sci 30:497, 1985

114. Wong B, Edwards FF, Kiehn TE, et al: Continuous high-grade *Mycobacterium avium-intracellulare* bacteremia in patients with the acquired immune deficiency syndrome. Am J Med 78:35, 1985

115. Chiu J, Nussbaum J, Bozzette S et al: Treatment of disseminated *Mycobacterium avium* complex infection in AIDS with amikacin, ethambutol, rifampin and ciprofloxacin. Ann Intern Med 113:358, 1990

116. Agins BD, Berman DS, Spicehandler D et al: Effect of combined therapy with ansomycin, clofazimine, ethambutol, and isoniazid for *Mycobacterium avium* infection in patients with AIDS. J Infect Dis 159:784, 1989

117. Bach MC: Treating disseminated *Mycobacterium avium*

intracellulare infection (letter). Ann Intern Med 110:169, 1989

118. Hirschel B, Chang HR, Mach N et al: Fatal infection with a novel, unidentified mycobacterium in a man with the acquired immunodeficiency syndrome. N Engl J Med 323:109, 1990

119. Wang HH, Tollerud D, Danar D et al: Another Whipple-like disease in AIDS? N Engl J Med 314:1577, 1986

120. Smith PD, Macher AM, Bookman MA et al: *Salmonella typhimurium* enteritis and bacteremia in the acquired immunodeficiency syndrome. Ann Intern Med 102:207, 1985

121. Baskin DH, Lax JD, Barenberg D: Shigella bacteremia in patients with acquired immune deficiency. Am J Gastroenterol 82:338, 1987

122. Pasternak J, Bolivar R, Hopfer RL et al: Bacteremia caused by *Campylobacter*-like organisms in two male homosexuals. Ann Intern Med 101:339, 1984

123. Laughon BE, Druckman DA, Vernon A et al: Prevalence of enteric pathogens in homosexual men with and without acquired immunodeficiency syndrome. Gastroenterology 94:984, 1988

124. Lake-Bakaar G, Quadros E, Beidas S et al: Gastric secretory failure in patients with the acquired immunodeficiency syndrome (AIDS). Ann Intern Med 109:502, 1988

125. Hornick RB, Musik SI, Wenzel R et al: The Broad St. pump revisited: Response of volunteers to ingested cholera vibrios. Bull NY Acad Med 47:1181, 1971

126. Easmon CSF, Crane JP: Uptake of ciprofloxacin by macrophages. J Clin Pathol 38:442, 1985

127. Neill MA, Opal SM, Heelan J et al: Failure of ciprofloxacin to eradicate convalescent fecal excretion after acute salmonellosis: Experience during an outbreak in health care workers. Ann Intern Med 114:195, 1991

128. Klein RS, Harris CA, Small CB et al: Oral candidiasis in high risk patients as the initial manifestation of the acquired immunodeficiency syndrome. N Engl J Med 311:354, 1984

129. Tom W, Aaron J: Esophageal ulcers caused by *Torulopsis glabrata* in a patient with AIDS. Am J Gastroenterol 82:766, 1987

130. Johnson PC, Khardorf N, Najjar AF et al: Progressive disseminated histoplasmosis in patients with acquired immunodeficiency syndrome. Am J Med 85:152, 1988

131. Bronnimann DA, Adam RD, Galgiani JN et al: Coccidioidomycosis in the acquired immunodeficiency syndrome. Ann Intern Med 106:372, 1987

132. Friedman-Kien AE, Laubenstein LJ, Marmor M et al: Kaposi's sarcoma and *Pneumocystis carinii* pneumonia among homosexual men—New York and California. MMWR 30:250, 1981

133. Beral V, Peterman TA, Berkelman RL et al: Kaposi's sarcoma among persons with AIDS: A sexually transmitted infection? Lancet 1:123, 1990

134. Saltz RK, Kurtz RC, Lightdale CJ: Kaposi's sarcoma: Gastrointestinal involvement and correlation with skin findings and immunologic function. Dig Dis Sci 29:817, 1984

135. Friedman SL, Wright TL, Altman DF: Gastrointestinal Kaposi's sarcoma in patients with acquired immunodeficiency syndrome: Endoscopic and autopsy findings. Gastroenterology 98:102, 1985

136. Laubenstein LJ, Krigel RL, Odajnyk CM et al: Treatment of Kaposi's sarcoma with etoposide or a combination of doxorubicin, bleomycin, and vinblastine. J Clin Oncol 2:1115, 1984

137. Winkler WP, Kotler DP, McCray RS: Nd:YAG laser palliation of Kaposi's sarcoma. Gastroenterol Endosc 35:98A, 1989

138. Ziegler JL, Beckstead JA, Volberding PA et al: Non-Hodgkin's lymphoma in 90 homosexual men: Relation to generalized lymphadenopathy and the acquired immunodeficiency syndrome. N Engl J Med 311:565, 1984

139. Harper ME, Kaplan MH, Marsell LM et al: Concomitant infection with HTLV-I and HTLV-III in a patient with T8 lymphoproliferative disease. N Engl J Med 315:1073, 1987

140. Farman J, Tavitian A, Rosenthal LE et al: Focal esophageal candidiasis in acquired immunodeficiency syndrome (AIDS). Gastrointest Radiol 11:213, 1986

141. Rosario MT, Raso CL, Comer GM, Clain DJ: Transnasal brush cytology for the diagnosis of *Candida* esophagitis in the acquired immunodeficiency syndrome. Gastrointest Endosc 35:102, 1989

142. Lake-Bakaar G, Tom W, Lake-Bekaar D et al: Gastropathy and ketoconazole malabsorption in the acquired immunodeficiency syndrome. Ann Intern Med 109:471, 1988

143. Alessi E, Berti E, Cusini M et al: Oral hairy leukoplakia. J Am Acad Dermatol 22:79, 1990

144. Newman C, Polk F: Resolution of oral hairy leukoplakia during therapy with 9-(1,3-dihydroxy-2-propoxymethyl) guanine (DHPG). Ann Intern Med 107:348, 1987

145. Winkler JR, Murray PA: Peridontal disease, a potential oral expression of AIDS may be a rapidly progressive peridontitis. Calif Dent Assoc J 15:20, 1987

146. Kotler DP, Wilson CS, Haroutounian G, Fox CH: Detection of HIV-1 RNA in solitary esophageal ulcers in two patients with the acquired immunodeficiency syndrome. Am J Gastroenterol 84:313, 1989

147. Kotler DP, Reka S, Orenstein JM, Fox CF: Chronic idiopathic esophageal ulceration in the acquired immunodeficiency syndrome: Characterization and treatment with corticosteroids. Unpublished manuscript, 1991

148. Rabenek L, Boyko WJ, McLean DM et al: Unusual esophageal ulcers containing enveloped virus-like particles in homosexual men. Gastroenterology 90:1881, 1986

149. Kitchen VS, Helbert M, Francis MD et al: Epstein-Barr virus-associated oesophageal ulcers in AIDS. Gut 31:1223, 1990

150. Bach MC, Howell DA, Valenti AJ et al: Aphthous ulceration of the gastrointestinal tract in patients with the acquired immunodeficiency syndrome. Ann Intern Med 112:465, 1990

151. Dretler RH, Rausher DB: Giant esophageal ulcer healed with steroid therapy in an AIDS patient. Rev Infect Dis 11:768, 1989

152. Tracey KJ, Wei H, Manogue KR: Cachectin/tumor necrosis factor induces cachexia, anemia and inflammation. J Exp Med 167:1211, 1988

153. Fong Y, Moldawer LL, Marono M et al: Cachectin/TNF or IL-1 alpha induces cachexia with redistribution of body proteins. Am J Physiol 256:R659, 1989

154. Sclafani A, Koopmans HS, Vasselli J, Reivhman M: Effects of intestinal bypass surgery on appetite, food intake, and body weight in obese and lean rats. Am J Physiol 234:E389, 1978

155. Gillin JS, Shike M, Alcock N et al: Malabsorption and mucosal abnormalities of the small intestine in the acquired immunodeficiency syndrome. Ann Intern Med 102:619, 1985

156. Smith PD, Lane C, Gill VJ et al: Intestinal infections in

patients with acquired immunodeficiency syndrome (AIDS). Ann Intern Med 108:328, 1988

157. Batman PA, Miller AR, Forster SM et al: Jejunal enteropathy associated with human immunodeficiency virus infection: Quantitative histology. J Clin Pathol 42:275, 1989

158. Griffin GE, Miller A, Batman P et al: Damage to jejunal intrinsic autonomic nerves in HIV infection. AIDS 2:379, 1988

159. Cummings AG, LaBrooy JT, Stanley DP et al: Quantitative histologic study of enteropathy associated with HIV infection. Gut 31:317, 1990

160. Mathan MM, Griffin GE, Miller A et al: Ultrastructure of the jejunal mucosa in human immunodeficiency virus infection. J Pathol 161:119, 1990

161. Greenson JK, Belitsos PC, Yardley JH, Bartlett JG: AIDS enteropathy: Occult enteric infections and duodenal mucosal alterations in chronic diarrhea. Ann Intern Med 114:366, 1991

162. Kotler DP, Gaetz HP, Klein EB et al: Enteropathy associated with the acquired immunodeficiency syndrome. Ann Intern Med 101:421, 1984

163. Quinones-Galvan A, Lifshitz-Guinzberg A, Ruiz-Arguelles GJ: Gluten-free diet for AIDS-associated enteropathy. Ann Intern Med 113:806, 1990

164. Hecker LM, Kotler DP: Gastrointestinal manifestations of AIDS. In Conn RB (ed): Current Diagnosis. Philadelphia, JB Lippincott (in press)

165. Rupstra AC, Canning EU, Van Ketel RJ et al: Use of light microscopy to diagnose small-intestinal microsporidiosis in patients with AIDS. J Infect Dis 157:827, 1988

166. Hashim SA, Bergen SS Jr, Krell K, Van Italie TB: Intestinal absorption and mode of transport in portal vein of medium chain fatty acids. J Clin Invest 43:1238, 1964

167. King AB, McMillan G, St. Arnaud J, Ward TT: Less diarrhea seen in HIV+ patients on a low fat elemental diet (abstr). In: Proceedings of the V International Conference on AIDS, 1989, Montreal, Canada p 466A

168. Kotler DP, Tierney AR, Wang J, Pierson RN Jr: Effect of home total parenteral nutrition upon body composition in AIDS. JPEN 14:454, 1990

169. Chatis PA, Miller CH, Schrager LE, Crumpacker CS: Successful treatment with foscarnet of an acyclovir-resistant mucocutaneous infection with herpes simplex virus in a patient with acquired immunodeficiency syndrome. N Engl J Med 320:297, 1989

170. Simonsen JN, Cameron W, Galinya MN et al: Human immunodeficiency virus infection among men with sexually transmitted disease. N Engl J Med 319:274, 1988

171. Hicks CB, Benson PM, Lupton GP, Tramont EC: Seronegative secondary syphilis in a patient infected with the human immunodeficiency virus (HIV) with Kaposi sarcoma. Ann Intern Med 107:492, 1987

172. Sulaiman MZ, Foster J, Pugh SF: Prevalence of *Chlamydia trachomatis* infection in homosexual men. Genitourin Med 63:179, 1987

173. Jones JM, Miller JN, George WL: Microbiological and biochemical characterization of spirochetes isolated from the feces of homosexual males. J Clin Microbiol 24:1071, 1986

174. Penn I: Cancers of the anogenital region in renal transplant recipients. Cancer 58:611, 1986

175. DePalo G, Rilke F, Zur Hausen H (eds): Herpes and Papilloma Viruses: Their role in the Carcinogenesis of the Lower Genital Tract, vol 2. New York, Raven Press, 1988

176. Frazer IH, Medley G, Crapper RM et al: Association between anorectal dysplasia, human papilloma virus and human immunodeficiency virus infection in homosexual men. Lancet 2:657, 1986

177. Cooper HS, Patchefsky AJ, Marks G: Cloacogenic carcinoma of the anorectum in homosexual men: An observation of four cases Dis Colon Rectum 22:557, 1979

178. Frank D, Raicht RF: Intestinal perforation associated with cytomegalovirus infection in patients with acquired immune deficiency syndrome. Am J Gastroenterol 79:201, 1984

179. Biggs BA, Crow SM, Lucas CR et al: AIDS related Kaposi's sarcoma presenting as ulcerative colitis and complicated by toxic megacolon. Gut 28:1302, 1987

180. Kuhlman JE, Fishman EK: Acute abdomen in AIDS: CT diagnosis and triage. RadioGraphics 10:621, 1990

181. Scannell KA: Surgery and human immunodeficiency virus disease. J AIDS 2:43, 1989

182. Robinson G, Wilson SE, Williams RA: Surgery in patients with acquired immunodeficiency syndrome. Arch Surg 122:170, 1987

183. Wexner SD, Smithy WB, Milsom JW, Dailey TH: The surgical management of anorectal diseases in AIDS and pre-AIDS patients. Dis Colon Rectum 29:719, 1986

184. Schneider PA, Abrams DI, Rayner AA, Hohn DC: Immunodeficiency associated thrombocytopenic purpura. Arch Surg 122:1175, 1987

185. Martin P, DiBisceglie AM, Kassianides C et al: Rapidly progressive non-A non-B hepatitis in patients with human immunodeficiency virus infection. Gastroenterology 97:1559, 1989

186. Soloman RE, Kaslow RA, Phair JP et al: Human immunodeficiency virus and hepatitis delta virus in homosexual men: A study of four cohorts. Ann Intern Med 108:51, 1988

187. Hagopian WA, Huseby JS: *Pneumocystis* hepatitis and choroiditis despite successful aerosolized pulmonary prophylaxis. Chest 96:949, 1989

188. Terada S, Reddy R, Jeffers LJ et al: Microsporidian hepatitis in the acquired immunodeficiency syndrome. Ann Intern Med 107:61, 1987

189. Czapar CA, Weldon-Linne CM, Moore DM, Rhone DP: Peliosis hepatitis in the acquired immunodeficiency syndrome. 110:611, 1986

190. Schwartz MS, Brandt LJ: The spectrum of pancreatic disorders in patients with the acquired immunodeficiency syndrome. Am J Gastroenterol 84:459, 1989

191. Bouchard P, Sai P, Reach G et al: Diabetes mellitus following pentamidine-induced hypoglycemia in humans. Diabetes 31:40, 1982

192. Kapembwa MS, Fleming SC, Griffin GE et al: Fat absorption and exocrine pancreatic function in human immunodeficiency virus infection. Q J Med 74:49, 1990

16

HIV Infection in Children

Karina M. Butler   *Philip A. Pizzo*

Of the many diseases and infections that can cause serious morbidity and mortality in children, infection with the human immunodeficiency virus (HIV) stands apart. It is among the most relentless of infections. Unlike the situation with childhood cancer, where one member of a family is ill, we routinely encounter entire families who are infected—infected parents who know that their children will be deprived of parents too soon, uninfected children who must cope with the tragedy of watching family members die, and families for whom the pain and suffering directly associated with infection are increased by the added burdens of secrecy and fear. Today, management issues encompass not only those pertaining to primary antiretroviral therapy and to the treatment and prophylaxis of secondary infections, but also the issues of improved psychosocial and community-based support for the family. In undertaking the management of children with HIV infection, emphasis must shift from the treatment of an acute or subacute illness to the management of a chronic condition. In designing therapeutic strategies, the family unit must be considered and, where possible, care of parents and children coordinated so that access to care can be optimized.

EPIDEMIOLOGY

The acquired immunodeficiency syndrome (AIDS) was first reported to occur in homosexual males[1-6] and intravenous (IV) drug users.[5] It was rapidly characterized as a syndrome of profound immunodeficiency that resulted in the development of unusual opportunistic infections,[4-9] unusual manifestations of more common infections,[6,9] and malignancy.[3,9,10] The casual mention of an infected woman in an editorial on opportunistic infections and Kaposi's sarcoma in homosexual men[11] gave little warning of the epidemic that was to afflict women

and children, as well as men, worldwide. One year later a new immune deficiency syndrome in infants that shared many of the features of the adult syndrome was described. The possibility of transmission of an infective agent from mother to infant was hypothesized[12] and subsequently validated.[13-15] Isolation of the human immunodeficiency virus (HIV-1) in 1983[16] and the development of culture and serodiagnostic techniques[17-20] allowed confirmation of HIV, then referred to as human T-cell lymphotropic virus type III (HTLV-III) or lymphadenopathy-associated virus (LAV), as the novel cause of AIDS. In the same period, the occurrence of AIDS in transfused infants brought recognition of the second most common mode of transmission of infection to children, transfusion of contaminated blood or blood products.[21-23]

Of the 2,963 cases of AIDS in children reported to the Centers for Disease Control (CDC) by March 31, 1991, 84% resulted from mother-to-infant transmission of infection (also referred to as perinatal or vertical transmission) and 391 cases (14%) developed following transfusion of contaminated blood or blood products. Other less common modes of transmission to children include child sexual abuse[24] and, rarely, breast-feeding.[25]

Additionally, 670 cases in adolescents have been reported to the CDC. In adolescents the predominant mode of transmission has been through the transfusion of contaminated blood or blood products; however, homosexual or bisexual contact accounts for about 30% of adolescent cases, particularly in the older age groups. As in adults, IV drug use and heterosexual transmission of infection are the other important categories of transmission in this age group.[26] The male–female ratio is correspondingly lower in infected adolescents than in adults, 3:1 *versus* 9:1. The higher percentage of females among infected adolescents further amplifies the problem. These are the individuals at greatest risk of becoming single teenage mothers and transmitting the infection to their infants, and who are least able to cope with taking care of an HIV-infected infant. As a group, adolescents, with their inherent sense of invulnerability, are least likely to modify their behavior in response to concerns of infection. It is alarming that a good factual knowledge of HIV infection is unlikely to alter the sexual behavior of hemophiliac adolescents.[27] This underscores the need for aggressive preventative intervention in this population.

Mother-to-Infant Transmission

Because mother-to-infant transmission accounts for the majority of infections in children, consideration of HIV infection in children must also include consideration of HIV-infected women. Although the 16,805 cases of AIDS in women, 77% of which were in women 20 to 45 years of age, represent just less than 10% of the 171,876 cases reported to the CDC as of March 31, 1991, these figures do not adequately reflect the risk of infection to future children. A national seroprevalence study has recently estimated the overall prevalence of HIV infection among childbearing women to be 0.15%.[28] This rate varies by race, ethnicity, and geographic location.[29-32] In selected urban hospitals in the northeastern United States, up to 7.8% of women seen during 1986–1989 for non-HIV-related causes were seropositive,[33] and in 1987, 3% of women attending a clinic for sexually transmitted diseases in Baltimore were seropositive,[34] whereas the overall seroprevalence rate for women students attending 19 universities throughout the United States was 0.02%.[35] In areas of high seroprevalence the relative proportion of infected women is greater, reflecting the growing importance of heterosexual transmission of infection.

Based on such studies, and on the incidence of AIDS (adjusted for reporting delays), it was estimated that 1,600 to 2,200 infected children would be born in 1991 alone,[28,36] and that in the next 3 years, 6,300 to 9,400 infected children would be born in the United States.[36] The marked overrepresentation of minority and disadvantaged women among HIV-infected women (52% of reported cases of AIDS occur in African-Americans and 21% in Hispanics) is reflected in the racial and ethnic distribution of HIV infection in children. Eighty-two percent of cases in children less than 5 years old reported to the CDC through 1990 were in African-American and Hispanic children.[37] Overall, 71% of cases of infection in women can be linked to IV drug use, either by the woman herself or by a sexual contact. A smaller number of cases are associated with sexual contact with an infected hemophiliac, bisexual or otherwise infected male, birth in a Pattern II country (*i.e.,* those countries where most of the reported cases are associated with heterosexual transmission and the male-to-female ratio is approximately 1:1), or transfusion. Although often heroic in their efforts to seek care for their children, infected women, who come predominantly from a background of poverty, drug use, and depen-

dency, are often poorly equipped to bring about the life-style changes necessary for their own and their families' needs.

HIV infection is significantly affecting the health of our children. Although reported cases of AIDS in children account for just about 2% of reported cases in the United States thus far, AIDS ranks among the top ten causes of death in infants, children, and adolescents. In New York and New Jersey it is the second leading cause of death of African-American children aged 1 to 4 years. Overall, it has surpassed all other infections as a cause of death and is likely to rank among the top five causes of death within the next several years. Furthermore, although the number of adolescents with AIDS is relatively small, the rapid increase in the number of affected individuals 20 to 29 years old, coupled with a median latency period after infection of 8 to 10 years, is indicative of acquisition of infection during adolescence.

The effect of HIV infection on children must also be considered on a global scale. HIV infection has reached pandemic proportions, with cases of AIDS reported from 152 countries worldwide. Seroprevalence rates in parts of Africa range from 5% to 30%,[38-40] and a rate of 10% has been reported from Haiti.[41] AIDS is contributing significantly to infant mortality in these developing countries, which are already beset by problems of poverty, poor nutrition, and diarrheal diseases. In a prospective study of perinatal transmission of HIV infection in Kinshasa, Zaire, 21% of infants born to seropositive mothers died in the first year of life, compared with 3.8% of infants born to seronegative mothers.[38] In a similar study in Haiti, the mortality rate for infants born to seropositive mothers was 23.4%, compared with 10.8% for infants born to seronegative women.[41]

One of the remarkable features to emerge from this epidemic is that not all infants born to infected mothers are infected. Although early reports suggested transmission rates of high as 40% to 50%,[42] the European Collaborative Group study (ECG) reported a transmission rate as low as 12.9% in infants born to HIV-infected mothers, 97% of whom did not have AIDS at the time of delivery.[43] In prior studies transmission rates clustered between 25% and 40%.[38,41,44-46] The higher rates in some of these studies might in part be explained by the greater number of symptomatic mothers participating—18% of the mothers in the study carried out by Ryder and colleagues had AIDS, compared with 2.8% of mothers participating in the ECSG[38,43]—or by the differing criteria accepted as confirmation of infection. Whereas some studies with high transmission rates accepted viral culture or polymerase chain reaction (PCR) results as clear evidence of infection,[47,48] in their 1991 report the ECSG did not.[43] Even after the different criteria are accounted for, however, the transmission rate determined in that study remains much lower than any previously determined. More information pertaining to the correct interpretation of positive viral culture or PCR results in an otherwise apparently healthy seroreverter will be gained as these children are monitored throughout childhood. As additional information on the vertical transmission of HIV infection becomes available, and as techniques of early diagnosis improve, it is likely that considerable variability in transmission rates, dependent on geographic location and stage of maternal disease, among other factors, will be found.

As yet we do not know the relative proportions of infants infected *in utero,* during delivery, or postpartum. This information is critical to the development of strategies aimed at interrupting vertical transmission. Evidence supporting *in utero* passage of the virus from the mother to the infant includes recovery of the virus from fetal tissue as early as 8 to 15 weeks' gestation,[49,50] recognition that placental cells can be infected,[51] detection of natural infection of the placenta by *in situ* hybridization techniques,[50] culture of virus from cord blood,[52] and detection of proviral sequences in the blood of newborn infants.[47,53-55] In addition, craniofacial dysmorphic features suggestive of an HIV-related embryopathy have been reported[56] but not confirmed.[43,57]

Undoubtedly, transmission can occur *in utero;* however, in a number of cases infection may not occur until delivery. During delivery the infant is exposed to considerable amounts of maternal blood and body fluids, and HIV has been recovered from cervical and vaginal secretions.[58,59] Thus, the infant may become infected in a manner analogous to the acquisition of hepatitis B infection. Although there are as yet no firm data to support this speculation, circumstantial evidence abounds. The spectrum of clinical manifestations in the perinatally infected child varies considerably. Some become ill rapidly and have a progressive course, often developing serious opportunistic infection within the first year of life. Others may remain asymptomatic for up to 10 years. It is possible that these different courses reflect different modes and timing of infection. This hypothesis is further strengthened by the failure of PCR techniques, a very sensitive method of viral detection, to detect proviral sequences in cord and peripheral blood of some neonates who subsequently prove to be infected.[55]

Transmission of HIV infection to an infant *via* breast milk has also been reported;[60] however, the importance of breast-feeding as a route of transmission of infection remains a matter of study. Despite anecdotal reports of infection occurring in this manner and the suggestion, from at least one prospective study, that breast-fed infants were at higher risk of infection than bottle-fed infants,[44] other studies have thus far failed to confirm a higher risk of infection.[38,61] However, the best group of mother-infant pairs in which to define those at risk for postpartum transmission may not have been incorporated into these studies. Anecdotal reports suggest that HIV transmission through breast milk may occur only when the mother is acutely infected and before maternal antibody has been generated. Focusing on a group of mothers who are seronegative at delivery but who are at high risk for infection may help determine this risk. This information is unlikely to be gathered in the United States, where breast-feeding by seropositive women is appropriately discouraged. However, recommendations differ in Third World countries because reliable milk substitutes are not as readily available. There, breast-feeding is encouraged because the increased mortality from diarrheal syndromes among bottle-fed infants is thought to outweigh any potential benefit derived from the lower risk of transmission of HIV.[25] As part of an ongoing study of perinatal transmission in Africa, attention is being directed to seronegative mother-infant pairs at high risk for conversion in the postpartum period; the study should provide important data on postpartum transmission.[62] In all likelihood transmission will eventually be proven to occur during many stages of pregnancy and delivery and during the postnatal period; however, determining the proportions of infants infected at each stage will help determine future therapeutic strategies.

It is equally important to determine those factors that might influence the rate of transmission. A number of studies that have attempted to answer this question are summarized in Table 16–1. As noted above, the precise role of breast-feeding remains to be determined. Factors that do not appear to influence transmission include the mode of delivery[44,61] and the ultimate residence of the infant.[44]

The potential importance of the maternal immune system in vertical transmission has led several investigators to assess the role of maternal antibodies in preventing transmission. The presence in serum of maternal HIV-neutralizing antibody[63,64] and maternal anti-p24 antibody[63] does not appear to influence transmission rates. Intense interest, however, has focused on the potential role of maternal antibody to a variety of epitopes within the envelope glycoprotein, including antibodies to epitopes in and around the principal neutralizing domain (PND), or the V3 hypervariable loop, in preventing transmission. Although some of these factors have correlated with transmission or a lack thereof, results have not been consistent between studies.[63,65,66] It is fair to say that the evidence supports a role for antibodies in transmission, but that the precise nature of that role remains undefined. Although a low maternal CD4 count had been postulated as one factor that might adversely influence transmission rates, results from different studies have not been uniformly consistent. The studies of Ryder *et al*[38] and Boue *et al*[67] tend to support the association of low maternal CD4 count and higher transmission rates, whereas that of Goedert *et al* does not.[63] However, one must take into account the overall distribution of CD4 counts within the enrolled population. Additional factors that may increase the risk of transmission include the level of maternal viremia[67] and p24 antigenemia.[67] Reports of uninfected siblings born to mothers who had previously delivered infected children,[68] and reports of discordance between twins,[57,69] indicate that the stage of maternal disease is not the only factor influencing the likelihood of disease transmission.

Of major importance in all studies of transmission

Table 16–1. Summary of Studies on Factors Potentially Influencing Maternal-Infant Transmission of HIV Infection

Factors That Might Influence Transmission	Effects			
	None	↑ Risk	↓ Risk	Undecided
Mode of delivery	1, 2, 3			4
Prematurity	3	2		
Breast-feeding	3	1		4
Infant's residence	1			
Maternal age	2, 5			
Route of maternal infection	1			
Maternal drug addiction	1			
Low CD4 count in mother	2	6, 7		1
Maternal viremia		7		
Maternal p24 antigenemia	8	7, 9		
Maternal antibody status:				
Low anti-HIV Ab		10		
Anti-p24 Ab	2			
High neutralizing Ab	2, 10			
High-affinity anti-gp120 Ab			2	
High-affinity anti-PND Ab			8	
Anti-PND Ab			11	

Code to reference articles:
1. Blanche et al[44]
2. Goedert et al[63]
3. Hutto et al[61]
4. Mock et al[262]
5. Halsey et al[41]
6. Ryder et al[38]
7. Boue et al[67]
8. Devash et al[66]
9. Borkowsky et al[263]
10. Krasinski et al[64]
11. Rossi et al[65]

is the lack of nonsexual transmission to other household contacts. This finding underscores the fact that in the absence of known risk behaviors, HIV infection is not a readily transmissable disease.[42,43,70]

DEFINITION OF AIDS IN CHILDREN

The AIDS case definition, as originally configured, required the presence of one or more of a number of highly specified opportunistic infections and malignancies, definitively diagnosed, which reliably reflected profound cellular immunodeficiency and for which no other cause could be established. The development of culture and serodiagnostic techniques for the identification of HIV infection resulted in modification of the initial reporting criteria in 1985 and in 1987. Emphasis is now placed on HIV testing as a component of the diagnostic process, and in the setting of confirmed HIV infection, a presumptive diagnosis of certain conditions is acceptable.[71] This modification also takes into account that period of an infant's life, 0 to 15 months, when testing may not yield definitive results, and recognizes the importance of recurrent bacterial infections and lymphocytic interstitial pneumonitis as indicator con-

ditions in children. Thus, establishing a diagnosis of AIDS, which represents only part of the spectrum of HIV infection, requires documentation of specific AIDS-defining illnesses according to CDC guidelines.[71] Although it is useful epidemiologically to determine whether a patient has AIDS, awareness of the full spectrum of HIV-associated illness is important for patient care. The CDC has also developed a definition and classification system covering the full spectrum of pediatric HIV infection.[72] P-0 represents indeterminate infection in children, usually less than 15 months old, in whom infection has neither been conclusively established nor excluded. Children in the P1 category have documented infection, are asymptomatic, and are classified based on immunologic parameters. Children with P2 disease have documented infection and signs and symptoms of infection. Many of the conditions in the P2 classification are AIDS indicator conditions, and the classification is further subdivided as P2B, P2C, P2D1, P2D2, and P2E1, reflecting those conditions, but not all manifestations of symptomatic HIV infection are included in the AIDS-defining conditions.

The CDC classification system is used both in Europe and the United States. In developing countries, where diagnostic facilities may be minimal, a case definition based on clinical findings is used.[73] It is recommended that, wherever possible, the definition based on clinical findings be used in conjunction with serologic testing to avoid overdiagnosing HIV infection.[39]

DIAGNOSIS

Infection is diagnosed either from recognition of a characteristic clinical syndrome accompanied by supporting, though not necessarily specific, laboratory data, from detection of viral antigens, from recovery of the virus from clinical specimens, or, as is most usual, from recognition of a specific pattern of serologic response. In adults and older children HIV infection can be reliably diagnosed if anti-HIV antibody is detected in the serum; however, the interpretation of such tests in the first 15 to 18 months of life is confounded by the presence of maternally derived antibody. Antibody testing is first carried out using the enzyme-linked immunosorbent assay (ELISA) and, if positive, is confirmed with the more specific immunoblot (Western blot) assay. Other less frequently used tests include radioimmunoprecipitation (RIA) and immunofluorescence assays (IFA). Because of its sensitivity and ease of application, the ELISA is used as a screening test. However, in achieving this measure of sensitivity, a margin of specificity is compromised, and false positive tests can occasionally occur, particularly when the ELISA is applied as a screening tool to a low-risk population. The sensitivity and specificity of ELISA testing can be enhanced by using recombinant proteins or synthetic peptides in place of the original mixture of HIV antigens.[74] This modification may replace the currently used ELISA in the future. A diagnosis of HIV infection should be made only when a positive test is repeated, found positive, and confirmed by Western blot techniques. In this way the overall specificity of the testing procedure is enhanced.[75] The Western blot detects antibodies to the various structural viral components: to the envelope (*env*) precursor glycoproteins, gp160; to the final envelope proteins, gp120 and gp41; to the core proteins or group-specific antigens (*gag*) p55, p24, and p17; to the polymerase gene products (*pol*), the reverse transcriptase enzymes p66 and p51; and to the endonuclease p31. Currently the CDC recommends using those criteria proposed by the Association of State and Territorial Public Health Laboratories Directors whereby a test is considered positive if any two of p24, gp41, or gp160/120 are present, recognizing that distinguishing gp160 from gp120 may be difficult and that for the purposes of interpretation they should be considered as one reactant.[76] Any test with identifiable bands but which fails to meet these criteria should be considered indeterminate and mandates careful clinical and serologic follow-up. Persons at low risk for HIV infection and with an indeterminate result persisting on repeated testing probably should be considered negative as they are "rarely if ever infected with either HIV-I or HIV-2."[77]

In adults and children who are infected by routes other than perinatal transmission, these tests are expected to reflect accurately the state of infection within months of exposure; however, seroconversion may be delayed, even up to 36 months, in some individuals.[78] Confirming the diagnosis in young, vertically infected children is more problematic.[79] We do not know when most vertically infected children acquire infection. Failure to diagnose infection in the first days or weeks of life may reflect acquisition of infection very late in gestation, during delivery, or during the postpartum period, rather than insensitivity of diagnostic methods. Furthermore, because of transplacental passage of maternal IgG antibody, detection of HIV-specific antibody in the infant only confirms potential exposure to infection; it does not prove infection in the infant. Therefore, either we must document the presence of antibody beyond the period of maternal antibody persistence (taken to be around 15 months), differentiate between antibody of maternal and fetal origin, or establish antibody-independent methods of diagnosis. The issue is further complicated by the persistence of maternally derived antibody beyond 15 months in a small number of infants,[43] the absence of detectable antibody in some infants with AIDS,[43,44,80,81] and seroreversion in some apparently healthy immunocompetent children despite previously positive viral culture and/or PCR results on more than one occasion.[43] It remains to be determined whether the latter children were truly infected, are in a latent phase of infection, or if they could have aborted infection. Using PCR and viral culture techniques, the CDC failed to confirm infection in any of a cohort of 120 seroreverters, four of whom had initially tested positive by PCR, and concluded that the phenomenon of virus-positive, antibody-negative children, although reported, is rare.[82] The opposite conclusion was drawn by Gabiano and colleagues,[83] who monitored a group of 32 seroreverters; viral antigens were identified in 19 children, ten of whom also had HIV DNA sequences detected by PCR; and in three additional children, the PCR was positive but viral antigens were not detected. The timing of detection of viral antigen in relation to the time of seroreversion was not stated in the preliminary report from this group. Only five of the children had mild symptoms, four of which were transitory and the rest asymptomatic. The authors concluded that a high proportion of clinically well seroreverters were likely to be infected, and on this conclusion based the suggestion that AIDS does not develop in the "nonresponder host." This will eventually be clarified as these children are monitored throughout childhood.

Various techniques have been used to improve the sensitivity and specificity of neonatal diagnosis.[74,79,84] In attempts to detect the specific antibody response of the infant to infection, anti-HIV antibodies of the IgM[45,85-87] and IgA classes,[87,88] which do not cross the placenta, have been sought. The transient nature of the IgM response and interference by the presence of abundant maternal IgG have hampered its use as a reliable diagnostic tool. Although modification of the initial assay system to deplete the specimen of IgG may overcome the first of these problems, the clinical utility of anti-HIV IgM assay as a diagnostic technique remains to be determined. Some investigators have proposed that anti-HIV IgA may be a more enduring marker of HIV infection in infants, since it was detected in 23 of 23 samples from HIV-infected infants over 12 months of age. In infants under 3 months of age, however, results were positive in only 3 of 13.[87] The detection of anti-HIV IgA in 10 of 12 infected infants, 5 of whom were 12 weeks or younger at first detection, is more encouraging.[88] IgA detection in saliva[89] and in tears[90] has also received consideration as a possible adjunct in the early diagnosis of HIV infection. Such methods, if reliable, would be particularly useful for large-scale screening in developing countries. Other methods to determine infant-derived antibody have included analysis of serial specimens by ELISA and Western blot techniques, looking for increasing levels of IgG antibody as measured by an increased optical density in the ELISA and by the emergence of new bands or an increased intensity in pre-existing bands in the immunoblot.[45]

As an alternative to detecting antibody formed in the infant, the *in vitro* antibody production assay detects antibody produced by infant lymphocytes *in vitro*. Lymphocytes obtained from the infant are cultured and the supernatant is screened for the presence of HIV-specific IgG by standard methods.[91,92] In a further modification of this method, the ELISPOT, antibody-producing cells are detected and enumerated in antigen-coated wells to which washed peripheral blood mononuclear cells (PBMC) are added, and the presence of HIV-specific antibody is subsequently determined.[93] These tests may provide a more sensitive and specific method of diagnosis in the early neonatal period.

The detection of viral antigens is a specific but less sensitive way of detecting infection. This may be the result of the abundance of maternal antibody, which allows antigen-antibody complexes to form. Commercially available HIV antigen assays detect core antigen (p24 antigen) and have proved useful diagnostically during the ''window'' prior to seroconversion[94] and in children too ill to generate an antibody response.[80] The p24 antigen levels are thought to correlate, albeit imperfectly, with viral burden and are more likely to be positive in advanced stages of disease;[95] however, they lack the sensitivity required of a diagnostic method. Use of acid hydrolysis may increase the sensitivity of this assay. When antigen is detectable, the quantifiable nature of this assay renders it a useful tool for monitoring disease activity and response to therapeutic intervention.

In most infections, isolation and recovery of the organism remains the gold standard by which infection is proved. Over the years the sensitivity of viral culture techniques have improved, so that HIV can be recovered from more than 98% of infected adults.[96] The use of viral culture in establishing an early diagnosis of infec-

tion in children with vertically acquired infection has not been so straightforward. Although some have reported success using microcultures of unfractionated whole blood,[97] a technique that may overcome the limitations of blood volume requirements, the isolation and growth of HIV remains too laborious, expensive, and potentially hazardous for routine diagnostic use. Furthermore, negative cultures in the first weeks of life do not correlate perfectly with the absence of vertically acquired infection,[48] and it remains to be determined whether the lower sensitivity rate for viral cultures in the first weeks of life is an inherent limitation of the assay system or reflects transmission of infection during the peripartum or postpartum period. Also confusing are the reports of positive cultures in children who subsequently became culture negative, seroreverted, and have remained immunologically healthy.[43,82] This raises the possibility that in at least some of these cases, recovery of the virus may represent contamination of the original specimen by maternal cells or contamination at a later stage in the isolation procedure. An alternative explanation posits the existence of a group of children who spontaneously abort infection. These are obviously critical issues pertaining to the proper evaluation of viral culture as a diagnostic technique in the newborn. In children older than 6 months of age, the sensitivity and specificity of viral cultures approach 100%, although they are still not cost- or time-efficient for routine use. However, in the research setting, quantitation of plasma viremia may facilitate the monitoring of response to antiretroviral agents.[98,99]

PCR is a technique whereby minute quantities of proviral nucleic acid sequences or viral RNA in PBMC can be amplified to a detectable level.[100] Such a sensitive test might revolutionize the diagnosis of HIV infection in infancy,[48,54,55,101] permitting the accurate identification of infected infants and facilitating therapeutic intervention. However, failure of this test to detect the virus in infants who subsequently proved to be infected has raised some important questions. Does this failure reflect test insensitivity, or is it confirmatory evidence of a subgroup of vertically infected children who acquire infection during delivery and thus have levels of viremia below the threshold of detection of the PCR technique? The reliability of the test as a diagnostic tool is further challenged by the observation that infants with a positive PCR test remain immunologically healthy and serorevert. An answer to this question will be obtained only as such children are monitored throughout childhood, as it is possible that the onset of symptomatic infection in this cohort may be considerably delayed. Initial PCR assays sought amplification of proviral DNA, and whereas a positive test confirms the presence of infection, it does not indicate whether infection is active or latent. Amplification of HIV RNA allows the detection of actively replicating virus. Escaich and colleagues have suggested that this can be used as an additional diagnostic and prognostic indicator in infants born to seropositive mothers. In their small series, the presence of viral RNA in newborns correlated with the early development of symptomatic infection.[48]

Although PCR and viral culture techniques approach 100% sensitivity by 6 months of age, these techniques are not readily available outside a research setting. In many infants, however, a diagnosis can be made by this time based on knowledge of the mother's serostatus and the infant's clinical symptoms and immunologic parameters. In the recent ECS,[43] when hypergammaglobulinemia, a low CD4/CD8 ratio, and/or clinical symptoms of HIV infection were sought, a diagnosis of infection could be made with 48% sensitivity and 100% specificity at 6 months of age. Seeking only the presence of hypergammaglobulinemia and a low CD4/CD8 ratio resulted in an increased sensitivity, to 79%, and a slight corresponding loss in specificity, to 96%. Although this may be an adequate basis on which to initiate therapy or to enroll the patient in a clinical trial, waiting until 6 months of age is not adequate for many children: in the same study 64% of infected children had clinical or immunologic symptoms by 3 months of age and 30% had developed AIDS by 6 months of age.

CLINICAL MANIFESTATIONS

Onset of Clinical Symptoms

Although many HIV-associated conditions are common to infected children and adults (Table 16–2), there are important differences in the rate of disease progression and in the incidence of some conditions. Among adults and young hemophiliacs, an inverse relationship between age at seroconversion and subsequent time to onset of clinical symptoms, with a longer incubation period for those infected at a younger age, has been demonstrated.[102] In one study, young hemophiliacs with low CD4 counts were less likely to progress to AIDS than older hemophiliacs with similar CD4 counts.[103] In contrast, in children infected by vertical transmission the incubation period is shorter and disease progresses more rapidly.[104] When this group of perinatally infected children is further analyzed, the onset of symptomatic disease appears to occur in a bimodal fashion.[105] Children who become symptomatic before 1 year of age frequently develop opportunistic infections and have HIV-related encephalopathy.[44,45,104] In this group, opportunistic infection, which manifests at a median patient age of 5 to 7 months, is strongly correlated with the presence of severe encephalopathy, which usually manifests at 9 to 15 months.[44,104] This pattern of disease presentation is associated with rapid progression and early mortality.[44,104] In contrast, children who do not develop opportunistic infection or severe encephalopathy during this period follow a less rapid decline and are significantly more likely to survive beyond 5 years of age.[44,104] The development of lymphocytic interstitial pneumonitis or recurrent bacterial infections as the pri-

Table 16–2. Signs and Symptoms of HIV Infection

Organ System Affected	Signs and Symptoms
General	Fever, malaise, failure to thrive, lymphadenopathy
Respiratory	Otitis, sinusitis, lymphocytic interstitial pneumonitis; pneumonias: bacterial, viral (CMV), protozoal (PCP), and fungal (*Candida* spp., *C. neoformans*)
Cardiovascular	Cardiomyopathy, pericarditis, arrhythmias, arteritis
Gastrointestinal	Anorexia, nausea, diarrhea, wasting, parotitis, oropharyngeal candidiasis, oral hairy leukoplakia, aphthous ulceration, gingivitis, HSV stomatitis, esophagitis (candidal, CMV, HSV), hepatitis, cholecystitis, pancreatitis, enteropathy, colitis (bacterial, viral, protozoal, fungal)
Renal	Nephrotic syndrome, acute nephritis, renal tubular dysfunction
Hematopoietic	Anemia, leukopenia, thrombocytopenia
Endocrine	Short stature, adrenal insufficiency
Central nervous	Loss of developmental milestones, impaired cognitive ability, acquired microcephaly, spastic paraparesis, extrapyramidal tract signs, aseptic meningitis
Ocular	Chorioretinitis (CMV, HSV, VZV, toxoplasmosis), cotton wool spots
Locomotor	Peripheral neuropathy, myopathy
Skin	*Infectious:* bacterial (*S. aureus*); viral (HSV, VZV, *M. contagiosum,* warts); fungal (*Candida* spp., tinea corporis, tinea capitis, *Malassezia* spp.); infestations (scabies) *Inflammatory:* seborrheic, eczematoid, and psoriatic eruptions; drug eruptions
Recurrent bacterial infections	*Sites:* otitis, sinusitis, pneumonia, meningitis, osteomyelitis, bacteremia, urinary tract, cellulitis, bacterial colitis *Common organisms:* *S. pneumoniae, H. influenzae, N. meningitides, Salmonella* spp., atypical mycobacteria
Malignancy	Lymphoma, Kaposi's sarcoma, leiomyoma, others

mary manifestation of HIV infection is associated with a better prognosis than is the development of opportunistic infection or encephalopathy.[44,104] The long-term prognosis for children who are less symptomatic during the early years of life is just unfolding. Although disease eventually appears to progress in most children within 5 years, in a few anecdotal cases perinatally infected children have remained symptom free for up to 10 years. The heterogenicity in both symptom expression and in time to onset of symptoms remains to be explained. Genetic factors, viral strains, cofactors, or timing of transmission of infection (early in pregnancy or during labor and delivery) may all contribute to this diversity.

One further important distinction between vertically infected children and adults has been noted. Whereas the development of serious opportunistic infection is associated with CD4 counts of less than 200 cells/mm^3 in adults, children with counts manyfold higher developed *Pneumocystis carinii* pneumonia.[106-108] Recognition of the importance of age-specific changes in CD4 counts among young children reminds us to be aware of the importance of age-related changes and their potential impact on the manifestations and course of infection in children.

GENERAL MANIFESTATIONS OF INFECTION

The initial manifestations of disease may be subtle and insidious—failure to thrive, lymphadenopathy, slowly progressive organomegaly, an increased incidence of common infections (otitis, sinusitis, pneumonia)—or dramatic: the development of an unusual infection such as *P. carinii* pneumonia. Symptomatic acute infection with a mononucleosis-like syndrome is rarely if ever recognized in children. Common clinical features include malaise, fevers, lymphadenopathy (which may often regress in later stages of disease), hepatosplenomegaly, respiratory tract infections, chronic persistent or recurrent diarrhea, failure to thrive, and persistent mucocutaneous candidiasis. A variety of nonspecific cutaneous manifestations have also been described, including seborrheic dermatitis and eczematoid eruptions.[109,110]

Recurrent Bacterial Infections

In children less than 13 years of age, the development of recurrent serious bacterial infections is an AIDS-defining condition. The increased susceptibility to bacterial infections is due to the multiple immune defects present, including B-cell, T-cell, macrophage, and neutrophil dysfunction.[111-114] Common invading organisms include *Streptococcus pneumoniae, Hemophilus influenzae, Staphylococcus aureus, Meningococcus,* and *Salmonella* spp. Other gram-negative pathogens, including *Pseudomonas* spp., and the coagulase-negative staphylococci assume importance in patients who are hospitalized, have central lines in place, or are

neutropenic. A variety of rare opportunistic bacteria have also been incriminated as pathogens in the HIV-infected host.[115-117] Intravenous immune globulin (IVIG) has been used in an effort to decrease the incidence of bacterial infections in HIV-infected children. Attempts to evaluate the clinical utility of this approach were frustrated by the use of historical controls in the early studies of the efficacy of IVIG. The impression of clinical effect was, however, sufficient to prompt initiation of a large randomized blinded multicenter trial to prospectively assess its impact on the incidence of bacterial infections. The results of this trial have not been published, but the data have been analyzed and a precis of the results disseminated. Although IVIG had no impact on mortality, the incidence of bacterial infection was decreased in the subgroup of symptomatic children with CD4 counts of 200 cells/mm^3 or greater and who received IVIG at a dosage of 400 mg/kg given every 4 weeks. IVIG was of no discernible benefit to children with CD4 counts less than 200 cells/mm^{3,3a}. Because this study was initiated prior to the availability of zidovudine, the impact that antiretroviral therapy might have on the incidence of infections cannot be optimally assessed. An ongoing study is evaluating the role of IVIG given to children receiving zidovudine. Although most clinicians agree with the administration of IVIG to the small subset of children with hypogammaglobulinemia, there is otherwise no consensus on the appropriate indications for therapy. Approaches range from the most liberal, administering it every 4 weeks to all HIV-infected children, to the more restrictive, reserving it for those with CD4 counts of 200 cells/mm^3 or greater and a documented history of recurrent bacterial infections. Although *Streptococcus pneumoniae* is one of the principal bacterial pathogens affecting HIV-infected children, and although the incidence of pneumonococcal infection among the HIV-infected exceeds that in children with sickle cell disease, little has been done to assess the impact of immunization and chemoprophylaxis on the incidence of pneumococcal infection in these children.

Atypical mycobacterial infections, usually with organisms of the *Mycobacterium avium-intracellulare* complex (MAI), contribute significantly to the morbidity and mortality of children with advanced AIDS. Although MAI are ubiquitous organisms and ready colonizers, disseminated disease rarely develops in the absence of profoundly depressed CD4 counts. Infection may present as localized lymphadenitis (a condition frequently encountered in young healthy hosts), asymptomatic bacteremia, or disseminated disease. Fever, anorexia, pneumonia, enteropathy, hepatitis, abdominal pain, and bone marrow suppression are common manifestations of systemic involvement. Meningitis is less frequently encountered. There is no standard therapy for systemic MAI infections. Standard antituberculous agents have been uniformly disappointing; however, the Pediatric Branch of the National Cancer Institute is currently conducting a Phase I/II study to evaluate the safety and activity of clarithromycin, a macrolide antibiotic, against

MAI infection. Other agents in current use include rifampin, rifabutine, ethambutol, etionamide, ciprofloxacin, clofazamine, and amikacin.

Respiratory Tract

Recurrent episodes of otitis and sinusitis are almost universally experienced by children with symptomatic HIV infection and are often the initial manifestation of symptomatic disease. Recurrent episodes of bacterial pneumonias with normal childhood pathogens are also problematic; however, lymphocytic interstitial pneumonitis (LIP) or its variant, pulmonary lymphoid hyperplasia, and *P. carinii* pneumonia are the pathologic processes most characteristic of HIV infection in children.

LIP, originally reported to develop in about half of children with AIDS,[15,118,119] was diagnosed in 20% of pediatric AIDS cases reported to the CDC in 1990.[120] The spectrum of clinical manifestations ranges from asymptomatic to severely symptomatic with progressive hypoxia and dyspnea. Digital clubbing, lymphadenopathy, parotitis, and hypergammaglobulinemia often complete the clinical picture. The definitive diagnosis depends on histologic examination of lung tissue, which reveals diffuse nodular aggregates of lymphocytes and plasma cells within the alveolar septa and peribronchial areas.[119] The typical radiographic appearance is that of a diffuse nodular infiltrate. Although on occasion this can be readily distinguished from the typical appearances of *P. carinii* pneumonia, the considerable overlap in the radiographic features of these two entities prevents their reliable differentiation based on radiographic appearance alone. LIP may be presumptively diagnosed in an HIV-infected child who has bilateral reticulonodular interstitial pulmonary infiltrates persisting for more than 2 months, without other explanation, and that do not respond to antibiotic therapy.[71] In severe cases, therapy with steroids, 2 mg/kg/day, followed by rapid tapering, may be beneficial.[121] On occasion refractory disease requires maintenance steroid therapy. Acute deterioration in respiratory function is more likely due to intercurrent infection than to LIP, and a search for pathogens should be concluded before steroid therapy is initiated. Both the Epstein-Barr virus (EBV) and HIV have been causally implicated in this syndrome; EBV VCA titers are typically elevated, and EBV-specific DNA has been detected in the lungs of affected children by *in situ* hybridization techniques.[122]

P. carinii pneumonia has been a leading cause of death in HIV-infected children. It is the most commonly reported opportunistic infection in HIV-infected children and was definitively diagnosed in 27% of children with AIDS reported to the CDC during 1990. Although *P. carinii* pneumonia can and does develop at any age, it may be the initial manifestation of HIV infection in the young, vertically infected infant, with an average age at onset of 5 to 13 months.[104,107,108,123] *P. carinii* pneumonia has been the presenting feature of HIV infection in more than 50% of children who developed AIDS within the first year of life.[124] Whereas *P. carinii* pneumonia in adults usually represents reactivation of prior infection, in infants the clinical disease is a manifestation of primary infection and is associated with a higher mortality, with a median survival of 1 to less than 12 months.[104,107,108,125]

P. carinii pneumonia can develop insidiously or acutely, with symptoms appearing within hours. It must always be considered among the diagnostic possibilities in the assessment of the tachypneic HIV-infected child. Tachypnea and cough are the key symptoms. Fever, though usually present, may be relatively low grade initially. Cyanosis, often unapparent at rest, may develop during bouts of coughing or exertion. When typical, the radiographic appearance of a diffuse interstitial pneumonitis is helpful in reaching a diagnosis. Radiographic changes may lag behind the clinical presentation, may be atypical, or may be confounded by the presence of chronic interstitial changes. Gallium scanning has been suggested as a useful adjunct in the diagnosis of *P. carinii* pneumonia in the patient with a normal chest radiograph; however, increased uptake is a nonspecific finding found in a number of conditions that may affect these patients and is not diagnostic. The definitive diagnosis rests on recovery of the organism. This has been greatly facilitated by the development of techniques of sputum induction with nebulized hypertonic saline, which leads to vigorous coughing and sputum production.[126,127] In our hands this technique has been diagnostic in children as young as 18 months. Failing this, bronchoalveolar lavage is a highly sensitive method of diagnosing *P. carinii* infection, with a sensitivity of 85% to 97% in adult patients.[128] Only rarely is it necessary to resort to open lung biopsy to establish the diagnosis in other than the very young patient, in whom the former techniques may not be applicable, or, as is more commonly the case, when it is necessary to ensure that there is no other concomitant process contributing to continued respiratory deterioration despite appropriate anti-*Pneumocystis* therapy. However, even this use of open lung biopsy must be carefully considered. In a retrospective study of open lung biopsies performed in 66 adult patients with AIDS, successful therapeutic change was possible in only one patient.[129] The impact of prophylactic agents such as aerosolized pentamidine on the sensitivity of these diagnostic procedures remains to be determined.

Trimethoprim-sulfamethoxazole (TMP-SMX) (20 mg/kg of the trimethoprim component in three to four divided doses) and parenteral pentamidine (4 mg/kg) can be used to treat *P. carinii* pneumonia, with overall survival rates in adults on the order of 75%. Survival in infants is lower. Because of the adverse effects associated with pentamidine, TMP-SMX is considered the agent of choice unless specifically contraindicated.[130] Additional drugs with anti-*Pneumocystis* activity include trimetrexate,[131,132] pyrimethamine-sulfadoxine, dapsone alone or in combination with trimethoprim, primaquine in combination with clindamycin, and a hydroxynaphtho-quinone, designated 566C80.[133] Recent recognition of the beneficial affect of adjunctive steroids in the management of *P. carinii* pneumonia has resulted in the recommendation that steroid therapy be initiated as early as possible in adult patients with moderate to severe *P. carinii* pneumonia.[134] As the pathogenesis of *P. carinii* pneumonia may differ in adults and children, with children experiencing primary rather than reactivation disease, the recommendations of the Consensus Panel were not extended to include children less than 13 years of age. As yet there are no data on the use of steroids in this particular setting. Nonetheless, given the outcome of *P. carinii* infection in younger children despite current standard therapy, we now initiate steroid therapy in those with moderate to severe *P. carinii* pneumonia, but will continue to carefully reevaluate the role of steroids as additional information becomes available.

The recommendations for prophylaxis in children have undergone extensive revision.[124] It is now apparent that normal infants and young children have CD4 counts that are significantly higher than those of normal adults (Table 16–3).[107,135,136] The importance of this finding is reflected in two studies that demonstrate the inadequacy of applying prophylactic strategies developed for adults to the pediatric population.[107,108] The current guidelines for *P. carinii* prophylaxis in children are based on the characteristics of *P. carinii* infection in infancy and the age-specific changes in CD4 cell count (Table 16–4).[124]

TMP-SMX and pentamidine are the two agents currently recommended for the prophylaxis of *P. carinii* pneumonia in adults. Although there have been no trials of TMP-SMX in HIV-infected children, it has documented efficacy as a prophylactic agent in children with cancer. Based on this and on information extrapolated from studies in adults, it is recommended as the agent of choice for the prophylaxis of *P. carinii* infection in children. A variety of regimens can be used.[124] In practice, we administer TMP-SMX (150 mg/m² of the trimethoprim component in two divided doses) on 3 consecutive days each week. To date we have encountered three failures with this regimen.[136a]

The feasibility of aerosolized pentamidine prophylaxis in young children is the subject of current study; however, it is well tolerated by older children and is a potential alternative to TMP-SMX for children less than 5 years old who are intolerant of TMP-SMX. Aerosolized pentamidine (300 mg given *via* Respirgard II inhaler) can be given on a monthly basis. It is significantly more expensive than TMP-SMX prophylaxis. If neither agent is tolerated, or for children less than 5 years old who are intolerant of TMP-SMX, dapsone (1 mg/kg/day, not to exceed 100 mg) can be used. As an alternative we have used parenteral pentamidine (4 mg/kg) as a single IV dose every 4 weeks.

Extrapulmonary infection with *P. carinii* can occur. Otitis, mastoiditis,[137] retinitis,[138] and disseminated disease[139] have been reported in adults, though not yet in children.

Although infection with *P. carinii* is the single most common cause of respiratory failure in children with AIDS, the importance of bacterial infections in contributing to respiratory compromise was highlighted by Vernon *et al* in their review of respiratory failure in HIV-infected children. Of 31 children with respiratory failure, 13 had *P. carinii* pneumonia, but nine had bacterial infection: five with *Pseudomonas aeruginosa* and one each with *Klebsiella pneumoniae, Staphylococcus aureus, Hemophilus influenzae,* and *Streptococcus pneumoniae.*[140]

The lungs may be involved by a variety of other infectious processes, including atypical and typical mycobacterial infections, viral infections (particularly with the herpesviruses), and fungal infection. The contribution of the normal childhood respiratory viruses to morbidity in HIV-infected children is just being assessed. Respiratory syncytial virus (RSV) is a common cause of bronchiolitis in children and can be associated with severe disease in the compromised host. RSV infection of the HIV-infected child is associated with an

Table 16–3. Age-Adjusted CD4+ Counts in Children, Compared With Adult Values

	Child's Age (mo)				Adults
	1–6	*7–12*	*13–24*	*25–74*	
Number tested	106	28	46	29	327
Absolute CD4 count					
Median (cells/mm³)	3,211	3,128	2,601	1,668	1,027
5th to 95th percentiles	1,153–5,285	967–5,289	739–4,463	505–2,831	237–1,817
Percentage of CD4 cells					
Median (%)	52	48	46	42	51
5th to 95th percentiles	36–67	33–63	31–60	32–52	35–67
CD4/CD8 ratio					
Median	2.2	2.1	2.0	1.4	1.7
5th to 95th percentiles	0.9–3.5	0.8–3.4	0.6–3.4	0.7–2.1	0.4–3.0

Adapted from information provided by the Centers for Disease Control.[124]

Table 16–4. CDC 1991 Guidelines for Prophylaxis Against *Pneumocystic carnii* Pneumonia

1. Any infant or child with a prior episode of *P. carinii* pneumonia.
2. Any child with a CD4 count less than 20% of the absolute lymphocyte count, regardless of the absolute CD4 count.
3. and:

Age	Indications
1–11 mo	CD4 count unknown in a) Infant or known HIV-infected mother b) Seropositive or infected infant
	or
	CD4 count <1,500 cells/mm³
12–23 mo	CD4 count <750 cells/mm³ *and* HIV seropositive or infected
2–5 yr	CD4 count <500 cells/mm³ *and* HIV infected
>6 yr	CD4 count <200 cells/mm³ *and* HIV infected

The reader is urged to consult the original CDC publication (reference 124) for amplification of these guidelines.

increased frequency of pneumonia, prolonged viral excretion, and an increased risk of superinfection. The mortality associated with RSV infection of the HIV-infected host appears to be similar to that observed with RSV infection of other compromised hosts.[141] Fatal adenoviral[142] and measles pneumonia[143,144] have been described in HIV-infected children.

Cardiovascular System

HIV-related cardiac abnormalities, first brought to attention by Fink *et al* in 1984,[145] are common in both adults[146,147] and children.[148,149] In children a wide spectrum of abnormalities has been described, including arrhythmias, abnormal contractility, lymphocytic pericarditis, pericardial effusion, dilated cardiomyopathy, and sudden death.[149] In a prospective study of the cardiovascular manifestations of HIV-infected children, Lipshultz, while acknowledging that five of 31 children followed were initially referred because of cardiac symptoms, documented an extremely high incidence of cardiac abnormalities: electrocardiographic (ECG) abnormalities were detected in 28 (93%) of 30, pericardial effusions in eight, and abnormalities of left ventricular function in 28 (93%) of 30.[149] These findings, which did not correlate with the stage of infection, are all the more striking in that 11 of these patients were designated as asymptomatic from HIV infection. This high rate of abnormalities, and their documentation in asymptomatic patients, contrast with the detection of cardiomyopathy in just 14% of perinatally infected chil-

dren followed prospectively by Scott *et al* and the presence of cardiomyopathy only in symptomatic children.[104] The differences between these two studies may well reflect the fact that in the latter study, the diagnosis of cardiomyopathy rested on the presence of heart failure, cardiac enlargement, left ventricular hypertrophy, and ST-T wave abnormalities. Serial noninvasive cardiac monitoring promotes the earlier detection of cardiac involvement, which explains the higher incidence of involvement reported in the former study. As yet little is known of the timing of onset of these abnormalities in the course of infection. In the cohort of children followed by Scott *et al*, cardiomyopathy was diagnosed at 1 to 2 years of age; however, Lipshultz's study suggests that subclinical involvement is an early manifestation of infection. The clinical diagnosis of cardiac involvement is often difficult to make, with disease recognized only at an advanced stage. Cardiac failure can be obscured by the presence of tachycardia, tachypnea, hepatomegaly, and edema, related to the myriad other problems that afflict these children. Noninvasive cardiac evaluation with ECG and echocardiography is a sensitive tool for the detection of these abnormalities and should become part of the routine evaluation of HIV-infected children.

The precise contribution of cardiac manifestations to HIV-related mortality remains to be determined, though cardiac abnormalities are commonly detected on postmortem examination in AIDS-related deaths. On pathologic examination a variety of abnormalities may be detected: nonspecific focal myocardial degeneration with cytoplasmic vacuolization, nuclear enlargement and pleomorphism, focal inflammatory changes, lymphocytic infiltration, focal necrosis, biventricular dilation, and hypertrophy.[148–150] Direct infection of the heart has been demonstrated with *in situ* hybridization techniques.[151,152] The precise cell infected was not determined, though the myocyte has been implicated, and correlation was not established between the presence of virus and either histopathologic or clinical evidence of myocarditis or cardiac muscle disease.[152] Thus, the pathogenesis of HIV-related cardiomyopathy has not been elucidated. It is probably multifactorial in etiology, with infection, immunologic factors, and nutritional deficiency all contributing. Therapy should be aimed at correcting nutritional deficiencies, improving pulmonary function, and treating infection where these are contributing factors. Therapy with inotropic agents and diuretics may also be helpful. In our experience antiretroviral therapy has neither exacerbated nor ameliorated cardiomyopathy in our patients. In addition to cardiomyopathy, an arteriopathy involving small and medium-sized arteries and resulting in aneurysm formation has been described in children with AIDS.[153,154]

Gastrointestinal Tract

The gastrointestinal (GI) tract is invariably involved during HIV infection. Malnutrition and emaciation typify the end stages of AIDS. Anorexia, dysphagia, odynophagia, malabsorption, chronic diarrhea, increased metabolic needs, and infections all contribute to the progressive debility and wasting. As the degree of nutritional deficiency experienced by these patients can be a cause of immunodeficiency *per se,* it is important to optimize nutrition at every stage of this infection. Supplemental enteral and parenteral feeding may be necessary.

Many of the infectious complications of HIV infection involve the GI tract. Oral candidiasis frequently heralds the onset of symptomatic disease. Nystatin suspension, clotrimazole troches, ketoconazole, and fluconazole can all be used to control infection. Esophageal involvement is suggested by the development of painful dysphagia or retrosternal pain; however, in the young child, anorexia may be the only clue to extensive involvement. Although ketoconazole or fluconazole can be used to treat candidal esophagitis, inability to take oral medications or failure to respond can necessitate IV amphotericin B therapy. Herpes simplex stomatitis, esophagitis, and perirectal ulceration also occur. Although herpes simplex infections are usually responsive to acyclovir, recurrence off therapy is common, and chronic prophylaxis may occasionally be necessary. The report of acyclovir resistance developing in patients who had received prolonged courses of therapy is alarming[155] and cautions against the unnecessary use of prophylaxis. The successful treatment of acyclovir-resistant herpes simplex viral infections with foscarnet has been reported,[156] and this agent promises to be useful for treating both herpes simplex and cytomegalovirus (CMV) infection. CMV is a less frequent cause of esophagitis in children and is more frequently implicated in the development of enteritis and colitis. Treatment with ganciclovir may be required. Oral hairy leukoplakia, possibly caused by EBV,[157] appears as a white rugose plaque on the tongue and is less common in children than in adults. Recurrent large painful aphthous ulcerations can also be problematic and may respond to steroid therapy.[158]

Abdominal pain, persistent or recurrent diarrhea, and colitis are all common symptoms in the HIV-infected child. Among the infectious causes, bacteria (*e.g., Salmonella, Shigella, Campylobacter,* or atypical mycobacteria, especially *C. difficile*), viruses (CMV, adenoviruses, rotaviruses), and protozoa (*Cryptosporidium, Isospora belli, Giardia,* and microsporidia) must all be considered in the differential diagnosis. More often no specific agent is identified and other noninfectious causes must be sought. HIV-infected children have a higher incidence of lactose intolerance, which manifests at an earlier age than in noninfected children, and symptomatic improvement can be obtained by eliminating lactose from the diet.[159] The term *AIDS enteropathy* has been coined to describe the syndrome of recurrent or persistent diarrhea in the absence of any identifiable pathogen. The etiology of this syndrome

has not been determined; however, occult enteric infection, direct invasion of the gut by HIV, and localized immune deficiency have all been implicated.[160]

The management of severe diarrhea is problematic. Where a specific treatment is available, it should be used; however, for the most troublesome of pathogens, such as MAI and cryptosporidia, there are no good therapies, and palliation of symptoms may be all that is possible.

Hepatitis in HIV-infected patients can result from infection or drug toxicity. Hepatitis, herpes virus infections, and adenovirus infections can all produce a clinical picture of hepatitis. MAI infection can also result in clinical hepatitis. In many cases no etiologic agent is identified and a direct relationship to HIV infection has been postulated. On histologic examination a pattern compatible with chronic active hepatitis has been described in children with hepatomegaly and without obvious opportunistic infection.[161]

Pancreatitis is a rare complication of HIV infection in children. In adults, it has developed in association with opportunistic infection by CMV, *Cryptococcus, Toxoplasma gondii, Mycobacterium tuberculosis,* and *Candida*[162] and as a side-effect of therapeutic agents. The development of pancreatitis among recipients of parenteral and aerosolized pentamidine,[163,164] dideoxyinosine (ddI),[165-168] and dideoxycytidine (Salgo and Liberman, pers. commun., 1991) has been observed. Pancreatitis unrelated to opportunistic infection or therapeutic intervention has also been described and may be caused directly by HIV infection.[169]

The Kidney

Disorders of fluid, electrolyte, and acid-base balance are common in children with advanced HIV infection. Hyponatremia is the most common abnormality of adult patients;[170] however, renal disease, adrenal cortical insufficiency, GI disease, drug toxicities, and acute intercurrent infection can all interact to produce virtually any pattern of electrolyte disorder.

Renal disease in adult patients has been subdivided into three main categories: acute renal failure secondary to acute tubular necrosis, a miscellany of vascular, tubulointerstitial, and glomerular disorders, and a specific HIV-related nephropathy characterized by the development of proteinuria associated with focal glomerulosclerosis and culminating in early renal failure.[170,171] Although the same spectrum of clinical disease can be seen in children, primary renal disease is a relatively infrequent manifestation of HIV infection, developing in 7% to 9% of children with symptomatic disease.[104,172] In one review that detailed the histopathologic findings and clinical course in 12 children, five had focal glomerulosclerosis and progressed to renal failure within 1 year, five had mesangial hypertrophy, one had segmental necrotizing glomerulonephritis, and one had minimal change disease.[172] Renal involvement progressed more slowly among these children than in adults, and deaths were primarily due to other AIDS-related conditions. There is no standard therapy for the management of AIDS-related nephropathy in children.

Hematopoietic System

The incidence of anemia and cytopenia correlates with disease progression.[173,174] Anemia, neutropenia, and thrombocytopenia can be due to dyshematopoiesis or to increased peripheral destruction of the hematopoietic cells. Dyshematopoiesis can result from infection of the bone marrow (infection with the HIV *per se* or with opportunists such as the mycobacteria, CMV, parvovirus, and *Histoplasma*), from immune dysregulation affecting the normal growth and differentiation of progenitor cells, from direct infiltration of the marrow by malignant processes, from drug toxicity, or from the nutritional deficiencies commonly experienced by patients with advanced disease. An increase in the peripheral destruction of hematopoietic cells is most often immunologically mediated; however, hypersplenism can also contribute.

Anemia is the most common hematologic abnormality encountered. Among adult patients, the incidence of anemia correlates with the disease severity and varies from 5% to 95% in different series. Detailed data regarding its etiology are lacking. The role of erythropoietin in reversing the anemia experienced by children receiving zidovudine is currently undergoing evaluation at the National Cancer Institute. Investigation of erythropoietin response in anemic recipients of ddI, an agent that is not associated with the same degree of myelosuppressive effects as zidovudine, and of the response of these patients both to endogenous and exogenous erythropoietin may be helpful in elucidating the pathogenesis of HIV-related anemia.

Infection with B19 parvovirus is a potentially treatable cause of anemia. B19 parvovirus has been recognized as the etiologic agent of erythema infectiosum (fifth disease) in children, aplastic crises in patients with hemoglobinopathies, and arthropathy in adults, and can cause nonimmune hydrops fetalis. Although infection in the immunocompetent host is usually self-limited, persistent infection in the immunocompromised host can cause severe anemia related to erythroid marrow failure and erythrocyte transfusion dependency. Persistent parvovirus infection in seven HIV-infected adults, six of whom were treated with IVIG with recovery of erythropoiesis.[175]

Leukopenia, generally correlating with disease severity, may be due to lymphopenia, granulocytopenia, or both. Lymphopenia, a major hematologic feature in infected adults, is also experienced by children. It is again important to emphasize that the normal CD4 counts of young children are severalfold higher than those in adults (see Table 16–3). Normalization for age is essential before due significance can be attached to a given count. Leukopathology is not confined to a re-duction in the numbers of circulating cells but also applies to disturbances in white cell function. Defects have been identified, in adults and children, in the cells of both the monocyte-macrophage and granulocyte lineages.[112–114,176] Defects in monocyte function include defective intracellular killing of microbes, antigen presentation, response to chemotaxis, interleukin-1 secretion, phagocytosis, and clearance functions. Defects in T-helper cell function can develop in asymptomatic seropositive patients, antedating significant reductions in CD4 cell numbers.[177] Similar defects have been described in children[178] and may play a critical role in determining susceptibility to infection. The functional defects of B cells in the HIV-infected patient are just now being unraveled. While the most obvious expression of B-cell dysfunction is the dysgammaglobulinemia, characteristic of HIV-infected children, recognition that B cells, like T cells and macrophages, can secrete cytokines, including tumor necrosis factor (TNF) and interleukin-6,[179] illustrates the complexity of cellular interactions in this infection. Unstimulated B cells from HIV-infected persons secrete high levels of TNF-α and can induce expression of HIV in coculture with chronically infected cell lines.[179] The function of granulocytes, which also have the capacity to secrete TNF (among other cytokines), may also be impaired.[114] Roilides and colleagues examined neutrophil function in 25 HIV-infected children. A range of defects including reduced chemotaxis in asymptomatic but not symptomatic children, and decreased bactericidal activity despite normal superoxide generation was detected. Of interest, the bactericidal defects were in part reversed by the addition of granulocyte-macrophage colony-stimulating factor (GM-CSF).[114] GM-CSF and G-CSF can also enhance neutrophil cytotoxicity to HIV-infected cells[180] and may prove important as adjunctive therapy, not just in increasing cell numbers but also in augmenting cellular function. The effects of three dideoxynucleosides on neutrophil function were examined by Roilides *et al,* who demonstrated significant enhancement of killing of *S. aureus* by neutrophils in the presence of dideoxyinosine but not dideoxycytidine or zidovudine.[181]

As early as 1982, thrombocytopenia was recognized as a common manifestation of AIDS. Although megakaryocytes have been shown to express viral RNA,[182] in most cases the thrombocytopenia has an autoimmune basis and is associated with the presence of circulating immune complexes and specific platelet autoantibodies.[183,184] Therapeutic approaches include specific antiretroviral therapy, IVIG, Rh$_o$(D)immune globulin, steroid administration, and, rarely, splenectomy.[185] Immune-mediated thrombocytopenia may be the initial manifestation of disease in children, preceding the development of other symptoms, occasionally by years. Increased levels of circulating immune complexes and the presence of platelet-associated IgG are related to its development, and in this situation there is no depletion of megakaryocytes within the bone marrow. Therapy with IVIG and steroids may be effective.[186] Improvement in thrombocytopenia in zidovudine recipients has been reported in adults.[187,188] In children, resolution of severe thrombocytopenia refractory to IVIG, steroids, and in one case splenectomy, has been observed following initiation of ddI therapy.[168] Thrombocytopenia is also common in children in the advanced stages of disease. Although immune mechanisms can continue to play a role here, often direct involvement of the bone marrow by opportunists such as CMV or MAI compounds the problem.

Examination of the bone marrow may reveal any of a variety of abnormalities, including alteration in cellularity; however the myeloid:erythroid ratio is usually normal. Myelodysplasia is common, and reticulin fibrosis, fat atrophy, and necrosis may all be encountered. Hemophagocytophagia, which is described in many viral infections, has been reported. Lymphoid aggregates, a typical feature in adults, are the most commonly identified abnormality in the bone marrow of infected children.[189] There is considerable overlap in the hematologic abnormalities encountered, and pancytopenia commonly develops as the disease advances. Hematologic abnormalities are not confined to disorders of cell number or cell function. Abnormal immunoglobulins that functionally resemble lupus anticoagulants have been described in a number of patients, both adults and children, but are rarely of clinical significance.[190-192]

Endocrine System

A variety of endocrine abnormalities, including dysfunction of the thyroid, adrenal, and gonadal axis, have been described in HIV-infected adults. Although involvement of the endocrine system in a variety of infectious and malignant processes has been demonstrated at autopsy, the clinical relevance of many of the subtler abnormalities of function that have been demonstrated in the clinically well HIV-infected patient remains to be determined.[193] Failure to thrive (including failure to grow) is very characteristic of HIV-infected children. Among HIV-infected hemophiliacs, deviation from normal growth curves has been suggested as an early sign of progression to symptomatic disease.[194] Although isolated growth hormone deficiency has been reported in at least one HIV-infected child,[195] detailed evaluation of the endocrine system of children with CDC class P2 diseases by two independent groups of researchers has so far failed to identify a single common defect responsible for growth failure.[196,197] Subtle abnormalities of thyroid function were detected by both groups and a relationship to impaired growth was postulated. Schwartz and colleagues found depressed somatomedin C levels in eight of 12 patients, despite normal growth hormone levels. In common with studies of endocrine function in adult patients, subtle abnormalities of adrenal function occur in HIV-infected children. Although cortisol and aldosterone responses are preserved,[196-198]

elevation of basal cortisol levels and the presence of an exaggerated response to adrenocorticotropin (ACTH) in some patients have been noted.[196,198] Abnormalities compatible with a selective deficiency of 17-desoxysteroid hormone production have also been observed.[198]

Central Nervous System

Central nervous system (CNS) involvement is one of the devastating features of HIV infection in children. Encephalopathy is part of the initial clinical presentation of AIDS in 11% to 16% of children.[37,43,44,104] These figures, however, may misrepresent the prevalence of encephalopathy among symptomatic children. Although in two European prospective studies, 27 (29%) of 94 and 2 (31%) of 16 perinatally infected children had neurologic dysfunction,[44,199] in one U.S.-based study, 90% of children with symptomatic HIV infection had neurologic impairment.[200] As children advance through their disease course, the incidence of neurologic abnormalities progressively increases.[200-203] Approximately 30% to 35% of symptomatic children enrolled in the trials of antiretroviral therapy conducted at the National Cancer Institute are encephalopathic.

Different patterns of progression of encephalopathy have been described. Some children follow a subacute progressive course, others a more indolent pathway, and yet others appear to have a static encephalopathy.[203] The manifestations of encephalopathy are age related. Young children suffer delays in attaining developmental milestones, lose those already acquired, and can develop secondary microcephaly, reflecting impaired brain growth. In older children, early signs of encephalopathy include a subtle loss of intellectual ability, difficulty in concentration, difficulty with schoolwork, and behavioral and emotional disturbances. In both age groups, motor involvement characterized by the presence of spastic paraparesis, may dominate the clinical picture. Extrapyramidal tract manifestations, cerebellar signs, peripheral neuropathy, and seizures can all be further evidence of CNS involvement. Brain imaging studies frequently show prominence of the ventricles and sulci with calcifications often, although not exclusively, confined to the basal ganglia area. Frank encephalopathy is easily recognized, but involvement can be subtle and then recognized only when detailed testing of neuropsychometric function is undertaken. The development of HIV-related encephalopathy within the first year of life is associated with a particularly poor prognosis.[44,104]

The exact pathogenesis of HIV encephalopathy has not been clearly elucidated. Macrophages may be the vehicle of dissemination to the CNS. Infection of the CNS, including the cerebrospinal fluid (CSF), spinal cord, and peripheral nerves has been demonstrated[204-209] and further supported by demonstration of intrathecal synthesis of specific anti-HIV IgG. Mounting evidence supports the concept that CNS involvement occurs early in the course of infection,[210,211] however, the precise origins of the infected cells remain controversial. Infection of capillary endothelial cells, mononuclear inflammatory cells, and giant cells occur,[207,209] but whether cells of neural origin become infected *in vivo* remains a matter of debate. Infection of the CNS usually is of low titer, and a direct relationship between all of the CNS manifestations of HIV infection and direct viral invasion is deemed unlikely. However, brain tissue from patients with HIV encephalitis has been found to contain high levels of unintegrated viral DNA,[212] and the level of P24 antigen in the CSF has been found to correlate with the presence of dementia in adults and progressive encephalopathy in children.[213] Thus, a direct correlation between level of infection and the onset of symptomatic disease may yet be confirmed. Immune dysregulation, the secretion of cytokines noxious to the CNS, direct neurotoxicity of some HIV proteins, and coinfections have all been postulated as additional mechanisms of neuropathology. In one prospective study of perinatally infected children, an inverse correlation between the presence of intrathecal anti-HIV antibody synthesis and encephalopathy was reported, suggesting that a failure of the immune system to patrol the presence of HIV might contribute to the development of clinical encephalopathy.[44] Cytokines that have been implicated but not yet convicted in the pathogenesis of encephalopathy include TNF[214] and quinolinic acid (Brouwers, pers. commun.), among others. Inevitably a combination of factors will be found responsible for the heterogenicity of clinical manifestations that have been expediently grouped and designated as HIV-related encephalopathy. Meanwhile, attempts at reversal or amelioration of HIV encephalopathy through the use of antiretroviral agents have been undertaken and improvements noted.[168,215,216]

Acute aseptic meningitis due to HIV occurs in adult patients but is rare in children. Abnormalities in the cerebrospinal fluid (CSF), though not unusual, are typically minor—a mild pleocytosis or elevated protein levels.[202,217] Marked changes in any of the CSF parameters—pleocytosis, elevated protein levels, or depressed glucose levels—should prompt a search for another process, infectious or neoplastic. It is equally important to note that infection of the CNS can be present even in the presence of an entirely normal CSF. Virus has been recovered from the CSF in this setting.[206] The p24 antigen can be detected in the CSF even in the absence of detectable levels in the serum.

A vacuolar myelopathy of the spinal cord causing a progressive spastic or ataxic paraparesis was first described in 1985 in HIV-infected adults, many of whom had clinical evidence of AIDS dementia.[218] HIV has been recovered from the spinal cord and a direct etiologic relationship postulated.[204] More recently, the spinal cords of HIV-infected children were examined at autopsy, and inflammatory infiltrates, characterized by the presence of inflammatory cells, multinucleated giant cells, and myelin pallor, were identified in nine of 16 studied.[209] Vacuolar myelopathy was noted in two cases

and attributed to HIV in only one. Children with spinal cord infiltrates frequently had coexisting brain infiltrates. HIV–nucleic acid sequences, demonstrated by *in situ* hybridization, appeared to be confined to the inflammatory and multinucleated giant cells and were not detected in nerve cells.

Involvement of the peripheral nervous system has been reported at all stages of infection in adults, whereas peripheral neuropathy in children is rare. Dalakas and Pezeshkpour have classified the neuropathies in adult patients into six subtypes: acute Guillain-Barré syndrome, chronic inflammatory demyelinating polyneuropathy, mononeuritis multiplex, an axonal sensory painful neuropathy, a sensory ataxic neuropathy, and an inflammatory polyradiculopathy presenting as cauda equina syndrome.[219] Now, however, as the use of dideoxynucleosides such as dideoxycytidine and dideoxyinosine expands, drug toxicity must be considered in the differential diagnosis of peripheral neuropathy.

Children are less likely than adults to develop opportunistic infection of the CNS, making HIV *per se* the most likely culprit in the development of encephalopathy. CNS toxoplasmosis, cryptococcosis, and CMV encephalitis can all occur but are rare. The incidence of CNS lymphoma is to date distinctly lower in children than in adults. As this may be an artifact of the shorter survival time of HIV-infected children, improvement in antiretroviral and other supportive therapies may result in an increase in the incidence of this and other malignancies.

Myopathy

Myopathy can contribute to impairment of neuromuscular function in children. Again, more information is available on HIV infection in adults than in children. This more likely reflects the relatively limited experience with infection in children compared with adults rather than any real difference in the incidence of myopathy. Myopathy occurs at all stages of HIV infection. An autoimmune myopathy resembling polymyositis may develop in the early stages of infection and resolve with advancing disease. It presents with proximal muscle weakness, elevated creatinine phosphokinase (CPK) levels, and perivascular inflammation on muscle biopsy. In the later stages of HIV infection the etiologies are more diverse and often overlapping: nutritional deficiency, infections, and myelotoxic therapies can all contribute. Symptoms of proximal myopathy can often be obscured by coexisting neuropathology. CPK levels are typically elevated. Differentiating HIV-related myopathy from the toxic myopathy now recognized as a side-effect of prolonged zidovudine therapy may be problematic. Although muscle biopsy can be helpful, discontinuation of zidovudine and observation may be necessary to confirm the diagnosis.

The Eye

As in adults, CMV is the most common cause of sight-threatening disease in HIV-infected children, although it appears to be significantly less common in children. CMV retinitis typically begins with uniocular involvement that progresses over time to involve both eyes. Associated with the presence of plasma viremia, involvement of other organs may be simultaneously identified. The retinitis is generally asymptomatic unless there is macular or optic nerve involvement. It is unusual for children to report symptoms before significant visual compromise has occurred. Early diagnosis, therefore, depends on routine funduscopic examination. In the absence of specific therapy CMV retinitis usually progresses within 1 month and can result in total retinal destruction within 6 months.[220,221] Ganciclovir (DHPG) is the current standard treatment of CMV retinitis; however the development of neutropenia, especially in children simultaneously receiving zidovudine, may be dose limiting.[222,223] Although individual regimens may vary, a typical approach involves a 2-week induction course of therapy, 10 mg/kg/day in two divided doses, followed by a maintenance regimen, given as a single daily dose of 5 mg/kg/day 5 to 7 days per week. Because ganciclovir is virustatic rather than virucidal, relapse is common and reinduction courses are often necessary to regain control of active disease, despite which, survival permitting, disease ultimately progresses in most cases.[224–226] Additional drugs are clearly required for the long-term control of CMV retinitis.

Foscarnet was first reported to be beneficial in the treatment of CMV retinitis in an HIV-infected patient in 1985,[227] and its *in vivo* activity against CMV has since been confirmed.[228–231] Although foscarnet is usually not myelosuppressive, difficulties with its formulation and the development of associated toxicity, notably nephrotoxicity, can limit its utility. Like ganciclovir, foscarnet is virustatic, and relapses have been observed both after the discontinuation of therapy and in patients receiving maintenance therapy.[229–232] Little is known of its safety or efficacy in children; however, in one child with retinitis that progressed despite sequential therapy with ganciclovir and foscarnet alone, the combination of ganciclovir and foscarnet together was successful, with remission of active disease for more than 7 months.[233]

Herpesviruses have been implicated in the pathogenesis of an acute retinal necrosis syndrome characterized by the development of retinal exudates, vitreous opacity, anterior uveitis, and ultimately retinal detachment.[234–236] At our institution VZV has been responsible for at least two and probably three cases of a similar syndrome, two in HIV-infected children and one in an adult. In two cases the retinal necrosis progressed rapidly to blindness despite therapy with acyclovir and steroids. Thus, VZV effects should be added to the differential diagnosis of retinal lesions in this population.

Other rarely involved organisms include *M. avium-intracellulare, Histoplasmosis capsulatum, Candida albicans, Cryptococcus neoformans, Toxoplasma gondii, P. carinii,* and HSV. Routine ophthalmologic evaluations should be part of the care of all HIV-infected children.

The Skin

Kaposi's sarcoma, the most notorious of skin conditions associated with HIV infection, is exceedingly rare in children. However, mucocutaneous involvement by a variety of infectious and noninfectious processes virtually always occur at some stage during the course of HIV infection. Among the common skin infections, staphylococcal impetigo and folliculitis can be very troublesome and may respond to antistaphylococcal antibiotics. *Candida* spp. are the most common fungal pathogens causing thrush, angular chelitis, diaper dermatitis, and onychomycosis. *Malassezia furfur* (also called *Pityrosporon ovale* or *P. orbiculare*) can cause a pruritic folliculitis that may respond to ketoconazole. Cryptococcosis has been reported to cause cutaneous lesions resembling those of *Molluscum contagiosum.*[237] Infections with *Aspergillus* spp. are more rarely encountered; however, cutaneous inoculation has resulted in extensive localized cutaneous disease in at least one patient.

Herpes simplex infection manifests as a grouped vesicular eruption typically involving the perioral area and oral cavity. Herpetic infection can be more severe and prolonged than in the immunocompetent host; however, treatment with oral acyclovir is usually effective. Primary varicella infection can follow a protracted and complicated course, as in other immunocompromised hosts. It is our policy to administer varicella immune globulin (VZIG) to those children with a history of exposure in whom there is no previous history of chickenpox, and to treat those developing signs of infection with IV acyclovir, 1,500 mg/m^2/day given in divided doses every 8 hours. Shingles is the most easily recognized manifestation of recurrent infection; however, atypical zoster with dissemination can occur. Chronic indolent, hyperkeratotic, nodular ulcers are a newly recognized manifestation of chronic VZV infection.[110,238] Treatment with IV acyclovir is useful; however, the emergence of viral resistance may result in clinically refractory disease.[238]

Additional cutaneous viral infections which, although not a serious threat to health, can be very extensive and troublesome include *Molluscum contagiosum* and papillomaviruses. Papillomavirus type 5 has recently been described in association with widespread flat warts in a 10-year-old boy.[239] HIV-infected children can develop condylomata acuminata, which on occasion may be an indication of sexual abuse and may be the first clue to the presence of HIV infection.

Nonspecific dermatitis with extremely dry skin is common and may respond to symptomatic treatment with emollients. Severe seborrheic dermatitis can be the first clue to the presence of HIV infection. Classically involving the nasolabial folds, eyebrows, scalp, and, in infancy, the diaper area, it can be more extensive in the infected patient. Atopic dermatitis, another common condition of childhood, is frequently encountered within this population, even in children without a family history of atopy. Treatment involves the use of emollients and topical steroids as necessary.

HIV-infected children are prone to all of the common dermatologic afflictions of childhood, including infestation with the mite *Sarcoptes scabiei*. As in other immunocompromised hosts infection may follow a severe course, the so-called Norwegian scabies, presenting as an extensive pruritic vesiculopapular eruption in which the thousands of mites inhabiting the skin produce a thickening of the skin that can mimic psoriasis. Secondary pyoderma, alopecia, and hyperpigmentation of the skin can all develop. A variety of treatment regimens are available, including lindane, crotamiton, and benzyl benzoate.

The spectrum of drug-related cutaneous eruptions in HIV-infected children is similar to that in immunocompetent children, but the incidence is much higher. Also unusual is the report of drug-induced erythema multiforme in a 2-month-old infant.[240] Pyoderma gangrenosum[241] and leukocytoclastic vasculitis have also been observed.[110] Finally, nutritional deficiencies must be considered in the differential diagnosis of unusual skin eruptions.

Malignancy

An increase in the incidence of Kaposi's sarcoma was one of the first indications of the arrival of the AIDS epidemic. In adults, Kaposi's sarcoma is primarily a disease of gay white men. The discrepancy in its incidence between this and other risk-factor groups has not been satisfactorily explained. Although described in children as early as 1983,[242] it remains a rarity.[243] HIV-associated lymphomas are also rare in children, in contrast to their rising incidence in adults.[244] Palliation with radiotherapy has been attempted, but the optimum therapy is not known.[245] Of over 200 children referred to the NIH, CNS lymphomas have been diagnosed in only two patients, both of whom succumbed within months of diagnosis. Two additional patients developed leiomyoma, one involving the GI tract and one involving the liver (report in progress). This, together with recognition of three cases (two leiomyomas, one leiomyosarcoma) reported by Gould Chadwick *et al,*[246] and, to the authors' knowledge, the existence of one additional patient with multifocal leiomyosarcoma, is intriguing. Because this number exceeds the number of leiomyomas that would be expected as a random phenomenon, a direct relationship between HIV infection and the development of these tumors is likely. Malignancies have not been a major problem in the management of HIV-infected children to date; however, as survival is prolonged, it is very likely that they will become a major management issue in the future.

VACCINES IN THE HIV-INFECTED CHILD

There are a number of issues to be considered in determining an appropriate vaccine strategy for the HIV-infected child. As in the normal host, the risk and consequences of infection must be determined and balanced against vaccine efficacy and the potential for adverse reactions to the vaccine. Vaccine efficacy has generally been demonstrated in the normal host, and data on efficacy in the HIV-infected child are being gathered. Efficacy is likely to depend not just on the presence of HIV infection but on the stage of immune depletion. All vaccines carry a small risk of adverse effect. In the immunocompetent host these are generally minor and the potential benefits of normal childhood immunization clearly outweigh the associated risks. This balance could potentially be upset in the HIV-infected child, and immune dysregulation might result in an increase in the incidence or severity of adverse reactions. There is little data to support this contention, and evidence to date suggests that HIV-infected children tolerate routine immunization well.[247]

Another consideration is the possibility of vaccine-related disease. Immunosuppression in children has been associated with the development of vaccine-related measles pneumonia[248] and poliomyelitis.[249] For this reason, immunization with live polio vaccine (OPV) is not recommended, and the inactivated polio virus (IPV) vaccine should be substituted. However, there have been no reports of paralytic disease among a number of children who received OPV before the diagnosis of HIV infection was made. For the three other commonly recommended live vaccines, measles, mumps and rubella (MMR), there are no satisfactory killed virus vaccines, and a balance of the potential risk against the risk of wild disease must be struck. The resurgence of wild measles within our communities in the past few years, with fatal infections in some HIV-infected children, has been a harsh reminder of our vulnerability to this infection. As the risk of infection has increased and the consequences are serious, the balance tips in favor of vaccination. Thus, whereas in 1986 the CDC recommended that live virus (MMR) and live bacterial (BCG) vaccines should not be given to HIV-infected immunosuppressed children,[250] the resurgence in measles activity prompted revision, with the recommendation that the MMR vaccine be given.[251] This recommendation was facilitated by the absence of reported serious adverse reactions to measles vaccine among HIV-infected children who had received MMR vaccine up to then.[247,252]

There is less concern regarding the use of inactivated bacterial vaccines—the diphtheria, pertussis, and tetanus (DPT) vaccine and the *Hemophilus* vaccines (HbCV). Their use has been routinely recommended. However, HIV replicates in the activated cell; and one potential concern, of relevance to all vaccines, is that vaccination *via* T-cell activation might stimulate HIV replication and negatively affect the overall course of

HIV infection. This is a hypothetical concern at this point but merits investigation, because if confirmed it would need to enter the balance before any future vaccine recommendations could be made.

CDC guidelines currently advise that DPT, IPV, and HbCV be given to all HIV-infected children. MMR should be given to asymptomatic children and considered for administration to symptomatic children. OPV should not be used. It is also recommended that pneumococcal and influenza vaccines be given to symptomatic children but not to asymptomatic children. Because the response to these vaccines is likely greatest in the earlier stages of infection, and because recurrent pneumococcal infection may be the first manifestation of symptomatic disease, this may not be the best recommendation. As information on vaccine efficacy, the risk of vaccine-related disease, and risks and consequences of the specific infection becomes available, recommendations for vaccination will have a more rational basis.

THERAPY

Although curative therapy is not yet available, some progress has been made, and the enormous amount of knowledge that has been amassed concerning the molecular biology of HIV and the pathogenesis of AIDS is directing the development of more effective management strategies. Although improved and alternative antiretroviral therapies are clearly needed, attention is also being directed toward improving therapies and prophylaxis for the secondary complications of HIV infection—the bacterial and opportunistic infections, cardiovascular and pulmonary dysfunction, and so forth. In 1991, the treatment options for the HIV-infected child are limited. Zidovudine and dideoxyinose (didanosine, ddI) are the only currently licensed antiretroviral agent; however, we can anticipate increased availability of antiretroviral agents with new and expanded indications for treatment and an enhanced ability to optimally use these agents, based on sound pharmacokinetic principles, in the 1990s. Furthermore, as the clinical relevance of surrogate markers of infection is better defined, therapeutic decisions will be made on a more rational basis, with ultimate improvement in the quality and duration of survival of the HIV-infected child. Treatment of the HIV-infected child is best undertaken by a multidisciplinary team so that the myriad medical and social problems encountered by these children and their families can be optimally addressed.

Primary Antiretroviral Therapy

Dideoxynucleosides remain the mainstay of treatment of HIV-infected children. These agents, by selective inhibition of virus-encoded reverse transcriptase and/or DNA chain termination, act early in the virus's life cycle to interrupt the critical transfer of information from RNA to DNA. They are not active against the virus once it has completed the reverse transcription process and become integrated into the cell's genome. Zidovudine, the prototypic agent in this category, is currently approved for symptomatic HIV-infected children over 3 months of age and for those who are asymptomatic with abnormal laboratory values indicating significant immunosuppression. Precisely what constitutes significant immunosuppression in children is not defined. Zidovudine is recommended for adults with an absolute CD4 count at or below 500 cells/mm^3, and although this may be a reasonable guideline for children 6 years of age or older, in whom the normal range of CD4 counts is similar to that in adults, it may not be appropriate for the younger child, in whom normal CD4 counts are severalfold those of adults.

Zidovudine was discovered to have *in vitro* activity against HIV in 1985. Just 5 months later clinical trials were initiated in adult patients, and it was found to be well absorbed orally, enter the CSF, and have a serum half-life of about 1 hour. It has been subsequently proved to significantly benefit HIV-infected patients. Trials evaluating the tolerance and toxicity of zidovudine in HIV-infected children and to determine whether the trends for efficacy were comparable to those in adults were initiated in 1987. At that time, because it was known that inhibition of HIV replication *in vitro* required constant exposure to zidovudine at concentrations above 1 μM and that zidovudine had a short half-life, the first trials of zidovudine in children was designed to optimize the potential for efficacy. At the National Cancer Institute, with a keen awareness of the potential importance of the pharmacodynamics of these agents, and based on the pharmacokinetic data derived from studies in adults, a trial of zidovudine delivered by continuous infusion was initiated. This delivery method allowed the maintenance of a continuous level of drug above that considered necessary for viral inhibition and simultaneously overcame the problems associated with oral administration, namely, frequent dose administration, the availability of zidovudine as fixed-dosage capsules only, and the potential for erratic compliance. Delivery *via* a Hickman-Broviac catheter connected to a portable programmable infusion pump ensured verifiable compliance, an important issue when one is seeking trends in efficacy. The Pancreatic Provider 2000+ pump used in this study was lightweight (660 g) and could be carried in a backpack, shoulder bag, or belt, so that this study could be conducted virtually entirely on an outpatient basis. The IV route of delivery has many drawbacks, including technical demands, cost, the risk of catheter-associated complications, and limited applicability; however, it was important to assess a steady-state antiretroviral exposure schedule early in the experience with antiretroviral agents. Though this trial was designed primarily to monitor the safety of zidovudine and patient tolerance, all patients were comprehensively evaluated by serial immunologic, virologic, and neurodevelopmental evaluations in addition to detailed pharmacokinetic assessments.[215]

Thirteen (62%) of the 21 children entering the study of continuous infusion zidovudine had evidence of neurodevelopmental abnormalities before therapy was initiated. All of the children who had neurodevelopmental abnormalities improved when receiving zidovudine by continuous infusion, with signs of improvement detectable as early as 1 to 3 weeks after the start of therapy. This included improvement in affect and activity as well as the reacquisition of lost developmental milestones or intellectual function. Because serial age-appropriate psychometric assessment was performed on these patients, we were able to demonstrate that after 3 and 6 months of continuous infusion zidovudine, there was a significant improvement in the IQ scores of the treated patients, with a mean increment of 15.3 ± 3.3 points. The increment in the IQ scores in the children who presented with neurodevelopmental abnormalities was accompanied by improvements in some abnormal CT scans and in positron emission tomographs (PET). In this study zidovudine administered by continuous infusion led to a significant and, in a number of patients, sustained improvement in AIDS-related encephalopathy.

At the same time a multicenter Phase I study of zidovudine given IV initially and followed by oral administration was also initiated. The beneficial effects of zidovudine were also demonstrated. In both of these studies, the side-effects of zidovudine in children were similar to those reported in clinical trials in adults. Neutropenia and anemia were the main dose-limiting toxic effects. Since then additional toxic effects have been recognized in children as well as in adults, including myopathy, headaches, nausea, and insomnia. Beneficial effects included weight gain, decreased organomegaly,[215,253] a reduction in hypergammaglobulinemia,[215,253] an increase in CD4 cells,[215] and improved neurocognitive functioning.[215] In some patients, however, there was a discordance in response, with improved neurodevelopmental function occurring at the same time that disease may have progressed at other organ sites. This suggests that the efficacy of antiretroviral agent may need to be determined on a site-specific basis, and that neurodevelopmental assessment is an important surrogate measure of antiretroviral activity in HIV-infected children.[215] Further studies have confirmed the benefit of zidovudine in the treatment of symptomatic children,[216,254] although the optimum route of administration and dosage remain to be determined. Studies in adults have documented equal efficacy and fewer toxic effects with "low-dose" zidovudine therapy.[255,256] Although lower dose therapy in children might be better tolerated than the dosages currently used (120–180 mg/m²/day), because of the high prevalence of neurologic involvement in symptomatic children, efficacy might be compromised. An NIH-sponsored multicenter trial that includes detailed neuropsychometric testing is evaluating two dosage regimens, 90 and 180 mg/m²/day, and should help resolve this issue. The relative merits of the IV and oral routes of administration of zidovudine

in encephalopathic children are being evaluated at the National Cancer Institute. Although the latter study is being performed in children, because of the similarity of the pharmacokinetics in children over 6 months of age and in adults,[257,258] if one method of delivery is determined to be superior, these results will also raise important questions for the treatment of adults.

Zidovudine clearly benefits HIV-infected children. Strategies to overcome the limitations of zidovudine therapy have included using zidovudine in combination with other agents of differing toxicity profile and the addition of agents (such as G-CSF and erythropoietin) to circumvent the associated hematologic toxic effects. Additional problems include the rapid emergence of viral resistance, demonstrated in HIV isolates after as little as 6 months of therapy with zidovudine. This *in vitro* resistance may eventually prove to correlate with disease progression.

Dideoxycytidine (ddC) is a reverse transcriptase inhibitor with potent *in vitro* activity against HIV. Although ddC is not associated with bone marrow toxicity, a peripheral neuropathy has developed in patients receiving it at high dosage or for a prolonged period of time. It is possible that by alternating ddC with zidovudine, antiretroviral activity could be sustained while the exposure to either agent alone was limited. This approach has proved safe and tolerable with little acute toxicity in the short term and warrants further investigation.[259] Studies evaluating ddC as salvage therapy for children who become intolerant of or refractory to zidovudine are currently being pursued by the AIDS Clinical Trials Group.

Dideoxyinosine (ddI, didanosine) is the third member of the dideoxynucleoside family to be evaluated in children. It has potent antiretroviral activity *in vitro* and a more favorable toxicity profile than zidovudine or ddC. Thus it is potentially important both in the initial therapy of HIV-infected children and in the rescue of those intolerant of or refractory to zidovudine. To date over 90 children enrolled in a phase I/II study, initiated at the National Cancer Institute in January 1989, have received ddI at dosages ranging from 60 to 540 mg/m²/day given orally in three divided doses. Results in the first 43 children enrolled and monitored for 24 weeks have been reported.[168] In addition to safety and tolerance, patients in this study were evaluated serially for changes in clinical, immunologic, virologic, and neurodevelopmental manifestations. Pancreatitis, the main toxic effect encountered, developed in three of 27 children enrolled at the two highest dose levels. Clinical benefits included weight gain, decreased organomegaly, and decreased lymphadenopathy. The median CD4 cell counts in 38 patients with paired counts (baseline and after 24 weeks of therapy) increased from 218 to 327 cells/mm³ (p = 0.001), and the median p24 antigen level declined from 272 to 77 pg/ml (p = 0.005) over the same period. Analysis of the data provided by this study is ongoing. Pancreatitis continues to be the major toxic effect observed to date. The development of non-sight-threatening retinal pigmentary abnormalities in three ddI recipients has been observed and may be related to therapy.[259a]

The results obtained from the study of ddI in children have highlighted the importance of pharmacokinetic principles in determining drug efficacy,[168] the relevance of which extends equally to adults. Data analysis failed to reveal a significant dose-related effect on clinical parameters, changes in CD4 count, or changes in neurocognitive functioning. However, there was marked interpatient variability in the bioavailability of this agent. Thus, although the plasma concentration of ddI, as determined by the area under the plasma concentration–time curve (AUC), is dose dependent, the marked interpatient variability observed could obscure significant dose-response relationships. This was exemplified by the results of neuropsychometric testing. Cognitive improvement did not correlate with the dose of ddI *per se* but did correlate with the ddI plasma concentration. The results of such pharmacokinetic analysis can strongly influence the interpretation of therapeutic responsiveness, and individualized adjustment of dose may be necessary to optimize response. The precise role of ddI in the pediatric armamentarium is undergoing definition. The relative benefits of zidovudine and ddI will be compared as part of a large three-armed randomized multicenter study to be initiated through the NIAID-sponsored AIDS Clinical Trials Group.

Despite their considerable benefits, it is unlikely that either zidovudine or ddI alone will effect durable suppression of viral activity. To avoid resistance and maximize treatment potential, combination regimens that are not cross-resistant, that prove additive or synergistic, and that may be free of dose-limiting toxic effects will be necessary. Thus, in a Phase I trial coordinated by the National Cancer Institute, a combination regimen using zidovudine and ddI is being evaluated, both as initial therapy and as a rescue regimen, with lower doses of zidovudine provided for those experiencing zidovudine-related hematologic toxicity. The relative merits of such a combination compared with either zidovudine or ddI alone will be evaluated as the third arm of the AIDS Clinical Trials Group study.

In attempts to improve potency and bioavailability, prolong half-life, enhance CNS penetration, decrease toxicity, and generally make more effective and less toxic agents, a variety of nucleoside analogues are under development, and this class of agents is likely to remain the cornerstone of anti-HIV therapy for the immediate future.

Preferable to the combination of two agents with a common site of activity would be the combination of agents active at different stages in the virus's life cycle. For this reason recombinant CD4 (rCD4), a truncated form of the native T-cell surface glycoprotein CD4 that is capable of blocking HIV infection of CD4+ cells *in vitro,* was of particular interest, since it intercepts the life cycle of HIV by a mechanism of action different from that of the dideoxynucleosides. Studies of rCD4 *in vivo* have been disappointing, and attention has shifted from this as a primary antiretroviral agent to the second generation of CD4 molecules. In these CD4 hybrid compounds, CD4 can be conjugated to a variety of peptides, some of which are inherently cytotoxic and some of which activate antibody-dependent cellular cytotoxicity (ADCC). The natural affinity of the CD4 molecule for gp120-expressing infected cells is exploited, with CD4 acting as the carrier molecule and directing the conjugated peptide to its target. These agents have yet to enter clinical trials in children.

A number of other stages in the virus's life cycle are potential targets for antiretroviral therapy. HIV-1 encodes a specific protease that is required for the expression of several viral genes, and a number of protease inhibitors have been developed and are in the preclinical stages of drug evaluation. These protease inhibitors have great potential and may be the next major group of agents to significantly alter the course of infection.

PREVENTION

Because most new cases of HIV infection in children result from mother-to-infant transmission of HIV, preventive efforts must be undertaken on two fronts, focusing on ways to decrease the incidence of infection in women and on ways to interrupt transmission. As maternal humoral immunity may prove to be a significant factor influencing transmission, attention has focused on ways in which it might be augmented. Consideration is being given both to mechanisms of active immunization, using gp120 subunit vaccines, and passive immunization, using hyperimmune anti-HIV immune globulin (HIVIG). HIVIG is a preparation of highly purified immunoglobulin containing high titers of antibody to HIV structural proteins and has considerable functional activity in virus neutralization and ADCC assays. By either inducing neutralizing antibodies or by passively administering them, it is hoped to potentially decrease the likelihood of transmission of infection. The alternative or perhaps complementary approach is to use antiretroviral agents in an attempt to decrease the maternal viral load and thus prevent transmission. Soluble rCD4 has been shown to block cellular infection by HIV *in vitro* but has been disappointing *in vivo*. Recently, hybrid CD4 molecules have been developed that exploit the natural affinity of the CD4 component for gp120, to target infected gp120-expressing cells. In one such hybrid, CD4 has been substituted for the Fab portion of IgG-producing CD4-Ig. Because the CD4-Ig attaches to the infected cells, it is hoped that actual killing of these cell *via* ADCC mechanisms might ensue. CD4-Ig mimics natural antibody and in a rhesus monkey model has demonstrated ability to cross the placenta. Whether giving CD4-Ig during pregnancy and delivery might decrease the rate of vertical transmission remains to be determined.

The success of such a chemoprophylaxis strategy, however, will rest heavily on when maternal-fetal transmission occurs. If in most cases transmission occurs early in gestation, and perhaps even if transmission occurs mainly during later gestation and delivery, antiretroviral agents such as zidovudine, by decreasing the maternal viral load, may be our most useful tool in decreasing the passage of virus from mother to infant. Early identification of the infected pregnant woman will be critical if this strategy is to succeed. Toxicity and pharmacokinetic studies of zidovudine have been carried out in pregnant women[260,261] and in newborns, and trials to evaluate its efficacy in decreasing transmission rates are currently being initiated.

As yet we do not have a cure for AIDS, nor do we have an effective vaccine. HIV infection, however, is a preventable disease. In focusing our efforts on ways in which to interrupt the passage of virus from mother to infant, we must not overlook those problems within our society that have resulted in women, and consequently their children, becoming one of the fastest growing segments of the HIV-infected population.

REFLECTIONS

Pediatric HIV infection is a tragedy that is daily affecting the lives of increasing numbers of people. Although incredible progress has been made—in part as the direct result of challenges from activists and advocates—much more work remains to be done. Of special concern is the changing face of this epidemic. It is taking root among those who have less access to medical care, and among children. It is up to all of us to continue to strive for advancement in the developing field of antiretroviral therapy, and even more so to focus on prevention of transmission of infection, as prevention remains the most effective cure in this epidemic.

REFERENCES

1. Centers for Disease Control: *Pneumocystis* pneumonia— Los Angeles. MMWR 30:250, 1981
2. Centers for Disease Control: Kaposi's sarcoma and *Pneumocystis* pneumonia. MMWR 30:305, 1981
3. Hymes KB, Cheung T, Greene JB et al: Kaposi's sarcoma in homosexual men: A report of eight cases. Lancet 2:598, 1981
3a. The National Institute of Child Health and Human Development Intravenous Immunoglobulin Study Group: Intravenous immune globulin for the prevention of bacterial infections in children with symptomatic human immunodeficiency virus infection. N Engl J Med 325:73, 1991
4. Gottlieb MS, Schroff R, Schanker HM et al: *Pneumocystis carinii* pneumonia and mucosal candidiasis in previously healthy homosexual men. N Engl J Med 305:1425, 1981
5. Masur H, Michelis MA, Greene JB et al: An outbreak of community-acquired *Pneumocystis carinii* pneumonia: Initial manifestation of cellular dysfunction. N Engl J Med 305:1431, 1981
6. Siegal FP, Lopez C, Hammer GS et al: Severe acquired immunodeficiency in male homosexuals, manifested by chronic perianal ulcerative herpes simplex lesions. N Engl J Med 305:1439, 1981
7. Follansbee SE, Busch DF, Wofsy CB et al: Outbreak of *Pneumocystis carinii* pneumonia in homosexual men. Ann Intern Med 96:705, 1982
8. Mildvan D, Mathur U, Enlow RW et al: Opportunistic infections and immune deficiency in homosexual men. Ann Intern Med 96:700, 1982
9. Centers for Disease Control: Special Report. Epidemiologic aspects of the current outbreak of Kaposi's sarcoma and opportunistic infections. N Engl J Med 306:248, 1982
10. Friedman-Kien AE, Laubenstein LJ, Rubinstein P et al: Disseminated Kaposi's sarcoma in homosexual men. Ann Intern Med 96:693, 1982
11. Durack DT: Opportunistic infections and Kaposi's sarcoma in homosexual men (editorial). N Engl J Med 305:1465, 1981
12. Centers for Disease Control: Unexplained immunodeficiency and opportunistic infections in children—New York, New Jersey, California. MMWR 31:665, 1982
13. Rubinstein A, Sicklick M, Gupta A et al: Acquired immunodeficiency with reversed T4/T8 ratios in infants born to promiscuous drug-addicted mothers. JAMA 249:2350, 1983
14. Oleske J, Minnefor A, Cooper R et al: Immune deficiency syndrome in children. JAMA 249:2345, 1983
15. Scott GB, Buck BE, Leterman JG et al: Acquired immunodeficiency syndrome in infants. N Engl J Med 310:76, 1984
16. Barre-Sinoussi F, Cherman JC et al: Isolation of a T-lymphotropic retrovirus from a patient at risk for acquired immunodeficiency syndrome. Science 220:868, 1983
17. Laurence J, Brun-Vezinet F, Schutzer SE et al: Lymphadenopathy-associated viral antibody in AIDS. N Engl J Med 311:1269, 1984
18. Popovic M, Sarngadharan MG, Read E, Gallo RC: Detection, isolation, and continuous production of cytopathic retroviruses (HTLV-III) from patients with AIDS and pre-AIDS. Science 224:497, 1984
19. Gallo RC, Salahuddin SZ, Popovic M et al: Frequent detection and isolation of cytopathic retroviruses (HTLV-III) from patients with AIDS and at risk for AIDS. Science 224:500, 1984
20. Sarngadharan MG, Popovic M, Bruch L et al: Antibodies reactive with human T-lymphotropic retroviruses (HTLV-III) in the serum of patients with AIDS. Science 224:506, 1984
21. Ammann AJ, Cowan MJ, Wara DW et al: Acquired immunodeficiency in an infant: Possible transmission by means of blood products. Lancet 1:956, 1983
22. Shannon K, Ball E, Wasserman R et al: Transfusion associated cytomegalovirus infection and acquired immune deficiency syndrome in an infant. J Pediatr 103:859, 1983
23. Church JA, Isaacs H: Transfusion-associated acquired immune deficiency syndrome in infants. J Pediatr 105:731, 1984
24. Gutman L, St Claire KK, Weedy C et al: Human immunodeficiency virus transmission by child sexual abuse. Am J Dis Child 145:137, 1991
25. Oxtoby MJ: Human immunodeficiency virus and other viruses in human milk: Placing the issues in broader perspective. Pediatr Infect Dis J 7:825, 1988

26. Gayle H, D'Angelo LJ: Epidemiology of AIDS and HIV infection in adolescents. Pediatr AIDS 1:38, 1991

27. Overby KJ, Lo B, Litt IF: Knowledge and concerns about acquired immunodeficiency syndrome and their relationship to behavior among adolescents with hemophilia. Pediatrics 83:204, 1989

28. Gwinn M, Pappaioanou M, George JR et al: Prevalence of HIV infection in childbearing women in the United States: Surveillance using newborn samples. JAMA 265:1704, 1991

29. Hoff R, Berardi V, Weiblen B et al: Seroprevalence of human immunodeficiency virus among childbearing women. N Engl J Med 318:525, 1988

30. Novick LF, Berns D, Stricof R et al: HIV seroprevalence in newborns in New York State. JAMA 261:1745, 1989

31. Gayle JA, Selik RM, Chu SY et al: Surveillance for AIDS and HIV infection among black and Hispanic children and women of childbearing age. MMWR 39:SS23, 1990

32. Matuszak DL, Panny SR, Patel J, Israel E: HIV antibody seroprevalence among childbearing women surveyed in Maryland. Public Health Rep 105:562, 1990

33. St. Louis M, Rauch K, Petersen L et al: Seroprevalence of human immunodeficiency virus infection at sentinel hospital in the United States. N Engl J Med 323:213, 1990

34. Quinn T, Glasser D, Cannon RO et al: Human immunodeficiency virus infection among patients attending clinics for sexually transmitted diseases. N Engl J Med 318:197, 1988

35. Gayle HD, Keeling R, Garcia-Tunon M et al: Prevalence of the human immunodeficiency virus among university students. N Engl J Med 323:1538, 1990

36. Centers for Disease Control: HIV prevalence estimates and AIDS case projections for the United States: Report based upon a workshop. MMWR 39:1, 1990

37. Centers for Disease Control: HIV/AIDS surveillance. Year End Edition, 1991, pp 1–22

38. Ryder R, Nsa W, Hassig S et al: Perinatal transmission of the human immunodeficiency virus type I to infants of seropositive women in Zaire. N Engl J Med 320:1637, 1989

39. Oxtoby M: Perinatally acquired HIV infection. Pediatr AIDS 1:3, 1990

40. Guay L, Mmiro F, Ndugwa C et al: Perinatal outcome in HIV-infected women in Uganda (abstr). In: Proceedings of the Sixth International Conference on AIDS, San Francisco, CA 1990, vol 1, p 144

41. Halsey N, Boulos R, Holt E et al: Transmission of HIV-1 infections from mothers to infants in Haiti. JAMA 264:2088, 1990

42. Friedland GH, Klein R: Transmission of the human immunodeficiency virus. N Engl J Med 317:1125, 1987

43. European Collaborative Study: Children born to women with HIV infection: Natural history and risk of transmission. Lancet 0:253, 1991

44. Blanche S, Rouzioux C, Moscato MG et al: A prospective study of infants born to women seropositive for human immunodeficiency virus type 1. N Engl J Med 320:1643, 1989

45. Johnson JP, Nair P, Hines SE et al: Natural history and serologic diagnosis of infants born to human immunodeficiency virus-infected women. Am J Dis Child 143:1147, 1989

46. Andiman W, Simpson J, Olson B et al: Rate of transmission of human immunodeficiency virus type 1 infection from mother to child and short term outcome of neonatal infection. Am J Dis Child 144:758, 1990

47. Paterlini P, Lallemant-Le Coeur S, Lallemant M et al: Polymerase chain reaction for studies of mother to child transmission of HIV-1 in Africa. J Med Virol 30:53, 1990

48. Escaich S, Wallon M, Baginski I et al: Comparison of HIV detection by virus isolation in lymphocyte cultures and molecular amplification of HIV DNA and RNA in offspring of seropositive mothers. J AIDS 4:130, 1991

49. Sprecher S, Soumenkoff G, Puissant F, Degueldre M: Vertical transmission of human immunodeficiency virus (HIV) in a 15 week fetus. Lancet 2:228, 1986

50. Lewis SH, Reynolds-Kohler C, Fox HE, Nelson JA: HIV-1 in trophoblastic and villous Hofbauer cells and haematological precursors in eight week fetuses. Lancet 335:565, 1990

51. Maury W, Potts B, Rabson AB: HIV-1 infection of first-trimester and term human placental tissue: A possible mode of maternal-fetal transmission. J Infect Dis 160:583, 1989

52. DiMaria H, Courpotin C, Rouzioux C et al: Transplacental transmission of human immunodeficiency virus. Lancet 2:215, 1986

53. Harnish DG, Hammerberg O, Walker IR et al: Early detection of HIV in a newborn. N Engl J Med 316:272, 1987

54. Laure F, Courgnaud V, Rouzioux C et al: Detection of HIV-1 DNA in infants by means of the polymerase chain reaction. Lancet 2:538, 1988

55. Rogers M, Ou C-Y, Rayfield M et al: Use of polymerase chain reaction for early detection of the proviral sequences of human immunodeficiency virus in infants born to seropositive mothers. N Engl J Med 320:1649, 1989

56. Marion RW, Wiznia AA, Hutcheon G, Rubinstein A: Human T-cell lymphotropic type III (HTLV-III) embryopathy. Am J Dis Child 140:638, 1986

57. Qazi QH, Sheikh TM, Fikrig S: Lack of evidence for craniofacial dysmorphism in perinatal human immunodeficiency virus infection. J Pediatr 112:7, 1988

58. Vogt MW, Witt DJ, Craven DE et al: Isolation of HTLV-III/LAV from cervical secretions of women at risk for AIDS. Lancet 1:525, 1986

59. Wofsy CB, Cohen JB, Hauer LB et al: Isolation of AIDS-associated retrovirus from genital secretions of women with antibodies to the virus. Lancet 1:527, 1986

60. Ziegler JB, Cooper DA, Johnson RO, Gold J: Postnatal transmission of AIDS-associated retrovirus from mother to infant. Lancet 1:896, 1985

61. Hutto C, Parks WP, Lai S et al: A hospital-based prospective study of perinatal infection with human immunodeficiency virus type I. J Pediatr 118:347, 1991

62. Van de Perre P, Simonon A, Hitimana DG et al: Mother to infant transmission of HIV: First immunologic and serologic features from an ongoing cohort study in Kigali, Rawanda. (abstr). In: Proceedings of the Sixth International Conference on AIDS, 1990, San Francisco, CA vol 1, p 144

63. Goedert JJ, Mendez H, Drummond JE et al: Mother-to-infant transmission of human immunodeficiency virus type I: Association with prematurity or low anti-gp120. Lancet 2:1351, 1989

64. Krasinski K, Cao Y-Z, Friedman-Kien A et al: Elevated maternal total and neutralizing antibody does not prevent perinatal HIV1 (abstr Th.C.45) In: Proceedings of the Sixth International Conference on AIDS, San Francisco, CA 1990, vol 2, p 145

65. Rossi P, Moschese V, Broliden PA et al: Presence of maternal antibodies to human immunodeficiency virus I en-

velope glycoprotein gp120 epitopes correlates with the uninfected status of children born to seropositive mothers. Proc Natl Acad Sci USA 86:8805, 1989

66. Devash Y, Calvelli T, Wood DG et al: Vertical transmission of human immunodeficiency virus is correlated with absence of high affinity/avidity maternal antibodies to the gp120 principal neutralizing domain. Proc Natl Acad Sci USA 87:3445, 1990

67. Boue F, Pons JC, Keros L et al: Risk for HIV I perinatal transmission varies with the mother's stage of infection (abstr). In: Proceedings of the Sixth International Conference on AIDS, San Francisco, CA 1990, vol 1, p 144

68. Scott GB, Fischl MA, Klimas N et al: Mothers of infants with the acquired immunodeficiency syndrome: Evidence for both symptomatic and asymptomatic carriers. JAMA 253:363, 1985

69. Young KY, Nelson RP, Good RA: Discordant human immunodeficiency virus infection in dizygotic twins detected by polymerase chain reaction. Pediatr Infect Dis J 9:454, 1990

70. Fischl MA, Dickinson GD, Scott G et al: Evaluation of heterosexual partners, children, and household contacts of adults with AIDS. JAMA 257:640, 1987

71. Centers for Disease Control: Revision of the CDC surveillance case definition for acquired immunodeficiency syndrome. MMWR 36:3S, 1987

72. Centers for Disease Control: Classification system for human immunodeficiency virus (HIV) infection in children under 13 years of age. MMWR 36:225, 1987

73. World Health Organization: Provisional WHO clinical case definition for AIDS. Weekly Epidemiol Rec 10:72, 1986

74. Rakusan T, Parrott RH, Sever JL: Limitations in the laboratory diagnosis of vertically acquired HIV infection. J AIDS 4:116, 1991

75. Burke DS, Brundage JF, Redfield RR et al: Measurement of the false positive rate in a screening program for human immunodeficiency virus infections. N Engl J Med 319: 961, 1988

76. Centers for Disease Control: Interpretation and use of the Western blot assay for serodiagnosis of human immunodeficiency virus type I infections. MMWR 38:S7, 1989

77. Brooks Jackson J, MacDonald KL, Cadwell J et al: Absence of HIV infection in blood donors with indeterminate Western blot tests for antibody to HIV-I. N Engl J Med 322:217, 1990

78. Imagawa DT, Lee MH, Wolinsky SM et al: Human immunodeficiency virus type I infection in homosexual men who remain seronegative for prolonged periods. N Engl J Med 320:1458, 1989

79. Husson RN, Comeau AM, Hoff R: Diagnosis of HIV infection in infants and children. Pediatrics 86:1, 1990

80. Borkowsky W, Krasinski K, Paul D et al: Human-immunodeficiency virus infections in infants negative for anti-HIV by enzyme-linked immunoassay. Lancet 1:1168, 1987

81. Goetz DW, Hall SE, Harbison R, Reid M: Pediatric acquired immunodeficiency syndrome with negative human immunodeficiency virus antibody response by enzyme-linked immunosorbant assay and Western blot. Pediatrics 81:356, 1988

82. Rogers M, Ou C, Abrams E et al: Lack of proviral sequences in children who have lost maternal antibody following birth to HIV(+) mothers (abstr Th.C.47). In: Proceedings of the Sixth International Conference on AIDS, San Francisco, CA 1990, vol 1, p 145

83. Gabiano C, Riva C, Palomba E et al: HIV antigen expression and viral DNA detection by PCR in mononuclear cells of seronegative at-risk children (abstr FA.358). In: Proceedings of the Sixth International Conference on AIDS, San Francisco, CA 1990, vol 2, p 165

84. Rogers MF, Ou C-Y, Kilbourne B, Schochetman G: Advances and problems in the diagnosis of HIV infection in infants. In Pizzo PA, Wilfert CM (eds): Pediatric AIDS, p 159. Baltimore, Williams & Wilkins, 1990

85. Parry JV, Mortimer PP: Place of IgM testing in HIV serology (letter). Lancet 2:979, 1986

86. Pyun KH, Ochs HD, Dufford MTW, Wedgwood RJ: Perinatal infection with human immunodeficiency virus: Specific antibody response by the neonate. N Engl J Med 317: 611, 1987

87. Weiblen B, Lee F, Cooper E et al: Early diagnosis of HIV infection in infants by detection of IgA HIV antibodies. Lancet 335:988, 1990

88. Martin N, Levy J, Legg H et al: Detection of infection with human immunodeficiency virus (HIV) type I in infants by an anti-HIV immunoglobulin A assay using recombinant proteins. J Pediatr, 118:354, 1991

89. Archibald DW, Johnson JP, Nair P et al: Detection of salivary immunoglobulin A antibodies to HIV-I in infants and children. AIDS, 4:417, 1990

90. Renom G, Bouquety JC, Lanckriet C et al: HIV-specific IgA antibodies in tears of children with AIDS or at risk of AIDS. Res Virol 141:355, 1990

91. Amadori A, De Rossi A, Giaquinto C et al: In-vitro production of HIV specific antibody in children at risk of AIDS. Lancet 1:852, 1988

92. Pahwa S, Chirmule N, Leombruno C: In vitro synthesis of human immunodeficiency-specific antibodies in peripheral blood lymphocytes of infants. Proc Natl Acad Sci USA 86:7532, 1989

93. Lee FK, Nahmias AJ, Lowery S et al: ELISPOT: A new approach to studying the dynamics of virus-immune system interaction for diagnosis and monitoring of HIV infection. AIDS Res Hum Retroviruses 5:517, 1989

94. Allain JP, Laurian Y, Paul D et al: Serological markers in the early stages of human immunodeficiency virus infection in hemophiliacs. Lancet 2:1168, 1986

95. Paul D, Falk L, Kessler HA et al: Correlation of serum HIV antigen and antibody with clinical status in HIV-infected patients. J Med Virol 22:357, 1987

96. Jackson JB, Coombs RW, Sannerud K et al: Rapid and sensitive viral culture method for human immunodeficiency virus type I. J Clin Microbiol 26:1416, 1988

97. Dilworth S, Fowler AK, Watkins ME et al: Isolation of HIV-I from microliter quantities of whole blood (abstr FA.340). In: Proceedings of the Sixth International Conference on AIDS, San Francisco, CA 1990, vol 2, p 161

98. Ho DD, Moudgil T, Alam M: Quantitation of human immunodeficiency virus type 1 in the blood of infected persons. N Engl J Med, 321:1621, 1989

99. Saag M, Decker D, Campbell S et al: Quantification of plasma viremia in HIV infected children and adults (abstr FA.346). In: Proceedings of the Sixth International Conference on AIDS, San Francisco, CA 1990, vol 2, p 162

100. Eisenstein BI: The polymerase chain reaction: A new method of using molecular genetics for medical diagnosis. N Engl J Med 322:178, 1990

101. Edwards JR, Ulrich PP, Weintraub PS et al: Polymerase chain reaction compared with concurrent viral cultures for rapid identification of human immunodeficiency virus

infection among high risk infants and children. J Pediatr 115:200, 1989

102. Goedert JJ, Kessler CM, Aldedort LM et al: A prospective study of human immunodeficiency virus type I infection and the development of AIDS in subjects with hemophilia. N Engl J Med 321:1141, 1989

103. Becherer PR, Smiley ML, Matthews TJ et al: Human immunodeficiency virus-I disease progression in hemophiliacs. Am J Hematol 34:204, 1990

104. Scott GB, Hutto C, Makuch RW et al: Survival in children with perinatally acquired human immunodeficiency virus type I infection. N Engl J Med 321:1791, 1989

105. Auger I, Thomas P, De Gruttola V et al: Incubation periods for pediatric AIDS patients. Nature 336:575, 1988

106. Leibovitz E, Rigaud M, Pollack H et al: *Pneumocystis carinii* pneumonia in infants infected with the human immunodeficiency virus with more than 450 CD4 T lymphocytes per cubic millimeter. N Engl J Med 323:531, 1990

107. Kovacs A, Frederick T, Church J et al: CD4 T-lymphocyte counts and *Pneumocystis carinii* pneumonia in pediatric HIV infection. JAMA 265:1698, 1991

108. Connor E, Bagarazzi M, McSherry G et al: Clinical and laboratory correlates of *Pneumocystis carinii* pneumonia in children infected with HIV. JAMA 265:1693, 1991

109. Straka BF, Whitaker DL, Morrison SH et al: Cutaneous manifestations of the acquired immunodeficiency syndrome in children. J Am Acad Dermatol 18:1089, 1988

110. Prose NS: HIV infection in children. J Am Acad Dermatol 22:1223, 1990

111. Pahwa S, Fikrig S, Mendez R, Pahwa R: Pediatric acquired immunodeficiency syndrome: Demonstration of B lymphocyte defects in vitro. Diagn Immunol 4:24, 1986

112. Bender BS, Davidson BL, Kline R et al: Role of the mononuclear phagocyte system in the immunopathogenesis of human immunodeficiency virus infection and the acquired immunodeficiency syndrome. Rev Infect Dis 10:1142, 1988

113. Ellis M, Gupta S, Galant S et al: Impaired neutrophil function in patients with AIDS or AIDS related complex: A comprehensive evaluation. J Infect Dis 158:1268, 1988

114. Roilides E, Mertins S, Eddy J et al: Impairment of neutrophil chemotactic and bactericidal function in HIV-infected children and partial reversal after in vitro exposure to granulocyte-macrophage colony-stimulating factor. J Pediatr 117:531, 1990

115. Relman D, Loutit JS, Schmidt TM et al: The agent of bacillary angiomatosis: An approach to the identification of uncultured pathogens. N Engl J Med 323:1573, 1990

116. Perkocha LA, Geaghan SM, Yen B et al: Clinical and pathological features of bacillary peliosis hepatis in association with human immunodeficiency virus infection. N Engl J Med 323:1581, 1990

117. Slater L, Welch D, Hensel D, Coody D: A newly recognized fastidious gram-negative pathogen as a cause of fever and bacteremia. N Engl J Med 323:1587, 1990

118. Rubinstein A, Morecki R, Silverman B et al: Pulmonary disease in children with acquired immunodeficiency syndrome and AIDS related complex. J Pediatr 108:498, 1986

119. Joshi VV, Oleske JM, Minnefor B et al: Pathologic findings in children with the acquired immunodeficiency syndrome. Hum Pathol 16:241, 1985

120. Centers for Disease Control: AIDS-indicator diseases diagnosed in patients reported in 1990, by age group, United States. HIV/AIDS Surveillance 1991, p 16

121. Rubinstein A, Berenstein LJ, Charytan M et al: Corticosteroid treatment for pulmonary lymphoid hyperplasia in children with the acquired immunodeficiency syndrome. Pediatr Pulmonol 4:13, 1988

122. Andiman WA, Martin K, Rubinstein A et al: Opportunistic lymphoproliferations associated with Epstein-Barr viral DNA in infants and children with AIDS. Lancet 2:1390, 1985

123. Bye M, Bernstein LJ, Glaser J, Kleid D. *Pneumocystis carinii* pneumonia in young children with AIDS. Pediatr Pulmonol 9:251, 1990

124. Centers for Disease Control: Guidelines for prophylaxis against *Pneumocystis carinii* pneumonia for children infected with human immunodeficiency virus infection/exposure. MMWR 40(RR-2):1, 1991

125. Bernstein LJ, Bye M, Rubinstein A: Prognostic factors and life expectancy in children with acquired immunodeficiency syndrome and *Pneumocystis carinii* pneumonia. Am J Dis Child 143:775, 1989

126. Bigby TD, Margolskee D, Curtis JL et al: The usefulness of induced sputum in the diagnosis of *Pneumocystis carinii* pneumonia in patients with the acquired immunodeficiency syndrome. Am Rev Respir Dis 133:515, 1986

127. Pitchenik AE, Ganjei P, Torres A et al: Sputum examination for the diagnosis of *Pneumocystis carinii* pneumonia in the acquired immunodeficiency syndrome. Am Rev Respir Dis 133:226, 1986

128. Hopewell PC: *Pneumocystis carinii* pneumonia: Diagnosis. J Infect Dis 157:1115, 1988

129. Bonfils-Roberts E, Nickodem A, Nealon TF: Retrospective analysis of the efficacy of open lung biopsy in acquired immunodeficiency syndrome. Ann Thorac Surg 49:115, 1990

130. Kovacs JA, Masur H: *Pneumocystis carinii* pneumonia: Therapy and prophylaxis. J Infect Dis 158:254, 1988

131. Allegra CJ, Chabne BA, Tuazon CU et al: Trimetrexate for the treatment of *Pneumocystis carinii* pneumonia in patients with the acquired immunodeficiency syndrome. N Engl J Med 317:978, 1987

132. Sattler FR, Allegra C, Verdegem TD et al: Trimetrexate-leucovorin dosage evaluation study for treatment of *Pneumocystis carinii* pneumonia. J Infect Dis 161:91, 1990

133. Hughes W, Kennedy W, Shenep J et al: Safety and pharmacokinetics of 566C80, a hydroxynaphthoquinone with anti-*P. carinii* activity (abstr 861). In: Program and Abstracts of the 30th ICAAC, 1990, p 229

134. Panel C: Consensus statement on the use of corticosteroids as adjunctive therapy for *Pneumocystis carinii* pneumonia in the acquired immunodeficiency syndrome. N Engl J Med 323:1500, 1990

135. Yanase Y, Tango T, Okumura K et al: Lymphocyte subsets identified by monoclonal antibodies in healthy children. Pediatr Res 20:1147, 1986

136. Denny TN, Niven P, Skuza C et al: Age-related changes in lymphocyte phenotypes in healthy children (abstr 916). Pediatr Res 27:155, 1990

136a. Mueller BU, Butler KM, Husson RN, Pizzo PA: *Pneumocystis carinii* pneumonia despite prophylaxis in children with HIV infection. J Pediatr (in press)

137. Gherman CG, Ward RR, Bassis ML: *Pneumocystis carinii* otitis media and mastoiditis as the initial manifestation of the acquired immunodeficiency syndrome. Am J Med 85:250, 1988

138. Kwok S, O'Donnell JJ, Wood IS: Retinal cotton wool spots

in a patient with *Pneumocystis carinii* infection. N Engl J Med 307:184, 1982

139. Grimes MM, LaPook JD, Bar MH et al: Disseminated *Pneumocystis carinii* infection in a patient with the acquired immunodeficiency syndrome. Hum Pathol 18:307, 1987

140. Vernon DD, Holzman BH, Lewis P et al: Respiratory failure in children with acquired immunodeficiency syndrome and acquired immunodeficiency syndrome-related complex. Pediatrics 82:223, 1988

141. Chandwani S, Borkowsky W, Krasinski K et al: Respiratory syncytial virus infection in human immunodeficiency virus–infected children. J Pediatr 117:251, 1990

142. Janner D, Petru AM, Belchis D, Azimi P: Fatal adenovirus infection in a child with the acquired immunodeficiency syndrome. Pediatr Infect Dis J 9:434, 1990

143. Markowitz LE, Chandler FW, Roldan EO et al: Fatal measles pneumonia without rash in a child with AIDS. J Infect Dis 158:480, 1988

144. Krasinski K, Borkowsky W: Measles and measles immunity in children infected with human immunodeficiency virus. JAMA 261:2512, 1989

145. Fink L, Reichek N St J, Sutton MJ: Cardiac abnormalities in acquired immunodeficiency syndrome. Am J Cardiol 54:1161, 1984

146. Cohen IS, Anderson DW, Virmani P et al: Congestive cardiomyopathy in association with the acquired immunodeficiency syndrome. N Engl J Med 315:628, 1986

147. Reilly JM, Cunnion R, Anderson DW et al: Frequency of myocarditis, left ventricular dysfunction and ventricular tachycardia in the acquired immunodeficiency syndrome. Am J Cardiol 62:789, 1988

148. Joshi VV, Gadol C, Connor E et al: Dilated cardiomyopathy in children with acquired immunodeficiency syndrome: A pathologic study of five cases. Hum Pathol 19:69, 1988

149. Lipshultz SE, Chanock S, Sanders SP et al: Cardiovascular manifestations of human immunodeficiency virus infection in infants and children. Am J Cardiol 63:1489, 1989

150. Steinhertz LJ, Brochstein JA, Robins J: Cardiac involvement in congenital acquired immunodeficiency syndrome. Am J Dis Child 140:1241, 1986

151. Lipshultz SE, Perez-Atayde AR, Sanders SP et al: Identification of human immunodeficiency virus-1 RNA and DNA in the heart of a child with cardiovascular abnormalities and congenital acquired immunodeficiency syndrome. Am J Cardiol 66:246, 1990

152. Grody WW, Cheng L, Lewis W: Infection of the heart by the human immunodeficiency virus. Am J Cardiol 66:203, 1990

153. Joshi V, Pawel B, Connor E et al: Arteriopathy in children with acquired immune deficiency syndrome. Padiatr Pathol 7:261, 1987

154. Kure K, Park Y, Kim T-S et al: Immunohistochemical localization of an HIV epitope in cerebral aneurysmal arteriopathy in pediatric acquired immunodeficiency syndrome (AIDS). Pediatr Pathol 9:65, 1989

155. Erlich KS, Mills J, Chatis P et al: Acyclovir-resistant herpes simplex virus infections in patients with the acquired immunodeficiency syndrome. N Engl J Med 320:293, 1989

156. Chatis PA, Miller CH, Schrager LE, Crumpacker CS: Successful treatment of an acyclovir-resistant mucocutaneous infection with herpes simplex virus in a patient with acquired immunodeficiency syndrome. N Engl J Med 320:297, 1989

157. De Souza Y, Greenspan D, Felton J et al: Localization of Epstein-Barr virus DNA in the epithelial calls of oral hairy leukoplakia by in situ hybridization (letter). N Engl J Med 320:1559, 1989

158. Bach MC, Howell DA, Valenti A et al: Aphthous ulceration of the gastrointestinal tract in patients with the acquired immunodeficiency syndrome (AIDS). Ann Intern Med 112:465, 1990

159. Yolken RH, Hart W, Oung I et al: Gastrointestinal dysfunction and disaccharide intolerance in children infected with human immunodeficiency virus. J Pediatr 118:359, 1991

160. Greenson J, Belitsos PC, Yardley J, Bartlett J: AIDS enteropathy: Occult enteric infections and duodenal mucosal alterations in chronic diarrhea. Ann Intern Med 114:366, 1991

161. Duffy LF, Daum F, Kahn E et al: Hepatitis in children with acquired immunodeficiency syndrome. Gastroenterology 90:173, 1986

162. Schwartz M, Brandt LJ: The spectrum of pancreatic disorders in patients with the acquired immune deficiency syndrome. Am J Gastroenterol 84:459, 1989

163. Hart CC: Aerosolized pentamidine and pancreatitis. Ann Intern Med 111:691, 1989

164. Murphy RL, Noskin GA, Ehrenpreis ED: Acute pancreatitis associated with aerosolized pentamidine. Am J Med 88: 53N, 1990

165. Yarchoan R, Mitsuya H, Thomas RV et al: In vivo activity against HIV and favorable toxicity profile of 2′,3′-dideoxy-inosine. Science 245:412, 1989

166. Lambert JS, Seidlin M, Reichman RC et al: 2′,3′-Dideoxy-inosine (ddI) in patients with the acquired immunodeficiency syndrome or the AIDS-related complex: A phase I trial. N Engl J Med 322:1333, 1990

167. Cooley TP, Kunches LM, Saunders CA et al: Once-daily administration of 2′,3′-dideoxyinosine (ddI) in patients with the acquired immunodeficiency syndrome or AIDS-related complex. N Engl J Med 322:1340, 1990

168. Butler KM, Husson RN, Balis FM et al: Dideoxyinosine in children with symptomatic human immunodeficiency virus infection. N Engl J Med 324:137, 1991

169. Torre D, Montanari M, Paola Fiori M et al: HIV and the pancreas (letter). Lancet 2:1212, 1987

170. Glassock RJ, Cohen AH, Danovitch G, Parsa KP: Human immunodeficiency virus (HIV) infection and the kidney. Ann Intern Med 112:35, 1991

171. Rao TKS, Friedman JA, Nicastri A: The types of renal disease in the acquired immunodeficiency syndrome. N Engl J Med 316:1062, 1987

172. Strauss J, Abitol C, Zilleruelo G et al: Renal disease in children with the acquired immunodeficiency syndrome. N Engl J Med 321:625, 1989

173. Perkocha LA, Rodgers GM. Hematologic aspects of human immunodeficiency virus infection: Laboratory and clinical considerations. Am J Hematol 29:94, 1988

174. Spivak JL, Barnes DC, Fuchs E, Quinn TC: Serum immunoreactive erythropoietin in HIV-infected patients. JAMA 261:3104, 1989

175. Frickhofen N, Abkowitz JL, Safford M et al: Persistent B19 parvovirus infection in patients infected with human immunodeficiency virus type I (HIV-I): A treatable cause of anemia. Ann Intern Med 113:926, 1990

176. Murphy PM, Lane C, Fauci A, Gallin JI: Impairment of neutrophil bactericidal capacity in patients with AIDS. J Infect Dis 158:627, 1988

177. Clerici M, Stocks NI, Zajac AC: Detection of three distinct

patterns of T helper cell dysfunction in asymptomatic human immunodeficiency virus–positive patients. J Clin Invest 84:1892, 1989

178. Roilides E, Clerici M, De Palma L et al: Helper T-cell responses in children infected with human immunodeficiency virus type 1. J Pediatr 118:724, 1991

179. Fauci A, Schnittman SM, Poli G et al: Immunopathogenic mechanisms in human immunodeficiency virus (HIV) infection. Ann Intern Med 114:678, 1991

180. Baldwin GC, Fuller ND, Roberts R et al: Granulocyte- and granulocyte-macrophage colony stimulating factors enhance neutrophil cytotoxicity toward HIV infected cells. Blood 74:1673, 1989

181. Roilides E, Venzon D, Pizzo PA, Rubin M: Effects of antiretroviral dideoxynucleosides on polymorphonuclear leukocyte function. Antimicrob Agents Chemother 34:1672, 1990

182. Zucker-Franklin D, Cao Y: Megakaryocytes of human immunodeficiency virus–infected individuals express virla RNA. Proc Natl Acad Sci USA 86:5595, 1989

183. Walsh CM, Nardi MA, Karpatkin S: On the mechanism of thrombocytopenic purpura in sexually active homosexual men. N Engl J Med 311:635, 1984

184. Van der Lelie J, Lange JM, Vos JJ et al: Autoimmunity against blood cells in human immunodeficiency virus (HIV) infection. Br J Haematol 67:109, 1987

185. Hoffman DM, Caruso RF, Mirando T: Human immunodeficiency virus–associated thrombocytopenia. DICP, Ann of Pharmacother 23:157, 1989

186. Ellaurie M, Burns ER, Bernstein LJ et al: Thrombocytopenia and human immunodeficiency virus in children. Pediatrics 82:905, 1988

187. Swiss Group for Clinical Studies on the Acquired Immunodeficiency Syndrome (AIDS): Zidovudine for the treatment of thrombocytopenia associated with human immunodeficiency virus (HIV): A prospective study. Ann Intern Med 109:718, 1988

188. Oksenhendler E, Bierling P, Ferchal F et al: Zidovudine for thrombocytopenic purpura related to human immunodeficiency virus (HIV) infection. Ann Intern Med 110:365, 1989

189. Sandhaus LM, Scudder R: Hematologic and bone marrow abnormalities in pediatric patients with human immunodeficiency virus (HIV) infection. Pediatr Pathol 9:277, 1989

190. Bloom EJ, Abrams DI, Rodgers G: Lupus anticoagulant in the acquired immunodeficiency syndrome. JAMA 256:491, 1986

191. Cohen AJ, Phillips TM, Kessler ZCM: Circulating coagulation inhibitors in the acquired immunodeficiency syndrome. Ann Intern Med 104:175, 1986

192. Burns ER, Krieger B, Bernstein L, Rubinstein A: Acquired circulating anticoagulants in children with the acquired immunodeficiency syndrome. Pediatrics 82:763, 1988

193. Merenich JA, McDermott MT, Asp AA et al: Evidence of endocrine involvement early in the course of human immunodeficiency virus infection. J Clin Endocrinol Metab 70:566, 1989

194. Brettler D, Forsberg A, Bolivar E et al: Growth failure as a prognostic indicator for progression to acquired immunodeficiency syndrome in children with hemophilia. J Pediatr 117:584, 1990

195. Jospe N, Powell K: Growth hormone deficiency in an 8-year-old girl with human immunodeficiency virus infection. Pediatrics 86:309, 1990

196. Laue L, Pizzo PA, Butler K, Cutler GB: Growth and neuroendocrine dysfunction in children with the acquired immunodeficiency syndrome. J Pediatr 117:541, 1990

197. Schwartz LJ, St Louis Y, Wu R et al: Endocrine function in children with human immunodeficiency virus infection. Am J Dis Child 145:330, 1990

198. Oberfield S, Kairam R, Bakshi S et al: Steroid response to adrenocorticotropin stimulation in children with human immunodeficiency virus infection. J Clin Endocrinol Metab 70:578, 1990

199. European Collaborative Study: Neurologic signs in young children with human immunodeficiency virus infection. Pediatr Infect Dis J 9:402, 1990

200. Belman A, Diamond G, Dickson D et al: Pediatric acquired immunodeficiency syndrome: Neurologic syndromes. Am J Dis Child 142:29, 1988

201. Epstein LG, Sharer L, Oleske J et al: Neurologic manifestations of human immunodeficiency virus infection in children. Pediatrics 78:678, 1986

202. Epstein G, Sharer LG, Goudsmit J: Neurological and neuropathological features of human immunodeficiency virus infection in children. Ann Neurol 23:S19, 1988

203. Brouwers P, Belman A, Epstein L: Central nervous system involvement: Manifestations and evaluation. Pediatr AIDS 1:318, 1990

204. Ho DD, Rota TR, Schooley RT et al: Isolation of HTLV-III from cerebrospinal fluid and neural tissues of patients with the acquired immunodeficiency syndrome. N Engl J Med 313:1493, 1985

205. Shaw GM, Harper ME, Hahn BH et al: HTLV-III infection in the brains of adults and children with AIDS encephalopathy. Science 227:117, 1985

206. Levy JA, Shimabukuro J, Hollander et al: Isolation of AIDS-associated retroviruses from cerebrospinal fluid and brain of patients with neurological symptoms. Lancet 2:586, 1985

207. Wiley CA, Schrier R, Nelson JA et al: Cellular localization of human immunodeficiency virus infection within brains of acquired immune deficiency syndrome patients. Proc Natl Acad Sci USA 83:7089, 1986

208. Epstein LG, Goudsmit J, Paul D et al: Expression of human immunodeficiency virus in cerebrospinal fluid of children with progressive encephalopathy. 21:397, 1987

209. Sharer LR, Dowling PC, Cook SD et al: Spinal cord disease in children with HIV-I infection: A combined molecular biological and neuropathological study. Neuropathol Appl Neurobiol 16:317, 1990

210. Shaunak S, Albright RE, Klotman ME et al: Amplification of HIV-1 provirus from cerebrospinal fluid and its correlation with neurologic disease. J Infect Dis 161:1068, 1990

211. Gallo P, De Rossi A, Amadore A et al: Central nervous system involvement in HIV infection. AIDS Research & Human Retroviruses 4:211, 1988

212. Pang S, Koyanagi Y, Miles S et al: High levels of unintegrated HIV-DNA in brain tissue of AIDS dementia patients. Nature 343:85, 1990

213. Portegies P, Epstein L, Hung STA et al: Human immunodeficiency virus type I antigen in cerebrospinal fluid. Arch Neurol 46:261, 1989

214. Mintz M, Rapaport R, Oleske J et al: Elevated serum levels of tumor necrosis factor are associated with progressive encephalopathy in children with acquired immunodeficiency syndrome. Am J Dis Child 143:771, 1989

215. Pizzo PA, Eddy J, Falloon J et al: Effect of continuous intravenous infusion zidovudine (AZT) in children with symptomatic HIV infection. N Engl J Med 319:889, 1988

216. McKinney RE, Maha MA, Connor EM et al: A multicenter trial of oral zidovudine in children with advanced human immunodeficiency virus disease. N Engl J Med 324:1018, 1991

217. Hollander H: Cerebrospinal fluid abnormalities in individuals infected with human immunodeficiency virus. J Infect Dis 158:855, 1988

218. Petito CK, Navia BCE-S, Jordan BD et al: Vacuolar myelopathy pathologically resembling subacute combined degeneration in patients with the acquired immunodeficiency syndrome. N Engl J Med 312:874, 1985

219. Dalakas M, Pezeshkpour GH: Neuromuscular disease associated with human immunodeficiency virus infection. Ann Neurol 23(suppl):S38, 1988

220. Bloom JN, Palestine AG: The diagnosis of cytomegalovirus retinitis. Ann Intern Med 109:963, 1988

221. Palestine AG, Rodrigues MM, Macher AM et al: Ophthalmic involvement in acquired immunodeficiency syndrome. Ophthalmology 91:1092, 1984

222. Millar AB, Miller RF, Patou G et al: Treatment of cytomegalovirus retinitis with zidovudine and ganciclovir in patients with AIDS: Outcome and toxicity. Genitourin Med 66:156, 1990

223. Hochster H, Dieterich D, Bozzette S et al: Toxicity of combined ganciclovir and zidovudine for cytomegalovirus disease associated with AIDS. Ann Intern Med 113:111, 1990

224. Holland GN, Sidikaro Y, Kreiger AE et al: Treatment of cytomegalovirus retinopathy with ganciclovir. Ophthalmology 94:815, 1987

225. Jacobson MA, O'Donnell JJ, Brodie HR et al: Randomized prospective trial of ganciclovir maintenance therapy for cytomegalovirus retinitis. J Med Virol 25:339, 1988

226. Buhles WC, Mastre BJ, Tinker AJ et al: Ganciclovir treatment of life- or sight-threatening cytomegalovirus infection: Experience in 314 immunocompromised patients. Rev Infect Dis 10:S495, 1988

227. Singer DRJ, Fallon TJ, Schulenburg WE et al: Foscarnet for cytomegalovirus retinitis. Ann Intern Med 103:962, 1985

228. Farthing CF, Dalgleish AG, Clark A et al: Phosphonoformate (foscarnet): A pilot study in AIDS and AIDS related complex. AIDS 1:21, 1987

229. Walmsley S, Chew E, Read SE et al: Treatment of cytomegalovirus retinitis with trisodium phosphonoformate hexahydrate (foscarnet). J Infect Dis 157:569, 1988

230. Lehoang P, Girard B, Robinet M et al: Foscarnet in the treatment of cytomegalovirus retinitis in the acquired immune deficiency syndrome. Ophthalmology 96:865, 1989

231. Fanning MM, Read SE, Benson M et al: Foscarnet therapy of cytomegalovirus retinitis in AIDS. J AIDS 3:472, 1990

232. Jacobson MA, O'Donnell JJ, Mills JF: Foscarnet treatment of cytomegalovirus retinitis in patients with the acquired immunodeficiency syndrome. Antimicrob Agents Chemother 33:736, 1989

233. Butler KM, de Smet M, Husson RN et al: Treatment of aggressive CMV retinitis with ganciclovir in combination with foscarnet in a child with human immunodeficiency virus infection. J Pediatr (in press)

234. Willerson D, Aaberg TM, Reeser FH: Necrotizing vaso-occlusive retinitis. Am J Ophthalmol 84:209, 1977

235. Young NJA, Bird AC: Bilateral acute retinal necrosis. Br J Ophthalmol 62:581, 1978

236. Matsuo T, Nakayama T, Koyama T et al: A proposed mild type of acute retinal necrosis syndrome. Am J Ophthalmol 105:579, 1988

237. Concus A, Helfand RF, Imber MJ et al: Cutaneous cryptococcosis mimicking *Molluscum contagiosum* in a patient with AIDS. J Infect Dis 158:897, 1988

238. Pahwa S, Biron K, Lim W et al: Continuous varicella-zoster infection associated with acyclovir resistance in a child with AIDS. JAMA 260:2879, 1988

239. Prose N, von Knebel-Doeberitz C, Miller S et al: Widespread flat warts associated with human papillomavirus type 5: A cutaneous manifestation of human immunodeficiency virus infection. J Am Acad Dermatol 23:978, 1990

240. Salomon D, Saurat J-H: Erythema multiforme major in a two-month-old child with human immunodeficiency virus infection. Br J Dermatol 123:797, 1990

241. Paller AS, Sahn E, Garen PD et al: Pyoderma gangrenosum in pediatric acquired immunodeficiency syndrome. J Pediatr 117:63, 1990

242. Buck BE, Scott GB, Valdes-Dapens M, Parks W: Kaposi sarcoma in two infants with acquired immune deficiency syndrome. J Pediatr 103:911, 1983

243. Connor E, Boccon-Gibod L, Joshi V et al: Cutaneous acquired immunodeficiency syndrome–associated Kaposi's sarcoma in pediatric patients. Arch Dermatol 126:791, 1990

244. Epstein LG, DiCarlo FJ, Joshi V et al: Primary lymphoma of the central nervous system in children with the acquired immunodeficiency syndrome. Pediatrics 82:355, 1988

245. Goldstein J, Dickson DW, Rubenstein A et al: Primary central nervous system lymphoma in a pediatric patient with acquired immune deficiency syndrome. Cancer 66:2503, 1990

246. Gould Chadwick E, Connor E, Guerra Hanson C et al: Tumors of smooth muscle origin in HIV-infected children. JAMA 263:3182, 1990

247. Onorato IM, Markowitz LE, Oxtoby M: Childhood immunization, vaccine-preventable diseases and infection with the human immunodeficiency virus. Pediatr Infect Dis J 6:588, 1988

248. Mitus A, Holloway A, Evans AE et al: Attenuated measles vaccine in children with acute leukemia. Am J Dis Child 103:243, 1962

249. Nkowane BM, Wassilak SGF, Orenstein WA: Vaccine associated paralytic poliomyelitis. JAMA 257:1335, 1987

250. Centers for Disease Control: Immunization of children infected with human T-lymphotropic virus type III/lymphadenopathy virus. MMWR 35:595, 1986

251. Centers for Disease Control: Immunization of children with human immunodeficiency virus—supplementary ACIP statement. MMWR 37:181, 1988

252. McLaughlin M, Thomas P, Onorato I et al: Live virus vaccines in human immunodeficiency virus–infected children: A retrospective survey. Pediatrics 82:229, 1988

253. McKinney RE, Pizzo PA, Scott GB et al: Safety and tolerance of intermittent intravenous and oral zidovudine therapy in human immunodeficiency virus–infected pediatric patients: A phase I study. J Pediatr 116:640, 1990

254. Blanche S, Caniglia M, Fischer A et al: Zidovudine therapy in children with the acquired immunodeficiency syndrome. Am J Med 85(suppl 2A):203, 1988

255. Collier AC, Bozzette S, Coombs RW et al: A pilot study of low-dose zidovudine in human immunodeficiency virus infection. N Engl J Med 323:1015, 1990

256. Fischl MA, Parker CB, Pettinelli C et al: A randomized controlled trial of a reduced daily dose of zidovudine in patients with acquired immunodeficiency syndrome. N Engl J Med 323:1009, 1990

257. Balis FM, Pizzo PA, Eddy J et al: Pharmacokinetics of zidovudine administered intravenously and orally in chil-

dren with human immunodeficiency virus infection. J Pediatr 114:880, 1989

258. Balis FM, Pizzo PA, Murphy R et al: The pharmacokinetics of zidovudine administered by continuous infusion in children. Ann Intern Med 110:279, 1989

259. Pizzo PA, Butler KM, Balis F et al: Dideoxycytidine alone and in an alternating schedule with zidovudine (AZT) in children with symptomatic HIV infection: A pilot study. J Pediatr 117:799, 1990

259a. Whitcup S, Butler KM, Caruso R et al: Retinal toxicity in HIV infected children treated with a 2'3'-dideoxyinosine (ddI). Am J Ophthalmol (in press)

260. Lopez-Anaya A, Unadkat J, Schumann LA, Smith AL: Pharmacokinetics of zidovudine (azidothymidine): 1. Transplacental transfer. J AIDS 3:959, 1990

261. Watts DH, Brown ZA, Tartaglione T et al: Pharmacokinetic disposition of zidovudine during pregnancy. J Infect Dis 163:226, 1991

262. Mok JQ, Giaquinto C, De Rossi A et al: Infants born to mothers seropositive for human immunodeficiency virus. Lancet 1:164, 1987

263. Borkowsky W, Papaevangelou V, Moore T et al: Maternal p24 antigenemia does not predict HIV transmission to offspring (abstr). In: Proceedings of the Sixth International Conference on AIDS, San Francisco, CA 1990, vol 2, p 448

Noninfectious Organ-Specific Complications of HIV Infection

17

Dermatologic Complications

Bijan Safai   Joseph J. Schwartz

The cutaneous manifestations of human immunodeficiency virus (HIV) infection are extensive, encompassing malignancies (Kaposi's sarcoma, lymphoma), a variety of infections (bacterial, viral, and fungal), and noninfectious complications. This chapter considers the noninfectious cutaneous manifestations of HIV infection.

The noninfectious cutaneous disorders are numerous (Table 17A–1) and may occur in all stages of HIV infection. Subtle findings, such as dry skin or telangiectasias, or severe reactions, such as an exacerbation of psoriasis or extensive seborrheic dermatitis, may be the first clues to the presence of HIV infection. As HIV infection progresses, these conditions occur with greater frequency and severity.[1,2]

Although none of the disorders reported in this group have been linked directly to an infectious agent, these conditions may be in part due to an abnormal host response to infectious agents other than HIV.

SEBORRHEIC DERMATITIS

Seborrheic dermatitis is a common skin condition characterized by erythematous, scaly patches of skin. It is most often seen in the malar region, nasolabial fold, eyebrows, scalp, chest, and behind the ears. The prevalence of seborrheic dermatitis in the general population is reported to be 3%.[3] Among HIV-infected persons, the prevalence ranges from 7% to 50%,[4–7] making seborrheic dermatitis the most common noninfectious skin disorder associated with HIV.

Features of HIV-Associated Seborrheic Dermatitis

Both the frequency and the severity of HIV-associated seborrheic dermatitis are closely related to the stage of HIV infection and, as a result, are inversely correlated with the absolute number of CD4+ (T-helper) cells.[7] In a large series,[8] the incidence of seborrheic dermatitis was reported to be 4.7% in patients classified as Walter Reed stage 1, with an upward rise to 26.7% in those with stage 6 disease. In another report,[9] seborrheic dermatitis was seen in 5 (42%) of 12 patients with AIDS-related complex (ARC) and 15 (83%) of 18 patients with AIDS, and was more severe in the latter group.

Most cases of HIV-associated seborrheic dermatitis have an ordinary clinical presentation. However, atypical features such as thick greasy scales on the scalp and face and involvement of the axillae, groin, genitalia, and perianal areas have been described.[9,10] Histologically, HIV-associated seborrheic dermatitis is usually identical to non-HIV-infected cases, although distinct features such as parakeratosis, keratinocyte necrosis, lymphoid clusters at the dermoepidermal junction, and a perivascular plasma cell infiltrate have been reported.[11]

Etiology

The cause of seborrheic dermatitis in persons with or without HIV infection remains unclear. The incidence of seborrheic dermatitis is increased in many neurologic disorders such as Parkinson's disease, epilepsy, poststroke encephalopathy, and central nervous system (CNS) malignancies.[9,12] Seborrheic dermatitis is also reported to occur with greater frequently in HIV-infected patients with AIDS-associated dementia.[13] A dysfunction in neurohormonal regulation with increased sebum production has been proposed to explain the association of seborrheic dermatitis and neurologic disorders.

The yeast-like fungus *Pityrosporon* (*P. ovale, P. orbiculare*), commonly found on the skin, is thought to play a role in the pathogenesis of seborrheic dermatitis.

Table 17A–1.   Noninfectious Cutaneous Manifestations of HIV Infection in Nine Groups of Patients

Cutaneous Finding	Kaplan et al[7] (N = 222) No. (%)	Goodman et al[4] (N = 117) No. (%)	Sindrup et al[2] (N = 150) No. (%)	Coldiron et al[5] (N = 100) No. (%)	Alessi et al[8] (N = 516) No. (%)	Pennys[60] (N = 1,124) No. (%)	Mathes et al[9] (N = 30) No. (%)	Matis et al[6] (N = 59) No. (%)	Duvic et al[65] (N = 40) No. (%)
Seborrheic dermatitis	11 (5)	37 (32)	28 (19)	49 (49)	41 (8)	122 (11)	20 (67)	21 (36)	
Xerosis/asteatosis	11 (5)		6 (4)	23 (23)					
Xerosis/ichthyosis		36 (31)							
Ichthyosis	3 (1)								
Psoriasis	3 (1)	1 (1)	5 (3)	5 (5)					
Papular eruption		2 (2)			12 (2)	22 (2)			
Telangiectasia	2 (1)								25 (63)
Yellow nails		10 (9)							
Erythroderma	2 (1)								
Hair disease			2 (1)						
Drug rash						22 (2)			

In one series,[11] excessive *Pityrosporon* organisms were found in only a minority of biopsy specimens from AIDS patients with seborrheic dermatitis. However, in another study[14] a correlation between the severity of clinical disease and the number of *Pityrosporon* organisms was observed on Giemsa-stained smears. Furthermore, two patients treated with 2% ketoconazole, a topical antifungal agent, exhibited rapid clearing with a reduction in the number of *Pityrosporon* organisms per keratinocyte. Additional evidence suggesting a role for *Pityrosporon* in seborrheic dermatitis comes from a report in which 22% of patients taking oral ketoconazole had seborrheic dermatitis compared with 36% of those not using the drug.[4] However, the absence of pityrospora in many other HIV-associated seborrheic dermatitis cases suggests that *Pityrosporon* yeasts are not the cause of seborrheic dermatitis but that their presence may aggravate this common skin condition.

Treatment

Seborrheic dermatitis is much more difficult to treat in patients with HIV infection than in non-HIV-infected individuals. There is a poor response to topical corticosteroids and other conventional modalities. In one series, topical ketoconazole was helpful in 25% of cases.[7] In general, as the condition of the patient worsens, the seborrheic dermatitis becomes more severe and refractory to treatment.

PSORIASIS

Psoriasis is a common skin disorder seen in 1% to 2% of the general population and affecting people of both sexes and all ages. Available data do not indicate an increased prevalence of psoriasis among HIV-infected individuals. In one report, 13 (1%) in more than 1,000

HIV-infected individuals were found to have psoriasis.[15] Another report described psoriasis in eight (2%) of 400 patients.[7] However, in smaller series, a prevalence of 3% to 5% has been reported.[2,5,10]

Features of HIV-Associated Psoriasis

Although the prevalence of psoriasis in HIV-seropositive persons is similar to that in the general population, there appears to be a strong relationship between the initial onset of psoriasis and HIV infection. Psoriasis has been reported as the first clinical manifestation of HIV infection[4,7]; the development of eruptive psoriasis or a sudden exacerbation of preexisting disease should suggest the possibility of HIV infection.[15,16]

The clinical features of psoriasis in HIV-infected individuals are often atypical. The lesions may be guttate in appearance (similar to the lesions characteristic of a psoriatic flair associated with streptococcal infection) and may appear on the groin, axillae, scalp, palms, and soles. Severe onychodystrophy and palmar/plantar keratoderma are often seen. Extensive exfoliative psoriasis with generalized erythroderma has also been reported.[15]

Histologically, psoriasis in HIV-infected persons is similar to the ordinary form of psoriasis. However, features such as fewer Monro's abscesses (an accumulation of pyknotic neutrophil nuclei within the epidermis), irregular acanthosis, slight spongiosis, and less suprapapillary thinning of the epidermis are reported to be more characteristic of HIV-associated psoriasis. Also seen is a moderate perivascular and diffuse mononuclear infiltrate that may contain abundant macrophages and occasional multinucleated giant cells.[13] This histologic appearance may also share features of HIV-associated seborrheic dermatitis. Interestingly, in one study, all 13 AIDS patients with psoriasis also had seborrheic dermatitis. The authors concluded that rather than representing distinct entities, there is a spectrum of disease, with seborrheic dermatitis being the least and psoriasis the most severe presentation.[15]

Etiology

It is likely that HIV-associated psoriasis shares features with common psoriasis, in which there is a genetically influenced host response. HLA loci studies indicate an association of HLA class I molecules (HLA-B13, -Bw16, -Bw17, -Bw37) and psoriasis. CD8+ (T-suppressor) cells can interact with cells bearing class I molecules, while CD4+ (T-helper) cells are restricted to interactions with cells bearing HLA class II molecules. This suggests an interaction between CD8+ cells and a putative psoriatic antigen and may in part account for the onset and severity of psoriasis in HIV infection, where there is usually a predominance of CD8+ cells.[17]

It is also possible that the T-cell stimulation and increased cytokine activity seen in HIV infection may play a role in the pathogenesis of HIV-associated psoriasis. For example, increased levels of interferon-α and interferon-γ have been reported in patients with AIDS[18–21]; both have been shown to exacerbate psoriasis.[22,23]

Infections such as streptococcal infections may also influence the development of psoriasis in HIV-infected persons. It is well documented that streptococcal pharyngitis can trigger the onset of guttate psoriasis, and monoclonal antibodies to streptococcal antigens have been found to cross-react with skin antigens.[24] In one series[15] five of 13 AIDS patients with psoriasis had positive skin or throat cultures for streptococcal infection. Multiple courses of antibiotic therapy, however, have produced little or no improvement. Complete remission in a group of patients treated with trimethoprim-sulfamethoxazole has been reported.[19]

Treatment

Most therapeutic modalities used in the treatment of severe forms of psoriasis have immunosuppressive effects, including ultraviolet light B (UVB), psoralens plus ultraviolet light A (PUVA), corticosteroids, methotrexate, and cyclosporin.[15,16,25,26] The use of methotrexate in the first reported cases of HIV-associated psoriasis led to worsening immune function and poor outcomes and is thus contraindicated in this group of patients. Phototherapy has been effective in the treatment of psoriasis, but it is reported to exacerbate Kaposi's sarcoma in some HIV-infected cases.[15] Conventional treatments such as tar and topical corticosteroids have been largely ineffective.

There have been reports of the successful use of zidovudine in the treatment of psoriasis in patients with HIV infection. In all cases the condition relapsed when the medication was discontinued.[27–29] The mechanism of action of zidovudine in these cases is unknown, but the authors postulated that the drug may act against a putative psoriasis retrovirus.[13]

REITER'S SYNDROME/KERATODERMA BLENNORRHAGICA

The classic triad of Reiter's syndrome consists of urethritis, conjunctivitis, and an additive oligoarticular arthritis, mainly of the large joints of the lower extremity. The skin manifestations include keratoderma blennorrhagica (acral, pustular, keratotic lesions with onychodystrophy), circinate balanitis, and painless oral ulcers.[15]

Recent data indicate a greater prevalence of Reiter's syndrome in patients with HIV infection than in the general population.[30,31] In one report, 10 of 101 patients were found to have Reiter's syndrome.[30] However, the overall prevalence among HIV-positive individuals is unknown.

In a review of 36 patients with Reiter's syndrome and HIV infection, nine had keratoderma blennorrhagica.[30] It is important to note that keratoderma is also seen in AIDS-associated psoriasis and acquired ichthyosis without any accompanying arthritic symptoms.[7] The differential diagnosis also includes syphilis and *Trichophyton rubrum* infection, which can produce a similar clinical picture.

Treatment

As with the treatment of psoriasis in patients with HIV infection, immunosuppressive therapies were associated with increased morbidity.[16,25] There is also a poor response to conventional therapy. The use of oral etretinate and topical corticosteroids has been described as an effective treatment for both the arthropathy and the cutaneous lesions of Reiter's syndrome in HIV-associated cases.[32,33]

ACQUIRED ICHTHYOSIS

Acquired ichthyosis has been reported in conjunction with a number of conditions such as lymphoma, carcinoma, classic Kaposi's sarcoma, leprosy, and sarcoidosis.[4,34] In patients with HIV infection, acquired ichthyosis has been described as severe and involving the lower extremities.[4,13] Treatment has focused on control of symptoms with the use of keratolytic agents such as lactic acid and urea compounds.[13]

PORPHYRIA CUTANEA TARDA

Porphyria cutanea tarda, although rare, is the most common of the porphyric diseases. The defect in porphyrin metabolism is due to a decrease in hepatic uroporphyrin decarboxylase activity, which leads to an increase in metabolic precursors.[35] Clinical manifestations consist of cutaneous photosensitivity as the major symptom, facial hypertrichosis, and generalized hyperpigmentation. Lesions are typically found on sun-exposed areas of skin and range from small white plaques to fluid-filled vesicles and bullae that may erode and heal slowly.

Several reports strongly suggest a temporal relationship between HIV infection and the development of porphyria cutanea tarda. Two brothers with hemophilia are reported to have developed porphyria cutanea tarda shortly after they became HIV seropositive.[36] In eight of nine other cases, symptoms of porphyria cutanea tarda heralded a rapid progression to AIDS.[35,37–40]

The role of HIV infection in the development of porphyria cutanea tarda remains unclear. However, the close temporal association between HIV infection and the onset of porphyric symptoms suggests a cause-and-effect relationship. Viral hepatitis, alcohol ingestion, use of certain drugs, and altered hormonal metabolism are known to exacerbate porphyria cutanea tarda. An increase in estrogens, seen in some patients with HIV infection, has been proposed as one possible factor.[37] Recently, abnormal porphyrin metabolism has been demonstrated in patients with HIV infection.[41] The authors speculate that anemia, commonly seen in HIV infection, can lead to an upregulation of porphyrin biosynthesis. In addition, a correlation was made between immune activation, as measured by increased urine neopterin levels, and increased levels of urine porphyrin and its precursors. Further investigation is needed to clarify the relationship between HIV infection and porphyria cutanea tarda.

Treatment

Avoidance of ultraviolet light is the most simple and effective therapeutic modality. Phlebotomy led to improvement of skin lesions in three cases,[35,39] but this therapy has obvious limitations in patients with HIV disease. The antimalarial Plaquenil (hyroxychloroquine sulfate) was used in one patient without benefit.[37]

ACUTE AND CHRONIC PHOTOSENSITIVITY

Increased photosensitivity in patients with HIV infection has been observed. It may result in increased pigmentation, especially in black patients. Two similar case reports describe HIV-seropositive patients who developed severe generalized erythroderma which began in sun-exposed areas. In neither case was a photosensitizing agent identified.[42,43] Another report describes a patient with HIV infection and extreme sensitivity to UVB who developed granuloma annulare restricted to sun-exposed areas.[44] It is speculated that an immune response to certain photoproducts may cause the generalized reactions described in these cases.

PAPULAR AND FOLLICULAR ERUPTIONS IN HIV INFECTION

Several reports have described papular and follicular eruptions in patients with HIV infection. Because of the lack of uniformity in the terminology used in the reports, is uncertain whether the conditions described represent distinct clinical entities or a spectrum of one disease process. The shared features include: (1) pruritus, (2) involvement of the head and neck, upper trunk, and proximal extremities, (3) a perivascular and/or perifollicular inflammatory infiltrate, and (4) an absence of infectious etiology. These eruptions can be classified into papular (chronic and acute), and chronic follicular (including eosinophilic folliculitis).

Papular Eruptions

A transient maculopapular eruption was reported in 41 (12.2%) of 219 HIV-positive cases.[45] The eruption occurred most frequently on the face and truck. The initial lesions healed in 4 to 6 weeks. Histologically, a lymphoplasmacytic angiitis was repeatedly observed in many of these cases.

A more chronic eruption, often pruritic, has also been described among patients with AIDS and ARC.[4,46,47] The eruption consists of multiple, discrete, 2- to 5-mm skin-colored papules distributed over the head, neck, and upper truck. The histologic features are said to be nonspecific. No correlation has been found between the severity of the eruption and the stage of HIV infection.

A chronic papulofollicular eruption has also been reported among HIV-infected individuals. The eruption is reported to consist of follicular papules, usually occurring on the limbs and trunk. A perifollicular neutrophilic infiltrate has been observed histologically. No evidence of bacterial or fungal elements has been reported. Treatment with antibiotics has not been effective.[1,8,48]

Eosinophilic Pustular Folliculitis (HIV-Associated Eosinophilic Folliculitis)

Eosinophilic pustular folliculitis, a rare disorder with less than 100 reported cases,[49] is now being reported in patients with HIV infection.[50–53] The eruption is characterized by multiple urticarial, pruritic, follicular papules, 1 to 4 mm in diameter, scattered on the trunk, face, neck, and proximal extremities. The papules may coalesce to form erythematous plaques. The main histologic feature is an eosinophilic infiltrate of the hair follicle.

In addition to the previously reported cases of HIV-associated eosinophilic pustular folliculitis, a recent report has used the term "HIV-associated eosinophilic folliculitis" to describe the same condition in 13 additional patients.[52] Of all the patients described to date, 19 had AIDS at the time of onset and three were classified as having ARC. In one study eosinophilic pustular folliculitis was noted to be associated with CD4 counts less than 250 to 300/mm^3, making the entity a manifestation of late-stage HIV infection.[52] A relative peripheral eosinophilia (>6%) was seen in 15 of the 19 reported HIV-associated cases. An elevated serum IgE level has also been reported.[52]

Etiology

The cause of these disorders remains obscure. One group of authors postulate that the eruption may represent an aberrant immunologic response to common skin antigens such as dermatophytes or the mite *Demodex folliculorum,* which has been seen in histologic sections of eosinophilic pustular folliculitis.[51] No other pathogens have been found despite multiple cultures and serologic tests.[51,52]

Treatment

Topical corticosteroids have been largely ineffective in controlling these conditions. In six patients treated with UVB phototherapy,[53] the size and number of lesions as well as the pruritus decreased but there was recurrence on discontinuation of the treatment. Use of the antihistamine astemizole has been moderately effective in some cases.[52]

GRANULOMA ANNULARE

Granuloma annulare is characterized by erythematous or flesh-colored papules seen in an annular "ring-shaped" grouping. Although there have been a number of reported cases,[54–57] it is difficult to make a strong association with HIV infection because granuloma annulare is a more common dermatosis. In one HIV-infected case, granuloma annulare reportedly disappeared after 4 weeks of zidovudine therapy.[56] This suggests a possible relationship between the development of granuloma annulare and HIV infection, or the resulting immune dysfunction. In two cases in which information is available, the absolute number of T-helper cells was 40 and 72, evidence of severe cellular immune impairment.[55,56]

The histology of granuloma annulare in HIV-infected cases is similar to that in non-HIV-infected cases, showing a focally altered collagen surrounded by a palisading granuloma. However, in contrast to the T-helper cell infiltrate seen in the classic form, granuloma annulare in AIDS cases shows a T-suppressor cell infiltrate.[55]

NAIL AND HAIR CHANGES

Yellow discoloration of the nails (not associated with any infectious agent) is reported among HIV-infected persons. In one report,[58] four of eight patients had yellow discoloration of the distal portion of the nails, and in another report ten of 117 patients were said to have yellow nail syndrome. The yellow nail syndrome was initially described in association with pulmonary disease and lymphedema. Although referred to as yellow nail syndrome, it must be noted that the cases described in HIV-infected persons may not fulfill the diagnostic criteria for yellow nail syndrome, which includes the absence of cuticles and a distinctive onychodystrophy.[59]

Many conditions other than HIV infection, such as diabetes, drugs reactions, and nail polish, have also been reported to cause a yellow discoloration of the nail plate.

Numerous abnormalities of the hair, from alopecia to hypertrichosis, have been reported in patients with HIV infection.[60] A diffuse thinning of the hair may be the most common abnormality observed. In some cases an underlying inflammatory cell infiltrate of the scalp has been reported.[61] An interesting finding reported in at least 50% of black patients with AIDS is the loss of curl and gradual straightening of the scalp hair. In one case the hair changes were noted 6 months prior to the diagnosis of AIDS.[62]

DRUG REACTIONS

Trimethoprim-Sulfamethoxazole Sulfonamides

Trimethoprim-sulfamethoxazole is the combination drug of choice for the prophylaxis and treatment of *Pneumocystis carinii* pneumonia. The frequency of toxic effects from this drug is much higher in patients with HIV infection than in background populations. Skin eruption, the most common toxic manifestation, was reported in 18 of 35 patients with AIDS who were treated with high doses of the drug (trimethoprim, 20 mg/kg/day)—a frequency 10 times higher than in non-AIDS patients.[63] The eruption has been described as a generalized erythematous, maculopapular rash occurring 8 to 12 days into treatment. Fever is often associated with the rash.

Six patients with AIDS taking standard doses of sulfonamides were reported to developed toxic epidermal necrolysis. The patients recovered after discontinuation of the medication. All patients had fever and mucosal lesions.[60]

Zidovudine

Patients taking zidovudine have been reported to develop an increased pigmentation of the fingernails and toenails, resulting in a bluish discoloration.[64] The discoloration progressed distally starting at the base of the fingernail. This side-effect was most commonly seen in patients receiving high-dose zidovudine (1,200 mg/day).

Glucan-Induced Keratoderma

This unusual cutaneous reaction has been reported in six of 20 patients with AIDS or ARC who were treated with the immunostimulant glucan. This oligosaccharide is derived from the inner cell wall of the yeast *Saccharomyces cerevisiae*. A symmetric, palmoplantar, thick yellow hyperkeratosis with fissuring of the skin developed during the first 2 weeks of therapy. The condition resolved over a 2- to 4-week period after treatment. There were no pustules or nail changes suggestive of the keratoderma blennorrhagica seen in HIV-associated psoriasis or Reiter's syndrome.[65] The etiology of this unusual reaction to the yeast antigen is not known.

BANAL SKIN FINDINGS IN HIV INFECTION

Along with severe cutaneous manifestations, a few mild cutaneous signs and symptoms are commonly reported in patients with HIV infection.

Xerosis

Dry and cracking skin (xerosis and asteatosis) is reported in some of the large series.[5,7] The dry skin is often pruritic. Antihistamines have been reported to be ineffective in controlling the pruritus,[13] and treatment should be directed toward the underlying xerosis.

Telangiectasia

Although not frequently reported in larger series, linear telangiectasias of the anterior chest were reported in one study[66] to occur in 25 (62%) of 40 HIV-seropositive homosexual men. The incidence increased as the stage of HIV infection advanced. Histologic studies reportedly showed dilated vessels and a perivascular infiltrate. The anterior chest telangiectasias described were felt to be distinct from those seen in any other disease. No etiology was offered, but a disregulation of hormonal metabolism may be involved.

REFERENCES

1. Lim W, Sadick N, Gupta A et al: Skin diseases in children with HIV infection and their association with degree of immunosuppression. Int J Dermatol 29:24, 1990
2. Sindrup JH, Weismann K, Petersen CS et al: Skin and oral mucosal changes in patients infected with human immunodeficiency virus. Acta Derm Venereol 68:440, 1988
3. Johnson M-LT, Roberts J: Prevalence of dermatological diseases among persons 1–74 years of age: United States. Publication No. (PHS) 79-1660. Washington, DC, US Public Health Service, 1977
4. Goodman DS, Teplitz ED, Wishner A et al: Prevalence of cutaneous disease in patients with acquired immunodeficiency syndrome (AIDS) or AIDS-related complex. J Am Acad Dermatol 17:210, 1987
5. Coldiron BM, Bergstresser PR: Prevalence and clinical spectrum of skin disease in patients infected with human immunodeficiency virus. Arch Dermatol 125:357, 1989
6. Matis WL, Triana A, Shapiro R et al: Dermatologic findings associated with human immunodeficiency virus infection. J Am Acad Dermatol 17:746, 1987
7. Kaplan MH, Sadick N, McNutt NS et al: Dermatologic findings and manifestations of acquired immunodeficiency syndrome (AIDS). J Am Acad Dermatol 16:485, 1987
8. Alessi E, Cusini M, Zerroni R: Mucocutaneous manifestations in patients infected with human immunodeficiency virus. J Am Acad Dermatol 19:290, 1988
9. Mathes BM, Douglas MC: Seborrheic dermatitis in patients with acquired immunodeficiency syndrome. J Am Acad Dermatol 13:947, 1985
10. Eisenstat BA, Wormer GP: Seborrheic dermatitis and butterfly rash in AIDS. N Engl J Med 311:189, 1984
11. Soeprono FF, Schinella RA, Cockerell CJ et al: Seborrheic-like dermatitis of acquired immunodeficiency syndrome. J Am Acad Dermatol 14:242, 1986
12. Binder RL, Jonelis FJ: Seborrheic dermatitis in neuroleptic-induced parkinsonism. Arch Dermatol 119:473, 1983
13. Sadick NS, Mcnutt NS, Kaplan MH: Papulosquamous dermatoses of AIDS. J Am Acad Dermatol 22:1270, 1990
14. Groisser D, Bottone EJ, Lebwohl M: Association of *Pityrosporum orbiculare* (*Malassezia furfur*) with seborrheic dermatitis in patients with acquired immunodeficiency syndrome (AIDS). J Am Acad Dermatol 20:770, 1989
15. Duvic M, Johnson TM, Rapini RP et al: Acquired immunodeficiency syndrome-associated psoriasis and Reiter's syndrome. Arch Dermatol 123:1622, 1987
16. Johnson TM, Duvic M, Rapini RP: AIDS exacerbates psoriasis. N Engl J Med 313:1415, 1985
17. Baadsgaard O, Fisher GJ, Voorhees JJ, Cooper KD. Interactions of epidermal cells and T cells in inflammatory skin diseases. J Am Acad Dermatol 23:1312, 1990
18. Fuchs D, Hausen A, Reibnegger G et al: Psoriasis, gamma-interferon, and the acquired immunodeficiency syndrome (letter). Ann Intern Med 106:165, 1987
19. Espinoza LR, Berman A, Vasey FB et al: Psoriatic arthritis and acquired immunodeficiency syndrome. Arthritis Rheum 31:1034, 1988
20. Eyster ME, Goedert JJ, Poon MC, Preble OT: Acid-labile alpha interferon: A possible preclinical marker for the acquired immunodeficiency syndrome in hemophilia. N Engl J Med 309:583, 1983
21. Fuchs D, Hausen A, Reibnegger G et al: Urinary neopterin in the diagnosis of acquired immunodeficiency syndrome. Eur J Clin Microbiol 3:70, 1984
22. Baker BS, Griffiths CEM, Fry L, Valdimarsson H: Psoriasis and interferon. Lancet 2:342, 1986
23. Quesada JR, Gutterman JV: Psoriasis and alpha-interferon. Lancet 1:1466, 1986
24. Swerlick RA, Cunningham MW, Hall NK: Monoclonal antibodies cross-reactive with group A streptococci and normal and psoriatic skin. J Invest Dermatol 87:367, 1986
25. Winchester R, Bernstein DH, Fischer HD et al: The co-occurrence of Reiter's syndrome and acquired immunodeficiency syndrome. Ann Intern Med 106:19, 1987
26. Noonan FP, Kripke ML, Pedersen GM et al: Suppression of contact hypersensitivity in mice by ultraviolet irradiation is associated with defective antigen presentation. Immunology 43:527, 1981
27. Kaplan MH, Sadick NS, Wieder J et al: Antipsoriatic effects of zidovudine in human immunodeficiency virus-associated psoriasis. J Am Acad Dermatol 20:76, 1989
28. Ruzicka T, Froschl M, Hohenleutner U et al: Treatment of HIV-induced retinoid-resistant psoriasis with zidovudine. Lancet 2:1469, 1987
29. Duvic M, Rios A: Remission of AIDS-associated psoriasis with zidovudine (letter). Lancet 2:627, 1987
30. Kaye BR: Rheumatologic manifestations of infection with human immunodeficiency virus (HIV). Ann Intern Med 111:158, 1989
31. Berman A, Espinosa LR, Diaz JD et al: Rheumatic manifestations of human immunodeficiency virus infection. Am J Med 85:59, 1988

32. Belz J, Breneman DL, Nordlund JJ, Solinger A: Successful treatment of a patient with Reiter's syndrome and acquired immunodeficiency syndrome using etretinate. J Am Acad Dermatol 20:898, 1989

33. Richman TB, Kerdel FA: Reiter's syndrome (letter). Arch Dermatol 124:1007, 1988

34. Brenner S: Acquired ichthyosis in AIDS. Cutis 39:421, 1987

35. Wissel PS, Sordillo P, Anderson KE et al: Porphyria cutanea tarda associated with the acquired immune deficiency syndrome. Am J Hematol 25:107, 1987

36. Hogan D, Card RT, Ghadially et al: Human immunodeficiency virus infection and porphyria cutanea tarda. J Am Acad Dermatol 20:17, 1989

37. Reynaud P, Goodfellow K, Svec F: Porphyria cutanea tarda as initial presentation of the acquired immunodeficiency syndrome in two patients (letter). J Infect Dis 161:1032, 1990

38. Lobata MN, Berger TG: Porphyria cutanea tarda associated with the acquired immunodeficiency syndrome. Arch Dermatol 124:1009, 1988

39. Conrad ME: AIDS and porphyria cutanea tarda (letter). Am J Hematol 28:207, 1988

40. Nip-Sakamoto CJ, Wong RHW, Izumi AK: Porphyria cutanea tarda and AIDS. Cutis 44:470, 1989

41. Fuchs D, Artner-Dworzak E, Hausen A et al: Urinary excretion of porphyrins is increased in patients with HIV-1 infection. AIDS 4:341, 1990

42. Toback AC, Longley J, Cardullo AC et al: Severe chronic photosensitivity in association with acquired immunodeficiency syndrome. J Am Acad Dermatol 15:1056, 1986

43. Herman LE, Kurban AK: Erythroderma as a manifestation of the AIDS-related complex. J Am Acad Dermatol 17:507, 1987

44. Cohen PR, Grossman ME, Silvers DN, DeLeo VA: Generalized granuloma annulare located on sun-exposed areas in a human immunodeficiency virus-seropositive man with ultraviolet B photosensitivity. Arch Dermatol 126:830, 1990

45. James WD, Redfield RR, Lupton GP et al: A papular eruption associated with human T cell lymphotropic virus type III disease. J Am Acad Dermatol 13:563, 1985

46. Warner LC, Fisher BK: Cutaneous manifestations of the acquired immunodeficiency syndrome. Int J Dermatol 25:337, 1986

47. Hira SK, Wadhawan D, Kamanga J et al: Cutaneous manifestations of human immunodeficiency virus in Lusaka, Zambia. J Am Acad Dermatol 19:451, 1988

48. Barlow RJ, Schulz EJ: Necrotizing folliculitis in AIDS related complex. Br J Dermatol 116:581, 1987

49. Takematsu H, Nakamura K, Igarashi M, Tagami H: Eosinophilic pustular folliculitis. Arch Dermatol 121:917, 1985

50. Jenkins D, Fisher BK, Chalvardjian A, Adam P: Eosinophilic pustular folliculitis in a patient with AIDS. Int J Dermatol 27:34, 1988

51. Soeprono FF, Schinella RA: Eosinophilic pustular folliculitis in patients with acquired immunodeficiency syndrome. J Am Acad Dermatol 14:1020, 1986

52. Rosenthal D, LeBoit PE, Klumpp L, Berger TG: Human immunodeficiency virus-associated eosinophilic folliculitis. Arch Dermatol 127:206, 1991

53. Buchness MR, Lim HW, Hatcher VA et al: Eosinophilic pustular folliculitis in the acquired immunodeficiency syndrome. N Engl J Med 318:1183, 1988

54. Bakos L, Hampe S, da Rocha JL et al: Generalized granuloma annulare in a patient with acquired immunodeficiency syndrome (AIDS). J Am Acad Dermatol 17:844, 1987

55. Huerter CJ, Bass J, Bergfeld WF, Tubbs RR: Perforating granuloma annulare in a patient with acquired immunodeficiency syndrome. Arch Dermatol 123:1217, 1987

56. Leenutaphong V, Erckenbrecht, Zuleger S, Plewig G: Remission of human immunodeficiency virus-associated generalized granuloma annulare under zidovudine therapy (letter). J Am Acad Dermatol 19:1126, 1988

57. Pennys NS, Hicks B: Unusual cutaneous lesions associated with acquired immunodeficiency syndrome. J Am Acad Dermatol 13:845, 1985

58. Chernosky ME, Finley VK: Yellow nail syndrome in patients with acquired immunodeficiency disease. J Am Acad Dermatol 13:731, 1985

59. Scher RK: Acquired immunodeficiency syndrome and yellow nails (letter). J Am Acad Dermatol 18:758, 1988

60. Pennys NS: Skin Manifestations of AIDS. London, Martin Dunitz, 1989

61. Friedman-Kien AE, DeVita VT, Krigel R et al: A Color Atlas of AIDS. Philadelphia, WB Saunders, 1989

62. Kinchelow T, Schmidt U, Ingato S: Changes in the hair of black patients with AIDS (letter). J Infect Dis 157:394, 1988

63. Gordin FM, Simon GL, Wofsy CB, Mills J: Adverse reactions to trimethoprim-sulfamethoxazole in patients with the acquired immunodeficiency syndrome. Ann Intern Med 100:495, 1984

64. Furth PA, Kazakis AM: Nail pigmentation changes associated with azothymidine (zidovudine) (letter). Ann Intern Med 107:350, 1987

65. Duvic M, Reisman M, Finley V et al: Glucan-induced keratoderma in acquired immunodeficiency syndrome. Arch Dermatol 123:751, 1987

66. Fallon T, Abell E, Kingsley L et al: Telangiectasias of the anterior chest in homosexual men. Ann Intern Med 105:679, 1986

Pulmonary Complications 17B

Stewart J. Levine *James H. Shelhamer*

Noninfectious disorders are increasingly recognized as common and important causes of lung disease in patients infected with the human immunodeficiency virus (HIV).[1] These noninfectious pulmonary complications include neoplastic processes (*i.e.,* Kaposi's sarcoma and non-Hodgkin's lymphoma), interstitial pneumonitis (*i.e.,* nonspecific and lymphocytic interstitial pneumonitis), and inflammatory disorders of the airways. This chapter reviews the pathology, clinical and radiographic presentation, diagnosis, natural history, and treatment of these noninfectious pulmonary complications of HIV infection.

NEOPLASTIC PULMONARY COMPLICATIONS OF HIV INFECTION

Kaposi's Sarcoma

Prior to the acquired immunodeficiency syndrome (AIDS) epidemic, Kaposi's sarcoma in the United States was a rare, indolent vascular neoplasm that most commonly involved the skin of the lower extremities of elderly men of Jewish and Mediterranean origin.[2,3] In contrast, Kaposi's sarcoma is the most common malignancy complicating AIDS and often results in significant morbidity.[2,4] AIDS-associated Kaposi's sarcoma tends to be a multifocal process involving the skin, mucocutaneous membranes, lymph nodes, and visceral organs, most commonly the respiratory and gastrointestinal (GI) systems.[2,4-7] Kaposi's sarcoma preferentially occurs in men from homosexual or bisexual risk groups and has a 50:1 male–female ratio.[2,4,7] In addition, it is uncommon in pediatric AIDS patients. This epidemiologic pattern has suggested a multifactorial etiology that includes infectious (*i.e.,* cytomegalovirus [CMV] or Epstein-Barr virus [EBV] infection), environmental (*i.e.,* amyl nitrite inhalation), or genetic cofactors in addition to HIV-related immunosuppression.[2,4,8] Despite the increase in the total number of AIDS patients since the onset of the AIDS epidemic, the incidence of Kaposi's sarcoma has been decreasing at both the local and national levels.[8-11] The declining incidence may reflect a decreased exposure of individuals at risk for Kaposi's sarcoma to potential etiologic cofactors.

PATHOLOGY

Pulmonary involvement by AIDS-associated Kaposi's sarcoma has been reported in 6% to 35% of autopsies on patients with Kaposi's sarcoma, although some series have reported frequencies as high as 40% to 75%.[5,6,12-15] Although pulmonary Kaposi's sarcoma is generally found in patients with previously documented cutaneous, nodal, or visceral disease, isolated intrathoracic lesions have been reported in approximately 11% of cases.[5,6,16-22] Furthermore, pulmonary Kaposi's sarcoma can progress despite limited or stable extrapulmonary disease.[23]

Intrathoracic Kaposi's sarcoma can involve the pulmonary parenchyma, airways, pleura, or mediastinal lymph nodes.[13,16,17,21,24-26] Pulmonary parenchymal involvement is multifocal and follows interstitial lymphatic pathways along bronchovascular bundles, interlobular septae, and the pleura.[13,14,19-21] Although tumor cells frequently completely dissect into and thicken the walls of airways and blood vessels, they generally do not compress these structures.[19,20,24] Disease progression may result in the formation of nodular masses that have a peribronchial or perivascular distribution.[14,20,21,24,26] Advanced parenchymal lesions may obliterate alveolar spaces, with resulting radiographic consolidation.[19,21]

Submucosal lesions of the trachea and bronchi have an appearance similar to that of the cutaneous lesions and appear grossly as erythematous, irregular, macular or papular lesions.[13,24,27,28] Multiple discrete lesions may be distributed throughout the tracheobronchial tree, but frequently they are located at the carinas of segmental orifices.[16,28] Endobronchial lesions correlate histologically with extensive submucosal infiltration by Kaposi's sarcoma cells that secondarily entrap and obliterate mucosal glandular structures, as well as denude the columnar epithelium.[24,29] Infrequently, extensive endobronchial tumor masses can compromise the luminal integrity of either the tracheobronchial tree or the upper airway.[14,18,30]

Pleural Kaposi's sarcoma involves only the visceral pleura, with resultant plaque formation secondary to infiltrating tumor cells.[21,24] The pleural surface, however, is not disrupted, and concomitant pleural effusions are frequently present.[16,21,23,24] Hilar or mediastinal lymph node involvement by Kaposi's sarcoma may result in either gross adenopathy or only microscopic evidence of tumor infiltration.[21] Of note, pleural or hilar/mediastinal lymph node involvement can occur independently without associated pulmonary parenchymal lesions.[21]

The histopathology of Kaposi's sarcoma reveals a vascular tumor composed of interstitial linear and nodular accumulations of plump to elongate spindle cells within an extracellular network of reticulin fibers.[3,7,14,16,20,23,31] These spindle cells form numerous vascular clefts which are filled with erythrocytes. The lesions of Kaposi's sarcoma are associated with varying amounts of acute and chronic hemorrhage, as evidenced by extravasated erythrocytes and hemosiderin-laden macrophages.[14,16,20,23] An inflammatory infiltrate composed of lymphocytes and plasma cells is often present and may vary in intensity from scarce to so extensive that the classic spindle cell lesions are almost completely obscured.[13,14,20,23,32] An early form of Kaposi's sarcoma may be characterized by lesions that have an extensive inflammatory component with nonspecific plump mesenchymal cells and few spindle cells. Consequently, sampling of this inflammatory type of lesion may result in an incorrect diagnosis of an organizing interstitial pneumonitis rather than Kaposi's sarcoma.[13,19] Although it is unclear whether the cell of origin of Kaposi's sarcoma is vascular or lymphatic, there is evidence suggesting that small lymphatic-venule channels may represent the initial site of neoplasia.[3,4,12,33–35]

Parenchymal interstitial and intra-alveolar hemorrhage, which may be extensive, can often be found in association with KS lesions.[13,14,19,36] Pulmonary hemorrhage occurs secondary to extravasation of erythrocytes from foci of Kaposi's sarcoma, especially in patients with underlying defects in hemostasis. Pulmonary hemosiderosis may also be present.[19] Focal lymphoid infiltrates in areas unassociated with Kaposi's sarcoma lesions have also been reported.[19]

CLINICAL PRESENTATION

The clinical signs and symptoms of pulmonary Kaposi's sarcoma are often nonspecific and may be difficult to distinguish from those of AIDS-related opportunistic infections. Dyspnea and cough are the most common clinical manifestations and may be present in 100% of patients.[16,20,23,24,29] Fever and sputum production are not characteristic of pulmonary Kaposi's sarcoma and should alert the clinician to the possible presence of an opportunistic infection.[13,16,17,20,23,29,37] Wheezing, reported in 18% of 11 patients in one report, represented either airways obstruction secondary to endobronchial disease or pulmonary edema caused by obstruction of lymphatic vessels.[24] Hemoptysis has been reported to occur in 11% to 18% of cases and may represent extensive intra-alveolar hemorrhage or bleeding from endobronchial lesions.[14,19,24,26] The development of stridor is a sign of laryngeal or tracheal obstruction by the lesions of Kaposi's sarcoma and may be exacerbated by secondary hemorrhage and intraluminal thrombus formation.[24,30] Hoarseness is suggestive of the presence of vocal cord lesions.[37] Indeed, the presence of either focal wheezing, stridor, or hemoptysis, especially in the setting of previously documented cutaneous Kaposi's sarcoma, should alert the clinician to the possibility of endobronchial or mucosal lesions. Pleuritic chest pain may suggest the presence of underlying pleural disease and has been reported in 9% to 30% of cases.[24]

The physical examination in patients with pulmonary Kaposi's sarcoma is often nonrevealing. In one series of 19 patients with pulmonary Kaposi's sarcoma, only 16% had evidence of bilateral crackles on lung auscultation; in all other patients the examination results were normal.[16] The presence of decreased breath sounds and dullness to percussion may be suggestive of a pleural effusion associated with Kaposi's sarcoma. Because the physical examination often yields nonspecific findings, it is important to document the presence of either cutaneous or mucocutaneous Kaposi's sarcoma lesions, which can then serve as markers of possible lung involvement.

Although arterial blood gas determinations and pulmonary function tests are frequently abnormal in the setting of pulmonary Kaposi's sarcoma, neither can be used to definitively differentiate Kaposi's sarcoma from opportunistic infections. Arterial blood gases usually reveal the presence of mild to moderate hypoxemia and an increased alveolar to arterial oxygen gradient (D_A–aO_2).[16,24,29,38,39] The response of the D_A–aO_2 to exercise testing is variable.[39] Results of pulmonary function testing may be consistent with the presence of either parenchymal or endobronchial disease. The diffusing capacity for carbon monoxide is frequently abnormal in patients with parenchymal Kaposi's sarcoma, with reported mean values ranging from 41% to 64% of predicted in two studies involving 27 patients.[38–40] Air flow obstruction, as evidenced by an FEV_1/FVC ratio of less than 75%, has been reported in 50% to 100% of patients with endobronchial Kaposi's sarcoma who did not have a concomitant history of cigarette smoking or atopic disease.[40] In addition, decreases in lung volumes, consistent with the presence of a restrictive pulmonary process, have been found in approximately 30% of patients.[24,39]

The radiographic manifestations of pulmonary Kaposi's sarcoma correlate well with the anatomic and histologic distribution of disease.[16,19,21,23,24,29,31,38,41,42] Parenchymal pulmonary involvement is characterized by patchy, multifocal, bilateral, perihilar infiltrates that are either interstitial, alveolar, or mixed alveolar-interstitial in nature. These infiltrates often radiate from abnormal hilar masses (Fig. 17B–1).[41,42] Computed tomography (CT) reveals perivascular and peribronchial extension of Kaposi's sarcoma lesions consistent with the histopathologic progression of disease along interstitial lymphatic pathways with secondary involvement of alveolar spaces (Fig. 17B–2).[41] Several studies, however, have not described this perihilar distribution but rather have noted diffusely distributed interstitial, alveolar, or alveolar-interstitial infiltrates.[19,23,29,31,38] In these studies, interstitial infiltrates had a reticular or reticulonodular appearance consistent with tumor involvement of the pulmonary interstitium and interlobular septa. With disease progression, these alveolar-interstitial infiltrates coalesced into large, poorly defined areas of nodular parenchymal opacification or consolidation.[21,31,41] Multiple pulmonary nodules and nodular-appearing alveolar infiltrates ranging in size from 0.5 to 3 cm in diameter are also common, having been reported in 24% of 167 patients in ten series (see Fig. 17B–2).[19,38,41] There has also been a case report describing multiple cavitary nodules that were thought to represent tumor necrosis.[43] Focal unilateral alveolar infiltrates, which may be associated with segmental consolidation, have been re-

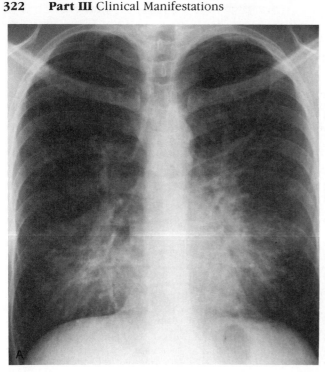
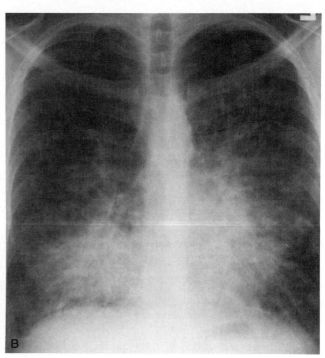

Figure 17B–1. (**A**) Typical chest radiographic manifestations of pulmonary Kaposi's sarcoma in a patient with bilateral patchy perihilar alveolar-interstitial infiltrates. (**B**) Follow-up chest radiograph after 1 month revealed progressive pulmonary Kaposi's sarcoma complicated by acute intra-alveolar hemorrhage. (Radiographs courtesy of Irwin Feuerstein, MD)

ported in 5% of patients. Occlusion of lobar orifices by endobronchial Kaposi's sarcoma mass lesions with secondary lobar atelectasis is rare.[18] Chest radiographs are normal in 5% of patients with pulmonary Kaposi's sarcoma and correspond to parenchymal lesions 2 mm to 1 cm in size.[19,21,38,41]

Unilateral or bilateral hilar or mediastinal lymphadenopathy, consistent with lymphatic involvement, has been described in 39% of 91 patients in six series.[38,41] However, one recent study of 24 patients found mediastinal adenopathy on only 2% of chest radiographs, although CT scans revealed spotty or 1+ adenopathy in 63% of patients.[41]

Nonloculated pleural effusions are a common radiographic finding. Pleural effusions, often bilateral and of variable size, have been reported in 45% of 167 cases in ten series.[15,19,38,41] Parenchymal infiltrates were found in association with pleural effusions in 90% of cases in one series involving 21 patients.[15] Thoracocentesis typically yields serous, serosanguineous, or frankly hemorrhagic exudative fluid.[16,19,23,24,29,38] Cytologic examination typically does not reveal any abnormalities predictive of Kaposi's sarcoma, and pleural biopsies are nondiagnostic, revealing either normal pleura or reactive mesothelial cells.[16,19,23,24,29,38] Pulmonary Kaposi's sarcoma has also been reported to result in bilateral chylous pleural effusions, which can be massive in size and represent sequelae of thoracic duct disruption by mediastinal disease.[44] In addition, a case of spontaneous pneumothorax complicating pleural Kaposi's sarcoma has been reported.[45]

Radionuclide scintigraphy, although not specific, may also provide suggestive evidence of pulmonary Kaposi's sarcoma. Because pulmonary Kaposi's sarcoma often does not label with ^{67}Ga citrate, a negative study in a patient with typical radiographic abnormalities and known Kaposi's sarcoma may be compatible with pulmonary involvement.[29,45–47] Even though pulmonary Kaposi's sarcoma may on occasion take up ^{67}Ga citrate, a positive study is more likely to indicate the presence of an opportunistic infection or another neoplastic process, such as lymphoma.[29,48] In contrast, thallium-201 scintigraphy may in the future prove to be useful in identifying pulmonary Kaposi's sarcoma, as the lesions appear to be thallium avid.[48,49,50]

DIAGNOSIS

Invasive diagnostic procedures such as fiberoptic bronchoscopy or open lung biopsy are necessary to definitively establish the diagnosis of pulmonary Kaposi's sarcoma, because clinical and radiographic findings are

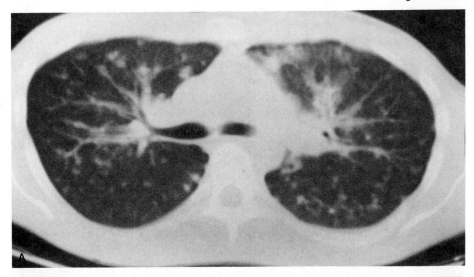

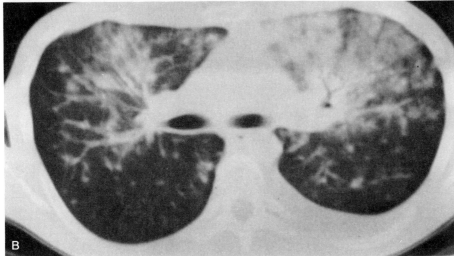

Figure 17B–2. Chest CT scans corresponding to Figures 17B–1A and 17B–1B. (**A**) Bilateral parenchymal nodules, as well as interstitial and alveolar infiltrates radiating from abnormal hilar masses. (**B**) Progressive pulmonary Kaposi's sarcoma with increased air space disease secondary to acute intra-alveolar hemorrhage. (CT scans courtesy of Irwin Feuerstein, MD)

nonspecific and thoracocentesis and pleural biopsy are nondiagnostic. The utility of fiberoptic bronchoscopy in establishing the diagnosis of pulmonary Kaposi's sarcoma is variable and is dependent on the type of pulmonary manifestation present. Inspection of the tracheobronchial tree alone may be sufficient for a presumptive diagnosis if characteristic erythematous, irregular, flat or slightly raised lesions, often at airway branch points, are seen.[16,24,37,49] Indeed, these lesions have been correlated with histologic evidence of Kaposi's sarcoma at autopsy.[29] When endobronchial biopsies have been attempted, the reported yields have been extremely variable, probably reflecting the submucosal location of this lesion. In eight small studies, the yield of endobronchial biopsy ranged from 0% to 83%, with an overall yield of 60%.[16,19,24,27,28,51–53] Because a presumptive diagnosis of endobronchial Kaposi's sarcoma is almost always adequate and because cases of excessive bleeding have been reported following attempts at en-

dobronchial biopsy, many clinicians do not employ this procedure in this setting. However, a careful visual examination of the nasal mucosa, oropharynx, larynx, and trachea should be performed because these areas are potential sites of involvement with endobronchial disease.

If endobronchial lesions are not identified, then histologic examination of the pulmonary parenchyma is necessary to establish the diagnosis. Unfortunately, the yield of transbronchial biopsy is quite low. This may reflect both sampling error, due to the multifocal nature of Kaposi's sarcoma, and the requirement for large pieces of tissue for pathologic examination, insofar as crush artifact, hemorrhage, and granulation tissue can mimic the lesions of Kaposi's sarcoma.[23] In ten small series involving 79 patients, transbronchial biopsies yielded a diagnosis of Kaposi's sarcoma in only 17% of cases.[12,16,20,23,25,28,36,53–55] In addition, clinicians should be aware of the possibility of significant pulmonary hemorrhage following transbronchial biopsy in patients with pulmonary Kaposi's sarcoma.[24] Although bronchoalveolar lavage (BAL) and transbronchial biopsy may not be useful in establishing the diagnosis of pulmonary Kaposi's sarcoma, fiberoptic bronchoscopy is indicated for patients with known pulmonary involvement who have a change in respiratory symptoms or radiographic infiltrates, to evaluate for the possibility of a concomitant opportunistic infection.

If fiberoptic bronchoscopy is nondiagnostic, an open lung biopsy may be necessary to establish the diagnosis.[12,23,56–58] The advantage of an open lung biopsy is that it provides the pathologist with a larger piece of tissue for examination, thereby minimizing the likelihood of crush artifact or sampling error.[12,23] However, even open lung biopsy is not 100% sensitive, and it, too, may be subject to sampling error because of the focal nature of the lesions.[16,23,49] For example, in one series of nine patients, open lung biopsy had a sensitivity of only 56%.[16]

NATURAL HISTORY

Pulmonary Kaposi's sarcoma is often a late, terminal manifestation of AIDS, with most studies reporting a life expectancy of less than 1 year, although instances of prolonged survival have also been reported.[16,38,49] The median survival time following the diagnosis of pulmonary Kaposi's sarcoma ranged from 1.1 to 12 months in three studies involving 60 patients.[16,24,29] Concurrent opportunistic pulmonary infections (*P. carinii,* CMV, fungi) were present in 52% of patients at the time of death and were associated with diminished survival. Progressive pulmonary Kaposi's sarcoma without concurrent pulmonary disorders may also result in respiratory failure and death.[13] Indeed, 36% of patients in three reports involving 45 patients died secondary to progressive hypoxemia resulting from extensive pulmonary Kaposi's sarcoma.[23,24,29] Other factors that may contribute to respiratory failure in patients with pulmonary Kaposi's sarcoma include associated alveolar hemorrhage and upper airway obstruction secondary to large endobronchial tumor masses. Factors that have been reported to be predictive of decreased survival have included the presence of pleural effusions and CD4 lymphocyte counts of less than 100/mm³.[38]

THERAPY

Therapeutic modalities that have been utilized in pulmonary Kaposi's sarcoma have included cytotoxic chemotherapy regimens, radiation therapy, and immunomodulatory therapy (interferon).[4] Unfortunately, none of these regimens have been effective in achieving a long-term cure in the setting of pulmonary Kaposi's sarcoma. However, therapeutic interventions may afford palliation and prolong survival.[4] Systemic chemotherapy has been used in patients with progressive pulmonary disease, and external radiation therapy and neodymium-

doped yttrium-aluminum-garnet (Nd:YAG) laser surgery have been used to alleviate obstructing intraluminal lesions.[18,38] However, systemic chemotherapeutic regimens have the potential for causing bone marrow suppression and neutropenia, which may place these patients at increased risk for infectious complications. Although most pleural effusions devolving from Kaposi's sarcoma do not require intervention, effusions that are large in size or produce symptoms may necessitate either intermittent therapeutic thoracocentesis, chest tube drainage, or pleural sclerosis.[49] However, in one series, neither systemic chemotherapy nor chest tube thoracostomy with tetracycline sclerosis was effective in controlling the pleural effusions of Kaposi's sarcoma.[15]

Because *P. carinii* pneumonia is a common infection in patients with pulmonary Kaposi's sarcoma, management of these patients should include anti-*Pneumocystis* prophylaxis therapy. Twice daily oral trimethoprim-sulfamethoxazole has been shown to an effective prophylactic agent in this setting and has been associated with prolonged survival.[59] Unfortunately, adverse reactions to trimethoprim-sulfamethoxazole are common, occurring in 50% of patients. Although aerosolized pentamidine is an effective prophylactic agent in AIDS patients, no data exist regarding its efficacy in the setting of pulmonary Kaposi's sarcoma.[60]

Non-Hodgkin's Lymphoma

HIV-infected patients are at increased risk for developing one of the non-Hodgkin's lymphomas.[33,61,62] Non-Hodgkin's lymphoma is the second most common malignancy complicating AIDS and, in contrast to Kaposi's sarcoma, does not appear to be confined to any particular risk group for HIV infection.[63–65] In addition, non-Hodgkin's lymphoma is considered an AIDS-defining illness by the Centers for Disease Control (CDC) when an HIV-seropositive patient develops an intermediate- or high-grade lymphoma of B-cell origin.[63] AIDS-associated non-Hodgkin's lymphoma is characterized by an aggressive pattern of behavior, with high-grade histologic features and advanced stage of disease at the time of presentation.[64–69] Furthermore, there is a predilection for dissemination and involvement of extranodal sites of disease, especially the central nervous system (CNS), gastrointestinal system, and bone marrow. Intrathoracic involvement is infrequent, having been reported in 7% of 469 patients in 11 series.[65–75] Although the pulmonary parenchyma is the most common intrathoracic site of disease, pleural and mediastinal lesions have also been reported. Intrathoracic disease may represent the solitary site of involvement by non-Hodgkin's lymphoma.[67,76]

PATHOLOGY

AIDS-associated non-Hodgkin's lymphoma is most frequently of B-cell lineage and can be categorized into three aggressive histopathologic groups: large cell immunoblastic, large noncleaved cell, and small non-cleaved cell, either Burkitt's or non-Burkitt's type.[33,62,63] Approximately 70% of AIDS patients with non-Hodgkin's lymphoma belong to the high-grade histologic groups, while 30% have intermediate-grade cell types.[33,65,66,68–70] Although low-grade cell types have also been reported in HIV-infected patients, it is not clear whether these represent a manifestation of AIDS.[63]

The pathogenesis of AIDS-associated non-Hodgkin's lymphoma is thought to be similar to that of lymphoid malignancies complicating other immunodeficiency states, such as immunosuppression in transplant recipients.[33] Polyclonal stimulation of B-cell populations by EBV infection, with subsequent *c-myc* gene activation, may mediate the malignant transformation of one of these B-cell clones into non-Hodgkin's lymphoma. However, insofar as only 40% of AIDS-associated non-Hodgkin's lymphomas contain EBV sequences or proteins, other viruses or oncogenes may be involved in the pathogenesis in a majority of cases.[33]

CLINICAL MANIFESTATIONS

Only a limited amount of information has been reported regarding the pulmonary manifestations of AIDS-associated non-Hodgkin's lymphoma. Pulmonary symptoms are often nonspecific and include dyspnea, cough, and chest pain, although patients may be completely asymptomatic.[67,72,76] In addition, nonspecific extrapulmonary B symptoms, such as fever, weight loss, or night sweats, are commonly present. Physical examination of the thorax may be normal or may reveal ronchi or evidence of a pleural effusion. The superior vena caval syndrome has been reported in a patient who presented with a large anterior mediastinal mass.[67] Generalized or focal extrapulmonary lymphadenopathy may also be present.

Radiographic manifestations of pulmonary parenchymal non-Hodgkin's lymphoma are most often characterized by noncavitary nodular lesions, which are often multiple and range in size from 0.5 to 3 cm in diameter, although a single 7-cm parenchymal nodule has been reported in a patient with isolated pulmonary disease (Fig. 17B–3).[72,76] Pulmonary non-Hodgkin's lymphoma has also been reported to manifest with diffuse interstitial infiltrates, suggesting the presence of lymphangitic involvement.[72] However, diffuse infiltrates may accompany nodular non-Hodgkin's lesions and be indicative of a concurrent opportunistic infection, such as *P. carinii* pneumonia.[72] Pleural effusions, which may be unilateral or bilateral, are the second most common radiographic manifestation of AIDS-associated non-Hodgkin's lymphoma.[49,65,71] Hilar or mediastinal lymphadenopathy is uncommon in this setting.[72,76]

DIAGNOSIS

The antemortem diagnosis of AIDS-associated pulmonary non-Hodgkin's lymphoma is extremely difficult to make. For example, although an autopsy series documented pulmonary involvement in eight cases, only three of the patients had been diagnosed prior to death.[77] Despite the limited amount of information that is available regarding the utility of fiberoptic bronchoscopy in this setting, it appears to be an extremely poor diagnostic method. In three series reporting on seven cases of pulmonary non-Hodgkin's lymphoma, transbronchial biopsy results were falsely negative in all cases.[25,72,76] Consequently, open lung biopsy is often necessary to establish the diagnosis. No information is available regarding the use of either transbronchial or percutaneous needle aspiration in this setting. Thoracocentesis should be performed if a pleural effusion is present and the specimen sent for cytologic analysis, which may yield the diagnosis.

NATURAL HISTORY

The prognosis for patients with AIDS-associated non-Hodgkin's lymphoma is generally poor, with median survival times ranging from 4 to 7 months in prior reports.[63,65,66,68,69,71] However, survival may be prolonged if a complete response to intensive, multidrug chemotherapeutic regimens is achieved.[69,71] Poor prognostic indicators include the presence of *P. carinii* pneumonia, a prior diagnosis of AIDS, extranodal lesions, CD4 T-lymphocyte counts of less than 100 cells/mm^3, and a low Karnofsky performance score.[68,69]

Little information is available regarding the survival of patients with pulmonary non-Hodgkin's lymphoma. In one series, three of four patients survived only 4 to 7 months after diagnosis, while one patient survived 16 months following multidrug chemotherapy and radiation therapy for pulmonary lesions.[72] However, a patient with primary pulmonary large cell immunoblastic lymphoma presenting as a nodular lesion reportedly survived for at least 8 months following resection alone.[76]

AIDS patients with lymphoma are at increased risk for pulmonary disease as compared to their counterparts without lymphoma.[73] Indeed, these patients can develop AIDS-related opportunistic infections, such as *P. carinii* pneumonia, as well as bacterial and fungal (*i.e., Aspergillus*) pneumonias secondary to chemotherapy-related neutropenia.[65,69,73,75,77,78] Consequently, prophylactic therapy for *P. carinii* pneumonia should be administered to all patients with AIDS-associated non-Hodgkin's lymphoma. Of interest, three of four patients in one series of pulmonary non-Hodgkin's lymphoma developed catheter-related *S. aureus* bacteremia, which was associated with a fatal diffuse pneumonitis in one patient.[72] Besides opportunistic infections, these patients may also develop interstitial pneumonitis secondary to cytotoxic chemotherapeutic agents.[73,75]

Hodgkin's Disease

Although Hodgkin's disease does not occur in increased frequency in AIDS patients and is not an AIDS-defining illness, its natural history in this setting appears to be significantly altered from that in non-HIV-infected pa-

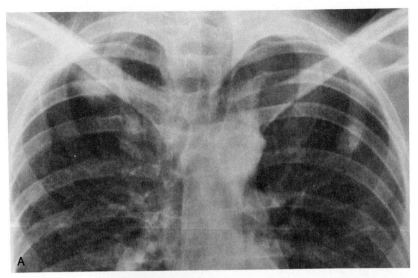

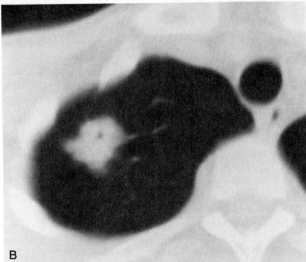

Figure 17B–3.   Chest radiograph (**A**) of a patient with pulmonary non-Hodgkin's lymphoma who presented with bilateral upper lobe nodular mass lesions. (**B**) The corresponding chest CT scan of the right upper lobe nodular lesion. (Courtesy of Irwin Feuerstein, MD)

tients.[65] AIDS-associated Hodgkin's disease is characterized by advanced stage (stage III or IV), the frequent presence of B symptoms, and extranodal involvement, typically of the bone marrow.[33,61,65,79,80] In addition, Hodgkin's disease may disseminate in a random, non-contiguous pattern, so that widespread disease may occur without hilar or mediastinal lymphadenopathy.[33,65] Pulmonary parenchymal involvement, which may appear radiographically as lobar infiltrates, may also occur without associated hilar or mediastinal lymphadenopathy.[81,82] Furthermore, it appears that hilar or mediastinal adenopathy occurs infrequently in AIDS-associated Hodgkin's disease, even in patients with nodular sclerosing histologic subtypes.[61,65,79–82] Although morphologic characteristics are similar in classic and AIDS-associated Hodgkin's disease, AIDS-associated lesions display high-grade histopathologic features.[33] In addition, AIDS-associated Hodgkin's disease has an ag-

gressive clinical course marked by progressive disease, concurrent opportunistic infections, and poor survival.[33,61,65,79,80]

INTERSTITIAL PNEUMONITIS

Lymphocytic Interstitial Pneumonitis

Lymphocytic interstitial pneumonitis (LIP) and pulmonary lymphoid hyperplasia (PLH) are important, potentially treatable causes of pulmonary disease in children with AIDS. LIP has been reported in as many as 43% to 48% of nonhemophiliac infants and children with AIDS and in 40% of pediatric AIDS patients who died or required lung biopsy for the diagnosis of pulmonary disease.[83–86] Furthermore, the presence of biopsy-proven LIP in an HIV-seropositive patient less than 13 years old is considered diagnostic of AIDS by CDC criteria.[87] In contrast to the situation in children, LIP infrequently complicates AIDS in adults and does not represent an AIDS-defining illness. The frequency of LIP in adult AIDS patients with pulmonary disease is estimated to be less than 1% to 2%, and only a few cases have been reported in the medical literature.[88] LIP in adults does not appear to be restricted to any particular AIDS risk group; however, black patients may be more predisposed than whites.[49] In addition, the diagnosis of adult LIP can either precede or follow the diagnosis of AIDS.[49]

PATHOLOGY

Although PLH and LIP were originally considered distinct disorders in pediatric patients, the term PLH/LIP complex is currently used to describe what is thought to represent a continuum or spectrum of pulmonary lymphoid lesions.[89,90] Both PLH and LIP are benign lymphocytic infiltrative disorders that differ in the predominant pattern and location of lymphoid aggregates.[89] In PLH, nodular lymphoid aggregates are localized to the bronchial mucosa and the adjacent interalveolar septa in a distribution corresponding to that of bronchial-associated lymphoid tissue.[83,89] These nodules are diffusely distributed throughout the pulmonary parenchyma and usually range in size from 0.5 to 2 mm in diameter.[83] Larger nodules, which can be 5 mm in diameter, may contain germinal centers and a thick-walled venule, consistent with hyperplastic bronchial-associated lymphoid tissue.[83,89] Microscopically these nodules are composed of aggregates of mature and immature lymphocytes and occasional plasma cells.[83,91]

LIP is characterized histologically by diffuse infiltration of the alveolar septa and peribronchiolar areas by lymphocytes, plasma cells, plasmacytoid lymphocytes, and immunoblasts.[84] LIP characteristically does not cause destruction of either the pulmonary vasculature or airways; however, alveolar consolidation secondary to lymphocytic infiltration has been reported in some adult cases.[91-93] Features of both PLH and LIP are often found concurrently in the same biopsy specimen, consistent with the hypothesis that these disorders represent a spectrum of the lymphocytic infiltrative process.[83,84,90] In addition, the degree of lymphoid infiltration in the PLH/LIP complex may range from mild to severe.[91]

Extrapulmonary sites of lymphoid infiltration have been documented in both children and adults with PLH/ LIP, suggesting that this process is part of a systemic, polyclonal B-cell lymphoid hyperplasia.[90,93] These extrapulmonary sites have included the liver, colon, thymus, spleen, kidneys, bone marrow, nasopharynx, skeletal muscle, and the parotid, adrenal, and salivary glands (with associated sicca syndrome). Furthermore, a diffuse infiltrative CD8 lymphocytosis syndrome has recently been described in adult HIV-infected patients.[94] This syndrome is characterized by a CD8 lymphocytosis with lymphocytic infiltration of the salivary and lacrimal glands and pulmonary parenchyma resulting in sicca

symptoms and LIP. Lymphocytic infiltrations of the liver, gastric mucosa, renal interstitium, and thymus also occurred. This disorder was associated with the presence of HLA-DR5, black race, and improvement after zidovudine therapy, which suggested that it represented a genetically predetermined host immune response to HIV infection.

Studies aimed at classifying the cell type of origin in PLH/LIP have yielded variable results.[12] The cellular composition of the lymphocytic infiltrates (i.e., lymphocytes, plasma cells, plasmacytoid lymphocytes, and immunoblasts) is consistent with a B-cell hyperplasia.[90,95] In addition, immunoperoxidase staining for κ and λ immunoglobulin light chains has revealed the lymphoid infiltrates to be polyclonal.[90,91,96,97] However, mixed B- and T-cell proliferation has been reported in a pediatric patient, with a predominance of OKT8+ cells.[96] Immunoperoxidase staining of cells from another pediatric LIP patient revealed a predominance of T8 and T11 cells, with occasional T4 and B cells.[98] Immunohistologic staining of lung biopsy specimens from two adults with LIP revealed T lymphocytes, with equal numbers of helper and suppressor cells in one case and essentially only suppressor cells in the other.[12,49,99]

Although the pathogenesis of AIDS-associated PLH/ LIP remains to be definitively determined, prior evidence has suggested an etiologic role for either EBV or HIV, or both.[12,49,90] EBV DNA was detected in the lungs of 80% of 15 patients with LIP in two studies, along with elevations in levels of antibodies to EBV capsid antigen.[83,98] EBV DNA has also been detected in peribronchiolar lymphocytic infiltrates, peripheral blood lymphocytes, and saliva from an infant with AIDS.[89,96] Consequently, the pathogenesis of the PLH/LIP complex may represent an atypical response to EBV infection by an immune system altered by HIV infection.[90] Indeed, EBV is known to be an independent, direct polyclonal B-cell activator without the requirement of T cells or macrophages.[12,96]

Other evidence has suggested that LIP may represent a sequela of pulmonary infection by HIV. Prior studies have noted the presence of HIV antigen and IgG antibody in BAL specimens from LIP patients, as well as the presence of HIV RNA (by *in situ* hybridization) within pulmonary lymphocytes and macrophages.[100-102] These HIV-infected cells may then be capable of inciting an inflammatory infiltrative pulmonary process by the release of cytokines or toxic viral products. Recently, HIV proviral DNA has been detected by polymerase chain reaction (PCR) techniques in alveolar fibroblasts and macrophages from patients with LIP.[103] In this study, both HIV-infected alveolar macrophages and fibroblasts were selectively killed *in vitro* by CD8 HIV-specific cytotoxic T lymphocytes, which suggested the involvement of cell-mediated cytotoxicity in the pathogenesis of LIP. This may also explain the predominance of suppressor-cytotoxic T lymphocytes in lung biopsy specimens from some patients with LIP. Although earlier studies suggested that identification of HIV in

BAL fluid or tissue specimens may be specific for LIP, recent studies have reported the culture of HIV from BAL fluid from AIDS patients without LIP.[104,105] In one of these studies, however, HIV p24 antigen was detected by immunoassay only from a patient with LIP.[105]

CLINICAL PRESENTATION

Pediatric PLH/LIP is a subacute or chronic disorder that is characterized by the insidious development of pulmonary disease that can potentially result in respiratory failure. Cough is the most common pulmonary symptom in this age group, being present in all 11 patients in one study, while fever and dyspnea are uncommon.[83,95] Failure to thrive was reported in all 21 patients in three series.[83,85,95] Physical examination is remarkable for the absence of tachypnea or adventitial lung sounds, whereas digital clubbing, salivary gland enlargement, and generalized lymphadenopathy are characteristic findings.[83] Indeed, the presence of fever, tachypnea, and adventitial lung sounds is more likely to represent an infectious process rather than PLH/LIP complex.[83] Arterial blood gas analysis generally reveals mild to moderate hypoxemia, with mean D_A–aO_2 gradients ranging from 24 to 40 mm Hg in two studies.[83,106] Although serum lactate dehydrogenase levels may be elevated in comparison with levels in healthy control subjects, they are significantly lower than levels found in the setting of *P. carinii* pneumonia.[83] Hypergammaglobulinemia in excess of what is found in *P. carinii* pneumonia is also common.[83] Chest radiographs reveal a diffuse pattern of 1- to 5-mm nodules in association with an underlying interstitial pulmonary infiltrate.[83] With disease progression, these nodules increase in size, and there is concomitant widening of the hilum and superior mediastinum suggestive of lymphadenopathy.[83,89,106] Gallium scans may reveal a diffuse pattern of uptake within the lungs that is indistinguishable from what is observed in *P. carinii* pneumonia.[89]

The clinical manifestations of adult LIP are also remarkable for the insidious development of pulmonary disease. Presenting complaints are often nonspecific and have included dyspnea, a nonproductive cough, fever, and weight loss.[92,93,99,107] Physical examination often reveals bilateral inspiratory crackles on lung auscultation, as well as diffuse lymphadenopathy.[93,99,107] Severe immunologic abnormalities consistent with AIDS, such as an inverted T4/T8 ratio, decreased T4 count, and polyclonal hyperimmunoglobulinemia, are commonly present.[93,108] Arterial blood gas values may be normal or may reveal hypoxemia, increased D_A–aO_2, and mild hypocapnia.[92,93,99,107] Pulmonary function tests may disclose restrictive impairments on spirometric testing and reductions in the diffusing capacity for carbon monoxide, which have been reported to be as low as 28% of predicted.[93,99,107] Chest radiographs characteristically reveal diffuse reticulonodular interstitial infiltrates, but patchy alveolar infiltrates are also seen.[93,99,107,108] In one study of 16 patients with LIP, 56% had combined reticulonodular interstitial and patchy alveolar infiltrates,

while the remainder had isolated interstitial infiltrates.[108] In this study, the nodules were as large as 5 mm in size. Radiographic evidence of mediastinal and hilar lymph node enlargement has also been reported.[107] Gallium-67 scans in adult patients with LIP have shown areas of increased activity within the pulmonary parenchyma.[99,107]

DIAGNOSIS

Histologic examination of the pulmonary parenchyma is necessary to establish a definitive diagnosis of LIP. Although a large sample of pulmonary parenchyma is better suited to establishing this diagnosis, transbronchial biopsies may be adequate when there is evidence of an interstitial lymphocytic and plasma cell infiltration.[92,99,101,107-109] In five small studies involving ten adult patients, transbronchial biopsies established the diagnosis of LIP in 50% of cases.[92,99,101,107,110] Open lung biopsy may be necessary if transbronchial biopsy fails to establish a diagnosis. Because LIP in adults is often an indolent process that may not require specific therapy, often the role of diagnostic procedures, such as fiberoptic bronchoscopy, is to exclude the presence of an opportunistic infection, which can have similar clinical and radiographic manifestations. This is important in patients with an established diagnosis of LIP who experience either a change in symptoms or radiographic infiltrates, especially if immunosuppressive therapy (corticosteroids) is being administered.

In pediatric patients an open lung biopsy is often necessary to establish a definitive histologic diagnosis of PLH/LIP complex.[49] In an attempt to avoid invasive diagnostic procedures in this patient population, it has been suggested that PLH/LIP complex can be discriminated from opportunistic infections, such as *P. carinii* pneumonia, on the basis of characteristic clinical and radiographic manifestations.[89] BAL, which has been shown to be effective for the diagnosis of *P. carinii* pneumonia in pediatric AIDS patients, should be considered to exclude the possibility of an infectious process if the diagnosis of PLH/LIP is established on clinical grounds alone.[49,111]

NATURAL HISTORY AND THERAPY

The natural history of PLH/LIP in children is variable, ranging from spontaneous resolution to slowly progressive pulmonary disease.[49,89] The typical course of pediatric PLH/LIP is characterized by the indolent development of hypoxemia, digital clubbing, and worsening radiographic infiltrates. Frank tachypnea and severe hypoxemia leading to respiratory failure may occur late in the course of disease.[89,112] Because of the variable course of PLH/LIP, therapy often is not required immediately and may be reserved until clinical evidence of disease progression occurs, such as worsening hypoxemia ($PaO_2 < 60$ mmHg).[112] Consequently, frequent and careful monitoring of disease activity is necessary in all patients.

If therapy is required, corticosteroids may be used, although limited data exist regarding their efficacy in this setting. In one study, all five patients experienced improvements in oxygenation and radiographic infiltrates after at least 3 months of therapy (prednisone, 2 mg/kg/day for 2 to 4 weeks until the PaO_2 increased by 20 mmHg, followed by 0.5 to 0.75 mg/kg on alternate days).[106] Neither the rate nor the severity of opportunistic infections increased; however, all patients received intravenous γ-globulin. The ten patients who did not receive corticosteroid therapy developed finger clubbing and progressive nodular infiltrates, while nine had progressive hypoxemia. Termination of corticosteroids in one patient was associated with worsening hypoxemia. Although relapses have been reported following termination of corticosteroids, stabile remissions following discontinuation of long-term corticosteroid therapy have also been described.[89,98] Intravenous γ-globulin has not been efficacious for this disorder, and no data are available regarding antiretroviral therapy for pediatric PLH/LIP.[49,89,106]

The prognosis for children with PLH/LIP is generally more favorable than for other pediatric AIDS patients. In five series involving 22 patients, 95% were alive at the conclusion of the follow-up period, which ranged from 6 months to 5.5 years.[83–85,95,97] In addition, these patients appear to be less likely to develop opportunistic infections.[83,98] Progression of PLH/LIP to frank lymphoma has not been a feature of pediatric PLH/LIP, although there has been one case of an infant who developed CNS lymphoma.[49,98] In addition, pediatric PLH/LIP has been found rarely to progress to a polyclonal B-cell lymphoproliferative disorder (PBLD).[113] PBLD is characterized by a polyclonal B-cell nodular infiltration of both nodal and extranodal sites that is thought to represent an intermediate portion of the spectrum of lymphoproliferative disorders, between PLH/LIP complex and malignant lymphoma.

Adult LIP also has a variable course that ranges from mild, stable disease to more severe pneumonitis resulting in significant dyspnea. The characteristic natural history of adult LIP is that of an insidious, chronic process with stable clinical manifestations that often does not require specific therapy. Spontaneous improvement in disease manifestations has also been reported.[92,93,109] When progressive dyspnea necessitates the institution of therapy, corticosteroids have been used, with varying results.[109] Although improvement in symptoms, hypoxemia, and radiographic infiltrates has occurred with oral prednisone therapy, relapses have been reported following discontinuation of therapy.[99] Adult LIP generally does not progress to respiratory failure or death, and most patients eventually succumb to other HIV-related complications, especially opportunistic infections.[49,99,107,109] Consequently, corticosteroids should probably be withheld unless severe dyspnea or hypoxemia is present. Only limited and conflicting data are available regarding the role of antiretroviral therapy in

this setting. Two patients were reported to improve following zidovudine therapy, while another patient did not respond to either zidovudine or high-dose acyclovir.[110,114] As in pediatric LIP/PLH, progression to lymphoma does not appear to occur.[108]

Nonspecific Interstitial Pneumonitis

Nonspecific interstitial pneumonitis (NIP) is a frequent but usually self-limited cause of pulmonary dysfunction in adult AIDS patients.[115] NIP has been documented in 5% to 38% of 240 AIDS patients in two series and was the cause of pneumonitis in 11% to 32% of patients with pulmonary disease.[39,115] In addition, NIP was present in 48% of 23 asymptomatic HIV-infected patients without *P. carinii* pneumonia in a recent prospective study.[116] Little information exists regarding NIP complicating pediatric HIV infection. Although early reports described desquamative interstitial pneumonitis (DIP) as a distinct entity, a later reappraisal found concurrent processes, such as LIP and *Aspergillus* and *Pneumocystis* infections, in these patients.[84,89,90] Consequently, it is unclear whether DIP in pediatric patients occurs secondary to other pulmonary disorders or represents a primary response to HIV or other infectious agents.[91]

PATHOLOGY

The histopathology of NIP is characterized by mild interstitial infiltration with lymphocytes and plasma cells.[115] Moderate edema, fibrin deposition, alveolar lining cell hyperplasia, and alveolar septal thickening are common.[115] Hyaline membranes, consistent with endothelial-epithelial damage, and interstitial lymphoid aggregates may also be present.[115] Histopathologic findings in asymptomatic patients with NIP are characterized by perivascular and peribronchial lymphocytic interstitial infiltrates and aggregates without associated edema, fibrin deposition, hyaline membranes, or alveolitis.[116]

The etiology of NIP is unclear. Although it has been suggested that NIP might represent an inflammatory response to HIV or EBV, no data exist to support this hypothesis.[115] In one report, *in situ* hybridization studies in ten patients failed to demonstrate the presence of HIV.[115] However, another study found that only one of 11 patients with NIP was receiving zidovudine, as compared to seven of 12 patients without pulmonary disease, which suggests a possible etiologic role for this virus.[116] In many patients NIP may be a consequence of prior pulmonary infections, concurrent pulmonary Kaposi's sarcoma, or exposure to potentially toxic recreational or therapeutic drugs.[115,117] However, NIP has also been documented in patients without any of these possible causes.[115]

CLINICAL AND RADIOGRAPHIC PRESENTATION

The clinical presentation of NIP is nonspecific and may be indistinguishable from that of other pulmonary complications of HIV infection, such as opportunistic infections.[115] Disease manifestations are characteristically mild in severity, with patients either being asymptomatic or complaining of fever or cough.[115,116] Physical examination may reveal diffuse, bilateral rales.[117] Arterial blood gas determinations characteristically reveal mild to moderate widening of the D_A–ao_2 gradient, which ranged from 11 to 32 mm Hg in 24 patients in two studies.[115,116] Exercise testing may reveal abnormal widening of the D_A–ao_2.[39] Pulmonary function testing of 14 patients in two series revealed normal mean diffusing capacities ranging from 82% to 85% of predicted, although individual patients had values as low as 66% of predicted.[39,116]

Radiographic manifestations are also often mild in severity and nonspecific in nature. Chest radiographs either reveal diffuse interstitial infiltrates or are normal.[39,115,117,118] These interstitial infiltrates may be either subtle or coarse in appearance and occasionally are unilateral in location or associated with pleural effusions.[118] Chest radiographs were normal in 44% to 100% of patients in three studies but in only one of seven patients in another series.[39,115,116,118] In one study involving 11 asymptomatic patients, ^{67}Ga citrate scans were commonly either normal or revealed mild 1+ pulmonary uptake; however, two patients had either 2+ or 3+ pulmonary uptake.[116]

NATURAL HISTORY

The natural history of NIP is characterized by a chronic, indolent course that commonly stabilizes or resolves without specific therapy.[39,115] Furthermore, patients can be completely asymptomatic, with only histopathologic evidence of subclinical disease.[116] Although NIP can result in ongoing lung injury, it does not result in respiratory failure or death, and its mild manifestations usually do not justify the institution of immunosuppressive therapy. Indeed, the clinical relevance of NIP is that its clinical presentation may be identical to that of an AIDS-related opportunistic infection, such as *P. carinii* pneumonia, that requires the institution of specific antimicrobial therapy.[115] Therefore, the role of diagnostic procedures in this setting is not to document the presence of NIP, but rather to exclude the presence of other potentially treatable pulmonary infections. As in LIP, fiberoptic bronchoscopy is indicated to rule out an opportunistic infection when a patient with known NIP has a change in symptoms or radiographic infiltrates.

Lymphocytic Alveolitis

Analysis of BAL cell populations from AIDS patients by various investigators has revealed increases in the proportion and number of lymphocytes consistent with the presence of a lymphocytic alveolitis.[119-121] Subtyping studies revealed these cells to be CD8+ cytotoxic T lymphocytes that were capable of recognizing and killing HIV-infected alveolar macrophages.[122,123] In a recent report, a CD8+ cytotoxic lymphocytic alveolitis was present in 72% of 22 HIV-infected patients without pulmonary infections or neoplasms, suggesting that it is a common finding in this setting.[123] Sixty-seven percent of these patients had pulmonary symptoms (nonproductive cough and dyspnea on exertion) and 36% had diffuse interstitial infiltrates that reflected the degree of lymphocytosis. In addition, 85% had abnormal pulmonary function test results with either a decreased diffusing capacity for carbon monoxide or abnormal widening of the D_A–ao_2 with exercise. Another recent study reported a significant correlation between the number and cytotoxic activity of CD8+/D44+ T lymphocytes against alveolar macrophages and the clearance of aerosolized technetium-labeled DTPA, which suggested disruption of the alveolar epithelium.[124] Open lung biopsy in four of the patients disclosed a diffuse lymphocytic infiltration involving lymphatic vascular channels but sparing the alveolar septa. Consequently, the authors have suggested that lymphocytic alveolitis may represent part of the spectrum of HIV-related pulmonary lymphoid infiltrative disorders, a spectrum that includes PLH/LIP and NIP.[123,124]

INFLAMMATORY AIRWAY DISORDERS

Bronchiolitis

Inflammatory disorders of the airways have been described in HIV-infected patients. Lymphocytic bronchiolitis was described in an adult patient with AIDS-related complex who presented with dyspnea, cough, diffuse micronodular infiltrates, mild obstructive and restrictive spirometric abnormalities, and a severely decreased carbon monoxide diffusing capacity.[125] BAL revealed a cytotoxic-suppressor T-cell lymphocytosis, and transbronchial biopsy revealed an intense peribronchiolar infiltration with lymphocytes and plasma cells. The patient was observed expectantly, without a change in disease manifestations. In a study of 33 patients with lymphocytic alveolitis, eight had spirometric evidence of small airways disease and three of four patients who underwent open lung biopsy had bronchiolitis.[123]

A case of corticosteroid-responsive bronchiolitis obliterans organizing pneumonia (BOOP) has also been reported in an HIV-positive patient.[126] Open lung biopsy established the diagnosis of BOOP and chronic interstitial pneumonitis after a nondiagnostic fiberoptic bronchoscopy. Presenting clinical manifestations included fever, nonproductive cough, dyspnea, bibasilar dry crackles, hypoxemia, progressive bilateral alveolar infiltrates, and a lymphocytic alveolitis, detected with BAL. In addition, another study reported the presence of bronchiolitis obliterans in 50% of 16 adult patients with LIP.[108] Consequently, lymphocytic bronchiolitis and bronchiolitis obliterans may represent part of the spectrum of HIV-related pulmonary lymphoid infiltrative processes. These inflammatory airways disorders may also contribute to the airways obstruction that has been documented in some AIDS patients.

CONCLUSION

Noninfectious pulmonary manifestations of HIV infection represent a spectrum of malignant and nonmalignant diseases. The accurate diagnosis of these disorders is important, for three reasons. First, specific therapy may be indicated in some clinical settings. Second, the short-term and long-term prognosis may be significantly altered. Third, these processes are frequently indistinguishable from infectious pulmonary complications of HIV infection which may require specific and immediate antimicrobial therapy.

REFERENCES

1. Murray JF, Garay SM, Hopewell PC et al: Pulmonary complications of the acquired immunodeficiency syndrome: An update. Report of the Second National Heart, Lung and Blood Institute Workshop. Am Rev Respir Dis 135:504, 1987
2. Steis RG, Longo DL: Clinical, biologic and therapeutic aspects of malignancies associated with the acquired immunodeficiency syndrome: Part 1. Ann Allergy 60:310, 1988
3. Cotran RS, Kumar V, Robbins SL (eds): Robbins' Pathologic Basis of Disease, p 1291. Philadelphia, WB Saunders, 1989
4. Krown SE: AIDS-associated Kaposi's sarcoma: Pathogenesis, clinical course and treatment. AIDS 2:71, 1988
5. Guarda LA, Luna MA, Smith JL et al: Acquired immune deficiency syndrome: Postmortem findings. Am J Clin Pathol 81:549, 1984
6. Niedt GW, Schinella RA: Acquired immunodeficiency syndrome: Clinicopathologic study of 56 autopsies. Arch Pathol Lab Med 109:727, 1985
7. Safai B, Johnson KD, Myskowski PL et al: The natural history of Kaposi's sarcoma in the acquired immunodeficiency syndrome. Ann Intern Med 103:744, 1985
8. Selik RM, Starcher ET, Curran JW: Opportunistic diseases reported in AIDS patients: Frequencies, associations and trends. AIDS 1:175, 1987
9. Des Jarlais DC, Stoneburner R, Thomas P et al: Declines in proportion of Kaposi's sarcoma among cases of AIDS in multiple risk groups in New York City. Lancet 2:1024, 1987
10. Rutherford GW, Schwarcz SK, Lemp GF et al: The epidemiology of AIDS-related Kaposi's sarcoma in San Francisco. J Infect Dis 159:569, 1989
11. Drew WL, Mills J, Haver LB et al: Declining prevalence of Kaposi's sarcoma in homosexual patients paralleled by a fall in CMV transmission. Lancet 1:66, 1988
12. Travis WD, Lack EE, Ognibene FP et al: Lung biopsy interpretation in the acquired immunodeficiency syndrome: Experience of the National Institutes of Health with literature review. Prog AIDS Pathol 1:51, 1989
13. Case records of the Massachusetts General Hospital: Case 1-1990. N Engl J Med 320:43, 1990
14. Nash G, Flefiel S: Pathologic features of the lung in the acquired immune deficiency syndrome: An autopsy study of seventeen homosexual males. Am J Clin Pathol 81:6, 1984
15. O'Brien RF, Cohn DL: Serosanguineous pleural effusions in AIDS-associated Kaposi's sarcoma. Chest 96:460, 1989
16. Garay SM, Belenko M, Fazzini E, Schinella R: Pulmonary manifestations of Kaposi's sarcoma. Chest 91:39, 1987
17. Bach MC, Bagwell SP, Fanninf JP: Primary pulmonary Kaposi's sarcoma in the acquired immunodeficiency syndrome: A cause of persistent pyrexia. Am J Med 85:274, 1988
18. Nathan S, Vaghaiwalla R, Mohsenifar Z: Use of Nd:YAG laser in endobronchial Kaposi's sarcoma. Chest 98:1299, 1990
19. Fouret PJ, Touboul JL, Mayaud CM et al: Pulmonary Kaposi's sarcoma in patients with acquired immune deficiency syndrome: A clinicopathological study. Thorax 42:262, 1987
20. Purdy LJ, Colby TV, Yousem SA, Battifora H: Pulmonary Kaposi's sarcoma: Premortem histologic diagnosis. Am J Surg Pathol 10:301, 1986
21. Davis SD, Henschke CI, Chamides BK, Westcott JL: Intrathoracic Kaposi sarcoma in AIDS patients: Radiographic-pathologic correlation. Radiology 163:495, 1987
22. Kornfield H, Axelrod JL: Pulmonary presentation of Kaposi's sarcoma in a homosexual patient. Am Rev Respir Dis 127:248, 1983
23. Ognibene FP, Steis RG, Macher AM et al: Kaposi's sarcoma causing pulmonary infiltrates and respiratory failure in the acquired immunodeficiency syndrome. Ann Intern Med 102:471, 1985
24. Meduri GU, Stover DE, Lee M et al: Pulmonary Kaposi's sarcoma in the acquired immune deficiency syndrome: Clinical, radiographic and pathologic manifestations. Am J Med 81:11, 1986
25. Marchevsky A, Rosen MJ, Chrystal G, Kleinerman J: Pulmonary complications of the acquired immunodeficiency syndrome: A clinicopathologic study of 70 cases. Hum Pathol 16:659, 1985
26. Misra DP, Sunderrajan EV, Hurst DJ, Maltby JD: Kaposi's sarcoma of the lung: Radiography and pathology. Thorax 37:155, 1982
27. Pitchenik AE, Fischl MA, Saldana MJ: Kaposi's sarcoma of the tracheobronchial tree: Clinical, bronchoscopic, and pathologic features. Chest 87:122, 1985
28. Hamm PG, Judson MA, Aranda CP: Diagnosis of pulmonary Kaposi's sarcoma with fiberoptic bronchoscopy and endobronchial biopsy: A report of five cases. Cancer 59:807, 1987
29. Kaplan LD, Hopewell PC, Jaffe J et al: Kaposi's sarcoma involving the lung in patients with the acquired immunodeficiency syndrome. J AIDS 1:23, 1988
30. Greenberg JE, Fischl MA, Berger JR: Upper airway obstruction secondary to acquired immunodeficiency syndrome–related Kaposi's sarcoma. Chest 88:638, 1985
31. Sivit CJ, Schwartz AM, Rockoff SD: Kaposi's sarcoma of the lung in AIDS: Radiologic-pathologic analysis. AJR 148:25, 1987
32. Santucci M, Pimpinelli N, Moretti S, Giannotti B: Classic and immunodeficiency-associated Kaposi's sarcoma. Arch Pathol Lab Med 112:1214, 1988
33. Knowles DM, Chadburn A: The neoplasms associated with AIDS. In Joshi VV (ed): Pathology of AIDS and Other Manifestations of HIV Infection, p 83. New York, Igaku-Shoin, 1990
34. Ziegler JL: Pathogenesis of AIDS-associated Kaposi's sarcoma. Lymphology 21:15, 1988
35. Dictor M, Andersson C: Lymphaticovenous differentiation in Kaposi's sarcoma: Cellular phenotypes by stage. Am J Pathol 130:411, 1988
36. Nash G, Flegiel S: Kaposi's sarcoma presenting as pul-

monary disease in the acquired immunodeficiency syndrome: Diagnosis by lung biopsy. Hum Pathol 15:999, 1984

37. Ognibene FP, Shelhamer JH: Kaposi's sarcoma. Clin Chest Med 9:459, 1988

38. Gill PS, Akil B, Colletti P et al: Pulmonary Kaposi's sarcoma: Clinical findings and results of therapy. Am J Med 87:57, 1989

39. Stover DE, White DA, Romano PA et al: Spectrum of pulmonary diseases associated with the acquired immune deficiency syndrome. Am J Med 78:429, 1985

40. Stover DE, Meduri GU: Pulmonary function tests. Clin Chest Med 9:473, 1988

41. Naidich DP, Tarras M, Garay SM et al: Kaposi's sarcoma: CT-radiographic correlation. Chest 96:723, 1989

42. Zibrak JD, Silvestri RC, Costello P et al: Bronchoscopic and radiologic features of Kaposi's sarcoma involving the respiratory system. Chest 90:476, 1986

43. Lai KK: Pulmonary Kaposi's sarcoma presenting as diffuse reticular nodular infiltrates with cavitary lesions. South Med J 83:1096, 1990

44. Pandya K, Lal C, Tuchschmidt J et al: Bilateral chylothorax with pulmonary Kaposi's sarcoma. Chest 94:1316, 1988

45. Floris C, Sulis ML, Turno R et al: Pneumothorax in pleuropulmonary Kaposi's sarcoma related to acquired immunodeficiency syndrome. Am J Med 87:123, 1989

46. Woolfenden JM, Carrasquillo JA, Larson SM et al: Acquired immunodeficiency syndrome: Ga-67 citrate imaging. Radiology 162:383, 1987

47. Kramer EL, Sanger JJ, Garay SM et al: Gallium-67 scans of the chest in patients with acquired immunodeficiency syndrome. J Nucl Med 28:1107, 1987

48. Golden JA, Sollitto RA: The radiology of pulmonary disease: Chest radiography, computed tomography and gallium scanning. Clin Chest Med 9:481, 1988

49. White DA, Matthay RA: Noninfectious pulmonary complications of infection with the human immunodeficiency virus. Am Rev Respir Dis 140:1763, 1989

50. Lee VW, Rosen MP, Baum A et al: AIDS-related Kaposi sarcoma: Findings on thallium-201 scintigraphy. AJR 151:1233, 1988

51. Lau K, Av J, Rubin A et al: Kaposi's sarcoma of the tracheobronchial tree. Chest 89:158, 1986

52. Au JP, Krauthammer M, Lau K, Rubin A: Kaposi's sarcoma presenting with endobronchial lesions. Heart Lung 15:411, 1986

53. Hanson PJV, Harcourt-Webster JN, Gazzard BG, Collins JV: Fiberoptic bronchoscopy in diagnosis of bronchopulmonary Kaposi's sarcoma. Thorax 42:269, 1987

54. Stover DE, White DA, Romano PA, Gellene RA: Diagnosis of pulmonary disease in acquired immune deficiency syndrome. Am Rev Respir Dis 130:659, 1984

55. Griffiths MH, Kocjan G, Miller RF, Godfrey-Faussett: Diagnosis of pulmonary infection in human immunodeficiency virus infection: Role of transbronchial biopsy and bronchoalveolar lavage. Thorax 44:554, 1989

56. Pass HI, Potter D, Shelhamer J et al: Indications for and diagnostic efficacy of open-lung biopsy in the patient with acquired immunodeficiency syndrome. Ann Thorac Surg 41:307, 1986

57. McKenna RJ, Campbell A, McMurtrey MJ, Mountain CF: Diagnosis for interstitial lung disease in patients with acquired immunodeficiency syndrome: A prospective comparison of bronchial washing, alveolar lavage, transbronchial lung biopsy, and open-lung biopsy. Ann Thorac Surg 41:318, 1986

58. Fitzgerald W, Bevelaqua FA, Garay SM, Aranda CP: The role of open lung biopsy in patients with the acquired immunodeficiency syndrome. Chest 91:659, 1987

59. Fischl MA, Dickinson GM, La Voie L: Safety and efficacy of sulfamethoxazole and trimethoprim chemoprophylaxis for *Pneumocystis carinii* pneumonia in AIDS. JAMA 259:1185, 1988

60. Leoung GS, Feigal DW, Montgomery AB et al: Aerosolized pentamidine for prophylaxis against *Pneumocystis carinii* pneumonia: The San Francisco community prophylaxis trial. N Engl J Med 323:769, 1990

61. Safai B, Lynfield R, Lowenthal DA, Koziner B: Cancers associated with HIV infection. Anticancer Res 7:1055, 1987

62. Raphael BG, Knowles DM: Acquired immunodeficiency syndrome–associated non-Hodgkin's lymphoma. Semin Oncol 17:361, 1990

63. Levine AM: Lymphoma in acquired immunodeficiency syndrome. Semin Oncol 104:12, 1990

64. Kaplan MH, Susin M, Pahwa SG et al: Neoplastic complications of HTLV-III infection: Lymphomas and solid tumors. Am J Med 82:389, 1987

65. Knowles DM, Chamulak GA, Subar M et al: Lymphoid neoplasia associated with the acquired immunodeficiency syndrome. Ann Intern Med 108:744, 1988

66. Ziegler JL, Beckstead JA, Volberding PA et al: Non-Hodgkin's lymphoma in 90 homosexual men: Relation to generalized lymphadenopathy and the acquired immunodeficiency syndrome. N Engl J Med 311:565, 1984

67. Levine AM, Meyer PR, Begandy MK et al: Development of B-cell lymphoma in homosexual men: Clinical and immunologic findings. Ann Intern Med 100:7, 1984

68. Kaplan LD, Abrams DI, Feigal E et al: AIDS-associated non-Hodgkin's lymphoma in San Francisco. JAMA 261:719, 1989

69. Bermudez MA, Grant KM, Rodvien R: Non-Hodgkin's lymphoma in a population with or at risk for acquired immunodeficiency syndrome: Indications for intensive chemotherapy. Am J Med 86:71, 1989

70. Levine AM, Gill PS, Meyer PR et al: Retrovirus and malignant lymphoma in homosexual men. JAMA 254:1921, 1985

71. Lowenthal DA, Straus DJ, Campbell SW et al: AIDS-related lymphoid neoplasia: The Memorial Hospital experience. Cancer 61:2325, 1988

72. Polish LB, Cohn DL, Ryder JW et al: Pulmonary non-Hodgkin's lymphoma in AIDS. Chest 96:1321, 1989

73. Sourour MS, Stover DE, Fels AOS: Pulmonary disease in AIDS patients with lymphoma. Am Rev Respir Dis 137:A168, 1987

74. Kalter SP, Riggs SA, Cabanillas F et al: Aggressive non-Hodgkin's lymphomas in immunocompromised homosexual males. Blood 66:655, 1985

75. Ioachim HL, Cooper MC, Hellman GC: Lymphomas in men at high risk for acquired immune deficiency syndrome. Cancer 56:2831, 1985

76. Poelzleitner D, Huebsch P, Mayerhofer S et al: Primary pulmonary lymphoma in a patient with the acquired immune deficiency syndrome. Thorax 44:438, 1989

77. Loureiro C, Gill PS, Meyer PR et al: Autopsy findings in AIDS-related lymphoma. Cancer 62:735, 1988

78. Ahmed T, Wormser GP, Stahl RE et al: Malignant lymphomas in a population at risk for acquired immune deficiency syndrome. Cancer 60:719, 1987

79. Prior E, Goldberg AF, Conjalka MS et al: Hodgkin's disease in homosexual men: An AIDS-related phenomenon? Am J Med 81:1085, 1986

80. Unger PD, Strauchen JA: Hodgkin's disease in AIDS com-

plex patients: Report of four cases and tissue immunologic marker studies. Cancer 58:821, 1986

81. Scheib RG, Siegel RS: Atypical Hodgkin's disease and the acquired immunodeficiency syndrome. Ann Intern Med 102:554, 1985

82. Schoeppel SL, Hoppe RT, Dorfman RF et al: Hodgkin's disease in homosexual men with generalized lymphadenopathy. Ann Intern Med 102:68, 1985

83. Rubinstein A, Morecki R, Silverman B et al: Pulmonary disease in children with acquired immune deficiency syndrome and AIDS-related complex. J Pediatr 108:498, 1986

84. Joshi VV, Oleske JM, Minnefor AB et al: Pathologic pulmonary findings in children with the acquired immunodeficiency syndrome: A study of ten cases. Hum Pathol 16:241, 1985

85. Scott GB, Buck BE, Leterman JG et al: Acquired immunodeficiency syndrome in infants. N Engl J Med 310:76, 1984

86. Jason JM, Stehr-Green J, Holman RC, et al, for the Hemophilia-AIDS Collaborative Study Group: Human immunodeficiency virus infection in hemophilic children. Pediatrics 82:565, 1988

87. Centers for Disease Control: Classification system for human immunodeficiency virus (HIV) infection in children under 13 years of age. MMWR 36:225, 1987

88. Cohn DL, Stover DE, O'Brien RF et al: Pulmonary complications of AIDS: Advances in diagnosis and treatment. Am Rev Respir Dis 138:1051, 1988

89. Rubinstein A, Morecki R, Goldman H: Pulmonary disease in infants and children. Clin Chest Med 9:507, 1988

90. Joshi VV, Oleske JM: Pulmonary lesions in children with the acquired immunodeficiency syndrome: A reappraisal based on data in additional cases and follow-up study of previously reported cases. Hum Pathol 17:641, 1986

91. Joshi VV: Pathology of acquired immunodeficiency syndrome in children. In Joshi VV (ed): Pathology of AIDS and Other Manifestations of HIV Infection, p 239. New York, Igaku-Shoin, 1990

92. Grieco MH, Chinoy-Acharya P: Lymphocytic interstitial pneumonia associated with the acquired immune deficiency syndrome. Am Rev Respir Dis 131:952, 1985

93. Solal-Celigny P, Couderc LJ, Herman D et al: Lymphoid interstitial pneumonitis in acquired immunodeficiency syndrome-related complex. Am Rev Respir Dis 131:956, 1985

94. Itescu S, Brancato LJ, Buxbaum J et al: A diffuse infiltrative CD8 lymphocytosis syndrome in human immunodeficiency virus infection: A host immune response associated with HLA-DR5. Ann Intern Med 112:3, 1990

95. Joshi VV, Oleske JM, Minnefor AB et al: Pathology of suspected acquired immune deficiency syndrome in children: A study of eight cases. Pediatr Pathol 2:71, 1984

96. Fackler JC, Nagel JE, Adler WH et al: Epstein-Barr virus infection in a child with acquired immunodeficiency syndrome. Am J Dis Child 139:1000, 1985

97. Boccon-Gibod L, Sacre JP, Just J et al: Lymphoid interstitial pneumonia in children with AIDS or AIDS-related complex. Pediatr Pathol 5:238, 1986

98. Kornstein MJ, Pietra GG, Hoxie JA, Conley ME: The pathology and treatment of interstitial pneumonitis in two infants with AIDS. Am Rev Respir Dis 133:1196, 1986

99. Morris JC, Rosen MJ, Marchevsky A, Teirstein AS: Lymphocytic interstitial pneumonia in patients at risk for the acquired immune deficiency syndrome. Chest 91:63, 1987

100. Ziza JM, Brun-Vezinet F, Venet A et al: Lymphadenopathy-associated virus isolated from bronchoalveolar lavage fluid in AIDS-related complex with lymphoid interstitial pneumonitis. N Engl J Med 313:183, 1985

101. Resnick L, Pitchenik AE, Fisher E, Croney R: Detection of HTLV-III/LAV-specific IgG and antigen in bronchoalveolar lavage from two patients with lymphocytic interstitial pneumonitis associated with AIDS-related complex. Am J Med 82:553, 1987

102. Chayt KJ, Harper ME, Marselle LM et al: Detection of HTLV-III RNA in lungs of patients with AIDS and pulmonary involvement. JAMA 256:2356, 1986

103. Plata F, Garcia-Pons F, Ryter A et al: HIV-1 infection of lung alveolar fibroblasts and macrophages in humans. AIDS Res Hum Retroviruses 6:979, 1990

104. Dean NC, Golden JA, Evans LA et al: Human immunodeficiency virus recovery from bronchoalveolar lavage fluid in patients with AIDS. Chest 93:1176, 1988

105. Linneman CC, Baughman RP, Frame PT, Floyd R: Recovery of human immunodeficiency virus and detection of p24 antigen in bronchoalveolar lavage fluid from adult patients with AIDS. Chest 96:64, 1989

106. Rubinstein A, Bernstein LJ, Charytan M et al: Corticosteroid treatment for pulmonary lymphoid hyperplasia in children with the acquired immune deficiency syndrome. Pediatr Pulmonol 4:13, 1988

107. Lin RY, Gruber PJ, Saunders R, Perla EN: Lymphocytic interstitial pneumonitis in adult HIV infection. NY State J Med 88:273, 1988

108. Oldham SAA, Castillo M, Jacobson FL et al: HIV-associated lymphocytic interstitial pneumonia: Radiologic manifestations and pathologic correlation. Radiology 170:83, 1989

109. Teirstein AS, Rosen MJ: Lymphocytic interstitial pneumonia. Clin Chest Med 9:467, 1988

110. Bach MC: Zidovudine for lymphocytic interstitial pneumonia associated with AIDS. Lancet 2:796, 1987

111. Bye MR, Bernstein L, Shah K et al: Diagnostic bronchoalveolar lavage in children with AIDS. Pediatr Pulmonol 3:425, 1987

112. Rubinstein A: Pediatric AIDS. Curr Prob Pediatr 16:364, 1986

113. Joshi VV, Kauffman S, Oleske JM et al: Polyclonal polymorphic B-cell lymphoproliferative disorder with prominent pulmonary involvement in children with acquired immune deficiency syndrome. Cancer 59:1455, 1987

114. Helbert M, Stoneham C, Mitchell D, Pinching AJ: Zidovudine for lymphocytic interstitial pneumonitis in AIDS. Lancet 2:1333, 1987

115. Suffredini AF, Ognibene FP, Lack EE et al: Nonspecific interstitial pneumonitis: A common cause of pulmonary disease in the acquired immunodeficiency syndrome. Ann Intern Med 107:7, 1987

116. Ognibene FP, Masur H, Rogers P et al: Nonspecific interstitial pneumonitis without evidence of *Pneumocystis carinii* in asymptomatic patients infected with human immunodeficiency virus. Ann Intern Med 109:874, 1988

117. Ramaswamy G, Jagadha V, Tchertkoff V: Diffuse alveolar damage and interstitial fibrosis in acquired immunodeficiency syndrome patients without concurrent pulmonary infection. Arch Pathol Lab Med 109:408, 1985

118. Simmons JT, Suffredini AF, Lack EE et al: Nonspecific interstitial pneumonitis in patients with AIDS: Radiologic features. AJR 149:265, 1987

119. White DA, Gellene RA, Gupta S et al: Pulmonary cell populations in the immunosuppressed patient: Bronchoalveolar lavage findings during episodes of pneumonitis. Chest 88:352, 1985

120. Wallace JM, Barbers RG, Oishi JS, Prince H: Cellular and

T-lymphocyte subpopulation profiles in bronchoalveolar lavage fluid from patients with acquired immunodeficiency syndrome and pneumonitis. Am Rev Respir Dis 130:786, 1984

121. Young KR, Rankin JA, Naegel GP et al: Bronchoalveolar lavage cells and proteins in patients with the acquired immunodeficiency syndrome: An immunologic analysis. Ann Intern Med 103:522, 1985

122. Plata F, Autran B, Pedroza Martins L et al: AIDS virus-specific cytotoxic T lymphocytes in lung disorders. Nature 328:348, 1987

123. Guillon JM, Autran B, Denis M et al: Human immuno-deficiency virus–related lymphocytic alveolitis. Chest 94:1264, 1988

124. Meignan M, Guillon JM, Denis M et al: Increased lung epithelial permeability in HIV-infected patients with isolated cytotoxic T-lymphocytic alveolitis. Am Rev Respir Dis 141:1241, 1990

125. Ettensohn DB, Mayer KH, Kessimian N, Smith PS: Lymphocytic bronchiolitis associated with HIV infection. Chest 93:201, 1988

126. Allen JN, Wewers MD: HIV-associated bronchiolitis obliterans organizing pneumonia. Chest 96:197, 1989

Renal Complications

17C

James E. Balow

Renal and electrolyte abnormalities regularly develop during the course of human immunodeficiency virus (HIV) infection and acquired immunodeficiency syndrome (AIDS).[1-4] Most of the abnormalities are secondary to the various components of AIDS and to complications of management of this disease. This chapter briefly examines fluid and electrolyte disorders, causes of renal dysfunction, types of glomerular lesions, tubulointerstitial diseases, and renal aspects of drug therapy in patients with AIDS.

FLUID AND ELECTROLYTE DISORDERS

Hyponatremia is one of the most common metabolic problems in patients with AIDS. Gastrointestinal salt losses from diarrhea, with only water repletion, are among the commonest causes of hyponatremia in these patients; management with volume repletion of appropriate crystalloid is generally straightforward.

In AIDS patients, it is important to consider rare causes of hyponatremia because specific fluid management may be necessary. Hyperkalemia and renal salt wasting help to distinguish the hypovolemic hyponatremia of adrenal insufficiency from other causes. Adrenal infections with cytomegalovirus, mycobacteria, or *Cryptococcus* are commonly found at autopsy, but functional adrenal insufficiency is relatively unusual.[1,2]

The syndrome of inappropriate antidiuretic hormone (SIADH) secretion is another uncommon cause of hyponatremia in AIDS. SIADH is most often due to infections or mass lesions (*e.g.,* tumor) in the brain or lungs of AIDS patients. SIADH is associated with euvolemic hyponatremia and is managed primarily by water restriction and the administration of vasopressin antagonists (*e.g.,* demeclocycline).

Other electrolyte disturbances, such as hypernatremia, hypocalcemia (due primarily to hypoalbuminemia), and hyperuricemia (primarily from volume depletion), are relatively common in AIDS patients, but these metabolic conditions rarely require specific therapy.[1,2]

RENAL FAILURE

Acute renal failure is common during the course of AIDS and its complications. Prerenal azotemia from volume depletion and sepsis is the most common form. The renal complications of drugs commonly used in AIDS patients are summarized in Table 17C–1. Trimethoprim-sulfamethoxazole can produce mild azotemia because it competes for tubular secretion of creatinine, but rarely does it cause a true depression of the glomerular filtration rate (GFR). Nephrotoxic agents, particularly pentamidine, amphotericin B, aminoglycosides, and radiologic contrast dye, are relatively common causes of azotemia.[5,6] Obstructive nephropathy may be extrinsic to the urinary tract, such as in lymphomas, or intrinsic,

Table 17C–1. Renal Complications of Drugs Commonly Used in AIDS Patients[5-8]

Drug	Complications
Amphotericin	Azotemia, acute renal failure, potassium and magnesium wasting, distal renal tubular acidosis, nephrocalcinosis
Pentamidine	Azotemia, acute renal failure
Sulfa drugs	Azotemia without change in GFR, sulfadiazine crystal–induced obstructive nephropathy, allergic interstitial nephritis
Acylovir	Acyclovir crystal–induced obstructive nephropathy
Aminoglycosides	Acute renal failure, magnesium wasting
Rifampin	Acute renal failure, Fanconi syndrome, renal tubular acidosis, nephrogenic diabetes insipidus, interstitial nephritis, glomerulonephritis
Foscarnet	Acute renal failure, nephrogenic diabetes insipidus

such as occurs with tubular precipitation of acyclovir[7] or sulfadiazine.[8] Careful attention to drug pharmacology is essential in AIDS patients because of the multisystem complications and the frequent need for multidrug regimens in this disease. An excellent review of the renal aspects of drug therapy for AIDS and its associated opportunistic infections is available.[5]

GLOMERULAR DISEASES

The various forms and relative frequencies of kidney lesions associated with AIDS, its associated conditions, and treatment are listed in Table 17C–2. The first reports of glomerular disease occurring in AIDS patients emanated from New York City in 1984. Gardenswartz and colleagues analyzed the cases of 32 patients with AIDS.[9] Renal abnormalities, seen in 13 patients, included several types of glomerular lesions, among them mesangial hyperplasia, membranoproliferative glomerulonephritis, and focal segmental glomerulosclerosis. The authors suggested that glomerular disease was relatively common in AIDS but that no specific type of lesion was characteristic.

Rao and colleagues reported nephropathy in 11 of 92 AIDS patients; the nephropathy was most frequently proteinuria due to focal segmental glomerulosclerosis.[10] Rapid deterioration of renal function was characteristic of AIDS patients with this lesion, as has been confirmed by others.[11] Rao was the first to suggest that focal segmental glomerulosclerosis was a characteristic AIDS-associated nephropathy.

Pardo and colleagues described clinical renal involvement in nearly half of their AIDS patients studied in Miami, Florida.[12] Mesangial, focal, and diffuse proliferative glomerulonephritis, as well as focal segmental glomerulosclerosis, were observed. Most patients were black, male, and drug abusers. Interestingly, hypertension has been rarely reported in AIDS patients with any form of glomerulopathy. Focal segmental glomerulosclerosis was also seen in pediatric AIDS patients in Miami.[13]

Focal segmental glomerulosclerosis has been suggested to be the prototypic HIV-associated nephropathy.[10-15] Focal segmental glomerulosclerosis in AIDS patients is accompanied by segmental collapse of glomerular capillaries, large numbers of tubuloreticular aggregates in glomerular endothelial cells, and striking degenerative changes in glomerular epithelial cells, as well as interstitial edema, tubular necrosis, cystic dilation of tubules, and protein casts.[10-18] Probes for the DNA of HIV hybridize *in vitro* to glomerular and tubular epithelial cells.[19] The kidneys of patients with focal segmental glomerulosclerosis are enlarged and echogenic on ultrasound studies.[20]

It had long been known that lesions of focal segmental glomerulosclerosis also occurred in patients with illicit intravenous (IV) drug abuse, but neither the New York[10] nor the Miami[12] groups could attribute all cases of focal segmental glomerulosclerosis in AIDS patients to concomitant IV drug–related glomerular disease.

The relatively common finding of glomerular disease in AIDS patients in New York[9-11,21] and Miami[12,13,22,23] (where there was a striking predominance of black males and IV drug–related HIV transmission) contrasts with experience reported in populations with different demographic characteristics and modes of HIV transmission. Thus, AIDS patients studied at the National Institutes of Health in Bethesda, Maryland,[24] at San Francisco General Hospital in San Francisco, California,[3] and in Europe,[2] in whom there was a predominance of white patients and homosexuality as the major risk factor for HIV transmission, showed little evidence of glomerular disease and extremely rarely had focal segmental glomerulosclerosis.

A definitive explanation is lacking for the discrepancy in prevalence rates of glomerular disease, particularly focal segmental glomerulosclerosis, in different groups of HIV-infected patients. However, it is clear that associated risk factors for the development of focal segmental glomerulosclerosis, such as black race and IV drug abuse, are important.[2,10-12] The premise that HIV *per se* produces a unique glomerular lesion remains controversial.

Small numbers of cases of other glomerular lesions, including minimal change disease,[13,15,25] membranous nephropathy,[15,19,26] other proliferative (including postinfectious) glomerulonephritides,[3,9,10,15,19] and thrombotic microangiopathy,[24,27] have been described (see Table 17C–2).

The management of glomerular disease in AIDS patients is not well defined. The effect of HIV-modulating drugs on focal segmental glomerulosclerosis is not certain but appears to be minimal.[2] These patients generally progress to end-stage renal failure at rates much faster than patients with non-AIDS forms of the disease. The survival of patients with full-blown AIDS in end-stage

Table 17C–2. Types and Relative Frequency of Kidney Pathology in AIDS Patients with Clinical Evidence of Renal Disease

A. Common renal lesions
 1. Acute tubular necrosis
 2. Mesangial hyperplasia
 3. Focal segmental glomerulosclerosis
 4. Interstitial nephritis
 5. Nephrocalcinosis
 6. Parenchymal and/or collecting system infections: viral, bacterial, fungal, protozoal

B. Unusual and rare renal lesions
 1. Minimal change nephropathy
 2. Post-infectious glomerulonephritis
 3. Membranous nephropathy
 4. Membranoproliferative glomerulonephritis
 5. Thrombotic microangiopathy
 6. Kaposi's sarcoma
 7. Lymphoma, infiltrative
 8. Carcinoma, renal cell or metastatic

renal failure is abysmal, and few patients are currently accepted into dialysis or renal transplant programs.[1,2,28]

TUBULOINTERSTITIAL DISEASE

Acute tubular necrosis (ischemic or nephrotoxic), focal nephrocalcinosis, chronic interstitial nephritis (due to antibiotics), urinary tract infection, and pyelonephritis are relatively common extraglomerular lesions in AIDS patients.[29] The nephrocalcinosis is most often related to amphotericin B therapy, *Mycobacterium avium-intracellulare,* or *Pneumocystis carinii* infection.[30] Granulomatous pyelonephritis, particularly due to candidal or mycobacterial infections, occurs. Other renal parenchymal infections include those caused by cytomegalovirus, *Nocardia, Histoplasma, Cryptococcus,* and *Pneumocystis carinii.* Secondary vasculitis with renal infarction has been seen. Metastatic foci of various types of lymphomas and carcinomas, as well as Kaposi's sarcoma, have been described in the kidney.

REFERENCES

1. Glassock R, Cohen A, Danovitch G, Parsa P: Human immunodeficiency virus (HIV) infection and the kidney. Ann Intern Med 112:35, 1990
2. Bourgoignie JJ: Renal complications of human immunodeficiency virus type 1. Kidney Int 37:1571, 1990
3. Mazbar SA, Schoenfeld PY, Humphreys MH: Renal involvement in patients infected with HIV: Experience at San Francisco General Hospital. Kidney Int 37:1325, 1990
4. O'Regan S, Russo P, Lapointe N, Rousseau E: AIDS and the urinary tract. J AIDS 3:244, 1990
5. Berns JS, Raphael RM, Stumacher RJ, Rudnick MR: Renal aspects of therapy for human immunodeficiency virus and associated opportunistic infections. J Am Soc Nephrol 1:1061, 1990
6. Lachaal M, Venuto R: Nephrotoxicity and hyperkalemia in patients with acquired immunodeficiency syndrome treated with pentamidine. Am J Med 87:260, 1989
7. Sawyer MH, Webb DE, Balow JE, Strauss SE: Acyclovir induced renal failure: Clinical course and histology. Am J Med 84:1067, 1988
8. Simon DI, Brosius FC, Rothstein DM: Sulfadiazine crystalluria revisited: The treatment of toxoplasma encephalitis in patients with acquired immunodeficiency syndrome. Arch Intern Med 150:2379, 1990
9. Gardenswartz MH, Lerner CW, Seligson GR et al: Renal disease in patients with AIDS: A clinicopathologic study. Clin Nephrol 21:197, 1984
10. Rao TK, Filippone EJ, Nicastri AD et al: Associated focal and segmental glomerulosclerosis in the acquired immunodeficiency syndrome. N Engl J Med 310:669, 1984
11. Carbone L, D'Agati V, Cheng J-T, Appel G: Course and prognosis of human immunodeficiency virus-associated nephropathy. Am J Med 87:389, 1989
12. Pardo V, Aldana M, Colton RM et al: Glomerular lesions in the acquired immunodeficiency syndrome. Ann Intern Med 101:429, 1984
13. Strauss J, Abitbol C, Zilleruelo G et al: Renal disease in children with the acquired immunodeficiency syndrome. N Engl J Med 321:625, 1989
14. Cohen A, Nast C: HIV-associated nephropathy: A unique combined glomerular, tubular, and interstitial lesion. Mod Pathol 1:87, 1988
15. D'Agati V, Suh J-I, Carbone L et al: Pathology of HIV-associated nephropathy: A detailed morphologic and comparative study. Kidney Int 35:1358, 1989
16. Seney FD, Burns DK, Silva FG: Acquired immunodeficiency syndrome and the kidney. Am J Kidney Dis 16:1, 1990
17. Soni A, Agarwal A, Chander P et al: Evidence for an HIV-related nephropathy: A clinico-pathological study. Clin Nephrol 31:12, 1989
18. Chander P, Agarwal A, Soni A et al: Renal cytomembranous inclusions in idiopathic renal disease as predictive markers for the acquired immunodeficiency syndrome. Hum Pathol 19:1060, 1988
19. Cohen A, Sun N, Shapshak P, Imagawa D: Demonstration of human immunodeficiency virus in renal epithelium in HIV-associated nephropathy. Mod Pathol 2:125, 1989
20. Schaffer R, Schwartz G, Becker J et al: Renal ultrasound in acquired immune deficiency syndrome. Radiology 153:511, 1984
21. Rao TK, Friedman EA, Nicastri AD: The types of renal disease in the acquired immunodeficiency syndrome. N Engl J Med 316:1062, 1987
22. Pardo V, Maneses R, Ossa L et al: AIDS-related glomerulopathy: Occurrence in specific risk groups. Kidney Int 31:1167, 1987
23. Bourgoignie JJ, Meneses R, Ortiz C et al: The clinical spectrum of renal disease associated with human immunodeficiency virus. Am J Kidney Dis 12:131, 1988
24. Balow JE, Macher AM, Rook AH: Paucity of glomerular disease in acquired immunodeficiency syndrome (abstr). Kidney Int 29:178, 1986
25. Singer DRJ, Jenkins AP, Gupta S, Evans DJ: Minimal change nephropathy in the acquired immune deficiency syndrome. Br Med J 291:868, 1985
26. Guerra IL, Abraham AA, Kimmel PL et al: Nephrotic syndrome associated with chronic persistent hepatitis B in an HIV antibody positive patient. Am J Kidney Dis 10:385, 1987
27. Charasse C, Michelet C, Le Tulzo Y et al: Thrombotic thrombocytopenic purpura with the acquired immunodeficiency syndrome: A pathologically documented case report. Am J Kidney Dis 17:80, 1991
28. Schoenfeld P, Feduska NJ: Acquired immunodeficiency syndrome and renal disease: Report of the National Kidney Foundation–National Institutes of Health Task Force on AIDS and Kidney Disease. Am J Kidney Dis 16:14, 1990
29. Kaplan MS, Wechsler M, Benson MC: Urologic manifestations of AIDS. Urology 30:441, 1987
30. Feuerstein IM, Francis P, Raffeld M, Pluda J: Widespread visceral calcifications in disseminated *Pneumocystis carinii* infection: CT characteristics. J Comput Assist Tomogr 14:149, 1990

Hematologic Complications of HIV Infection

17D

Donald W. Northfelt   *Ronald T. Mitsuyasu*

Clinically significant hematologic abnormalities are common in persons with human immunodeficiency virus (HIV) infection. Impaired hematopoiesis, immune-mediated cytopenias, and altered coagulation mechanisms have all been described in HIV-infected individuals. These abnormalities may occur as a result of HIV infection itself, as sequelae of HIV-related opportunistic infections or malignancies, or as a consequence of therapies employed for HIV infection and associated conditions. In this chapter we review the clinical manifestations, etiology, diagnosis, and treatment of common hematologic problems encountered in patients with HIV infection.

ANEMIA

Anemia is a common finding in patients with HIV infection, particularly in those with more advanced HIV-related disease. In a study of patients receiving no myelosuppressive therapies,[1] 8% of asymptomatic HIV-seropositive patients, 20% of patients with AIDS-related conditions (ARC), and 71% of patients with AIDS were anemic. Investigation of a cohort from a longitudinal study of HIV disease,[2] found anemia in 18% of HIV-seropositive patients, 50% of patients with ARC, and 75% of those with AIDS. The Multicenter AIDS Cohort Study found that 3.2% of HIV-seropositive patients with mean CD4+ T-lymphocyte counts of greater than 700 cells/mm^3 were anemic, whereas anemia was present in 20.9% of those with mean CD4+ T-lymphocyte counts less than 249 cells/mm^3.[3]

Anemia associated with HIV infection usually features normocytic and normochromic erythrocytes. Microcytosis is uncommon in this setting and is said to be an unreliable predictor of bone marrow iron stores. Most patients with advanced HIV disease have at least mild changes in red blood cell size and shape.[4]

There are a number of possible etiologies of anemia in patients with HIV infection (Table 17D–1). From the data reviewed above, it is clear that HIV infection alone may produce anemia in some patients. A study of serum immunoreactive erythropoietin in HIV-infected patients showed that levels of the hormone failed to rise commensurately with increasing anemia, suggesting that insufficient amounts of erythropoietin may be one cause of anemia in this setting.[3] Other studies have suggested that soluble factors in the serum of HIV-infected patients may inhibit hematopoiesis, or that direct infection of marrow progenitor cells may play a role in producing anemia and other hematologic abnormalities associated with HIV infection.[5,6]

Drug-induced Anemia

Zidovudine therapy is probably the most common cause of anemia in HIV-infected patients at the present time. In the original phase II clinical trial that demonstrated the efficacy of zidovudine in patients with HIV infection, statistically significant reductions in hemoglobin levels occurred in 34% of zidovudine-treated subjects following 6 weeks of therapy.[7] This fall in hemoglobin was accompanied by the progressive rise in erythrocyte mean corpuscular volume that has now become familiar to physicians treating patients with zidovudine. Thirty-one percent of zidovudine-treated subjects in the trial required red blood cell transfusions while receiving the drug. Marrow erythroid hypoplasia, aplasia, and megaloblastic maturation have all been shown to develop as

Table 17D–1. Causes of Peripheral Blood Cytopenias in Patients With HIV Infection

BONE MARROW INFECTIONS
HIV
B19 parvovirus
Mycobacterium avium complex
Mycobacterium tuberculosis
Histoplasma capsulatum
Coccidioides immitis
Cryptococcus neoformans
Pneumocystis carinii
Leishmania donovani

MEDICATIONS
Zidovudine
Trimethoprim-sulfamethoxazole
Dapsone
Sulfadiazine
Pyrimethamine
Amphotericin B
5-Flucytosine
Ganciclovir
Antineoplastics
Interferon-α

NEOPLASMS
Non-Hodgkin's lymphoma
Hodgkin's disease

a result of zidovudine therapy.[8] Subsequent studies have demonstrated that anemia is less common with reduced dosages of zidovudine,[9,10] but many patients receiving the drug in clinical practice will still require occasional transfusions or drug "holidays" to ameliorate this toxicity.

Effective therapy for zidovudine-induced anemia is available in the form of recombinant human erythropoietin. A double-blind, placebo-controlled study[11] demonstrated that recombinant human erythropoietin (100 U/kg thrice weekly by intravenous [IV] bolus) reduced the transfusion requirements of zidovudine-treated AIDS patients whose serum levels of endogenous erythropoietin were less than 500 IU/L. Significantly fewer erythropoietin-treated patients received transfusions, and those who were transfused received significantly fewer units of red blood cells than placebo-treated patients.

Antimicrobial and antineoplastic agents used for treatment or prophylaxis against HIV-related conditions also cause anemia. For example, the use of dapsone for the treatment or prevention of *Pneumocystis carinii* pneumonia may cause hemolytic anemia or generalized myelosuppression,[12] and anemia routinely occurs as part of the overall myelosuppressive effect of chemotherapy for AIDS-related non-Hodgkin's lymphoma.

Anemia Caused by Bone Marrow Infections

Infection with *Mycobacterium avium* complex is another common cause of anemia in AIDS. This infection, diagnosed in up to 18% of patients with AIDS during the course of their illness,[13] causes high-grade bacteremia and widely disseminated infection, usually involving the bone marrow. In such patients, anemia tends to occur out of proportion to other cytopenias.[14] A recent study at San Francisco General Hospital examined the relationship between *M. avium* complex bacteremia and transfusion requirements: it was demonstrated that patients with positive blood cultures for *M. avium* complex had a relative risk of 5.23 (p < 0.001) for receiving red blood cell transfusions, compared to patients with negative blood cultures.[15]

There is controversy regarding the benefit of the antimycobacterial therapies that are currently available for *M. avium* complex infection. Although some treatment studies have demonstrated a reduction in symptoms such as fever in conjunction with a reduction in the number of organisms in the blood,[16,17] no study of antimycobacterial therapy for *M. avium* complex infection has shown improvement of the associated anemia.

Two recent reports have highlighted the role of B19 parvovirus infection in the development of anemia in HIV-infected patients.[18,19] The etiologic agent of the childhood exanthem, fifth disease (erythema infectiosum), B19 parvovirus has been recognized for some time as a cause of severe chronic anemia in immuno-

compromised persons. Parvovirus DNA has now been detected in the serum and/or bone marrow of several patients with HIV infection and severe anemia. The anemia of parvovirus infection can be alleviated with infusions of immunoglobulin.

Other conditions associated with HIV infection can cause anemia as a result of direct involvement of the bone marrow (see Table 17D–1). Tuberculosis, histoplasmosis, cryptococcosis, pneumocystosis, and non-Hodgkin's lymphoma can all infiltrate the bone marrow,[20] generally causing pancytopenia.

Other Causes of Anemia

Anti-erythrocyte antibodies produce a positive direct antiglobulin test in approximately 20% of HIV-infected patients with hypergammaglobulinemia.[21,22] Although not well characterized, these antibodies behave as polyagglutinins, and it is unclear whether they are directed against specific cell-surface antigens or merely represent nonspecific attachment. Hemolytic anemia in the setting of an HIV-related positive direct antiglobulin test is rare.

Gastrointestinal bleeding should also be considered in the evaluation of HIV-infected patients with anemia. In addition to all of the usual causes of gastrointestinal blood loss, HIV-related infections such as cytomegalovirus colitis, and malignancies such as Kaposi's sarcoma and non-Hodgkin's lymphoma, may produce clinically significant bleeding.

THROMBOCYTOPENIA

Thrombocytopenia is frequently associated with HIV infection. In the Multicenter AIDS Cohort Study, platelet counts were measured in over 1,500 HIV-seropositive participants without AIDS; 6.7% of participants had platelet counts below 150,000 cells/mm^3 on at least one semiannual visit, and 2.6% of participants had platelet counts below 150,000 cells/mm^3 on two successive semiannual visits.[3] In a Swiss study, platelet counts less than 100,000 cells/mm^3 were noted in 9% of 321 HIV-seropositive IV drug users and in 3% of 359 HIV-seropositive homosexuals.[23] A smaller study from London reported platelet counts less than 150,000 cells/mm^3 in 30% (6/20) of patients with AIDS and in 8% (5/59) of patients with persistent generalized lymphadenopathy.[24]

There are a number of possible etiologies of thrombocytopenia in patients with HIV infection, including immune-mediated destruction, thrombotic thrombocytopenic purpura, impaired hematopoiesis, and toxic effects of medications. In many instances, however, thrombocytopenia is a relatively isolated hematologic abnormality, associated with a normal or increased number of megakaryocytes in the bone marrow, and therefore presents as the clinical syndrome of immune thrombocytopenic purpura (ITP).

HIV-related Immune Thrombocytopenic Purpura

Morris *et al* described a cluster of 11 cases of ITP in homosexual men in New York City in 1982.[25] The demographic characteristics and immunologic profiles of the patients were similar to those described in patients with AIDS. Subsequently ITP was reported in narcotic addicts, hemophiliacs, transfusion recipients, and children with HIV infection.[26] ITP is therefore recognized as a condition that is clearly associated with HIV infection.

A patient can be said to have true HIV-related ITP only if he or she has no other condition, and is receiving no treatment, that could cause thrombocytopenia. Most such patients are otherwise well. In fact, HIV-related ITP is most often an early manifestation of HIV infection, occurring before the development of any AIDS-defining condition.[23] CD4+ lymphocyte counts in reported series of patients with HIV-ITP have averaged between 300 and 600 cells/mm^3. HIV-related ITP is therefore commonly included among those conditions characterizing ARC,[27] and is included within Group II in the Centers for Disease Control classification of HIV-related illness.[28]

Several hypotheses have been advanced to explain the pathogenesis of HIV-related ITP. One theory holds that circulating immune complexes are nonspecifically deposited on platelet membranes, resulting in reticuloendothelial clearance.[29,30] Recent studies have shown that these immune complexes contain anti-HIV gp120 and complementary anti-idiotypic antibody.[31] Another hypothesis states that a specific IgG antiplatelet antibody binds to a 25-kilodalton antigen on the platelet membrane, resulting in platelet destruction.[32] Regardless of the actual mechanism responsible for platelet destruction, thrombocytopenia in HIV-infected patients may be compounded by impaired ability to produce platelets in sufficient numbers.[33]

Other workers sought to define a more central role for HIV itself in the pathogenesis of HIV-related ITP after noting the improvement seen in platelet counts of HIV-ITP patients treated with zidovudine (see below).[34] They performed ultrastructural analysis of bone marrow megakaryocytes from patients with HIV-related ITP and demonstrated unique structural aberrations. In addition, HIV RNA was shown by *in situ* hybridization to be expressed within the cells. The authors suggested that direct infection of megakaryocytes by HIV may impair platelet production and contribute to thrombocytopenia.

The classic approach to the diagnosis of ITP is to consider it a diagnosis of exclusion, meaning that any other cause of low platelet production or peripheral platelet destruction must be excluded before the diagnosis of ITP can be applied to a patient with a low platelet count. The same general approach should be taken in cases of possible HIV-related ITP. Bone marrow biopsy should be performed to exclude cytotoxic or alcohol-related drug effects. The marrow should be examined for the presence of lymphoma or opportunistic infections such as fungi or mycobacteria that would result in reduced megakaryocyte numbers and hence reduced platelet production. Other causes of peripheral platelet destruction must also be sought, including splenic sequestration resulting from liver disease with portal hypertension, drug-induced ITP, lymphoma-associated ITP, thrombotic thrombocytopenic purpura, or disseminated intravascular coagulation. The finding of platelet-associated immunoglobulin or immune complexes strengthens the diagnosis of HIV-related ITP but is neither sufficient nor necessary for the diagnosis.

A variety of therapeutic approaches are employed for the treatment of ITP in patients without HIV infection. Therapy with corticosteroids, cytotoxic agents, the attenuated androgen danazol, IV immune globulin infusions, plasmapheresis, interferon-α, and splenectomy have all been used with varying degrees of success. Many of these modalities have also been used for the treatment of ITP in patients with HIV infection. However, therapy for HIV-related ITP has been relatively unsatisfactory.

Walsh *et al*[35] treated 17 patients with HIV-related ITP using standard prednisone therapy for ITP. Platelet counts increased from a mean of 21,000 to above 100,000 cells/mm^3 in eight, and to above 50,000 cells/mm^3 in eight others, but 13 patients relapsed when the prednisone was tapered. Six of 26 patients treated with prednisone by Oksenhendler *et al*.[36] had sustained responses following tapering of therapy, while 11 did not respond at all. Abrams *et al*[37] observed sustained normalization of platelet counts in two of 24 patients after a tapered course of prednisone therapy. Theoretical concerns regarding the immunosuppressive effects of corticosteroid therapy in patients with HIV infection have never been objectively addressed.

The response rate to splenectomy in patients with HIV-related ITP has been variably reported as 60% to 100%,[36,38–40] with low rates of surgical morbidity. Concerns have been raised regarding the possible immunosuppressive effect of splenectomy in patients with HIV infection.[41] In addition, some surgeons hold the opinion that wound healing is impaired by HIV infection and are therefore reluctant to recommend operation.

Treatment of HIV-related ITP with high-dose IV immune globulin produced initial responses in 12 of 17 patients in one report, but the response was sustained in only one.[36] Anti-Rh immunoglobulin infusions have also been used, with similar success.[36] These relatively unimpressive results, as well as the extremely high cost of IV immune globulin therapy, have limited its use.

In a number of the early studies of zidovudine therapy for HIV infection, platelet counts were noted to rise during treatment. These observations led the Swiss Group for Clinical Studies on AIDS to conduct a prospective, placebo-controlled, blinded study of zidovudine therapy for HIV-related ITP.[42] Platelet counts increased from 1.1-fold to 3.8-fold in all patients over the 8-week course of zidovudine treatment; no change in platelet count was noted during placebo treatment. Zidovudine therapy in this study consisted of 2 g/day for 2 weeks, followed by 1 g/day for 6 weeks; one patient could tolerate only 250 mg/day because of leukopenia, but still had a twofold rise in platelet count.

Three case reports[43-45] have described treatment of HIV-related ITP using interferon-α in low doses. Side-effects were tolerable, and clinically meaningful elevations in platelet counts were observed. In an ongoing clinical trial reported at the 6th International Conference on AIDS,[46] nine HIV-seropositive patients with mucosal bleeding and/or hemorrhage associated with HIV-related ITP were treated with interferon-α2b, 3 million units given subcutaneously three times weekly. The mean platelet count for the group, 20,000 cells/mm^3, rose to 45,000 cells/mm^3 following 4 weeks of therapy and was maintained at 47,000 cells/mm^3 following 12 weeks of therapy. Bleeding resolved in seven of the nine patients, and side-effects of the treatment (transient flu-like symptoms) were tolerable.

Treatment of HIV-related ITP should probably be reserved for patients with clinically significant symptoms such as recurrent epistaxis, gingival or subconjunctival bleeding, or gastrointestinal hemorrhage. Therapy is also recommended for hemophiliacs with HIV-related ITP because of the substantial morbidity and mortality associated with bleeding in this group.[47] Only in these situations does it seem worthwhile to subject HIV-infected patients to the troublesome toxicity and questionable efficacy of most standard therapies for ITP. In contrast, zidovudine and interferon-α therapy can raise the platelet count while simultaneously providing antiretroviral activity, and therefore are the most attractive of the currently available treatments for HIV-related ITP.

Thrombotic Thrombocytopenic Purpura

Thrombotic thrombocytopenic purpura (TTP) is a clinical syndrome characterized by the classic pentad of fever, neurologic dysfunction, renal dysfunction, microangiopathic hemolytic anemia, and thrombocytopenia. The diagnosis is supported by the finding of hyaline microvascular thrombi in tissue biopsy specimens. An abnormal interaction between platelets and endothelium is thought to be responsible for the clinical and pathologic findings, but the mechanism accounting for this observation remains undefined. Plasmapheresis is generally accepted as standard therapy for TTP, although plasma infusions, exchange transfusions, antiplatelet drug therapy, corticosteroids, and splenectomy have all been used, with varying degrees of success.[48]

A number of cases of TTP occurring in patients with HIV infection have been described in the medical literature.[49-55] Data from one center have been interpreted as showing a statistically significant association of TTP with HIV infection.[51] In most of the reported cases, there was no diagnosis of AIDS prior to the development of TTP, although several patients had symptomatic HIV disease (persistent lymphadenopathy, oral candidiasis)

at presentation. This observation, along with the relatively high CD4 lymphocyte counts or CD4/CD8 lymphocyte ratios reported in some of the cases, suggests that TTP, like HIV-related ITP, is an early manifestation of HIV infection. The etiology of TTP in patients with HIV infection has not been established.

Most patients with HIV-related TTP have been successfully treated with plasmapheresis in conjunction with antiplatelet agents or corticosteroids, or both. Because HIV-infected patients with TTP appear to have relatively well-preserved immune function, and good response to plasmapheresis can be expected, prompt diagnosis and appropriate therapy are essential.

Other Causes of Thrombocytopenia in HIV Disease

Any of the infectious or neoplastic conditions that involve the bone marrow and any of the medications that cause generalized myelosuppression in patients with HIV infection can produce thrombocytopenia (see Table 17D–1). HIV-infected patients are also susceptible to developing thrombocytopenia for reasons unrelated to HIV infection, such as alcohol use, splenomegaly and liver disease, or drug effects (heparin, quinidine); these possibilities must always be considered in evaluating the thrombocytopenic HIV-infected patient.

GRANULOCYTOPENIA AND ABNORMAL GRANULOCYTE FUNCTION

Granulocytopenia is commonly encountered in patients with HIV infection. Although low granulocyte counts usually reflect the toxicity of therapies for HIV infection or associated conditions, studies of untreated patients have also shown a high incidence of granulocytopenia, particularly in patients with more profound immunodeficiency. For example, the Multicenter AIDS Cohort Study found that 0.8% of HIV-seropositive patients with mean CD4+ T-lymphocyte counts greater than 700 cells/mm^3 had abnormally low granulocyte counts, whereas granulocytopenia was present in 13.4% of those with mean CD4+ T-lymphocyte counts below 249 cells/mm^3.[3] Zon and Groopman noted low granulocyte counts in 13% of asymptomatic HIV-seropositive patients and in 44% of those with frank AIDS.[1]

The pathogenesis of granulocytopenia in patients with HIV infection is multifactorial (see Table 17D–1). An autoimmune mechanism involving antigranulocyte antibodies,[24,56] and impaired granulopoiesis[5,6] have been postulated to account for granulocytopenia in some patients, but the clinical importance of these observations has not been clearly established. Any infiltrative process involving the bone marrow (infection, malignancy) may also produce granulocytopenia. In clinical practice, however, drug toxicity is responsible for most of the granulocytopenia seen in patients with HIV infection.

Drug-induced Granulocytopenia

Zidovudine therapy is probably the most common cause of low granulocyte counts in patients with HIV infection. Severe granulocytopenia (<500 cells/mm³) developed in 16% of zidovudine-treated patients in the original placebo-controlled study of zidovudine therapy for AIDS and ARC[7]; only 2% of placebo-treated patients became granulocytopenic to this degree (p < 0.001). Despite the relatively high frequency of zidovudine-induced granulocytopenia, there were no reported episodes of bacterial infection or sepsis in the study group, nor have subsequent studies of zidovudine therapy at similar or lower doses[9,10,57] reported bacterial infections complicating zidovudine-induced granulocytopenia. The low observed risk of bacterial infection may be a reflection of the brief duration of zidovudine-induced granulocytopenia; in these studies, the dosage of zidovudine was reduced or discontinued when the granulocyte count fell below 500 to 1,000 cells/mm³. Granulocyte recovery is generally prompt following discontinuation of zidovudine therapy.

Shaunak and Bartlett described their experience in treating 30 patients with severe, recurrent (three or more episodes) zidovudine-induced granulocytopenia.[58] The total follow-up time was 493 months (41.1 patient-years) and the granulocyte count was less than 1,000 cells/mm³ for 41% of that time. Zidovudine therapy was reduced or discontinued when the granulocyte count fell below 500 to 1,000 cells/mm³. Patients with granulocyte counts below 500 cells/mm³ had a 230% higher incidence of bacterial infection than patients with granulocyte counts of 500 to 1,000 cells/mm³ (seven infections in 40 months vs. nine infections in 169 months; p < 0.016). The authors concluded that zidovudine therapy can be continued despite granulocytopenia without a major increase in the incidence of bacterial infection provided that the granulocyte count is not below 500 cells/mm³.

Ganciclovir therapy for symptomatic cytomegalovirus infection is another common cause of granulocytopenia in patients with AIDS. Jacobson et al[59] observed absolute granulocyte counts below 800 cells/mm³ in 10 of 32 patients receiving chronic daily maintenance ganciclovir therapy. Four patients developed central venous catheter–associated bacteremia; all had granulocyte counts above 1200 cells/mm³ when bacteremia occurred. In other studies reviewed by Jacobson,[60] bacterial infection was a very rare complication of ganciclovir-induced granulocytopenia. As with zidovudine therapy, the low observed risk of bacterial infection may reflect the brief duration of ganciclovir-induced granulocytopenia. In clinical practice, the dosage of ganciclovir is usually reduced or discontinued when the

granulocyte count falls below 500 to 1000 cells/mm³, and recovery is generally prompt.

A number of other medications commonly employed in the setting of HIV infection can cause granulocytopenia. Trimethoprim-sulfamethoxazole and pentamidine are standard therapy for most patients with P. carinii pneumonia. Granulocytopenia has been reported in a high percentage of patients receiving these antibiotics in clinical trials, but bacterial infections have not occurred as a consequence.[61–63] Interferon therapy, both alone[64,65] and in combination with zidovudine,[66] can also cause granulocytopenia.

Antineoplastic chemotherapy is probably the most common cause of low granulocyte counts in patients without HIV infection. Granulocytopenia secondary to cancer chemotherapy also complicates the treatment of HIV-infected patients, perhaps to an even greater extent as a result of impaired bone marrow function. However, there are few reports describing the types or incidence of granulocytopenia-related infections in this setting. Gill et al[67] recently reported on their experience with a relatively aggressive combination chemotherapy regimen (doxorubicin + bleomycin + vincristine, or ABV) in the treatment of advanced AIDS-related Kaposi's sarcoma. In their series, granulocytopenia (<1,000 cells/mm³) occurred in 11 of 33 patients, and bacterial infections developed in five. At San Francisco General Hospital, patients with AIDS-related non-Hodgkin's lymphoma frequently require hospitalization for empirical antibiotic therapy when granulocytopenia (<500 cells/mm³) and fever develop following chemotherapy.[68] In a review of 99 such hospitalizations,[69] 23 episodes of bacteremia were identified. This frequency of bacteremia is similar to that seen in cancer patients without HIV infection who develop granulocytopenia following chemotherapy.[70]

In summary, drug-induced granulocytopenia is common in patients with HIV infection, but the risk of bacterial infection is not extraordinary. Only when the granulocyte count falls below 500 cells/mm³ does the risk of infection and sepsis appear to be great, an observation in accord with similar findings in other disease states. Therefore, empirical antibiotic therapy need not be prescribed in cases of mild granulocytopenia resulting from drug therapy or underlying disease states. Rather, antibiotics are reserved for those situations in which frank evidence of bacterial infection is present, or the granulocyte count is below 500 cells/mm³ and expected to remain at that level for a prolonged period of time, as in the aftermath of chemotherapy for HIV-associated malignancies.

Defective Granulocyte Function

Qualitative functions of granulocytes from patients with HIV infection have been studied in vitro, and a number of abnormalities have been noted. Defective chemotaxis, deficient degranulation responses, and ineffective phagocytosis and killing have all been reported.[71-73] The clinical importance of these observations has not been clearly established.

USES OF HEMATOPOIETIC GROWTH FACTORS IN HIV DISEASE

As detailed above, anemia and granulocytopenia frequently result from the use of medications prescribed for the treatment of HIV infection and related conditions. Such treatment is often limited primarily by the development of these cytopenias. The use of erythropoietin to ameliorate the anemia occurring with zidovudine therapy was described earlier and is an example of the use of a hematopoietic growth factor to alleviate bone marrow toxicity and permit continued use of a critical therapy for the HIV-infected patient. Similarly, efforts have been made to alleviate the granulocytopenia in HIV-infected patients with the use of myeloid growth factors.

The first human trial of a myeloid growth factor was conducted in patients with AIDS and granulocytopenia, who received granulocyte-macrophage colony-stimulating factor (GM-CSF) in doses ranging from 0.5 to 8 mg/kg/day by continuous infusion.[74] A rapid, dose-related increase in granulocytes, monocytes, and eosinophils was seen, accompanied by increases in total marrow cellularity. Toxic manifestations included fever, facial flushing, skin rash, and phlebitis at infusion sites. Improvement in bacterial phagocytosis and intracellular killing by granulocytes was noted.[75] Long-term subcutaneous administration of GM-CSF in HIV-infected patients resulted in similar but sustained effects.[76]

Early studies of therapy for AIDS-related non-Hodgkin's lymphoma demonstrated that standard chemotherapy for lymphoma is poorly tolerated by patients with HIV infection, owing to severe myelosuppression. Therefore, two clinical trials have assessed the ability of GM-CSF to decrease the myelosuppressive effects of such chemotherapy. In one study[77] successive cohorts of patients with AIDS-related non-Hodgkin's lymphoma were given GM-CSF along with escalating doses of the m-BACOD (methotrexate, bleomycin, Adriamycin, cyclophosphamide, Oncovin, dexamethasone) regimen. Myelotoxicity was acceptable in all groups, including the final (standard-dose m-BACOD) group, whose mean granulocyte nadir was 1,227 cells/mm^3. In the second study,[68] patients with AIDS-related non-Hodgkin's lymphoma were treated with a minor modification of the standard CHOP (cyclophosphamide, hydroxydaunorubicin, Oncovin, prednisone) chemotherapy regimen. Half of the patients were randomized to receive additional therapy with GM-CSF. The group treated with GM-CSF had higher mean granulocyte nadirs, a shorter mean duration of granulocytopenia, fewer chemotherapy cycles complicated by granulocytopenia and fever, fewer days of hospitalization, and fewer dose reductions or

delays in chemotherapy administration. These studies demonstrate that chemotherapy for AIDS-related non-Hodgkin's lymphoma can be given at standard dosage with less toxicity when accompanied by therapy with GM-CSF to reduce myelosuppression.

Ongoing clinical trials are assessing the efficacy of GM-CSF in reducing the myelosuppressive effects of other treatments commonly employed in patients with HIV infection. GM-CSF therapy has alleviated granulocytopenia induced by zidovudine,[78] ganciclovir,[79] and interferon plus zidovudine.[80] The toxicities of GM-CSF (fever, rash, bone pain, myalgias) were similar in all of these studies.

The effect of GM-CSF therapy on HIV expression has not been fully clarified. Several studies have shown no consistent change in HIV p24 antigen serum levels or ability to recover virus from peripheral blood mononuclear cells of patients treated with GM-CSF.[74,75,81] However, Kaplan *et al*[68] reported that the median serum HIV p24 antigen level rose to 234% of baseline 1 week after administration of GM-CSF to patients being treated for AIDS-related non-Hodgkin's lymphoma, whereas the median level in control patients fell to 18% of baseline. They cautioned that GM-CSF appears to stimulate HIV replication.

Granulocyte colony-stimulating factor (G-CSF) has also been used in an attempt to overcome the myelosuppression induced by zidovudine. This growth factor has been shown to have no stimulatory effect on HIV replication in macrophages *in vitro*.[82] In a recent clinical trial, erythropoietin and G-CSF were given simultaneously to 20 patients who were divided into cohorts receiving various doses of zidovudine.[83] Six patients were removed from the study after developing transfusion-requiring anemia, but all were maintained with acceptable granulocyte counts (>1,500 cells/mm^3). Toxicities were insignificant, and no significant changes in HIV replication were noted.

In summary, hematopoietic growth factors are likely to play a significant role in the treatment of patients with HIV infection. They have proved useful both in reversing cytopenias due to HIV infection itself and in ameliorating the toxicity of zidovudine and other therapies given for HIV-related conditions. Concerns regarding the stimulatory effect of GM-CSF on HIV replication must be addressed before this agent can be more widely employed.

HEMOSTATIC ABNORMALITIES

Prolonged activated partial thromboplastin times (aPTT) are occasionally detected in patients with HIV infection. A number of studies have been performed to evaluate this finding, and antiphospholipid antibodies have been detected in such patients.

Antiphospholipid antibodies, including lupus anticoagulants and anticardiolipin antibodies, have been detected in a variety of disorders. These IgG or IgM antibodies are directed against phospholipid moieties, and therefore interfere *in vitro* with the action of the thromboplastin used in the aPTT test. Antiphospholipid antibodies are rarely associated with clinical bleeding, but, paradoxically, have been implicated in thrombotic disease.[84]

Although lupus anticoagulants and anticardiolipin antibodies have been detected with high frequency in selected cohorts of HIV-infected patients,[85–88] no associated thrombotic or hemorrhagic tendencies have been noted. One group of investigators[89] has noted that thrombotic skin lesions may occur in HIV-infected patients with antiphospholipid antibodies; the lesions grossly resemble the lesions of Kaposi's sarcoma but have distinct histopathologic features.

SUMMARY

Hematologic abnormalities are among the most frequent complications of HIV infection. A variety of pathogenic mechanisms have been identified that account for these findings. The toxicity of several frequently used treatments is responsible for producing hematologic abnormalities in many patients with HIV infection. Opportunistic infections, neoplasms, and autoimmune phenomena also create hematologic abnormalities in HIV-infected patients. Hematopoietic growth factors may correct some of the abnormalities seen in these patients, and may also permit continued use of essential therapies whose application would otherwise be limited by hematologic toxicities.

ACKNOWLEDGEMENT

Work supported in part by grants from the USPHS. NIH-NIAID, AI-27660; USPHS NIH, M01-RR0865; and State of California, University-wide AIDS Research Program, 90R-CC 86 LA.

REFERENCES

1. Zon L, Groopman J: Hematologic manifestations of the human immunodeficiency virus. Semin Hematol 25:208, 1988
2. Spivak JL, Barnes DC, Fuchs E, Quinn TC: Serum immunoreactive erythropoietin in HIV-infected patients. JAMA 261:3104, 1989
3. Kaslow RA, Phair JP, Friedman HB et al: Infection with the human immunodeficiency virus: Clinical manifestations and their relationship to immune deficiency. Ann Intern Med 107:474, 1987
4. Perkocha LA, Rodgers GM: Hematologic aspects of human immunodeficiency virus infection: Laboratory and clinical considerations. Am J Hematol 29:94, 1988
5. Stella CC, Ganser A, Hoelzer D: Defective *in vitro* growth of the hematopoietic progenitor cells in the acquired immunodeficiency syndrome. J Clin Invest 80:286, 1987
6. Folks TM, Kessler SW, Orenstein JM et al: Infection and replication of HIV-1 in purified progenitor cells of normal human bone marrow. Science 242:919, 1988
7. Richman DD, Fischl MA, Grieco MH et al: The toxicity of azidothymidine (AZT) in the treatment of patients with AIDS and AIDS-related complex. N Engl J Med 317:192, 1987
8. Walker RE, Parker RI, Kovacs JA et al: Anemia and erythropoiesis in patients with the acquired immunodeficiency syndrome and Kaposi sarcoma treated with zidovudine. Ann Intern Med 108:372, 1988
9. Volberding PA, Lagakos SW, Koch MA et al: Zidovudine in asymptomatic human immunodeficiency virus infection. N Engl J Med 322:941, 1990
10. Fischl MA, Richman DD, Hansen N et al: The safety and efficacy of zidovudine (AZT) in the treatment of subjects with mildly symptomatic human immunodeficiency virus type I (HIV) infection. Ann Intern Med 112:727, 1990
11. Fischl M, Galpin JE, Levine JD et al: Recombinant human erythropoietin for patients with AIDS treated with zidovudine. Ann Intern Med 322:1488, 1990
12. Medina I, Mills J, Leoung G et al: Oral therapy for *Pneumocystis carinii* pneumonia in the acquired immune deficiency syndrome. N Engl J Med 323:776, 1990
13. Hawkins CC, Gold JWM, Whimbey E et al: *Mycobacterium avium* complex infections in patients with the acquired immunodeficiency syndrome. Ann Intern Med 105:184, 1986
14. Bogner JR, Gathof B, Heinrich A et al: Erythrocyte antibodies in AIDS are associated with mycobacteriosis and hypergammaglobulinemia. Klin Wochenschr 68:1050, 1990
15. Jacobson MA, Peiperl L, Volberding PA et al: Red blood cell transfusion therapy for anemia in patients with AIDS and ARC: Incidence, associated factors, and outcome. Transfusion 30:133, 1990
16. Chiu J, Nussbaum J, Bozzette S et al: Treatment of disseminated *Mycobacterium avium* (MAI) infection in AIDS with amikacin, ethambutol, rifampin, and ciprofloxacin. Ann Intern Med 113:358, 1990
17. Hoy J, Mijch A, Sandland M et al: Quadruple-drug therapy for *Mycobacterium avium-intracellulare* bacteremia in AIDS patients. J Infect Dis 161:801, 1990
18. Mitchell SA, Welch JM, Weston-Smith S et al: Parvovirus infection and anaemia in a patient with AIDS: Case report. Genitourin Med 66:95, 1990
19. Frickhofen N, Abkowitz JL, Safford M et al: Persistent B19 parvovirus infection in patients infected with human immunodeficiency virus type 1 (HIV-1): A treatable cause of anemia in AIDS. Ann Intern Med 113:926, 1990
20. Northfelt DW, Mayer A, Kaplan LD et al: The usefulness of diagnostic bone marrow examination in patients with human immunodeficiency virus (HIV) infection. J AIDS 4:659, 1991
21. McGinniss M, Macher A, Rook A et al: Red cell autoantibodies in patients with acquired immunodeficiency syndrome. Transfusion 26:405, 1986
22. Toy PTCY, Reid ME, Burns M: Positive direct antiglobulin test associated with hyperglobulinemia in acquired immunodeficiency syndrome. Am J Hematol 19:145, 1985
23. Jost J, Tauber MG, Luthy R, Siegenthaler W: HIV-assoziierte Thrombozytopenie. Schweiz Med Wochenschr 118:206, 1988
24. Murphy MF, Metcalfe P, Waters AH et al: Incidence and mechanism of neutropenia and thrombocytopenia in pa-

tients with human immunodeficiency virus infection. Br J Haematol 66:337, 1987

25. Morris L, Distenfeld A, Amorosi E, Karpatkin S: Autoimmune thrombocytopenic purpura in homosexual men. Ann Intern Med 96:714, 1982

26. Ratner L: Human immunodeficiency virus-associated autoimmune thrombocytopenic purpura: A review. Am J Med 86:194, 1989

27. Abrams DI: The pre-AIDS syndromes: Asymptomatic carriers, thrombocytopenic purpura, persistent generalized lymphadenopathy, and AIDS-related complex. In Sande MA, Volberding PA (eds): The Medical Management of AIDS, p 91. Philadelphia, WB Saunders, 1988

28. Centers for Disease Control: Revision of the CDC surveillance case definition for acquired immunodeficiency syndrome. MMWR 36:3S, 1987

29. Walsh CM, Nardi MA, Karpatkin S: On the mechanism of thrombocytopenic purpura in sexually active homosexual men. Ann Intern Med 311:635, 1984

30. Karpatkin S, Nardi M, Lennette ET et al: Anti-human immunodeficiency virus type 1 antibody complexes on platelets of seropositive thrombocytopenic homosexuals and narcotic addicts. Proc Natl Acad Sci USA 85:9763, 1988

31. Karpatkin S, Nardi M: Cross-reactive anti-idiotype antibody vs anti-HIVgp120 in HIV-1-thrombocytopenia: Correlation with thrombocytopenia (abstr). Blood 74(suppl 1):128a, 1989

32. Stricker RB, Abrams DI, Corash L, Shuman MA: Target platelet antigen in homosexual men with immune thrombocytopenia. N Engl J Med 313:1375, 1985

33. Ballem P, Belzberg A, Chambers H, Spruston B: Platelet production in HIV infection: Evidence for a compensated thrombolytic state enhanced by AZT (abstr; Presented at the V International Conference on AIDS, Montreal, 1989 poster T.B.P. 270:332).

34. Zucker-Franklin D, Cao Y: Megakaryocytes of human immunodeficiency virus-infected individuals express viral RNA. Proc Natl Acad Sci USA 86:5595, 1989

35. Walsh C, Krigel R, Lennette E, Karpatkin S: Thrombocytopenia in homosexual patients: Prognosis, response to therapy, and prevalence of antibody to the retrovirus associated with the acquired immunodeficiency syndrome. Ann Intern Med 103:542, 1985

36. Oksenhendler E, Bierling P, Farcet J-P et al: Response to therapy in 37 patients with HIV-related thrombocytopenic purpura. Br J Haematol 66:491, 1987

37. Abrams DI, Kiprov DD, Goedert JJ et al: Antibodies to human T-lymphotrophic virus type III and development of the acquired immunodeficiency syndrome in homosexual men presenting with immune thrombocytopenia. Ann Intern Med 104:47, 1986

38. Schneider PA, Abrams DI, Rayner AA, Hohn DC: Immunodeficiency-associated thrombocytopenic purpura (IDTP): Response to splenectomy. Arch Surg 122:1175, 1987

39. Ravikumar TS, Allen JD, Bothe A, Steele G: Splenectomy: The treatment of choice for human immunodeficiency virus-related immune thrombocytopenia? Arch Surg 124:625, 1989

40. Ferguson CM: Splenectomy for immune thrombocytopenia related to human immunodeficiency virus. Surg Gynecol Obstet 167:300, 1988

41. Barbui T, Cortelazzo S, Minetti B et al: Does splenectomy enhance risk of AIDS in HIV positive patients with chronic thrombocytopenia? Lancet 2:342, 1987

42. Swiss Group for Clinical Studies on the Acquired Immunodeficiency Syndrome: Zidovudine for the treatment of thrombocytopenia associated with human immunodeficiency virus: A prospective study. Ann Intern Med 109:718, 1988

43. Northfelt DW, Kaplan LD, Abrams DI: Continuous, low-dose therapy with interferon-α for human immunodeficiency virus (HIV)-related immune thrombocytopenic purpura. Am J Hematol, in press

44. Ellis ME, Neal KR, Leen CLS: Alpha-2a recombinant interferon in HIV associated thrombocytopenia. Br J Med 295:1519, 1987

45. Lever AML, Brook MG, Yap I, Thomas HC: Treatment of thrombocytopenia with alpha interferon. Br J Med 295:1519, 1987

46. Luzzati R, DiPerri G, Malena M et al: Alpha-interferon in treatment of severe HIV-related thrombocytopenia (TP) (abstr; poster F.B.512). Presented at the VI International Conference on AIDS, San Francisco, 1990

47. Ragni MV, Bontempo FA, Myers DJ et al: Hemorrhagic sequelae of immune thrombocytopenic purpura in human immunodeficiency virus-infected hemophiliacs. Blood 75:1267, 1990

48. Shepard KV, Bukowski RM: The treatment of thrombotic thrombocytopenic purpura with exchange transfusions, plasma infusions, and plasma exchange. Semin Hematol 24:178, 1987

49. Jokela J, Flynn T, Henry K: Thrombotic thrombocytopenic purpura in a human immunodeficiency virus-seropositive homosexual man. Am J Hematol 23:341, 1987

50. Meisenberg BR, Robinson WL, Mosley CA et al: Thrombotic thrombocytopenic purpura in human immunodeficiency virus (HIV)-seropositive males. Am J Hematol 27:212, 1988

51. Leaf AN, Laubenstein LJ, Raphael B et al. Thrombotic thrombocytopenic purpura associated with human immunodeficiency virus type 1 (HIV-1) infection. Ann Intern Med 109:194, 1988

52. Nair JM, Bellevue R, Bertoni M, Dosik H: Thrombotic thrombocytopenic purpura in patients with the acquired immunodeficiency syndrome (AIDS)-related complex. Ann Intern Med 109:209, 1988

53. Botti AC, Hyde P, DiPillo F: Thrombotic thrombocytopenic purpura in a patient who subsequently developed the acquired immunodeficiency syndrome (AIDS). Ann Intern Med 109:242, 1988

54. Platanias LC, Paiusco D, Bernstein S, Murali MR: Thrombotic thrombocytopenic purpura as the first manifestation of human immunodeficiency virus infection. Am J Med 87:699, 1989

55. Besalduch J, Altes J, Morey M, Villalonga C: Thrombotic thrombocytopenic purpura and infection by the human immunodeficiency virus. Med Clin (Barc) 92:795, 1989

56. Van der Lelie J, Lange JMA, Voss JJE et al: Autoimmunity against blood cells in human immunodeficiency virus infection. Br J Haematol 67:109, 1987

57. Pinching AJ, Helbert M, Peddle B et al: Clinical experience with zidovudine for patients with acquired immune deficiency syndrome and acquired immune deficiency syndrome-related complex. J Infect 18:33, 1989

58. Shaunak S, Bartlett JA: Zidovudine-induced neutropenia: Are we too cautious? Lancet 1:91, 1989

59. Jacobson MA, O'Donnell JJ, Porteous D et al: Retinal and gastrointestinal disease due to cytomegalovirus in patients with acquired immune deficiency syndrome: Prevalence,

natural history, and response to ganciclovir therapy. Q J Med 254:473, 1988

60. Jacobson MA: Ganciclovir therapy for opportunistic cytomegalovirus disease in AIDS. In Volberding P, Jacobson MA (eds): AIDS Clinical Review 1990, chap 9. New York, Marcel Dekker, 1990

61. Gordin FM, Simon GL, Wofsy CB, Mills J: Adverse reactions to trimethoprim-sulfamethoxazole in patients with the acquired immunodeficiency syndrome. Ann Intern Med 100:495, 1984

62. Wharton JM, Coleman DL, Wofsy CB et al: Trimethoprim-sulfamethoxazole or pentamidine for *Pneumocystis carinii* pneumonia in the acquired immunodeficiency syndrome. Ann Intern Med 105:37, 1986

63. Sattler FM, Cowan R, Nielsen DM, Ruskin J: Trimethoprim-sulfamethoxazole compared with pentamidine for treatment of *Pneumocystis carinii* pneumonia in the acquired immunodeficiency syndrome. Ann Intern Med 109:280, 1988

64. Rios A, Mansell PWA, Newell GR et al: Treatment of acquired immunodeficiency syndrome-related Kaposi's sarcoma with lymphoblastoid interferon. J Clin Oncol 3:506, 1985

65. Real FX, Oettgen HF, Krown SE: Kaposi's sarcoma and the acquired immunodeficiency syndrome: Treatment with high and low doses of recombinant leukocyte A interferon. J Clin Oncol 4:544, 1986

66. Kovacs JA, Deyton L, Davey R et al: Combined zidovudine and interferon-α in patients with Kaposi's sarcoma and the acquired immunodeficiency syndrome (AIDS). Ann Intern Med 111:280, 1989

67. Gill PS, Rarick MU, Espina B et al: Advanced acquired immune deficiency syndrome-related Kaposi's sarcoma: Results of pilot studies using combination chemotherapy. Cancer 65:1074, 1990

68. Kaplan LD, Kahn JO, Crowe S et al: Clinical and virologic effects of recombinant human granulocyte-macrophage colony-stimulating factor (rGM-CSF) in patients receiving chemotherapy for HIV-associated non-Hodgkin's lymphoma: Results of a randomized trial. J Clin Oncol 9:929, 1991

69. Northfelt D, Hambleton J, Aragon T et al: Outcome of febrile neutropenia in patients with AIDS-related non-Hodgkin's lymphoma (abstr). Blood 76(suppl 1):491a, 1990

70. Schimpff SC: Empiric antibiotic therapy for granulocytopenic cancer patients. Am J Med 80(suppl 5C):13, 1986

71. Ellis M, Gupta S, Galant S et al: Impaired neutrophil function in patients with AIDS or AIDS-related complex: A comprehensive evaluation. J Infect Dis 158:1268, 1988

72. Valone FH, Payan DG, Abrams DI, Goetzl EJ: Defective polymorphonuclear leukocyte chemotaxis in homosexual men with persistent lymph node syndrome. J Infect Dis 150:267, 1984

73. Murphy P, Lane HC, Fauci AS et al: Impairment of neutrophil bactericidal capacity in patients with AIDS. J Infect Dis 158:627, 1988

74. Groopman JE, Mitsuyasu RT, DeLeo MJ et al: Effect of recombinant human granulocyte-macrophage colony-stimulating factor on myelopoiesis in the acquired immunodeficiency syndrome. N Engl J Med 317:593, 1987

75. Baldwin CG, Gasson JC, Quan SG et al: GM-CSF enhances neutrophil function in AIDS patients. Proc Natl Acad Sci USA 85:2763, 1988

76. Mitsuyasu R, Levine J, Miles SA et al: Effects of long-term subcutaneous (SC) administration of recombinant granulocyte-macrophage colony-stimulating factor (GM-CSF) in patients with HIV-related leukopenia (abstr). Blood 72(suppl 1):357, 1988

77. Walsh C, Wernz J, Laubenstein L et al: Phase 1 study of m-BACOD and GM-CSF in AIDS-associated non-Hodgkin's lymphoma (NHL): Preliminary results (abstr). Blood 74(suppl 1):126a, 1989

78. Levine JD, Allan JD, Tessitore JH et al: Granulocyte-macrophage colony-stimulating factor ameliorates the neutropenia induced by azidothymidine in AIDS/ARC patients (abstr). Proc Am Soc Clin Oncol 8:1, 1989

79. Grossberg HS, Bonnem EM, Buhles WC: GM-CSF with ganciclovir for the treatment of CMV retinitis in AIDS. N Engl J Med 320:1560, 1989

80. Scadden D, Bering H, Levine J et al: Combined AZT/interferon-alpha/GM-CSF for AIDS-associated Kaposi's sarcoma (KS) (abstr). Blood 74(suppl 1):127a, 1989

81. Krown SE, O'Boyle K, Gold JWM et al: Recombinant human granulocyte-macrophage colony-stimulating factor: A phase 1 trial in neutropenic AIDS patients (abstr W.B.P.309). Presented at the Fifth International Conference on AIDS, Montreal, 1989

82. Koyanagi Y, O'Brien WA, Zhao JQ et al: Cytokines alter production of HIV-1 from primary mononuclear phagocytes. Science 241:1673, 1988

83. Miles S, Mitsuyasu R, Fink N et al: Recombinant G-CSF and recombinant erythropoietin may abrogate the neutropenia and anemia of AIDS and may allow resumption of AZT (abstr M.C.P.52). Presented at the Fifth International Conference on AIDS, Montreal, 1989

84. Love PE, Santoro SA: Antiphospholipid antibodies: Anticardiolipin and the lupus anticoagulant in systemic lupus erythematosus (SLE) and in non-SLE disorders. Ann Intern Med 112:682, 1990

85. Bloom EJ, Abrams DI, Rodgers GM: Lupus anticoagulant in the acquired immunodeficiency syndrome. JAMA 256:491, 1986

86. Cohen AJ, Philips TM, Kessler CM: Circulating coagulation inhibitors in the acquired immunodeficiency syndrome. Ann Intern Med 104:175, 1986

87. Stimmler MM, Quismorio FP, McGehee WG et al: Anticardiolipin antibodies in the acquired immunodeficiency syndrome. Arch Intern Med 149:1833, 1989

88. Cohen H, Mackie IJ, Anagnostopoulos N et al: Lupus anticoagulant, anticardiolipin antibodies, and human immunodeficiency virus in haemophilia. J Clin Pathol 42:629, 1989

89. Smith KJ, Skelton HG, James WD et al: Cutaneous histopathologic findings in "antiphospholipid syndrome." Correlation with disease, including human immunodeficiency virus disease. Arch Dermatol 126:1176, 1990

18

Psychiatric and Psychosocial Aspects of HIV Infection

Jimmie C. Holland   *Paul Jacobsen*   *William Breitbart*

The diagnosis of acquired immunodeficiency syndrome (AIDS) carries with it the same psychological burden as that of many other life-threatening diseases.[1] An AIDS diagnosis, however, has far greater social consequences related to discrimination and stigmatization. Added to these significant liabilities is that the individual may develop central nervous system (CNS) complications that impair mental acuity and the ability to cope with the stresses. As a result, the frequency of psychiatric and neuropsychiatric disorders is high. This chapter outlines the factors that contribute to psychological distress and adjustment and describes the common psychiatric and neuropsychiatric disorders and their management. Figure 18–1 shows the interactive nature of psychosocial, psychiatric, and neurologic factors that complicate the clinical picture of human immunodeficiency virus (HIV) infection.

FACTORS IN ADAPTATION TO AIDS

How an individual adapts psychologically to illness depends on three factors: (1) *society-derived* attitudes and beliefs about the disease and those who develop it, (2) *patient-derived* factors such as coping skills and prior emotional stability, and the social supports available, and (3) *illness-derived* factors, which are the actual manifestations of disease, clinical course, and symptoms which the patient must confront and tolerate.[2] AIDS uniquely, as a disease, causes a profound burden in this triad, requiring a high level of resiliency to adapt to the disease and its consequences. Table 18–1 outlines the issues in each area as they apply to HIV and AIDS.

A major factor that complicates adjustment to AIDS is sociocultural: the meaning that society attaches to the disease and to the individuals who have it. HIV is the most feared disease in our society. The fact that it is transmitted by exchange of body fluids, most often by sexual transmission and intravenous (IV) drug use, adds to the stigma. The diagnosis of AIDS also commonly identifies the individual in two of the most stigmatized minorities in the United States—gay men and IV drug users. These issues may cause the individual to experience discrimination in housing, job, and health care. Anger, suspiciousness, and despair become understandable. Society has taken strong steps during this first decade of the AIDS epidemic to protect the rights and confidentiality of HIV-infected individuals.

The second factor influencing adaptation to AIDS is what the patient brings to the illness: personality, coping skills, prior psychological problems antedating illness, and the availability of individuals to support the patient during illness.

Personality, ability to cope with stress, and level of emotional maturity influence adaptation. The coping skills the person brings to deal with illness are critically important, particularly as the person faces the diagnosis and progressive illness.[3] Prior psychiatric disorders predict poorer adjustment; IV drug users frequently present serious behavioral problems such as noncompliance with treatment and psychological problems that complicate their care, such as drug-seeking actions.

Finally, the HIV-infected person needs social supports that are known to substantially buffer the stresses of serious illness.[4] Knowledge of positive HIV status or an AIDS diagnosis may lead family and friends to withdraw. For gay men, the diagnosis of AIDS may lead to the disclosure of illness and a life-style previously unknown to the family of origin. Individuals who have abused drugs frequently have alienated their family and

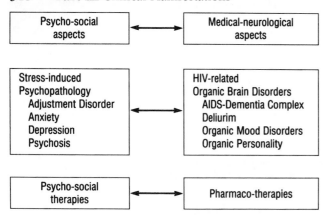

Figure 18–1. Complex nature of neuropsychiatric disturbances in HIV-spectrum diseases.

friends. Their difficulty in compliance with treatment does not engender empathy from health care providers, which presents additional problems.

The individual who develops HIV frequently has also already lost one or more friends to AIDS, resulting in cumulative bereavement. Chronic AIDS-related bereavement was studied in the New York City gay community.[5] Of 624 men studied, each could name an average of 6.2 men they knew who had died of AIDS. Among those who had suffered bereavement in the preceding 3 years, 50% were antibody positive and 27% had symptoms of AIDS. The bereaved had elevated scores on traumatic stress response, demoralization, sleep disturbance, disillusionment, and discontinuity.

The third factor in psychological adjustment is what

Table 18–1. Primary Factors Affecting Psychological Adjustment to AIDS

Societally derived
  Meaning society attaches to AIDS
    Stigma of contagious disease
    Assumption of stigmatized minority group status
  Discrimination in housing, job, health care
Patient factors
  Intrapersonal
    Personality/psychiatric history
    Coping skills to deal with life-threatening illness
  Interpersonal
    Availability of social support
    Withdrawal of others
    Death of friends/family with AIDS; cumulative
      bereavement
Illness-related factors
  Nature of HIV manifestations, complications and clinical
    course
  Presence of CNS complications
  Presence of pain
  Degree of debilitation; changes in life-style
  Management by health care staff

the person must react to: the nature of the HIV manifestations, complications, and clinical course. It is here that the societal meaning attached to HIV takes on personal meaning (Table 18–2). Uncertainty becomes the central issue of daily life as each body sensation is analyzed for evidence of progression or new infection. Concerns about losing mental acuity related to CNS complications is also a pervasive fear. Pain is a common symptom that adds to the stress. The changes in physical ability, appearance, and dependence on others are additional losses, coming with inability to work and to maintain a prior life-style.

These combined stresses may result in symptoms of demoralization, anxiety, depression, and hopelessness that are collectively called *anticipatory grieving* for the losses of health and future. Preoccupation with mortality and a sense of helplessness and vulnerability are typical. Symptoms of anxiety and depression vary within a spectrum of intensity, ranging from normal expected reactions to severe psychiatric symptoms.

The range of stressors experienced by all HIV-infected individuals suggests the need for early inclusion of psychosocial assessment. Particular attention should be given to identifying social, psychological, and financial support, as well as counseling about community resources and self-help organizations. Early psychiatric evaluation is useful to provide ongoing monitoring for signs of cognitive impairment and significant psychiatric symptoms. The psychosocial aspect often is a critical variable in the ability to provide adequate care.

An early discussion should assess patients' understanding of HIV infection and provide accurate information about the disease and outcome. Assessment of ability to work, maintain independent living, and manage personal affairs requires ongoing monitoring. Writing a will and identifying a health care proxy should also be discussed. These issues must be addressed because conflicts often arise between the family of origin and the significant other at a time when the patient no longer has capacity to make decisions.

PSYCHIATRIC DISORDERS

Prevalence

Given the co-occurring stressors outlined above, how many HIV-infected patients develop psychiatric disorders? When? Who is at greatest risk? How can psychiatric symptoms be distinguished from symptoms of HIV infection (*e.g.,* depression *vs.* HIV-related fatigue, and apathy *vs.* early dementia)?

In terms of prevalence, Tross and Hirsch found that 76% of patients with AIDS-related complex (ARC) met criteria for a psychiatric disorder; about half the patients with AIDS and about one fourth of asymptomatic gay men had a diagnosable psychiatric disorder.[6] Adjustment disorder with depressed and/or anxious features accounted for two thirds of the diagnoses. Table 18–3 lists the common psychiatric disorders. These data support

Table 18–2. Meanings Attached to AIDS Diagnosis

Fatal disease; no cure
Progressive debilitation
Progressive dependency
Possible loss of mental acuity
Loss of social and work role
Withdrawal of friends
Possible social discrimination
Change in life-style to protect others
Expectation of similar clinical course leading to death, as
   seen in friends

the view that individuals who fear progression to frank AIDS experience greater distress than those who already have an AIDS diagnosis. These data are similar to observations in cancer patients: some patients successfully treated and without sign of disease are unable to function because of their fear of recurrence.[2] When the recurrence occurs, distress diminishes; the feared event *has* happened.

With regard to anxiety disorders, Atkinson and colleagues found that 36% of AIDS patients, 39% of ARC patients, and 18% of asymptomatic HIV-seropositive patients had suffered from anxiety disorders in the 6 months preceding their evaluation; generalized anxiety disorder was the most common prior and current diagnosis.[7] Most prevalence data are based on studies of homosexual men. Less is known about the prevalence of psychiatric disorders in HIV-infected IV drug users, but it is likely to be even higher because IV drug users (including those in treatment) have a higher rate of psychiatric disorder than the general population.[7]

At least 50% of HIV-infected patients will experience a psychiatric disorder during the course of their illness. Most will have a mixture of reactive anxiety and depressive symptoms (adjustment disorder) common to other life-threatening and serious illnesses.[8] About

Table 18–3. Common Psychiatric Disorders in Patients with HIV Infections

       Adjustment disorders
         With anxious and depressed mood
       Anxiety disorders
         Panic disorder
         Generalized anxiety disorder
       Major depression
       Organic mental disorders
         Dementia (AIDS dementia complex)
         Delirium
         Organic mood disorders
         Organic personality disorder
         Organic hallucinosis
         Organic delusional disorder
       Substance abuse disorders
         Alcohol
         IV drug abuse

one fourth will develop symptoms of major depression. Rapkin and colleagues found that among a group of well-educated HIV-positive men, most were able to preserve a sense of hope and faith in the future despite their risk of AIDS.[9] This fact seemed to account for the surprisingly low level of syndromal depressive disorder and depressive symptoms.

A study of hemophiliacs with HIV infection helped to establish who is at greater risk of developing a psychiatric disorder.[10] Similar to cancer patients, the most distressed were those with a personal or family psychiatric history, lower education, low social support, and experience of a concurrent loss.

The boundary between normal and pathologic levels of psychological distress and psychiatric symptoms as found in the prevalence studies described above is often blurred, especially in HIV infection. Emotional distress and psychiatric symptoms are best understood from the perspective of a continuum that extends from normal distress to symptoms of a psychiatric disorder, depending on the severity and constellation of symptoms. In addition, attention to the intensity, duration, and nature of onset of symptoms helps to distinguish normal from abnormal types of distress.

Response to Diagnosis

For many individuals, the diagnosis of HIV positivity occurs in the context of being in a risk group and already having significant fears about developing HIV infection. Preoccupation with minor physical symptoms and situational anxiety and depression are common. Acute concern about illness may be precipitated by news of death of a friend or by other AIDS-related information.[11] Reassurance by a physical examination or HIV testing with counseling is sufficient to return most HIV-negative but high-risk individuals to their usual levels of coping and well-being.

When patients are first notified of HIV infection (following HIV antibody testing) or experience early symptoms of AIDS, they show a characteristic emotional response: a period of shock and disbelief, then a period of turmoil in which anxiety, depressive symptoms, irritability, disruption of appetite and sleep, and inability to concentrate and work are common. Intrusive thoughts about the diagnosis and its ominous implications for the future occur often.[12]

These symptoms usually resolve gradually over a 7- to 10-day period, particularly if the patient receives support from family and friends and from a supportive physician who outlines a treatment plan that offers hope.[13] Unless symptoms of emotional distress interfere with functioning or are prolonged or intolerable, professional intervention usually is not required beyond that provided by the empathic physician, nurse, social worker, or clergy for this expected emotional distress which accompanies the diagnosis of any serious life-threatening disease.

Anxiety Disorders

By far the most common emotion in individuals with HIV infection is uncertainty about the future and fears of illness. At some point, depending on intensity, duration, and time of onset, these normal concerns become a diagnosable anxiety disorder requiring evaluation and treatment. The degree of distress (*e.g.,* disruption of usual activities) and the number of signs and symptoms of anxiety that are present are identified (Table 18–4). The persistence of normal transient anxiety for weeks to months is reason for intervention. The sudden onset of anxiety symptoms in the HIV-infected patient, in the absence of a stressful event or of a preexisting history of psychiatric disorder, may be related to a change in medical status: metabolic imbalance, side-effects of medications (particularly zidovudine, corticosteroids, interferon), or withdrawal from alcohol, sedative-hypnotics, or narcotics. In the drug user, withdrawal is always a major consideration.[14]

Symptoms of moderate anxiety that interfere with social and occupational functioning suggest the common form of reactive anxiety or adjustment disorder. This form of anxiety typically occurs during a crisis or transitional point in the illness, such as notification of positive anti-HIV antibody test results, the diagnosis of AIDS, or the development of a complication later in the course of disease that signifies progression. An adjustment disorder may remit without treatment, as the crisis passes, but with HIV infection, severe and persistent symptoms of anxiety usually merit treatment.

Anxiety of greater intensity and duration suggests a generalized anxiety disorder, a panic disorder, or phobia. A careful history will usually reveal that the anxiety symptoms antedated the diagnosis of HIV infection and were exacerbated by illness. Severe anxiety can seriously compromise medical treatment; it may be necessary to control the anxiety symptoms before treatment can be undertaken (*e.g.,* a needle phobia or claustrophobia precluding treatment).

Supportive psychotherapy and counseling are central to helping patients cope with distress and anxiety. This means giving patients accurate information in a reassuring manner about HIV-related disease and treatment, and rehearsing what may occur during a feared anticipated procedure or event. Counseling should be built into medical management from the beginning. Cognitive-behavioral interventions that engage the patient in techniques that are self-applied are useful in reducing the anxiety associated with notification of anti-HIV antibody test results. In one recent study, stress prevention training, which combines education about HIV infection, risk reduction, and health-promoting behaviors with training in techniques for managing challenging situations (assertiveness) and preventing disruptive emotional arousal (relaxation training), was found superior to standard HIV seropositivity counseling for reducing distress following notification of anti-HIV antibody test results.[15] Relaxation training is also helpful in allowing phobic patients to tolerate anxiety-inducing diagnostic and treatment procedures.[16]

Pharmacologic interventions for anxiety are necessary when rapid control is desired, such as during a panic attack or an acute anxiety attack prior to a scheduled treatment procedure. Severe chronic anxiety also requires medication, especially when CNS involvement precludes other psychological interventions. Drugs used for HIV-infected patients with anxiety are benzodiazepines, azapirones, neuroleptics, antihistamines, β blockers, and antidepressants. Neuroleptics (*e.g.,* chlorpromazine, haloperidol) are useful in extreme agitation or anxiety accompanying delirium, but the risk of extrapyramidal symptoms is greater in HIV-seropositive patients.[17] Antihistamines (*e.g.,* hydroxyzine) are used when there is concern for respiratory function. β blockers (*e.g.,* propranolol) are useful in the treatment of mild situational anxiety in which peripheral autonomic symptoms (sweating, tachycardia) are prominent, though hypotension is a greater risk.[14] Antidepressants (*e.g.,* imipramine) are primarily used with anxious patients in the treatment of panic and severe phobic states.

Table 18–4. Signs and Symptoms of Anxiety

Appearance and behavior
  Flushed face
  Tense, worried expression
  Motor restlessness
  Nail biting
  Chain smoking
  Sweaty palms
  Diaphoresis
  Tremulousness
Subjective complaints
  Excessive monitoring of body functions
  Preoccupation with minor physical symptoms
  Little interest in usual activities
  Irritability
  Dizziness; headaches
  Weakness; exhaustion
  Tingling sensation in extremities
  Muscle tension, achiness, soreness
Cardiovascular
  Palpitations
  Sinus tachycardia
  Elevated systolic blood pressure
  Precordial pain
Respiratory
  Dyspnea; feeling of suffocation
  Hyperventilation
Gastrointestinal
  Anorexia; nausea
  Diarrhea
  Heartburn
  Air swallowing
Gynecologic/genitourinary
  Reduced sexual arousal
  Urinary urgency and frequency
  Dysurea
  Menstrual changes or pain

Benzodiazepines are the most commonly used medication in the treatment of anxiety in HIV-infected patients. All are effective, and the choice of a specific agent depends on the half-life of the drug. In general, anxiolytics with short half-lives (oxazepam, lorazepam) or intermediate half-lives (alprazolam) are preferable to those with long half-lives (diazepam, chlordiazepoxide) because steady-state plasma concentrations are reached rapidly and metabolites are eliminated rapidly. Lorazepam in doses of 0.5 to 1.0 mg three or four times a day controls anxiety. Lorazepam can be given IV if needed. It also controls the akathesias associated with neuroleptics given for antiemesis, which often present as anxiety. Alprazolam is useful in the treatment of adjustment disorders with single or mixed emotional features, "minor" depression, mixed features of reactions to stress and distress, and panic disorder. The dosage begins with 0.5 mg t.i.d. to 1.0 mg q.i.d. for severe symptoms. Longer-acting anxiolytics such as chlordiazepoxide are used in drug and alcohol withdrawal states. However, all should be given within a time-limited mode because of the risk of dependence. Patients with early or unrecognized dementia will experience greater sedation and confusion. Bedtime sedation (*e.g.,* triazolam, temazepam) may be helpful for anxiety-related insomnia.

Buspirone has far fewer sedating effects than the benzodiazepines and does not produce significant cognitive or psychomotor impairment.[18] The azaspirones have little or no potential for abuse, are not associated with physical or psychological dependence, and do not potentiate the CNS-depressant effects of alcohol or sedative-hypnotic drugs. Two recent studies demonstrated that buspirone is a safe and effective agent for the treatment of anxiety in HIV-infected individuals (P. Jacobsen, pers. commun.).[19] Both reports found that buspirone was well tolerated by HIV-infected patients taking zidovudine, and reduced anxiety. The major disadvantage of buspirone is the delay in therapeutic effect until the second week of therapy, making it a good choice for chronic anxiety. Short-acting benzodiazepines remain the treatment of choice for acute situational anxiety.

Depressive Disorders

On the continuum of sadness to depression, normal sadness accompanies awareness of life-threatening illness. More significant distress appears as demoralization: a sense of helplessness and dysphoria. Situational depression related to illness, with or without anxiety (adjustment disorder), is the most common depressive diagnosis in HIV patients. More severe symptoms indicate a diagnosis of major depression: depressed mood, dysphoria, low self-esteem, hopelessness, worthlessness, guilt, helplessness, and suicidal ideation. The physical signs relied on to diagnose depression in healthy individuals, such as fatigue, anorexia, insomnia, weakness, and diminished libido, are likely related to

HIV infection and should not be used to diagnose depression.

Another major diagnostic issue in depression in HIV is the fact that apathy, withdrawal, mental slowing, and avoidance of complex tasks are the early symptoms of cognitive impairment from the AIDS dementia complex. It may be difficult to differentiate the etiology of these symptoms from depression or AIDS dementia complex. Perry *et al* suggest that careful history and clinical examination can differentiate these two entities.[13] A correlation between neuropsychological impairment and depression has not been found.

Depression and HIV-related organic mood disorders with depressive symptoms can be difficult to differentiate and indeed can occur together, because the prevalence of both is high in HIV-infected patients.[13] Organic mood disorders often manifest with depressive symptoms and may be related to delirium associated with metabolic disturbance, to fever, or to the subcortical dementing process.

The management of depression entails (1) supportive psychotherapy; (2) the control of distressing physical symptoms, especially pain, with analgesics; (3) adjunctive measures such as behavioral interventions; and (4) psychopharmacologic measures. Although the tricyclic antidepressants are the most widely used, fluoxetine, psychostimulants, and alprazolam are also of value. Tricyclic antidepressants, especially imipramine or amitriptyline, are effective for bedtime sedation and pain control as well. A tricyclic with a more stimulatory side-effect profile, such as desipramine, is useful for management of depressive symptoms characterized by apathy and withdrawal. When sedating effects are desirable, amitriptyline, doxepine, or imipramine is chosen. As in cancer patients, the initial dosage should be low. HIV-seropositive patients often respond to doses of 10 to 25 mg at bedtime. The dosage should be increased by 10 to 20 mg over 2- to 3-day periods. Psychostimulants are useful in withdrawn, apathetic states: dextroamphetamine, 2.5 mg, or methylphenidate, 2.5 mg, in the morning. Pemoline, used similarly, is a non-controlled substance that, in doses of 18.75 mg to 37.5 mg, is effective for these symptoms. These psychostimulants are effective in the treatment of depression occurring with AIDS dementia complex. Fluoxetine, 20 mg given in the morning, is useful for the depressive symptoms of withdrawal and apathy. It may be increased to 20 mg b.i.d., given in the morning and at noon. Alprazolam is useful for control of combined anxiety and depressive symptoms (0.5 mg b.i.d. or t.i.d.). Lithium carbonate should be continued in patients in whom manic depressive disorder is present, although the risk of confusion may be enhanced in patients receiving zidovudine.[14] Control of mania secondary to ziduvodine treatment may be attempted with lithium.[20]

In a study of drug efficacy, Hintz and colleagues (1990) found that imipramine and fluoxetine had the most favorable efficacy and least side-effects ratings.[21] HIV-seropositive patients responded better than those with ARC or AIDS.

Depression and Suicide

As with other life-threatening illnesses such as cancer, AIDS is associated with a heightened frequency of suicidal ideation, suicide attempts, and suicides.[22,23] However, in suicidal patients with AIDS, a history of suicide attempts antedating medical illness is common. A study of men with AIDS in New York City found a risk of suicide 36 times greater than for men without AIDS, and 66 times greater than the risk for the general population. By comparison, the risk of suicide in cancer patients is twice the average in the general population.[23]

Depression is the most important factor in AIDS-related suicide, as it is in suicide in general.[13,16,22] Hopelessness is the usual link between the two. Guilt about past behavior, multiple bereavements, absent or inadequate social supports, isolation from family and friends, and hopelessness are also common factors.[24] Substance abuse and preexisting psychiatric disorders heighten the risk of suicide, which is already 10 to 20 times higher than in the general population. In a psychiatric clinic for HIV-seropositive IV drug users and their sexual partners, extremely high rates of suicidal thoughts and attempts were found: 80% of asymptomatic seropositive patients and patients with ARC had a history of suicidal thoughts, and half had made suicide attempts.[25] Atkinson and colleagues found suicidal thoughts or attempts to be elevated among both HIV-positive and HIV-negative homosexual men.[26]

Suicidal ideation is uncommon in the HIV testing setting when intensive pretest and posttest counseling is offered.[12] Suicidal ideation occurred equally among those who were seropositive or seronegative and was related to level of mood disturbance rather than to HIV antibody status *per se.* Suicidal ideation stayed at pretest levels (27.1%) 1 week after notification of seropositivity but fell to 16% 2 months later, comparable to the rate in the seronegative group.[14]

Methods of suicide or attempted suicide in AIDS are similar to those used by cancer patients: drug overdose, hanging, and jumping. Disease-related factors, especially pain and debilitating physical symptoms, appear to play a role in suicide, although this has not been studied.

Early and sustained counseling of high-risk individuals can avert suicide. Allowing the patient to discuss suicidal thoughts often decreases the risk of suicide. Patients often reconsider the idea of suicide when the physician acknowledges the legitimacy of that option and the patient's need to retain a sense of control over life and death. Evaluation requires search for the meaning of suicidal thoughts and for seriousness of the intent. The quality of internal (cognitive) and external (family, support system) controls is important. A discussion should include the patient, lover, spouse, or family, as there is often pressure on family members and lovers to assist in plans for suicide.

Identification and treatment of organic mental disorders and depression and control of pain are essential.

Analgesics, neuroleptics, and antidepressant drugs should be used to treat pain, agitation, delirium, psychosis, and depression. Initiation of a crisis intervention–oriented psychotherapeutic approach, mobilizing the patient's support system, is important. Consultants familiar with substance abuse and its management should be called in when relevant. Pastoral counseling, hospices, and voluntary support services for AIDS patients all play critical roles in helping provide increased support and comfort. The goal of intervention should be to prevent a suicide that is driven by poorly controlled psychological and physical symptoms.

Organic Mental Disorders

There are two major forms of organic mental disorders, delirium and dementia. Delirium is often superimposed on the AIDS dementia complex in advanced disease. Chapter 17 reviewed the cognitive changes caused by AIDS dementia complex, which relate to the direct effects of the HIV virus on the CNS. This section outlines the neuropsychiatric dysfunction resulting from CNS complications from a range of causes. In fact, delirium most often has multiple etiologic factors. It is estimated that the prevalence of organic mental disorders occurring at some time in the clinical course in patients with AIDS approaches 65%.[13] In terminal stages the likelihood reaches 90%, primarily for the development of delirium. Other clinical manifestations of organic mental disorders are organic anxiety disorder, organic personality disorder, organic hallucinosis, and organic delusional disorder.

Delirium occurs with greater frequency in advanced disease owing to organ system failure (*e.g.,* hypoxia, metabolic disturbance, septicemia, bleeding). In HIV-infected patients opportunistic CNS infections are common, as are CNS lymphomas and progressive multifocal leukoencephalopathy. Neurotoxic side-effects occur with the range of antiviral, antineoplastic, and antibiotic agents. Delirium is characterized by a fluctuating level of consciousness, misperceptions, delusions, sleep-wake cycle loss, and agitation or withdrawal. The underlying cause should be established and treatment started to correct it. Unfortunately, this is sometimes not possible in advanced AIDS, and the etiology may be related to several factors. One must initiate one-to-one observation, provide a reassuring environment, and use medication as needed for control of behavior and distress. A low-dose neuroleptic such as haloperidol (0.5 to 1.0 mg b.i.d. or t.i.d.) or lorazepam to combat agitation or restlessness is effective. However, careful attention is needed because of the increased risk of extrapyramidal side-effects with the potent neuroleptics such as halperidol, which is commonly used to control delirium. Dystonias, parkinsonian symptoms, and neuroleptic malignant syndrome have been reported with dosages as low as 10 mg/day.[17] Ongoing research by Breitbart and colleagues suggests that most patients can be managed on very low doses of haloperidol or chlorpromazine (*e.g.,* haloperidol, 0.5–1.0 mg/day, and chlorpromazine, 40–80 mg/day) given by mouth.[17] Extrapyramidal side-effects are quite uncommon at these dose levels. More severely agitated patients need higher doses and close observation.

Organic mood disorders caused by brain changes occur with delirium and the AIDS dementia complex, making depression a common concurrent problem. Poor impulse control leads to suicide attempts in these patients. Corticosteroids and analgesics are common drug offenders, as are interferon and chemotherapeutic agents. Paranoid states or manic symptoms requiring management may develop. Low-dose thioridazine (10 mg t.i.d. or q.i.d.) is effective in reducing distress. Lower potency neuroleptics are safer for use in patients with subcortical HIV disease.

PAIN AND AIDS

Pain is a significant, sometimes neglected problem in HIV-infected patients that contributes to psychological morbidity.[27-29] One study of hospitalized patients with AIDS revealed that 50% of patients required treatment for pain.[27] Chest pain, headache, oral cavity pain, abdominal pain, and peripheral neuropathy are most common. Pain was present in 53% of patients with advanced AIDS; the accompanying conditions included peripheral neuropathy, abdominal pain, headaches, and Kaposi's sarcoma. The prevalence was 43% in HIV-infected persons receiving outpatient care.[29] Painful sensory neuropathy accounted for 50% of pain diagnoses, and lower extremity pain with Kaposi's sarcoma occurred in 45% of patients. Patients with pain were more depressed and more functionally impaired than those without pain. In uncontrolled pain, psychological distress is likely the *consequence* of the pain.

The psychiatric management of HIV-related pain involves the use of psychotherapeutic, cognitive-behavioral, and psychopharmacologic techniques.[30] Short-term supportive psychotherapy based on a crisis intervention model provides emotional support, continuity of care, information about pain management, and assistance to patients and families. Relaxation, hypnosis, and biofeedback are effective as part of a multimodal approach.

Psychotropic drugs, particularly the tricyclic antidepressants and the psychostimulants, are useful in enhancing the pain-blocking properties of analgesics in the pharmacologic management of HIV-related pain. The tricyclic antidepressants (amitriptyline, clomipramine, imipramine, nortriptyline, desipramine, doxepine, trazodone, and fluoxetine) have potent analgesic properties and are widely used to treat chronic pain syndromes, particularly the peripheral neuropathies commonly seen with HIV infection. Antidepressants have direct analgesic effects and the capacity to enhance the analgesic effects of morphine. Psychostimulants are helpful in diminishing sedation secondary to narcotic analgesics and enhance their analgesic effects. Opiate analgesics, the mainstay of treatment for moderate to severe pain, may worsen dementia or cause treatment-limiting sedation, confusion, or hallucinations in patients with neurologic complications of AIDS. The judicious use of psychostimulants to diminish sedation and of neuroleptics to clear confusion can be quite helpful.

Fears of addiction regarding drug abuse affect both patient compliance and physician management of narcotic analgesics and often lead to undermedication of HIV-infected patients with pain. Studies of chronic narcotic analgesic use in patients with cancer, however, have demonstrated that although tolerance and physical dependence commonly occur, addiction, psychological dependence, or drug abuse are rare and almost never occur in individuals who do not have histories of drug abuse. More problematic is managing pain in HIV-infected patients who are actively using IV drugs. Drug-seeking manipulative behavior, unreliable histories, and poor compliance make these patients difficult to treat. Physicians who believe they are being manipulated by drug-seeking patients often hesitate to use adequate doses of narcotic analgesics to control pain. Physicians must set clear limits on behavior. As much as possible, pain management should deal directly with the problems of opiate withdrawal and drug treatment. Clinicians should err on the side of believing patients' complaints of pain and should utilize knowledge of specific HIV-related pain syndromes to corroborate the report of a patient perceived as being unreliable.[31]

In summary, reactive anxiety, with or without depressive symptoms, is the most prevalent symptom in HIV-infected individuals. More severe generalized anxiety occurs less often. Major depression with hopelessness predicts suicidal behavior and requires monitoring of risk. Delirium and dementia produce changes in mood from medication side-effects, metabolic disturbances, organ failure, and CNS infection. These aspects of HIV infection frequently complicate the diagnosis and management of HIV-seropositive patients, who are at high risk of developing psychiatric disorders.

REFERENCES

1. Holland JC, Tross S: The psychosocial and neuropsychiatric sequelae of the acquired immunodeficiency syndrome and related disorders. Ann Intern Med 103:760, 1985
2. Holland JC: Clinical course of cancer. In Holland JC, Rowland JH (eds): Handbook of Psychooncology: Psychological Care of the Patient with Cancer, p 95. New York, Oxford University Press, 1989
3. Rowland JH: Intrapersonal resources: Coping with illness. In Holland JC, Rowland JH (eds): Handbook of Psychooncology: Psychological Care of the Patient with Cancer, p 44. New York, Oxford University Press, 1989
4. Rowland JH: Interpersonal resources: Social support. In Holland JC, Rowland JH (eds): Handbook of Psychoon-

cology: Psychological Care of the Patient with Cancer, p 58. New York, Oxford University Press, 1989

5. Dean L, Hall WE, Martin JL: Chronic and intermittent AIDS-related bereavement in a panel of homosexual men in New York City. J Palliat Care 4:54, 1988

6. Tross S, Hirsch D: Psychological distress and neuropsychological complications of HIV and AIDS. Am Psychol 43:929, 1988

7. Atkinson JH, Grant I, Kennedy CJ et al: Prevalence of psychiatric disorders among men infected with human immunodeficiency virus. Arch Gen Psychiatry 45:859, 1988

8. Derogatis LR, Morrow GR, Fetting J et al: The prevalence of psychiatric disorders among cancer patients. JAMA 249:751, 1983

9. Rapkin JC, Williams JBW, Nengebauer R et al: Maintenance of hope in HIV spectrum homosexual men. Am J Psychiatry 147:1322, 1990

10. Dew MA, Ragni MV, Nimorwicz P: Infection with human immunodeficiency virus and vulnerability to psychiatric distress: A study of men with hemophilia. Arch Gen Psychiatry 47:737, 1990

11. Tross S: Acquired immunodeficiency syndrome. In Holland JC, Rowland JH (eds): Handbook of Psychooncology: Psychological Care of the Patient with Cancer, p 254. New York, Oxford University Press, 1989

12. Jacobsen PB, Perry SW, Hirsch DA: Behavioral and psychological responses to HIV antibody testing. J Consult Clin Psychol 58:31, 1990

13. Perry SW: Organic mental disorders caused by HIV: Update on early diagnosis and treatment. Am J Psychiatry 147:696, 1990

14. Fernandez F, Levy JK: Psychiatric diagnosis and pharmacotherapy of patients with HIV infection. In Tasman A, Goldfinger SM, Kaufmann CA (eds): Review of Psychiatry, vol 9, p 614. Washington, DC, American Psychiatric Press, 1990

15. Perry SW, Fishman B, Jacobsberg L et al: Effectiveness of psychoeducational interventions in reducing emotional distress after human immunodeficiency virus antibody testing. Arch Gen Psychiatry 48:143, 1991

16. Loscalzo M, Jacobsen P: Practical behavioral approaches to the effective management of pain and distress. J Psychosoc Oncol 8:139, 1990

17. Breitbart W, Marotta RF, Call P: AIDS and neuroleptic malignant syndrome. Lancet 2:1488, 1988

18. Moskowitz H, Smiley A: Effects of chronically administered buspirone and diazepam on driving-related skills and performance. J Clin Psychiatry 43:45, 1982

19. Batki SL: Buspirone in drug users with AIDS or AIDS-related complex. J Clin Psychopharmacol 10:111S, 1990

20. O'Dowd MA, McKegney FP: Manic syndrome associated with zidovudine. JAMA 260:3587, 1988

21. Hintz S, Kuck J, Peterkin JJ et al: Depression in the context of human immunodeficiency virus infection: Implications for treatment. J Clin Psychiatry 51:497, 1990

22. Marzuk PM, Tierney H, Tardiff K et al: Increased risk of suicide in persons with AIDS. JAMA 259:1333, 1988

23. Frierson RL, Lippman SB: Suicide and AIDS. Psychosomatics 29:226, 1988

24. Breitbart W: Suicide in cancer patients. Oncology 1:49, 1987

25. Orr D, O'Dowd MA, McKegney FP, Natali C: A comparison of self reported suicidal behaviors in different stages of HIV infection (abstr). Presented at the VI International AIDS Conference, San Francisco, June 20–24, 1990

26. Atkinson H, Gutierrez R, Cohler L et al: Suicide (abstr). In: AIDS 90 Summary: A Practical Synopsis of the VI International Conference, June 20–24, 1990, San Francisco, p 255. Philadelphia: Philadelphia Sciences Group, 1991

27. Lebovits AK, Lefkowitz M, McCarthy D et al: The prevalence and management of pain in patients with AIDS: A review of 134 cases. Clin J Pain 5:245, 1989

28. Newshau G, Wainapel S, Schmitz D: Pain related syndromes and their treatment in persons with AIDS (abstr). Presented at the Eighth Annual Scientific Meeting of the American Pain Society, Phoenix, Ariz, 1989

29. Breitbart W, Passik S, Bronaugh T et al: Pain in the ambulatory AIDS patient: Prevalence and psychosocial correlates (abstr). Presented at the Thirty-eighth Annual Meeting of the Academy of Psychosomatic Medicine, Atlanta, October 17–20, 1991

30. Chuang H: Psychiatry (abstr). In: AIDS 90 Summary: A Practical Synopsis of the VI International Conference, June 20–24, 1990, San Francisco, p 253. Philadelphia, Philadelphia Sciences Group, 1991

31. Temoshok L, Baum A: Psychosocial Perspectives on AIDS: Etiology, Prevention and Treatment. Hillsdale, NJ, Lawrence Erlbaum Associates, 1990

IV

Treatment of the HIV Infection

19

Strategies and Progress in the Development of Antiretroviral Agents

Margaret I. Johnston   John J. McGowan

This chapter outlines the strategies employed in the discovery and development of new antiviral agents specific for the human immunodeficiency virus (HIV), the causative agent of the acquired immunodeficiency syndrome (AIDS). Specific advances that show promise for the future will be highlighted.

In the past 8 years, since the discovery of HIV, an unprecedented search to find effective antiviral therapies has taken place. This search has been fueled by the seriousness of the pandemic, prodded by patient interest groups, encouraged by federal funding, nurtured by collaborations between government, academic, and pharmaceutical sectors of the research community, and based on knowledge accumulated from previous and ongoing basic research efforts. Advances in nucleoside chemistry, biochemistry, retrovirology, molecular biology, cell biology, and immunology, as well as developments in the applied areas of scale-up synthesis, drug formulation, and drug delivery, have all contributed to the discovery and development of therapies to treat HIV infection and the opportunistic infections associated with AIDS.

Methods being pursued to discover new active "lead" compounds are numerous. Traditionally, the empirical screening of large numbers of chemically diverse classes of compounds and natural products for their ability to inhibit replication of the pathogen or cancer in question has been the most successful approach to the discovery of new lead compounds. In 1987, the National Cancer Institute established a contract-based screening program that evaluates over 10,000 agents yearly for their ability to inhibit HIV replication in a cell culture screening assay. Active agents that have

been discovered in this program include carbovir[1] and a class of oxathiin benzoic acid esters and derivatives.[2]

At the other end of the spectrum of approaches, rational drug design is also being pursued. Perhaps the best-known example is the design of a soluble form of the CD4 receptor that serves as the major attachment site for HIV on the surface of susceptible cells. Soluble CD4, shown to be active in blocking HIV infection of cultured cells, is undergoing clinical evaluation. Another example is the more recent discovery of haloperidol as a weak inhibitor of the HIV protease. The ability to exploit this finding to design more potent, non-peptide-based inhibitors of HIV protease may herald a new approach to the discovery of new lead compounds.

A third general approach to the identification of lead inhibitors is the targeting of specific, critical steps of viral replication. In this now widely employed strategy, *in vitro* biochemical assays for specific viral functions (*e.g.,* reverse transcriptase, protease) are employed to screen tens of thousands of compounds for activity. Compounds for testing are selected empirically on the basis of their chemical diversity or rationally because they represent analogues of active compounds known to inhibit that step of viral replication. Rational drug design and targeted drug discovery have been supported through investigator-initiated research grants, including the National Cooperative Drug Discovery Group program funded by the National Institute of Allergy and Infectious Diseases and a structural biology program of the National Institute of General Medical Sciences.

Elucidation of the replication cycle of HIV permits identification of numerous points of possible intervention, many of which are being exploited in the drug discovery process (Fig. 19–1). These are outlined briefly here (the numbers refer to the steps in viral replication indicated in Figure 19–1). (1) Soluble CD4 as an inhibitor of virus binding to the cell surface has already been mentioned and will be described in detail elsewhere in this volume. The fusion process is inhibited by peptide analogues of the fusion domain of gp41.[3] (2) Uncoating is being pursued through studies aimed at understanding the structure of the p24 capsid protein.[4] This promising approach was used successfully to identify inhibitors of picornavirus replication.[5,6] (3–5) Production of proviral DNA includes several possible targets, including binding of the primer tRNA, production of DNA from RNA by reverse transcriptase (RT), degradation of viral RNA by the RNAse H domain of RT, and

second-strand DNA synthesis by RT. (6–7) Proviral DNA, transported into the nucleus by mechanisms not fully understood, undergoes specific cleavages at the 5' and 3' termini and is integrated into the host DNA through action of the viral integrase. In 1990, soluble assays for integration were reported; these will serve as the basis for development of high throughput assays suitable for inhibitor evaluation (R. Craigie *et al,* unpubl. observ.).[7] (8–10) Once integrated, the proviral DNA lies dormant until the viral long terminal repeat (LTR) is activated by viral or cellular proteins. The activity of both the viral Tat and Rev proteins is critical for viral replication, whereas the function of other regulatory proteins, including Nef, Vif, Vpu, and Vpr, is not completely understood. Assays for Tat and Rev have been established,

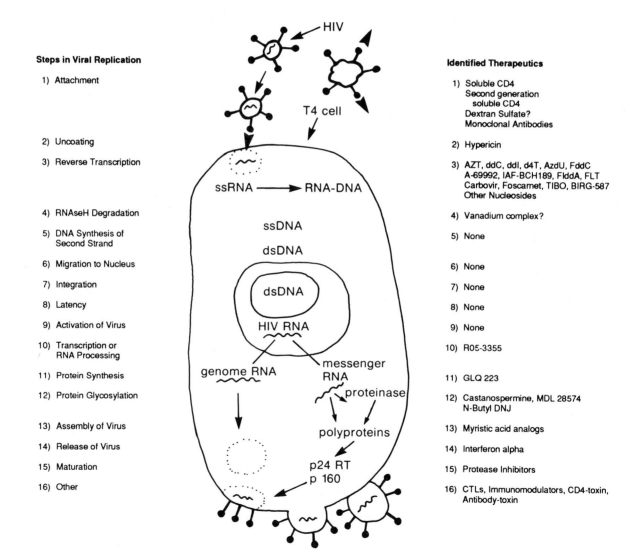

Steps in Viral Replication

1) Attachment

2) Uncoating

3) Reverse Transcription

4) RNAseH Degradation

5) DNA Synthesis of Second Strand

6) Migration to Nucleus

7) Integration

8) Latency

9) Activation of Virus

10) Transcription or RNA Processing

11) Protein Synthesis

12) Protein Glycosylation

13) Assembly of Virus

14) Release of Virus

15) Maturation

16) Other

Identified Therapeutics

1) Soluble CD4
   Second generation soluble CD4
   Dextran Sulfate?
   Monoclonal Antibodies

2) Hypericin

3) AZT, ddC, ddI, d4T, AzdU, FddC
   A-69992, IAF-BCH189, FlddA, FLT
   Carbovir, Foscarnet, TIBO, BIRG-587
   Other Nucleosides

4) Vanadium complex?

5) None

6) None

7) None

8) None

9) None

10) R05-3355

11) GLQ 223

12) Castanospermine, MDL 28574
    N-Butyl DNJ

13) Myristic acid analogs

14) Interferon alpha

15) Protease Inhibitors

16) CTLs, Immunomodulators, CD4-toxin, Antibody-toxin

Figure 19–1. The life cycle of HIV-1. Column on left indicates possible points of therapeutic intervention. Column on right lists examples of agents proposed to inhibit HIV-1 replication at the indicated steps.

and the first anti-Tat agent is expected to enter clinical trial in 1991. (11–12) Viral RNA is transported out of the nucleus and is translated, in the case of mRNA, or incorporated into new virions, in the case of genomic RNA. Frameshifting during the translation of viral mRNA is essential for the production of proteins encoded by the *pol* gene (protease, RT, and integrase).[8] Certain viral proteins undergo glycosylation, which has been pursued as a target for possible intervention.[9–12] (13–15) Assembly, budding, and maturation of infectious virions is dependent on the action of (*a*) cellular *N*-protein myristoyl transferase, which adds myristic acid to the N-terminus of *gag* and *gag-pol* viral polyprotein precursors, a critical step in assembly,[13] and (*b*) an aspartyl protease encoded by the *pol* gene and responsible for cleavage of the *gag* and *gag-pol* precursors into mature proteins.[14–16] (16) Several immune-based methods, such as sCD4-PE40 and cytotoxic T cells (CTL), rely on expression of viral epitopes on the surface of infected cells.

Once a lead active agent has been identified, regardless of the process used in its discovery, additional studies are conducted to improve the characteristics of the agent until a suitable candidate for clinical evaluation is identified. Such studies usually include elucidating the structure-activity relationship of the molecule to improve its potency and selectivity. Improving stability, solubility, and bioavailability may also be necessary to turn an active lead into a clinical candidate. Selection of a clinical candidate is usually followed by scale-up synthesis, formulation, and rigorous pharmacology and toxicology studies to support the Investigational New Drug (IND) application.

The following sections describe three recent promising approaches based on nonnucleoside RT inhibitors, an inhibitor of Tat, and protease inhibitors. Finally, potential therapeutic approaches that rely on gene therapy will be reviewed.

REVERSE TRANSCRIPTASE

Basic research on retroviruses led to the discovery and characterization of RT and laid the cornerstone for a new understanding of the molecular biology of viruses inside the eukaryotic cell. Research on animal retroviruses also provided the base of information needed to rapidly advance our understanding of HIV. In particular, the discovery of RT revolutionized molecular biology. The tools for cloning genes opened the door to understanding retroviral replication and, in the 1970s, stimulated development of therapies targeted to this unique enzyme.[17–19] In therapeutic areas, the study of retroviral RT also led to the development of enzymatic, cellular, and animal model systems to study gene regulation, cellular processes, and oncogenesis.[20] It is not surprising that compounds to inhibit RT were identified before it was known that the HIV RT was formed by viral protease–mediated cleavage of the *gag-pol* polyprotein to form either a 66-kDa or a 51-kDa subunit (both share the same N-termini but have different C-termini).[19–22] These two subunits form the active enzyme, which exists as a heterodimer under physiologic conditions. Yet the purified (denatured and refolded) 66-kDa monomeric subunit is equal in activity to the heterodimer when assayed *in vitro*.[23,24] Perhaps use of this monomer or of selected peptide domains will facilitate crystallization and elucidation of the three-dimensional structure of the HIV RT.

RT has been a prominent target in the discovery and development of therapies to suppress or prevent HIV infection and related diseases.[25,26] The first drug shown to be clinically effective and licensed for the treatment of HIV infection in humans (3′-azido-2′,3′-dideoxythymidine [zidovudine, or AZT]) was initially tested for its potential as an anticancer compound.[27–30] Indeed, many pyrimidine and purine nucleoside analogues have been shown to inhibit replication and the pathogenic effects of a wide range of animal and human retroviruses (Fig. 19–2). Most nucleosides are progressively phosphorylated by cytoplasmic enzymes to nucleoside 5′-triphosphates that compete with the natural substrate for binding to cellular DNA polymerase and the viral RT.[31,32] It is assumed that most nucleosides are incorporated into the viral DNA and prevent the continued polymerization of the DNA chain. The termination of DNA chain synthesis results in prevention of viral replication.[32,33] Other mechanisms of action are possible. Because of the unique metabolic and pharmacologic properties of each nucleoside analogue, it is hazardous to generalize with regard to mechanism of action, toxicity, or efficacy of any nucleoside analogue (Table 19–1).[34] Clearly, nucleoside analogues delay HIV disease progression.[35] Because drug-resistant strains are likely to emerge in individuals treated with AZT, alternative nucleosides are needed.[36–40] Perhaps these drugs will be used simultaneously or sequentially to treat the disease and potentially delay the appearance of isolates resistant to one compound. Several comprehensive reviews on nucleoside analogues tested for anti-HIV activity have been published.[34,41,42]

Benzodiazepinones, anthraquinones, phosphonoformic acid, HPA-23, suramin, flavonoids, and catechin derivatives are among the nonnucleoside compounds that are thought to inhibit HIV.[43–46] In contrast to nucleoside analogues, the nonnucleoside compounds need not be phosphorylated to be active, nor do they necessarily interfere with nucleoside binding to RT or cellular DNA polymerases. Most nonnucleoside analogues were identified through targeted drug discovery programs. Several examples are discussed below.

Flavonoids were initially found active against HIV by comparing their ability to inhibit the HIV RT with their ability to inhibit cellular DNA polymerases (α, β, and γ).[43,44] Addition of 5′-hydroxyl groups to the parent compounds maximized the observed inhibition. The unsaturated pyrone ring was also critical for antiviral activity.[43] Compounds like catechin, similar in structure to flavonoids but lacking the pyrone ring, were much

Dideoxynucleosides in Clinical Trials

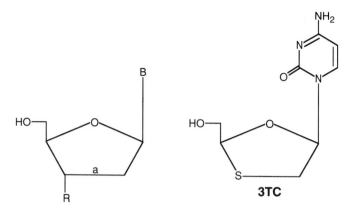

Drug	B	R	Clinical Status
AZT	Thymine	N_3	Approved adults and children
FLT	Thymine	F	Phase I
AZdU (CS-87)	Uracil	N_3	Phase I
ddC	Cytosine	H	Phase I/II
D4T	Thymine (a=double bond)	H	Phase I/II
5-F-ddC	5-Fluorocytosine	H	Phase I
ddI	Hypoxanthine	H	Phase II/III Approved for AZT intolerant adults and children
3TC			Phase I

Figure 19–2.   Structures and current clinical status of the nucleoside analogs.

less active against the HIV RT.[41] The most active compound in this class was 5,6,7,-trihydroxyflavone (baicalein) (Fig. 19–3). Baicalein was also found to have the least effect on cellular DNA polymerase (γ).[44,47] Quercetin and myricetin were found active against the viral RT but were also potent inhibitors of the cellular α and β DNA polymerases. The flavonoids did not appear to compete with nucleoside triphosphates for binding to RT. A competitive effect was observed with respect to polynucleotide template binding, but this effect was not complete.[43,44] As with other nonnucleoside analogues (suramin, for example), the mechanism of inhibition is still not fully understood. Unfortunately, the lead compound baicalein and the other flavonoids tested appear to have a cytotoxic effect against lymphocytes in cell culture. These toxic effects have not been reported

Table 19–1.   Principal Toxic Effects, Measures to Counteract Toxicity, and Degree of Cross-Resistance to Azidothymidine Exhibited by Nucleoside Analogues in Clinical Evaluation

Nucleoside	Principal Toxic Effect	Countermeasures	Resistance
Zidovudine (AZT)	Anemia, myelotoxicity	Alter dose/schedule erythropoietin combinations	Less sensitive isolates (≥ 100-fold) after 12 mo of treatment
Dideoxycytidine (ddC)	Peripheral neuropathy	Alter dose/schedule combinations	Not cross-resistant to AZT *in vitro*
Didehydrodideoxythymidine (D4T)	Peripheral neuropathy, elevated liver enzymes	Alter dose/schedule combinations	Variable sensitivity to AZT-resistant isolates
Dideoxyinosine (ddI)	Peripheral neuropathy, pancreatitis, diarrhea	Alter dose/schedule combinations Change formulation	Not cross-resistant to AZT *in vitro*
Azidouridine (AzDu)	Nausea/headache	Phase I ongoing; dose-limiting toxicity not attained	Cross-resistant *in vitro* in AZT-resistant isolates
3-Fluoro thymidine (FLT)	Potential anemia, myelotoxicity	Early Phase I trial; dose-limiting toxicity not attained	Not cross-resistant *in vitro* to AZT-resistant isolates

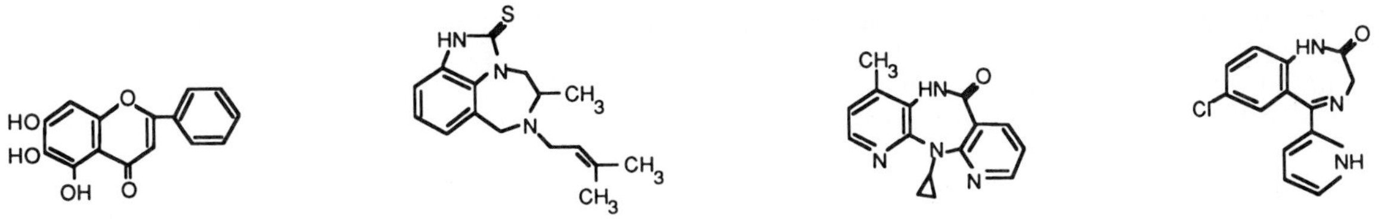

Figure 19–3. Structures of the non-nucleoside analog known to inhibit the HIV RT. Ro 5-3335 is an inhibitor of HIV Tat, but is shown here because of the similarity to other benzodiazepines.

in previous animal or human tests of flavonoids. Further analysis of these compounds in an animal model system is warranted to determine their potential use in the treatment of retroviral infections.

A series of structurally distinct compounds that are related to benzodiazepines were perhaps the most intriguing new compounds to be reported in 1990 (see Fig. 19–3). Several discovery teams within companies (Jansen Pharmaceuticals, Boehringer Ingelheim Pharmaceutical, UpJohn Company, Merck, and Hoffman–La Roche), working with academicians in some cases, discovered compounds that are now undergoing preclinical or clinical evaluation. Through structure-activity analysis, medicinal chemists have maximized the anti-HIV and pharmacokinetic profiles of these compounds. For example, the activity profile reported by Merluzzi and co-workers[48] was dibenzo < monopyrido < dipyrido-diazepinones, with 11-cyclopropyl-7-methyl-dipryido [2,3-b:3′,3′-f]1,4-diazepin-6H-5-one (BI-RG-587) as their lead compound. Pauwels *et al*[49] were the first to report the activity of a series of tetrahydro-imidazol[4,5,1-jk][1,4]-benzodiazepin-2(1H)-one and -thione derivatives (TIBO). A change in the C2 position of the imidazole ring resulted in a 450-fold increase in HIV activity. Additional compounds have been synthesized with the aim of increasing activity while eliminating or minimizing unwanted pharmacologic activities (*i.e.,* muscarinic or benzodiazepine effects) associated with other compounds in this class.[48,49] The mechanism of action of this series of compounds is still not fully understood. Both TIBO and BI-RG-587 bind to the same site on RT, are noncompetitive inhibitors, and have little or no effect on RT from HIV-2 or simian immunodeficiency virus (SIV). Interestingly, TIBO-related compounds appear to be significantly more effective in blocking RT activity when a natural template-primer substrate is used than when a synthetic template-primer pair is utilized (L. E. White *et al,* unpubl. observ.). Resistance to this class of compounds appears to develop quickly *in vitro* and *in vivo*. Therefore, the potential utility and clinical development of this class of compounds remains unknown.

The anthraquinone dimer hypericin was the first and most notable anthraquinone found active in inhibiting HIV replication in cell culture and in retroviral infections in animals.[50–52] Structure-activity analysis has been performed by several groups.[50,52] The effects of hydroxy, amino, halogen, carboxylic acid, or sulfonate groups in increasing the ability of these compounds to inhibit HIV was determined. Polyphenolic- and polysulfonate-substituted compounds were the most active.[42] Lavie *et al* reported that removal of carbonyl groups resulted in a significant loss of activity.[52] The authors concluded that the quinone structure was vital for antiviral activity. The mechanism of action of this unique group of compounds is not clear, but at least three possibilities exist. First, quinones are known to form free radicals that can intercalate with nucleic acids.[50] Second, hypericin and 1,2,5,8,-tetrahydroanthraquinone appear to have a selective effect on HIV RT *in vitro*.[51,52] Finally, these agents might bind virion cores and prevent uncoating. Despite an unknown mechanism of action, this group of compounds continues to hold promise in the treatment of HIV-induced disease.

Tat

HIV-directed research has led to an increased understanding of the complexities of viral gene expression and regulation. The insights gained with HIV have broad implications for targeting therapies that interrupt the regulation processes of other infectious diseases or cancer. At present, no drugs or treatments that inhibit a specific regulatory gene are in clinical trial. Thus, innovative research that has led to potential drugs which block gene expression has brought a cautious optimism.

The two required regulatory genes are *tat* and *rev*.[53–56] Evidence continues to mount that a third protein, Nef, also serves to regulate HIV expression.[57] Other accessory proteins have been identified (Vif, Vpu, and Vpr).[58–60] These less understood accessory proteins may be important in HIV regulation *in vivo* but are not essential for the virus when passaged in tissue culture.[60–62]

Tat has been the most extensively studied of the HIV regulatory proteins.[63–65] Tat is a robust *trans-*

activator that stimulates the transcription of genes under the control of the HIV LTR and affects their subsequent translation.[65] Indeed, Tat has a positive effect on its own expression.[64] Tat mRNA, spliced from two exons, is translated to form the 86-amino acid protein (Fig. 19–4).[53,63,66,67] The first exon precedes the *env* gene and codes for the first 72 amino acids.[65] At least three functional domains have been described within the first exon (see Fig. 19–4).[65,68–71] These domains have been mapped using synthetic peptides and site-directed mutagenesis.[69,72,73] Amino acids 49–57 are required for nuclear localization, while the first 58 amino acids are functional *in vitro* in *trans*-activating assays.[71,73]

Trans-activation by Tat is pivotal to the viral life cycle.[64] Tat's potential effect on HIV pathogenesis is less well understood. Purified Tat protein added exogenously to uninfected cells can have an immunosuppressive effect.[52,73] This immunosuppressive effect could result from binding to receptors (*e.g.,* dipeptidylpeptidase IV) or adhesion molecules on the cell surface (W. Bachovchin, pers. commun.). Alternatively, Tat could *trans*-activate heterologous genes inside the cell (*e.g.,* TNF-β, IL-6) that cause the dysfunctional production of cytokines and hormones that regulate the immune system.[74–76]

The precise mechanism of Tat action(s) is still unclear. Current data suggest that *de novo* mRNA synthesis is required[77] whereas *de novo* protein synthesis is not required for Tat *trans*-activation.[77,78] Tat does not appear to act directly on mRNA stability or translation. Tat appears to increase the rate of transcription initiation (or elongation) by relieving a block in the *cis*-acting Tat-responsive element known as TAR.[79–82] Tat can bind TAR directly either as a nascent RNA transcript or through one of several host cell proteins that interact to form a complex that allows Tat to initiate viral transcription at the TAR site in the viral genome (see Fig. 19–4).[83–85] Although binding of Tat to DNA cannot be excluded, most data favor the direct or indirect binding (with a host protein) to TAR RNA.[86–88] TAR is a fundamental element required for HIV replication. Downstream from transcription initiation, TAR is localized at +10 to +44 nucleotides of the viral genome and appears to function in its natural orientation.[81,89] It is present within the viral LTR and at the 5′-terminus of all HIV transcripts.[83,90–92] TAR forms a stable stem-loop structure. Tat binds to the stem and the bulge of TAR, whereas the loop may be bound by host proteins.[86,93] Nucleotide changes in the stem do not appear to affect activity if base pairing is maintained.[94,95] Yet small changes in the loop and bulge region greatly reduce TAR activity.[73,89,94,95]

Tat is a good target for potential drug intervention because it represents an early target in viral replication in latently infected cells, and also because less drug might be needed to inhibit this more highly conserved regulatory protein than to inhibit other enzymes (RT or proteinase) or other structural proteins produced in larger amounts inside the infected cell. Several years ago, Hoffman–La Roche, in collaboration with researchers at the Roche Institute, St. Luke's Hospital, NY, and Rockefeller University, embarked on a drug discovery effort using a highly specific screen for compounds that interfere with Tat activity (M. C. Hsu *et al,* unpubl. observ.).[96] A high-capacity cell-based assay was used as a random screen of compounds in the Hoffman–La Roche repository. Briefly, a secretable alkaline phosphatase under control of the HIV-1 LTR was used in parallel with other systems using the same or different reporter genes under the control of other murine retroviral LTRs.[97] Similar rapid quantitative bioassays have been developed by others.[97,98] An active lead compound was discovered on random screening of the first 200 classes of compounds in the repository (see Fig. 19–3). The anti-HIV activity of a lead compound (Ro 5-3335) was confirmed in assays when added to cells at the time of infection with HIV, cells transfected with recombinant HIV DNA, or cells chronically infected with HIV. In each case the compound specifically inhibited viral replication at concentrations that were not toxic to uninfected cells. These findings are highly significant because AZT does not inhibit chronically infected cells and because Ro 5-3335 is active against AZT-resistant isolates.[99]

Ro 5-3335 is a benzodiazepine but is distinct from other benzodiazepines identified as RT inhibitors. Unlike TIBO and BI-RG-587, Ro 5-3335 does not bind to HIV RT and is active against HIV-2 in cell culture assays. Like TIBO and BI-RG-587, Ro 5-3335 has no significant effect on the central nervous system. Preliminary evidence indicates that Ro 5-3335 is active in inhibiting HIV replication when added at the time of transcription initiation, but not after elongation has begun. The compound is reported to have an 85% bioavailability in dogs, with a plasma half-life of 2 hours and a peak serum level of approximately 0.8 μM after oral dosing of 1 mg/kg.[99] Other chemical analogues are being analyzed to ensure that the best compound is selected for clinical development. If successful, it will prove to be the first antiviral compound to specifically inhibit a viral regulatory gene product, which will open new doors to the treatment of infectious diseases, inflammatory diseases, and cancer.

PROTEASE

One of the most promising targets being pursued at this time is the virally encoded protease.[100–102] During translation of viral mRNA, viral structural proteins encoded by the *gag* gene (CA, MA, NC) and enzymes encoded by the *pol* gene (RT/RNAse H, IN, PR) are produced as *gag* and *gag-pol* polyproteins. These polyproteins are cleaved by the viral protease (PR) into mature proteins. Activation of protease appears to coincide with budding and maturation of new virions. Maturation is accompanied by a change in morphology from a particle with no central capsid to a particle with the characteristic dense cone-shaped core under electron microscopy. If

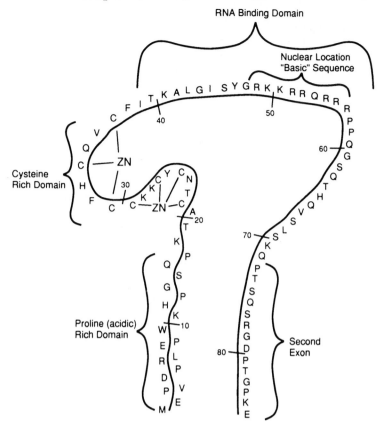

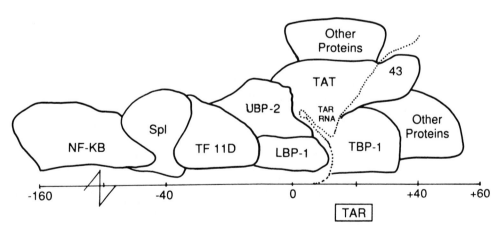

Figure 19–4. A theoretical structure of the HIV Tat. The amino acid sequence is represented by one letter symbols. The three identified functional domains of the protein, and the two exons spliced to form the mRNA, are indicated. A theoretical representation of some of the known protein binding sites associated with the viral LTR are shown.

protease is inactive as a result of a point or deletion mutation, viral particles fail to mature morphologically and are not infectious.[14-16,103] This suggests that inhibition of protease would be useful in blocking production of infectious virions from chronically infected cells, with the concomitant hope that such an inhibitor would have an impact on viral burden and the course of the disease in infected individuals.

Relative to other viral targets, with the exception of RT, research on protease was accomplished with great speed as a result previous basic research done on similar viral and cellular proteases. Sequencing of the gene for this 99-amino acid protein demonstrated that the protease contains a conserved aspartyl-threonine/serine-glycine active site characteristic of aspartyl proteases.[14] Although the sites cleaved by protease do not contain a strict amino acid specificity, preferences for certain amino acids at certain sites have been described.[104,105] Previous research on aspartyl proteases had revealed that aspartyl proteases cleave through a tetrahedral intermediate,[106,107] which suggested that peptides containing modifications of the scissile bond that mimic the tetrahedral hydrated amide species (hydroxyethylene isosteres, hydroxyethyamines, reduced amide, phosphinates, α,α-difluoroketones) might inhibit enzyme activity. Several groups employed this approach to design inhibitors of renin, an aspartyl protease that cleaves angiotensinogen in the pathway to production of angiotensin II, a potent vasoconstrictor.[108] Researchers were thus poised to evaluate these types of inhibitors for activity against the HIV protease.

HIV protease was chemically synthesized.[109,110] Recombinant protease was also available once procedures for controlling the expression of protease in bacteria were developed, since high levels of expression of the protease were found to be toxic to bacteria.[111-113] The three-dimensional structure of aspartyl protease from Rous sarcoma virus was already known,[114] and the structure of protease from HIV was quickly deciphered.[115-117] This was followed very closely by elucidation of the structure of HIV protease–peptide inhibitor complexes.[118,119] Development of simple, rapid assays to detect protease inhibitors contributed to the speed with which structure-activity relationships could be determined.[120-126] Thus, as a result of combined approaches, including mechanistic studies, protein synthesis, cloning and purification, development of enzyme assays, and elucidation of enzyme structure, potent peptide-based inhibitors of HIV replication were reported in a relatively short period of time (Fig. 19–5).[127-132] In addition, a

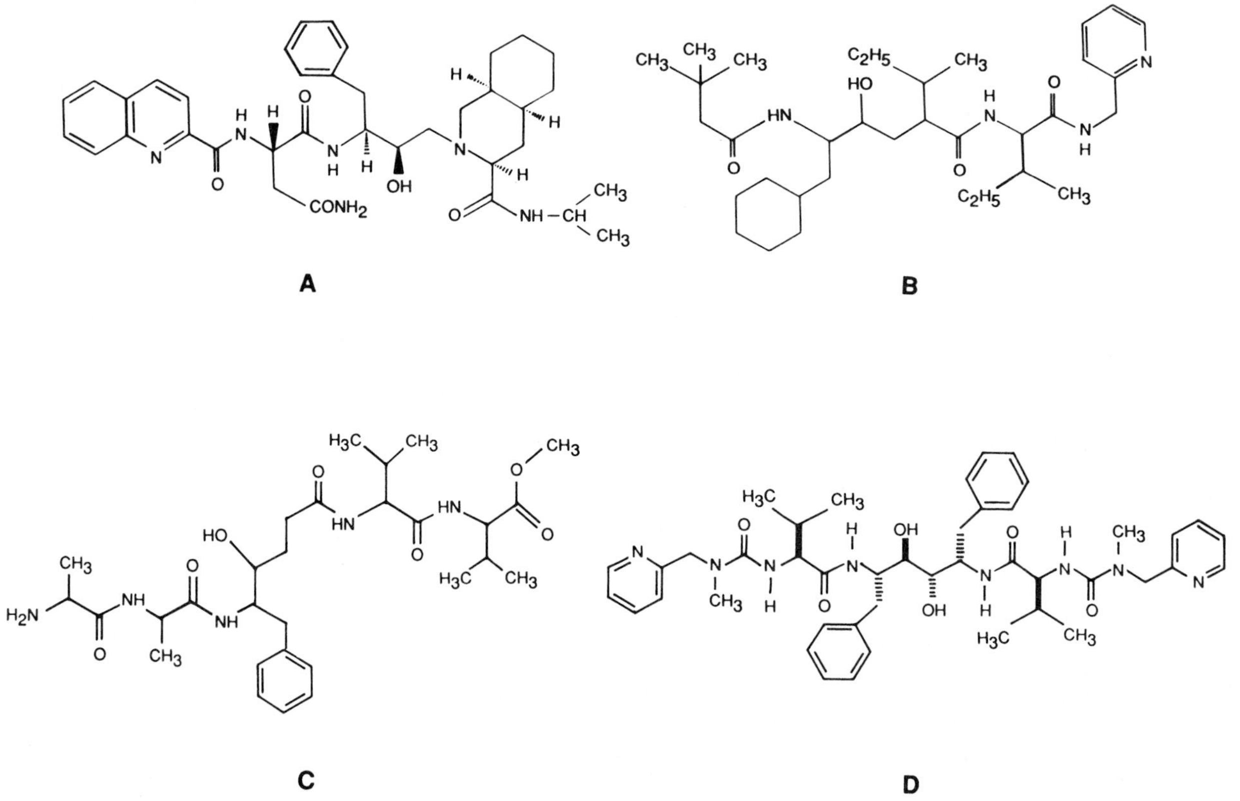

Figure 19–5. Representative inhibitors of HIV protease from Roberts *et al*[127] (**A**), from McQuade *et al*[130] (**B**), from Meek *et al*[128] (**C**) and from Paul *et al*[138a] (**D**).

lead natural product, cerulenin, was reported to inhibit HIV protease.[133] Synthetic analogues of cerulenin that show less cytotoxicity have been reported.[134]

The optimal peptide length for inhibition of the HIV protease appears to be about 6 to 7 amino acids. Previous research has suggested problems with the use of peptide-based drugs, including degradation by proteolytic enzymes (leading to short duration of action), rapid excretion by the liver, and poor bioavailability when taken orally. Modifications to improve these properties will be necessary. In addition, the long-term effects of these inhibitors need to be carefully evaluated, because one *in vitro* study concluded that inhibitor-induced block in HIV maturation was reversed by incubation of the immature particles in drug-free solution for several hours.[130]

In addition to the peptide-based approaches, other strategies are being pursued in the design of protease inhibitors. Erickson and collaborators at Abbott Laboratories exploited the C2 symmetry of the protease target to design an inhibitor with C2 symmetry.[135,136] The lead compound is somewhat less peptide-like, containing two peptide N-termini but no C-terminus. This agent was found to bind to and inhibit the enzyme while retaining the symmetry of both the enzyme and the inhibitor. Activity against HIV in cell culture was comparable to that observed with peptide analogues.

A novel computer-based approach was pursued by DesJarlais *et al*, who searched three-dimensional data bases to identify agents with a similar three-dimensional structure that would "fit" the protease active site.[137] The computer program DOCK was used to evaluate the coordinates of 10,000 molecules in the Cambridge Crystallographic Database. Compounds were ranked and then visually evaluated for key bonding interactions. Bromperidol was identified as a possible inhibitor, and its commercially available analogue, haloperidol, was evaluated. Haloperidol was found to have a K_i for HIV protease of about 100 μM. At 500 μM, haloperidol inhibited replication of HIV in cultured cells. These concentrations are several logs higher than what can be attained *in vivo* without unacceptable toxicities. Nonetheless, this non-peptide-based lead compound can be subjected to rigorous structure-activity studies in hopes of designing a more potent, selective, non-peptide-based inhibitor of HIV protease. If successful, the structure-based approach to the discovery of lead compounds active against HIV as well as other targets for which the crystal structure is known may be greatly stimulated.

Unlike mammalian and fungal aspartyl proteases, which are composed of a single polypeptide comprised of two equivalent domains that probably arose from gene duplication, the HIV protease is smaller and functionally active when a dimer. Dissociation of the dimer form, or prevention of dimer association during virus assembly, are additional targets for blocking protease action that have not yet been fully exploited. Previous research demonstrating that dissociation of herpesvirus hetero-

dimeric ribonucleotide reductase by peptides corresponding to the C-terminus of the small subunit leads to inactivation suggests that this approach is worthy of pursuit.[138-140] Recently, Babé and co-workers in Craik's laboratory demonstrated that recombinant protease composed of defective monomers or nonidentical subunits were catalytically defective.[141] This supports the postulate that inhibition of HIV-1 protease dimer formation is an attractive target for intervention strategies.

OTHER TARGETS

Other targets in the HIV replication cycle are being avidly pursued. These include myristoylation, where lead compounds have been identified and shown to be active in blocking HIV replication.[142,143] Novel fatty acid, heteroatom-containing substrates of the myristoyl-CoA: protein N-myristoyl-transferase (NMT) were prepared and evaluated. The heteroatom substitutions produced a significant reduction in the hydrophobicity of the substrate without altering the chain length or specificity of addition. These substrates were added to viral proteins, and their reduced hydrophobicity resulted in redistribution of the fatty acid–modified proteins from membrane to cytosolic fractions. Importantly, these modified substrates were incorporated into only a subset of cellular proteins that are normally myristoylated. The key to specificity resulted from cooperativity between the NMT, acylCoA, and the peptide binding site; specifically, the length of the bound acylCoA was found to influence what peptide substrate was bound by the enzyme. Certain analogues were relatively effective in inhibiting replication of HIV in cell culture at nontoxic concentrations.[143]

A potentially important target that initially proved somewhat more difficult to pursue is the virally encoded integrase. Until recently, knowledge of the integration process for any retrovirus was rather limited. It is now clear that the viral integrase is the only protein needed to generate the recessed 3' ends that are the precursor for integration and to insert this viral proviral DNA into target DNA.[7] A rapid *in vitro* assay for integrase activity has been devised (R. Craigie *et al*, unpubl. observ.). Such assays will facilitate the search for agents that prevent integration in cells infected with HIV.

GENE THERAPY

Now that research to block various critical stages of viral replication is under active pursuit, several laboratories are turning their attention to a longer range goal—the application of gene therapy techniques to the treatment of HIV infection. Gene therapy approaches being pursued fall into two general categories: cellular immunotherapy, sometimes referred to as "intracellular immunization,"[144] and antiviral gene therapy.

It has been demonstrated previously that allogeneic bone marrow transplantation has not been successful in reconstituting the immune system of infected individuals, probably because the transplanted cells can become infected with HIV.[145] The goal of cellular immunotherapy is to reconstitute the immune system of HIV-infected individuals with functional bone marrow hematopoietic stem cells that have been genetically altered to confer on the cells resistance to infection by HIV. At least initially, this approach will involve the removal of autologous bone marrow cells, genetic manipulation of these cells to confer resistance to HIV infection, and administration of the altered cells to the patient. Eventually it may be possible to transplant nonautologous cells. Research activities in this area are currently focused on identifying and optimizing approaches that would confer resistance to HIV infection. These approaches include introduction of a gene that results in production of (1) a polyribonucleotide (anti-sense or ribozyme) that inhibits the function of a critical portion of the viral genomic RNA or DNA, or one or more viral mRNAs[146]; (2) a viral gene product (protein or RNA) that interferes with normal viral replication or assembly; (3) a product that blocks expression of CD4 on the cell surface or results in expression of an altered CD4 molecule that renders the cells resistant to HIV infection; or (4) introduction of a gene that activates only on infection with HIV and, once activated, results in production of a toxin lethal to that cell.

Another general gene therapy approach may be termed antiviral gene therapy. The goal of antiviral gene therapy is to genetically alter the patient's cells to produce high levels of a molecule with direct antiviral activity, such as soluble CD4, the soluble form of the cell receptor for HIV. When the antiviral protein is released from the cell, it would protect surrounding cells from HIV infection. Researchers are currently working to increase the level of expression of soluble CD4 by genetically altered cells so that blood levels that effectively block HIV entry into noninfected cells are attained *in vivo*.[147] The ability of various isolates of HIV to be inhibited by this process needs to be more fully explored to determine the potential usefulness of this approach. Results from ongoing clinical trials with soluble CD4 given intravenously will be helpful in determining the potential efficacy and safety of this approach and the level of soluble CD4 needed to observe a clinical response.

Each of these approaches depends on the further development of appropriate retroviral or other vectors or other methods to deliver the gene of interest safely to the target cell and to ensure that appropriate levels of expression are maintained and controlled. Most promising to date are recombinant, infectious retroviruses that express the transferred gene after integration but do not result in production of virions capable of a subsequent round of infection. Recombinant retroviruses are generally produced by introduction of a replication-defective virus (containing the gene to be transferred but lacking the genes for structural viral proteins) in a packaging cell line that contains helper retroviral genome(s) (lacking the packaging sequence but capable of providing required structural proteins). Numerous challenges remain. Retroviral vectors generally produce low titers of recombinant viruses and express low levels of the gene(s) of interest in primary hemopoietic cells. Further, the nonreplicating status of retroviral vectors needs to be ensured in order to limit the chances of generating malignancies by unintentional activation of oncogenes.

While much of the ongoing work is proceeding with retroviral vectors used in other types of gene transfer experiments, researchers are also exploring the possible use of HIV vectors for delivery to HIV-infected individuals.[148] This approach has several potential advantages. The mechanism by which HIV replicates (*e.g., trans*-activation) may allow higher levels of gene expression and higher titers of recombinant viruses than have been possible for the oncogenic retroviruses utilized to date. Second, the desired genes would be targeted to cells that are infectable by HIV, thus sparing other cells from possible negative effects. Finally, exogenously introduced genes would be primarily dependent on expression of HIV proteins; the HIV regulatory proteins needed to activate the HIV gene control elements within the inserted DNA would only be present should the cell become infected with HIV. Possible disadvantages include pathogenic properties of the modified virus; these properties could probably be eliminated through appropriate design of the inserted DNA. The activation of the HIV control elements by certain other viruses or cellular proteins also would have to be minimized or eliminated. Potential immunotoxicity must also be addressed; the effect of expression of HIV genes on T-cell immune function needs to be carefully evaluated to ensure that cells modified by the HIV vectors retain their normal immune function.

One of the limitations in the use of retroviral vectors in gene therapy has been the concern that the random integration process employed by retroviruses could result in disruption of the function of a critical gene or the activation of cellular oncogenes. Recently, an efficient adeno-associated virus (AAV) vector that integrates into a specific site in the human genome has been described.[149] An AAV vector containing an anti-sense to the TAR region found on all HIV mRNAs was designed and used to transfect T cells.[150] T cells producing the TAR anti-sense RNA were permanently resistant to HIV replication. Because AAV is nonpathogenic, efficiently infects and integrates into host cells, and integrates into a single site, it may come to surpass retroviral vectors in gene therapy applications.

The application of gene therapy may not depend on the use of viral vectors to deliver the gene of interest. Several research groups have reported that functional genes can be administered by direct injection into living animals.[151-154] This approach, at least conceptually, would be technically easier, faster, and safer than the use of retroviral vectors, and may also be reversible. These considerations, combined with the long-term expression observed in other systems, suggest that this potential approach for the synthesis and release of therapeutic proteins *in vivo* should be pursued further.

Researchers are utilizing *in vitro* cell culture systems to evaluate the effectiveness and safety of gene therapeutic approaches for the treatment of HIV-infected individuals. The possible toxic effects of genetically altered cells will need to be carefully evaluated in animals. Experiments in animal models of HIV infection are planned for the future. Clear evidence of efficacy will be necessary prior to the development of protocols for evaluation of gene therapeutic approaches in HIV-infected individuals.

Acknowledgments: The authors thank Nancy Brown, Bernadette Monacelli, and Dr. Mohamed Nasr for assistance in preparation of this chapter, and Dr. Nava Sarver for a critical reading.

REFERENCES

1. Vince R, Hua M, Brownell J, Daluge S: Potent and selective activity of a new carbocyclic nucleoside analog (carbovir NSC 614846) against human immunodeficiency virus *in vitro*. Biochem Biophys Res Commun 156:1046, 1988
2. Schultz RJ, Narayanan VL, Pierce JL et al: Oxathiin carboxanilide (NSC 61585), a novel new anti-HIV agent. Proc Am Assoc Cancer Res 33:409, 1990
3. Owens RJ, Tanner CC, Mulligan MJ et al: Oligopeptide inhibitors of HIV-induced syncytium formation. AIDS Res Human Retroviruses 6:1289, 1990
4. Rossman MG: Antiviral agents targeted to interact with viral capsid proteins and a possible application to human immunodeficiency virus. Proc Natl Acad Sci USA 85:4625, 1988
5. Smith TJ, Kremer MJ, Luo M et al: The site of attachment in human retrovirus 14 for antiviral agents that inhibit uncoating. Science 233:1286, 1989
6. Diana GD, Pevear DC, Otto MJ et al: Inhibitors of viral uncoating. Pharmacol Ther 42:289, 1989
7. Bushman FD, Craigie R: Activities of human immunodeficiency virus (HIV) integration protein *in vitro:* specific cleavage and integration of HIV DNA. Proc Natl Acad Sci USA 88:1, 1991
8. Jacks T, Power MD, Masiarz FR et al: Characterization of ribosomal frameshifting in HIV-1 *gag-pol* expression. Nature 331:280, 1988
9. Johnson VA, Walker BD, Barlow MA et al: Synergistic inhibition of human immunodeficiency virus type 1 and type 2 replication *in vitro* by castanospermine and 3'-azido-3'-deoxythymidine. Antimicrob Agents Chemother 33:53, 1989
10. Hansen JE, Clausen H, Nielsen C et al: Inhibition of human immunodeficiency virus (HIV) infection *in vitro* by anticarbohydrate monoclonal antibodies: Peripheral glycosylation of HIV envelope glycoprotein gp120 may be a target for virus neutralization. J Virol 64:2833, 1990
11. Fenouillet E, Gluckman JC, Bahraoui E: Role of N-linked glycans of envelope glycoproteins in infectivity of human immunodeficiency virus type 1. J Virol 64:2841, 1990
12. Ruprecht RM, Mullaney S, Andersen J, Bronson R: *In vivo* analysis of castanospermine, a candidate antiretroviral agent. J AIDS 2:149, 1989
13. Gottlinger HG, Sodroski JG, Haseltine WA: Role of the capsid precursor processing and myristoylation in morphogenesis and infectivity of human immunodeficiency virus type 1. Proc Natl Acad Sci USA 86:5781, 1989
14. Kohl NR, Emini EA, Schleif WA et al: Active human immunodeficiency virus protease is required for viral infectivity. Proc Natl Acad Sci USA 85:4686, 1988
15. Loeb DD, Swanstrom R, Everitt L et al: Complete mutagenesis of the HIV-1 protease. Nature 340:397, 1989
16. Peng C, Ho BK, Chang TW, Chang NT: Role of human immunodeficiency virus type 1-specific protease in core protein maturation and viral infectivity. J Virol 63:2550, 1989
17. Gilboa E, Mitra SW, Goff SP, Baltimore D: A detailed model of reverse transcription and tests of crucial aspects. Cell 18:93, 1980
18. Goff SP: Retroviral reverse transcriptase: Synthesis, structure and function. J AIDS 3:817, 1990
19. Lightfoote MM, Coligan JE, Folks TM et al: Structural characterization of reverse transcriptase and endonuclease polypeptide of the acquired immunodeficiency syndrome retrovirus. J Virol 60:771, 1986
20. Chandra P, Vogel A, Gerber T: Inhibitors of retroviral DNA polymerase: Their implication in the treatment of AIDS. Cancer Res 45(suppl):4677, 1985
21. di Marzo Veronese FD, Copeland TD, DeVico AL et al: Characterization of highly immunogenic p66/p51 as the reverse transcriptase of HTLV-III/LAV. Science 231:1289, 1986
22. Prasad VR, Goff SP: Structure-function studies of HIV reverse transcriptase. Proc Natl Acad Sci USA 616:11, 1990
23. Clark PK, Ferris AL, Miller DA et al: HIV-1 reverse transcriptase purified from a recombinant strain of *Escherichia coli*. AIDS Res Hum Retroviruses 6:753, 1990
24. Deibel MR, Jr, McQuade TJ, Brunner DP, Tarpley WG: Denaturation/refolding of purified recombinant HIV reverse transcriptase yields monomeric enzyme with high enzymatic activity. AIDS Res Hum Retroviruses 6:329, 1990
25. Mitsuya H, Broder S: Inhibition of the *in vitro* infectivity and cytopathic effects of human T-lymphotrophic virus type III/lymphadenopathy-associated virus (HTLV-III/LAV) by 2',3'-dideoxynucleosides. Proc Natl Acad Sci USA 83:1911, 1986
26. Mitsuya H, Broder S: Strategies for antiviral therapy in AIDS. Nature 325:773, 1987
27. Ostertag W, Roesler G, Krieg CJ et al: Induction of endogenous virus and of thymidine kinase by bromodeoxyuridine in cell cultures transformed by Friend virus. Proc Natl Acad Sci USA 71:4980, 1974
28. Dube SK, Pragnell IB, Kluge N et al: Induction of endogenous and of spleen focus-forming viruses during dimethylsulfoxide-induced differentiation of mouse erythroleukemia cells transformed by spleen focus-forming virus. Proc Natl Acad Sci USA 72:1863, 1975
29. Mitsuya H, Weinhold KJ, Furman PA et al: 3'-Azido-3'-deoxythymidine (BW A509U): An antiviral agent that inhibits the infectivity and cytopathic effect of human T-lymphotropic virus type III/lymphadenopathy-associated virus *in vitro*. Proc Natl Acad Sci USA 82:7096, 1985
30. Fischl MA, Richman DD, Grieco MH et al: The efficacy of azidothymidine (AZT) in the treatment of patients with AIDS and AIDS-related complex: A double-blind, placebo-controlled trial. N Engl J Med 317:185, 1987

31. Cooney DA, Ahluwalia G, Mitsuya H et al: Initial studies on the cellular pharmacology of 2′,3′-dideoxyadenosine, an inhibitor of HTLV-III infectivity. Biochem Pharmacol 36:1765, 1987

32. Johnson MA, Ahluwalia G, Connelly MC et al: Metabolic pathways for the activation of the antiretroviral agent 2′,3′-dideoxyadenosine in human lymphoid cells. J Biol Chem 263:15354, 1988

33. Furman PA, Fyfe JA, St Clair MH et al: Phosphorylation of 3′-azido-3′-deoxythymidine and selective interaction of the 5′-triphosphate with human immunodeficiency virus reverse transcriptase. Proc Natl Acad Sci USA 83:8333, 1986

34. Nasr M, Litterst C, McGowan J: Computer-assisted structure-activity correlations of dideoxynucleoside analogs as potential anti-HIV drugs. Antiviral Res 14:125, 1990

35. Broder S: Clinical applications of 3′-azido-2′,3′-dideoxythymidine (AZT) and related dideoxynucleosides. Med Res Rev 10:419, 1990

36. Yarchoan R, Mitsuya H, Broder S: Strategies for the combination therapy of HIV infection. J AIDS 3(suppl 2):S99, 1990

37. Mitsuya H, Yarchoan R, Broder S: Molecular targets for AIDS therapy. Science 249:1533, 1990

38. McGowan J, Tomaszewski JE, Cradock J et al: Overview of the preclinical development of an antiretroviral drug, 2′,3′-dideoxyinosine. Rev Infect Dis 12(suppl 5):S513, 1990

39. Larder BA, Darby G, Richman DD: HIV with reduced sensitivity to zidovudine (AZT) isolated during prolonged therapy. Science 243:1731, 1989

40. Richman DD: Susceptibility to nucleoside analogues of zidovudine-resistant isolates of human immunodeficiency virus. Am J Med 88:8S, 1990

41. Marquez VE: Design, synthesis, and antiviral activity of nucleoside and nucleotide analogues. ACS Symp Series 401:140, 1989

42. Balzarini J, Cooney DA, Dalal M et al: 2′,3′-Dideoxycytidine: Regulation of its metabolism and anti-retroviral potency by natural pyrimidine nucleosides and by inhibitors of pyrimidine nucleotide synthesis. Mol Pharmacol 32:798, 1987

43. Ono K, Nakane H, Fukushima M et al: Differential inhibitory effects of various flavonoids on the activities of reverse transcriptase and cellular DNA and RNA polymerases. Eur J Biochem 190:469, 1990

44. Nakane H, Ono K: Differential inhibitory effects of some catechin derivatives on the activities of human immunodeficiency virus reverse transcriptase and cellular deoxyribonucleic and ribonucleic acid polymerases. Biochemistry 29:2841, 1990

45. Schinazi RF, Chu CK, Babu JR et al: Anthraquinones as a new class of antiviral agents against human immunodeficiency virus. Antiviral Res 13:265, 1990

46. Schinazi RF, Eriksson BF, Hughes SH: Comparison of inhibitory activities of various antiretroviral agents against particle-derived and recombinant human immunodeficiency virus type 1 reverse transcriptases. Antimicrob Agents Chemother 33:115, 1989

47. Ono K, Nakane H, Fukushima M et al: Inhibition of reverse transcriptase activity by a flavonoid compound, 5,6,7,-trihydroxyflavone. Biochem Biophys Res Commun 160:982, 1989

48. Merluzzi VJ, Hardgrave KD, Labadia M et al: Inhibition of HIV-1 replication by a non-nucleoside reverse transcriptase inhibitor. Science 250:1411, 1990

49. Pauwels R, Andries K, Desmyter J et al: Potent and selective inhibition of HIV-1 replication *in vitro* by a novel series of TIBO derivatives. Nature 343:470, 1990

50. Lavie G, Valentine F, Mazur B et al: Studies of the mechanisms of action of the antiretroviral agents hypericin and pseudohypericin. Proc Natl Acad Sci USA 86:5963, 1989

51. Meruelo D, Lavie G, Lavie D: Therapeutic agents with dramatic antiretroviral activity and little toxicity at effective doses: Aromatic polycyclic diones hypericin and pseudohypericin. Proc Natl Acad Sci USA 85:5230, 1988

52. Lavie G, Mazur Y, Lavie D et al: Hypericin as an antiretroviral agent: Mode of action and related analogues. Proc Natl Acad Sci USA 616:556, 1990

53. Arya SK, Guo C, Josephs SF, Wong-Staal F: Trans-activator gene of human T-lymphotropic virus type III (HLTV-III). Science 229:69, 1985

54. Feinberg MB, Jarret RF, Aldovini A et al: HTLV-III expression and production involve complex regulation at the levels of splicing and translation of viral RNA. Cell 46:807, 1986

55. Allen JS, Coligan JE, Lee TH et al: A new HTLV-III/LAV encoded antigen detected by antibodies from AIDS patients. Science 230:810, 1985

56. Franchini G, Robert-Guroff M, Ghrayeb J et al: Cytoplasmic localization of the HTLV-III 3′ Orf protein in cultured T cells. Virology 155:593, 1986

57. Lee TH, Coligan JE, Allan JS et al: A new HTLV-III/LAV protein encoded by a gene found in cytopathic retroviruses. Science 231:1546, 1986

58. Ogawa K, Shibata R, Kiyomasu T et al: Mutational analysis of the human immunodeficiency virus *vpr* open reading frame. J Virol 63:4110, 1989

59. Cohen EA, Terwilliger EF, Sodroski JG, Haseltine WA: Identification of a protein encoded by the *vpu* gene of HIV-1. Nature 334:532, 1988

60. Fisher AG, Ensoli B, Ivanoff L et al: The *sor* gene of HIV-1 is required for efficient virus transmission *in vitro*. Science 237:888, 1987

61. Cohen EA, Terwilliger EF, Jalinoos Y et al: Identification of HIV-1 *vpr* product and function. J AIDS 3:11, 1990

62. Strebel K, Klimkait T, Martin MA: A novel gene of HIV-1, *vpu,* and its 16-kilodalton product. Science 241:1221, 1988

63. Fisher AG, Aldovini A, Debouck C et al: The transactivator gene of HTLV-II is essential for virus replication. Nature 320:367, 1986

64. Dayton AI, Sodroski JG, Rosen CA et al: The transactivator gene of the human T cell lymphotropic virus type III is required for replication. Cell 44:941, 1986

65. Sodroski J, Patarca R, Rosen C et al: Location of the trans-activating region on the genome of human T-cell lymphotropic virus type III. Science 229:74, 1985

66. Aldovini A, Debouck C, Feinberg MB et al: Synthesis of the complete trans-activation gene product of human T-lymphotropic virus type III in *Escherichia coli*: Demonstration of immunogenicity *in vivo* and expression *in vitro*. Proc Natl Acad Sci USA 83:6672, 1986

67. Goh WC, Rosen C, Sodroski J et al: Identification of a protein encoded by the trans-activator gene tat III of human T-cell lymphotropic retrovirus type III. J Virol 59:181, 1986

68. Rappaport J, Lee SJ, Khalili K, Wong-Staal F: The acidic amino-terminal region of the HIV-1 Tat protein constitutes an essential activating domain. New Biol 1:101, 1989

69. Sadaie MR, Rappaport J, Benter T et al: Missense mutations in an infectious human immunodeficiency viral genome:

Functional mapping of *tat* and identification of the *rev* splice acceptor. Proc Natl Acad Sci USA 85:63, 1988

70. Ruben S, Perkins A, Purcell R et al: Structural and functional characterization of human immunodeficiency virus Tat protein. J Virol 63:1, 1989

71. Frankel AD, Bredt DS, Pabo CO: Tat protein from human immunodeficiency virus forms a metal-linked dimer. Science 240:70, 1988

72. Garcia JA, Harrich D, Soultanakis E et al: Human immunodeficiency virus type 1 LTR Tat and Tar region sequences required for transcriptional regulation. EMBO J 8:765, 1989

73. Frankel AD, Biancalana S, Hudson D: Activity of synthetic peptides from the Tat protein of human immunodeficiency virus type 1. Proc Natl Acad Sci USA 86:7397, 1989

74. Ensoli B, Barillarti G, Salahuddin SZ et al: Tat protein of HIV-1 stimulates growth of cells derived from Kaposi's sarcoma lesions of AIDS patients. Nature 345:84, 1990

75. Breen EC, Rezai AR, Nakajima K et al: Infection with HIV associated with elevated IL-6 levels and production. J Immunol 144:480, 1990

76. Kekow J, Wachsman W, McCutchan JA et al: Transforming growth factor-β and suppression of humoral immune responses in HIV infection. J Clin Invest 87:1010, 1991

77. Gentz R, Chen CH, Rosen CA: Bioassay for trans-activation using purified human immunodeficiency virus Tat-encoded protein: Trans-activation requires mRNA synthesis. Proc Natl Acad Sci USA 86:821, 1989

78. Jeang KT, Shank PR, Kumar A: Transcriptional activation of homologous viral long terminal repeats by the human immunodeficiency virus type 1 or the human T-cell leukemia virus type 1 Tat protein occurs in the absence of *de novo* protein synthesis. Proc Natl Acad Sci USA 85:8291, 1988

79. Cullen BR: Trans-activation of human immunodeficiency virus occurs via a bimodal mechanism. Cell 46:973, 1986

80. Braddock M, Chambers A, Wilson A et al: HIV-1 Tat activates presynthesized RNA in the nucleus. Cell 58:269, 1989

81. Rosen CA, Sodroski JG, Haseltine WA: The location of *cis*-acting regulatory sequences in the human T cell lymphotropic virus type III (HTLV-III/LAV) long terminal repeat. Cell 41:813, 1985

82. Muesing MA, Smith DH, Capon DJ: Regulation of mRNA accumulation by a human immunodeficiency virus trans-activator protein. Cell 48:691, 1987

83. Laspia MF, Rice AP, Mathews MB: HIV-1 Tat protein increases transcriptional initiation and stabilizes elongation. Cell 59:283, 1989

84. Peterlin BM, Luciw PA, Barr PJ, Walker MD: Elevated levels of mRNA can account for the trans-activation of human immunodeficiency virus. Proc Natl Acad Sci USA 83:9734, 1986

85. Selby MJ, Peterlin BM: Trans-activation by HIV-1 Tat via a heterologous RNA binding protein. Cell 62:769, 1990

86. Marciniak RA, Garcia-Blanco MA, Sharp PA: Identification and characterization of a HeLa nuclear protein that specifically binds to the trans-activation-response (Tar) element of human immunodeficiency virus. Proc Natl Acad Sci USA 87:3624, 1990

87. Dingwall C, Ernberg I, Gait MJ et al: Human immunodeficiency virus 1 Tat protein binds trans-activation-responsive region (Tar) RNA *in vitro*. Proc Natl Acad Sci USA 86:6925, 1989

88. Roy S, Delling U, Chen CM et al: A bulge structure in HIV-1 Tar RNA is required for Tat binding and Tat-mediated trans-activation. Genes Dev 4:1365, 1990

89. Selby MJ, Bain ES, Luciw PA, Peterlin BM: Structure, sequence, and position of the stem-loop in Tar determine transcriptional elongation by Tat through the HIV-1 long terminal repeat. Genes Dev 3:547, 1989

90. Schwartz S, Felber BK, Fenyo EM, Pavlakis GN: Env and Vpu proteins of human immunodeficiency virus type 1 are produced from multiple bicistronic mRNAs. J Virol 64:5448, 1990

91. Jacobovits A, Smith DH, Jacobovits EB, Capon DJ: A discrete element 3' of human immunodeficiency virus 1 (HIV-1) and HIV-2 mRNA initiation sites mediates transcriptional activation by an HIV trans-activator. Mol Cell Biol 8:2555, 1988

92. Kao SY, Calman A, Luciw PA, Peterlin BM: Anti-termination of transcription within the long terminal repeat of HIV-1 by *tat* gene product. Nature 330:489, 1987

93. Berkhout B, Silverman RH, Jeang KT: Tat trans-activates the human immunodeficiency virus through a nascent RNA target. Cell 59:273, 1989

94. Hauber J, Cullen BR: Mutational analysis of the trans-activation-responsive region of the human immunodeficiency virus type 1 long terminal repeat. J Virol 62:673, 1988

95. Feng S, Holland EC: HIV-1 Tat trans-activation requires the loop sequence within Tar. Nature 334:165, 1988

96. Sim IS: The human immunodeficiency virus Tat protein: A target for antiviral agents. Proc Natl Acad Sci USA 616:64, 1990

97. Berger J, Hauber J, Hauber R et al: Secreted placental alkaline phosphatase: A powerful new quantitative indicator of gene expression in eukaryotic cells. Gene 66:1, 1988

98. Hasler JM, Weighous TF, Pitts TW et al: A rapid quantitative bioassay based on the human immunodeficiency virus trans-activator. AIDS Res Hum Retroviruses 5:507, 1989

99. Hsu MC: Tat inhibitors. Presented at a conference on HIV Disease, Pathogenesis and Therapy, Grenelefe, Fla, March 13–14, 1991

100. Debouck C, Metcalf BW: Human immunodeficiency virus protease: A target for AIDS therapy. Drug Dev Res 21:1, 1990

101. Dunn BM, Kay J: Targets for antiviral chemotherapy: HIV-proteinases. Antiviral Chem Chemother 1:3, 1990

102. Johnston MI, Allaudeen HS, Sarver N: HIV proteinase as a target for drug action. Trends Pharmacol Sci 10:305, 1989

103. Louis JM, Smith CA, Wondrak EM et al: Substitution mutations of the highly conserved arginine 87 of HIV-1 protease result in loss of proteolytic activity. Biochem Biophys Res Commun 164:30, 1989

104. Kotler M, Katz RA, Danho W et al: Synthetic peptides as substrates and inhibitors of a retroviral protease. Proc Natl Acad Sci USA 85:4185, 1988

105. Pearl LH, Taylor WR: Sequence specificity of retroviral protease. Nature 328:482, 1987

106. Rich DH, Bernatowicz MS, Agarwal NS et al: Inhibition of aspartic proteases by pepstatin and 3-methylstatine derivatives of pepstatin: Evidence for collected substrate enzyme inhibition. Biochemistry 24:3165, 1985

107. Rich DH, Sun ETO: Mechanism of inhibition of pepsin by pepstatin. Biochem Pharmacol 29:2205, 1980

108. Sham HL: Renin inhibitors: Design and synthesis of a new class of conformationally restricted analogues of angiotensinogen. J Med Chem 31:284, 1988

109. Schnieder J, Kent S: Enzymatic activity of a synthetic 99-residue protein corresponding to the putative HIV-1 protease. Cell 54:363, 1988

110. Nutt RF, Brady SF, Darke PL et al: Chemical synthesis and enzymatic activity of a 99-residue peptide with a sequence proposed for the immunodeficiency virus protease. Proc Natl Acad Sci USA 85:7129, 1988

111. Debouck C, Gorniak JG, Strickler JE et al: Human immunodeficiency virus protease expressed in *Escherichia coli* exhibits autoprocessing and specific maturation of the *gag* precursor. Proc Natl Acad Sci USA 84:8903, 1987

112. Barr PJ, Power MD, Lee-Ng CT et al: Expression of active human immunodeficiency virus reverse transcriptase in *Saccharomyces cerevisiae*. Biotechnology 5:486, 1987

113. Farmerie WG, Loeb DD, Casavant NC et al: Expression and processing of the AIDS virus reverse transcriptase in *Escherichia coli*. Science 236:305, 1987

114. Miller M, Jaskolski M, Rao JK et al: Crystal structure of a retroviral protease proves relationship to aspartic protease family. Nature 337:576, 1989

115. Navia MA, Fitzgerald PM, McKeever BM et al: Three-dimensional structure of aspartyl protease from human immunodeficiency virus HIV-1. Nature 337:615, 1989

116. Wlodawer A, Miller M, Jaskolski M et al: Conserved folding in retroviral proteases: Crystal structure of a synthetic HIV-1 protease. Science 245:616, 1989

117. Lapatto R, Blundell T, Hemmings A et al: X-ray analysis of HIV-1 proteinase at 2.7 A resolution confirms structural homology among retroviral enzymes. Nature 342:299, 1989

118. Miller M, Schneider J, Sathyanarayana BK et al: Structure of complex of synthetic HIV-1 protease with a substrate-based inhibitor at 2.3 A resolution. Science 246:1149, 1989

119. Swain AL, Miller MM, Green J et al: X-ray crystallographic structure of a complex between a synthetic protease of human immunodeficiency virus 1 and a substrate-based hydroxyethylamine inhibitor. Proc Natl Acad Sci USA 87:8805, 1990

120. Tomaszek TA, Magaard VW, Bryan HG et al: Chromophoric peptide substrates for the spectrophotometric assay of HIV-1 protease. Biochem Biophys Res Commun 168:274, 1990

121. Hyland LJ, Dayton BD, Moore ML et al: A radiometric assay for HIV-1 protease. Anal Biochem 188:408, 1990

122. Phylip LH, Richards AD, Kay J et al: Hydrolysis of synthetic chromogenic substrates by HIV-1 and HIV-2 proteinases. Biochem Biophys Res Commun 171:439, 1990

123. Tamburini PP, Dreyer RN, Hansen J et al: A fluorometric assay for HIV-protease activity using high-performance liquid chromatography. Anal Biochem 186:363, 1990

124. Richards AD, Phylip LH, Farmeri WG et al: Sensitive, soluble chromogenic substrates for HIV-1 proteinase. J Biol Chem 265:7733, 1990

125. Matayoshi ED, Wang GT, Krafft GA, Erickson J: Novel fluorogenic substrates for assaying retroviral proteases by resonance energy transfer. Science 247:954, 1990

126. Billich A, Winkler G: Colorimetric assay of HIV-1 proteinase suitable for high-capacity screening. Peptide Res 3:274, 1990

127. Roberts NA, Martin JA, Kinchington D et al: Rational design of peptide-based HIV proteinase inhibitors. Science 248:358, 1990

128. Meek TD, Lambert DM, Dreyer GB et al: Inhibition of HIV-1 protease in infected T-lymphocytes by synthetic peptide analogues. Nature 343:90, 1990

129. Rich DH, Green J, Toth MV et al: Hydroxyethylamine analogues of the p17/p24 substrate cleavage site are tight-binding inhibitors of HIV protease. J Med Chem 33:1285, 1990

130. McQuade TJ, Tomasselli AG, Liu L et al: A synthetic HIV-1 protease inhibitor with antiviral activity arrests HIV-like particle maturation. Science 247:454, 1990

131. Ashorn P, McQuade TJ, Thaisrivongs S et al: An inhibitor of the protease blocks maturation of human and simian immunodeficiency viruses and spread of infection. Proc Natl Acad Sci USA 87:7472, 1990

132. Dreyer GB, Metcalf BW, Tomaszek TA et al: Inhibition of human immunodeficiency virus 1 protease in vitro: Rational design of substrate analogue inhibitors. Proc Natl Acad Sci USA 86:9752, 1989

133. Moelling K, Schulze T, Knoop MT et al: *In vitro* inhibition of HIV-1 proteinase by cerulenin. FEBS Lett 261:373, 1990

134. Blumenstein JJ, Copeland TD, Oroszlan S, Michejda CJ: Synthetic nonpeptide inhibitors of HIV protease. Biochem Biophys Res Commun 163:980, 1989

135. Kempf DJ, Norbeck DW, Codacovi L et al: Structure-based, C2 symmetric inhibitors of HIV protease. J Med Chem 33:2687, 1990

136. Erickson J, Neidhart DJ, VanDrie J et al: Design, activity and 2.8 A crystal structure of a C2 symmetric inhibitor complexed to HIV-1 protease. Science 249:527, 1990

137. DesJarlais RL, Seibel GL, Kuntz ID et al: Structure-based design of nonpeptide inhibitors specific for the human immunodeficiency virus 1 protease. Proc Natl Acad Sci USA 87:6644, 1990

138. Dutia BM, Frame MC, Subak-Sharpe JH et al: Specific inhibition of herpes virus ribonucleotide reductase by synthetic peptides. Nature 321:439, 1986

138a. Paul D, Knigge M, Mack D et al: Anti-HIV activity of protease inhibitors in vitro. J Cellular Biochem 15E:104, 1991

139. Cohen EA, Gaudreau P, Brazeau P, Langelier Y: Specific inhibition of herpes virus ribonucleotide reductase by a nonpeptide derived from the carboxy terminus of subunit 2. Nature 321:441, 1986

140. McClements W, Yamanaka G, Garsky V et al: Oligopeptides inhibit the ribonucleotide reductase of herpes simplex virus by causing subunit separation. Virology 162:270, 1988

141. Babé L, Pichuatnes S, Craik CS: Inhibition of HIV protease activity by heterodimer formation. Biochemistry 30:106, 1991

142. Heuckeroth RO, Jackson-Machelski E, Adams SP et al: Novel fatty acyl substrates for myristoyl-CoA:protein N-myristoyl-transferase. J Lipid Res 31:1121, 1990

143. Bryant ML, Heukeroth RO, Kimata JT et al: Replication of human immunodeficiency virus 1 and Moloney murine leukemia virus is inhibited by different heteroatom-containing analogs of myristic acid. Proc Natl Acad Sci USA 86:8655, 1989

144. Baltimore D: Intracellular immunization. Nature 335:395, 1988

145. Fauci AS, Lane HC: Antiretroviral therapy and immunologic reconstitution in AIDS. Ann Inst Pasteur Immunol 138:261, 1987

146. Sarver N, Cantin E, Chang P et al: Ribozymes as potential anti-HIV-1 therapeutic agents. Science 247:1222, 1990

147. Morgan RA, Looney DJ, Muenchau DD et al: Retroviral vectors expressing soluble CD4: A potential gene therapy for AIDS. AIDS Res Hum Retroviruses 6:183, 1990

148. Poznansky M, Lever A, Bergeron L et al: Gene transfer into human lymphocytes by a defective human immunodeficiency virus type 1 vector. J Virol 65:532, 1991

149. Kotin RM, Siniscalco M, Samulski RJ et al: Site-specific integration by adeno-associated virus. Proc Natl Acad Sci USA 87:2211, 1990

150. Chatterjee S, Wong KK, Rose J, Johnson P: Transduction of intracellular resistance to HIV production by an adeno-associated virus-based antisense vector. In Channock RM, Ginsberg H, Brown F, Lerner RA (eds): Vaccines 91: Modern Approaches to New Vaccines, Including the Prevention of AIDS, p 85. Cold Spring Harbor, New York, Cold Spring Harbor Laboratory, 1991

151. Nabel EG, Plautz G, Nabel G: Site-specific gene expression *in vivo* by direct gene transfer into the arterial wall. Science 249:1285, 1990

152. Lin H, Parmacek MS, Morle G et al: Expression of recombinant genes in myocardium *in vivo* after direct injection of DNA. Circulation 82:2217, 1990

153. Johnston SA: Biolistic transformation: Microbes to mice. Nature 346:776, 1990

154. Wolfe JA, Malone RW, Williams P et al: Direct gene transfer into mouse muscle *in vivo*. Science 247:1465, 1990

20

Antiretroviral Therapy

Azidothymidine and Other Deoxynucleoside Analogues

Douglas D. Richman

An effective antiretroviral drug was identified and licensed only 5 years after the first published description of AIDS and only 3 years after the isolation of the etiologic agent, human immunodeficiency virus (HIV). The unprecedented speed of this medical achievement is gratifying. This drug, azidothymidine (AZT, zidovudine), is neither completely suppressive of disease nor free from toxicity. The impetus for more and better drugs thus has been great. AZT and the majority of the first promising candidate compounds for the treatment of HIV infection have been nucleoside analogues. That this class of compounds should become the first antiretroviral drugs should not be surprising.

The art and science of the synthesis of nucleoside analogues have flourished for decades in the occasionally successful search for anticancer and antiviral drugs. Most such syntheses are reported as accomplishments of organic chemistry but fail to result in a therapeutically useful compound. For example, Horwitz *et al* in 1964[1] and later Lin and Prusoff in 1978[2] reported the synthesis of 3'-azido-3'-deoxythymidine (AZT), which failed to find a role in cancer chemotherapy. The synthesis of 2',3'-dideoxynucleosides[3,4] resulted in the generation of reagents useful for the performance of the Sanger DNA sequencing technique.[5] Nevertheless, with the experience in nucleoside synthesis and the success in identifying effective inhibitors of herpesvirus DNA polymerases, reverse transcriptase was not surprisingly the first target in the replicative cycle of HIV for which an effective compound was identified. Dozens of nucleoside analogues have been shown to inhibit HIV *in vitro*; however, only a small fraction of these successfully overcome the many hurdles between *in vitro* efficacy and clinical utility.

The potential of any candidate compound to be a useful drug depends on the ratio of specific activity (*e.g.,* antiviral) and toxicity. Although factors such as ease of synthesis, stability, and pharmacokinetics are all important, the therapeutic index of a deoxynucleoside analogue as an antiretroviral drug is a function primarily of its intracellular nucleotide metabolites. The drug itself thus represents an extracellular prodrug.

The efficacy (antiretroviral activity) of the deoxynucleoside analogue is a function of two variables: (1) the ability of the cell to transport the drug across its membrane and anabolically phosphorylate the compound to its triphosphate, and (2) the capacity of the deoxynucleoside triphosphate to inhibit the viral reverse transcriptase activity. For example, 2',3'-dideoxythymidine (ddT) triphosphate is as potent an inhibitor of reverse transcriptase activity as is AZT triphosphate[6-8]; however it is approximately 1,000-fold less potent as an antiretroviral agent.[7,9,10] Both AZT and ddT readily diffuse into the host cell.[11] Host cell enzymes recognize AZT as its physiologic deoxynucleoside thymidine; however, ddT is very poorly phosphorylated by host cells.[9] The viral reverse transcriptase in the infected host cell thus does not get exposed to ddT triphosphate.

The toxicity, like the efficacy, of the deoxynucleoside analogues is a function of the ability of the host cell to transport and anabolically phosphorylate the compound. In contrast to efficacy, however, toxicity depends on the capacity of these nucleotides to inhibit host cell enzymes, in contrast to the viral polymerase. A number of potential host cell targets exist. For example, AZT monophosphate inhibits thymidylate kinase.[12] Dideoxycytidine (ddC) competes with ddC-choline metabolism.[13] The host cell DNA polymerases, however, are the prime candidates for host cell targets for toxicity with drugs of this class.

3'-AZIDO-3'-DEOXYTHYMIDINE (ZIDOVUDINE)

In vitro Pharmacology

AZT is a white to off-white, odorless, bitter, crystalline solid with a molecular weight of 267.24 daltons. It is soluble to 25 mg/ml in water at 25° C. It has a pK$_a$ of 9.68 and is relatively stable in solution or at room temperature in crystalline form. AZT is an analogue of thymidine in which the 3'-hydroxyl (−OH) is replaced by an azido (−N$_3$) group (Fig. 20A–1). Because the term thymidine designates a 2'-deoxynucleoside, the term 3'-deoxythymidine or its derivatives designate a 2',3'-

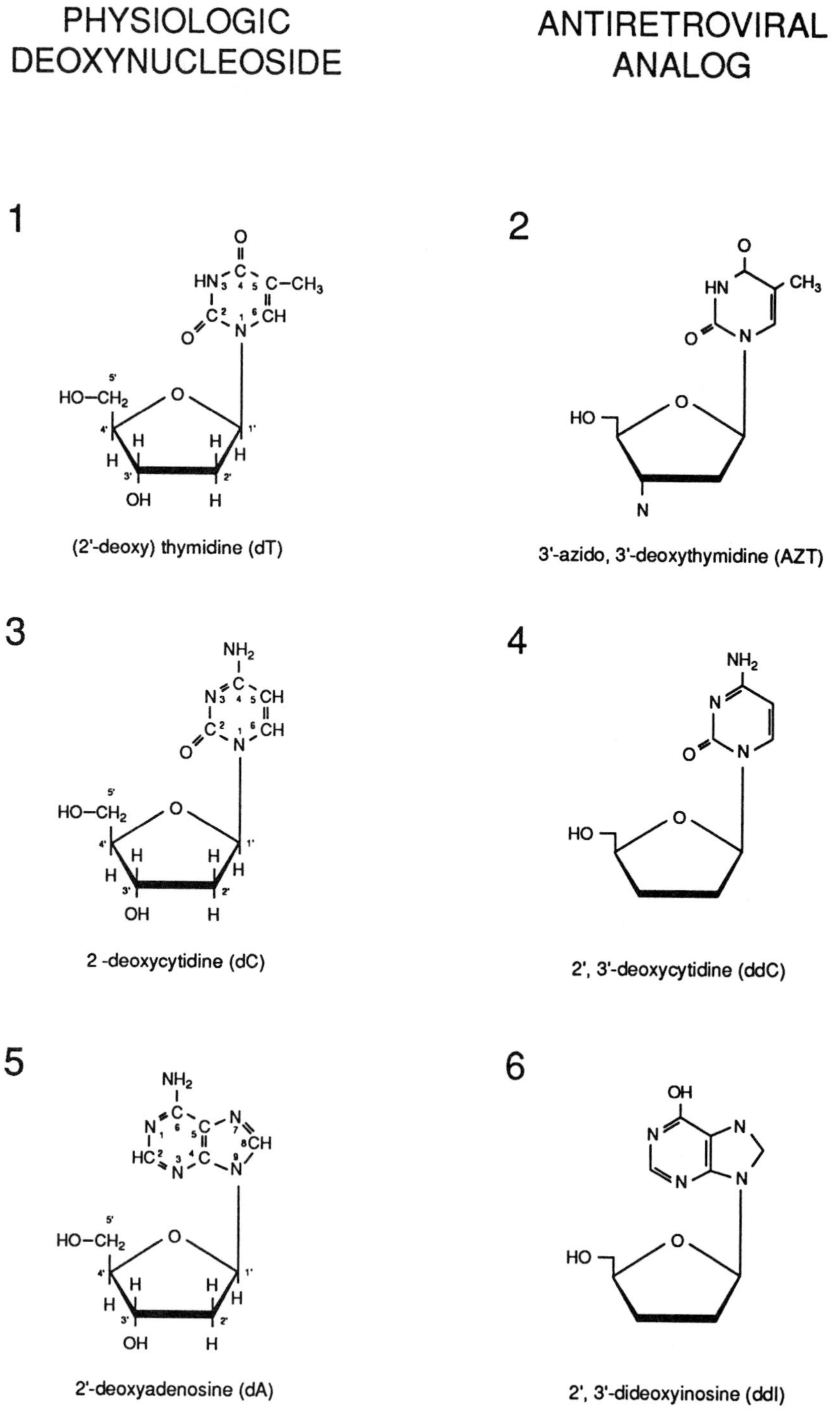

PHYSIOLOGIC
DEOXYNUCLEOSIDE

ANTIRETROVIRAL
ANALOG

1

(2'-deoxy) thymidine (dT)

2

3'-azido, 3'-deoxythymidine (AZT)

3

2-deoxycytidine (dC)

4

2', 3'-deoxycytidine (ddC)

5

2'-deoxyadenosine (dA)

6

2', 3'-dideoxyinosine (ddI)

Figure 20A–1. Chemical structures of nucleoside analogs with extensive clinical use compared to the structure of their corresponding physiologic deoxynucleosides.

dideoxynucleoside. The generic designation for AZT is zidovudine (occasionally abbreviated as ZDV). This term conveys no information, whereas AZT or azidothymidine indicates the structure of the compound and represents the designation in common usage by patients, physicians, and researchers.

In 1985 Mitsuya and colleagues reported that AZT inhibited the replication of HIV in peripheral blood mononuclear cells (PBMC) and several T-cell lines at concentrations of 1 μM, approximately 100-fold less than the toxic concentration for these cells.[14,15] These first assays were performed at high multiplicities of infection and for prolonged periods of infection. With most other assay systems utilizing a variety of cell lines and virus isolates, 50% inhibitory concentrations tend to fall between 0.01 and 0.05 μM.[14,16-20] Many other groups have confirmed similar levels of efficacy with toxicity appearing at 100- to 1,000-fold higher concentrations in human cells with reported exceptions. AZT at concentrations as low as 1 to 10 μM appears to be toxic *in vitro* to normal human erythroid granulocyte-macrophage and primitive hematopoietic progenitor cells[21,22] and to inhibit mitogen-stimulated growth DNA repair in human peripheral lymphocytes.[23] These concentrations approach the peak levels attained in serum. This hypersensitivity to the effects of AZT in marrow cells is reversed by uridine but not thymidine.[17] Both the mechanisms and potential applications of these observations await future investigations.

Unlike the physiologic deoxynucleosides, which are transported across cell membranes, AZT appears to enter cells by nonfacilitated diffusion.[24] The lipophilic 3'-azido group imparts this membrane permeability. Cellular thymidine kinase converts AZT into its monophosphate (Fig. 20A–2).[12] Cellular thymidylate kinase converts the monophosphate into the diphosphate, which is further converted to the triphosphate (AZT-TP), the active antiviral compound, by other cellular enzymes.[12] This anabolic phosphorylation of AZT, an inactive compound, to the active metabolite, AZT-TP, by host cell enzymes indicates the potential host cell influences on antiviral activity. The predominance of AZT monophosphate (AZT-MP) in human cells exposed to AZT[12,25] suggests that thymidylate kinase is the rate-limiting enzyme in the synthesis of the active AZT-TP, which represents only about 1% to 5% of intracellular drug.[12,26] The half-life of intracellular AZT-TP after removal of AZT from the culture medium is approximately 200 minutes.[26] AZT-MP presumably inhibits thymidylate kinase, resulting in this anabolic block and also resulting in the inhibition of phosphorylation of thymidine in cells treated with AZT.[12] This impact on intracellular nucleotide pools has consequences for cell toxicity and antagonism or synergy with other nucleoside drugs.[27-29] This block does not appear to occur in murine cells, in which AZT appears to be more effective both *in vitro* and *in vivo*.[25,30,31] The addition of thymidine reverses both the efficacy and toxicity of AZT, indicating the competition of these drugs for thymidine kinase and the competition of their triphosphates for viral reverse transcriptase and for host DNA polymerases.[14,17,32,33]

AZT-TP, as an analogue of thymidine triphosphate, inhibits the reverse transcriptase of HIV-1 and other lentiviruses *in vitro*.[7,8,33-36] Inhibition of host cell DNA

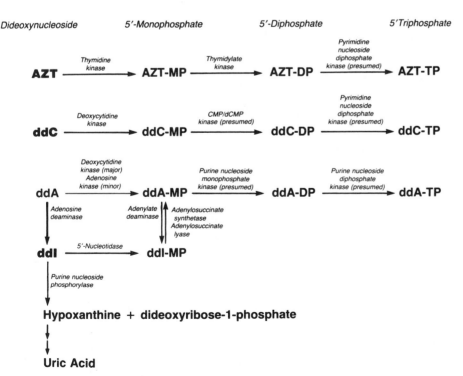

Figure 20A–2. Pathways for anabolic phosphorylation (from[290] with permission).

polymerases α, β, and δ is considerably weaker, presumably accounting for its therapeutic ratio.[6,33,34,37,38] Of note, mitochondrial DNA synthesis appear to be extremely sensitive to AZT-TP *in vitro*,[39] despite one report of low susceptibility of DNA polymerase γ.[38] This sensitivity has been postulated to account for some of the toxicity produced by AZT, especially the myositis.

The DNA polymerase of hepatitis B virus (HBV) is also inhibited by AZT-TP, although with less potency than for retroviral polymerases.[40] Of interest, inhibition by AZT-TP of the DNA polymerase of many gram-negative bacteria results in antibacterial activity.[41] Bacterial resistance readily develops as a consequence of loss of thymidine kinase activity; nevertheless, toxicologic studies of AZT that were undertaken in animals would later prove time-saving in its development as an antiviral agent. Chain termination has been demonstrated with the *E. coli* DNA polymerase.[41,42] Studies *in vitro* with reverse transcriptase and the synthetic template, poly(rA)-oligo(dT),[12–18] have demonstrated chain termination with AZT-TP[34]; however, enzyme kinetic studies have suggested that AZT-TP acts as a competitive substrate inhibitor with respect to thymidine triphosphate.[36] With the incorporation of AZT-TP, a 3′-OH group is no longer available to form a 3′-5′-phosphodiester bond to permit the addition of another nucleotide triphosphate to the DNA chain. The relative importance of chain termination and competition with thymidine triphosphate as the mechanism of action of AZT-TP remains to be determined.

The inhibition of reverse transcriptase prevents the normal production of viral DNA, with a resulting inhibition of transcription and translation. These effects have been documented with several laboratory strains of HIV-1 in PBMC and in many continuous cell lines utilizing as end points cytopathology, the production of reverse transcriptase or of viral antigens, or even T-cell functions.[18] Despite the variation in assay systems, inhibition is observed at concentrations as low as 0.01 μM.[14,16–20] Clinical isolates from patients never administered AZT display little variation in susceptibility to AZT.[20] Other retroviruses examined to date also are inhibited by AZT *in vitro*. These include HTLV-I,[43] avian leukosis virus,[44] several murine retroviruses,[30,45,46] feline leukemia virus,[47] equine infectious anemia virus,[30] simian immunodeficiency virus (SIV),[48] and feline immunodeficiency virus.[49] No antiviral activity has been observed against a broad range of human viruses from other families[50] with the exception of one of the human herpesviruses, Epstein-Barr virus (EBV), for which the 50% effective dose appears to be between 1 and 10 μM.[51]

Although AZT effectively inhibits the replication of cell-free HIV-1, it appears not to inhibit virus production by chronically infected cells or transmission of infection to uninfected cells by syncytium formation.[19,52–54] Two studies, however, have discerned quantitative effects of AZT on chronically infected cells that merit further analysis.[55,56] The addition of AZT after the initial step of reverse transcription has been completed can have a significant impact on virus replication in that cell. Infectious progeny virus can reinfect already infected cells. These reinfections of already infected cells proceed through a step of reverse transcription, producing the accumulation of unintegrated viral DNA and resulting in cytopathology in T lymphocytes.[57] This process of reinfection induces in CD4 lymphocytes programmed cell death, as indicated by endonucleolytic activity of host cell chromosomes known as apoptosis.[58] Extremely low concentrations of AZT inhibit these reinfections and convert a cytolytic infection into a chronic one.[57,58]

Animal Pharmacology and Toxicology

In preclinical toxicologic studies, the median lethal dose of AZT in mice and rats is greater than 750 mg/kg intravenously (IV) and greater than 3,000 mg/kg orally.[59] The IV administration of up to 150 mg/kg/day of AZT for 4 weeks in rats and of up to 85 mg/kg/day for 2 weeks in dogs resulted in no recognized toxicity.[59] Oral administration of 500 mg/kg AZT to beagle dogs produces vomiting and bloody stools. Oral administration of 30 to 100 mg/kg/day of AZT to mice, rats, or monkeys will produce a macrocytic anemia over a period of a month or more.[31,59] Mutagenicity can be detected at 1,000 to 5,000 μg/ml in the L5178Y mouse lymphoma cell mutagenicity assay.[59] Chromosomal aberrations in human lymphocytes cultured in 3 μg/ml AZT and transformation of T3 mouse cells in 0.5 μg/ml occur. No genetic toxicology has been documented in the bacterial mutagenicity assay (Ames test), the marrow cytogenetics of rats assay, or in teratogenicity studies in rats and rabbits.[59]

Use in Animal Models

The expeditious introduction of AZT into clinical trials and the documentation of efficacy preceded the evaluation of AZT in animal models of retrovirus infection. As a consequence, the clinical experience with AZT is being used as the standard by which animal models are being validated, rather than the animal models being used to validate the efficacy of a drug prior to clinical evaluation. AZT administered intraperitoneally or in drinking water from the time of virus inoculation is effective in treating mice infected with the Rauscher murine leukemia virus complex as measured by spleen weight, infectious spleen cells, infectivity titers in plasma, or mortality.[31] The injection of a murine type C retrovirus (designated Cas-Br-E) into embryos produces a progressive neurologic disease in the newborns that is inhibited by administering AZT in the drinking water of the pregnant mothers.[60] This transplacental delivery of drug is encouraging for the potential of treating congenital HIV infection, as well as the treatment of central nervous system (CNS) disease produced by retroviruses. Virus replication and disease are also restricted in models of Friend virus complex and LP-BM5 murine leukemia viruses (murine AIDS) in mice[61,62] and SIV associated with type D retrovirus.[63] AZT administered at or before the time of inoculation can prevent the establishment of infections with feline leukemia viruses,[47,64] and can retard but not prevent infection of cynomologous monkeys with SIV,[65] which supports the possible application of AZT in the postexposure prophylaxis of health care workers. Also of possible clinical relevance, the antibacterial activity of AZT has been translated into *in vitro* efficacy in models of *E. coli* urinary tract infection in mice and *Salmonella dublin* infection in calves.[66]

Clinical Experience

PHASE 1 STUDY AND PHARMACOKINETICS

AZT was the first drug demonstrated to be clinically effective and licensed for use for the treatment of HIV infection. It was first administered to patients in 1985 within only 6 months of the demonstration of its efficacy *in vitro*.[14] In a Phase I dose escalation study in 19 adults with severe HIV infection,[67] AZT was rapidly absorbed from the gastrointestinal tract, with mean peak serum levels attained in about 1 hour. Dose-independent kinetics occurred at doses up to 10 mg/kg every 4 hours. Approximately 60% of ingested drug is bioavailable because of first-passage glucuronidation by the liver.[68] Glucuronidation is mediated effectively by human UDP-glucuronosyltransferase but poorly by the rat enzyme, suggesting why this metabolism occurs in humans but not in some animal models.[69] The glucuronidated metabolite has no apparent toxicity or antiviral activity and, like AZT, is excreted almost exclusively by the kidneys, with a mean half-life of 1 hour. The mean peak serum concentration of AZT in an adult administered 200 mg is approximately 1.5 to 10 μM, with significant individual variability.[68,70] Peak levels are lower but absorption is more prolonged when AZT is ingested with fatty meals.[71] The renal clearance of AZT is approximately 350 ml/min/70 kg, and total body clearance is approximately 1900 ml/min/70 kg at doses of up to 5 mg/kg.[72] In patients with impaired renal function, the half-life of AZT is only slightly prolonged because of rapid hepatic glucuronidation.[73] The glucuronide of AZT (GAZT) does accumulate in patients with reduced creatinine clearance.[74] Toxic effects resulting from chronically elevated levels of GAZT have not been appreciated. Mild to moderate impairment of liver function associated with hepatitis in hemophiliacs had little significant impact on AZT pharmacokinetics.[75] The rate of glucuronidation is significantly reduced and the half-life is thus significantly prolonged in proportion to the degree of hepatic impairment in cirrhotics.[76] Dosage adjustments may thus be indicated in such patients.

The half-life of AZT is prolonged by co-administration of probenecid, which competes both for hepatic glucuronidation and for renal tubular secretion.[77,78] Pharmacokinetic interactions with several other drugs, including acetaminophen, co-trimoxazole, ganciclovir, acyclovir, and ddC, have not been documented.[79–83]

AZT penetrates into the cerebrospinal fluid (CSF) well, with CSF-plasma ratios of 50% to 100% at least 4 hours after the first dose.[68,80] The excellent transport into the CSF may result from the lipophilicity of AZT, which permits nonfacilitated diffusion across cell membranes.[11,24] Semen concentrations of AZT ranged from 1.3- to 20-fold higher than serum levels when studied in six patients, suggesting pH-dependent trapping of AZT, which is a weak base (pK$_a$ = 9.68).[84] There is no evidence for a concomitant reduction in virus titers in semen. AZT also crosses the placenta in mice and monkeys[60,85] and enters the milk of mice,[60] encouraging investigation of its use in pregnant women. Slight differences in pharmacokinetic parameters appear to occur in pregnant women antepartum and postpartum.[86] Umbilical cord levels just exceed maternal serum levels.[86,87]

In addition to pharmacokinetic data, the Phase I study generated anecdotal evidence of some toxic effects during the 6-week regimen (headaches and leukopenia), which were manageable. Therapeutic benefits were also suggested in several patients, including weight gain, improved sense of well-being, improved CD4 lymphocyte counts, and return of delayed-type hypersensitivity skin test reactions. These observations prompted the design of a multicenter, randomized, placebo-controlled, double-blind study.[88,89]

EFFICACY

Two hundred eighty-two patients with either a first episode of *Pneumocystis carinii* pneumonia diagnosed within 120 days or with advanced AIDS-related complex (ARC) were stratified according to CD4 lymphocyte counts and then randomly assigned to receive either placebo or 250 mg of AZT orally every 4 hours for 24 weeks. One hundred forty-five subjects receiving AZT and 137 receiving placebo entered the study between February and June of 1986. The study was terminated on September 18, 1986, by an independent monitoring board because 19 placebo recipients and one AZT recipient had died (p < 0.001). At that time 27 subjects had completed 24 weeks of study, 152 had completed 16 weeks, and the remainder had completed at least 8 weeks. In addition to prolonging survival, AZT therapy reduced the frequency and severity of opportunistic infections, improved body weight, prevented deterioration in the Karnofsky performance score, increased peripheral CD4 lymphocyte counts, and reversed skin test anergy in many patients. Of note, the rates of opportunistic infections in the AZT and placebo groups did not begin to diverge until after 6 to 8 weeks of therapy, which suggests that the recovery of some immune function may be independent of and delayed with respect to recovery of CD4 lymphocyte counts.

An elevation in CD4 lymphocyte counts, a reduction in p24 antigenemia, increased platelet counts, weight gain, improved neurologic function, and an improved sense of well-being may all occur within the first 2 weeks of therapy. CD4 lymphocyte counts rise to a median of

30 to 50 cells above pretherapy values, attaining peak values within 2 to 4 weeks,[89-93] then gradually fall to baseline values over a period of 16 to 40 weeks, the shorter periods occurring in populations with more advanced disease. Of note, responses show great interindividual variation, with some patients showing no elevation of counts, and in others, counts increasing by 100 to 200 cells/mm^3 or more. In patients with more than 500 CD4 cells/mm^3 before receiving AZT, the CD4 count tends not to increase in response to AZT therapy.[91] Study populations with no symptoms or with advanced disease responded no better to 1,200 to 1,500 mg AZT/day than to 500 to 600 mg/day.[90,92] In a study with limited numbers of study subjects, 50 mg, 100 mg, and 200 mg given every 4 hours all appeared to produce similar CD4 cell responses.[93] In another small study utilizing concurrent ddC, 50 mg, 100 mg, and 200 mg of AZT given every 8 hours appeared to result in a dose-response effect on CD4 cell number, and 50 mg every 8 hours of AZT alone appeared to induce a real but suboptimal response.[83]

Of note, data are accumulating to suggest that only a small part of the clinical benefit observed with AZT therapy can be attributed to CD4 elevations (A. Tsiatis and M. Fischl, pers. commun.). Thus, either CD4 cell function or other parameters of immune function that we do not now assay are ameliorated by AZT therapy. This observation is consistent with the dissociation in the original study of the appearance of CD4 cell count elevations and impact on opportunistic infections and death.[88] Several nonspecific serum markers of mononuclear cell activation, like β_2-microglobulin, neopterin, serum immunoglobulins, soluble CD8, and soluble CD4 levels, return toward normal with AZT therapy.[94-96]

With regard to virus replication, AZT does not reduce isolation rates from PBMC,[89,93,97,98] although it does appear to reduce virus infectivity titers in the CSF[98] and in plasma by approximately 90%.[93,99] Much investigation is being directed toward identifying useful assays to quantitate HIV replication. Until these are developed and validated, the enzyme-linked immunosorbent assay (ELISA) for p24 antigen in serum or plasma remains a useful assay of antiretroviral drug activity. The assay is highly standardized and reproducible; however, p24 antigenemia is present in only a proportion of patients, and its biologic significance is not well delineated.

In the original placebo-controlled study, viral p24 antigenemia was significantly reduced by AZT therapy.[88] This reduction in p24 antigenemia with AZT administration and its rise following withdrawal of drug has been observed by several investigators.[97,100-104] In some patients the level of p24 antigenemia may increase even though the patient continues to ingest drug. The mechanism by which this occurs is unknown.

In parallel with CD4 cell responses, p24 responses have not appeared to be dose related between 1,500 and 300 mg/day[90,92,93]; however, 50 mg given orally every 8 hours to a small number of patients with advanced stages of HIV infection appeared to reduce p24 anti-

genemia in a smaller proportion of patients than did the higher doses.[83] AZT also has consistently cleared p24 antigen from the CSF in a high proportion of patients.[97,103,105,106]

The administration of AZT has been associated with anecdotal reports of significant neurologic improvement.[107-109] These observations have been supported by neuropsychological assessments of the subjects participating in the placebo-controlled study. AZT partially reversed and delayed further deterioration in cognitive dysfunction, as assessed by tests of memory and attention, for example.[110] No improvement was appreciated on measures of affective symptoms. The remarkable neuropsychological benefits in adults and children with more advanced disease is also encouraging,[101,109,111,112] as is the observation that AZT therapy has significantly reduced the incidence of AIDS dementia complex.[113]

Thrombocytopenia may be another specific complication of HIV infection to respond to the administration of AZT. Although AZT is toxic to cells of the erythroid and granulocytic series, slight mean increases were observed in platelet counts in the Phase II study.[89] Several case reports have appeared describing significant improvements in thrombocytopenia associated with the administration of AZT.[114-116] Prospective placebo-controlled studies of patients with thrombocytopenia documented an impressive impact of AZT on this condition.[98,117] Neither the mechanism of the thrombocytopenia nor how AZT reverses it has been elucidated. A beneficial response of HIV-associated nephropathy has also been reported.[118]

On a greater scale, however, the introduction of AZT administration to patients with advanced HIV infection in 1986 and 1987 appears to have been associated in a number of epidemiologic studies with significant reductions in the incidence of new cases with AIDS-defining opportunistic events and of AIDS-related mortality.[113,119-122] A favorable response to AZT has been reported in a patient with advanced disease due to HIV-2 infection.[123] Despite some *in vitro* activity against hepadnaviruses, no activity against chronic HBV infection has been observed.[124]

TOXICITY

Although significant clinical benefit has been documented with AZT, serious adverse clinical reactions occur, particularly bone marrow suppression.[89] In the Phase II, placebo-controlled trial, nausea, myalgia, insomnia, and severe headaches were reported more frequently by recipients of AZT.[89] These adverse symptoms usually resolve over the first 1 to 4 months if the patient can tolerate sustained therapy.[125] The symptoms are occasionally, but not usually, worse or more frequent at higher doses.[90,125]

Anemia with hemoglobin levels below 7.5 g/dl developed in 24% of AZT recipients and in 4% of placebo recipients (p < 0.001) of the original patient population with advanced infection.[89] These patients had an increased requirement for transfusions with packed red blood cells. Macrocytosis developed within weeks in most of the AZT group. Of note, not all patients with macrocytosis developed anemia, and not all episodes of anemia were macrocytic. Erythropoietin levels are increased in the presence of red cell hypoplasia.[126] Neutropenia (<500 cells/mm^3) occurred in 15% of AZT recipients, as compared with 2% of placebo recipients ($p < 0.001$). Subjects who entered the study with low CD4 lymphocyte counts, low serum vitamin B12 levels, anemia, or low neutrophil counts were more likely to have hematologic side-effects. Prolonged marrow failure has been associated with AZT administration.[127] Although marrow toxicity with AZT is more likely the more severe the underlying disease, no absolute predictors of susceptibility to toxic side-effects are available.[89] Moreover, the underlying mechanism of marrow insufficiency in HIV infection remains obscure.

An apparent increased association of hematologic toxic effects with acetaminophen administration[89] may not hold up with further scrutiny. No other association of drug interactions was appreciated in the Phase II study.[89] Ganciclovir (DHPG), a drug in widespread use in a number of patients with AIDS, has significant additive toxicity on granulocytes with AZT to the extent that the two drugs often cannot be safely co-administered at AZT doses as low as 300 mg/day.[82] This toxicity cannot be accounted for by pharmacokinetic interaction.[82]

A myositis-like syndrome, characterized by parathesias, myalgias, muscle edema, muscle wasting, and elevations in serum lactate dehydrogenase and creatinine phosphokinase levels, has also been associated with prolonged AZT administration,[128-132] although a similar syndrome also occurs in untreated patients infected with HIV.[133-139] Accumulating clinical experience indicates that prolonged AZT therapy produces weakness and muscle wasting in a proportion of patients, especially those with more advanced HIV disease. The muscles of AZT-treated patients with myositis display ragged-red fibers indicative of mitochondrial degeneration and loss.[129] This pathology has not been readily distinguishable from the myositis associated with HIV infection,[129] and the two conditions may in fact have additive effects. Depletion of mitochondrial DNA in patients with AZT-induced myopathy may be due to inhibition of mitochondrial DNA polymerase γ.[140]

Anecdotal reports of infrequent toxic effects, for example seizures, have also been published. These reports are always difficult to interpret. Seizures occur in patients with AIDS, even in the absence of neuroradiologic abnormalities that are suggestive of cerebral toxoplasmosis or malignancy. The question is whether AZT adds an additional, but small, risk for seizures. Although none of the original 282 study patients, 127 of whom received drug for more than 1 year, were reported to have had seizures, several case reports of seizures temporarily associated with administration of AZT were reported once thousands of patients were receiving drug.[141-143] Anec-

dotal reports of other effects such as post-AZT withdrawal meningitis[144] have not yet been confirmed by others.

The initial report of nail pigmentation in a black patient taking AZT[145] has been confirmed with general experience.[146] With tens of thousands of patients having been administered AZT, anecdotal reports of adverse experiences such as macular edema[147] and hepatotoxicity[148] are difficult to interpret. Many patients referred for AZT-associated hepatotoxicity have proved to have mycobacterial or cytomegaloviral disease (unpubl. observ.). Esophageal ulceration associated with nighttime administration without water[149] may be obviated by three or five times daily regimens. Several significant overdoses of AZT (7 to 36 g) with suicidal intent have been remarkably well tolerated,[150-155] with one measured serum level as high as 185 μM.[150] One of these patients experienced seizures with no long-term sequelae after a dose of 36 g.[153]

EXPANDED CLINICAL EXPERIENCE

The monitoring of the Phase II study patients suggested continued benefit with prolonged therapy.[156] Survival rates of patients treated with AZT were higher than might have been expected from previous experience with similar patients. Patients continued to experience episodes of opportunistic infections; however, these infections were either of decreased severity or were more responsive to conventional therapy. Hematologic toxic effects continued to be the major laboratory abnormality associated with drug administration; however, new or more frequent toxic effects were not observed with more prolonged therapy.[156] Progressive bone marrow suppression did not appear to be associated with prolonged administration.

Additional experience has extended and confirmed these observations on efficacy and toxicity in patient populations with HIV infection. These populations included 4,805 patients in the compassionate plea program following the placebo-controlled study; patients in France, Canada, and Australia; and inner-city populations that include minorities and IV drug users.[125,157-160]

Three large multicenter trials of the AIDS Clinical Trials Group (ACTG) of the National Institute of Allergy and Infectious Diseases (NIAID) have yielded data with important implications, not only for the use of AZT but for antiretroviral chemotherapy in general. These important implications involve the application of therapy to patients with HIV infection before significant disease develops and the principle that efficacy does not continue to accrue as the dose of drug is escalated. ACTG study 016 demonstrated that patients with 200 to 500 CD4 lymphocytes/mm^3 and one or two symptoms of ARC were less likely to experience disease progression if they were administered the originally licensed dose of 200 mg orally every 4 hours than if they were given a placebo (Table 20A–1).[91] The probability of disease

Table 20A–1. Correlation of Risk of Progression With CD4 T-Lymphocyte Count Before Treatment and With AZT Treatment

CD4 T-Lymphocyte Count Before Treatment	No. of Subjects in Whom Disease Progressed*			
	Overall	Placebo Group	Zidovudine Group	p Value†
Total subjects, n	711	351	360	
200–300 cells/mm³, n/n	19/140	12/64	7/76	0.04
300–400 cells/mm³, n/n	15/209	12/101	3/108	0.01
400–500 cells/mm³, n/n	12/168	10/90	2/78	0.06
>500 cells/mm³, n/n	5/194	2/96	3/98	0.63

* Number of subjects in whom disease progressed/total number of subjects.
† By log rank tests.
Data indicate both the correlation of risk to progression of disease with CD4 lymphocyte count and the impact of AZT therapy on that risk in patients with CD4 lymphocyte counts below 500 cells/mm³. In this study, AIDS Clinical Trials Group protocol 016, subjects with one or two symptoms of AIDS-related complex were randomized to AZT (200 mg every 4 hours) or placebo. Progression was defined as AIDS or new symptoms and a CD4 cell count below 200 cells/mm³.
Data reproduced with permission from Fischl *et al.*[91]

progression in the placebo recipients was inversely related to the CD4 T-lymphocyte count at entry into the study. In subjects with more than 500 CD4 cells/mm³, the probability of progression during the 2-year observation period was so small that no benefit of therapy could be discerned. In subjects with fewer than 500 CD4 cells/mm³, however, the risk of progression was reduced by just over 50%, regardless of the probability of progression at entry based on such predictions of risk as CD4 cell count, symptoms, or HIV p24 antigenemia (see Table 20A–1). Serious anemia and neutropenia occurred respectively in 5% and 4% of AZT recipients. These levels of toxicity were significantly lower than those described in subjects with more advanced stages of infection, an indication that underlying HIV disease diminishes the margin of tolerance for many drug toxic effects.

ACTG study 019 was conducted in asymptomatic subjects seropositive for HIV.[90] The study reinforced the conclusions that AZT delayed the progression of disease with acceptable levels of toxicity in patients infected with HIV and less than 500 CD4 lymphocytes/mm³ (Fig. 20A–3). In the population with more than 500 CD4 lymphocytes/mm³, no benefit was discernible for the first 2 years of observation, and that component of the study has continued. ACTG study 019 also examined the issue of drug dose. Subjects were randomized to a placebo arm, a high-dose AZT arm of 300 mg orally every 4 hours while awake (equivalent to the total daily dose of 1,500 mg in the original Phase II study), or a low-dose AZT arm of 100 mg five times daily. The subjects in both the high- and low-dose arms had lower rates of disease progression than the placebo recipients, and the lower rates mirrored the benefits observed in ACTG 016. The he-

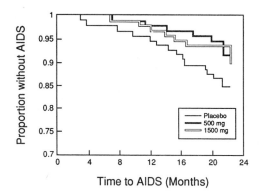

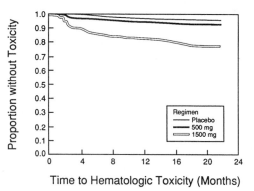

Figure 20A–3. Effect of two different doses of AZT on progression of HIV disease and on drug toxicity. In AIDS Clinical Trials Group protocol 019 asymptomatic, HIV-infected study subjects with less than 500 CD4 lymphocytes/mm³ were randomized to 500 mg AZT daily, 1500 mg AZT daily, or placebo. (**A**) Progression of disease was reduced equivalently by both doses of AZT. (**B**) Hematologic toxicity did occur at 1500 mg AZT orally per day, but the rates in subjects receiving 500 mg daily approached those on placebo. (From [90] with permission.)

matologic toxic effects of the low dose (500 mg/day) were barely increased over those seen in the placebo recipients, while the toxic effects of the higher dose resembled those seen with the 1,200-mg dose in the ACTG 016 study. Two major conclusions were thus generated by ACTG study 019. First, AZT can delay the progression to disease in asymptomatic patients with fewer than 500 CD4 cells/mm³. Second, toxicity, but not benefit, increases with an increasing daily dose of AZT.

ACTG study 002 reinforced these conclusions regarding dose in patients with AIDS.[92] Five hundred twenty-four patients who had experienced one episode of *P. carinii* pneumonia were randomized to either 250 mg orally every 4 hours or 200 mg every 4 hours for 1 month, followed by 100 mg every 4 hours. The higher dose represented the regimen in the original Phase II placebo-controlled study. The recipients of the lower dose fared at least as well as those given the higher dose, and experienced less toxicity. ACTG studies 002 and 019 thus indicate that the chemotherapy of HIV might not reflect the paradigm developed for oncologic chemotherapy, in which benefit is thought to accrue until the maximally tolerated dose is approached. Both ACTG study 002 and ACTG study 019 indicated that AZT had been administered in doses that were too high, and that less toxicity and perhaps longer and more sustained therapy will be possible in the future, with little if any loss of efficacy, at doses of only 500 to 600 mg/day. This lower dosage will also benefit combination drug regimens.

Concerns have been raised regarding the possibility that AZT might not work in ethnic or racial minorities[161] and that it might be associated with increased rates of non-Hodgkin's lymphoma.[162] A Veterans Administration cooperative study was undertaken to examine the ability of AZT to prevent the progression of disease in a specific racial or ethnic population. As was seen in ACTG protocol 016, blacks and Hispanic whites who were treated early with AZT fared worse than those treated late.[161] Many suspect that this observation resulted from a statistical fluke from a *post hoc* analysis of the study not designed to address this question. Two analyses of other study populations have not been able to confirm any racial or ethnic differences in clinical effects.

The National Cancer Institute's experience with the prolonged use of AZT in a highly selected study population showed a high rate of non-Hodgkin's lymphoma.[162] Many clinicians are appreciating a higher prevalence of lymphoma in patients with advanced HIV infection. This experience is probably not due to cumulative exposure to AZT *per se*.[163] It is probable that more lymphomas are seen because AZT prolongs the lifetime of patients with advanced immunosuppression and because chemoprophylaxis reduces the incidence of opportunistic infections in this population.

AZT therapy can delay both disease and death. Despite the cost of the drug, estimates of the cost-effectiveness for of AZT in the treatment of both ad-

vanced and asymptomatic HIV infection have been favorable.[164,165] The specter of AZT increasing the pool of potential transmitters of disease[166] or of increasing viral resistance to drug therapy cannot be invoked to discourage treatment of the individual who seems likely to benefit.

PEDIATRIC USE

The pharmacokinetics of AZT are similar in adults and children, although younger children tend to have increased rates of clearance.[101,111,167] This observation, and the potential benefit of sustained drug levels, prompted studies of the delivery of AZT by continuous infusion.[101,167] Children also appear to tolerate the drug at least as well as adults. A similar beneficial impact of AZT on weight gain, p24 antigenemia, and CD4 lymphocyte counts occurs in children.[101,111] One of the noteworthy aspects of HIV infection in children is its remarkable impact on the developing nervous system. This frequent complication of pediatric HIV infection has permitted the documentation of the beneficial impact of AZT on dementia and delayed developmental milestones in children.[101,111,112] The published experience and a number of issues unique to the chemotherapy of HIV infection in the pediatric population are addressed in detail elsewhere.[168]

MANAGEMENT OF TOXIC EFFECTS

Although suppression of p24 antigenemia has not been proven to correlate with clinical outcome, the return of p24 antigenemia within a week or 2 of a significant reduction in or withdrawal of AZT therapy argues that AZT should be conceived of as a suppressive regimen.[104] This problem raises the issue of the proper management of toxic drug effects. Adverse reactions, including nausea, insomnia, and headaches, occur in many patients taking AZT. Most endure these symptoms because of the potential benefit and find that the reactions subside with time.[125] Occasionally a patient will find the symptoms intolerable and elect to discontinue treatment.

The management of hematologic toxic effects is a more frequent problem. Many physicians have treated anemia alone with packed red blood cell transfusions while maintaining therapy with AZT. With a hemoglobulin below 10 that is still dropping, the dose of AZT should probably be reduced to 100 mg every 8 hours. Erythropoietin clearly will benefit some patients, but its proper use requires further definition at this early stage in its use.[169,170] The appropriate time to switch to an alternative nucleoside is also a matter of judgment that will benefit from additional data. Some patients with anemia can be maintained on AZT therapy at reduced doses for long periods; for others, anemia is the harbinger of granulocytopenia.

Granulocytopenia requires dose reduction. Once again, there are no data to argue a best method for dose reduction. The magnitude of fall from baseline granulocyte counts and the rate of fall influence modification. One guideline is to reduce the dosage to 100 mg every 8 hours if the neutrophil count falls below 800 cells/mm³ and to discontinue the drug at a count of 400 to 500 cells/mm³. The co-administration of other drugs like ganciclovir, co-trimoxazole, or pyrimethamine may contribute to granulocytopenia, and alternatives should be considered. If AZT must be withdrawn on two or three occasions, then the potential harm, effort, and cost of further attempts to administer AZT should be avoided. Similarly, if a serious opportunistic infection develops (*e.g.,* serious CMV retinitis) for which a treatment is deemed necessary (ganciclovir), then AZT should be discontinued rather than the indicated treatment delayed. As with the management of anemia, the timing of administration and the role of granulocyte-macrophage colony-stimulating factor (GM-CSF),[171,172] granulocyte colony-stimulating factor (G-CSF),[173] or alternative nucleoside therapy require judgment that will benefit from additional data. The recognition and management of myopathy have not been precisely defined. Whether to monitor for signs and symptoms or to assay quarterly for elevated creatinine phosphokinase levels has been debated. Nonsteroidal anti-inflammatory drugs and steroids have been recommended,[129,130] but these would be expected to affect the myositis associated with HIV more than the drug-induced mitochondrial toxicity. Controlled studies have not been reported. The benefit of alternative nucleosides has not been investigated, although one should be concerned that these also inhibit mitochondrial DNA polymerase γ (see below).

RESISTANCE

The emergence of AZT resistance in patients with AIDS or ARC has raised new considerations in regard to the use of the drug and the design of new drug regimens.[20] Little variation in AZT sensitivity was seen in isolates from patients never treated with AZT. No reduction in sensitivity was documented during the first 6 months of treatment. After 6 months, most isolates replicate in the presence of higher concentrations of AZT. Many isolates exhibit more than 100-fold increases in resistance and replicate at drug concentrations not attainable with normal doses of drug. Mutations in 4-amino acid residues of the reverse transcriptase gene of HIV have to date been associated with AZT resistance, and the progressive accumulation of mutations is associated with a stepwise increase in the degree of resistance.[174] Although the emergence of resistance has not yet been demonstrated to be associated with diminished drug efficacy, this is a reasonable concern.[175]

It is encouraging that AZT-resistant isolates retain their susceptibilities to most other agents. Only nucleosides with 3'-azido moieties, for example, 3'-azido-3'-deoxyuridine (AZdU) and 3'-azido-3'-deoxyguanosine (AZG), have so far been shown to have diminished inhibitory activity against AZT-resistant isolates. Cross-resistance to other nucleosides or to compounds of other classes with antiretroviral activity has not yet been observed.[176]

An extension of the study of isolates from patients on prolonged AZT therapy to isolates from subjects administered AZT at earlier stages of disease, specifically the subjects in ACTG studies 016 and 019, has indicated that in the latter patients, resistance develops significantly more slowly than in patients with AIDS or advanced ARC.[177] The likelihood that resistant virus will emerge under the selective pressure of prolonged therapy increases as the CD4 lymphocyte count falls. The emergence of resistance is a function of mutation rate and replication rate. It is increasingly apparent that the level of viral replication ("virus load") increases as the immune status diminishes.[99,178] It is also encouraging that the lower dose regimens utilized in ACTG studies 002 and 019 did not select for resistant virus more readily than the higher dose regimens.[177]

The likelihood that resistance will develop after 1 year of therapy in a patient with AIDS or advanced ARC is 90%. By contrast, isolates from a patient with 200 to 500 CD4 lymphocytes/mm³ and few or no symptoms indicate a 30% likelihood of measurably diminished susceptibility to AZT.[177] The clinical significance of drug resistance may depend on the quantitative reduction of sensitivity. If a greater than 100-fold reduction in susceptibility to AZT is looked for, it is found within 12 months in one third of isolates from the higher risk patients, but the same degree of reduction in susceptibility to AZT is found only occasionally in patients with earlier stage disease after 2 years of therapy.[177,179]

The impact of drug resistance on the responses to antiretroviral chemotherapy and the consequences of other drugs and drug combinations on these responses will require further investigation.

DIDEOXYCYTIDINE (ddC)

In vitro Pharmacology

Dideoxycytidine is the 3'-deoxy analogue of the physiologic deoxynucleoside, 2'-deoxycytidine. The cellular metabolism of ddC appears even less complicated than that of AZT. It enters the cell by the nucleoside transport system and is anabolized to the triphosphate by deoxycytidine kinase and subsequent cellular enzymes in the phosphorylation of deoxycytidine (see Fig. 20A–2).[13,180–182] Of note, the requirement for facilitated transport across cell membranes may account for the limited entry of ddC into the CSF.[11] A high proportion of intracellular nucleotide is ddC-TP.[13,183,184] In contrast to AZT, ddC is poorly phosphorylated by murine cells.[13,25] The mouse may thus be a poor model with which to evaluate ddC.[185] As with AZT, the physiologic nucleoside (deoxycytidine in the case of ddC) competes with both the efficacy and the toxicity of ddC *in vitro*.[13,181,183,185,186] The addition of thymidine to cells significantly enhances the phosphorylation of ddC,[181] presumably by reducing the intracellular nucleotide pools.

This is the basis for the well-documented potential for synergy or antagonism between combinations of nucleoside analogues.[27,28] Cells do not appear able to deaminate ddC enzymatically; however, metabolism of some drug to ddC-choline does occur.[13]

ddC-TP inhibits reverse transcriptase to confer its antiviral activity.[187] Chain termination does occur *in vitro*.[42] The selectivity of ddC is based on the lower susceptibility of human DNA polymerase α and β to ddC-TP.[183,188] Of note, mitochondrial DNA polymerase γ is as sensitive as reverse transcriptase,[183,189] which with ddC treatment *in vitro* results in cytotoxicity and selective loss of mitochondrial DNA.[189,190] The mechanisms of the distinctive and often nonoverlapping toxic effects of the deoxynucleoside analogues, such as AZT and ddC, are as yet poorly characterized. For example, either ddC-choline inhibition of myelination or ddC-TP inhibition of mitochondrial DNA polymerase γ could theoretically produce neuropathy.

ddC was selected for clinical development before ddA and ddI for several reasons. It is more potent than AZT *in vitro,* with activity demonstrable at concentrations as low as 0.01 μM in some assay systems,[15] although it is less sensitive in other assay systems, with 50% inhibitory concentrations between 0.1 and 1 μM.[9,20] It is also resistant to deamination[13,183] and phosphorolytic cleavage of base from sugar. It was well absorbed from the GI tract, had uncomplicated pharmacokinetics in pilot animal studies, and appeared nontoxic in animals.[42,191]

Animal Pharmacology and Toxicology

No toxic effects of ddC were identified in rodents at any single dose that could be administered, or with 1,000 mg/kg administered orally three times daily for 5 days, or with peritoneal infusions of 47 mg/kg/day for 1 week. The only toxic effect seen was some decrease in bone colony-forming units cultured *in vitro* from mice receiving the infusion. In dogs receiving constant IV infusions for 5 days, soft, blood-tinged stools became apparent at a dosage of 3.53 mg/kg/hr. In dogs, oral or parenteral doses approaching 100 mg/kg/day for 4 weeks resulted in similar toxic GI effects and moderate thrombocytopenia and anemia. It must be remembered that nucleoside anabolism varies significantly among species, and that has important implications for the use of animals models to determine efficacy and toxicity. Following the first clinical trials of ddC, high-dose oral administration of drug to *Cynomolgus* monkeys resulted in peripheral neuropathy (W. Soo, pers. commun.). Some macaques administered 15 to 30 mg/kg IV developed neuropathy; all exhibited lethargy and hematologic toxic effects.[192]

The pharmacokinetics of ddC in mouse, dog, and rhesus monkey indicate some species variation. Oral bioavailability is 100% in monkeys and dogs, but 30% to 50% in mice.[193] The elimination half-life is 2 hours in monkeys and dogs but 1 hour in mice.[193] The total body clearance rate is 9.5 to 12 ml/min/kg in the monkey, 5 to 6 ml/min/kg in the dog, and 30 to 50 ml/min/kg in the mouse. Penetration of ddC into the CSF is 3% to 4% of the plasma level in monkeys.[193] The drug is excreted, predominantly as the parent compound, in the urine.[193]

Use in Animal Models

High-dose prophylactic administration of ddC to cats delayed the onset of antigenemia following inoculation with feline leukemia virus and suppressed disease expression until drug therapy was withdrawn.[194,195] The drug delayed the onset of antigenemia but did not prevent infection with SIV in cynomolgus monkeys[65] or with simian retrovirus type 2 in pigtail macaques.[192] Although susceptible *in vitro,*[63] ddC even at toxic levels had no inhibitory activity in naturally infected macaques.[192] The triphosphate of ddC is a potent inhibitor of the DNA polymerase of duck HBV and its animal relatives.[196] ddC inhibited virus replication of HBV in the Peking duck model.[197]

Clinical Experience

The peak concentration of ddC is roughly proportional to the administered dose, and a peak concentration of 0.5 μM was observed after a 1-hour infusion of 0.06 mg/kg.[198] The peak concentration was 8 ng/ml after ingestion of a 0.5-mg tablet.[199] The serum levels thus attained with standard doses were much lower than the 50% inhibitory concentration *in vitro.* Consequently the Phase I study started with a dose that proved too high, and the explanation for the activity of the dose that is in current use (0.75 mg orally q.8h.) is elusive. The plasma half-life was approximately 1 to 2 hours, with renal clearance accounting for drug elimination.[198,199] Oral bioavailability was 70% to 80%. CSF concentrations of drug were 9% to 37% of concurrent plasma levels 2 to 3.5 hours after an IV infusion.[198] No evidence of metabolism of ddC has been noted.

The Phase I studies also indicated that ddC decreased circulating p24 antigenemia, as does AZT; however, at dosages of 0.03 to 0.09 mg/kg every 4 hours, it produced a moderate dermatitis and mucositis in the first few weeks of therapy, some neutropenia and thrombocytopenia, and, more important, a severe peripheral neuropathy in the second or third month of therapy.[198] In a study with a larger dosage range, 0.06 and 0.03 mg/kg given orally every 4 hours produced a diffuse erythematous rash and aphthous stomatitis during the first weeks of therapy; these effects resolved without necessitating interruption of drug administration.[200] Hematologic toxic effects were notably rare. Peripheral sensory neuropathy occurred in all patients at these doses between week 4 and week 14 and improved slowly in most patients after discontinuation of ddC. Serum p24 antigen levels fell significantly (by more than

70%) in most patients during therapy. CD4 cell numbers tended to rise transiently on study; however, no clear difference in skin test positivity or rate of HIV isolation from blood coculture positivity was seen. At dosages of 0.01 and 0.005 mg/kg given orally every 4 hours, skin rashes and aphthous stomatitis were mild or absent. Peripheral neuropathy, which occurred by weeks 12 to 14 in all patients taking 0.01 mg/kg orally every 4 hours, was less severe and resolved more quickly than at higher doses. Significant suppression of serum p24 antigen levels was seen in many patients taking 0.01 mg/kg orally every 4 hours. Thus, ddC therapy has clear dose-related toxic effects and dose-related effects on CD4 lymphocyte counts and p24 antigenemia.[201] Several Phase I/II studies were necessary to identify a dosage (0.75 mg every 8 hours) that appeared to retain the drug's effects on viral and immunologic markers with a tolerable frequency of toxic effects.[201] At this dosage, approximately 10% to 20% of patients will experience a mild peripheral sensory neuropathy that resolves with prompt cessation of therapy.

Although these initial studies indicated that ddC may have a limited role as a single drug for the treatment of HIV infection, several encouraging observations prompted the evaluation of alternating and combination regimens of ddC and AZT.[83,198,202] First, ddC significantly reduced p24 antigenemia, an effect seen previously only with AZT. Second, ddC resulted in little hematologic toxicity. Thus, these two dideoxynucleosides with favorable effects on p24 antigenemia and CD4 lymphocyte counts have significant but nonoverlapping toxic effects. These observations form the rationale for protocols with alternating and combination regimens of AZT and ddC: the goal is to reduce toxic effects while maintaining antiviral benefits. The clinical role of ddC will be more clearly defined when results become available from a number of Phase II/III studies in progress that are evaluating ddC therapy alone or combined with AZT in several patient populations.

DIDEOXYINOSINE (ddI, DIDANOSINE)

In vitro Pharmacology

Dideoxyinosine is the deaminated 3'-deoxy analogue of the physiologic deoxynucleoside, 2'-deoxyadenosine. HIV-1 replication is inhibited in most continuous cell lines at 1 to 10 μM ddI and in primary macrophage cultures at 0.1 to 1 μM.[9,15,176] The generation of active triphosphates from ddA and ddI is much more complicated than for AZT or ddC (see Fig. 20A–2). Adenosine deaminase, which is abundant in serum and cells, rapidly deaminates ddA to ddI.[203,204] Intracellular ddI is then converted to the monophosphate, ddI-MP,[204,205] and ddI-MP is then aminated to ddA-MP.[205] The active triphosphate is then generated by a series of enzymatic steps that convert ddI-MP to ddA-TP *via* ddA-MP and ddA-DP.[206] These pathways may thus be subject to variability

among different cells[207,208] and to complex interactions with other nucleosides. As with AZT-TP and ddC-TP, ddA-TP inhibits the activity of reverse transcriptase of HIV,[42,187] other lentiviruses,[30] and host cell DNA polymerases,[188,203] as well as duck hepadnavirus DNA polymerase.[196] The half-life of ddA-TP in cells after removal of ddI or ddA from the culture medium appears to be quite long—8 to 24 hours.[209] This long half-life provided the rationale for evaluating ddI in Phase I trials in once- or twice-daily regimens.

Animal Pharmacology and Toxicology

Continuous IV infusions of ddA in dogs at 31 mg/kg/hr resulted in steady-state plasma levels of 1.5 μg/ml (6 μM) ddA and 25 μg/ml (95 μM) ddI. No toxic effects were observed during 10 days of infusion at these levels, which exceed the antiviral levels by at least an order of magnitude. Higher infusion levels produce hypotension and tachycardia.

ddA is deaminated completely to ddI in minutes in the dog, rat, and mouse.[210] In the dog the elimination half-life of ddI is 73 minutes and the total body clearance rate is 4 to 5 ml/kg/min. Orally administered ddA produces gastric irritation and undergoes hydrolysis to base and sugar unless it is administered with a buffer.[210] Reliable oral bioavailability data will thus depend on formulation. In rats and dogs, high doses of ddA given orally result in the generation of a nephrotoxic catabolite in the gut. Large doses in animals result in anemia and leukopenia.[211] In dogs, chronic administration of large doses produces toxic effects in multiple organs, including the liver, heart, kidney, and pancreas. Because ddI and ddA appear to be interconverted by cellular metabolism and yield equivalent levels of the active ddA-triphosphate, ddI has been selected between the two for clinical evaluation.

Clinical Experience

Even when ddA is administered by IV infusion it is deaminated so rapidly and quantitively to ddI that only ddI is detectable in the serum.[212] Because of its acid lability, orally administered ddI must be buffered. Approximately 25% to 40% of buffered ddI is orally bioavailable.[212,213] The peak plasma concentrations attained with the currently administered doses are approximately 4 to 8 μM.[213] The serum half-life is 60 to 90 minutes[213]; however, as noted earlier, the intracellular half-life of the active metabolite ddA-TP is sufficiently long to justify oral administration once or twice a day. The CSF concentration after an IV infusion was 21% of the plasma level.[212] Approximately 36% of an IV dose was recovered unchanged in the urine,[212] with the remaining drug presumably metabolized to hypoxanthine and uric acid. Serum uric acid levels rise approximately 1 to 3 mg, as do serum triglyceride levels, in subjects administered ddI chronically.[214]

Three Phase I/II studies have been reported involving 129 adults with AIDS or ARC.[213-216] These escalating-dose studies suggest that elevations of CD4 lymphocyte counts and a reduction in p24 antigenemia begin to occur at daily oral doses of 3 to 4 mg/kg.[214]

Daily doses above 10 to 12 mg/kg result in painful peripheral neuropathy and pancreatitis in a majority of patients.[213,215,216] As with ddC, the interval to onset and the intensity of symptoms of the neuropathy appear to be dose dependent with ddI.[213] Not surprisingly, ddC-induced neuropathy is exacerbated by ddI therapy.[217] Very little hematologic toxicity has been observed. Approximately 20% of patients develop diarrhea that is attributed to the osmotic load of the buffering agent, 5.2 g of citrate-phosphate buffer, in the sachet formulation rather than to the nucleoside itself.

Pancreatitis is the most serious toxic effect of ddI and is occasionally fatal. At the doses under investigation in Phase II/III studies and in the expanded access program (167 to 375 mg given orally twice a day), approximately 3% to 6% of patients develop clinical pancreatitis and elevated serum amylase levels; however, insufficient data have been published to define precisely the incidence rates and relative risk factors. Asymptomatic elevations in amylase levels may serve as a warning to discontinue therapy. The one clear risk factor for the development of pancreatitis, and a contraindication to the prescription of ddI, is a prior history of pancreatitis. Amylasemia associated with parotitis may also occur with the administration of ddI. The mechanism of these toxic effects has not been established.

The licensure of ddI in late 1991 provided an alternative antiretroviral for general clinical use. The initial clinical indications were for patients intolerant of AZT or who were clinically failing on AZT. Informed judgments regarding the relative roles of AZT and ddI must await the controlled clinical trials of the AIDS Clinical Trials Group, which are scheduled for completion in 1992.

OTHER DEOXYNUCLEOSIDE ANALOGUES

Dozens of nucleoside analogues have been shown to inhibit the replication of HIV selectively or, as the triphosphate, to inhibit reverse transcriptase activity *in vitro*. Several of these analogues will be entering clinical trials. Because assay systems for antiviral activity and cell toxicity vary with each investigator, strict comparisons are difficult. Hundreds of analogues have been synthesized and tested for antiretroviral activity. Analysis of structure-activity relationships have elucidated some patterns, at the very least identifying structures that are associated with inactivity.[218]

Dideoxynucleosides with activity against HIV also include dideoxyguanosine (ddG).[9] The 3'-azido derivatives of deoxyguanosine (AZG) and several pyrimidines, such as azidodeoxyuridine, are promising *in vitro*,[219-223] as are the 3'-fluoro derivatives of ddT and ddG but not of ddA or ddC.[222,224-230] 2,6-Diaminopurine and 2',3'-deoxyriboside and its 3'-fluoro and 3'-azido derivatives are effective *in vitro*.[225,231,232]

Compounds with selective activity against HIV include the unsaturated 2',3'-didehydro derivatives of ddC and ddT, termed 2',3'-didehydrodideoxycytosine (ddeC or d4C) and 2',3'-didehydrodideoxythymidine (ddeT or d4T).[10,224,233-238] The 2',3'-didehydropurines are relatively ineffective[219,232,239,240]; however, carbovir, the carbocyclic equivalent of didehydrodideoxyguanosine, has a promising selectivity index against HIV-1 *in vitro*.[6,241-244]

Oxytanocin, a nucleoside with a 4-membered sugar ring, and its derivatives also appear to inhibit the replication of HIV *in vitro*.[245-247] With the success of acyclovir and ganciclovir, effective antiherpes nucleoside drugs with acyclic sugar analogues, compounds of this class have been screened for antiretroviral activity. Among the most promising are 9-phosphonylmethoxyethyl derivatives of adenine (PMEA) and its related derivatives.[248-250] Analogous to acyclovir and its relatives, these compounds may structurally resemble a physiologic, cyclic nucleoside and undergo phosphorylation at a carbon resembling the 5'-carbon.[251] Another series of compounds with an acyclic component instead of sugar are 9-(4,-hydroxy-1',2'-butadienyl)adenine (termed adenallene) and its cytosine equivalent (termed cytallene).[252]

Properties in addition to antiviral activity may be incorporated into drug design. For example, one possible limitation to the use of ddA and ddI is their susceptibility to gastric acid–catalyzed hydrolysis of the glycosidic bond. The derivative 2'-fluoro-ddA is more resistant to this acid-catalyzed hydrolysis; however, most antiretroviral activity is lost.[253] Its stereoisomer 2'-fluoro-ara-ddA is resistant to hydrolysis and retains antiretroviral activity comparable to that of ddA,[253,254] as do several other 2'-halo-containing pyrimidines.[255,256]

Factors in addition to *in vitro* potency and toxicity, such as preclinical animal toxicology and constraints on synthesis and pharmacokinetics, may dictate which nucleosides progress to clinical trial. In addition to AZT, ddC, and ddI, AZdU and d4T have entered Phase I/II clinical trials. D4T appears to be less inhibitory than AZT when monophosphorylated on thymidylate kinase and to produce less toxicity in certain *in vitro* and animal models.[26,257,258]

By early 1992, at least three nucleosides in addition to AZT, ddI, and ddC were in clinical trial. D4T was shown in studies not yet published to be active in increasing CD4 lymphocyte counts and reducing p24 antigenemia. It also, like ddC and ddI but not like AZT, produced a dose-dependent, toxic peripheral neuropathy. Further studies were planned to identify a regimen with a satisfactory ratio of activity to toxicity and to compare this regimen in larger trials to AZT.

Two other nucleosides were in phase I/II clinical

evaluation, 3'-fluoro-ddT and 2'-deoxy-3'-Thiacytidine.[259] The (−) enantiomer of the latter compound, which is known as 3TC and is substantially less toxic but equally effective to the (+) enantiomer *in vitro*, is in phase I/II clinical evaluation.

COMBINATION THERAPY WITH NUCLEOSIDES

Because of the complexity and severity of advanced HIV infection, polypharmacy has become a necessary component of therapy. In addition to the treatment of opportunistic infections and malignancies, reasons for adding drugs to nucleoside therapy include prophylaxis for infection, amelioration of drug toxicity, and immunomodulation. Acyclovir was originally proposed for use because of data suggesting that it might enhance the *in vitro* activity of AZT[239]; however, this effect has not been well substantiated *in vitro* and *in vivo*.[93] It is the prophylactic activity of acyclovir against herpesvirus that has generated more recent investigation, to a large extent based on the early encouraging study from Europe and Australia.[267] The two drugs have been shown to have independent pharmacokinetics.[80,81] Erythropoietin, GM-CSF, and G-CSF are of interest for their potential to ameliorate the hematologic toxic effects of AZT.[169–173] Interleukin-2 has been considered as an immunomodulator that might enhance the benefits of AZT. Documentation of its role will require further investigation.

It is the combinations of nucleosides with each other and with other antiretrovirals that may have the greatest impact on the chemotherapy of HIV infection. Analogous to the chemotherapy of tuberculosis and malignancies, such combinations may provide additive or synergistic efficacy and delay the emergence of resistant virus.

In vitro Studies

With nucleosides being among the first antiretrovirals accessible, it is important to assess their combined effects *in vitro*. Because of their interaction on phosphorylation rates and nucleotide pools, antagonism or synergy is possible. For example, ribavirin was early demonstrated to antagonize the activity of AZT, although it enhances the activity of dideoxypurines.[27,28] The combination of AZT and ddC that has entered clinical trials is additive or slightly synergistic.[27,185,268] AZT has also been reported to be synergistic *in vitro* with other reverse transcriptase inhibitors, including nucleosides,[269] foscarnet,[270] and the nonnucleoside BI-RG-587, which resulted in a combination index for synergy below 0.2.[265] By contrast, no effect was observed with ansamycin (rifabutine) at clinically attainable concentrations, although the AZT-ansamycin combination has some activity at very high concentrations.[271]

Drugs that have activity at the earliest steps of virus replication, binding, and penetration have consistently shown synergy with AZT. These drugs include the polyanionic polymers, among them dextran sulfate[272–276] and recombinant soluble CD4 and its derivatives.[277,278] Other reports of *in vitro* antiretroviral studies of combinations have shown synergy of ampligen and AZT,[279] synergy of AZT and the glycosylation inhibitor castanospermine,[280] and lack of interaction of AZT and isoprinosine.[281]

The first drug shown to have synergy with AZT *in vitro* was the recombinant interferon-α (IFN-α).[282] With the clinical availability of these two compounds, the most extensive experience with combination chemotherapy has been with AZT and IFN-α.

Clinical Studies

The encouraging synergy *in vitro* between AZT and IFN-α has been nicely confirmed in a mouse model with a quantitative assay for viremia with Rauscher leukemia virus.[283] The combinations permitted significant dose reductions to maintain efficacy while diminishing drug toxicity. Moreover, with this model of postexposure prophylaxis, when the drugs were given 4 hours after virus challenge, disease was prevented and protective immunity was induced. After cessation of therapy, animals were resistant to rechallenge with infectious virus. The addition of human IFN-α to AZT also had encouraging effects for both prophylactic and therapeutic use for short periods in cats infected with feline leukemia virus, although neutralizing antibodies to the human protein developed after several weeks of therapy.[62,284]

Human clinical experience with the combination was undertaken initially for the treatment of Kaposi's sarcoma.[285–287] A pilot study of 12 asymptomatic patients using AZT and lymphoblastoid IFN-α suggested additive toxicity, but the study design did not permit definite conclusions to be drawn about toxicity or efficacy end points.[288] The larger studies in patients with Kaposi's sarcoma have defined the limits of tolerance with the combination.[285–287] Interferon did not appear to affect AZT pharmacokinetics. At 600 mg/day of AZT, over one half of patients could not tolerate IFN-α at doses of more than 10 million units/day. Neutropenia was the primary toxic effect, but anemia, fatigue, and hepatotoxicity were also dose limiting in some patients. In one study the addition of IFN-α appeared to delay virus isolation from PBMC[285]; however, studies specifically designed to assess virologic and immunologic markers will be needed to assess the potential of the combination as antiretroviral therapy.

A Phase I/II study of 56 patients receiving various regimens of AZT and ddC in combination indicated the lack of pharmacokinetic interaction, no toxicity unexpected from either drug alone, and effects on CD4 cells and p24 antigen levels suggestive of responses greater in magnitude and duration than with AZT alone.[83] A Phase II/III study is in progress to assess these impressions. The combination of AZT and the CD4-IgG hybrid molecule,[289] despite encouraging *in vitro* synergy, has failed to show additive effects on virologic or immunologic markers (unpub. observ.).

The era of antiretroviral combination chemotherapy has just begun, and nucleoside analogues will almost certainly represent basic components of such regimens.

REFERENCES

1. Horwitz JP, Chua J, Noel M: Nucleosides: V. The monomesylates of 1-(2'-deoxy-β-D-lyxofuranosyl) thymine. J Organ Chem 29:2076, 1964
2. Lin T-S, Prusoff WH: Synthesis and biological activity of several amino analogues of thymidine. J Med Chem 21:109, 1978
3. Robins MJ, Robins RK: The synthesis of 2',3'-dideoxyadenosine from 2'-deoxyadenosine. J Am Chem Soc 86:3585, 1964
4. Horwitz JP, Chua J, Noel M, Donatti JT: Nucleosides: XI. 2',3'-dideoxycytidine. J Organ Chem 32:817, 1967
5. Sanger F, Nicklen S, Coulson AR: DNA sequencing with chain-terminating inhibitors. Proc Natl Acad Sci USA 74:5463, 1987
6. Parker WB, White EL, Shaddix SC et al: Mechanism of inhibition of human immunodeficiency virus type 1 reverse transcriptase and human DNA polymerase α, β, and γ by the 5'-triphosphates of carbovir, 3'-azido-3'-deoxythymidine, 2',3'-dideoxyguanosine, and 3'-deoxythymidine. J Biol Chem 266:1754, 1991
7. Frank KB, McKernan PA, Smith RA, Smee DF: Visna virus as an in vitro model for human immunodeficiency virus and inhibition by ribavirin, phosphonoformate, and 2',3'-dideoxynucleosides. Antimicrob Agents Chemother 31:1369, 1987
8. Prasad VR, Myrick K, Haseltine W, Goff SP: Expression of enzymatically active reverse transcriptase of simian immunodeficiency virus in bacteria: Sensitivity to nucleotide analogue inhibitors. Virology 179:896, 1990
9. Mitsuya H, Broder S: Inhibition of the in vitro infectivity and cytopathic effect of human T-lymphotrophic virus type III/lymphadenopathy-associated virus (HTLV-III/LAV) by 2',3'-dideoxynucleosides. Proc Natl Acad Sci USA 83:1911, 1986
10. Hamamoto Y, Nakashima H, Matsui T et al: Inhibitory effect of 2',3'-didehydro-2',3'-dideoxynucleosides on infectivity, cytopathic effects, and replication of human immunodeficiency virus. Antimicrob Agents Chemother 31:907, 1987
11. Domin BA, Mahony WB, Zimmerman TP: 2',3'-dideoxythymidine permeation of the human erythrocyte membrane by nonfacilitated diffusion. Biochem Biophys Res Commun 154:825, 1988
12. Furman PH, Fyfe JA, St. Clair MH et al: Phosphorylation of 3'-azido-3'-deoxythymidine and selective interaction of the 5'-triphosphate with human immunodeficiency virus reverse transcriptase. Proc Natl Acad Sci USA 83:8333, 1986
13. Cooney DA, Dalal M, Mitsuya H et al: Initial studies on the cellular pharmacology of 2',3'-dideoxycytidine, an inhibitor of HTLV-III infectivity. Biochem Pharmacol 35:2065, 1986
14. Mitsuya H, Weinhold KJ, Furman PA et al: 3'-azido-3'-deoxythymidine (BW A509U): An antiviral agent that inhibits the infectivity and cytopathic effect of human T-lymphotropic virus type III/lymphadenopathy-associated virus in vitro. Proc Natl Acad Sci USA 82:7096, 1985
15. Perno C-F, Yarchoan R, Cooney DA et al: Inhibition of human immunodeficiency virus (HIV-1/HTLV-IIIBa-L) replication in fresh and cultured human peripheral blood monocytes/macrophages by azidothymidine and related 2',3'-dideoxynucleosides. J Exp Med 168:1111, 1988
16. Richman DD, Kornbluth RS, Carson DA: Failure of dideoxynucleosides to inhibit human immunodeficiency virus replication in cultured human macrophages. J Exp Med 166:1144, 1987
17. Sommadossi JP, Carlisle R, Schinazi RF, Zhou Z: Uridine reverses the toxicity of 3'-azido-3'-deoxythymidine in normal human granulocyte-macrophage progenitor cells in vitro without impairment of antiretroviral activity. Antimicrob Agents Chemother 32:997, 1988
18. Lyerly HK, Cohen OJ, Weinhold KJ: Transmission of HIV by antigen presenting cells during T-cell activation: Prevention by 3'-azido-3'-deoxythymidine. AIDS Res Hum Retroviruses 3:87, 1987
19. Nakashima H, Matsui T, Harada S et al: Inhibition of replication and cytopathic effect of human T cell lymphotropic virus type III/lymphadenopathy-associated virus by 3'-azido-3'-deoxythymidine in vitro. Antimicrob Agents Chemother 30:933, 1986
20. Larder BA, Darby G, Richman DD: HIV with reduced sensitivity to zidovudine (AZT) isolated during prolonged therapy. Science 243:1731, 1989
21. Sommadossi JP, Carlisle R: Toxicity of 3'-azido-3'-deoxythymidine and 9-(1,3-dihydroxy-2-propoxymethyl)guanine for normal human hematopoietic progenitor cells in vitro. Antimicrob Agents Chemother 31:452, 1987
22. Dainiak N, Worthington M, Riordan MA et al: 3'-azido-3'-deoxythymidine (AZT) inhibits proliferation in vitro of human haematopoietic progenitor cells. Br J Haematol 69:299, 1988
23. Munch-Petersen B: Azidothymidine inhibits mitogen stimulated growth and DNA-repair in human peripheral lymphocytes. Biochem Biophys Res Commun 157:1369, 1988
24. Zimmerman TP, Mahony WB, Prus KL: 3'-azido-3'-deoxythymidine. J Biol Chem 262:5748, 1987
25. Balzarini J, Pauwels R, Baba M et al: The in vitro and in vivo anti-retrovirus activity, and intracellular metabolism of 3'-azido-2',3'-dideoxythymidine and 2',3'-dideoxycytidine are highly dependent on the cell species. Biochem Pharmacol 37:897, 1988
26. Ho H-T, Hitchcock MJM: Cellular pharmacology of 2',3'-dideoxy-2',3'-didehydrothymidine, a nucleoside analog active against human immunodeficiency virus. Antimicrob Agents Chemother 33:844, 1989
27. Baba M, Pauwels R, Balzarini J et al: Ribavirin antagonizes inhibitory effects of pyrimidine 2',3'-dideoxynucleosides but enhances inhibitory effects of purine 2',3'-dideoxynucleosides on replication of human immunodeficiency virus in vitro. Antimicrob Agents Chemother 31:1613, 1987
28. Vogt MW, Hartshorn KL, Furman PA et al: Ribavirin antagonizes the effect of azidothymidine on HIV replication. Science 235:1376, 1987
29. Frick LW, Nelson DJ, St. Clair MH et al: Effects of 3'-azido-3'-deoxythymidine on the deoxynucleotide triphosphate pools of cultured human cells. Biochem Biophys Res Commun 154:124, 1988
30. Dahlberg JE, Mitsuya H, Blam SB et al: Broad spectrum antiretroviral activity of 2',3'-dideoxynucleosides. Proc Natl Acad Sci USA 84:2469, 1987

31. Ruprecht RM, O'Brien LG, Rossoni LD et al: Suppression of mouse viremia and retroviral disease by 3'-azido-3'-deoxythymidine. Nature 323:467, 1986

32. Szebeni J, Patel SS, Hung K et al: Effects of thymidine and uridine on the phosphorylation of 3'-azido-3'-deoxythymidine (zidovudine) in human mononuclear cells. Antimicrob Agents Chemother 35:198, 1991

33. Huang P, Farquhar D, Plunkett W: Selective action of 3'-azido-3'-deoxythymidine 5'-triphosphate on viral reverse transcriptases and human DNA polymerases. J Biol Chem 265:11914, 1990

34. St. Clair MH, Richards CA, Spector T et al: 3'-azido-3'-deoxythymidine triphosphate as an inhibitor and substrate of purified human immunodeficiency virus reverse transcriptase. Antimicrob Agents Chemother 31:1972, 1987

35. Vrang L, Oberg B, Lower J, Kurth R: Reverse transcriptases from human immunodeficiency virus type 1 (HIV-1), HIV-2, and simian immunodeficiency virus (SIV mac) are susceptible to inhibition by foscarnet and 3'-azido-3'-deoxythymidine triphosphate. Antimicrob Agents Chemother 32:1733, 1988

36. Reardon JE, Miller WH: Human immunodeficiency virus reverse transcriptase. J Biol Chem 265:20302, 1990

37. Vrang L, Bazin H, Remaud G et al: Inhibition of the reverse transcriptase from HIV by 3'-azido-3'-deoxythymidine triphosphate and its threo analogue. Antiviral Res 7:139, 1987

38. Cheng Y-C, Dutschman GE, Bastow KF et al: Human immunodeficiency virus reverse transcriptase. J Biol Chem 262:2187, 1987

39. Simpson MV, Chin CD, Keilbaugh SA et al: Studies on the inhibition of mitochondrial DNA replication by 3'-azido-3'-deoxythymidine and other dideoxynucleoside analogs which inhibit HIV-1 replication. Biochem Pharmacol 36:1033, 1989

40. Nordenfelt E, Löfgren B, Chattopadhyaya J, Öberg B: Inhibition of hepatitis B virus DNA polymerase by 3'-azido-3'-deoxythymidine triphosphate but not by its threo analog. J Med Virol 22:231, 1987

41. Elwell LP, Ferone R, Freeman GA et al: Antibacterial activity and mechanism of action of 3'-azido-3'-deoxythymidine (BW A509U). Antimicrob Agents Chemother 31:274, 1987

42. Mitsuya H, Jarrett RF, Matsukura M et al: Long-term inhibition of human T-lymphotropic virus type III/lymphadenopathy-associated virus (human immunodeficiency virus) DNA synthesis and RNA expression in T cells protected by 2',3'-dideoxynucleosides in vitro. Proc Natl Acad Sci USA 84:2033, 1987

43. Matsushita S, Mitsuya H, Reitz MS, Broder S: Pharmacological inhibition of in vitro infectivity of human T lymphotropic virus type 1. J Clin Invest 80:394, 1987

44. Olsen JC, Furman P, Fyfe JA, Swanstrom R: 3'-azido-3'-deoxythymidine inhibits the replication of avian leukosis virus. J Virol 61:2800, 1987

45. Ostertag W, Roesler G, Krieg CJ et al: Induction of endogenous virus and of thymidine kinase by bromodeoxyuridine in cell cultures transformed by Friend virus. Proc Natl Acad Sci USA 71:4980, 1974

46. Krieg CJ, Ostertag W, Clauss U et al: Increase in intracisternal A-type particles in Friend cells during inhibition of Friend virus (SFFV) release by interferon or azidothymidine. Exp Cell Res 116:21, 1978

47. Tavares L, Roneker C, Johnston K et al: 3'-azido-3'-deoxythymidine in feline leukemia virus-infected cats: A model for therapy and prophylaxis of AIDS. Cancer Res 47:3190, 1987

48. Mitsuya H, Broder S: Inhibition of infectivity and replication of HIV-2 and SIV in helper T-cells by 2',3'-dideoxynucleosides in vitro. AIDS Res Hum Retroviruses 4:107, 1988

49. Remington KM, Chesebro B, Wehrly K et al: Mutants of feline immunodeficiency virus resistant to 3'-azido-3'-deoxythymidine. J Virol 65:308, 1991

50. De Clercq E, Balzarini J, Descamps J, Eckstein F: Antiviral, antimetabolic and antineoplastic activities of 2'- or 3'-amino or -azido-substituted deoxyribonucleosides. Biochem Pharmacol 29:1849, 1980

51. Lin JC, Zhang ZX, Smith MC et al: Anti-human immunodeficiency virus agent 3'-azido-3'-deoxythymidine inhibits replication of Epstein-Barr virus. Antimicrob Agents Chemother 32:265, 1988

52. Smith MS, Brian EL, Pagano JS: Resumption of virus production after human immunodeficiency virus infection of T lymphocytes in the presence of azidothymidine. J Virol 61:3769, 1987

53. Nakashima H, Tochikura TS, Kobayashi N et al: Effect of 3'-azido-2',3'-dideoxythymidine (AZT) and neutralizing antibody on human immunodeficiency virus (HIV)–induced cytopathic effects: Implication of giant cell formation for the spread of virus in vivo. Virology 159:169, 1987

54. Poli G, Orenstein JM, Kinter A et al: Interferon-α but not AZT suppresses HIV expression in chronically infected cell lines. Science 244:575, 1989

55. Pincus SH, Wehrly K: AZT demonstrates anti-HIV-1 activity in persistently infected cell lines: Implications for combination chemotherapy and immunotherapy. J Infect Dis 162:1233, 1990

56. Rooke R, Tremblay M, Wainberg MA: AZT (zidovudine) may act postintegrationally to inhibit generation of HIV-1 progeny virus in chronically infected cells. Virology 176:205, 1990

57. Pauza CD, Galindo JE, Richman DD: Reinfection results in accumulation of unintegrated viral DNA in cytopathic and persistent HIV-1 infection of CEM cells. J Exp Med 172:1035, 1990

58. Terai C, Kornbluth RS, Pauza CD et al: Apoptosis as a mechanism of cell death in cultured T lymphoblasts acutely infected with HIV. J Clin Invest 87:1710, 1991

59. Ayers KM: Preclinical toxicology of zidovudine. Am J Med 85:186, 1988

60. Sharpe AH, Jaenisch R, Ruprecht RM: Retroviruses and mouse embryos: A rapid model for neurovirulence and transplacental antiviral therapy. Science 236:1671, 1987

61. Ohnota H, Okada Y, Ushijima H et al: 3'-azido-3'-deoxythymidine prevents induction of murine acquired immunodeficiency syndrome in C57BL/10 mice infected with LP-BM-5 murine leukemia viruses, a possible animal model for antiretroviral drug screening. Antimicrob Agents Chemother 34:605, 1990

62. Morrey JD, Warren RP, Okleberry KM et al: Effects of zidovudine on friend virus complex infection in rfv-$3^{r/s}$ genotype–containing mice used as a model for HIV infection. J AIDS 3:500, 1990

63. Tsai C-C, Follis KE, Benveniste RE: Antiviral effects of 3'-azido-3'-deoxythymidine, 2',3'-dideoxycytidine, and 2',3'-dideoxydenosine against simian acquired immunodeficiency syndrome–associated type D retrovirus in vitro. AIDS Res Hum Retroviruses 4:359, 1989

64. Zeidner NS, Rose LM, Mathiason-DuBard CK et al: Zidovudine in combination with alpha interferon and interleukin-2 as prophylactic therapy for FeLV-induced

immunodeficiency syndrome (FeLV-FAIDS). J AIDS 3:787, 1990

65. Lundgren B, Ljungdahl-Ståhle E, Böttiger D et al: Acute infection of cynomolgus monkeys with simian immunodeficiency virus (SIV$_{SM}$) as a model to evaluate antiviral compounds: Effects of 3'-azido-3'-deoxythymidine, foscarnet and 2',3'-dideoxycytidine. Antiviral Chem Chemother 1:299, 1990

66. Keith BR, White GC, Wilson HR: In vivo efficacy of zidovudine (3'-azido-3'-deoxythymidine) in experimental gram-negative-bacterial infections. Antimicrob Agents Chemother 33:479, 1989

67. Yarchoan R, Klecker RW, Weinhold KJ et al: Administration of 3'-azido-3'-deoxythymidine, an inhibitor of HTLV-III/LAV replication, to patients with AIDS or AIDS-related complex. Lancet 1:575, 1986

68. Klecker KW Jr, Collins JM, Yarchoan R et al: Plasma and cerebrospinal fluid pharmacokinetics of 3'-azido-3'-deoxythymidine: A novel pyrimidine analog with potential application for the treatment of patients with AIDS and related diseases. Clin Pharmacol Ther 41:407, 1987

69. Resetar A, Spector T: Glucuronidation of 3'-azido-3'-deoxythymidine: Human and rat enzyme specificity. Biochem Pharmacol 38:1389, 1989

70. Laskin OL, de Miranda P, Blum MR: Azidothymidine steady-state pharmacokinetics in patients with AIDS and AIDS-related complex. J Infect Dis 159:745, 1989

71. Unadkat JD, Collier AC, Crosby SS et al: Pharmacokinetics of oral zidovudine (azidothymidine) in patients with AIDS when administered with and without a high-fat meal. AIDS 4:229, 1990

72. Blum MR, Liao SHT, Good SS, de Miranda P: Pharmacokinetics and bioavailability of zidovudine in humans. Am J Med 85:189, 1988

73. Singlas E, Pioger JC, Taburet AM et al: Zidovudine disposition in patients with severe renal impairment: Influence of hemodialysis. Clin Pharmacol Ther 46(2):190, 1990

74. Pioger JC, Taburet AM, Fillastre JP, Singlas E: Pharmacokinetics of zidovudine (AZT) and its glucuronide in healthy volunteers and in uremic patients. Presented at the 28th Interscience Conference on Antimicrobial Agents and Chemotherapy, Los Angeles, October 24, 1988

75. Morse GD, Olson J, Portmore A et al: Pharmacokinetics of orally administered zidovudine among patients with hemophilia and asymptomatic human immunodeficiency virus (HIV) infection. Antiviral Res 11:57, 1989

76. Taubret A-M, Naveau S, Zorza G et al: Pharmacokinetics of zidovudine in patients with liver cirrhosis. Clin Pharmacol Ther 47:731, 1990

77. de Miranda P, Good SS, Yarchoan R et al: Alteration of zidovudine pharmacokinetics by probenecid in patients with AIDS or AIDS-related complex. Clin Pharmacol Ther 46:494, 1990

78. Kornhauser DM, Hendrix CW, Nerhood LJ et al: Probenecid and zidovudine metabolism. Lancet 2:473, 1989

79. Steffe EM, King JH, Inciardi JF et al: The effect of acetaminophen on zidovudine metabolism in HIV-infected patients. J AIDS 3:691, 1990

80. Surbone A, Yarchoan R, McAtee N et al: Treatment of the acquired immunodeficiency syndrome (AIDS) and AIDS-related complex with a regimen of 3'-azido-2',3'-dideoxythymidine (azidothymidine or zidovudine) and acyclovir. Ann Intern Med 108:534, 1988

81. Hollander H, Lifson AR, Maha M et al: Phase I study of low-dose zidovudine and acyclovir in asymtomatic human immunodeficiency virus seropositive individuals. Am J Med 87:628, 1989

82. Hochster H, Dieterich D, Bozzette S et al: Toxicity of combined ganciclovir (DHPG) and zidovudine (AZT) with the therapy of AIDS-related CMV disease: Results of a NIAID AIDS Clinical Trials Group Phase I study (ACTG 004). Ann Intern Med 113:111, 1990

83. Meng TC, Fischl MA, Boota AM et al: Combination therapy with zidovudine and dideoxycytidine in patients with advanced HIV infection: A phase I/II study. Ann Int Med 116, 1992, (in press)

84. Henry K, Chinnock BJ, Quinn RP et al: Concurrent zidovudine levels in semen and serum determined by radioimmunoassay in patients with AIDS or AIDS-related complex. JAMA 259:3023, 1988

85. Lopez-Anaya A, Unadkat JD, Schumann LA, Smith AL: Pharmacokinetics of zidovudine (azidothymidine): I. transplacental transfer. J AIDS 3:959, 1990

86. Watts DH, Brown ZA, Tartaglione T et al: Pharmacokinetic disposition of zidovudine during pregnancy. J Infect Dis 163:226, 1991

87. Liebes L, Mendoza S, Wilson D, Dancis J: Transfer of zidovudine (AZT) by human placenta. J Infect Dis 161:203, 1989

88. Fischl MA, Richman DD, Grieco MH et al: The efficacy of azidothymidine (AZT) in the treatment of patients with AIDS and AIDS-related complex: A double-blind, placebo-controlled trial. N Engl J Med 317:185, 1987

89. Richman DD, Fischl MA, Grieco MH et al: The toxicity of azidothymidine (AZT) in the treatment of patients with AIDS and AIDS-related complex: A double-blind, placebo-controlled trial. N Engl J Med 317:192, 1987

90. Volberding PA, Lagakos SW, Koch MA et al: Zidovudine in asymptomatic human immunodeficiency virus infection: A controlled trial in persons with fewer than 500 CD4-positive cells per cubic millimeter. N Engl J Med 322:941, 1990

91. Fischl MA, Richman DD, Hansen N et al: The safety and efficacy of zidovudine (AZT) in the treatment of subjects with mildly symptomatic human immunodeficiency virus type 1 (HIV) infection: A double-blind, placebo-controlled trial. Ann Intern Med 112:727, 1990

92. Fischl MA, Parker CB, Pettinelli C et al: A randomized controlled trial of a reduced daily dose of zidovudine in patients with the acquired immunodeficiency syndrome. N Engl J Med 323:1009, 1990

93. Collier AC, Bozzette S, Coombs RW et al: A pilot study of low-dose zidovudine in human immunodeficiency virus infection. N Engl J Med 323:1015, 1990

94. Jacobson MA, Abrams DI, Volberding PA et al: Serum beta$_2$-microglobulin decreases in patients with AIDS or ARC treated with azidothymidine. J Infect Dis 159:1029, 1989

95. Reddy MM, Vodian M, Grieco MH: Effect of azidothymidine on soluble CD4 levels in patients with AIDS or AIDS-related complex. J Clin Lab Anal 4:396, 1990

96. Reddy MM, McKinley G, Englard A, Grieco MH: Effect of azidothymidine (AZT) on HIV p24 antigen, beta$_2$-microglobulin, neopterin, soluble CD8, soluble interleukin-2 receptor and tumor necrosis factor alpha levels in patients with AIDS-related complex or AIDS. Int J Immunopharmacol 12:737, 1990

97. Spector SA, Kennedy C, McCutchan JA et al: The antiviral effect of zidovudine and ribavirin in clinical trials and the use of p24 antigen levels as a virologic marker. J Infect Dis 159:822, 1989

98. Lane HC, Falloon J, Walker RE et al: Zidovudine in patients with human immunodeficiency virus (HIV) infection and Kaposi sarcoma. Ann Intern Med 111:41, 1989

99. Ho DD, Moudgil T, Alam M: Quantitation of human immunodeficiency virus type 1 in the blood of infected persons. N Engl J Med 321:1621, 1989

100. Chaisson RE, Leuther MD, Allain JP et al: Effect of zidovudine on serum human immunodeficiency virus core antigen levels: Results from a placebo-controlled trial. Arch Intern Med 148:2151, 1988

101. Pizzo PA, Eddy J, Falloon J et al: Effect of continuous intravenous infusion of zidovudine (AZT) in children with symptomatic HIV infection. N Engl J Med 319:889, 1988

102. Jackson GG, Paul DA, Falk LA et al: Human immunodeficiency virus (HIV) antigenemia (p24) in the acquired immunodeficiency syndrome (AIDS) and the effect of treatment with zidovudine (AZT). Ann Intern Med 108:175, 1988

103. De Wolf F, Goudsmit J, De Gans J et al: Effect of zidovudine on serum human immunodeficiency virus antigen levels in symptom-free subjects. Lancet 1:373, 1988

104. Spear JM, Benson CA, Pottage JC Jr et al: Rapid rebound of serum human immunodeficiency virus antigen after discontinuing zidovudine therapy. J Infect Dis 158:1132, 1988

105. Kennedy CJ, Teschke RS, Hesselink JR et al: Clinical evaluation of the central nervous system in HIV infected patients on azidothymidine (AZT) (abstr). Presented at the III International Conference on AIDS, Washington, DC, June 1987

106. De Gans J, Lange JMA, Derix MMA et al: Decline of HIV antigen levels in cerebrospinal fluid during treatment with low-dose zidovudine. AIDS 2:37, 1988

107. Fiala M, Cone LA, Cohen N et al: Responses of neurologic complications of AIDS to 3'-azido-3'-deoxythymidine and 9-(1,3-dihydroxy-2-propoxymethyl)guanine: I. Clinical features. J Infect Dis 2:250, 1988

108. Yarchoan R, Berg G, Brouwers P et al: Response of human-immunodeficiency-virus–associated neurological disease to 3'-azido-3'-deoxythymidine. Lancet 1:132, 1987

109. Yarchoan R, Thomas RV, Grafman J et al: Long-term administration of 3'-azido-2',3'-deoxythymidine to patients with AIDS-related neurological disease. Ann Neurol 23(suppl):S82, 1988

110. Schmitt FA, Bigley JW, McKinnis R et al: Neuropsychological outcome of zidovudine (AZT) treatment of patients with AIDS and AIDS-related complex. N Engl J Med 319:1573, 1988

111. McKinney RE Jr, Maha MA, Connor EM et al: A multicenter trial of oral zidovudine in children with advanced human immunodeficiency virus disease. N Engl J Med 324:1018, 1991

112. DiCarli C, Fugate L, Falloon J et al: Brain growth and cognitive improvement in children with human immunodeficiency virus–induced encephalopathy after 6 months of continuous infusion zidovudine therapy. J AIDS 4:585, 1991

113. Portegies P, deGans J, Lange JMA et al: Declining incidence of AIDS dementia complex after introduction of zidovudine treatment. Br Med J 299:819, 1989

114. Hymes KB, Greene JB, Karpatkin S: The effect of azidothymidine on HIV-related thrombocytopenia. N Engl J Med 318:516, 1988

115. Oksenhendler E, Bierling P, Ferchal F et al: Zidovudine for thrombocytopenic purpura related to human immunodeficiency virus (HIV) infection. Ann Intern Med 110:365, 1989

116. Gottlieb MS, Wolfe PR, Chafey S: Case report: Response to AIDS-related thrombocytopenia to intravenous and oral azidothymidine (3'-azido-3'-deoxythymidine). AIDS Res Hum Retroviruses 3:109, 1987

117. Swiss Group for Clinical Studies on AIDS: Zidovudine for the treatment of HIV-associated thrombocytopenia: A placebo-controlled prospective study. Ann Intern Med 109:718, 1988

118. Lam M, Park MC: HIV-associated nephropathy: Beneficial effect of zidovudine therapy. N Engl J Med 323:1775, 1990

119. Gail MH, Rosenberg PS, Goedert JJ: Therapy may explain recent deficits in AIDS incidence. J AIDS 3:296, 1990

120. Lemp GF, Payne SF, Neal D et al: Survival trends for patients with AIDS. JAMA 263:402, 1990

121. Solomon PJ, Wilson SR, Swanson CE, Cooper DA: Effect of zidovudine on survival of patients with AIDS in Australia. Med J Aust 153:254, 1990

122. Moore RD, Hidalgo J, Sugland BW, Chaisson RE: Zidovudine and the natural history of the acquired immunodeficiency syndrome. N Engl J Med 324:1412, 1991

123. Dawson SG, Chapel HM, Eglin RP: Zidovudine and HIV-2 disease. AIDS 4:933, 1990

124. Marcellin P, Pialoux G, Girard P-M et al: Absence of effect of zidovudine on replication of hepatitis B virus in patients with chronic HIV and HBV infection. N Engl J Med 321:1758, 1989

125. Gelmon K, Montaner JSG, Fanning M et al: Nature, time course and dose dependence of zidovudine-related side effects: Results from the Multicenter Canadian Azidothymidine Trial. AIDS 3:555, 1989

126. Walker RE, Parker RI, Kovacs JA et al: Anemia and erythropoiesis in patients with the acquired immunodeficiency syndrome (AIDS) and Kaposi sarcoma tested with zidovudine. Ann Intern Med 108:372, 1988

127. Streeter DF, Witkowski JT, Khare GP et al: Mechanism of action of 1-beta-delta-ribofuranosyl-1,2,4-triazole-3-carboxamide (Virazole), a new broad-spectrum antiviral agent. Proc Natl Acad Sci USA 20:1174, 1973

128. Bessen LJ, Greene JB, Louie E et al: Severe polymyositis-like syndrome associated with zidovudine therapy of AIDS and ARC. N Engl J Med 318:708, 1988

129. Dalakas MC, Illa I, Pezeshkpour GH et al: Mitochondrial myopathy caused by long-term zidovudine therapy. N Engl J Med 322:1089, 1990

130. Till M, MacDonell KB: Myopathy with human immunodeficiency virus type 1 (HIV-1) infection: HIV-1 or zidovudine? Ann Intern Med 113:492, 1990

131. Gertner E, Thurn JR, Williams DN et al: Zidovudine-associated myopathy. Am J Med 86:814, 1989

132. Helbert M, Fletcher T, Peddle B et al: Zidovudine-associated myopathy. Lancet 2:689, 1988

133. Dalakas MC, Pezeshkpour GH, Gravell M, Sever JL: Polymyositis associated with AIDS retrovirus. JAMA 256:2381, 1986

134. Bailey RO, Turok DI, Jaufmann BP, Singh JK: Myositis and acquired immunodeficiency syndrome. Hum Pathol 18:749, 1987

135. Simpson DM: Myopathy associated with human immunodeficiency virus (HIV) but not zidovudine. Ann Intern Med 109:842, 1988

136. Chad DA, Smith TW, Blumenfeld A et al: Human immunodeficiency virus (HIV)–associated myopathy: Immu-

nocytochemical identification of an HIV antigen (gp 41) in muscle macrophages. Ann Neurol 28:579, 1990

137. Gonzales MF, Olney RK, So YT et al: Subacute structural myopathy associated with human immunodeficiency virus infection. Arch Neurol 45:585, 1988

138. Simpson DM, Bender AN: Human immunodeficiency virus–associated myopathy: Analysis of 11 patients. Ann Neurol 24:79, 1988

139. Nordstrom DM, Petropolis AA, Giorno R et al: Inflammatory myopathy and acquired immunodeficiency syndrome. Arthritis Rheum 32:475, 1989

140. Arnaudo E, Dalakas M, Shanske S et al: Depletion of muscle mitochondrial DNA in AIDS patients with zidovudine-induced myopathy. Lancet i:508, 1991

141. Stites DP, Casavant CH, McHugh TM et al: Flow cytometric analysis of lymphocyte phenotypes in AIDS using monoclonal antibodies and simultaneous dual immunofluorescence. Clin Immunol Immunopathol 38:161, 1986

142. Hagler DN, Frame PT: Azidothymidine neurotoxicity. Lancet 2:1392, 1986

143. Harris PJ, Caceres C: Azidothymidine in the treatment of AIDS. N Engl J Med 318:250, 1988

144. Helbert M, Peddle B, Kocsis A et al: Acute meningo-encephalitis on dose reduction of zidovudine. Lancet 1:1249, 1988

145. Furth PA, Kazakis AM: Nail pigmentation changes associated with azidothymidine (zidovudine). Ann Intern Med 107:350, 1987

146. Don PC, Fusco F, Fried P et al: Nail dyschromia associated with zidovudine. Ann Intern Med 112:145, 1990

147. Lalonde RG, Deschênes JG, Seamone C: Zidovudine-induced macular edema. Ann Intern Med 114:297, 1991

148. Dubin G, Braffman MN: Zidovudine-induced hepatotoxicity. Ann Intern Med 110:85, 1989

149. Edwards P, Turner J, Gold J, Cooper DA: Esophageal ulceration induced by zidovudine. Ann Intern Med 112:65, 1990

150. Hargreaves M, Fuller G, Costello C, Gazzard B: Zidovudine overdose. Lancet 2:509, 1988

151. Pickus OB: Overdose of zidovudine. N Engl J Med 318:1206, 1988

152. Spear JB, Kessler HA, Nusinoff-Lehrman S, de Miranda P: Zidovudine overdosage. Ann Intern Med 109:76, 1988

153. Routy JP, Prajs E, Blanc AP et al: Seizure after zidovudine overdose. Lancet 1:384, 1989

154. Selwyn PA, Iezza A: Zidovudine overdose in an intravenous drug user. AIDS 4:822, 1990

155. Terragna A, Mazzarello G, Anselmo M et al: Suicidal attempts with zidovudine. AIDS 4:88, 1990

156. Fischl MA, Richman DD, Causey DM et al: Prolonged zidovudine therapy in patients with AIDS and advanced AIDS-related complex. JAMA 262:2405, 1990

157. Creagh-Kirk T, Doi E, Andrews S et al: Survival experience among patients with acquired immunodeficiency syndrome receiving zidovudine therapy. JAMA 260:3009, 1988

158. Dournon E, Rozenbaum W, Michon C et al: Effects of zidovudine in 365 consecutive patients with AIDS or AIDS-related complex. Lancet 1:1297, 1988

159. Swanson CE, Cooper DA: Factors influencing outcome of treatment with zidovudine in patients with AIDS in Australia. AIDS 4:749, 1990

160. Samuels JE, Hendrix J, Hilton M et al: Zidovudine therapy in an inner city population. J AIDS 3:877, 1990

161. Hamilton JD, Hartigan PM, Simberkoff MS, VA Cooperative Group: Early versus later zidovudine treatment of symptomatic HIV infection: Results of a VA cooperative study. Clin Res 39:216A, 1991

162. Pluda JM, Yarchoan R, Jaffe ES: Development of non-Hodgkin's lymphoma in a cohort of patients with severe human immunodeficiency virus (HIV) infection on long-term antiretroviral therapy. Ann Intern Med 113:276, 1990

163. Moore RD, Kessler H, Richman DD et al: Non-Hodgkin lymphoma in patients with advanced HIV-infection treated with zidovudine. JAMA 266:2208, 1991

164. Scitovsky AA, Cline MW, Abrams DI: Effects of the use of AZT on the medical care costs of persons with AIDS in the first 12 months. J AIDS 3:904, 1990

165. Schulman KA, Lynn LA, Glick HA, Eisenberg JM: Cost effectiveness of low-dose zidovudine therapy for asymptomatic patients with human immunodeficiency virus (HIV) infection. Ann Intern Med 114:798, 1991

166. Anderson RM, Gupta S, May RM: Potential of community-wide chemotherapy or immunotherapy to control the spread of HIV-1. Nature 350:356, 1991

167. Balis FM, Pizzo PA, Murphy RF et al: The pharmacokinetics of zidovudine administered by continuous infusion in children. Ann Intern Med 110:279, 1989

168. Pizzo PA, Wilfert CM: Treatment considerations for children with HIV infection. In Pizzo PA, Wilfert CM (eds): Pediatric AIDS, p 478. Baltimore, Williams & Wilkins, 1991

169. Fischl M, Galpin JE, Levine JD et al: Recombinant human erythropoietin for patients with AIDS treated with zidovudine. N Engl J Med 322:1488, 1990

170. DaCosta NA, Hultin MB: Effective therapy of human immunodeficiency virus–associated anemia with recombinant human erythropoietin despite high endogenous erythropoietin. Am J Hematol 36:71, 1991

171. Baldwin GC, Gasson JC, Quan SG et al: Granulocyte-macrophage colony-stimulating factor enhances neutrophil function in acquired immunodeficiency syndrome patients. Proc Natl Acad Sci USA 85:2763, 1988

172. Groopman JE, Mitsuyasu R, DeLeo MJ et al: Effect of recombinant human granulocyte-macrophage colony-stimulating factor on myelopoiesis in the acquired immunodeficiency syndrome. N Engl J Med 317:593, 1987

173. Kimura S, Matsuda J, Ikematsu S et al: Efficacy of recombinant human granulocyte colony-stimulating factor on neutropenia in patients with AIDS. AIDS 4:1251, 1990

174. Larder BA, Kemp SD: Multiple mutations in HIV-1 reverse transcriptase confer high-level resistance to zidovudine (AZT). Science 246:1155, 1989

175. Richman DD: Zidovudine resistance of human immunodeficiency virus. Rev Infect Dis 12:S507, 1990

176. Larder BA, Chesebro B, Richman DD: Susceptibilities of zidovudine-susceptible and -resistant human immunodeficiency virus isolates to antiviral agents determined by using a quantitative plaque reduction assay. Antimicrob Agents Chemother 34:436, 1990

177. Richman DD, Grimes JM, Lagakos SW: Effect of stage of disease and drug dose on zidovudine susceptibilities of isolates of human immunodeficiency virus. J AIDS 3:743, 1990

178. Coombs RW, Collier AC, Allain J-P et al: Plasma viremia in human immunodeficiency virus infection. N Engl J Med 321:1626, 1989

179. Richman DD, Guatelli JC, Grimes J et al: Detection of mutations associated with zidovudine resistance in human immunodeficiency virus by use of the polymerase chain reaction. J Infect Dis 164:1075, 1991

180. Eriksson B, Vrang L, Bazin H et al: Different patterns of

inhibition of avian myeloblastosis virus reverse transcriptase activity by 3′-azido-3′-deoxythymidine 5′-triphosphate and its threo isomer. Antimicrob Agents Chemother 31: 600, 1987

181. Balzarini J, Cooney DA, Dalal M et al: 2′,3′-dideoxycytidine: Regulation of its metabolism and anti-retroviral potency by natural pyrimidine nucleosides and by inhibitors of pyrimidine nucleotide synthesis. Mol Pharmacol 32:798, 1987

182. Ullman B, Coons T, Rockwell S, McCartan K: Genetic analysis of 2′,3′-dideoxycytidine incorporation into cultured human T lymphoblasts. J Biol Chem 263:12391, 1988

183. Starnes MC, Cheng Y-C: Cellular metabolism of 2′,3′-dideoxycytidine, a compound active against human immunodeficiency virus in vitro. J Biol Chem 262:988, 1987

184. Hao Z, Cooney DA, Hartman NR et al: Factors determining the activity of 2′,3′-dideoxynucleosides in suppressing human immunodeficiency virus in vitro. Mol Pharmacol 34: 431, 1988

185. Tornevik Y, Eriksson S: 2′,3′-dideoxycytidine toxicity in cultured human CEM T lymphoblasts: Effects of combination with 3′-azido-3′-deoxythymidine and thymidine. Mol Pharmacol 38:237, 1990

186. Bhalla KN, Gongrong L, Grant S et al: The effect in vitro of 2′-deoxycytidine on the metabolism and cytotoxicity of 2′,3′-dideoxycytidine. AIDS 4:427, 1990

187. Chen MS, Oshana SC: Inhibition of HIV reverse transcriptase by 2′,3′-dideoxynucleoside triphosphates. Biochem Pharmacol 36:4361, 1987

188. Waqar MA, Evans MJ, Manly KF et al: Effects of 2′,3′-dideoxynucleosides on mammalian cells and viruses. J Cell Physiol 121:402, 1984

189. Zimmermann W, Chen SM, Bolden A, Weissbach A: Mitochondrial DNA replication does not involve DNA polymerase α. J Biol Chem 255:11847, 1980

190. Chen C-H, Cheng Y-C: Delayed cytotoxicity and selective loss of mitochondrial DNA in cells treated with the anti-human immunodeficiency virus compound 2′,3′-dideoxycytidine (abstr). J Biol Chem 264:11934, 1989

191. Mitsuya H, Broder S: Strategies for antiviral therapy in AIDS. Nature 325:773, 1987

192. Tsai C-C, Follis KE, Yarnall M, Blakley GA: Toxicity and efficacy of 2′,3′-dideoxycytidine in clinical trials of pigtailed macaques infected with simian retrovirus type 2. Antimicrob Agents Chemother 33:1908, 1989

193. Kelley JA, Litterst CL, Roth JS et al: The disposition and metabolism of 2′,3′-dideoxycytidine, an *in vitro* inhibitor of human T-lymphotropic virus type III infectivity, in mice and monkeys. Drug Metab Dispos 15:595, 1987

194. Hoover EA, Zeidner NS, Perigo NA et al: Feline leukemia virus–induced immunodeficiency syndrome in cats as a model for evaluation of antiretroviral therapy. Intervirology 30(suppl 1):12, 1989

195. Polas PJ, Swenson CL, Sams R et al: In vitro and in vivo evidence that the antiviral activity of 2′,3′-dideoxycytidine is target cell dependent in a feline retrovirus animal model. Antimicrob Agents Chemother 34:1414, 1990

196. Lee B, Luo W, Suzuki S et al: In vitro and in vivo comparison of the abilities of purine and pyrimidine 2′,3′-dideoxynucleosides to inhibit duck hepadnavirus. Antimicrob Agents Chemother 33:336, 1989

197. Kassianides C, Hoffnagle JH, Miller RH et al: Inhibition of duck hepatitis B virus replication by 2′,3′-dideoxycytidine: A potent inhibitor of reverse transcriptase. Gastroenterology 97:1275, 1989

198. Yarchoan R, Perno CF, Thomas RV et al: Phase studies of 2′,3′-dideoxycytidine in severe human immunodeficiency virus infection as a single agent and alternating with zidovudine (AZT). Lancet 1:76, 1988

199. Gustavson LE, Fukuda EK, Rubio FA, Dunton AW: A pilot study of the bioavailability and pharmacokinetics of 2′,3′-dideoxycytidine in patients with AIDS or AIDS-related complex. J AIDS 3:28, 1990

200. Merigan TC, Skowron G, Bozzette S et al: Circulating p24 antigen levels and responses to dideoxycytidine in human immunodeficiency virus (HIV) infections: A phase I and II study. Ann Intern Med 110:189, 1989

201. Merigan TC, ddC Study Group of the AIDS Clinical Trials Group of the NIAID: Safety and tolerance of dideoxycytidine as a single agent. Am J Med 88(suppl 5B):11S, 1990

202. Skowron G, Merigan TC: Alternating and intermittent regimens of zidovudine (3′-azido-3′-deoxythymidine) and dideoxycytidine (2′,3′-dideoxycytidine) in the treatment of patients with acquired immunodeficiency syndrome (AIDS) and AIDS-related complex. Am J Med 88(suppl 5B):20S, 1990

203. Montefiori DC, Mitchell WM: Infection of the HTLV-II–bearing T-cell line C3 with HTLV-III/LAV is highly permissive and lytic. Virology 155:726, 1986

204. Cooney DA, Ahluwalia G, Mitsuya H et al: Initial studies on the cellular pharmacology of 2′,3′-dideoxyadenosine, an inhibitor of HTLV-III infectivity. Biochem Pharmacol 36:1765, 1987

205. Johnson MA, Fridland A: Phosphorylation of 2′,3′-dideoxyinosine by cytosolic 5′-nucleotidase of human lymphoid cells. Mol Pharmacol 36:291, 1989

206. Ahluwalia G, Cooney DA, Mitsuya H et al: Initial studies on the cellular pharmacology of 2′,3′-dideoxyinosine, an inhibitor of HIV infectivity. Biochem Pharmacol 36:3797, 1987

207. Carson DA, Haertle T, Wasson DB, Richman DD: Biochemical genetic analysis of 2′,3′-dideoxyadenosine metabolism in human T lymphocytes. Biochem Biophys Res Commun 151:788, 1988

208. Agarwal RP, Busso ME, Mian AM, Resnick L: Uptake of 2′,3′-dideoxyadenosine in human immunodeficiency virus-infected and noninfected human cells. AIDS Res Hum Retroviruses 5:541, 1989

209. Ahluwalia G, Johnson MA, Fridland A et al: Cellular pharmacology of the anti-HIV agent 2′,3′-dideoxyadenosine (abstr). Proc Am Assoc Cancer Res 29:349, 1988

210. Russell JW, Klunk LJ: Comparative pharmacokinetics of new anti-HIV agents: 2′,3′-dideoxyadenosine and 2′,3′-dideoxyinosine. Biochem Pharmacol 38:1385, 1989

211. McGowan JJ, Tomaszewski JE, Cradock J et al: Overview of the preclinical development of an antiretroviral drug, 2′,3′-dideoxyinosine. Rev Infect Dis 12:S513, 1991

212. Hartman NR, Yarchoan R, Pluda JM et al: Pharmacokinetics of 2′,3′-dideoxyadenosine and 2′,3′-dideoxyinosine in patients with severe human immunodeficiency virus infection. Clin Pharmacol Ther 47:647, 1990

213. Lambert JS, Seidlin M, Reichman RC et al: 2′,3′-dideoxyinosine (ddI) in patients with the acquired immunodeficiency syndrome or AIDS-related complex. N Engl J Med 322:1333, 1990

214. Yarchoan R, Mitsuya H, Thomas RV et al: In vivo activity against HIV and favorable toxicity profile of 2′,3′-dideoxyinosine. Science 245:412, 1989

215. Cooley TP, Kunchies LM, Saunders CA et al: Once-daily administration of 2′,3′-dideoxyinosine (ddI) in patients with the acquired immunodeficiency syndrome or AIDS-related complex. N Engl J Med 322:1340, 1990

216. Yarchoan R, Pluda JM, Thomas RV et al: Long-term toxicity/activity profile of 2′,3′-dideoxyinosine in AIDS or AIDS-related complex. Lancet ii:526, 1990

217. LeLacheur SF, Simon GL: Exacerbation of dideoxycytidine-induced neuropathy with dideoxyinosine. J AIDS 4:538, 1991

218. Nasr M, Litterst C, McGowan J: Computer-assisted structure-activity correlations of didexoynucleoside analogs as potential anti-HIV drugs. Antiviral Res 14:125, 1990

219. Baba M, Pauwels R, Balzarini J et al: Selective inhibition of human immunodeficiency virus (HIV) by 3′-azido-2′,3′-dideoxyguanosine in vitro. Biochem Biophys Res Commun 145:1080, 1987

220. Lin T-S, Chen MS, McLaren C et al: Synthesis and antiviral activity of various 3′-azido, 3′-amino, 2′,3′-unsaturated, and 2′,3′-dideoxy analogues of pyrimidine deoxyribonucleosides against retroviruses. J Med Chem 30:440, 1987

221. Lin T-S, Guo JY, Schinazi RF et al: Synthesis and antiviral activity of various 3′-azido analogues of pyrimidine deoxyribonucleosides against human immunodeficiency virus (HIV-1, HTLV-III/LAV). J Med Chem 31:336, 1988

222. Balzarini J, Baba M, Pauwels R et al: Anti-retrovirus activity of 3′-fluor- and 3′-azido-substituted pyrimidine 2′,3′-dideoxynucleoside analogues. Biochem Pharmacol 37:2847, 1988

223. Eriksson BFH, Chu CK, Schinazi RF: Phosphorylation of 3′-azido-2′,3′-dideoxyuridine and preferential inhibition of human and simian immunodeficiency virus reverse transcriptases by its 5′-triphosphate. Antimicrob Agents Chemother 33:1729, 1989

224. Matthes E, Lehmann C, Scholz D et al: Inhibition of HIV-associated reverse transcriptase by sugar-modified derivatives of thymidine 5′-triphosphate in comparison to cellular DNA polymerases alpha and beta. Biochem Biophys Res Commun 1:78, 1987

225. Balzarini J, Baba M, Pauwels R et al: Potent and selective activity of 3′-azido-2,6-diaminopurine-2′,3′-dideoxyriboside, 3′-fluoro-2,6-diaminopurine-2′,3′-dideoxyriboside, and 3′-fluoro-2′,3′-dideoxyguanosine against human immunodeficiency virus. Mol Pharmacol 33:243, 1988

226. Herdewijn P, Pauwels R, Baba M et al: Synthesis and anti-HIV activity of various 2′- and 3′-substituted 2′,3′-dideoxyadenosines: A structure-activity analysis. J Med Chem 30:2131, 1987

227. Herdewijn P, Balzarini J, Baba M et al: Synthesis and anti-HIV activity of different sugar-modified pyrimidine and purine nucleosides. J Med Chem 31:2040, 1988

228. Matthew E, Lehmann C, Scholz D et al: Phosphorylation, anti-HIV activity and cytotoxicity of 3′-fluorothymidine. Biochem Biophys Res Commun 153:825, 1988

229. Hartmann H, Vogt MW, Durno AG et al: Enhanced in vitro inhibition of HIV-1 replication by 3′-fluoro-3′-deoxythymidine compared to several other nucleoside analogs. AIDS Res Hum Retroviruses 4:457, 1988

230. Koshida R, Cox S, Harmenberg J et al: Structure-activity relationships of fluorinated nucleoside analogs and their synergistic effect in combination with phosphonoformate against human immunodeficiency virus type 1. Antimicrob Agents Chemother 33:2083, 1989

231. Balzarini J, Robins MJ, Zou RM et al: The 2′,3′-dideoxyriboside of 2,6-diaminopurine and its 2′,3′-didehydro derivative inhibit the deamination of 2′,3′-dideoxyadenosine, an inhibitor of human immunodeficiency virus (HIV) replication. Biochem Biophys Res Commun 145:277, 1987

232. Balzarini J, Pauwels R, Baba M et al: The 2′,3′-dideoxyriboside of 2,6-diaminopurine selectively inhibits human immunodeficiency virus (HIV) replication in vitro. Biochem Biophys Res Commun 145:269, 1987

233. Lin T-S, Schinazi RF, Chem MS et al: Antiviral activity of 2′,3′-dideoxycytidin-2′-ene (2′,3′-dideoxy-2′,3′-didehydrocytidine) against human immunodeficiency virus in vitro. Biochem Pharmacol 36:311, 1987

234. Balzarini J, Pauwels R, Herdewijn P et al: Potent and selective anti-HTLV-III/LAV activity of 2′,3′-dideoxycytidinene, the 2′,3′-unsaturated derivative of 2′,3′-dideoxycytidine. Biochem Biophys Res Commun 140:735, 1986

235. Lin T-S, Schinazi RF, Prusoff WH: Potent and selective in vitro activity of 3′-deoxythymidin-2′-ene (3′-deoxy-2′,3′-didehydrothymidine) against human immunodeficiency virus. Biochem Pharmacol 36:2713, 1987

236. Chu CK, Schinazi RF, Arnold BH et al: Comparative activity of 2′,3′-saturated and unsaturated pyrimidine and purine nucleosides against human immunodeficiency virus type 1 in peripheral blood mononuclear cells. Biochem Pharmacol 37:3543, 1988

237. Mansuri MM, Starrett JE Jr, Ghazzouli I et al: 1-(2,3-Dideoxy-beta-delta-glycero-pent-2-enofuranosyl)thymine: A highly potent and selective anti-HIV agent. J Med Chem 32:461, 1989

238. Marongiu ME, August EM, Prusoff WH: Effect of 3′-deoxythymidin-2′-ene (d4T) on nucleoside metabolism in H9 cells. Biochem Pharmacol 39:1523, 1990

239. Mitsuya H, Matsukura M, Broder S: Rapid in vitro systems for assessing activity of agents against HTLV-III/LAV. In Broder S (ed): AIDS: Modern Concepts and Therapeutic Challenges, p 303. New York, Marcel Dekker, 1987

240. Baba M, Pauwels R, Herdewijn P et al: Both 2′,3′-dideoxythymidine and its 2′,3′-unsaturated derivative (2′,3′-dideoxythymidinene) are potent and selective inhibitors of human immunodeficiency virus replication in vitro. Biochem Biophys Res Commun 142:128, 1987

241. Marquez VE, Tseng CK-H, Treanor SP, Driscoll JS: Synthesis of 2′,3′-dideoxycyclopentenyl carbocyclic nucleosides as potential drugs for the treatment of AIDS. Nucleosides Nucleotides 6:239, 1987

242. Yeom Y-H, Remmel RP, Huang S-H et al: Pharmacokinetics and bioavailability of carbovir, a carbocyclic nucleoside active against human immunodeficiency virus, in rats. Antimicrob Agents Chemother 33:171, 1989

243. Vince R, Hua M, Brownell J et al: Potent and selective activity of a new carbocyclic nucleoside analog (carbovir: NSC 614846) against human immunodeficiency virus in vitro. Biochem Biophys Res Commun 156:1046, 1988

244. Coates JAV, Inggall HJ, Pearson BA et al: Carbovir: The (−) enantiomer is a potent and selective antiviral agent against human immunodeficiency virus in vitro. Antiviral Res 15:161, 1991

245. Seki J-I, Shimada N, Takahashi K et al: Inhibition of infectivity of human immunodeficiency virus by a novel nucleoside, oxetanocin, and related compounds. Antimicrob Agents Chemother 33:773, 1989

246. Norbeck DW, Kern E, Hayashi S et al: Cyclobut-A and Cyclobut-G: Broad-spectrum antiviral agents with potential utility for the therapy of AIDS. J Med Chem 33:1281, 1990

247. Hayashi S, Norbeck DW, Rosenbrook W et al: Cyclobut-A and Cyclobut-G, carbocyclic oxetanocin analogs that inhibit the replication of human immunodeficiency virus in T cells and monocytes and macrophages in vitro. Antimicrob Agents Chemother 34:287, 1990

248. Pauwels R, Balzarini J, Schols D et al: Phosphonylmethoxyethyl purine derivatives, a new class of anti-human

immunodeficiency virus agents. Antimicrob Agents Chemother 32:1025, 1988

249. Balzarini J, Naesens L, Herdewijn P et al: Marked in vivo antiretrovirus activity of 9-(2-phosphonylmethoxyethyl)adenine, a selective anti-human immunodeficiency virus agent. Proc Natl Acad Sci USA 86:332, 1989

250. Votruba I, Travnicek M, Rosenberg I et al: Inhibition of avian myeloblastosis virus reverse transcriptase by diphosphates of acyclic phosphonylmethyl nucleotide analogues. Antiviral Res 13:287, 1990

251. Balzarini J, Hao Z, Herdewun P et al: Intracellular metabolism and mechanism of anti-retrovirus action of 9-(2-phosphonylmethoxyethyl)adenine, a potent anti-human immunodeficiency virus compound. Proc Natl Acad Sci USA 88:1499, 1991

252. Hayashi S, Phadtare S, Zemlicka J et al: Adenallene and cytallene: Acyclic nucleoside analogues that inhibit replication and cytopathic effect of human immunodeficiency virus in vitro. Proc Natl Acad Sci USA 85:6127, 1988

253. Marquez VE, Tseng CK-H, Kelley JA et al: 2',-3'-dideoxy-2'-fluoro-ARA-A: An acid-stable purine nucleoside active against human immunodeficiency virus (HIV). Biochem Pharmacol 36:2719, 1987

254. Hitchcock MJM, Woods K, De Boeck H, Ho H-T: Biochemical pharmacology of 2'-fluoro-2',3'-dideoxyarabinosyladenine, an inhibitor of HIV with improved metabolic and chemical stability over 2',3'-dideoxyadenosine. Antiviral Chem Chemother 1:319, 1991

255. Sterzycki RZ, Ghazzouli I, Brankovan V et al: Synthesis and anti-HIV activity of several 2'-fluoro–containing pyrimidine nucleosides. J Med Chem 33:2149, 1990

256. Martin JA, Bushnell DJ, Duncan IB et al: Synthesis and antiviral activity of monofluoro and difluoro analogues of pyrimidine deoxyribonucleosides against human immunodeficiency virus (HIV-1). J Med Chem 33:2138, 1990

257. Zhu Z, Ho H-T, Hitchcock MJM, Sommadossi J-P: Cellular pharmacology of 2',3'-didehydro-2',3'-dideoxythymidine (D4T) in human peripheral blood mononuclear cells. Biochem Pharmacol 39:R15, 1991

258. Mansuri MM, Hitchcock MJM, Buroker RA et al: Comparison of in vitro biological properties and mouse toxicities of three thymidine analogs active against human immunodeficiency virus. Antimicrob Agents Chemother 34:637, 1990

259. Soudeyns H, Yao H-J, Gao Q et al: Anti-human immunodeficiency virus type 1 activity and in vitro toxicity of 2'-deoxy-3'-thiacytidine (BCH 189), a novel heterocyclic nucleoside analogue. Antimicrob Agents Chemother 35:1386, 1991

260. Richman DD, Rosenthal AS, Skoog M et al: BI-RG-587 is active against zidovudine-resistant human immunodeficiency virus type 1 and synergistic with zidovudine. Antimicrob Agents Chemother 35:305, 1991

261. Fiddian AP, European/Australian Collaborative Study Group: Zidovudine plus or minus acyclovir in patients with AIDS or ARC (abstr). Presented at the 28th Interscience Conference on Antimicrobial Agents and Chemotherapy, Los Angeles, October 24, 1988

262. Eron JJ, Hirsch MS, Merrill DP et al: Synergistic inhibition of HIV-1 by the combination of zidovudine (AZT) and 2',3'-dideoxycytidine (ddC) *in vitro* (abstr). Presented at the VII International Conference on AIDS, Florence, Italy, June 16–21 1991

263. Harmenberg J, Akesson-Johansson A, Vrang L, Cox S: Synergistic inhibition of human immunodeficiency virus

replication in vitro by combinations of 3'-azido-3'deoxythymidine and 3'-fluoro-3'deoxythymidine. AIDS Res Hum Retroviruses 6:1197, 1990

264. Eriksson BFH, Schinazi RF: Combinations of 3'-azido-3'-deoxythymidine (zidovudine) and phosphonoformate (foscarnet) against human immunodeficiency virus type 1 and cytomegalovirus replication in vitro. Antimicrob Agents Chemother 33:663, 1989

265. Birch C, Tachedjian G, Lucas CR, Gust ID: In vitro effectiveness of a combination of zidovudine and ansamycin against human immunodeficiency virus. J Infect Dis 158:895, 1988

266. Ueno R, Kuno S: Dextran sulfate, a potent anti-HIV agent in vitro having synergism with zidovudine (letter). Lancet 1:1379, 1987

267. Hayashi S, Fine RL, Chou T-C et al: In vitro inhibition of the infectivity and replication of human immunodeficiency virus type 1 by combination of antiretroviral 2',3'-dideoxynucleosides and virus-binding inhibitors. Antimicrob Agents Chemother 34:82, 1990

268. Anand R, Nayyar S, Pitha J, Merril CR: Sulphated sugar alpha-cyclodextrin sulphate, a uniquely potent anti-HIV agent, also exhibits marked synergism with AZT, and lymphoproliferative activity. Antiviral Chem Chemother 1:41, 1990

269. Busso ME, Resnick L: Anti-human immunodeficiency virus effects of dextran sulfate are strain dependent and synergistic or antagonistic when dextran sulfate is given in combination with dideoxynucleosides. Antimicrob Agents Chemother 34:1991, 1990

270. Anand R, Nayyar S, Galvin TA et al: Sodium pentosan polysulfate (PPS), an anti-HIV agent, also exhibits synergism with AZT, lymphoproliferative activity, and virus enhancement. AIDS Res Hum Retroviruses 6:679, 1990

271. Johnson VA, Barlow MA, Chou T-C et al: Synergistic inhibition of human immunodeficiency virus type 1 (HIV-1) replication in vitro by recombinant soluble CD4 and 3'-azido, 3'-deoxythymidine. J Infect Dis 159:837, 1989

272. Ashorn P, Moss B, Weinstein JN et al: Elimination of infectious human immunodeficiency virus from human T-cell cultures by synergistic action of CD4-pseudomonas exotoxin and reverse transcriptase inhibitors. Proc Natl Acad Sci USA 87:8889, 1990

273. Flad HD, Ernst M, Kern P: A phase I/II trial of recombinant interleukin-2 in AIDS/ARC: Alterations of phenotypes of peripheral blood mononuclear cells. Lymphokine Res 5(suppl 1):S171, 1986

274. Johnson VA, Walker BD, Barlow MA et al: Synergistic inhibition of human immunodeficiency virus type 1 and type 2 replication in vitro by castanospermine and 3'-azido-3'-deoxythymidine. Antimicrob Agents Chemother 33:53, 1989

275. Schinazi RF, Cannon DL, Arnold BH et al: Combinations of isoprinosine and 3'-azido-3'-deoxythymidine in lymphocytes infected with human immunodeficiency virus type 1. Antimicrob Agents Chemother 32:1784, 1988

276. Hartshorn KL, Vogt MW, Chou T-C et al: Synergistic inhibition of human immunodeficiency virus in vitro by azidothymidine and recombinant alpha A interferon. Antimicrob Agents Chemother 31:168, 1987

277. Ruprecht RM, Chou T-C, Chipty F et al: Interferon-α and 3'-azido-3'-deoxythymidine are highly synergistic in mice and prevent viremia after acute retrovirus exposure. J AIDS 3:591, 1990

278. Zeidner NS, Myles MH, Mathiason-DuBard CK et al: Alpha interferon (2b) in combination with zidovudine for the treatment of presymptomatic feline leukemia virus–induced immunodeficiency syndrome. Antimicrob Agents Chemother 34:1749, 1990

279. Krown SE, Gold JWM, Niedzwiecki D et al: Interferon-alpha with zidovudine: Safety, tolerance and clinical and virologic effects in patients with Kaposi sarcoma associated with the acquired immunodeficiency syndrome (AIDS). Ann Intern Med 112:812, 1990

280. Kovacs JA, Deyton L, Davey R et al: Combined zidovudine and interferon alpha therapy in patients with Kaposi sarcoma and the acquired immunodeficiency syndrome (AIDS). Ann Intern Med 111:280, 1989

281. Fischl MA, Uttamchandani RB, Resnick L et al: A phase I study of recombinant human interferon-α₂ₐ or human lymphoblastoid interferon-αₙ₁ and concomitant zidovudine in patients with AIDS-related Kaposi's sarcoma. J AIDS 4:1, 1991

282. Orholm M, Pedersen C, Mathiesen L et al: Suppression of p24 antigen in sera from HIV-infected individuals with low-dose alpha interferon and zidovudine: A pilot study. AIDS 3:97, 1989

283. Capon DJ, Chamow SM, Mordenti J et al: Designing CD4 immunoadhesins for AIDS therapy. Nature 337:525, 1989

284. Yarchoan R, Mitsuya H, Myers CE, Broder S: Clinical pharmacology of 3′-azido-2′,3′-dideoxythymidine (zidovudine) and related dideoxynucleosides. N Engl J Med 321:726, 1989

Interferon-α in HIV Infection

20B

Robert E. Walker   *H. Clifford Lane*

The interferons were among the first agents to be considered in the immunopathogenesis and potential therapeutics of human immunodeficiency virus (HIV) infection. Two fundamental observations have contributed to their importance: interferons exhibit antimicrobial and antiproliferative effects *in vitro* against a diverse array of pathogens and cell types; and blood levels of interferons are known to fluctuate in association with progressive immunologic decline in patients with acquired immunodeficiency syndrome (AIDS) or AIDS-related complex (ARC).

Although endogenous interferons cannot as yet be directly implicated in viral pathogenesis, exogenously produced interferons have been used to treat numerous human viral infections and proliferative states. In some settings, such as hairy cell leukemia, interferon therapy may be curative. Coupled with what is known about the antiviral activities of the interferons are advances in molecular biology and recombinant DNA technology that allow for relative ease in producing pharmacologic quantities of these agents. The scientific rationale for investigating the role of interferons, in conjunction with the availability of these compounds, has generated much interest in the potential use of interferons as therapy for HIV infection.

The interferons are a family of naturally occurring peptide cytokines, classically described as immunomodulators yet serving a multitude of biologic functions. The precise mechanisms by which they regulate immune function are unknown. Structurally and functionally they can be divided into three major subclasses, α, β, and γ, also called respectively leukocyte, fibroblast, and immune interferon. Interferon-α (IFN-α) is itself a family of polypeptides consisting of at least 24 human subtypes,[1] produced by white blood cells and fibroblasts in response to viral infection and in response to challenge with double-stranded RNAs. Much is known about the protein structure and molecular biology. The IFNs-α contain 165 to 166 amino acid residues, are rich in leucine, glutamate, and glutamine, and have molecular weights ranging from 16 to 27 kilodaltons (kDa).[2] The degree of heterogeneity between different IFN-α molecules may approach 40% at the amino acid level.[1,2] Most are nonglycosylated. The human IFN-α gene has been cloned and sequenced and is known to lie on the short arm of chromosome 9.[2]

Three forms of human IFN-α are currently available for clinical use: recombinant α₂ₐ (also called αA or Roferon-A) and recombinant α₂ᵦ (α2 or Intron A), which differ by only a single arginine/lysine substitution at position 23; and lymphoblastoid IFN (αN1 or Wellferon), the purified, naturally occurring product.

IFN-β defines a distinctly different subclass of interferons. Like IFN-α, IFN-β is produced by leukocytes and fibroblasts and can be induced by viruses and double-stranded RNAs. The IFN-β subclass, however, contains primarily a single, N-glycosylated species, and its amino acid homology with IFN-α ranges from 30% to 75%.[2,3] Both IFN-α and IFN-β share the same high-affinity cell receptor.[4]

As distinct from IFN-α and IFN-β, IFN-γ is produced by T lymphocytes, primarily in response to antigens and mitogens, and binds to a unique cell surface receptor. One polypeptide species predominates, but many different N-glycosylated glycoproteins in this subclass result from posttranslational modifications.[3] IFN-γ has minimal if any amino acid homology with IFNs-α and -β.[2–4]

Numerous other interferons exist, although their precise physiologic roles, degrees of chemical relatedness, and mechanisms of action remain largely unknown. In the context of HIV disease, the therapeutic potential of IFNs-α and -γ has been studied most intensively, and IFN-α has been shown to be the most active member of this cytokine family.[5,6]

ENDOGENOUS INTERFERON AND HIV INFECTION

Most studies examining the relationship between interferon production in HIV-infected patients and the course of disease have revealed an apparent paradox: whereas serum levels of IFN-α generally increase with disease progression, *in vitro* production of interferon by leukocytes declines. One group found that 100% of 76 patients with AIDS or ARC had circulating levels of interferon, compared with one of 86 HIV-negative controls and five of ten HIV-negative patients with varicella-zoster virus infection.[7] These investigators used a bioassay for interferons that did not distinguish between subclasses. Another group, using a radioimmunoassay specific for IFN-α, found measurable levels in the sera of 18 of 141 HIV-positive patients, 17 of whom had AIDS.[8] These same investigators showed the transient appearance of IFN-α in the sera of some patients during acute HIV infection as well.

Serum IFN-α levels may even predict progression to AIDS. In a 2-year study of 99 asymptomatic homosexual men, 14 had increasing or persistently elevated (>48 IU/ml) levels of IFN-α, and all 14 developed ARC or AIDS over the study period.[9] In six patients for whom data were available, the mean time between the appearance of interferon in the serum and clinical progression was 6.5 months. None of the other study subjects with low or undetectable levels of serum interferon progressed in the follow-up period. In the setting of AIDS-related Kaposi's sarcoma, serum IFN-α may have similar prognostic significance. In 28 AIDS patients receiving IFN-α therapy for Kaposi's sarcoma, circulating levels of IFN-α prior to the initiation of therapy identified a subset of patients in whom the tumor progressed despite treatment.[10]

Numerous investigators have looked closely at the physicochemical properties of the IFN-α species that appears in the sera of patients with HIV disease, postulating that alterations might explain the apparent loss of protection afforded by this endogenous molecule with antiviral activity. As early as 1982, for example, one group found that the IFN-α species recovered from six of eight homosexual patients with either Kaposi's sarcoma or persistent lymphadenopathy was inactivated at acid pH.[11] A second report extended the finding to patients with hemophilia and AIDS.[12] Acid-labile IFN-α had been previously described in autoimmune diseases such as systemic lupus erythematosus,[13] and its occurrence in AIDS was initially cited as evidence that AIDS may be an autoimmune disease.

Investigators studying the natural history of HIV infection soon began to explore the role of acid-labile IFN-α as a predictor of clinical progression. In one re-port, sustained elevations in serum acid-labile interferon proved to be more specific for full-blown AIDS than β_2-microglobulin, HTLV-III antibody testing, and lymphocyte subset determinations.[14] The authors of the study also observed that elevations in acid-labile interferon preceded the onset of clinical deterioration in two patients with ARC. A second group tested the acid stability of the IFN-α species detected in patients who progressed to AIDS and found two patterns of development.[9] In some patients, the relative proportion of acid-labile IFN-α increased gradually over time, while in others a relatively rapid change occurred. The rapid increase in acid-labile interferon levels correlated with marked clinical deterioration in some patients, including three who died during the 2-year study period.

In vitro testing for IFN-α production by leukocytes from HIV-infected patients has revealed the converse: deficient interferon production correlates with clinical progression. In an assay system measuring interferon production in response to challenge with herpesvirus-infected fibroblasts, peripheral blood mononuclear cells (PBMC) from patients with AIDS manifested by opportunistic infections with or without Kaposi's sarcoma produced up to 1,000-fold less IFN-α than cells from either patients with AIDS-related Kaposi's sarcoma alone, patients with lymphadenopathy, homosexual controls, or heterosexual controls.[15] This study did not address whether the interferon deficiency antedated the occurrence of opportunistic infections, nor were the patients followed through resolution of their infection, so it is impossible to discriminate the effects of HIV infection from those of opportunistic infections on interferon production in this series. A subsequent prospective study utilizing the same assay system found that a deficit in interferon production preceded the development of opportunistic infection, although the interferon deficit did not achieve statistical significance as an independent predictor.[16]

A quantitative deficiency in IFN-α production has been confirmed by others using similar *in vitro* systems. For example, nonadherent leukocytes recovered from seropositive patients, regardless of clinical stage, produced significantly reduced levels of IFN-α in response to exposure to influenza A virus or to a leukemia cell line, compared to cells from uninfected donors.[17] Somewhat different results were obtained when IFN-α production from PBMC of HIV-infected patients was measured after exposure to vesicular stomatitis virus, herpes simplex type 1, and Newcastle disease virus.[18] Whereas patients with CDC Stages III and IV disease had marked reductions in IFN-α production that were highly statistically significant, PBMC from asymptomatic seropositive patients (CDC Stage II) produced normal amounts of IFN-α. Increased circulating levels of IFN-α in later stages of disease were also reported in this study.

In summary, serum levels of IFN-α appear to correlate with disease progression in some patients, and the presence of interferon may serve as a marker of poor prognosis. The specific species of circulating interferon is unique in its acid lability. Despite elevated serum levels, IFN-α production by PBMC from infected individuals is markedly reduced. No tenable hypothesis has been offered to explain this apparent inconsistency of reduced cellular production in the setting of increased serum levels as clinical illness progresses.

INTERFERON AS TREATMENT FOR KAPOSI'S SARCOMA

All interferons exhibit antiproliferative activity.[19] Growth inhibition has been demonstrated in erythroid precursors, lymphoid cells, regenerating hepatocytes, fibroblasts, as well as tumor cells.[19-21] The mechanisms by which interferons exert their inhibitory effects are unknown but most likely involve depression of DNA and protein synthesis, interruption of polyribosome formation, prolongation of the intermitotic phase, and alterations in cytokinesis.[22-26] Interferons as cytoreductive therapy have been evaluated in numerous clinical trials and have been shown to induce regressions of hairy cell leukemia, lymphoma, multiple myeloma, breast cancer, and osteosarcoma.[19,27]

IFN-α also displays a wide range of immunoregulatory effects, including enhanced natural killer (NK) cell activity, induction of T-cell–mediated cytotoxicity, and altered macrophage function.[28] Thus, the combined antitumor and immunoenhancing activities of this agent made it a particularly attractive early candidate for the treatment of AIDS-related Kaposi's sarcoma. Conventional cytotoxic agents for treating this neoplasm, such as etoposide and vinblastine, are associated with high rates of tumor response—in excess of 80% in some series.[29] However, the response duration is generally less than 1 year,[29] and these agents may further suppress immune function in HIV-infected patients and increase the likelihood that opportunistic infections will develop. In addition, experience in patients with Kaposi's sarcoma due to other causes of immunosuppression—for example, in the setting of corticosteroid therapy—had demonstrated that this tumor frequently regresses when the inciting factor (e.g., steroids) is removed. The regression accompanying immune restoration also suggested that immunostimulants might be of therapeutic benefit. IFN-α does not lead to further immunosuppression and is now licensed by the Food and Drug Administration and considered the treatment of choice for AIDS-related Kaposi's sarcoma in patients with CD4 counts greater than 200 cells/mm³ in whom systemic therapy is believed to be warranted.[30,31]

The results of a selected series of clinical trials of IFN-α in the treatment of Kaposi's sarcoma are summarized in Table 20B–1. One of the earliest studies[32] documented a 42% major response rate (25% complete responses, 17% partial responses) in 12 patients with AIDS-related Kaposi's sarcoma. Recombinant IFN-α_{2a} was administered intramuscularly (IM) at doses of 36 or 54 million units/day for 1 month, then thrice weekly. Responses were judged by reductions in measurable

lesions of the skin, lymph nodes, and gastrointestinal (GI) tract and were confirmed by biopsy. Of note, in some patients who had either minor responses or stable disease during the first month, the Kaposi's sarcoma progressed when the interferon dosing interval was reduced to thrice weekly.

Although absolute CD4 counts were not reported, the OKT4/OKT8 ratios before treatment ranged from 0 to 1.61 (mean, 0.63). All four patients with progressive disease in the study had pretreatment ratios of 0.56 or less, whereas all but one major responder had ratios of 0.82 or above. The authors noted an association between either a normal T-lymphocyte response to phytohemagglutinin prior to therapy or an improved response during therapy and a clinical response, although this association did not attain statistical significance in the 12-patient series. The mean OKT4/OKT8 ratio was also noted to rise from 0.63 to 0.96 after 3 weeks of daily interferon treatment.

Side-effects occurring in this study were those commonly ascribed to interferon: fever, chills, anorexia, headache, myalgias, arthralgias, hair loss, paresthesias, leukopenia, and reversible transaminase elevations. Only two patients required dose reductions, one because of hypotension and weakness, the other because of fatigue and neutropenia.

In a series reported by the group at San Francisco General Hospital, a total of 60 patients were treated with varying doses of recombinant IFN-α administered intravenously (IV) or subcutaneously (SC).[33,34] Half of the patients received an induction period of daily dosing for 5 days per week every other week for 2 months, followed by a maintenance phase at the same or a reduced dosing interval. The other 30 patients received interferon thrice weekly throughout. The daily dosages initially employed in this study were relatively low (1 to 5 million units per m² of body surface area), and only 10% of patients experienced a complete response. The investigators noted that no significant changes in T4/T8 ratios occurred with interferon. No new or life-threatening toxic effects were reported in this trial.

Subsequent reports from San Francisco General Hospital have looked at IFN-α_{2b} given SC at 30 million units/m² thrice weekly for 8 weeks, a regimen that yielded complete and partial response rates of approximately 40%.[34] On the basis of their accumulated experience, the San Francisco investigators concluded that (1) higher doses of interferon produce greater antitumor efficacy, (2) a response to interferon is associated with improved survival, and (3) during the study period, fewer opportunistic infections were reported in responders than in nonresponders.

Additional small to moderate-size studies have helped to refine the role of interferon in treating Kaposi's sarcoma.[35-39] In one study of 30 treated patients, pretherapy CD4 counts correlated significantly with clinical response.[35] Although the major response rate in this trial was only 13%, the chance of responding was approximately 70% for a patient with a pretherapy CD4 count above 200 cells/mm³, a total lymphocyte count above

Table 20B–1. Selected Clinical Studies of Interferon-α in the Treatment of AIDS-Related Kaposi's Sarcoma

IFN Type	Starting Dose (×1,000,000 Units)	Route	Initial Frequency	Duration of Treatment (wk)	Immune Status	No. of Evaluable Patients	Response Rate (%)*	Reference
SINGLE AGENT STUDIES								
rIFN-α_{2a}	36–54	IM	q.d.	7–48	T4/T8 = 0.63, (range, 0–1.6)	12	42	32
rIFN-α_{2a} or -α_{2b}	1–5/m²	SC or IV	q.d. × 5 d. q.o.w.	≥8	T4/T8 = 0.5 (range, 0.2–1.1)	30	47	33
rIFN-α_{2b}	1–50/m²	SC or IV	q.d. × 5 d. q.o.w.	≥8	T4/T8 = 0.62, (range, 0.2–1.9)	20	30	37
Lymphoblastoid	7.5–25/m²	IM	q.d.	4–32	Mean CD4 = 59	30	13	35
Lymphoblastoid	20	IM	q.d.	7–28	Mean CD4 = 270	12	66	39
rIFN-α_{2a}	3.0–54	IM	q.d.	4–88	T4/T8 = 0.43	70	27	38
rIFN-α_{2a}	27–36	SC	q.d.	8–40	Mean CD4: responders, 368; nonresponders, 217	26	46	36
rIFN-α_{2b}	35	SC	q.d.	1–92	Mean CD4: complete responders, 408; partial responders, 386; nonresponders, 154	21	38	40
COMBINATION STUDIES								
Lymphoblastoid	5.0 + ZDV	SC	q.d.	12–58	Mean CD4 = 552	22	50	49
rIFN-α_{2a} or lymphoblastoid	4.5–18 + ZDV	IM	q.d.	8	Mean CD4 = 236	37	46	50
rIFN-α_{2a} or lymphoblastoid	9.0–27 + ZDV	IM	q.d.	8–48	CD4 range: 169–206	43	47	51

rIFN = recombinant interferon, KS = Kaposi's sarcoma, m² = square meter, ZDV = zidovudine, q.o.w. = every other week, IM = intramuscular, SC = subcutaneous, IV = intravenous.
* Response rate is the sum of complete and partial responses.

1,500/mm³, no cytomegaloviremia, and no history of opportunistic infection. A second study corroborated the association of a relatively intact immune system with response to therapy.[36] Among 28 patients with Kaposi's sarcoma, 46% had either complete or partial responses. Responders had higher initial CD4 counts than nonresponders (mean ± SD: 368 ± 179 vs. 217 ± 169 cells/mm³), although this difference did not reach statistical significance. Responders did, however, have a significant rise in CD4 counts during the course of treatment (mean increase of 90 cells/mm³), compared with no change in the CD4 counts of nonresponders. In this and other studies, the stage and duration of Kaposi's sarcoma did not significantly influence tumor response rates.

Other reports have come to several similar conclusions, the most important of which may be that tumor response to IFN-α in patients with HIV infection depends on a critical number of functioning T cells (Fig. 20B–1). Of 21 patients with AIDS-related Kaposi's sarcoma treated at the National Institutes of Health (NIH) with up to 35 million units/day of IFN-α_{2b} given SC, five patients (24%) had a complete clinical response and histologic tumor regression, and three (14%) had partial responses (Fig. 20B–2).[40] Tumor response was closely correlated with immune function as measured by CD4 counts; the mean CD4 counts (cells/mm³ ± SEM) for

complete responders, partial responders, and nonresponders were 408 ± 96, 386 ± 116, and 154 ± 33, respectively. Additionally, all five patients with pretreatment CD4 counts above 400 cells/mm³ showed significant tumor responses, as compared with none of seven patients with pretreatment CD4 counts below 150 cells/mm³.

Despite interferon's effect on tumor burden, no significant immunologic changes were observed during this study, in contrast to the findings of others.[36] Specifically, in the NIH study, CD4 percentages in peripheral blood, NK cell numbers and activity, and blast transformation to antigen and mitogen were not significantly altered even after 1 year of daily IFN-α treatment. Thus, although the antiproliferative activity of IFN-α in Kaposi's sarcoma is clearly dependent on immune status, prolonged high-dose IFN-α administration did not produce measurable improvement in immunologic function in this group of HIV-infected patients.

INTERFERON AS ANTIVIRAL THERAPY

Studies of IFN-α in patients with AIDS-related Kaposi's sarcoma demonstrate antiretroviral activity as well. One study, for example, found an association between clin-

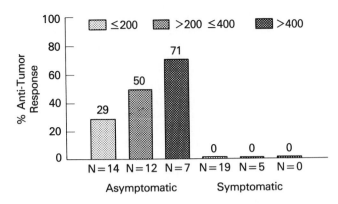

Figure 20B–1. Kaposi's sarcoma tumor response rates by pretherapy CD4 lymphocyte counts in cohorts of patients treated with IFNα. Interferon was administered SC at dosages of 30 million units/m² thrice weekly or 35 million units/day. (Reprinted with permission of Schering-Plough.)

ical response and decline in HIV antigenemia.[36] In this series, all seven responders with Kaposi's sarcoma and initial antigenemia showed a 50% or greater decline in detectable antigen levels over the course of the study; only one of five nonresponders with antigenemia

showed a comparable decrement. In another study, anti-HIV properties were detected both by HIV cocultures of patient PBMC with uninfected, stimulated lymphoblasts and by serum p24 antigen assays.[40] Persistently reduced HIV activity in cultures was found in three patients after 16 to 48 weeks of therapy. Additionally, nine of 13 responders with Kaposi's sarcoma demonstrated a greater than 75% reduction in p24 antigenemia; among the eight nonresponders, no significant decreases in p24 antigenemia were detected. As was true for Kaposi's sarcoma response, anti-HIV effects occurred only in patients with relatively intact immune function (*i.e.,* CD4 counts above 500 cells/mm³) and only after long-term, high-dose interferon therapy. In all four patients with pretreatment CD4 counts above 500 cells/mm³, HIV cultures became persistently negative and serum p24 levels became undetectable. In contrast, in the 17 patients with CD4 counts below 500 cells/mm³, no significant changes in culture or p24 levels were seen. Thus, by 1988 two small but carefully performed clinical trials of IFN-α in patients with AIDS-related Kaposi's sarcoma had generated the important observation that interferon could inhibit HIV replication in the subset of patients with still-preserved immune function.

Supportive information for a potential antiviral role for interferon came from concurrent *in vitro* work. One study demonstrated that recombinant IFN-α$_{2a}$ inhibited

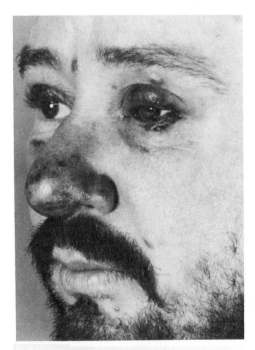 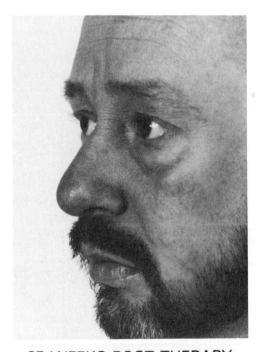

PRE-THERAPY   35 WEEKS POST THERAPY

Figure 20B–2. Effects of IFN-α on facial lesions of Kaposi's sarcoma. The pretherapy CD4 count in this case was 559 cells/mm³. (Reprinted with permission of Lane HC et al: Anti-retroviral effects of interferon-alpha in AIDS-associated Kaposi's sarcoma. Lancet 2:1218, 1988.) (See also Color Fig. 4, Color insert.)

HIV replication in PBMC in a dose-dependent fashion and that complete inhibition was possible at drug concentrations achievable *in vivo*.[5] A second study showed that zidovudine and IFN-α act in synergistic fashion to inhibit viral replication.[41] In other work that used lymphocytic and promonocytic cell clones chronically infected with HIV, IFN-α was shown to inhibit posttranscriptional stages of the viral life cycle.[42] Whereas zidovudine targets the early event of reverse transcription and successfully prevents acute HIV infection of susceptible cells, IFN-α appears to interfere with the assembly and release of progeny virions from the chronically or permanently infected cell. This series of experimental observations provided a theoretical construct for understanding the *in vitro* synergy of interferon and zidovudine and provided additional support for clinical trial designs using drug combinations.

Laboratory and clinical studies of interferon have also complemented one another in understanding the rebound effect seen after withdrawal of interferon. HIV replication *in vitro* increases markedly when interferon is removed from the culture media.[43] Earlier work in a murine retrovirus system had demonstrated the so-called post-budding effect, whereby interferon inhibits release of preformed virions from the cell, leading to the formation of clusters of virions on the outer plasma membrane.[44] Electron microscopic studies of HIV infection reveal an abundance of intracellular virions in interferon-treated cells, which strongly suggests that interferon acts in part by blocking viral release.[42] Some investigators have postulated that the accumulation of virus on the outer cell membrane might lead to the release of increased numbers of preformed virus particles once interferon is withdrawn.[42]

Although extensive clinical studies addressing a possible rebound effect have not been performed, serum p24 antigen levels and HIV culture data from several patients with HIV infection participating in interferon trials support an associated rebound effect *in vivo*.[40,45] For example, one patient[45] with asymptomatic HIV infection received 25 to 35 million units of IFN-α by daily SC injection and experienced a dramatic p24 antigen response. Initial antigen levels of 111 pg/ml fell to undetectable levels during 12 weeks of interferon therapy, then rebounded to over 10,000 pg/ml several months after interferon was stopped (Fig. 20B–3). A second patient[40] with Kaposi's sarcoma attained a complete tumor response after 10 weeks of daily SC IFN-α, with a corresponding fall in serum p24 antigen levels from approximately 600 pg/ml to 100 pg/ml. Serum p24 antigen levels rose again after interferon was discontinued. This patient received extended periods of interferon therapy on two subsequent occasions, with associated declines in p24 antigenemia during each course of therapy and prompt rises in p24 antigen levels each time interferon was stopped. When interferon was finally discontinued (in this case because of cardiotoxicity), serum p24 antigen levels rose to nearly 800 pg/ml, exceeding even pretreatment levels. Although it is difficult to equate with certainty the rebound effect in the laboratory with that seen clinically, the mere existence of the phenomenon suggests that interferon as a single agent probably has a very limited role in treating HIV infection.

Two randomized, placebo-controlled trials have evaluated IFN-α as single-agent antiviral therapy in HIV disease.[45,46] In a multicenter trial comparing two doses of recombinant IFN-α_{2a} with placebo in 67 patients with advanced HIV infection as evidenced by a history of an

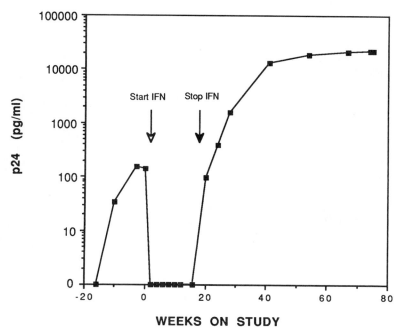

Figure 20B–3. Response of serum p24 antigen level to IFN-α in a patient with asymptomatic HIV infection. Pretherapy CD4 count was 775 cells/mm^3. (Reprinted with permission from Lane HC et al: Interferon-alpha in patients with asymptomatic human immunodeficiency virus (HIV) infection: A randomized, placebo-controlled trial. Ann Intern Med 112:805, 1990.)

opportunistic infection, no measurable benefit could be discerned.[46] In that study, patients were randomly assigned to receive placebo or interferon thrice weekly by SC or IM injection at a dose of either 3 or 36 million units. The results in the 37 patients who were able to complete 12 weeks of therapy revealed no significant differences between the three groups in CD4 counts, p24 antigen levels, number of opportunistic infections during the study period, or median survival. The patient population in this study, however, differed from that in other comparative trials in several key respects. These patients all had advanced disease, as evidenced by their history of opportunistic infections and their median CD4 counts, which ranged from 47 to 62 cells/mm³ between the treatment groups. Therefore the apparent lack of benefit from interferon in this study may be attributable to the profound immune deficiency already present in the patients.

In a second study, 34 asymptomatic, seropositive patients with CD4 counts of 400 cells/mm³ or higher and positive PBMC cultures for HIV were randomly assigned to receive IFN-α_{2b} or placebo by daily SC injection.[45] The study period ranged from 12 to 36 weeks, and the mean daily dose for those taking interferon was 17.5 million units. PBMC cultures became persistently negative in seven (64%) of 11 patients who took interferon for 12 or more weeks, but in only two (12%) of the 17 patients given placebo. The mean time to culture negativity was 11 weeks. Only two patients assigned to receive interferon were p24 antigenemic; one withdrew from the study after 3 weeks, while the other had a marked reduction in antigen levels that was closely related to interferon administration and dosage (see Fig.

20B–3). All five antigenemic patients assigned to the placebo group remained antigenemic throughout the study.

Immunologic parameters followed in these patients suggested an additional benefit conferred by interferon. Insofar as interferon therapy is associated with leukopenia and reductions in total numbers of circulating leukocyte subpopulations, the percentage of circulating lymphocytes that are CD4 positive (*i.e.,* the CD4%) may be a more reliable marker of immune function than absolute CD4 counts in HIV-infected patients receiving interferon.[47,48] The CD4% in patients receiving interferon was either stable or increased slightly, whereas it declined slightly over the study period in patients given placebo (Fig. 20B–4).[45]

In addition to the more favorable virologic and immunologic profiles seen in patients treated with IFN-α, the treated group fared better with regard to clinical end points at long-term follow-up. Over a 24-month period, opportunistic infections occurred in five (29%) patients on placebo but in none of the interferon-treated patients. Similarly, death from an AIDS-related illness occurred in three (18%) placebo-treated patients and no interferon-treated patients. Kaposi's sarcoma developed in one patient several weeks after interferon was stopped. The clinical differences between the two groups could not be accounted for by the use of zidovudine, anti-*Pneumocystis* prophylaxis, other investigational agents, or entry CD4 counts. However, the authors of the study raised the concern that p24 antigenemia may have been inequitably distributed despite randomization, since five of the seven antigenemic patients on study were assigned to placebo. Thus the

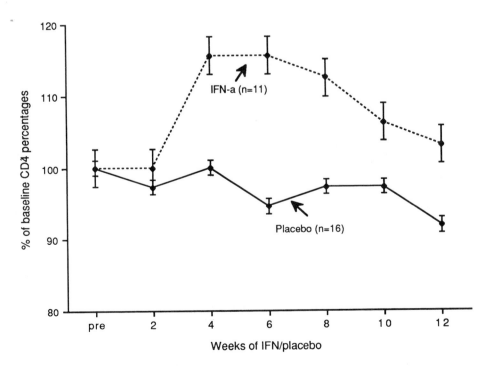

Figure 20B–4. Changes in mean CD4 percentages in patients during 12 weeks of IFN-α therapy (*n* = 11; *broken line*) or placebo (*n* = 16; *solid line*). Data were normalized by assigning the determination obtained before study a value of 100% and are expressed as mean ± SE. (Reprinted with permission from Lane HC et al: Ann Intern Med 112:805, 1990.)

results of this study, while provocative and potentially of great importance, require confirmation.

INTERFERON AS PART OF COMBINATION THERAPY

Once the safety and antiviral activity of IFN-α in HIV-infected patients had been established, the next logical step proved to be combining interferon with one or more other agents active against HIV. Combination therapy for treating HIV infection has a number of theoretical advantages, including synergistic efficacy, the potential for reduced dosages and less toxicity, and the ability to thwart the emergence of resistant viral isolates. The combination of zidovudine with IFN-α has been the most extensively studied to date, primarily because of the accumulated clinical experience with each agent as monotherapy. Supportive *in vitro* work came from the demonstration that the combination allowed 100- to 600-fold reductions in concentrations of these agents while producing antiviral activity equivalent to that seen with either agent alone.[38]

Three simultaneously conducted, randomized Phase I studies have evaluated this combination, all yielding similar results albeit with some intriguing differences.[49-51] One study conducted at the NIH looked at 37 evaluable patients with Kaposi's sarcoma and CD4 counts ranging from 83 to over 1,500 cells/mm³ (mean, 552 cells/mm³).[49] Patients were assigned to one of three zidovudine dose levels for 6 weeks—either 50, 100, or 250 mg every 4 hours—after which lymphoblastoid IFN-α was begun at 5 million units/day by SC injection and increased as tolerated to a daily maximum of 35 million units. Once a maximum tolerated dose was determined for each patient, this dosage was continued for another 12 weeks. Twenty-two of the 37 patients completed the full 12 weeks of therapy. The major dose-limiting toxic effects included neutropenia, thrombocytopenia, and transaminase elevations in the higher zidovudine dosage groups, while fatigue was the most prevalent toxic effect in those taking the lowest zidovudine dose and 15 million units or more of interferon.

The authors concluded that the combination of zidovudine and IFN-α can be safely administered to patients with AIDS-related Kaposi's sarcoma, although the degree and extent of toxic effects seen in the patient sample were greater than anticipated from experience with these agents as monotherapy. The optimal regimen for long-term administration proved to be 100 mg of zidovudine every 4 hours and 5 to 10 million units of IFN-α daily. Despite this reduction in interferon dose compared with that used in previous clinical trials, the antitumor efficacy of the combination was equivalent to prior experience: a major response rate of 50% with one complete response and ten partial responses (of 22 patients). Mean CD4 counts decreased over the course of the study from 552 to 450 cells/mm³, although the mean

CD4% remained stable at 35%. Of the six p24 antigenemic patients, three (50%) developed undetectable levels; 16 of 16 remained antigen negative. Thus the combination appeared to have antitumor and antiviral efficacy *in vivo*, based on these preliminary Phase I data.

A second study evaluated the combination in a group of patients with Kaposi's sarcoma and a mean CD4 count of 236 cells/mm³.[50] As in the first study, neutropenia was the major dose-limiting toxic effect; other major toxic effects included anemia, transaminase elevations, thrombocytopenia, and constitutional symptoms. The maximum tolerated doses in this study were 18 million units of recombinant IFN-α_{2a} by daily IM injection and 100 mg of zidovudine every 4 hours, or 4.5 million units of IFN-α_{2a} daily and 200 mg of zidovudine every 4 hours.

A major tumor response was seen in 46% of patients, with no significant difference between dose levels. Although 65% of patients with more than 200 CD4 cells/mm³ at entry demonstrated a tumor response, a substantial proportion of patients (30%) with fewer than 200 CD4 cells/mm³ at entry also showed regression of tumor, which suggested enhanced activity of the combination compared to interferon alone. In contrast to the declines in CD4 counts reported in the NIH study, some patients in this series did have an increase in CD4 counts. Modest rises in CD4 numbers were associated with an initial CD4 count below 200 cells/mm³ and the lowest interferon dosage (4.5 million units/day). Patients with initial CD4 counts above 200/mm³ or those on higher interferon doses experienced stable or slight decreases in absolute CD4 numbers.

Of the nine patients with p24 antigen levels of 25 pg/ml or higher, eight showed declines of 50% or more during therapy, and no patient who was negative at the start of study became positive on the combination. The authors of this study also analyzed data from peripheral blood HIV cultures and were able to correlate progressive increases in time to culture positivity (a possible marker for viral load) with tumor response. Culture data obtained 3 weeks after combination therapy was discontinued showed a return of time to culture positivity to the pretherapy baseline level for patients whose tumors regressed during treatment. These observations provided additional evidence of antiviral activity of this regimen.

A third study examined the combination in 56 patients with Kaposi's sarcoma whose CD4 counts ranged from 42 to 386 cells/mm³.[51] Patients were assigned to one of three dose levels of interferon—9, 18, or 27 million units by daily IM injection—plus zidovudine, initiated at 100 mg every 4 hours and increased if tolerated to 200 mg every 4 hours. Forty-three patients successfully completed 8 weeks of combined treatment. As in the previous studies, neutropenia was the major dose-limiting toxic effect. The maximum tolerated dose was 100 mg of zidovudine every 4 hours and 18 million units of interferon daily. Neutropenia occurred in 44% of patients in the study and was more marked than anticipated from the toxicity profile of each drug administered alone.

Other toxic effects encountered with the combination included serious anemia, which developed in 18% of patients in the study and did not differ in severity with the different dose levels, and transaminase elevations, which were moderate to severe in 22% of patients. Patients receiving the highest dose of both drugs experienced toxic hepatic effects that were particularly severe and rapid in onset.

Potential synergistic efficacy of the combination was seen in several immunologic, virologic, and tumor growth parameters. CD4 counts in this series remained stable or increased during the first several weeks, and the increases in counts were maintained longer than would be expected with zidovudine alone. Levels of p24 antigen declined by 50% or more in 70% of patients with detectable p24 antigenemia, the more marked responses occurring in patients receiving the highest doses. Rebound increases in p24 levels after 31 to 55 weeks of therapy were seen in 25% of patients who initially responded. Interestingly, these investigators compared viral isolates obtained pretreatment and after 12 months of combination therapy in a small number of patients and found no difference in sensitivity to zidovudine. The major response rate for Kaposi's sarcoma was 47% in this series. Although tumor response was associated with a CD4 count of 200 cells/mm³ or greater, 45% of responders had fewer than 200 CD4 cells/mm³, suggesting enhanced antiproliferative activity of the combination.

Thus, the results of three Phase I trials evaluating the combination demonstrate that the regimens studied can be tolerated for prolonged periods and have antiretroviral and antitumor activity. However, certain toxic effects, among them neutropenia, thrombocytopenia, and hepatic dysfunction, occurred with a much greater frequency than was anticipated from experience with each drug as single-agent therapy. Important questions regarding this combination remain, including long-term safety, optimal dosing regimen for efficacy, whether or not true synergistic efficacy exists, and the subpopulations least likely to develop toxicity and most likely to benefit. Subsequent nonrandomized trials have produced inconclusive results, however.[52,53] A prospective, randomized study comparing the combination with either agent alone is currently underway at the NIH; a second trial conducted by the AIDS Clinical Trials Group of the National Institute of Allergy and Infectious Diseases is analyzing different dosing regimens of concurrent and delayed combination therapy. The results of these investigations should answer many of these remaining questions.

Other interferon-containing combination regimens under evaluation attempt to minimize toxicity while preserving the efficacy of this cytokine. For example, one approach has been to combine growth factors such as granulocyte-macrophage colony-stimulating factor (GM-CSF) with interferon and zidovudine in order to prevent or reverse myelotoxicity while maintaining moderate to high interferon doses. One recent study reported on 19 patients who developed neutropenia on combined zidovudine and interferon, all of whom experienced reversal of neutropenia within 7 days of starting GM-CSF.[54] At an initial dosage of 125 mg/m² given by daily SC injection, GM-CSF accounted for only minimal additional toxicity. No adverse effect on tumor response, CD4 cell count, or p24 antigen level was demonstrated. In a study of 24 patients treated at the NIH, GM-CSF effectively reversed the neutropenia induced by combined interferon and zidovudine therapy at a mean minimum effective dose of 0.30 µg/kg/day by SC injection, without adverse effects on p24 antigen level.[55] Thus it appears likely that GM-CSF and perhaps other growth factors will be important adjuncts in marrow-toxic combination regimens.

TOXICITY OF INTERFERON

The safety of IFN-α given systemically is now well established, as this agent has been studied in over 1,400 patients with a variety of malignancies, representing more than 4,000 patient-months of exposure.[56] With rare exceptions, the toxic effects encountered when IFN-α was given to individuals with HIV infection were identical to those described in published oncology series. Nearly all patients who receive systemic therapy will experience some adverse effects. For the majority, this will mean a constellation of flulike symptoms, including fever (96% of patients), fatigue (66%), rigors (51%), and anorexia (42%).[56] These symptoms are dose dependent, often respond to symptomatic therapy with acetaminophen, and generally subside within 1 to 2 days after therapy is reduced or discontinued. Most patients will become tolerant of these effects as therapy is continued.

Major organ system involvement, in order of frequency, include GI, central nervous, hematopoietic, skin, and cardiovascular effects. Nausea and vomiting occur in approximately 40%, though only 5% of cases are severe, and diarrhea afflicts 20%. Asymptomatic hepatic transaminase elevations develop in 10% of patients and usually resolve within 1 week after interferon is discontinued. Mild confusion and somnolence may each occur in 10% of patients, are usually part of the initial flulike illness, and may not reverse for up to 2 weeks after therapy is modified or discontinued. Depression and anxiety may also manifest, particularly in individuals with a history of psychiatric disturbances. Leukopenia and neutropenia, which accounted for 50% to 60% of dose-limiting toxic effects in interferon plus zidovudine combination trials, account for approximately 20% of dose-modifying toxic effects in single-agent series. Despite this incidence of myelotoxicity, infections are reported in only about 6% of patients taking interferon and are rarely severe. Thrombocytopenia and anemia are uncommon complications. Dermatologic side-effects include transient rashes (4%), pruritus (4%), and hair loss, which is usually reversible. Proteinuria in the non-nephrotic range occurred in nearly 30% of HIV-infected patients in one series[40] and also responds to dose modification; frank azotemia and glomerulonephritis are not associated with IFN-α therapy.

Cardiovascular toxicity is unusual, and one recent review of the literature reported a total of 36 patients exhibiting cardiac effects in response to IFN-α therapy.[57] Toxic effects include arrhythmias, myocardial ischemia and infarction, and cardiomyopathy; the single most important risk factor is a history of cardiac disease. A second report[58] described three patients with AIDS-related Kaposi's sarcoma who developed reversible congestive cardiomyopathy presenting as acute congestive heart failure after 11 to 100 weeks of daily high-dose IFN-α. Cardiac function improved in all patients after interferon was stopped, and two of the patients tolerated rechallenge with interferon at reduced dosages. The authors postulated that cardiotoxicity in AIDS patients may be due to synergy between HIV and interferon.

Certain biochemical and serologic indices may be altered by interferon treatment. Anecdotal reports describe hypertriglyceridemia in association with IFN-α therapy in patients with and without AIDS,[59] and our experience treating patients at the NIH with interferon alone and in combination with zidovudine or dideoxyinosine supports this observation. The mechanism for this alteration in lipid metabolism may be multifactorial, insofar as hypertriglyceridemia occurring with progressive HIV infection in the absence of interferon therapy is well documented.[60] In addition, interferons induce surface expression of class I major histocompatibility complex antigens, including β_2-microglobulin.[2] Circulating levels of β_2-microglobulin, shown to be predictive of progression of HIV disease to an AIDS-defining illness,[61,62] are therefore potentially misleading and of limited utility in evaluating patients receiving interferon.

Although the list of potential adverse effects is formidable, the toxic effects of IFN-α are rarely life-threatening and can usually be controlled by modifying the dosage or stopping the drug. Despite the substantial numbers of patients who might be expected to experience side-effects, only about 10% of patients treated for malignancy with interferon require termination of therapy owing to toxicity.[56] In an ongoing NIH trial comparing zidovudine and IFN-α alone and in combination in HIV-infected patients with CD4 counts above 500 cells/mm³, only three (2%) of 180 patients enrolled to date have developed severe toxic effects necessitating termination of therapy. However, approximately 15% of patients receiving interferon alone or in combination with zidovudine have discontinued participation in the study, citing impaired quality of life due to subjective side-effects such as fatigue, depressed mood, and difficulty concentrating. Thus, for asymptomatic HIV-infected patients, the discomforts associated with interferon, rather than objective toxic effects, may be the most important obstacle to the wider use of this agent. In addition, as experience with long-term administration in HIV-infected patients continues to accumulate, particularly in the context of multidrug regimens, additional toxic effects may be encountered.

FUTURE DIRECTIONS

IFN-α is the treatment of choice for AIDS-related Kaposi's sarcoma in patients with CD4 counts above 200 cells/mm³. Over the past decade of intense clinical investigation in HIV infection, interferon has proved to be relatively safe and effective at inhibiting HIV replication. Ongoing studies may help to identify predictors of clinical response to guide the rational use of this potent cytokine. It appears unlikely that a single agent will emerge as definitive therapy for HIV infection. Combination regimens such as those currently under evaluation will most likely replace monotherapy. Interferon is an attractive adjunct to the reverse transcriptase inhibitors because of its different mechanism of action, potential for synergy, and safety profile. With the advent of readily available recombinant growth factors, some of the major dose-limiting toxic effects associated with combination therapies may be ameliorated. Thus, IFN-α will be an important component of future multi-agent strategies. As further insights are gained into the molecular mechanisms of HIV pathogenesis and latency, greater logic can be brought to bear on the selection and use of this and other promising agents.

REFERENCES

1. Laurence J: Immunology of HIV infection: I. Biology of the interferons. AIDS Res Human Retroviruses 6:1149, 1990
2. Pestka S, Langer JA, Zoon KC, Samuel CE: Interferons and their actions. Annu Rev Biochem 56:727, 1987
3. Zoon KC: Human interferons: Structure and function. Interferon 9:1, 1987
4. Pestka S, Kelder B, Familletti PC et al: Molecular weight of the functional unit of human leukocyte, fibroblast, and immune interferons. J Biol Chem 258:9706, 1983
5. Ho DD, Rota TR, Kaplan JC et al: Recombinant human interferon alfa-A suppresses HTLV-III replication in vitro. Lancet 1:602, 1985
6. Brinchmann JE, Gaudernack G, Vartdal F: In vitro replication of HIV-1 in naturally infected CD4+ T cells is inhibited by rIFN alpha2 and by a soluble factor secreted by activated CD8+ T cells, but not by rIFN beta, rIFN gamma, or recombinant tumor necrosis factor-alpha. J AIDS 4:480, 1991
7. Ambrus JL, Poiesz BJ, Lillie MA et al: Interferon and interferon inhibitor levels in patients with varicella-zoster virus, acquired immunodeficiency syndrome, acquired immunodeficiency syndrome-related complex, or Kaposi's sarcoma, and in normal individuals. Am J Med 87:405, 1989
8. Skidmore SJ, Mawson SJ: Alpha-interferon in anti-HIV positive patients. Lancet 1:520, 1987

9. Buimovici-Klein E, Lange M, Klein RJ et al: Long-term follow-up of serum-interferon and its acid-stability in a group of homosexual men. AIDS Res 2:99, 1986

10. Preble OT, Rook AH, Steis R et al: Interferon-induced 2′-5′ oligoadenylate synthetase during interferon alpha therapy in homosexual men with Kaposi's sarcoma: Marked deficiency in biochemical response to interferon in patients with the acquired immunodeficiency syndrome. J Infect Dis 152:457, 1985

11. DeStefano E, Friedman RM, Friedman-Kien AE et al: Acid-labile human leukocyte interferon in homosexual men with Kaposi's sarcoma and lymphadenopathy. J Infect Dis 146:451, 1982

12. Eyster ME, Goedert JJ, Poon M-C et al: Acid-labile interferon: A possible preclinical marker for the acquired immunodeficiency syndrome in hemophilia. N Engl J Med 309:583, 1983

13. Preble OT, Black RJ, Friedman RM et al: Systemic lupus erythematosus: Presence in human serum of an unusual acid-labile leukocyte interferon. Science 216:429, 1982

14. Calabrese LH, Proffitt MR, Gupta MK et al: Serum β_2-microglobulin and interferon in homosexual males: Relationship to clinical findings and serologic status to the human T lymphotropic virus (HTLV-III). AIDS Res 1:423, 1984–85

15. Lopez C, Fitzgerald PA, Siegal FP: Severe acquired immune deficiency syndrome in male homosexuals: Diminished capacity to make interferon-alpha in vitro associated with severe opportunistic infections. J Infect Dis 148:962, 1983

16. Siegal FP, Lopez C, Fitzgerald PA et al: Opportunistic infections in acquired immune deficiency syndrome result from synergistic defects of both the natural and adaptive components of cellular immunity. J Clin Invest 78:115, 1986

17. Abb J, Peichowiak H, Zachoval R et al: Infection with human T-lymphotropic virus type III and leukocyte interferon production in homosexual men. Eur J Clin Microbiol 5:365, 1986

18. Rossol S, Voth R, Laubenstein HP et al: Interferon production in patients infected with HIV-1. J Infect Dis 159:815, 1989

19. Kronenberg LH: Cellular effects of interferon. In Stiehm ER (mod): Interferon: Immunobiology and Clinical Significance. Ann Intern Med 96:80, 1982

20. Ortega JA, Ma A, Shore NA et al: Suppressive effect of interferon on erythroid cell proliferation. Exp Hematol 7:145, 1979

21. Jahiel RI, Taylor D, Rainford N et al: Inducers of interferon inhibit the mitotic response of liver cells to partial hepatectomy. Proc Natl Acad Sci USA 68:740, 1971

22. Gewert DR, Clemens MJ: Inhibition by interferon of thymidine uptake and deoxyribonucleic acid synthesis in human lymphoblastoid cells. Biochem Soc Trans 8:353, 1980

23. Creasey AA, Bartholomew JC, Merigan TC: Role of G_0-G_1-arrest in the inhibition of tumor cell growth by interferon. Proc Natl Acad Sci USA 77:1471, 1980

24. Pfeffer LM, Murphy JS, Tamm I: Interferon effects on the growth and division of human fibroblasts. Exp Cell Res 121:111, 1979

25. Brouty-Boye D, Macieira-Coelho A, Fiszman M et al: Interferon and cell division: VIII. Effect of interferon on macromolecular synthesis in L1210 cells in vitro. Int J Cancer 12:250, 1973

26. O'Shaughnessy MV, Easterbrook KB, Lee SH et al: Interferon inhibition of autogenously induced virions (C particles) in synchronized L-929 cell cultures. JNCI 53:1687, 1974

27. Pomerantz RJ, Hirsch MS: Interferon and human immunodeficiency virus infection. Interferon 9:113, 1987

28. Borden EC, Ball LA: Interferons: Biochemical, cell growth inhibitory, and immunological effects. Prog Hematol 12:299, 1981

29. Krown SE: AIDS-associated Kaposi's sarcoma: Pathogenesis, clinical course and treatment. AIDS 2:71, 1988

30. Groopman JE, Scadden DT: Interferon therapy for Kaposi sarcoma associated with the acquired immunodeficiency syndrome (AIDS). Ann Intern Med 110:335, 1989

31. Food and Drug Administration: Press release, November 21, 1988

32. Krown SE, Real FX, Cunningham-Rundles SC et al: Preliminary observations on the effect of recombinant leukocyte A interferon in homosexual men with Kaposi's sarcoma. N Engl J Med 308:1071, 1983

33. Volberding P, Valero R, Rothman J et al: Alpha interferon therapy of Kaposi's sarcoma in AIDS. Ann NY Acad Sci 437:439, 1984

34. Abrams DI, Volberding PA: Alpha interferon therapy of AIDS-associated Kaposi's sarcoma. Semin Oncol 14(suppl 2):43, 1987

35. Gelmann EP, Preble OT, Steis R et al: Human lymphoblastoid interferon treatment of Kaposi's sarcoma in the acquired immune deficiency syndrome: Clinical response and prognostic parameters. Am J Med 78:737, 1985

36. De Wit R, Boucher CAB, Veenhof KHN et al: Clinical and virological effects of high-dose recombinant interferon-alpha in disseminated AIDS-related Kaposi's sarcoma. Lancet 2:1214, 1988

37. Groopman JE, Gottlieb MS, Goodman J et al: Recombinant alpha-2 interferon therapy for Kaposi's sarcoma associated with the acquired immunodeficiency syndrome. Ann Intern Med 100:671, 1984

38. Real FX, Oettgen HF, Krown SE: Kaposi's sarcoma and the acquired immunodeficiency syndrome: Treatment with high and low doses of recombinant leukocyte A interferon. J Clin Oncol 4:544, 1986

39. Rios A, Mansell PWA, Newell GR et al: Treatment of acquired immunodeficiency syndrome-related Kaposi's sarcoma with lymphoblastoid interferon. J Clin Oncol 3:506, 1985

40. Lane HC, Feinberg J, Davey V et al: Anti-retroviral effects of interferon-alpha in AIDS-associated Kaposi's sarcoma. Lancet 2:1218, 1988

41. Hartshorn KL, Vogt MW, Chou T-C et al: Synergistic inhibition of human immunodeficiency virus in vitro by azidothymidine and recombinant alpha A interferon. Antimicrob Agents Chemother 31:168, 1987

42. Poli G, Orenstein JM, Kinter A et al: Interferon-alpha but not AZT suppresses HIV expression in chronically infected cell lines. Science 244:575, 1989

43. Yamamoto JK, Barre-Sinoussi F, Bolton V et al: Human alpha and beta interferon but not gamma suppress the in vitro replication of LAV, HTLV-III and ARV-2. J Interferon Res 6:143, 1986

44. Pitha PM, Wivel NA, Fernie BF et al: Effect of interferon on murine leukemia virus infection: IV. Formation of non-infectious virus in chronically infected cells. J Gen Virol 42:467, 1979

45. Lane HC, Davey V, Kovacs JA et al: Interferon-alpha in

patients with asymptomatic human immunodeficiency virus (HIV) infection: A randomized, placebo-controlled trial. Ann Intern Med 112:805, 1990

46. Interferon Alpha Study Group: A randomized placebo-controlled trial of recombinant human interferon alpha 2a in patients with AIDS. J AIDS 1:111, 1988

47. Taylor JM, Fahey JL, Detels R et al: CD4 percentage, CD4 number, and CD4:CD8 ratio in HIV infection: Which to choose and how to use. J AIDS 2:114, 1989

48. Masur H, Ognibene FP, Yarchoan R et al: CD4 counts as predictors of opportunistic pneumonias in human immunodeficiency virus (HIV) infection. Ann Intern Med 111:223, 1989

49. Kovacs JA, Deyton L, Davey R et al: Combined zidovudine and interferon alpha therapy in patients with Kaposi sarcoma and the acquired immunodeficiency syndrome (AIDS). Ann Intern Med 111:280, 1989

50. Krown SE, Gold JWM, Miedzwiecki D et al: Interferon alpha with zidovudine: Safety, tolerance, and clinical and virologic effects in patients with Kaposi sarcoma associated with the acquired immunodeficiency syndrome (AIDS). Ann Intern Med 112:812, 1990

51. Fischl MA, Uttamchandani RB, Resnick L et al: A phase I study of recombinant human interferon alpha 2a or human lymphoblastoid interferon alpha n1 and concomitant zidovudine in patients with AIDS-related Kaposi's sarcoma. J AIDS 4:1, 1991

52. Orholm M, Pedersen C, Mathiesen L et al: Suppression of p24 antigen in sera from HIV-infected individuals with low-dose alpha-interferon and zidovudine: A pilot study. AIDS 3:97, 1989

53. De Wit R, Danner SA, Bakker PJM et al: Combined zidovudine and interferon-alpha treatment in patients with AIDS-associated Kaposi's sarcoma. J Intern Med 229:35, 1991

54. Scadden DT, Bering HA, Levine JD et al: Granulocyte-macrophage colony-stimulating factor mitigates the neutropenia of combined interferon alfa and zidovudine treatment of acquired immune deficiency syndrome–associated Kaposi's sarcoma. J Clin Oncol 9:802, 1991

55. Davey RT, Davey VJ, Metcalf JA et al: A phase I/II trial of zidovudine, interferon-alpha, and granulocyte-macrophage colony-stimulating factor in the treatment of human immunodeficiency virus type 1 infection. J Infect Dis 164:43, 1991

56. Spiegel RJ: The alpha interferons: clinical overview. Semin Oncol 14(suppl 2):1, 1987

57. Sonnenblick M, Rosin A: Cardiotoxicity of interferon: A review of 44 cases. Chest 99:557, 1991

58. Deyton LR, Walker RE, Kovacs JA et al: Reversible cardiac dysfunction associated with interferon alfa therapy in AIDS patients with Kaposi's sarcoma. N Engl J Med 321:1246, 1988

59. Olsen EA, Lichtenstein GR, Wilkinson WE: Changes in serum lipids in patients with condylomata acuminata treated with interferon alpha-n1 (Wellferon). J Am Acad Dermatol 19:286, 1988

60. Grunfeld C, Kotler DP, Hamadeh R et al: Hypertriglyceridemia in the acquired immunodeficiency syndrome. Am J Med 86:27, 1989

61. Fahey JL, Taylor J, Detels R et al: The prognostic value of cellular and serologic markers in infection with human immunodeficiency virus type 1. N Engl J Med 322:166, 1990

62. Anderson RE, Lange W, Shiboski S et al: Use of β_2-microglobulin level and CD4 lymphocyte count to predict development of acquired immunodeficiency syndrome in persons with human immunodeficiency virus infection. Arch Intern Med 150:73, 1990

Soluble CD4, Immunomodulators, Immunotoxins, and Other Approaches to Anti-HIV Therapy

20C

Peter J. Gomatos   *Nicholas M. Stamatos*   *Robert T. Schooley*

CD4+ T cells and cells of mononuclear phagocytic lineage are the major targets for the human immunodeficiency virus (HIV).[1-3] Virus replicates in both cell types.[1,2,4-9] Several lines of evidence have clearly established CD4 as the major receptor for HIV. HIV envelope glycoprotein, gp120, binds specifically to the CD4 molecule present on the cell surface.[1,2,8,10-12] Identification of the CD4-gp120 interaction as the initial step in viral infection has provided the basis for antiviral strategies.

CD4 is expressed in a broad range of cell types but is present predominantly in cells of the thymus, spleen, and brain.[13] The CD4 molecule normally facilitates helper T-cell recognition of antigens presented by class II major histocompatibility complex (MHC) molecules.[8,13-16] The mature CD4 molecule consists of a 372-amino acid extracellular segment with four tandem immunoglobulin (Ig)–like domains (V1V2V3V4), a 23-amino acid transmembrane region, and a 38-amino acid, highly charged, cytoplasmic domain.[13,17-19]

The region of CD4 critical for interaction with class II MHC molecules is distinct from but overlapping with the region that binds gp120.[14,15,20] The gp120 binding site is present within residues 41 to 55 in the V1 region (the amino-proximal Ig-like domain of CD4).[14,17,21-24]

However, both termini of the V1 region are critical for maintaining the conformational integrity of the gp120 binding site within residues 41 to 55.[21,25,26] The lack of N-linked glycans in V1V2 suggests that these sugar residues have little or no importance in the CD4-HIV gp120 interaction.[27] Productive infection of cells expressing truncated forms of CD4 confirmed that the binding site for HIV was within the V1V2 domains.[28] Thus, if additional molecules are required for virus entry, their interaction with the cytoplasmic, transmembrane, or membrane-proximal extracellular regions of CD4 is not a requirement for successful infection.

The amino acid sequence of gp120 is highly variable among HIV-1 strains, but hypervariable regions of gp120 are interspersed with highly conserved regions in a manner reminiscent of antibody molecules.[29] Insofar as all HIV strains utilize CD4 as a receptor, it would appear that some or all of these conserved regions contribute to the interaction between gp120 and CD4.[8] A gp120-specific monoclonal antibody (mAb) that blocks interaction between gp120 and CD4 recognized an epitope contained within amino acids 397–439.[30] With *in vitro* mutagenesis, it was found that deletion of 12 amino acids from this region of gp120 resulted in complete loss of binding.[31] Moreover, a single amino acid substitution in this region resulted in significantly decreased binding to CD4.[31,32]

Although the interaction between CD4 and gp120 is a major determinant of infection, some cell lines were susceptible to productive infection by HIV-1 *in vitro via* CD4-independent mechanisms. Human primary chondrocytes, foreskin fibroblasts, and synovial cells, which do not express CD4, supported low but significant levels of infection by HIV-1 or HIV-2 strains.[33] Five hepatoma cell lines were also susceptible to infection by HIV-1 strains despite the absence of CD4 on their cell surfaces.[34] These studies demonstrate the complexity of the interaction between HIV and its host cells and emphasize the importance of evaluating potential antiviral agents in a variety of experimental systems.

The association of HIV-1 with antibody provides another CD4-independent mechanism for entry of virus into cells.[35,36] Antibody-dependent enhancement of HIV-1 infectivity is mediated by the FcRIII receptor on human macrophages and possibly another Fc receptor on human CD4+ lymphocytes.[37] Although enhancement of HIV-1 infection in CD4+ lymphocytes could not be blocked by anti-FcRIII antiserum, it was inhibited in these lymphocytes by the addition of human IgG aggregates. These results do not exclude the possibility that HIV-1, in association with antibody, can also enter monocytes or macrophages through CD4 receptors.[38,39] An additional mechanism for entry of antibody-bound HIV into cells utilizes complement receptors.[35,40]

RECOMBINANT SOLUBLE CD4 (rsCD4)

Inhibition of the virus-receptor interaction provides an attractive approach to therapeutic intervention against HIV.[41–45] It was proposed that because of its essential role, the interaction of gp120 and cellular CD4 would not be significantly affected by genetic variation among HIV-1 isolates. Thus, a soluble form of CD4 potentially could bind to both virus and infected cells and protect uninfected cells. It is also possible that rsCD4 could exert its effects not by preventing binding but by interfering with later steps, *i.e.,* uncoating or proper orientation for reverse transcription.

Several groups independently developed rsCD4 derivatives.[41–45] Soluble secreted forms of CD4 were produced that lacked its transmembrane and cytoplasmic domains. The rsCD4 bound gp120 with an affinity and specificity comparable to that of cellular CD4 binding. The finding that sera from AIDS patients coprecipitated the rsCD4 polypeptide only if recombinant gp120 (rgp120) was included in the binding reaction suggests that rsCD4 had assumed the appropriate configuration. Most rsCD4 molecules contain the four Ig-like domains (V1V2V3V4), but a fragment containing only the two amino-terminal domains (V1V2) was almost as inhibitory to viral replication as the whole extracellular portion.[22,26,46–48] Of particular importance was that class II–specific T-cell interactions were not inhibited by rsCD4.[43]

The infectivity of the laboratory strain HTLV-IIIB was blocked equally well by rsCD4 and OKT4A, an anti-CD4 mAb that blocks gp120 binding to CD4. In contrast, the infectivity of HIV-2 and simian immunodeficiency virus (SIV) strains was more refractory to inhibition by rsCD4.[49,50] The dose levels of rsCD4 required to produce 50% inhibition of infectivity of HIV-2 and SIV ranged from 50- to 400-fold higher and from 5- to 20-fold higher, respectively, than for HIV-1 laboratory strains.[51] Markedly higher concentrations of rsCD4 were also required to inhibit infectivity of two low-passage monocyte-tropic strains of HIV-1 that had been recently isolated from patients and grown only in monocytes.[52] The relative inefficiency of rsCD4 for inhibition of HIV infection in monocytes was a property of the virion and not of the target cell. HIV isolates that infected both monocytes and T cells required similarly high levels of rsCD4 (100–200 μg/ml) for inhibition of infection, yet the use of specific antibodies supports the conclusion that the receptor on monocytes is in fact CD4.

The infectivity in lymphocytes of primary isolates of HIV-1 was also more refractory to inhibition by rsCD4 than that of laboratory strains.[53] It was suggested that the laboratory strains of HIV-1 represented one extreme and were selected in the laboratory on the basis of a greater affinity for CD4. Despite the large variation in sensitivity to inhibition by rsCD4, the rgp120 derived from cloning of the primary clinical HIV-1 isolates bound equally well to rsCD4 as did the rgp120 of the laboratory strains.[54] In striking contrast, the rgp120 derived from HIV-2 or SIV had significantly lower affinity for rsCD4.[55] Thus, some other explanation is needed to explain the differential sensitivities of the HIV-1 strains to rsCD4.

Clinical Use of Soluble rsCD4

Successful use of rsCD4 in man depends in part on its immunogenicity, its effect on cellular immunity, and its pharmacokinetics. If the host recognizes rsCD4 as foreign and develops an immune response against it, would the clearance of rsCD4 be increased or would the immune system be modulated in a way that results in more immunosuppression?

Infection with HIV-1 has been associated with autoantibodies to CD4. Indeed, high titers of antibodies to rsCD4 were found in the sera of up to 12.6% of HIV-1–infected individuals.[56–58] None were found in normal human sera or in sera from HIV-2–infected individuals. These anti-rsCD4 antibodies bound to a different epitope from that bound by OKT4A. In addition, they had no immediate effect on CD4+ T cell count or on progression of HIV-1 disease, which suggests no causal relationship with increased immune suppression. Although a variable proportion of these autoantibodies reacted with rsCD4 by recognizing epitopes on the V3V4 domains, none bound to human cellular CD4.[56,58] This result suggests that HIV-1 infection generates antibodies directed against a region of CD4 distinct from the virus-binding domain and the domain that interacts with MHC class II receptors. A possible anti-idiotypic origin of these antibodies was unlikely.

The safety and pharmacokinetics of rsCD4 were evaluated in patients with acquired immunodeficiency syndrome (AIDS) or AIDS-related complex (ARC).[59,60] When rsCD4 was administered by rapid intravenous (IV) infusion, the initial volume of distribution was essentially equivalent to plasma volume and the serum half-life was approximately 45 to 60 minutes. Bioavailability was 51% following intramuscular (IM) injection and 46% after subcutaneous (SC) injection. The mean peak concentration of rsCD4 after IM or SC injection occurred 2 to 6 hours after administration. After the initial phase of each study was completed, patients were allowed to continue on maintenance therapy, with rsCD4 administered IM or SC 3 or 7 days per week. Zidovudine was permitted only during the maintenance portion of the study. Preliminary data suggest that zidovudine did not alter the pharmacokinetics of rsCD4: the half-life, maximum concentration, and clearance of rsCD4 in patients receiving dual therapy were nearly identical to those in a group of subjects treated solely with rsCD4.[59]

No significant differences in hepatic, renal, or hematologic measurements were noted during therapy with rsCD4 at any dosage. The development of anti-CD4 antibodies in a few patients receiving rsCD4 was not associated with adverse clinical or immunologic events. No consistent or sustained changes were observed in the relative or absolute number of CD4+ T cells. Whereas the p24 antigen levels did not change in patients receiving lower doses of rsCD4, there was an average decline of 23% from baseline value of p24 in patients receiving 30 mg/day. There was little change in plasma viral titer or in the amount of virus that could be cultivated from 10^6 cells while patients were on therapy.[53,60] No significant toxic effects were observed in another Phase I trial in which rsCD4 was given at doses of up to 1 mg/kg.[61] Because the maximum tolerated dose in humans was not determined in any of the studies, further trials with higher doses of rsCD4 were planned.

The therapeutic effect of human rsCD4 was also assessed in SIVmac-infected rhesus monkeys.[62] A single IM injection of rsCD4 resulted in peak plasma levels in monkeys within 2 hours and yielded an estimated rsCD4 serum half-life of about 6 hours. Four SIVmac-infected rhesus monkeys were given a 50-day course of daily IM injections. During treatment, no changes were noted in the relative distribution or function of peripheral blood lymphocytes (PBL) or in serum assessment of liver or renal function. SIVmac could not be isolated from the second week of treatment until 1 month after completion of therapy. Functional abnormalities reflecting SIVmac-induced disease also improved in these animals.

The therapeutic response to rsCD4 in SIVmac-infected rhesus monkeys was attributed to the production of an anti-human rsCD4 antibody.[50] Surprisingly, the plasma of these animals also contained an antibody that reacted with the rhesus monkey rsCD4 molecule and that bound to monkey CD4+ PBL. Thus, the expected immunologic tolerance to rhesus monkey cell surface CD4 had been overcome by the daily administration of human rsCD4. Of note, the extracellular portion of the rhesus monkey CD4 differs from its human homologue at 33 of 375 amino acids.[50]

Future plans include a Phase I study of the safety and pharmacokinetics of rsCD4 in infants and children infected with HIV or at risk for HIV infection. Additional protocols include the use of combination therapies to detect possible synergy between rsCD4 and other antiretroviral or immunomodulating agents.

IMMUNOADHESINS

Therapy based on the use of rsCD4 as a single agent is unsatisfactory. Recombinant sCD4 acted merely as a passive shield. Binding of rsCD4 to gp120, wherever it occurred, did not destroy infected cells or virus. In addition, it was difficult to sustain adequate antiviral concentrations of rsCD4 because of its short half-life *in vivo*. Modification of this therapeutic approach was clearly needed.

Immunoadhesins were designed to combine the binding specificity of CD4 with the effector domain of an Ig.[47,63,64] Genetically engineered immunoadhesins contained either V1V2 or all four Ig-like domains, V1V2V3V4 of CD4 fused to the Fc domain of IgG1.[47,63] The IgG1 subtype, because of its long half-life, was deliberately chosen to supply Fc and complement binding sites. The immunoadhesins were disulfide-linked dimers that contained two gp120 binding sites that were not sterically hindered. These hybrids demonstrated high-affinity binding both to Fc receptors and to gp120. Disappointingly, though, they did not bind to the first component, C1q, in the complement pathway.

At concentrations comparable to those used for rsCD4, the immunoadhesins prevented cell killing by HIV without concomitant inhibition of cell proliferation. They also facilitated the destruction of HIV-infected cells by phagocytosis or antibody-dependent cell-mediated cytotoxicity (ADCC).[65] Moreover, there was no evidence of enhancement of infection by immunoadhesins in cells that expressed high-affinity Fc receptors. The half-life of immunoadhesins in humans was expected to be comparable to that of human IgG1. Indeed, the immunoadhesin constructs had a circulating half-life nearly 200 times longer than that of rsCD4. Transplacental transfer of the CD4-containing immunoadhesins was an important bonus of the strategy.[63] Thus, the engineering of immunoadhesins yielded designer immune molecules with maximum anti-HIV activity.

To expand the capabilities of the immunoadhesin constructs, molecules that combined the specificity of CD4 with the effector functions of other Ig subclasses were generated.[64] Plasmids were constructed in which the exons encoding the V1V2 domains of CD4 were linked to all but the V_H1 and C_H1 domains of the mouse μ or γ2a heavy chains. Both constructs bound to HIV gp120. In contrast to the immunoadhesins constructed with the Fc portion of IgG1, these constructs bound complement in addition to binding to Fc receptors. The pentameric CD4-IgM chimera was at least 1,000-fold more active than its dimeric CD4-IgG2a counterpart in syncytium inhibition assays.

Clinical Trials With Immunoadhesins

Patients with AIDS or ARC were entered into clinical trials.[66–69] The rsCD4-IgG1 construct was administered by continuous IV infusion, by IV bolus weekly, by IM injection weekly, or by SC injection three times a week. After completion of the initial phase, most patients received the agent by IM injections once or twice a week.

rsCD4-IgG1 was well tolerated when given IV or IM and had a much more favorable pharmacokinetic profile than rsCD4. No significant changes were observed in hematologic or serum chemical parameters. When given IV, the clearance of rsCD4-IgG1 was 15 times lower than that for rsCD4, and its median terminal elimination half-life was 33 hours. After IM injection, the bioavailability was 18% to 46% and the serum half-life was approximately 32 hours. After SC injection, the serum half-life was 34 to 46 hours. In regard to serum half-life, none of the routes of administration had a distinct advantage.

In patients receiving rsCD4-IgG1, the absolute number of lymphocytes, including CD4+ and CD8+ T cells remained stable. Analysis of the effects of rsCD4-IgG1 on p24 antigen levels and plasma viremia is pend-

ing. At the time of reporting, none of the subjects had developed detectable antibodies against rsCD4-IgG1. Trials using larger amounts and more frequent dosing regimens are needed to establish the maximally tolerated dose and the effectiveness of this agent.

A study is being developed to evaluate the safety, tolerance, and pharmacokinetics of rsCD4-IgG1 in HIV-1–infected pregnant women. The study will also determine the degree of transfer of this construct across the placenta by measuring drug levels in newborns. The results will have significant therapeutic implications for the perinatal transmission of HIV.

IMMUNOTOXINS

Immunotoxins consist of cell-reactive ligands (antibodies, hormones, or growth factors) coupled to plant or bacterial toxins or their toxic subunits.[70,71] Plant toxins (*e.g.*, ricin) usually consist of a ribosome-inactivating A chain linked by a disulfide bond to a galactose-specific lectin (B chain) that promotes cell binding. The A and B chains of plant toxins can be separated following reduction, and the A chain, once purified, can be chemically linked to different ligands (*e.g.*, CD4) to generate a conjugate with cell specificity. It was postulated that after the ligand attached to gp120 on the cell surface, the toxin-CD4 complexed to gp120 would enter the cell by endocytosis and be released into the cytoplasm, where its A chain would inhibit protein synthesis. This immunotoxin would theoretically reduce the number of HIV-infected cells *in vivo* and thereby slow the progression of disease.

Immunotoxins Containing Ricin

The deglycosylated A chain of ricin, dgA, was coupled to rsCD4[72,73] and the resulting conjugate, rsCD4-dgA, was separated from free dgA by high-pressure liquid chromatography. The rsCD4-dgA had gp120 binding activity comparable to 25% to 50% that of native rsCD4. Deglycosylation of the ricin A chain significantly reduced hepatotoxicity in mice by preventing the conjugate from homing to liver cells and resulted in more effective delivery to target cells. The LD_{50} of the conjugate in mice was equivalent to 1 g of rsCD4-dgA administered to a 70-kg human. The relatively low toxicity of rsCD4-dgA in mice, coupled with its potent *in vitro* cytotoxicity ($IC_{50} = 10 \times 10^{-10}$ M) to HIV-infected H9 human cells and its lack of interaction with class II antigens, suggested that it would be a safe and specific drug for the treatment of patients infected with HIV.

Alternatively, the dgA of ricin was conjugated to either of two human IgG-κ mAbs specific for the HIV envelope protein, gp41.[74] Monoclonal antibodies with this specificity were chosen as ligands for ricin because gp41 is expressed only by infected cells and is highly conserved. Both immunotoxins containing antibodies to gp41 killed 50% of infected H9 and U937 cells at 1.5

$\times\ 10^{-9}$ and 5×10^{-9} M, respectively. Addition of chloroquine to U937 cultures lowered the dosage required for killing of 50% of infected cells (IC_{50}) 100-fold. The specificity of killing was confirmed by the observation that the effect of both immunotoxins was blocked by rgp160 but not by rgp120 or human IgG. Neither immunotoxin was cytotoxic for MHC class II–expressing Daudi cells below 10^{-7} M. gp120-positive cells from seropositive subjects were susceptible *in vitro* to an immunotoxin containing the ricin A chain and a murine mAb against gp120.[75] Use of murine mAbs as ligands is not ideal. Their potential to generate a host immune response will preclude their repeated use.

Immunotoxins Containing *Pseudomonas* Exotoxin

A variety of techniques were used to link a variable portion of *Pseudomonas* exotoxin (PE) A, a bacterial toxin, to proteins that would deliver the toxin to specific cells.[76] CD4(178)-PE 40 is a recombinant protein in which the cell recognition region (domain 1) of PE A toxin is replaced with the amino-terminal 178 amino acids of human CD4 containing the gp120 binding region. The segment of PE remaining in the hybrid protein contained domains II and III, which are responsible for translocation across the cell membrane and adenosine diphosphate ribosylation of elongation factor 2, with resulting inhibition of protein synthesis. A substantially pure, monomeric form of CD4(178)-PE40 was obtained.

The specificity and efficacy of CD4(178)-PE40 were analyzed in cells infected with a gp160-producing recombinant vaccinia virus and in HIV-infected cells.[46,77,78] The CD4(178)-PE40 hybrid toxin was found to be an extremely potent cytotoxic agent, selectively killing HIV-infected cells with IC_{50} values around 100 pM. The IC_{50} values for both cell killing and inhibition of virus production were at least an order of magnitude below the reported K_d value for CD4-gp120 binding. This finding may reflect that the hybrid toxin acts catalytically in the cytosol. The toxicity of the immunotoxin toward cells expressing the HIV envelope glycoprotein was neutralized by OKT4A antibody, which blocks the CD4-gp120 interaction. Because OKT4A had no effect on the toxicity of native PE, specificity was thus conferred on the immunotoxin by the CD4 moiety. A latently infected human T-cell line, in which expression of HIV was inducible, was sensitive to CD4(178)-PE40 only after virus induction. A high concentration of CD4(178)-PE40 did not inhibit protein synthesis in Raji cells, a B-cell line that expresses relatively large amounts of MHC class II molecules.

These results support the therapeutic potential of the CD4(178)-PE 40 in the treatment of HIV-infected individuals. However, inhibition of HIV replication *in vitro* by CD4-PE constructs was incomplete.[79] In a coculture of HIV-infected and -uninfected cells, the hybrid toxin delayed HIV-induced cell killing and suppressed production of free virus, but did not prevent the eventual death of most cells. CD4-PE constructs also delayed but did not inhibit HIV replication in human PBL. Viral replication occurred following removal of the CD4-PE constructs from these cultures. A major potential problem with hybrid toxins arises from the fact that latently infected T cells or monocytes may lack HIV envelope proteins on their surface and thus may not be susceptible to killing by immunotoxins. When cells do express gp120 on their surface, they become targets for ADCC or cytotoxic T lymphocytes (CTL). If such immunotoxins are to be useful, it will only be as adjuncts to other modalities of treatment in later stages of disease as the host becomes more immunosuppressed.

FUTURE DIRECTIONS WITH CD4-BASED THERAPY

Unfavorable pharmacokinetic properties and limited scope of action make rsCD4 unsuitable for use as a single agent against HIV. Maintenance of an antiviral inhibitory concentration of rsCD4 would likely require continuous administration. Latently infected cells are not its targets, nor is it known if rsCD4 crosses the blood-brain barrier. Effective use of rsCD4 may occur in combination with other agents that act at different stages of the HIV replicative cycle. Synergism with zidovudine or with zidovudine/interferon-αA was demonstrated *in vitro*.[80,81] Replication of HIV-1 in acutely infected cells was inhibited for an extended period, but eventually occurred despite the continued presence of the three drugs.[81] Moreover, the two- or three-drug combinations were ineffective in inhibiting viral infection in persistently infected cells.

The need for agents with longer half-life and extended capacity led to the development of second-generation compounds, the immunoadhesins and immunotoxins. This approach augments blocking activity by directing a cellular or chemical attack against gp120-bearing cells. As 0.002% of circulating mononuclear cells in asymptomatic seropositive patients and 0.25% in symptomatic patients are expressing viral gp120 at any one time,[82] it is unlikely that even these second-generation drugs will be effective in diminishing the viral burden. Moreover, it is likely that the antigenicity of the immunotoxins and of those immunoadhesins in which murine mAb is an integral component will preclude their repeated usage. It remains to be established that the immunoadhesins cross the human placenta and prevent maternal transmission of HIV to the fetus.

We are now witnessing the design of third-generation agents. Three innovative, CD4-based approaches utilizing gene therapy offer hope for halting progression of HIV-1 disease: (1) expression of rsCD4 by retroviral vectors,[83] (2) alteration of CD4 such that it traps gp120 intracellularly,[84] and (3) priming of CTL to destroy cells expressing HIV-1 envelope proteins.[85]

The first approach takes advantage of the finding

that most replicating cells can be transduced *in vitro* by retrovirus vectors and can continuously express the integrated genes. The soluble CD4 produced by the transduced cells would be secreted locally, and thereby HIV entry into that cell would be inhibited. Ideally, bone marrow transplantation of transduced pluripotent hematopoietic cells would reconstitute a functional immune system. As an alternative to bone marrow transplantation, cell implants could be used as *in vivo* factories for the continuous production of rsCD4.

In the second approach, protection against HIV would be achieved intracellularly by introducing a gene for a mutated form of CD4 with a specific retention signal for the endoplasmic reticulum. In HeLa cells that expressed the mutated forms of CD4 along with gp120 or gp160, the viral proteins were trapped complexed to mutated CD4 within the lumen of the endoplasmic reticulum and were not expressed at the cell surface. If this approach is to be developed further, it will be necessary to show that wild-type HIV replication can be suppressed in cells expressing the mutated CD4, and that the function of native CD4 is not impaired in these cells.

In the third approach, chimeric proteins containing the extracellular domain of CD4 and signal-transducing polypeptides of the T cell or Fc receptor were stably expressed at the cell surface. Theoretically, CTL could be transfected with these chimeric genes, expanded in culture with interleukin-2, and reinfused into the patient. These cells would thus be primed to recognize and kill cells expressing HIV gp120. Under appropriate conditions, cells expressing the CD4 chimeras could be stimulated *in vivo* by interaction with HIV-1, and thus could respond dynamically to the viral burden.

FUTURE DIRECTIONS OF OTHER APPROACHES

This section briefly discusses several other antiviral agents. Some have been under investigation for several years; others are in early stages of clinical development.

Isoprinosine/Inosine Pranobex

Isoprinosine is a synthetic immunostimulatory agent with minimal or no direct antiviral activity against HIV.[86,87] In one of two placebo-controlled clinical trials, its use delayed progression to AIDS in HIV-infected individuals.[87] No serious side-effects were observed. This beneficial effect occurred even though isoprinosine did not stem the decline in CD4+ T cell numbers or result in any change in p24 levels during its use. Because the second clinical trial reported that isoprinosine was not effective in delaying progression to AIDS, an additional study is mandatory before claims of efficacy can be accepted.[88]

The future clinical trials can be expected to include the simultaneous use of zidovudine. In combination therapy, isoprinosine caused a doubling in the area under the serum concentration–time curve and an increase in the mean half-life of zidovudine.[89] The advantages of combined treatment could include: (1) possible immunoenhancement resulting from isoprinosine, (2) a lower dose of zidovudine needed to maintain a therapeutic level, and (3) a longer interval between individual zidovudine doses.

Imuthiol/Diethyldithiocarbamate (DTC)

DTC, a metabolite of Antabuse (disulfuram), is another immunorestorative agent that has no direct effect on HIV replication.[90] It is an antioxidant that inhibits production of prostaglandin E_2 (PGE_2) in macrophages, thus potentially reversing downregulation of T-cell responses by PGE_2. In a placebo-controlled clinical trial, DTC appeared active in reducing the number of opportunistic infections and other events relating to progression to ARC and AIDS. Hematologic, liver, and renal functions remained normal.[91] There were no significant differences in the number of CD4+ T cells between treated and control groups. The effectiveness of DTC awaits confirmation in ongoing and future trials.

Thiols

Cellular reducing systems were reported to have a role in preventing activation of HIV in latently infected cells.[92] *N*-acetylcysteine (NAC) suppressed the induction of HIV gene expression in latently infected cells stimulated with tumor necrosis factor-α or interleukin-6. Additionally, nontoxic concentrations of ascorbate suppressed virus production and cell fusion in HIV-infected T-lymphocytic cell lines.[93] Moreover, 2-mercaptoethanol or NAC enhanced T-cell colony formation *in vitro* in cells from patients with AIDS or ARC. 2-Mercaptoethanol was more effective in this capacity but is too toxic to be administered *in vivo*.[94]

The underlying premise of this therapeutic approach is that thiols given exogenously will raise the intracellular glutathione levels and keep HIV quiescent. NAC has already been used systemically for the treatment of acetaminophen poisoning and for its protective effect against damage produced by free radicals during cancer chemotherapy. Only clinical trials will determine if any of these agents will be safe and effective.

Compound Q

Trichosanthin, or Compound Q, an extract from root tubers, has been used as treatment for tumors and as an abortifacient.[95] GLQ 223, a highly purified form of compound Q, selectively killed cells infected *in vitro* with HIV-1.[96] A treatment protocol raised concerns about the toxicity of Compound Q.[97,98] Most patients developed side-effects, including fever, rash, violent dreams, or coma, and three patients (all in an advanced stage of disease) died after taking the drug. Patients treated at two sites showed an increase in absolute number of CD4+ T cells and a decline in p24 antigen levels. Two Phase I trials of highly purified GLQ 223 are currently being conducted.

Hypericin

Hypericin, an aromatic polycyclic dione, has been chemically synthesized.[95] It strongly inhibited retroviral infection *in vitro* and protected mice from infection with Friend leukemia virus. Potential mechanisms of action include interference with the uncoating or disassembly of HIV after entry into cells, or interference with viral assembly or shedding from infected cells.[99,100] Hypericin has been claimed to cross the blood-brain barrier in humans, and has been used as an antidepressant. A dose escalation Phase I trial of synthetic hypericin is ongoing.

BI-RG-587

BI-RG-587, a dipyridodiazepinone, was selected from a program involving the synthesis of muscarinic receptor antagonists.[101] It does not have peripheral muscarinic or central benzodiazepine activities. It inhibited the growth of laboratory and primary HIV-1 isolates with an IC_{50} in the nanomolar range but had no activity against HIV-2 or SIV reverse transcriptases or DNA polymerases. Cytotoxicity studies showed a high therapeutic index in culture of greater than 8,000. In chimpanzees, plasma levels in excess of 600 times the IC_{50} were observed after single oral doses of 20 mg/kg. BI-RG-587 crosses the blood-brain barrier effectively. An early open-label, staggered dose escalation study is being developed to assess the safety, tolerance, and activity of this promising agent alone or in combination with zidovudine.

TIBO

The tetrahydro-imidazo(4,5,1-jk)(1,4)-benzodiazepin-2(1*H*)-one and -thione (TIBO) derivatives inhibited HIV-1 replication *in vitro* at nanomolar concentrations that were 100-fold lower than their cytotoxic concentration.[102] TIBO compounds did not block replication of HIV-2 or any other RNA- or DNA-containing viruses. The TIBO derivatives share some structural features with the classic dihydrobenzodiazepines, but they contain a unique tricyclic system and were devoid of diazepam-like effects in rodents. There was no anti-HIV-1 activity in a large variety of classic benzodiazepines tested. The TIBO derivatives prevented acute HIV-1 infection *in vitro,* whereas in persistently infected cells there was little or no inhibition. In six healthy males, plasma levels exceeding the anti-HIV-1 IC_{50} were maintained for 24 hours. The TIBO compound was well tolerated, with no significant changes in hematological, biochemical, or cardiovascular parameters. Clinical development of this class of agents is proceeding.

Protease Inhibitors

The HIV protease presents a crucial virus-specific target for new therapies. In principle, inhibition of the protease within HIV-1 and other retroviruses should abrogate the maturation of both the virion core and the processing of retroviral enzymes. Both peptide and symmetric, nonpeptidic inhibitors were synthesized.[103–106] Both classes of compounds when used at nanomolar concentrations exerted a potent and highly specific antiretroviral activity against HIV-1 in multiple cell systems. In their presence, the released virus particles contained mostly p55 and other *gag* precursors, but not p24. The released particles had aberrant morphology and were noninfectious. Some of these analogues inhibited both HIV-1 and HIV-2 proteases, with little effect on the structurally related human aspartyl proteases. Initial experiments in rodents indicated that concentrations exceeding those required for *in vitro* anti-HIV activity could be maintained for several hours without any visible signs of toxicity. This class of compounds may have a wide therapeutic margin, which holds promise for the treatment of HIV infection in patients.

Anti-*tat* Inhibitors

The *tat* gene product markedly enhances the expression of viral genes.[107] Thus, inhibitors blocking its functions can be expected to inhibit viral replication. Elucidation of the structure of its binding site(s) and of its mechanism(s) of action will permit the development of drugs to inhibit its multiple functions. Evaluation of these drugs in clinical trials will follow.

Acknowledgment: John A. Wohlhieter and Sibyl Goode assisted in the research and preparation of this chapter.

REFERENCES

1. Dagleish AG, Beverley PC, Clapham PR et al: The CD4 (T4) antigen is an essential component of the receptor for the AIDS retrovirus. Nature 312:763, 1985
2. Klatzmann D, Champagne E, Chamaret S et al: T-lymphocyte T4 molecule behaves as a receptor for human retrovirus LAV. Nature 312:767, 1984
3. McDougal JS, Mawle A, Cort SP et al: Cellular tropism of the human retrovirus HTLV-III/LAV. J Immunol 135:3151, 1985
4. Asjo BA, Ivhed I, Gidlund M et al: Susceptibility to infection by the human immunodeficiency virus (HIV) correlates with T4 expression in a parental monocytoid cell line and its subclones. Virology 157:359, 1987
5. Collman R, Godfrey B, Cutilli J et al: Macrophage-tropic strains of human immunodeficiency virus type 1 utilize the CD4 receptor. J Virol 64:4468, 1990
6. Meltzer MS, Skillman DS, Gomatos PJ et al: Role of mononuclear phagocytes in the pathogenesis of human immunodeficiency virus infection. Annu Rev Immunol 8: 169, 1990

7. Pauza CD, Price TM: Human immunodeficiency virus infection of T cells and monocytes proceeds via receptor-mediated endocytosis. J Cell Biol 107:959, 1988

8. Sattentau QJ, Weiss RA: The CD4 antigen: Physiological ligand and HIV receptor. Cell 52:631, 1988

9. Sodroski J, Goh WC, Rosen C et al: Role of the HTLV-III/LAV envelope in syncytium formation and cytopathicity. Nature 322:470, 1986

10. Lyerly HK, Matthews TJ, Langlois AJ et al: Human T-cell lymphotropic virus IIIb glycoprotein (gp120) bound to CD4 determinants on normal lymphocytes and expressed by infected cells serves as target for immune attack. Proc Natl Acad Sci USA 84:4601, 1987

11. Maddon PJ, Dalgleish AG, McDougal JS et al: The T4 gene encodes the AIDS virus receptor and is expressed in the immune system and the brain. Cell 47:333, 1986

12. McDougal JS, Kennedy MS, Sligh JM et al: Binding of HTLV-III/LAV to T4+ T cells by a complex of the 110 K viral protein and the T4 molecule. Science 231:382, 1986

13. Klatzmann DR, McDougal JS, Maddon PJ: The CD4 molecule and HIV infection. Immunodefic Rev 2:43, 1990

14. Bowman MR, MacFerrin KD, Schreiber SL, Burakoff SJ: Identification and structural analysis of residues in the V1 region of CD4 involved in interaction with human immunodeficiency virus envelope glycoprotein gp120 and class II major histocompatibility complex molecules. Proc Natl Acad Sci USA 87:9052, 1990

15. Clayton LK, Sieh M, Pious DA, Reinherz EL: Identification of human CD4 residues affecting class II MHC versus HIV-1 gp120 binding. Nature 339:548, 1989

16. Doyle C, Strominger JL: Interaction between CD4 and class II MHC molecules mediates cell adhesion. Nature 330:256, 1987

17. Arthos J, Deen KC, Chaikin MA et al: Identification of the residues in human CD4 critical for the binding of HIV. Cell 57:469, 1989

18. Clark SJ, Jefferies WA, Barclay AN et al: Peptide and nucleotide sequences of rat CD4 (W3/25) antigen: Evidence for derivation from a structure with four immunoglobulin-related domains. Proc Natl Acad Sci USA 84:1649, 1987

19. Maddon PJ, Littman DR, Godfrey M et al: The isolation and nucleotide sequence of cDNA encoding the T cell surface protein T4: A new member of the immunoglobulin gene family. Cell 42:93, 1985

20. Lamarre D, Ashkenazi A, Fleury S et al: The MHC-binding and gp120-binding functions of CD4 are separable. Science 245:745, 1989

21. Ashkenazi A, Presta LG, Marsters SA et al: Mapping the CD4 binding site for human immunodeficiency virus by alanine-scanning mutagenesis. Proc Natl Acad USA 87:7150, 1990

22. Chao BH, Costopoulos DS, Curie T et al: A 113-amino acid fragment of CD4 produced in *Escherichia coli* blocks human immunodeficiency virus–induced cell fusion. J Biol Chem 264:5812, 1989

23. Jameson BA, Rao PE, Kong LI: Location and chemical synthesis of a binding site for HIV-1 on the CD4 protein. Science 240:1336, 1988

24. Mizukami T, Fuerst TR, Berger EA, Moss B: Binding region for human immunodeficiency virus (HIV) and epitopes for HIV-blocking monoclonal antibodies of the CD4 molecule defined by site-directed mutagenesis. Proc Natl Acad Sci USA 85:9273, 1988

25. Arthos J, Deen KC, Shatzman A et al: The genetic analysis of the HIV envelope binding domain on CD4. Ann NY Acad Sci 616:116–24, 1990

26. Clayton LK, Hussey RE, Steinbrich R et al: Substitution of murine for human CD4 residues identifies amino acids critical for HIV-gp120 binding. Nature 335:363, 1988

27. Ibegbu CC, Kennedy MS, Maddon PJ et al: Structural features of CD4 required for binding to HIV. J Immunol 142:2250, 1989

28. Bedinger P, Moriaty A, von Borstel RC II et al: Internalization of the human immunodeficiency virus does not require the cytoplasmic domain of CD4. Nature 334:162, 1988

29. Coffin JM: Genetic variation in AIDS viruses. Cell 46:1, 1986

30. Lasky LA, Nakamura G, Smith DH et al: Delineation of a region of the human immunodeficiency virus type 1 gp120 glycoprotein critical for interaction with the CD4 receptor. Cell 50:975, 1985

31. Olshevsky U, Helseth E, Furman C et al: Identification of individual human immunodeficiency virus type 1 gp120 amino acids important for CD4 receptor binding. J Virol 64:5701, 1990

32. Hemming A, Bomlstedt A, Flodby P et al: Cystein 402 of HIV gp120 is essential for CD4-binding and resistance of gp120 to intracellular degradation. Arch Virol 109:269, 1989

33. Ikeuchi K, Kim S, Byrn RA et al: Infection of nonlymphoid cells by human immunodeficiency virus type 1 or type 2. J Virol 64:4226, 1990

34. Cao YZ, Friedman-Kien AE, Haung YX et al: CD4-independent, productive human immunodeficiency virus type 1 infection of hepatoma cell lines in vitro. J Virol 64:2553, 1990

35. Robinson DC, Montefiori DC, Mitchell WM: Antibody-dependent enhancement of human immunodeficiency virus type 1 (HIV) infection. Lancet 1:790, 1988

36. Takeda A, Tuazon CU, Ennis FA: Antibody-enhanced infection by HIV-1 via Fc receptor–mediated entry. Science 242:580, 1988

37. Homsy J, Meyer M, Tateno M et al: The Fc receptor and not CD4 receptor mediates antibody enhancement of HIV infection in human cells. Science 244:1357, 1989

38. Perno CF, Baseler MW, Broder S, Yarchoan R: Infection of monocytes by human immunodeficiency virus type 1 blocked by inhibitors of CD4-gp120 binding, even in the presence of enhancing antibodies. J Exp Med 171:1043, 1990

39. Zeira M, Byrn RA, Groopman JE: Inhibition of serum-enhanced HIV-1 infection of U937 monocytoid cells by recombinant soluble CD4 and anti-CD4 monoclonal antibody. AIDS Res Hum Retroviruses 6:629, 1990

40. Robinson Jr, WE, Montefiori DC, Mitchell WM: Complement-mediated antibody-dependent enhancement of HIV-1 infection requires CD4 and complement receptors. Virology 175:600, 1990

41. Deen KC, McDougal JS, Inacker R et al: A soluble form of CD4 (T4) protein inhibits AIDS virus infection. Nature 331:82, 1988

42. Fisher RA, Bertonis JM, Meier W et al: HIV infection is blocked in vitro by recombinant soluble CD4. Nature 331:76, 1988

43. Hussey RE, Richardson NE, Kowalski M et al: A soluble CD4 protein selectively inhibits HIV replication and syncytium formation. Nature 331:78, 1988

44. Smith DH, Byrn RA, Marsters SA et al: Blocking of HIV-1

infectivity by a soluble, secreted form of the CD4 antigen. Science 238:1704, 1987

45. Traunecker A, Lüke W, Karjalainen K: Soluble CD4 molecules neutralize human immunodeficiency virus type 1. Nature 331:84, 1988

46. Ashorn P, Moss B, Weinstein JN, Chaudhary VK et al: Elimination of infectious human immunodeficiency virus from human T-cell cultures by synergistic action of CD4-*Pseudomonas* exotoxin and reverse transcriptase inhibitors. Proc Natl Acad Sci USA 87:8889, 1990

47. Capon DJ, Ward RH: Antiviral effects of CD4 derivatives. Curr Opin Immunol 2:433, 1989–90

48. Garlick RL, Kirschner RJ, Eckenrode FM et al: *Escherichia coli* expression, purification, and biological activity of a truncated soluble CD4. AIDS Res Hum Retroviruses 6:465, 1990

49. Clapham PR, Weber JN, Whitby D et al: Soluble CD4 blocks the infectivity of diverse strains of HIV and SIV for T cells and monocytes but not for brain and muscle cells. Nature 337:368, 1989

50. Watanabe M, Chen ZW, Tsubota H et al: Soluble human CD4 elicits an antibody response in rhesus monkeys that inhibits simian immunodeficiency virus replication. Proc Natl Acad Sci USA 88:120, 1991

51. Looney DJ, Hayashi S, Nicklas M et al: Differences in the interaction of HIV-1 and HIV-2 with CD4. J AIDS 3:649, 1990

52. Gomatos PJ, Stamatos NM, Gendelman HE et al: Relative inefficiency of soluble recombinant CD4 for inhibition of infection by monocyte-tropic HIV in monocytes and T cells. J Immunol 144:4183, 1990

53. Daar ES, Li XL, Moudgil T, Ho DD: High concentrations of recombinant soluble CD4 are required to neutralize primary human immunodeficiency virus type 1 isolates. Proc Natl Acad Sci USA 87:6574, 1990

54. Brighty DW, Rosenberg M, Chen ISY, Ivey-Hoyle M: Envelope proteins from clinical isolates of HIV-1 which are refractory to neutralization by sCD4 possess high affinity for the CD4 receptor. Proc Natl Acad Sci USA 88:7802-5, 1991

55. Ivey-Hoyle M, Culp JS, Chaikin MA et al: Envelope glycoproteins from biologically diverse isolates of immunodeficiency viruses have widely different affinities for CD4. Proc Natl Acad Sci USA 88:512, 1991

56. Kowalski M, Ardman B, Basiripour L et al: Antibodies to CD4 in individuals infected with human immunodeficiency virus type 1. Proc Natl Acad Sci USA 86:3346, 1989

57. Moore JP, Sattentau QJ, Clapham PR: Enhancement of soluble CD4-mediated HIV neutralization and gp120 binding by CD4 autoantibodies and monoclonal antibodies. AIDS Res Hum Retroviruses 6:1273, 1990

58. Thiriart C, Goudsmit J, Schellekens P et al: Antibodies to soluble CD4 in HIV-1-infected individuals. AIDS 2:345, 1988

59. Kahn JO, Allan JD, Hodges TL et al: The safety and pharmacokinetics of recombinant soluble CD4 (rCD4) in subjects with the acquired immunodeficiency syndrome (AIDS) and AIDS-related complex: A phase 1 study. Ann Intern Med 112:254, 1990

60. Schooley RT, Merigan TC, Gaut P et al: Recombinant soluble CD4 therapy in patients with the acquired immunodeficiency syndrome (AIDS) and AIDS-related complex: A phase I–II escalating dosage trial. Ann Intern Med 112:247, 1990

61. Sun W, Virani N, Hawkes C et al: High dose continuous IV infusions of soluble CD4 (sCD4) (abstr 2177). Presented at the VI International Conference on AIDS, San Francisco, June 20–23, 1990

62. Watanabe M, Reimann KA, Delong PA et al: Effect of recombinant soluble CD4 in rhesus monkeys infected with simian immunodeficiency virus of macaques. Nature 337:267, 1989

63. Capon DJ, Chamow SM, Mordenti J et al: Designing CD4 immunoadhesins for AIDS therapy. Nature 337:525, 1989

64. Traunecker A, Schneider J, Kiefer H, Karjalainen K: Highly efficient neutralization of HIV of recombinant CD4-immunoglobulin molecules. Nature 339:68, 1989

65. Byrn RA, Mordenti J, Lucas C et al: Biological properties of a CD4 immunoadhesin. Nature 344:667, 1990

66. Collier A, Katzenstein D, Coombs R et al: Safety and pharmacokinetics of intravenous recombinant CD4 immunoadhesin (rCD4-IgG) (AIDS Clinical Trials Group Protocol 121) (abstr S.B.480). Presented at the VI International Conference on AIDS, San Francisco, June 20–23, 1990

67. Davey R Jr, Davey V, Polis M et al: A phase I trial of recombinant human CD4-immunoglobulin (rCD4-IgG) in HIV-1 infection (abstr S.B.481). Presented at the VI International Conference on AIDS, San Francisco, June 20–23, 1990

68. Hodges TL, Kahn J, Kaplan L et al: Phase I study of the safety and pharmacokinetics of recombinant human CD4 immunoglobulin (rCD4-IgG) administered by intramuscular (IM) injection in patients with AIDS and ARC (abstr S.B.478). Presented at the VI International Conference on AIDS, San Francisco, June 20–23, 1990

69. Yarchoan R, Pluda JM, Adamo D et al: Phase I study of rCD4-IgG administered by continuous intravenous (IV) infusion to patients with AIDS or ARC (abstr S.B.479). Presented at the VI International Conference on AIDS, San Francisco, June 20–23, 1990

70. Vitetta ES: The development of immunotoxins for the therapy of cancer, AIDS, and immune dysfunctions. Int Symp Princess Takamatsu Cancer Res Fund 19:333, 1988

71. Vitetta ES, Fulton RJ, May RD et al: Redesigning nature's poisons to create anti-tumor reagents. Science 238:1098, 1987

72. Ghetie V, Till MA, Ghetie MA et al: Large scale preparation of an immunoconjugate constructed with human recombinant CD4 and deglycosylated ricin A chain. J Immunol Methods 126:135, 1990

73. Ghetie V, Till MA, Ghetie M-A et al: Preparation and characterization of conjugates of recombinant CD4 and deglycosylated ricin A chain using different cross-linkers. Bioconjugate Chem 1:24, 1990

74. Till MA, Zolla-Pazner S, Gorny MK et al: Human immunodeficiency virus–infected T cells and monocytes are killed by monoclonal human anti-gp41 antibodies coupled to ricin A chain. Proc Natl Acad Sci USA 86:1987, 1989

75. Matsushita S, Koito A, Maeda Y et al: Selective killing of HIV-infected cells by anti-gp120 immunotoxins. AIDS Res Hum Retroviruses 6:193, 1990

76. Chaudhary VK, Mizukami T, Fuerst TR et al: Selective killing of HIV-infected cells by recombinant human CD4-*Pseudomonas* exotoxin hybrid protein. Nature 335:369, 1988

77. Berger EA, Chaudhary VK, Clouse KA et al: Recombinant CD4-*Pseudomonas* exotoxin hybrid protein displays HIV-

specific cytotoxicity without affecting MHC class II–dependent functions. AIDS Res Hum Retroviruses 6:795, 1990

78. Berger EA, Clouse KA, Chaudhary VK et al: CD4-*Pseudomonas* exotoxin hybrid protein blocks the spread of human immunodeficiency virus infection in vitro and is active against cells expressing the envelope glycoproteins from diverse primate immunodeficiency retroviruses. Proc Natl Acad Sci USA 86:9539, 1989

79. Tsubota H, Winkler G, Meade HM et al: CD4-*Pseudomonas* exotoxin conjugates delay but do not fully inhibit human immunodeficiency virus replication in lymphocytes in vitro. J Clin Invest 86:1684, 1990

80. Hayashi S, Fine RL, Chou TC et al: In vitro inhibition of the infectivity and replication of human immunodeficiency virus type 1 by combination of antiretroviral 2′,3′-dideoxynucleosides and virus-binding inhibitors. Antimicrob Agents Chemother 34:82, 1990

81. Johnson VA, Barlow MA, Merrill DP et al: Three-drug synergistic inhibition of HIV-1 replication in vitro by zidovudine, recombinant soluble CD4, and recombinant interferon-alpha A. J Infect Dis 161:1059, 1990

82. Ho DD, Moudgil T, Alam M: Quantitation of human immunodeficiency virus type 1 in the blood of infected persons. N Engl J Med 321:1621, 1989

83. Morgan RA, Looney DJ, Muenchau DD et al: Retroviral vectors expressing soluble CD4: A potential gene therapy for AIDS. AIDS Res Hum Retroviruses 6:183, 1990

84. Buonocore L, Rose JK: Prevention of HIV-1 glycoprotein transport by soluble CD4 retained in the endoplasmic reticulum. Nature 345:625, 1990

85. Romeo C, Seed B: Cellular immunity to HIV activated by CD4 fused to T cell or Fc receptor polypeptides. Cell 64:1037, 1991

86. Tsang KY, Johnson EA, La Via MF: Anti-p24 antibody reactivity in the acquired immunodeficiency syndrome (AIDS)–related complex treated with isoprinosine (letter). Ann Intern Med 109:595, 1988

87. Pedersen C, Sandström E, Petersen CS et al: The efficacy of inosine pranobex in preventing the acquired immunodeficiency syndrome in patients with human immunodeficiency virus infection: The Scandinavian Isoprinosine Study Group. N Engl J Med 322:1757, 1990 [Comment in: N Engl J Med 322:1807, 1990; erratum published in: N Engl J Med 323:1360, 1990]

88. Kweder SL, Schnur RA, Cooper EC: Inosine pranobex—is a single positive trial enough? (editorial). N Engl J Med 322:1807, 1990 [Comment on: N Engl J Med 322:1757, 1990]

89. De Simone C, Ferrazzi M, Bitonti F et al: Pharmacokinetics of zidovudine and concomitant inosine-pranobex in AIDS patients. Immunopharmacol Immunotoxicol 10:437, 1988

90. Hersh EM, Funk CY, Petersen EA, Mosier DE: Biological activity of diethyldithiocarbamate (Ditiocarb, Imuthiol) in an animal model of retrovirus-induced immunodeficiency disease and in clinical trials in patients with HIV infection: The Ditiocarb Study Group. Dev Biol Stand 72:355, 1990

91. Hersh EM, Brewton G, Abrams D et al: A randomized, double-blind, placebo-controlled trial of diethyldithiocarbamate (Ditiocarb, Imuthiol) in patients with ARC and AIDS (abstr S.B.489). Presented at the VI International Conference on AIDS, San Francisco, June 20–23, 1990

92. Kalebic T, Kinter A, Poli G et al: Suppression of human immunodeficiency virus expression in chronically infected monocytic cells by glutathione, glutathione ester, and *N*-acetylcysteine. Proc Natl Acad Sci USA 88:986, 1991

93. Harakeh S, Jariwalla RJ, Pauling L: Suppression of human immunodeficiency virus replication by ascorbate in chronically and acutely infected cells. Proc Natl Acad Sci USA 87:7245, 1990

94. Wu J, Levy EM, Black PH: 2-Mercaptoethanol and *N*-acetylcysteine enhance T cell colony formation in AIDS and ARC. Clin Exp Immunol 77:7, 1989

95. Abrams DI: Alternative therapies in the treatment of HIV infection. In Rhein RW, Goodwin SJ (eds): AIDS Reference Guide ¶1315:1–2. Washington, DC, Atlantic Information Services, 1989

96. McGrath MS, Hwang KM, Caldwell SE et al: GLQ223: An inhibitor of human immunodeficiency virus replication in acutely and chronically infected cells of lymphocyte and mononuclear phagocyte lineage. Proc Natl Acad Sci USA 86:2844, 1989

97. Gershon D: Compound Q: AIDS drug trial resumes. Nature 344:183, 1990

98. Buderi R: Row over controversial new AIDS drug. Nature 341:267, 1989

99. Mitsuya H, Yarchoan R, Broder S: Molecular targets for AIDS therapy. Science 249:1533, 1990

100. Sandström E: Antiviral therapy in human immunodeficiency virus infection. Drugs 38:417, 1989

101. Merluzzi VJ, Hargrave KD, Labadia M et al: Inhibition of HIV-1 replication by a nonnucleoside reverse transcriptase inhibitor. Science 250:1411, 1990

102. Pauwels R, Andries K, Desmyter J et al: Potent and selective inhibition of HIV-1 replication in vitro by a novel series of TIBO derivatives. Nature 343:470, 1990

103. Meek TD, Lambert DM, Dreyer GB et al: Inhibition of HIV-1 protease in infected T-lymphocytes by synthetic peptide analogues. Nature 343:90, 1990

104. Erickson J, Neidhart DJ, VanDrie J et al: Design, activity, and 2.8 A crystal structure of a c2 symmetric inhibitor complexed to HIV-1 protease. Science 249:527, 1990

105. Ashorn P, McQuade TJ, Thaisrivongs S et al: An inhibitor of the protease blocks maturation of human and simian immunodeficiency viruses and spread of infection. Proc Natl Acad Sci USA 87:7472, 1990

106. McQuade TJ, Tomasselli AG, Liu L et al: A synthetic HIV-1 protease inhibitor with antiviral activity arrests HIV-like particle maturation. Science 247:454, 1990

107. Haseltine WA: Development of antiviral drugs for the treatment of AIDS: Strategies and prospects. J AIDS 2:311, 1989

21

Therapeutic Approach to the HIV-Seropositive Patient

Stephen L. Boswell   *Martin S. Hirsch*

In the decade since the acquired immunodeficiency syndrome (AIDS) epidemic was first recognized, much has been learned about the management of human immunodeficiency virus (HIV) infection and its consequences. Information has inundated practitioners who are struggling to care for HIV-seropositive individuals. The information is voluminous, rapidly changing, and at times contradictory. This chapter attempts to help physicians develop a systematic approach to managing the HIV-seropositive patient, based on the accumulated information.

The Centers for Disease Control (CDC) has estimated that approximately 1 million Americans are currently infected with HIV and that approximately 40,000 new infections are occurring each year.[1] Further, approximately 600,000 HIV-seropositive persons in the United States may have T-helper lymphocyte counts below 500/mm³. Based on current guidelines for the use of zidovudine, these individuals are candidates for antiretroviral therapy (Table 21–1). Unfortunately, only a small fraction of those infected know of their HIV seropositivity, and of those who know, a smaller fraction still have sought medical care. Identifying those at risk for HIV infection, encouraging them to be tested, and encouraging those with positive results to seek medical care are significant challenges not only for the public health community but for all health care providers. The first step to providing good HIV care is to identify those who may be infected.

PREVENTING COMPLICATIONS OF HIV INFECTION

Careful evaluation and early intervention are essential to preventing complications of HIV infection. It is important that the health care provider identify those aspects of a patient's daily activities and medical history that may pose problems for the individual patient. Included in this assessment should be a review of the patient's sexual behavior, recreational drug use, support systems, and psychiatric history.

As their disease progresses, individuals who are HIV seropositive become increasingly susceptible to secondary infections. Many of these infections can be prevented with proper intervention. These efforts are warranted when three criteria are met: the organism represents a significant threat (it is both common and results in significant morbidity), an intervention can result in a meaningful decrease in this threat, and the intervention is acceptable to the patient. Table 21–2 lists the relative frequencies of various infectious agents and the anatomic sites most commonly affected by the agents. There is significant geographic variation in the prevalence of many of these secondary infections. Further, the significance of the threat posed by each of the infections varies among patients, especially in relation to possible interventions. Thus, efforts to prevent secondary infections among HIV-seropositive patients must be tailored to individual situations.

Preventing Exposure to Infectious Agents

Among the protozoa that cause significant morbidity in HIV-seropositive individuals is *Toxoplasma gondii.* IgG antibodies to *T. gondii* are detected in 40% to 50% of healthy young adults in the United States. By comparison, approximately 20% of British adults and 90% of French adults are infected.[2,3] Within the United States there is great geographic variation in the prevalence of toxoplasmosis, with approximately three times more

Table 21–1. Spectrum of Immunologic Deficiency as Measured by T-Cell Distributions Among Adults in the United States

Investigator	Years	Absolute T-Cell Range (Cells/mm³)		
		<200	200–500	>500
Army	1985–89	17%	41%	42%
Navy	1985–89	19%	45%	36%

Data from Brundage,[89] for the U.S. Army Retrovirus Research Group.

cases reported in Florida than in other states.[4] Persons with AIDS who were born in Haiti are at increased risk of developing cerebral toxoplasmosis in comparison with groups with risk factors for HIV infection—12.4% *versus* 1.7% (p < 0.001) in one study.[4] Hispanics, too, appear to be at increased risk of developing toxoplasmosis when compared with non-Haitian, non-Hispanic patients.[4] It has been suggested that the increased incidence of toxoplasmosis among these populations is in large part due to the higher prevalence of *T. gondii* in tropical areas.[5] The risk of experiencing active toxoplasmosis has been estimated to be as high as 30% among persons with HIV infection who are also seropositive for *T. gondii*.[6]

The predominant routes of transmission of *T. gondii* are oral and congenital. It has been estimated that 25% of lamb and pork samples in the United States contain tissue cysts.[7] These cysts are rarely isolated from beef.

Transmission by unpasteurized goat milk, eggs, and poorly washed vegetables is also suspected.[8–10] Congenital transmission occurs almost exclusively when the mother acquires infection during gestation.[3] For all patients, but especially for patients who are anti-*T. gondii* antibody negative, it is reasonable to explain the importance of thoroughly cooking meat, especially lamb and pork. Cysts in meat are made noninfectious by heating the meat to 66° C, by smoking or curing it, or by freezing it to −20° C. Careful hand washing after handling raw meat or vegetables is essential. Eggs should not be eaten raw (raw eggs may be in many foods, such as Hollandaise sauce). In some areas where it is popular to feed infants unpasteurized milk, HIV-seropositive mothers should be advised against this practice. The careful washing of all vegetables should be encouraged.

Contact with cat feces should be avoided by HIV-seropositive individuals. Gloves should be worn while disposing of cat litter. To avoid coming into contact with animal feces elsewhere, HIV-seropositive individuals should wear gloves during any activity, such as gardening, that places them in contact with soil. Serologic testing of cats is of little value because testing does not reveal whether the cat is excreting oocyts.

Cryptosporidium and *Isospora belli* are protozoa that cause diarrheal illness in HIV-seropositive individuals. As with many secondary infectious agents, they most frequently affect individuals in more advanced stages of HIV infection, when immunocompromise becomes pronounced. These infections have decreased in frequency among HIV-seropositive individuals in the United States over the past several years. Their decreas-

Table 21–2. HIV-Associated Infectious Agents by Location and Relative Frequency

	CNS	Lungs	GI Tract	Disseminated
Very common	Cyptococcus neoformans Toxoplasma gondii	Pneumocystis carinii Streptococcus pneumoniae Hemophilus influenzae	Candida albicans Mycobacterium avium-intracellulare Cytomegalovirus Herpes simplex Salmonella spp.	Mycobacterium avium-intracellulare Cryptococcus neoformans Cytomegalovirus
Common (not in all geographic/demographic subgroups)	Coccidioides immitis	Mycobacterium tuberculosis Staphylococcus aureus Histoplasma capsulatum	Cryptosporidium Isospora belli Strongyloides stercoralis	Mycobacterium tuberculosis Histoplasma capsulatum C. immitis
Rare or very rare	Mycobacterium tuberculosis Cytomegalovirus JC virus Aspergillus spp. Histoplasma capsulatum Listeria monocytogenes Nocardia spp.	Mycobacterium avium-intracellulare Nocardia spp. Rhodococcus equi Mycobacterium kansasii Aspergillus spp. Legionella pneumophilia		S. stercoralis Mycobacterium kansasii Leishmania spp. Cat-scratch disease bacillus

ing incidence may result from several factors, such as counseling patients to avoid activities that may put them at high risk for acquiring the infections. For example, counseling individuals to avoid oral-anal contact during sex may significantly decrease their risk of acquiring both *Cryptosporidium* and *I. belli*. As with *T. gondii,* careful washing of vegetables may also play a role in decreasing the incidence of these infections. The second reason why many of these infections may be diminishing among HIV-seropositive individuals is the improved treatment of AIDS. The widespread use of antifolates for *Pneumocystis carinii* pneumonia prophylaxis and the treatment of toxoplasmosis may have played a role in decreasing the incidence of isosporiasis.

Clinically significant *Salmonella* infections occur with increased frequency among HIV-seropositive individuals.[11] Estimates suggest that one third of these infections may occur before the onset of clinical AIDS.[11] Most frequently, humans acquire *Salmonella* by ingesting contaminated food and water. Raw milk, undercooked poultry, eggs, and meat are most frequently implicated. Acquisition may also occur through sexual contact, especially oral-anal contact. Thus, counseling that emphasizes proper food preparation and safe sexual practices plays a significant role in minimizing the risk of exposure.

Clinical tuberculosis is also more common in HIV-seropositive individuals. HIV-seropositive individuals should avoid situations where the likelihood of exposure to *Mycobacterium tuberculosis* is increased. One such situation occurs when aerosolized pentamidine is administered outside of appropriately designed facilities. The use of aerosolized pentamidine may induce coughing and thereby facilitate transmission of undiagnosed pulmonary tuberculosis from HIV-seropositive patients to persons sharing the same breathing space during or after treatment. The potential for transmission of tuberculosis depends on the prevalence of tuberculosis in the HIV-seropositive population being served, as well as on such factors as room ventilation, the number of infectious droplet nuclei generated by the patient, and the duration of exposure. For these reasons, home administration of aerosolized pentamidine should be avoided. Recommendations to deal with the risk of tuberculosis in aerosolized pentamidine facilities are summarized in Table 21-3.

Herpes group viruses cause significant morbidity and mortality among those who are HIV seropositive. Herpes simplex virus (HSV), cytomegalovirus (CMV), and Epstein-Barr virus (EBV) can all be transmitted in oral and genital secretions. Although most adults with HIV infection are seropositive for these viruses, some are not. Moreover, it is likely that secondary infections can occur in the most profoundly immunocompromised. A frank discussion about sexual practices and the use of condoms may help prevent the transmission of these viruses.

CMV-related disease may also be minimized by better transfusion practices. Steps should be taken to avoid

Table 21–3. Recommendations to Reduce the Chance of Airborne Tuberculosis Transmission from HIV-Seropositive Patients

1. All HIV-seropositive patients should be screened for tuberculosis infection or disease before starting pentamidine aerosol therapy. Screening should include a history and physical examination, modified Mantoux skin test (including control antigens), chest x-rays, sputum examination, and other diagnostic tests where appropriate.
2. Patients with a history of previous PPD positivity or with current PPD reactions greater than 5 mm with no evidence of tuberculosis should receive INH preventive therapy, regardless of age, as per current CDC/ATS guidelines.[43]
3. Whenever possible the use of aerosolized pentamidine in the home setting should be discouraged. Specially designed treatment centers are the most appropriate setting for aerosolized pentamidine treatment. Further, proper supervision of therapy may improve its overall effectiveness.
4. Regardless of PPD status, patients receiving aerosol treatment should be reevaluated for tuberculosis if they develop persistent cough, fever, or symptoms compatible with tuberculosis. Aerosol therapy should be suspended pending the result of diagnostic tests.
5. Treatment centers serving patients in high-risk groups for tuberculosis infection (intravenous drug users, Haitians and others from endemic areas for tuberculosis, prisoners, homeless) should rescreen patients and staff for tuberculosis every 6 months. If tuberculosis infection is known to be unusual among the patient population served, rescreening of patients and staff may be less frequent. However, all patients and staff must be screened initially and at least annually thereafter.

Reproduced with permission from Tuberculosis Program, Massachusetts Department of Public Health: Guidelines to Reduce the Chance of Airborne Tuberculosis Transmission from HIV-Seropositive Patients, 1989.

the use of blood products from CMV-seropositive donors in HIV-seropositive, CMV-seronegative individuals. These steps alone, however, may not be sufficient. There is growing evidence that CMV-seropositive, HIV-seropositive persons may also be at risk for transfusion-transmitted CMV. Several instances of immunocompromised individuals infected with multiple CMV strains have been reported.[12-16] This suggests that prior exposure to one CMV strain may not confer complete protection against infection by other strains in the immunosuppressed host. Therefore, steps may be needed to reduce the risk of transfusion in the much larger number of individuals who are both CMV seropositive and HIV seropositive, particularly when they are profoundly immunocompromised, by using CMV-seronegative blood and components.

In some cases it may be impractical to depend solely on the use of CMV-seronegative units in this larger population, especially in regions with particularly high CMV seroprevalence rates or if an unusual blood group is required for transfusion. In such situations, consideration should be given to other options that involve the removal of leukocytes likely to transmit CMV from red cell preparations. The use of frozen, deglycerolized red blood cells,[17] saline-washed red blood cells,[18] and perhaps leukocyte filtration[19] can decrease the risk of CMV transmission in red cell transfusion. Peritransfusion CMV prophylaxis currently is an impractical option because of toxicity and expense. All of these options involve additional societal costs but must be considered in the light of the significance of CMV disease among HIV-seropositive individuals.

Additional efforts to screen or minimize platelet transfusions to HIV-seropositive patients may also be appropriate. Avoiding unnecessary transfusions can play a significant role in decreasing the morbidity and mortality of CMV among HIV-positive individuals.

Chemoprophylaxis of Secondary Infections

An important factor contributing to improved longevity and quality of life among HIV-seropositive individuals is the appropriate use of infection prophylaxis. Numerous drugs are available to limit the development of many secondary infections. Most commonly used are agents to prevent *P. carinii* pneumonia, such as trimethoprim-sulfamethoxazole (TMP-SMX, cotrimoxazole), aerosolized pentamidine, and dapsone. Other infections amenable to chemoprophylaxis include HSV infections, candidiasis, and tuberculosis. Research is currently underway to ascertain whether chemoprophylaxis may prevent additional infections as well. Table 21–4 lists several drugs under consideration as potential prophylactic agents.

One of the most frequent decisions regarding chemoprophylaxis comes in considering drugs to prevent *P. carinii* pneumonia. The United States Public Health Service currently recommends prophylaxis for adults with a prior history of *P. carinii* pneumonia, an absolute CD4 cell count of 200 cells/mm³ or below, or a CD4 cell count that has fallen to 20% or less of the total lymphocyte count.[20] It may also be appropriate to start *P. carinii* prophylaxis earlier if certain clinical signs are present. For example, the presence of thrush or fever in an individual with an absolute CD4 cell count between 200 and 300 cells/mm³ is indicative of an increased risk of developing *P. carinii* pneumonia.[21]

Among HIV-seropositive children the use of CD4 cell counts to assess the need for anti-*Pneumocystis* prophylaxis is more complicated. *P. carinii* pneumonia has been frequently reported in children with CD4 cell counts above 500/mm³.[22] The CD4 cell count in healthy children is often above 3,000/mm³ in infancy and declines with age.[23] This age-related variation in CD4 cell count may contribute to the wide variation of these counts among children who develop *P. carinii* pneumonia. As a result of this variation recommendations for anti-*Pneumocystis* prophylaxis for children change as a function of age. Table 21–5 lists guidelines for the initiation of anti-*Pneumocystis* prophylaxis in children.[24]

Once it has been determined that anti-*Pneumocystis* prophylaxis is necessary, there are several regimens from which to choose. Controlled trials are underway to directly compare the efficacy and toxicities of these regimens in adults. Several factors should enter into the treatment decision. Systemic therapy may have certain advantages over local therapy. TMP-SMX (cotrimoxazole) may decrease the rate of recurrence not only of *P. carinii* pneumonia but also of other infections, such as isosporiasis and perhaps toxoplasmosis. The presence of intrinsic lung disease may adversely affect the distribution of aerosolized pentamidine. Nonuniform distribution of aerosolized pentamidine may contribute to upper lobe pneumonitis with and without pneumothorax.[25,26] In addition, rare cases of extrapulmonary *P. carinii* infections may occur more commonly in those receiving local therapy.

The toxicity of individual agents may also affect their use in specific situations, and may vary with stage of

Table 21–4.   Examples of Drugs Currently Available or Under Study for Chemoprophylaxis of Several Secondary Infections in HIV-Infected Patients

Infectious Organism	*Potential Chemoprophylaxis*	*Population Under Consideration*
Mycobacterium avium-intracellulare	Rifabutin, clarithromycin	CD4 cell count ≤ 200 cells/mm³
Herpes simplex virus	Acyclovir	Recurrent HSV outbreaks
Cytomegalovirus	Acyclovir, oral ganciclovir	CD4 cell count ≤ 200 cells/mm³, CMV seropositive
Mycobacterium tuberculosis	Isoniazid	Modified Mantoux positive*
Toxoplasma gondii	Pyrimethamine, clarithromycin	*Toxoplasma* IgG seropositive
Candida albicans (oral, vaginal)	Chlorhexidine gluconate, clotrimazole, nystatin, fluconazole	Secondary prophylaxis *or* CD4 cell count ≤ 200 cells/mm³
Pneumocystis carinii	Trimethoprim-sulfamethoxazole, aerosolized pentamidine, dapsone, 566 C80	CD4 cell count ≤ 200 cells/mm³

* 5 TU of intradermal injection into the forearm; interpretation is positive if the area of induration is ≥5 mm.

Table 21–5. Recommendations for Initiation of *P. carinii* Pneumonia Prophylaxis for Children Who Are Either HIV Infected, HIV Seropositive, or <12 Months Old and Born to an HIV-Infected Mother

Age	CD4 Cell Count (Cells/mm³) Below Which PCP Prophylaxis Is Recommended*
1–11 mo	1,500
12–23 mo	750
24 mo–5 yr	500
≥6 yr	200

* If the percent of CD4 lymphocytes is less than 20%, regardless of age or absolute CD4 cell count, then anti-*Pneumocystis* prophylaxis should be initiated.

illness. Cotrimoxazole may be well tolerated in early HIV disease but become less tolerable as disease advances. Little is known about the teratogenicity of aerosolized pentamidine. Trimethoprim is teratogenic in animals, whereas dapsone appears safe in pregnancy.[27,28] Consequently, if a sexually active, HIV-seropositive woman is in need of prophylaxis, dapsone may be a good choice for prophylaxis. Dapsone is inexpensive and because of its long half-life is dosed infrequently. Care should be taken when using dapsone in combination with dideoxyinosine (ddI), however. Because dapsone is absorbed more effectively in an acid environment, the current ddI sachet formulation, which is designed to neutralize gastric acidity, may interfere with absorption of dapsone. A high incidence of *P. carinii* pneumonia has been noted in patients receiving dapsone prophylaxis concomitantly with ddI. It has been recommended that patients who are receiving both ddI and dapsone be advised to take dapsone 2 hours prior to ddI.[29] This concern may be diminished by a new formulation of ddI that is currently under development. Aerosolized pentamidine requires administration once per month but is frequently costly. Compliance may be improved by matching patient preferences to the medication employed. Thus, the process of choosing chemoprophylaxis should be thought of as a dynamic one in which several agents may be used at different stages of illness in a single patient. Table 21–6 lists typical dosages, estimates of adverse reactions, and additional information for dapsone, aerosolized pentamidine (300 mg monthly using a Respirgard II nebulizer), and TMP-SMX in adults with HIV infection.

Figure 21–1 depicts one paradigm for these choices. Although this model is not intended to encompass all of the considerations germane to the decision to initiate anti-*Pneumocystis* therapy with specific agent(s), it does provide several generalizations. TMP-SMX is the initial regimen preferred by many physicians. If a patient is allergic to TMP-SMX, dapsone can frequently be used because cross-sensitivity is uncommon. Significant glucose-6-phosphate dehydrogenase (G-6-PD) deficiency may discourage the use of dapsone and TMP-SMX in some patients. The highest prevalence of this deficiency in the United States is among African-American males (11%), females (3%; 20% are heterozygous), and indi-

Table 21–6. Commonly Used Dosages, Adverse Reaction Rates, and Estimates of Relapse Rates for Three Commonly Used Agents for *P. carinii* Pneumonia Prophylaxis

Agent	Dosage	Estimates of Adverse Reaction Rate*	Points to Consider
Dapsone	50–100 mg/day	17%[91]	May be particularly useful in pregnancy Long half-life may improve compliance Drug reaction to trimethoprim-sulfamethoxazole does not necessarily indicate that a patient cannot take dapsone Concomitant administration with ddC or ddI may increase risk of developing peripheral neuropathy If taken concomitantly with ddI, dapsone should be taken 2 hours prior to ddI
Aerosolized pentamidine	300 mg/mo	5.6%	Intrinsic lung disease may decrease effectiveness Once monthly treatment may improve compliance Use may alter radiographic appearance of recrudescent disease and may decrease yield of bronchoalveolar lavage[26] Positioning of patient during therapy may affect overall effectiveness[92]
Trimethoprim-sulfamethoxazole	1 DS tab b.i.d.†	13%[91]	Is often difficult to use concomitantly with zidovudine, especially in patients with more advanced disease

* Necessitating discontinuation of medication.
† Lower doses or less frequent dosing may be equally effective and have less toxicity.

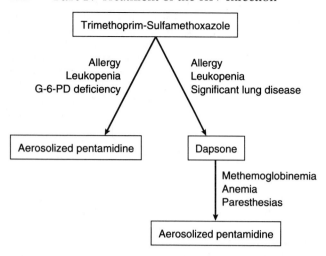

```
          ┌──────────────────────────────┐
          │ Trimethoprim-Sulfamethoxazole │
          └──────────────────────────────┘
            ╱                        ╲
      Allergy                    Allergy
      Leukopenia                 Leukopenia
      G-6-PD deficiency          Significant lung disease
         ╱                            ╲
  ┌───────────────────────┐     ┌──────────┐
  │ Aerosolized pentamidine │   │ Dapsone  │
  └───────────────────────┘     └──────────┘
                                      │
                              Methemoglobinemia
                              Anemia
                              Paresthesias
                                      │
                          ┌───────────────────────┐
                          │ Aerosolized pentamidine │
                          └───────────────────────┘
```

Figure 21–1. Decision paradigm for *P. carinii* pneumonia prophylaxis.

viduals of Greek, Japanese, Indian, Southeast Asian, and Sephardic Jewish ancestry.

Although no studies of chemoprophylactic regimens for *P. carinii* pneumonia among HIV-infected children have been performed, extrapolation from experience with drugs used for anti-*Pneumocystis* prophylaxis in children with other diseases is possible. Based on safety information, ease of administration, and proven efficacy in children with cancer and in adult AIDS patients, TMP-SMX is the drug of choice for anti-*Pneumocystis* prophylaxis of HIV-infected or HIV-exposed children 1 month of age or older.

The recommended dosage for *P. carinii* pneumonia prophylaxis in children is 150 mg trimethoprim + 750 mg sulfamethoxazole/m²/day, 3 days per week. These dosages should be adjusted upward as the child grows. The total daily dose should not exceed 320 mg trimethoprim and 1,600 mg sulfamethoxazole.

For HIV-infected children 5 years of age or older, aerosolized pentamidine is recommended if TMP-SMX cannot be tolerated. The dose and delivery system recommended for adults—300 mg every 4 weeks *via* a Respirgard II jet nebulizer—have also been used for children, although no pharmacokinetic or efficacy data supporting this regimen for children are available. For children less than 5 years old who cannot tolerate TMP-SMX, or for children 5 years old or older who cannot tolerate either TMP-SMX or aerosolized pentamidine, dapsone may be used for anti-*Pneumocystis* prophylaxis. The recommended dosage is 1 mg/kg body weight/day, given orally. The total daily dose should not exceed 100 mg/day. Although dapsone is not available in a liquid preparation, the tablets can be crushed and given with or in food. For children receiving either TMP-SMX or dapsone, monthly complete blood cell counts with differential and platelet count are suggested.

P. carinii pneumonia is not the only infection that can be prevented with chemoprophylaxis. Reactivation HSV infections are common, and although these infections are usually self-limiting early in the course of HIV infection, they may produce extensive and persistent ulcerative disease in individuals in whom immunocompromise is more advanced. Thus, in individuals who have frequent bouts of overt HSV, suppressive therapy with acyclovir may be warranted.[30]

The prolonged use of acyclovir has been associated with acyclovir-resistant HSV in clinical isolates, particularly in immunocompromised hosts.[31,32] It remains unclear whether prolonged continuous HSV suppression with acyclovir is more likely than intermittent use for acute episodes to lead to the development of resistant strains. Among HIV-seropositive individuals who suffer frequent and severe episodes of HSV infections, acyclovir suppression should be considered. If lesions recur or persist despite acyclovir suppression, the possibility of acyclovir resistance should be considered.

Oral candidiasis occurs in most HIV-seropositive individuals at some point during their illness. It may be worsened by the increased use of antibiotics. Oral candidiasis is sometimes subtle and difficult to diagnose. In addition to the classic appearance of pseudomembranous candidiasis (thrush), it can also appear as smooth red patches throughout the oral mucosa. *Candida* cheilitis is frequently seen as well. Chemoprophylaxis has been shown to decrease the risk of oral candidiasis among renal transplant recipients, patients with solid malignant neoplasms, and patients with acute leukemia. Nystatin, clotrimazole, chlorhexidine gluconate, ketoconazole, and fluconazole are among the agents that have been shown to be effective.[33–37] Although studies involving the use of these agents to prevent oral candidiasis in HIV-seropositive individuals are lacking, it appears that the frequency can be reduced with the appropriate use of chemoprophylaxis. Chemoprophylaxis should be considered in patients after their first bout of oral candidiasis and when symptomatic HIV-seropositive individuals are given antibiotics to treat bacterial infections.

The long-term use of ketoconazole for the prophylaxis of oral candidiasis, although often effective, is problematic because of the often inconsistent absorption of the drug, its potential liver toxicity, and because of the adrenal suppression that sometimes accompanies its use.[38] Although it is not subject to the same erratic absorption as ketoconazole, fluconazole is quite costly and may have as yet unrecognized toxic effects. Topical agents for the prophylaxis of oral candidiasis are frequently effective and well tolerated. One 10-mg clotrimazole troche may be held in the mouth for 15 to 30 minutes three times each day and is preferred over oral nystatin suspension.[35] Chlorhexidine gluconate may be useful in this role, especially in patients with significant gingivitis and periodontitis.[37] Nystatin is available in either an oral suspension or as a pastille. Nystatin oral pastilles (200,000 units), one pastille taken three times each day, or nystatin suspension (100,000 U/mL), a 15-ml swish-and-swallow six times per day, can also be used.

Vulvovaginal candidiasis is a frequent problem in HIV-seropositive women. The problem tends to occur earlier in HIV infection than does oral candidiasis.[39] Again, several agents are available for prophylaxis. These include clotrimazole and nystatin suppositories and miconazole and clotrimazole creams. Although controlled trials are lacking, the use of a one of these agents several times each week may decrease the frequency of vulvovaginal candidiasis.

Toxoplasmosis may also be a preventable opportunistic infection in HIV-seropositive individuals. Although there are currently no chemoprophylactic regimens of proven efficacy, several agents are under study. In deciding which agent to use for the prevention of *P. carinii* pneumonia, the clinician must weigh the *Toxoplasma* serostatus of the individual patient. Cotrimoxazole is not only one of the most effective drugs for preventing *P. carinii* pneumonia, it may have anti-*T. gondii* activity as well. Therefore, among individuals who are *T. gondii* IgG seropositive and who have no contraindications to the use of TMP-SMX, this drug may be the ideal choice for *P. carinii* prophylaxis. Several other drugs or drug combinations (*e.g.,* pyrimethamine-sulfamethoxazole or clarithromycin) are currently under study for *Toxoplasma* prophylaxis.

Another infection increasingly found in HIV-seropositive individuals is *M. tuberculosis.* As in the case of *T. gondii,* most individuals who are infected with *M. tuberculosis* are asymptomatic, and disease most frequently represents recrudescence of infection. It is estimated that over 90% of persons reported to have clinical disease have harbored *M. tuberculosis* infection for a year or more.[40] The risk of developing active tuberculosis appears to be elevated in HIV-seropositive individuals.[41] Screening for *M. tuberculosis* is essential in order to identify infected persons at high risk of developing disease, because many of these individuals would benefit from preventive therapy. Further, screening can identify persons with clinical disease in need of treatment. Although screening should probably include all HIV-seropositive individuals, it is particularly important for the homeless and for residents of long-term care facilities, such as nursing homes, correctional institutions, mental institutions, and the like.

Tuberculin skin testing is the most common method of identifying persons infected with *M. tuberculosis.* The administration of 5 units of purified protein derivative (PPD) tuberculin intracutaneously (Mantoux test) is the recommended method. The test is considered positive if the diameter of induration is greater than or equal to 5 mm.[42] However, among individuals who show symptoms characteristic of HIV infection, both skin testing and screening chest radiography should be performed.[43] This combination is recommended because of the

higher probability of a false-negative skin test result in this population. An HIV-seropositive individual of any age whose tuberculin skin test is deemed positive or who has a history of a positive skin test and was untreated should receive preventive therapy for 12 months. Before this therapy is initiated, sputum should be obtained for culture to exclude active pulmonary tuberculosis. The usual preventive therapy is isoniazid (10 mg/kg/day for children, 300 mg/day for most adults). In settings where the prevalence of isoniazid-resistant organisms is high, alternative chemoprophylaxis regimens should be considered.

Other common infections found in HIV-seropositive individuals include *M. avium-intracellulare, C. neoformans, Salmonella* spp., and CMV. Studies are currently underway using various chemoprophylactic agents to prevent infections with these organisms. At present, chemoprophylaxis outside of these controlled trials cannot be recommended.

Immunizations

Individuals who are HIV seropositive should be properly immunized. Whenever possible, immunization should occur early in the course of HIV infection to improve the response rates. Tables 21–7 and 21–8 list immunization recommendations for HIV-seropositive adults and children, respectively. Passive immunotherapy with immune serum globulin has been shown to reduce the frequency of bacterial infection in certain HIV-seropositive children.[44,45] The routine use of immune globulin in adults is not currently recommended. For HIV-seropositive adults who are traveling to developing countries, immune serum globulin should be given to diminish the risk of acquiring hepatitis A infection. Because immune globulin can interfere with the response to live vaccines, it should be given either 2 weeks after or 3 months before live measles or measles-mumps-rubella (MMR) vaccine.[46] If an HIV-seropositive child is receiving intravenous (IV) immune globulin for the prophylaxis of serious bacterial infections, the MMR vaccination schedule should be adjusted accordingly.

Several contraindications to the use of vaccines should be noted. Because of the theoretical risk to the

Table 21–7. Recommendations for Vaccination of HIV-Seropositive Children

Vaccine	Asymptomatic	Symptomatic
DTP	Yes	Yes
OPV	No	No
IPV	Yes	Yes
MMR	Yes	Yes
Hemophilus B	Yes	Yes
Pneumococcal	No	Yes
Influenza virus	No	Yes

Table 21–8.   Recommendations for Vaccination of HIV-Seropositive Adults

Vaccine	Recommendations
DTP	All patients: booster every 10 years
IPV	Persons who have never been immunized: three doses of enhanced-potency inactivated vaccine
	Persons previously immunized who are traveling to developing countries; the patient should receive one dose of the inactivated vaccine
MMR	Persons who were born after 1956 and
	(1) who have not been immunized or
	(2) were immunized before 1980 and who have neither serologic evidence of infection nor a history of physician-diagnosed measles
Hemophilus B	All patients: single dose early in HIV infection
Pneumococcal	All patients: single dose early in HIV infection
Influenza virus	All patients: yearly
Hepatitis B	Patients who do not demonstrate antibody or antigen: series of 3 injections
Typhoid	Patients traveling to developing countries: inactivated parenteral typhoid vaccine, booster doses every 3 years
Meningococcus	Patients traveling to areas with recognized epidemics or to regions where such disease is endemic, especially if prolonged contact with the populace is anticipated
Plague	Patients traveling to areas where there is a high probability of exposure
Japanese encephalitis	Patients traveling to endemic or epidemic areas
Cholera	Rarely indicated for patients traveling to developing countries, may be required by destination country
Rabies	Patients anticipating contact with uncommon wild animals or living for prolonged times in areas where rabies is prevalent
Yellow fever	Contraindicated
BCG	Contraindicated
Live oral typhoid	Contraindicated
Live oral polio	Contraindicated

HIV-seropositive woman and the developing fetus, pregnant women or women likely to become pregnant within 3 months after vaccination should not be given live attenuated virus vaccines (MMR).[47] In general, vaccination of pregnant women should occur in the second and third trimesters of pregnancy to minimize the risk of teratogenicity. Because of the risk of exposure to live polio virus from persons recently immunized, oral polio vaccine should not be given to anyone living in the household of an HIV-seropositive individual. There is no substantive evidence of risk to the fetus or HIV-seropositive woman from the use of inactivated virus or bacteria vaccines or toxoids.[47]

Sexually active women account for a growing number of HIV-seropositive patients. Pregnant women should be tested for immunity to rubella. Susceptible women should be immunized immediately after delivery. Newborns of pregnant carriers of HBV should receive hepatitis B immune globulin (HBIG) and the HBV vaccine series shortly after delivery.

Knowledge of a child's HIV status is not necessary before decisions regarding immunization are made. Inactivated childhood vaccines should be given to HIV-infected children, regardless of whether or not they are symptomatic. If a child is known to be HIV infected or if the child's household has a member who is HIV infected, then inactivated polio virus vaccine (IPV) should be used. The MMR vaccine should be given to all HIV-infected children.

Nutrition

HIV-seropositive individuals often experience significant nutritional deficiencies and progressive weight loss during the course of their illness. In fact, a 10% body weight loss in conjunction with more than 30 days of constitutional symptoms in an HIV-seropositive individual is sufficient for the diagnosis of AIDS.[48] In central Africa, AIDS is known as "slim disease" for the profound wasting that often accompanies it. Evidence suggests, however, that malnutrition in HIV-seropositive individuals is not confined to the terminal stages of disease but is an early manifestation of HIV infection in many patients. A CDC study of Stage III subjects has shown that up to 67% of HIV-seropositive subjects have at least one nutritional deficiency, and 36% of this cohort have multiple nutritional abnormalities.[49]

Nutritional deficiencies and weight loss may be a consequence of several factors. Inadequate intake, altered metabolism, and malabsorption may play roles, either independently or in concert. The importance of each of these factors varies among individuals and with the stage of illness. Therefore, proper nutritional therapy for an HIV-seropositive patient will change as disease progresses.

In addition to protein and calorie malnutrition, deficiencies in a variety of specific nutrients have been observed. Among these are zinc, selenium, folic acid, vitamin B6, and vitamin B12.[50-54] Many of these deficiencies have been linked to immune function abnormalities, as demonstrated by protein and calorie deprivation in the setting of famine, which increases the risk of infection and overall mortality.[55] Mechanisms may include a reduction in the number of T lymphocytes, impaired cell-mediated immunity, impaired secretory immunity, reduced complement secretion, altered phagocytic function, and decreased natural killer cell activity.[56–59] In addition, there is substantial evidence that overall protein-calorie status as well as specific nutrient status play an important role in the functioning of the nervous system.[60]

Among the many postulated causes of nutritional deficiencies in HIV-seropositive patients is hypermetabolism associated with infection. Evidence for this has been found in studies of the treatment of opportunistic viruses and HIV infection itself. For example, ganciclovir treatment of serious CMV infection has been associated with an increase in body weight, lean body mass, body fat, and serum albumin.[61] Treatment of HIV infection itself may improve energy balance, according to the results of early trials involving zidovudine therapy in which a 3-kg weight gain was observed during therapy.[62] Thus, treatment of HIV and its attendant infections may slow or reverse the wasting process and is central to managing nutritional deficiencies in HIV-seropositive patients.

Simple feeding strategies have often been ineffective for increasing lean body mass. As has been observed in cancer patients, aggressive feeding, if it increases mass at all, results in fat deposition rather than improvement of tissue function or an increase in lean body mass.[63,64] No published studies have demonstrated that significant benefit accrues from total parenteral nutrition, enteral support, or dietary interventions alone in HIV-seropositive individuals. Research is currently attempting to elucidate the role of appetite stimulants, anti-cytokine therapies, anabolic agents, and metabolic inhibitors in treating nutritional deficiencies and weight loss in HIV-seropositive individuals.

Of these therapeutic possibilities, appetite stimulants have received the most attention. One of these, megestrol acetate, is being used by some practitioners to treat AIDS-associated weight loss.[65,66] The first published report of the clinical benefit of this agent was based on studies of breast cancer patients.[67] Preliminary observations of its use in HIV-seropositive individuals suggest that while it may increase body mass in some situations, it produces a larger increase in body fat than in lean tissue.[68] Its ultimate role in the management of HIV-associated weight loss and nutritional deficiencies has yet to be delineated.

Another common nutritional deficiency among HIV-seropositive patient is vitamin B12. Persons with AIDS frequently have lower than normal serum vitamin B12 levels. Multiple causes for this have been suggested, including altered vitamin B12 transport proteins, malabsorption due to chronic diarrhea, and HIV enteropathy involving the terminal ileum.[69,70] Occult vitamin B12 deficiencies may contribute to the immunologic, neu-

rologic, and hematologic abnormalities seen in HIV-seropositive individuals. Vitamin B12 levels should be checked periodically, especially in individuals who have clinical or laboratory abnormalities consistent with vitamin B12 deficiency. In individuals with borderline and low serum vitamin B12 levels, parenteral administration of vitamin B12 is warranted.

Deficiencies in other essential nutrients (vitamin B6, zinc) have also been reported in HIV-seropositive individuals. These reports have led many who are HIV seropositive to increase their dietary intake of certain nutrients. Harmless as this practice may seem, reports of individuals taking high, even toxic, doses of vitamins, minerals, and other nutrients have started to appear. Such megadose therapy should be discouraged as premature and potentially dangerous.

Current therapeutic options for the treatment of nutritional deficiencies and weight loss in HIV-seropositive individuals remain empirical. They consist of dietary adjustments or supplements, treatment of underlying diseases, and, rarely, parenteral alimentation. Careful surveillance of certain nutritional markers (*e.g.,* weight, albumin, iron, vitamin B12) may allow the early correction of some nutritional deficiencies. However, data linking aggressive nutritional therapy to improved clinical outcomes are lacking.

DISEASE MONITORING

History and Physical Examination

HIV infection is increasingly being viewed as a chronic disease. Providers have begun to shift their focus from the treatment of acute problems to the management of chronic HIV infection, the anticipation of emerging problems, and early intervention. Central to this approach is the careful monitoring of infected individuals.

A periodic detailed history and physical examination are indispensable to managing HIV-seropositive patients. The history should include a general review of symptoms and a series of more detailed questions tailored to the individual's stage of illness. Further, a careful sexual history should be periodically obtained to assess the potential for exposure to infection and as a means of reviewing and reinforcing safe sexual practices. In addition, a substance abuse history should be sought on a periodic basis. If the patient is chemically dependent, concrete treatment options should be offered. Methadone maintenance treatment programs have resulted in lower AIDS incidence and a lower AIDS-specific mortality among those who use opiates and who enter treatment soon after starting drug use.[71] A greater cessation of IV drug use and less needle sharing in patients on methadone maintenance have also been reported.[72] No pharmacologic treatments have proved effective for alcoholism and cocaine addiction. Several nonpharmacologic therapies for addiction exist. They include individual counseling, support groups, Alcoholics Anonymous, Narcotics Anonymous, and various forms of group or individual psychotherapy. Recognition of the temporal nature of many of the signs and symptoms of HIV infection can be quite helpful in managing the HIV-seropositive individual. Table 21–9 relates the relative frequency of symptoms attributable to HIV infection by stage of illness. Although this description is an oversimplification of the complexity of this disease, it serves a useful purpose by identifying certain symptoms and signs that may be unusual during one stage of illness while quite common in another. This information can be helpful in diagnosing problems and in reassuring patients frightened by symptoms unrelated to their HIV infection. In general, the symptoms and signs that occur during earlier stages of HIV infection frequently occur in later stages as well. Thus, as the disease progresses, the number of signs and symptoms attributable to HIV infection increases. Certain symptoms, such as depression, can occur at any stage of illness. Any individual who is told that he or she is HIV seropositive is at significantly increased risk of depression. In fact, several studies have demonstrated a high risk of suicide among HIV-seropositive individuals.[73] Careful attention to social withdrawal, apathy, weight change, anhedonia, sleep disturbances, and mood and behavior changes is essential. Should depression develop, early counseling and, if appropriate, psychopharmacologic intervention may be crucial.

The physical examination should be tailored to the individual patient and the stage of illness. Although a detailed review of the physical examination of the HIV-seropositive individual is beyond the scope of this chapter, several features unique to the examination will be considered. Common clinical findings are listed in Table 21–10.

One of the most frequently missed signs of HIV infection is oral hairy leukoplakia, and therefore a careful oral examination for this and other oral lesions (e.g., thrush, Kaposi's sarcoma, mucosal petechiae, aphthous stomatitis, gingivitis, warts) should be conducted. Early recognition of oral pathology can play a significant part in decreasing morbidity among HIV-seropositive individuals.

The skin is probably the most commonly affected organ that is accessible to routine examination. Kaposi's sarcoma (especially prevalent in HIV-seropositive homosexual men), warts, molluscum contagiosum, herpes simplex, herpes zoster, psoriasis, seborrheic dermatitis, and fungal infections of the toes and fingernails are especially common. A skin rash may be the first manifestation of numerous other problems, among them syphilis, cat-scratch disease, and other systemic bacterial or fungal infections. Familiarity with the appearance and treatment of these dermatologic manifestations of HIV infection is an important part of care.

Another important part of the examination should be a careful inspection and documentation of lymphadenopathy, particularly if there are unusual features. Persistent generalized lymphadenopathy, a common feature of HIV infection, frequently occurs early in HIV infection. It is characterized by small (≤ 1 cm), shotty, nontender extrainguinal lymph nodes that change little over extended periods of time (usually more than 3 months). However, if large firm, tender nodes develop, these can be signs of new and significant disease, such as lymphoma or disseminated infection with mycobacteria or *T. gondii.*

Funduscopy and tests of visual acuity should be conducted periodically in the HIV-seropositive individual. Cotton wool spots are seen frequently and should be differentiated from CMV retinitis. CMV retinitis is found in a large number of HIV-seropositive individuals at autopsy (>20% in some studies), often without a history of previous symptoms. Because the drugs (ganciclovir and foscarnet) used to treat CMV infection are frequently toxic and must be given parenterally, treatment should be reserved for symptomatic individuals or those with lesions impinging on the macula. Thus, screening fundal photography in asymptomatic individuals has little bearing on clinical care.

Genital and rectal examinations should be con-

Table 21–9. Symptoms and Signs Characteristic of HIV Infection by Stage of Illness

Stage of Illness	Symptoms and Signs
Early (CD4 cell count > 500/mm³)	Rashes (seborrheic dermatitis, herpes zoster, psoriasis, folliculitis, Kaposi's sarcoma) Pruritus (usually related to xeroderma) Oral hairy leukoplakia Oral ulcers Rhinorrhea Lymphadenopathy (persistent shotty nodes) Mononeuritides (e.g., Bell's palsy)
Middle (CD4 cell count 200–500/mm³)	Pseudomembranous thrush Sore tongue (thrush) Oral ulcers (aphthous stomatitis) Anorexia Weight loss Nausea Vomiting Diarrhea Malaise Recurring fever Night sweats
Late (CD4 cell count ≤ 200/mm³)	Memory problems Cognition difficulties Mood and behavioral changes Paresthesias Focal weakness Ataxia Odynophagia Cough Wheeze Dyspnea on exertion Visual problems (scotomata, floaters)

Table 21–10.   Frequent Clinical Findings in the HIV-Seropositive Patient

Examination	Clinical Finding	Potential Clinical Significance
Vital signs and appearance	Weight loss	HIV-related wasting syndrome
	Muscle wasting	
	Fever	If no localizing symptoms, consider infections with MAI, TB, CMV, and occult sinusitis or prostatitis
Eye	White indistinct retinal spots	Cotton wool spots; no known significance
	White retinal exudates and hemorrhages	CMV retinitis
	Visual field defects	Unilateral: optic neuritis, CMV or toxoplasma retinitis
		Bilateral: CNS mass lesion (lymphoma, toxoplasmosis, PML)
Oral cavity	White plaques	Oral candidiasis, oral hairy leukoplakia
	Oral ulcers	HSV, CMV, aphthous ulcers, disseminated histoplasmosis
	Gingivitis/periodontitis	HIV-associated gingivitis/periodontitis
	Purple lesion	Kaposi's sarcoma
Lymph nodes	Persistent (>3 mo) generalized (two or more extrainguinal sites) lymphadenopathy (PGL)	Persistent generalized lymphadenopathy
	Lymphadenopathy in which individual nodes are either tender, large, or inflamed	Lymphoma, toxoplasmosis, tuberculosis, syphilis
Abdomen	Hepatosplenomegaly	MAI, tuberculosis, lymphoma, histoplasmosis
	Perirectal ulcer	HSV, CMV, histoplasmosis
Genitalia	Genital sores	Syphilis, HSV, chancroid, warts
Nervous system	Cognitive difficulties	HIV encephalopathy, stroke, depression, vitamin B_{12} deficiency
	Sensory-motor deficits	CNS lymphoma, CNS toxoplasmosis, cryptococcal meningoencephalitis, syphilis, progressive multifocal leukoencephalopathy, HIV-associated neuropathy, nucleoside toxicity
Skin	Purple macule or papule	Kaposi's sarcoma, cat-scratch disease
	Scaling rash	Seborrheic dermatitis, fungal infection, psoriasis
	Purpura	HIV-associated thrombocytopenia
	Vesicular rash	Herpes zoster, HSV, drug reaction

ducted in all HIV-seropositive individuals on a regular basis. This includes a routine Papanicolaou test in women. Studies suggest a correlation between HIV infection and cervical dysplasia.[74,75] Whether this represents a causal relationship or is a manifestation of other sexually transmitted infections is not yet known. Persistent rectal or anal lesions that do not respond to treatment should be biopsied. Lymphoma and rectal cancer have been reported to occur with increased frequency among those who are HIV seropositive. Sigmoidoscopy and/or colonoscopy with biopsy may be required to discover the cause of chronic diarrhea, which may be due to lymphoma or bowel infections caused by CMV, HSV, and MAI.

Neurologic examinations should be conducted frequently. A baseline neuropsychiatric evaluation when the patient is asymptomatic is often quite useful. Formal neuropsychiatric testing may help in detecting subtle changes in mental status that are not easily detected on routine mental status examinations. However, these tests demand a significant time commitment and can be expensive. As a consequence, current research efforts are directed toward developing new testing methods that are more sensitive and specific, simpler to administer, and less costly.

Laboratory Testing

HIV infection predisposes individuals to anemia, neutropenia, and thrombocytopenia either as a consequence of the disease itself or of the drugs used to treat it. Periodic evaluation of blood counts is essential. The frequency of these evaluations should increase as disease progresses and drug therapy is initiated. Table 21–11 lists many of the laboratory tests commonly performed in the initial evaluation of an HIV-seropositive patient. A suggested follow-up laboratory evaluation is described in Table 21–12. If abnormalities in the complete blood cell count (CBC) arise, it is important to evaluate these, including the assessment of iron, folate, and vitamin B12 levels when appropriate. A chemistry profile, including lactate dehydrogenase, can be helpful in diagnosing problems attributable to nutritional deficiency, liver disease, muscle disease, *P. carinii* pneumonia, and

Table 21–11.   Initial Laboratory Evaluation
of an HIV-Seropositive Patient

Complete blood cell count with differential
T-cell subsets
Electrolytes
Liver function tests, creatinine, BUN
Urinalysis
Syphilis serology
HB$_s$Ag, HB$_c$Ab, HB$_s$Ab
Posteroanterior and lateral chest radiographs
PPD (modified Mantoux) with anergy control
Serum *T. gondii* IgG antibody titer

---

lymphoma. In patients receiving pentamidine (aerosolized or IV) and ddI, periodic measurement of serum lipase or amylase levels is appropriate, as clinical and subclinical pancreatitis has been attributed to both drugs.

Serologic testing for syphilis is essential because co-infections are common and the treatment of syphilis is likely to be more effective if initiated earlier in HIV infection than later. The natural history of syphilis is altered by HIV infection, and therefore careful attention to the past history and treatment for syphilis is necessary for proper management. In an individual who is rapid plasma reagent and treponemal antibody positive and in whom a prior history of syphilis cannot be documented, further workup, including a lumbar puncture, should be considered. *Toxoplasma* IgG serology is advocated by some physicians in the hope that if neurologic abnormalities occur in the course of HIV infection, a second set of serologies may help to determine if toxoplasmosis is involved. Further, approximately one third of individuals who have positive IgG serology will develop symptomatic disease. As discussed earlier, chemoprophylaxis may be useful for those who have been previously exposed to *T. gondii.* CMV serology and cultures currently have little role in managing the HIV-positive, asymptomatic patient. However, if the patient needs transfusion, the use of CMV serology to assess the patient's antibody status may be employed. HBV serologies should be evaluated when the patient first enters medical care; if the patient does not demonstrate previous infection, he or she should be vaccinated. A baseline chest radiograph obtained when the patient is asymptomatic can be helpful in detecting subsequent subtle pulmonary abnormalities.

Assessing Prognosis

Several indicators are available for identifying those at risk of developing complications of HIV infection, such as *P. carinii* pneumonia or toxoplasmosis. They include *selected* symptoms and signs, as well as several laboratory tests. These indicators have come to be called "surrogate markers" because they are meant to substitute for the end points of disease that have been used extensively in AIDS clinical trials. Surrogate markers have many potential uses and, if interpreted cautiously, may help guide individual treatment, as well as help identify promising new agents for therapy.

It is important, however, to point out some of the difficulties associated with interpreting prognostic indicators. Many studies that have looked at these indicators have used different predictive end points. For example, the most commonly used end point is "AIDS-defining illness", although other studies have used *P.*

Table 21–12.   Suggested Laboratory Evaluation of HIV-Seropositive Patients

Test	*Use*	*Typical Frequency*
Complete blood cell count	Diagnosis of anemia, leukopenia, thrombocytopenia associated with HIV or related infections and medications	Asymptomatic individuals: every 6–12 mo Symptomatic individuals: every 3–6 mo (may need to be more frequent if the patient is taking zidovudine or other marrow toxic medications)
T-cell subsets	Treatment decisions regarding initiation of antiretroviral therapy and *P. carinii* prophylaxis Assessment of prognosis	Every 3–6 months
Chemistry	Diagnosis of complications of HIV infection and treatment	Every 2–6 mo in symptomatic patients
	Assessment of nutritional status (*e.g.,* albumin, iron, vitamin B12, *etc.*)	Every 12 mo
Syphilis serology	Diagnosis of syphilis	Every 6–12 mo and as indicated by history
CMV serology	Prevention of transfusion-transmitted CMV infections among CMV-seronegative patients	Prior to anticipated transfusions of cellular blood products
Toxoplasma IgG antibody	Diagnosis of Toxoplasmosis	Every 12 mo in previously seronegative patients
Purified protein derivative and anergy panel	Diagnosis of latent tuberculosis Guides choice of agent for *P. carinii* pneumonia prophylaxis	Every 12 mo until patient is anergic on two consecutive occasions

carinii pneumonia and death. Although there is some correlation among these end points, they clearly are different. Thus, the prognosis as estimated from these different end points may be quite different. Further, there are problems with using "AIDS-defining illness" in evaluating surrogate markers. If one uses this definition, an individual whose AIDS-defining illness is Kaposi's sarcoma would be treated in the same fashion as an individual whose AIDS-defining illness is *P. carinii* pneumonia, although the prognosis following these two illnesses is markedly different.

It is, however, possible to make some generalizations regarding the prognosis of HIV-seropositive patients. Several clinical markers are useful in identifying individuals at high risk of progression. The commonly cited clinical predictors of progression to AIDS are thrush, oral hairy leukoplakia, constitutional symptoms (sustained weight loss, fatigue, night sweats, persistent diarrhea), anergy, and herpes zoster. Persistent generalized lymphadenopathy was once thought to predict progression to AIDS in HIV-seropositive homosexual men, but more recent studies suggest that this is not the case.[76] Herpes zoster, while correlating with disease progression, has little predictive power. Thus, 2-year progression rates to clinical AIDS for men with herpes zoster is approximately 22%.[77] This rate is only slightly higher than the rate in asymptomatic HIV-seropositive men.[78] Thrush and oral hairy leukoplakia occur later in the disease course than herpes zoster and tend to be better predictors of progression to AIDS. Among the San Francisco General Hospital cohort of HIV-seropositive men, 39% and 42% of patients with thrush and oral hairy leukoplakia, respectively, progressed to AIDS over a 2-year period.[77] In the same cohort, virtually all patients with constitutional symptoms developed AIDS within 2 years. Anergy, another late manifestation of HIV infection, is a significant predictor of progression to AIDS, especially for patients with CD4 cell counts less than $400/mm^3$.[79] It should be emphasized that most data on disease prognosis have been collected in studies whose participants were predominantly homosexual men. Extrapolation to other risk groups must be done cautiously.

The laboratory findings that seem to be of most value in assessing prognosis in HIV-seropositive individuals are the absolute CD4 cell count (or percentage of CD4 lymphocytes and CD4/CD8 ratio), serum β_2-microglobulin levels (β_2-microglobulin is a cell surface glycoprotein that is believed to be elevated in rapid lymphocyte turnover), and serum neopterin levels.[80] Of the various predictive laboratory measurements, the CD4 cell count is currently the best single indicator of disease progression. Approximately 30% of patients with a cell count less than $200/mm^3$ develop AIDS-defining illness within 1 year of such a finding. It is estimated that 50% of patients with a cell count between $200/mm^3$ and $400/mm^3$ develop AIDS within 3 years. Individuals with cell counts above $400/mm^3$ have about a 15% chance of developing AIDS within 3 years.

Proper interpretation of the CD4 cell count requires an understanding of its biologic variation. A diurnal increase in the CD4 count of approximately 60 cells/mm^3 between 8 A.M. and 10 P.M. blood samples has been reported in individuals with Walter Reed stages 1 through 5 infection.[81] Although this fluctuation is significantly blunted in comparison with the approximately 500 cells/mm^3 change observed in HIV-seronegative individuals, it should be taken into account when evaluating CD4 measurements. Great variation can often exist within and among laboratories with regard to assessments of CD4 cell counts. This variation must always be considered when these laboratory markers are used in making clinical decisions. In general, significant decisions about clinical care should not be made on the basis of a single T-cell subset analysis, and evaluation of changes should be made using the same laboratory.

Serum HIV p24 antigen levels have also been used to assess prognosis. Several commercial assays are available to measure HIV p24 antigen. Each is slightly different, and this difference may play a role in assessing the value of this marker as a predictor of disease progression.[82] In general, detectable serum HIV p24 antigen can be found in 10% to 20% of HIV-seropositive individuals.[77,83] It is often present in the days to weeks prior to seroconversion, then disappears, only to reappear late in infection. Among a cohort of homosexual men followed for several years, p24 antigenemia developed in approximately 5% to 7% per year.[84] Although the presence or absence of p24 antigenemia does independently predict progression to AIDS, the quantitative antigen level does not correlate well with progression. Thus, if it is to be used in clinical decision-making, a very high p24 antigen level should be given no more weight than a moderately elevated p24 antigen level. Overall, the p24 antigen level is a poorer predictor of prognosis than the CD4 cell count, β_2-microglobulin level, or neopterin level. Other viral markers, such as plasma viremia or HIV nucleic acid measurements by polymerase chain reaction technology, are not sufficiently standardized for general use.

ANTIRETROVIRAL THERAPY

Zidovudine (azidothymidine, Retrovir) has been clearly demonstrated to prolong survival in patients with AIDS or advanced AIDS-related complex, and to delay progression to AIDS in patients with fewer than 500 CD4 cells/mm^3 in peripheral blood. Current recommendations in the United States are to use dosages of 500 to 600 mg/day in divided doses at all stages of infection for individuals with fewer than 500 CD4 cells/mm^3. No clear benefit has yet been seen in persons with baseline CD4 cell counts above 500 cells/mm^3.

Available data do not answer the question of whether zidovudine should be recommended for all individuals with mildly symptomatic or asymptomatic HIV infection. Whether such early intervention increases overall survival and quality of life for all who are HIV seropositive is unclear. Nor have the optimal dose regimens been clearly defined. Because the intracellular half-life of phosphorylated zidovudine is considerably longer than its serum half-life, the original 4-hour zidovudine regimen has been questioned. The recognition of this fact has led to the elimination by many of the early morning dose of zidovudine. Some centers have begun to study 8-hour dosing of zidovudine, with encouraging results.[85] However, these studies have involved small numbers of individuals and have focused on surrogate marker performance. More study is needed in larger numbers of individuals and focusing on clinical outcome data before the use of these longer dosing intervals can be recommended. The toxicity of the 4- and 8-hour dosing regiments appears similar.

During zidovudine therapy, laboratory-demonstrated resistance to the drug develops frequently, particularly in patients with advanced infection. By 12 months of treatment, an estimated 89% of persons with late-stage HIV infection have resistant isolates, compared with 31% with early-stage infection. High-level zidovudine resistance occurs almost exclusively in late-stage disease but does not appear related to zidovudine dosage. The clinical significance of zidovudine resistance is unclear, although clinical failure is frequently associated with it. Large-scale epidemiologic studies currently underway may further clarify the association.

Cross-resistance has been observed to other agents containing an azido group (*e.g.,* azidouridine) but not to agents that have no azido group (*e.g.,* ddI, ddC). It is reasonable to consider these latter agents in patients in whom zidovudine fails. However, decisions to change antiretroviral therapy based on *in vitro* data must be weighed carefully. Providers should inform patients that there are as yet no data to support a correlation between reduced *in vitro* sensitivity and clinical outcomes. Patients who are tolerating zidovudine well must weigh the potential for adverse reactions to new antiretroviral therapy. Clinical trials designed to answer these questions are in progress.

The principal adverse reactions associated with zidovudine result from bone marrow toxicity (Table 21–13). Anemia and neutropenia occur most frequently; both tend to be more severe in more advanced stages of disease and are dose related. In most situations, especially in individuals who began taking zidovudine while asymptomatic, the anemia is quite mild. It is frequently accompanied by an elevation in the mean corpuscular volume of as much as 30 to 40 mm^3/cell. A relatively small percentage of treated individuals, disproportionately represented by those with more advanced disease, may experience a more severe anemia. Evaluation of this anemia typically discloses a depressed reticulocyte count, normal serum folate level, and a normal serum vitamin B12 level. Bone marrow evaluation shows a low number of red cell precursors. Erythropoietin levels are usually elevated. This anemia may respond to zidovudine dose reduction. However, patients may require blood transfusion.

Table 21–13. Estimates of Frequencies of Adverse Reactions Associated with Use of Antiretroviral Therapies in Adults

Drug (Typical Dosage)	Adverse Reaction	Time Course	Prevalence*
Zidovudine (AZT) (500 mg/day)	Insomnia	<2 wk	B
	Fever or rash	<2 wk	A
	Nausea	<1 mo	D
	Macrocytosis	>1 mo	E
	Anemia	>1 mo	B–C
	Neutropenia	>1 mo	B–C
	Nail pigmentation†	>1 mo	D
	Myopathy	>6 mo	B
ddI (167–375 mg b.i.d.)	Nausea/vomiting	<2 wk	B
	Hyperuricemia	<1 mo	A
	Pancreatitis	>2 mo	B
	Neuropathy	>3 mo	B–C‡
ddC (0.375–0.75 mg t.i.d.)	Fever	<4 wk	B
	Rash	<4 wk	B
	Oral ulcers	<4 wk	B
	Neuropathy	>3 mo	C‡

* A: <1%. B: 1%–5%. C: 6%–25%. D: 26%–50%. E: 51%–100%.
† Occurs with increased frequency among black and Asian individuals.
‡ Peripheral neuropathy varies as a function of dosage schedule and duration of therapy.

Studies evaluating the use of erythropoietin in persons with AIDS have found a reduction in transfusion requirements among those whose endogenous erythropoietin levels at baseline were less than or equal to 500 IU/L.[86] For individuals with baseline endogenous erythropoietin levels above 500 IU/L, no reduction in transfusion requirement was observed. Data on the use of erythropoietin in earlier stages of HIV infection are not yet available. Therefore, erythropoietin therapy should be reserved for persons with AIDS-associated anemia who have low endogenous erythropoietin levels.

The neutropenia associated with zidovudine use is dose related and becomes more significant in advanced disease. It is generally associated with high doses and occurs after the first 3 months on the drug. The neutropenia is often worsened when a patient is placed on additional medications that also cause neutropenia. This is most frequently seen when patients develop CMV retinitis requiring ganciclovir therapy. Zidovudine therapy is usually discontinued while induction ganciclovir therapy is begun. Once maintenance ganciclovir therapy is started, it is possible in some patients to slowly reinstitute zidovudine therapy.

At present, zidovudine and ddI are approved by the Food and Drug Administration for the treatment of HIV infection. One other drug, ddC, is available in clinical trials or through expanded access programs. Several other drugs with antiretroviral activity *in vitro* are undergoing study in clinical trials.

It is likely that combinations of antiretroviral agents will be used with increasing frequency over the next few years. Combinations may attack the virus at different replicative sites, allow dose reduction of individual agents, and reduce the emergence of drug resistance. *In vitro* studies suggest that synergistic interactions are seen with certain combinations (*e.g.,* zidovudine with interferon-α, zidovudine with ddI or ddC), whereas antagonism is seen with others (*e.g.,* zidovudine with ribavirin). Agents with overlapping toxicities (*e.g.,* ddC and ddI) should be avoided in combination. Clinical trials of various antiretroviral combinations are in progress.

REFERENCES

1. Centers for Disease Control: HIV prevalence estimates and AIDS case projections for the United States: Report based upon a workshop. MMWR 16:1, 1990
2. World Health Organization: Toxoplasmosis surveillance. Weekly Epidemiol Rec WHO 59:162, 1984
3. McCabe RE, Remington JS: *Toxoplasma gondii.* In Mandell GL, Douglas RG, Bennett JE (eds): Principles and Practice of Infectious Diseases, p. 2090. New York, Churchill Livingstone, 1990
4. Levy RM et al: Neuroepidemiology of acquired immunodeficiency syndrome. In Rosenblom ML, Levy RM, Bredesen DE (eds): AIDS and the Nervous System. New York, Raven Press, 1988
5. Feldman HA: Toxoplasmosis: An overview. Bull NY Acad Med 50(2):110, 1974
6. Grant IH, Gold JMW, Armstrong D: Risk of CNS toxoplasmosis in patients with AIDS (abstr 441). Presented at the 26th Interscience Conference on Antimicrobial Agents and Chemotherapy, New Orleans, 1986
7. Dubey JP: A review of toxoplasmosis in pigs. Vet Parasitol 19:181, 1986
8. Riemann HP et al: Toxoplasmosis in an infant fed unpasteurized goat milk. J Pediatr 87:573, 1975
9. Sacks JJ, Roberto RR, Brooks NF: Toxoplasmosis infection associated with raw goat's milk. JAMA 248:1728, 1982
10. Swartzberg JE, Remington JS: Transmission of *Toxoplasma.* Am J Dis Child 129:777, 1975
11. Celum CL et al: Incidence of salmonellosis in patients with AIDS. J Infect Dis 156:998, 1987
12. Spector SA, Hirata KK, Newman TR: Identification of multiple cytomegalovirus strains in homosexual men with acquired immunodeficiency syndrome. J Infect Dis 150:953, 1984
13. Collier AC et al: Identification of multiple strains of cytomegalovirus in homosexual men. J Infect Dis 159:123, 1989
14. Chou SW: Reactivation and recombination of multiple cytomegalovirus strains from individual organ donors. J Infect Dis 160:11, 1989
15. Chou SW: Acquisition of donor strains of cytomegalovirus by renal-transplant recipients. N Engl J Med 314:1418, 1986
16. Chandler SH, Handsfield HH, McDougall JK: Isolation of multiple strains of cytomegalovirus from women attending a clinic for sexually transmitted disease. J Infect Dis 155:655, 1987
17. Tolkoff-Rubin NA et al: Cytomegalovirus infection in dialysis patients and personnel. Ann Intern Med 89:625, 1978
18. Luban NL et al: Low incidence of acquired cytomegalovirus infection in neonates transfused with washed red blood cells. Am J Dis Child 141:416, 1987
19. Gilbert GL et al: Prevention of transfusion-acquired cytomegalovirus infection in infants by blood filtration to remove leucocytes. Neonatal Cytomegalovirus Infection Study Group [see comments]. Lancet 1:1228, 1989
20. Centers for Disease Control: Guidelines for prophylaxis against *Pneumocystis carinii* pneumonia for persons infected with human immunodeficiency virus. MMWR 5:1, 1989
21. Phair J et al: The risk of *Pneumocystis carinii* pneumonia among men infected with human immunodeficiency virus type 1. Multicenter AIDS Cohort Study Group. N Engl J Med 322:161, 1990
22. Leibovitz E et al: *Pneumocystis carinii* pneumonia in infants infected with the human immunodeficiency virus with more than 450 CD4 T lymphocytes per cubic millimeter. N Engl J Med 323:531, 1990
23. Denny TN, Niven P, Skuza C: Age-related changes of lymphocyte phenotypes in healthy children. Pediatr Res 27:155, 1990
24. Centers for Disease Control: Guidelines for prophylaxis against *Pneumocystis carinii* pneumonia for children infected with human immunodeficiency virus. MMWR 40(RR-2):1, 1991
25. Abd AG et al: Bilateral upper lobe *Pneumocystis carinii* pneumonia in a patient receiving inhaled pentamidine prophylaxis. Chest 94:329, 1988
26. Jules EKM et al: Aerosolized pentamidine: Effect on diagnosis and presentation of *Pneumocystis carinii* pneumonia. Ann Intern Med 112:750, 1990
27. Kahn G: Dapsone is safe during pregnancy (letter). J Am Acad Dermatol 13(5 pt 1):838, 1985
28. Tuffanelli DL: Successful pregnancy in a patient with dermatitis herpetiformis treated with low-dose dapsone (letter). Arch Dermatol 118:876, 1982
29. Safety Memo 013: Safety information about dapsone and ddI: Potential interaction between dapsone and ddI. AIDS Clinical Trials Group and Jacobus Pharmaceutical Company, 1991
30. Kaplowitz LG et al: Prolonged continuous acyclovir treatment of normal adults with frequently recurring genital herpes simplex virus infection. The Acyclovir Study Group. JAMA 265:747, 1991
31. Sacks SL et al: Progressive esophagitis from acyclovir-resistant herpes simplex: Clinical roles for DNA polymerase mutants and viral heterogeneity? Ann Intern Med 111:893, 1989
32. Englund JA et al: Herpes simplex virus resistant to acyclovir: A study in a tertiary care center. Ann Intern Med 112:416, 1990
33. Brincker H: Prevention of mycosis in granulocytopenic patients with prophylactic ketoconazole treatment. Mykosen 26:242, 1983
34. Owens NJ et al: Prophylaxis of oral candidiasis with clotrimazole troches. Arch Intern Med 144:290, 1984
35. Gombert ME et al: A comparative trial of clotrimazole troches and oral nystatin suspension in recipients of renal transplants: Use in prophylaxis of oropharyngeal candidiasis. JAMA 258:2553, 1987
36. Bodey GP, Samonis G, Rolston K: Prophylaxis of candidiasis in cancer patients. Semin Oncol 17(suppl 6):24, 1990
37. Ferretti GA et al: Chlorhexidine for prophylaxis against

oral infections and associated. J Am Dent Assoc 114:461, 1987

38. Best TR et al: Persistent adrenal insufficiency secondary to low-dose ketoconazole therapy. Am J Med 82:676, 1987

39. Imam N et al: Hierarchical pattern of mucosal candida infections in HIV-seropositive women. Am J Med 89:142, 1990

40. Centers for Disease Control: Screening for tuberculosis and tuberculous infection in high-risk populations: Recommendations of the Advisory Committee for Elimination of Tuberculosis. MMWR 8:1, 1990

41. Sande MA, Volberding PA (eds): The Medical Management of AIDS. Philadelphia, WB Saunders, 1990

42. Centers for Disease Control: The use of preventive therapy for tuberculous infection in the United States: Recommendations of the Advisory Committee for Elimination of Tuberculosis. MMWR 8:9, 1990

43. Centers for Disease Control: Tuberculosis and human immunodeficiency virus infection: Recommendations of the Advisory Committee for the Elimination of Tuberculosis (ACET). MMWR 38:236, 1989

44. National Institute of Child Health and Human Development: Investigator Physician Information Release: Intravenous immunoglobulin for prophylaxis of serious bacterial infections in symptomatic HIV-infected children. Washington, DC, National Institute of Child Health and Human Development, 1991

45. Calvelli TA, Rubinstein A: Intravenous gamma-globulin in infant acquired immunodeficiency syndrome. Pediatr Infect Dis 5:S207, 1986

46. Centers for Disease Control: Health information for international travel. Atlanta, Centers for Disease Control, 1990

47. Centers for Disease Control: General recommendations on immunization. MMWR 38(13):205, 1989

48. Council of State and Territorial Epidemiologists; AIDS Program, Center for Infectious Disease, Centers for Disease Control: Revision of the CDC surveillance case definition for acquired immunodeficiency syndrome. MMWR 36(suppl 1):1S, 1987

49. Javier JJ et al: Nutritional abnormalities associated with HIV infection. Neurosci Abs 16:614, 1990

50. Falutz J, Tsoukas C, Gold P: Zinc as a cofactor in human immunodeficiency virus-induced immunosuppression (letter). JAMA 259:2850, 1988

51. Shoemaker JD, Millard MC, Johnson PB: Zinc in human immunodeficiency virus infection (letter). JAMA 260:1881, 1988

52. Dworkin BM et al: Selenium deficiency in the acquired immunodeficiency syndrome. JPEN 10:405, 1986

53. Baum MK: Association of vitamin B6 status with parameters of immune function in early HIV-1 infection. J AIDS 4:1122, 1991

54. Smith I et al: Folate deficiency and demyelination in AIDS (letter). Lancet 2:215, 1987

55. Burkes RL et al: Low serum cobalamin levels occur frequently in the acquired immune deficiency syndrome and related disorders [see comments]. Eur J Haematol 38:141, 1987

56. Kotler DP et al: Magnitude of body-cell-mass depletion and the timing of death from wasting in AIDS. Am J Clin Nutr 50:444, 1989

57. Keusch CT, Orrutia JJ, Fernandez R: Humoral and cellular aspects of intracellular bacteria killing in Guatemalan children with protein-calorie malnutrition. In Suskind RM

(ed): Malnutrition and the Immune Response. New York, Raven Press, 1977

58. Chandra RK: Mucosal immune responses in malnutrition. Ann NY Acad Sci 409:345, 1983

59. Souba WW, Wilmore DW: Postoperative alteration of arteriovenous exchange of amino acids across the gastrointestinal tract. Surgery 94:342, 1983

60. Chandra RK: Serum complement and immunoconglutinin in malnutrition. Arch Dis Child 50:225, 1975

61. Saxena QB, Saxena RK, Alder WH: Effect of protein calorie malnutrition on the levels of natural and inducible cytotoxic activities in mouse spleen cells. Immunology 51:727, 1985

62. Dreyfus PM: Diet and nutrition in neurologic disorders. In Shils ME, Young VR (eds): Modern Nutrition in Health and Disease, p 1458. Philadelphia, Lea & Febiger, 1988

63. Kotler DP et al: Body mass repletion during ganciclovir treatment of cytomegalovirus infections in patients with acquired immunodeficiency syndrome. Arch Intern Med 149:901, 1989

64. Yarchoan R et al: Administration of 3'-azido-3'-deoxythymidine, an inhibitor of HTLV-III/LAV replication, to patients with AIDS or AIDS-related complex. Lancet 1:575, 1986

65. Shike M et al: Changes in body composition in patients with small-cell lung cancer: The effect of total parenteral nutrition as an adjunct to chemotherapy. Ann Intern Med 101:303, 1984

66. Cohn SH et al: Changes in body composition of cancer patients following combined nutritional support. Nutr Cancer 4:107, 1982

67. von Roenn JH, Murphy RL, Wegener N: Megestrol acetate for treatment of anorexia and cachexia associated with human immunodeficiency virus infection. Semin Oncol 17(6 suppl 9):13, 1990

68. von Roenn JH et al: Megestrol acetate for treatment of cachexia associated with human immunodeficiency virus (HIV) infection. Ann Intern Med 109:840, 1988

69. Tchekmedyian NS et al: High-dose megestrol acetate: A possible treatment for cachexia. JAMA 257:1195, 1987

70. Hellerstein MK et al: Current approach to the treatment of human immunodeficiency virus-associated weight loss: Pathophysiologic considerations and emerging management strategies. Semin Oncol 17(6 suppl 9):17, 1990

71. Harriman GR et al: Vitamin B12 malabsorption in patients with acquired immunodeficiency syndrome. Arch Intern Med 149:2039, 1989

72. Herbert V et al: Low holotranscobalamin II is the earliest serum marker for subnormal vitamin B12 (cobalamin) absorption in patients with AIDS. Am J Hematol 34:132, 1990

73. Hartel D et al: Methadone maintenance treatment (MMTP) and reduced risk of AIDS and AIDS-specific mortality in intravenous drug users (IVDU's) (abstr 8546). Presented at the IV International Conference on AIDS, Stockholm, 1988

74. Ball JC, Lange WR, Meyers CP: The effectiveness of methadone maintenance in reducing IV drug use and needle sharing among heroin addicts at risk for AIDS (abstr 8503). Presented at the IV International Conference on AIDS, Stockholm, 1988

75. Marzuk PM et al: Increased risk of suicide in persons with AIDS. JAMA 259:1333, 1988

76. Schafer A et al: The increased frequency of cervical dysplasia-neoplasia in women infected with the human

immunodeficiency virus is related to the degree of immunosuppression. Am J Obstet Gynecol 164:593, 1991

77. Centers for Disease Control: Risk for cervical disease in HIV-infected women—New York City. MMWR 39:846, 1990

78. Osmond D et al: Lymphadenopathy in asymptomatic patients seropositive for HIV (letter). N Engl J Med 317:246, 1987

79. Moss AR et al: Seropositivity for HIV and the development of AIDS or AIDS related condition: Three year follow up of the San Francisco General Hospital cohort. Br Med J 296:745, 1988

80. Greenspan D et al: Relation of oral hairy leukoplakia to infection with the human immunodeficiency virus and the risk of developing AIDS. J Infect Dis 155:475, 1987

81. MacDonell KB et al: Prognostic usefulness of the Walter Reed staging classification for HIV infection. J AIDS 1:367, 1988

82. Fahey JL et al: The prognostic value of cellular and serologic markers in infection with human immunodeficiency virus type 1. N Engl J Med 322:166, 1990

83. Malone JL et al: Sources of variability in repeated T-helper lymphocyte counts from human immunodeficiency virus type 1-infected patients: Total lymphocyte count fluctuations and diurnal cycle are important. J AIDS 3:144, 1990

84. Bremer JW et al: Which HIV antigen EIA do you use? Your therapeutic and clinical evaluations may depend upon the choice (abstr SB540). Presented at the VI International Conference on AIDS, San Francisco, 1990

85. de Wolf F et al: Risk of AIDS related complex and AIDS in homosexual men with persistent HIV antigenaemia. Br Med J 295:569, 1987

86. Polk BF et al: Predictors of the acquired immunodeficiency syndrome developing in a cohort of seropositive homosexual men. N Engl J Med 316:61, 1987

87. Collier AC et al: A pilot study of low-dose zidovudine in human immunodeficiency virus infection. N Engl J Med 323:1015, 1990

88. Fischl M et al: Recombinant human erythropoietin for patients with AIDS treated with zidovudine. N Engl J Med 322:1488, 1990

89. Brundage JF et al: The current distribution of CD4+ T-lymphocyte counts among adults in the United States with human immunodeficiency virus infections: Estimates based on the experience of the U.S. Army. U.S. Army Ret-

rovirus Research Group [published erratum appears in J AIDS 3:837, 1990]. J AIDS 3:92, 1990

90. Guidelines to reduce the chance of airborne tuberculosis transmission from HIV-infected patients. Tuberculosis Program, Massachusetts Department of Public Health, 1989

91. Lang OW, Kessinger JM, Tucker RM: Low dose dapsone prophylaxis of *Pneumocystis carinii* pneumonia. (abstr T.B.05). Presented at the V International Conference on AIDS, Montreal, 1989

92. Baskin MI, Abd AG, Ilowite JS: Regional deposition of aerosolized pentamidine: Effects of body position and breathing pattern. Ann Intern Med 113:677, 1990

93. Fischl MA, Dickinson GM, La VL: Safety and efficacy of sulfamethoxazole and trimethoprim chemoprophylaxis for *Pneumocystis carinii* pneumonia in AIDS. JAMA 259:1185, 1988

94. Richman DD et al: The toxicity of azidothymidine (AZT) in the treatment of patients with AIDS and AIDS-related complex: A double-blind, placebo-controlled trial. N Engl J Med 317:192, 1987

95. Fischl MA et al: The safety and efficacy of zidovudine (AZT) in the treatment of subjects with mildly symptomatic human immunodeficiency virus type 1 (HIV) infection: A double-blind, placebo-controlled trial. The AIDS Clinical Trials Group. Ann Intern Med 112:727, 1990

96. Volberding PA et al: Zidovudine in asymptomatic human immunodeficiency virus infection: A controlled trial in persons with fewer than 500 CD4-positive cells per cubic millimeter. The AIDS Clinical Trials Group of the National Institute of Allergy and Infectious Diseases. N Engl J Med 322:941, 1990

97. Bristol-Myers Squibb Co: Didanosine Quarterly Safety Summary. Wallingford, CT, Bristol-Myers Squibb Co, 1990

98. Dalakas MC et al: Mitochondrial myopathy caused by long-term zidovudine therapy. N Engl J Med 322:1098, 1990

99. Don PC et al: Nail dyschromia associated with zidovudine. Ann Intern Med 112:145, 1990

100. Merigan TC, Skowron G: Safety and tolerance of dideoxy-cytidine as a single agent: Results of early-phase studies in patients with acquired immunodeficiency syndrome (AIDS) or advanced AIDS-related complex. Study Group of the AIDS Clinical Trials Group of the National Institute of Allergy and Infectious Diseases. Am J Med 88:11S, 1990

22

Counseling of HIV-Infected Individuals, Their Families, and Their Partners

Jimmie C. Holland   William Breitbart   Hindi Mermelstein

Physicians' counseling is a critical component of their total care of individuals infected with the human immunodeficiency virus (HIV), their families, and their sexual partners. Counseling about the common psychosocial and psychiatric disorders encountered in persons with HIV infection is discussed elsewhere in this book. However, physicians' responsibilities also extend to the public health issues the HIV epidemic has raised: how to provide information about risk behaviors and how to encourage reduction of them; how to counsel about the need for HIV testing in those for whom HIV infection must be considered in the differential diagnosis; and how to counsel individuals at high risk about the benefits of early diagnosis of HIV infection.[1] This chapter focuses on the public health aspect of counseling by the physician that is critical to containment of the acquired immunodeficiency syndrome (AIDS) epidemic. Although many physicians are pessimistic about their ability to change behaviors of patients by counseling, the degree of change achieved recently in dietary habits, exercise, and smoking suggests that it can be done. All studies point to the central role of physicians' advice in promoting change. With regard to the HIV epidemic, primary care physicians must become as comfortable in discussing sexual and drug-taking behaviors with young patients, especially the black and Hispanic populations at highest risk, as they are in discussing smoking and other risks, if there is to be any impact on the prevention of AIDS.[1]

Moreover, research is moving rapidly in relation to health education methods to reach the groups at highest risk for AIDS, and techniques to reduce high-risk behaviors and encourage safe sex are actively under study.

The physician must stay abreast of current information in these areas to counsel most effectively. However, negative personal attitudes of physicians must also be examined, insofar as they impact adversely on ability to counsel effectively. Patients with the dual diagnoses of substance abuse and an AIDS-related condition are often believed to be unlikely to change their behavior in any appreciable way. Nevertheless, studies have found that patients in a methadone maintenance clinic significantly reduced the numbers of sexual partners and the frequency of needle sharing to prevent HIV infection after counseling.[2] Negative attitudes toward patients whose HIV exposure resulted from homosexual practices can prevent the physician from functioning as an effective counselor for these individuals.

This chapter provides information needed for counseling about HIV and antibody testing, partner notification procedures, the special issues raised by pregnant women and infants, and health education strategies needed to contain the HIV epidemic. The guidelines provided for HIV counseling and testing are derived from the New York City Department of Health Guidelines for Physicians on HIV Counseling and Testing, 1989,[3] to which the reader is referred.

COUNSELING ABOUT HIV TESTING

Who Should Be Counseled?

HIV testing is currently the most effective means of identifying individuals who can transmit HIV infection and whose behavior is critical to preventing spread. There are many reasons to vigorously encourage early

HIV testing. The beneficial effect of treatment of HIV-seropositive asymptomatic individuals with zidovudine is reason to encourage individuals to be tested.[4] Aerosolized pentamidine is now proven prophylaxis for *Pneumocystis carinii*. Other infections, such as tuberculosis and syphilis, are best treated early. Preventing exposure of spouses or offspring to HIV should become an increasingly compelling reason for HIV testing as the epidemic grows.

Physicians are urged, as a part of routine care, to consider which of their patients are at risk for HIV infection and to offer HIV testing to them. Patients who may be unaware of any risk factors but who need to know of possible HIV infection because of their medical status, such as pregnancy, should also be offered testing. However, because a positive test result forces confrontation with mortality and threatens relationships with others, counseling before and after HIV testing is essential.[5] Current guidelines recommend counseling and testing of the following high-risk individuals[3]:

1. Men who have had sex with men
2. Intravenous (IV) drug users who have shared needles
3. Sexual partners of those in items (1) or (2)
4. Individuals treated for other sexually transmitted diseases

Those who should be counseled and strongly encouraged to be tested are the following:

1. Persons who have had multiple sexual partners of unknown serologic status, especially prostitutes
2. Recipients of blood or blood products between 1978 and 1985
3. Sexual partners of those in items (1) and (2)
4. Individuals with heavy crack usage (related to greatly increased sexual activity)

How Should Counseling About the HIV Antibody Test Be Done?

Considerable experience gained at test sites has led to the development of protocols for pre- and post-test counseling by physicians and their support staff. The steps ensure that all medical, legal, and educational aspects are covered (Table 22–1).

PRE-TEST COUNSELING

Step 1.　*Engagement*—Put the patient at ease.

Step 2.　*Reason for Testing*—When the patient asks for antibody testing, it is important to know the reason for the request, because it may affect immediate management (*e.g.,* development of a symptom; death of a friend).

When the physician recommends antibody testing, it is likely that a risk history (sexual or drug) or a medical finding leads to the recommendation for testing.

Table 22–1.　Steps in HIV Counseling and Testing

PRE-TEST COUNSELING	POST-TEST COUNSELING
Place person at ease	Present test results
Review reason for testing	Allow time to absorb
Assess current health status	Express emotions
Assess risk behaviors	Review priorities
Review risk reduction/ changes/barriers	Clarify meaning of test
Clarify meaning of test	Develop medical care plan
Plan for test results	Outline risk reduction
Plan for contact notification	Implement contact notification
Discuss confidentiality	Review confidentiality issues
Summarize	Identify social support
Ask decision about testing	Plan referral and follow-up
Obtain informed consent	

Modified from the New York City Department of Health Guidelines for Physicians on HIV Counseling and Testing, 1989.

Step 3.　*Current Health Assessment*—Review patient's concerns and assess for symptoms of HIV or other sexually transmitted diseases.

Step 4.　*Risk Assessment*—Assessing risk involves asking questions about sex and drug use that are difficult for some physicians to ask and for many patients to answer. A nonjudgmental, open manner will set the patient at ease. The AMA Physician Guidelines (1988) outline areas that should be covered, either systematically in the medical history or informally, whichever the physician finds easier[3]:

1. History of sexually transmitted diseases
2. Current and past sexual practice, partners, including known or suspected HIV-positive individuals
3. Sexual activity with prostitutes (male or female), IV drug users, bisexual males
4. Sexual practices: condom use; penile-vaginal; oral-genital; oral-anal; anal-genital
5. Drug use history: alcohol, marijuana, barbiturates, amphetamines, hallucinogens, cocaine, heroin

These questions about life-style that may have put the person at risk permit an assessment of risk while also allowing the clinician an opportunity to explain how each behavior or practice may put the person at risk. It is important to correct misinformation about transmission routes and to assure the person about the safety of casual contacts.

Step 5.　*Risk Reduction*—Go over what practices need to change to reduce HIV risk. Drug use? Sexual practices? Partner attitudes? Refer to proper community resources for help.

Step 6.　*Clarify Meaning of Test*—The interpretation of a negative or positive antibody test should be given, including false positives and negatives. Encourage the patient to describe what a positive test result would mean personally. Correct that personal meaning based on the reality of test results.

Step 7. *Plan for Test Results*—What life-style changes will the patient make following a positive or negative test result? Help patients anticipate the level of distress they may feel later, on hearing the results. Explore their sources of support. Assess their psychiatric status and obtain a psychiatric consultation if suicidal risk seems likely.

Step 8. *Plan for Contact Notification*—Discuss the importance of notifying sexual and needle-sharing partners if the test is positive, and options available for help in doing so, if needed (see post-testing counseling session, below).

Step 9. *Discuss Confidentiality*—Discuss the possibilities of discrimination if confidentiality of test results should be breached. Offer the option of confidential testing, in which information is in the chart for use by physicians and nurses, *versus* the anonymous testing option, in which the person is identified only by a number.

Step 10. *Summary of Session*—Review the patient's understanding of the test's significance, likely response to news, and ability to follow medical advice. Discuss referrals; explore risk assessment and concerns.

Step 11. *Discuss Decision About Testing*—Point out that the decision to take the test is patient's own.

Step 12. *Informed Consent*—Sign the appropriate consent form, draw blood and make an appointment for counseling about the results.

Following these well-defined steps is a way to become familiar with the needed information to be reviewed and discussed with the patient and to ensure that all points have been covered in a counseling session. A checklist has been developed in some centers to ensure adherence to the medical and legal aspects of the counseling mandated to be done with antibody testing.

POST-TEST COUNSELING

A session should be scheduled as early as possible after HIV antibody testing has been done and the results are available. Waiting for results is an anxiety-ridden period during which some individuals find it difficult to function.

Step 1. *Present Test Results*—In a calm and relaxed manner, give the test results immediately, directly, and clearly. Engaging in small talk before giving the results only adds to anxiety. The news should always be given in a face-to-face session, never by telephone. The interpretation of positive and negative results should be given, with an explanation of what they mean in terms of exposure, antibody formation, and the relationship to developing AIDS.

Step 2. *Allow the Patient Time To Absorb the Information*—A negative result is good news, but the patient must be told that exposure in the prior 6 months may not show up on the antibody test just done. Positive results may elicit feelings on a spectrum ranging from expression of strong emotions to stoic silence. It is best to observe the response first, and then determine the type of support the patient needs.

Step 3. *Express Initial Reactions*—Encourage the patient to describe how he or she feels and to examine the meaning of the findings in relation to the patient's future (*e.g.,* childbearing potential). Correct misinformation about immediate goals and plans. Ask about suicidal thoughts and plans. Refer for psychiatric evaluation, if needed.

Psychological distress after notification of seropositivity has been studied. Significant distress occurred in over half the individuals notified.[6-8] Severe anxiety, depression, and preoccupation with AIDS were greatest in those who felt they had had least opportunity to discuss the meaning of the test results.[9] Perry and colleagues in a prospective study found that prior to notification, both seropositive and seronegative individuals scored high on anxiety and depression.[9] Notification of seronegativity resulted in immediate reduction of distress. Those who tested seropositive did not experience an increase in distress on notification, perhaps because of the ceiling effect on measures of distress. By week 10, levels of distress in seropositive and seronegative subjects were comparable. Despite fears of grave distress, individuals appeared to tolerate the information remarkably well. These data parallel the responses of patients to news of a positive biopsy for cancer.[10] The reduction in distress that was seen among the seropositive patients studied, however, may have been related to the intensive pre-test and post-test counseling provided. Clearly, with appropriate counseling, notification of HIV seropositivity does not lead to irreversible psychological damage. Additionally, the fear that many individuals would become acutely suicidal on notification of seropositivity has not been borne out by clinical experience or research. Perry and colleagues also found that suicidal ideation was surprisingly uncommon during the HIV testing period and when present, it tended to be mild.[11] Suicidal ideation appeared equally among those who were seropositive or seronegative and appeared to be a function of depression rather than HIV status.

Step 4. *Establish Priorities*—Have the patient start thinking of the decisions to be made in light of the test results. Concerns may seem overwhelming in the first few days; the patient should focus on only the most pressing decisions.

Step 5. *Clarify Meaning of Test Result.*—Review what the test means to the person and clarify the actual meaning of a positive, negative, or inconclusive result, based on current knowledge. Point out the speed with which earlier treatment is becoming possible and the delay in progression to disease symptoms. Hope is critical at this stage. In fact, Rapkin and colleagues found hope to be well sustained by a group of seropositive gay men, despite the prognosis for developing a fatal illness.[12]

Step 6. *Develop a Medical Follow-up Plan*—Arrange HIV medical care, explain the immunologic work-up, provide reproductive counseling and TB screening, and outline treatment options. Encourage the patient to become well informed about HIV. Tell the patient about resources and support groups. Review the need for use of condoms and safe sex practices. Plan health maintenance in relation to nutrition and avoidance of sexually transmitted disease.

Step 7. *Review Risk-Reduction Guidelines*—Go over risk behaviors and the need to change life-style. Review types of contacts that are risky and those that are not dangerous to others (casual physical contact). Provide literature about HIV. Review the patient's current potential contacts that add to risk (*e.g.,* an untested boyfriend).

Step 8. *Implement Contact Notification Plan*—After attention to the patient's concerns, turn the discussion to others who might have been exposed, and how the patient wishes to inform them of their risk in view of the positive HIV test. Point out alternatives to personal notification that can be used to protect confidentiality.

Although a reduction in high-risk sexual behaviors occurred in gay men before testing for the HIV antibody was widely available, several large studies have demonstrated that risk behavior changes with knowledge of serostatus: those notified of seropositivity generally reduce risk behaviors more than untested individuals, unnotified seropositive individuals, or those notified of seronegative status.[13,14] In fact, an increase in high-risk behavior among some informed of HIV-seronegative status has been noted.

Needle use risk reduction has taken place among IV drug users in drug treatment programs; however, sexual behavior risk reduction is still problematic.[6,15,16] An alarmingly small percentage of pregnant IV drug users who learn of their own HIV seropositivity decide to electively terminate a pregnancy that may result in an HIV-seropositive newborn.[17] Less is known about the impact of HIV testing on heterosexuals; however, in one study of heterosexual IV drug users, 80% of those who initiated condom use in their sexual activity lost their partners because of forced disclosure of seropositivity.[6] These data reflect the need for more research on promotion of behavioral change.

Step 9. *Review Confidentiality Issues*—Consider with the patient the meaning of the positive results, allowing him or her to think about how the information might be used in a discriminatory way (*e.g.,* job security) and how those issues affect others who should know.

Step 10. *Mobilize a Support System*—Review what the patient will do in the next 24 hours, because the level of distress may be disorganizing for a short period. The person may feel numb and unable to plan. Identify and call a person to help. Give the patient the telephone numbers of community resources and appropriate support groups and health education programs.

Step 11. *Summarize Referral and Follow-up*—Write out plans that include medical care, social support,

risk reduction plans, and notification of partners. Schedule a follow-up visit or clear referral. Indicate availability by telephone if needed.

In summary, the post-test counseling session reviews all the points made in pre-test counseling, but addresses each within the framework of the actual test results. The personal issues predominate, but of special concern are those public health issues raised in step 8—notification of sexual partners or those who may have shared needles with the individual, issues pertinent to the patient's responsibility to others.

Who Should Be Notified, and How?

A major ethical dilemma that has arisen in the HIV epidemic is the right to confidentiality of the HIV-positive person *versus* the right of others to know they have been exposed to HIV. The usual public health measures of reporting all cases and notifying those exposed as a means of curtailing an epidemic has had limited applicability in the HIV epidemic because of the potential for discrimination against HIV-infected individuals and the inappropriate use of information about serostatus. Guidelines have evolved to aid the physician in considering options that provide maximum confidentiality while also permitting contact notification.

The importance of notifying contacts must be addressed in both pre- and post-test counseling (step 8 in both procedures above). The individual must understand that partner notification reduces the risk of spread to noninfected persons, reduces reinfection exposure of those who are HIV positive, and allows persons to take these issues into account in their health care, especially reproductive-age women. Because it may be difficult to face friends or partners with this information, counseling about why a seropositive patient must inform and how to do it, even while respecting confidentiality, becomes critical. The pre-test counseling session should review who has been exposed and the importance of telling them. This exploration of the area begins the patient thinking about it and permits review of the problems likely to be encountered. The New York City Department of Health has printed a brochure, "Sometimes Words Don't Come Easily . . . Informing Your Contacts," which can be requested for assisting the patient in telling others.

The post-test counseling session deals with notification of contacts in light of the patient's seropositive status, examining now the time frame within which partners have been exposed and the details of who must be notified. There are several options to be considered for contact notification:

1. The patient accepts responsibility and agrees to notify contacts directly; however, the physician must assess the likelihood of the patient's actually doing so.
2. The patient asks for help in notification. This may require additional sessions or bringing a partner in for joint counseling.

3. The patient asks that the physician or a third party notify. In New York City, a third-party notification program permits referral to a special public health office.

A combination of the three ways may be most desirable, with different approaches used for different contacts. For example, the patient may want to tell a current partner directly and may ask that the physician or public health facility notify past contacts.

In addition, New York and some other states recognize "permission to warn" in certain circumstances, or to notify a public health officer who may do so. The circumstances are as follows: (1) when the physician feels it is medically appropriate and there is a significant risk to the contact, and (2) when the patient has been counseled to notify and the physician believes he or she will not. In such a case, the physician must notify the patient of his plan to notify a contact; the patient may express a preference for whether the physician or a public health officer will notify, but he or she cannot refuse to permit notification. Notification of contacts is always done in person and using the counseling procedure outlined earlier for pre-test counseling. The identity of the contact is kept confidential by excluding the name and any identifying information, such as the time of testing, that might disclose identity. Although the physician has no legal obligation to notify contacts, the circumstances outlined above permit the "opportunity to warn" in particularly distressing circumstances of unknown exposure.

COUNSELING PREGNANT WOMEN ABOUT HIV

In no other segment of the population is the impact of HIV more evident than in childbearing women who have had sexual or drug use contacts that put them at risk, because not only the mother but the fetus is at risk of developing a fatal disease. Pediatric AIDS is now the most common fatal congenitally acquired infection in the United States, and 80% of cases are the result of perinatal transmission.[18] The number varies, but presently it is believed that the fetal infection rate is about 40% in HIV-positive mothers. In some cities, such as New York and Miami, the percentage of births to HIV-positive mothers varies from about 1.0% to 3.5% of all births. For these reasons, the New York City Department of Health recommends that both men and women who have engaged in risk behavior be urged to consider antibody testing before making childbearing decisions.[3] HIV-positive women should defer pregnancy. A seropositive pregnant woman should be provided with information about risks to herself and the fetus. Options, including abortion, should be included in counseling. Although women studied by Holman and colleagues usually informed their partners or the father of the child, 20% did not, out of fear of abandonment.[18]

Pre- and post-testing counseling is of critical importance in this group. The pregnant mother must know the risk to her unborn child. However, a seropositive HIV test in children less than 18 months old reflects maternal antibody that has crossed the placenta and does not necessarily indicate HIV infection in the child. Children should be retested periodically to determine definitely whether they are infected. A negative antibody test at birth likely means that the child is not infected.

Although the protocol outlined above is applicable to pre- and post-test counseling of pregnant women, they have a greater need for ongoing medical and psychological support, especially if they must care for an infected infant. Holman and colleagues have developed a special counseling protocol to ensure that all areas of concern in this group are covered in counseling sessions.[18] Research is needed to develop effective support programs aimed at helping young women who are HIV positive, and at preventing transmission among women of childbearing age.

NEED FOR MORE COUNSELING

Public health officials are urgently pointing out the need for better use of existing educational measures to stem HIV transmission in the United States.[1,16] Examples of opportunities to improve education are numerous. Strategies are needed to reach the high-risk population in communities. Testing sites, for example, are likely not reaching the populations at highest risk.[16] Greater effort should be made to identify and develop outreach programs for those at highest risk. Table 22–2 outlines sites that must be more aggressively targeted for educational, support, and counseling activities, such as storefront clinics, prenatal and sexually transmitted diseases clinics, and physicians offices in high-risk areas of practice. Project TRUST, in Boston, is an example of an effort to increase the counseling of IV drug users.[19] The project has nurses, counselors, and recovered IV drug users who work as outreach workers. It is located in a neighborhood with known drug users. It offers free anonymous testing after counseling, and advises about the use of bleach to disinfect needles and the use of condoms for safe sex. Pregnancy testing, tuberculosis

Table 22–2. Sites for Increased HIV Counseling and Risk Assessment

Clinic-based counseling linked to:
    Chemical dependency treatment programs
    Sexually transmitted disease clinics
Third-party partner notification program
Outreach programs
    Street workers
    Storefront services
Family planning centers
Prenatal clinics
Child health centers
Physicians' offices or clinics in high-risk areas

testing, and other services are provided on site. Referrals to Spanish- or English-language support programs and drug and alcohol treatment and social services are offered. Similar efforts are needed in cities with high rates; the efforts should take into account the cultural factors of those at risk and tailor interventions to ensure applicability.

SUMMARY

The best means of containing the HIV epidemic is education. Physicians have a key role to play as counselors for individuals at risk of HIV by providing information not only on medical care but about the virus, how it is transmitted, and how each individual has a responsibility to reduce risk behaviors for the sake of himself or herself, and others. Counseling about the public health aspects of HIV begins when a request for testing occurs or when an indication for HIV antibody testing is noted in an individual.[20] Experience has led to the development of protocols for pre- and post-test counseling that, when followed, ensure that all medical and legal points are covered: what the virus is and how it is transmitted; behaviors that have or will put the person at risk; ways to reduce risk; what the test means in relation to treatment; and how to plan for notification of contacts, medical follow-up, and life-style changes. The right of the physician to warn a contact at high risk in a medically appropriate situation may be exercised when the patient is informed that notification will occur. Special attention is needed to counsel the pregnant woman about her health and that of her fetus. Physicians' roles as counselors in the HIV epidemic will only expand. The ability to take a careful risk assessment history, which includes sexual practices and drug use history, and to counsel high-risk individuals is critically important to limiting the spread of HIV infection.

REFERENCES

1. Drotman DP: Earlier diagnosis of human immunodeficiency virus (HIV) infection and more counseling. Ann Intern Med 110:680, 1989
2. Curtis JL, Crummey FC, Baker SN et al: HIV screening and counseling for intravenous drug abuse patients: Staff and patient attitudes. JAMA 261:258, 1989
3. New York City Department of Health: Guidelines for Physicians in HIV Counseling and Testing and Related Documents. New York, New York City Department of Health, Bureau of Public Health Education, 1989
4. Volberding PA, Lagakos SW, Koch MA et al: Zidovudine in asymptomatic human immunodeficiency virus infection: A controlled trial in persons with fewer than 500 CD-4 positive cells per cubic millimeter. N Engl J Med 322:941, 1990
5. Jacobsen PB, Perry SW, Hirsch DA: Behavioral and psychological responses to HIV antibody testing. J Consult Clin Psychol 58:37, 1990
6. Casadonte PP, DesJarlais D, Friedman S, Rotrosen J: Psychological and behavioral impact of learning HIV test results in IV drug users (abstr). Presented at the IV International Conference on AIDS, Stockholm, Sweden, 1988
7. Jacobsen PB, Perry SW, Hirsch DA et al: Psychological reactions of individuals at risk from AIDS during an experimental drug trial. Psychosomatics 29:182, 1988
8. Ostrow DG, Joseph JH, Kessler R et al: Disclosure of HIV antibody status: Behavioral and mental health characteristics. AIDS Educ Prev 1:1, 1989
9. Perry SW, Jacobsberg L, Fishman B et al: Psychological responses to serological testing for HIV. AIDS 4:145, 1990
10. Holland JC, Rowland JH (eds): Handbook of Psychoncology: Psychological Care of the Patient with Cancer. New York, Oxford University Press, 1989
11. Perry SW, Jacobsberg L, Fishman B: Suicidal ideation and HIV testing. JAMA 263:679, 1990
12. Rapkin JC, Williams JBW, Nengebauer R et al: Maintenance of hope in HIV spectrum homosexual men. Am J Psychiatry 147:1322, 1990
13. Coates TJ, Morin SF, McKusick L: Behavioral consequences of AIDS antibody testing among gay men. JAMA 258:1889, 1987
14. Fox R, Odaka NJ, Brookmeyer R, Polk BF: Effect of antibody disclosure on subsequent sexual activity in homosexual men. AIDS 1:241, 1987
15. DesJarlais DC, Friedman SR, Hopkins W: Risk reduction for the acquired immunodeficiency syndrome among intravenous drug users. Ann Intern Med 103:755, 1985
16. Danila RN, Schultz JM, Osterholm MT et al: HIV-1 counseling and testing sites, Minnesota: Analysis of trends in clinical characteristics. Am J Public Health 80:419, 1990
17. Selwyn PA, Carter RJ, Hartel D et al: Elective termination of pregnancy among HIV seropositive and seronegative intravenous drug users (abstr). Presented at the IV International Conference on AIDS, Stockholm, Sweden, June 1988
18. Holman S, Berthaud M, Sunderland A et al: Women infected with human immunodeficiency virus: Counseling and testing during pregnancy. Semin Perinatol 13:7, 1989
19. Centers for Disease Control: Counseling and testing intravenous drug users for HIV infection—Boston. MMWR 38:489, 1989
20. Perry SW, Markowitz JC: Counseling for HIV testing. Hosp Commun Psychiatry 39:731, 1988

V

Prevention and Public Health

23

Prevention of the Sexual Transmission of HIV

Thomas A. Peterman   *Willard Cates, Jr.*
Judith N. Wasserheit

Over 95% of Americans feel that they are at little or no risk of developing the acquired immunodeficiency syndrome (AIDS).[1] Some have based their assessments on realistic consideration of their sexual and drug use behaviors; and in this respect they have accomplished one of the most important steps in preventing transmission. Others may have not thought about it carefully or may not recognize their risk, and so are unlikely to be taking the steps necessary to protect themselves.

Because of the prevalence of human immunodeficiency virus (HIV) infection and its high associated morbidity, many persons in the United States should consider changing their sexual behavior. These persons include an estimated 10 million men who have had sex with men,[2] 1 million current users of injectable drugs,[2] 12 million individuals who acquire a sexually transmitted disease (STD) each year,[3] and millions of others who will have sex with one or more new partners. For persons living in other Western countries, the risks for acquiring HIV infection and the need for behavior change are similar to those in the United States. In some African and Caribbean countries, because of the prevalence of HIV infection in the general population, virtually everyone must consider the need for changing sexual behavior.

Preventing sexual transmission of HIV requires more than a list of options for personal protection. Additional support is needed from individual counselors, health departments, and society as a whole. Many persons should consider counseling their friends, associates, or clients about AIDS. Health departments must continue to monitor the epidemic to provide accurate information about risks, effective ways to avoid them, and methods to help persons at risk. Finally, everyone in society should consider changes needed to facilitate realistic discussion of HIV risk behavior and to provide an environment that promotes the health of persons at risk.

PERSONAL PROTECTION

To be effective, HIV prevention efforts must ultimately influence individual decisions. Many approaches to personal protection are possible. Choosing the best options will depend on the individual's value system and the relative effectiveness of the change. To reduce the risk of acquiring HIV, sexually active persons must either lower their risk of having sexual intercourse with an infected partner or lower the risk of transmission during intercourse.

Most of us are looking for ways to balance the risk of acquiring infection with the benefits of sexual pleasure. An individual can eliminate the risk of sexually acquired HIV infection by never having sex, but only a small percentage of people choose that option for a lifetime. By age 19, 75% of all adolescent women will have experienced sexual intercourse, an increase of 8% since the AIDS epidemic began.[4] It may be easier to change sexual practices than to stop having sex altogether. For example, women in college surveyed in 1975 and 1989 had similar numbers of sex partners (21% had had three or more partners in the previous year), but the proportion who regularly used condoms increased from 12% to 41%.[5] Similarly, many gay men have switched from anal intercourse to safer sexual practices.[6] Each individual has many options for risk reduction, with benefits that are increasingly quantifiable. However, the cost to an individual of changing sexual behavior will ultimately depend on a complex set of personal needs for sexual intimacy.

Avoiding Infected Partners

If an uninfected person chooses only uninfected sex partners, there is no risk of acquiring infection. Choosing the right partner is an important strategy for avoiding infection,[7] but the difficulty of this task is often underestimated. For one thing, partner selection is determined by social networks and geographic proximity. Moreover, most people with HIV infection are asymptomatic: they look like uninfected people. Thus, a key part of risk reduction through careful partner selection is knowing partners well before having sex with them.

The characteristics of persons with the highest HIV prevalence are well known (Table 23–1). Men should consider potential sex partners as probably infected if they are either other men or users of injectable drugs. Somewhat lower HIV prevalence rates occur among women who have had sex with bisexual men or with injectable drug users, women who received transfusions between 1978 and 1985, and women from countries where heterosexual transmission is common. In the United States, as a rule of thumb, a woman with more than 10 lifetime sex partners might unknowingly have had one who was either bisexual or an injectable drug user.

Women should consider potential sex partners as probably infected if they are bisexual men, injectable drug users, or men with hemophilia. Somewhat lower HIV prevalence rates occur in men who have had sex with women who used injectable drugs, with men who received transfusions between 1978 and 1985, and with men from countries where heterosexual transmission is common. Although the number is arbitrary, men who have had more than 20 lifetime sex partners may have unknowingly had one who was infected and should also be considered potentially infected with HIV.

Nearly everyone can identify high-risk behavior in a questionnaire,[1] but few studies have assessed the ability to identify risk in a potential sex partner under real-world conditions. Among 422 sexually active college students, 32% of the men and 23% of the women were sexually involved with more than one person, and in over 60% of cases the partner did not know about it.[8] Among female partners of infected bisexual men, 20 (38%) of 52 women did not know that their partner was bisexual, even though many were in long-term relationships.[9]

Other clues may indicate that a partner could be infected. Persons previously infected with other STDs, particularly syphilis, have a greater likelihood of also having HIV infection than those who have never had an STD.[10] Crack cocaine use has been associated with trading sex for money or cocaine, anonymous sex with multiple partners, and high rates of syphilis and perhaps HIV.[11,12] Infection is much more common in some geographic areas than others. In 1989, one in every 200 women giving birth in New York State was HIV infected, compared to none of 17,273 in New Hampshire.[13] Within states, HIV is often concentrated in certain cities, and within those cities, in particular neighborhoods. A serosurvey in one U.S. hospital found HIV antibody in one in every five men aged 25 to 44 years admitted with a non-AIDS-related illness.[14] Persons who live in areas with a high prevalence of AIDS should consider all partners as potentially infected.

If a partner could be infected, both members of the couple should undergo HIV testing before initiating sexual intercourse without a condom. Ideally, all de-

Table 23–1. Factors Influencing the Likelihood That a Sexual Partner in the United States is HIV Infected

Characteristic	HIV Prevalence (%)	Relative Prevalence
Partner's HIV transmission-risk history		
None[7]	0.01	1 (referent)
Transfusion recipient (one unit, 1984)[76]	0.04	4
IV drug user, Los Angeles[71]	3	300
IV drug user, New York[71]	34	3,400
Man who had sex with men, San Francisco[71]	30	3,000
Man with hemophilia[77]	62	6,200
Geographic variation		
Childbearing women		
New Mexico[13]	0.01	1 (referent)
New York[13]	0.58	58
Hospitalized men ages 25–44, U.S.		
Hospital 23[14]	0.4	1 (referent)
Hospital 1[14]	21.7	54
HIV antibody test results		
HIV negative	0.004	1 (referent)
HIV untested[2]	0.4	100
HIV positive (with confirmatory Western blot)[2,43]	98	24,500

cisions related to types of sexual activities should be guided by the results of the HIV test. Monogamous couples with negative HIV antibody tests need not observe any precautions to prevent HIV transmission.[15] For monogamous couples in which both partners are HIV infected, there are theoretical concerns about repeated exposure to HIV or exposure to different strains, but no increased risk has been demonstrated. Increasing numbers of persons are seeking antibody testing to help with decisions about sexual relationships. Antibody status is now even included in ads in the ''Personal'' section of some newspapers.

The vast majority of infected persons are identifiable with an antibody test. However, a small proportion of recently infected persons may be tested in the window period during which they are infectious but have a negative HIV antibody test. The importance of the window period is a function of the incidence, time to develop antibody, and prevalence. For example, if 40,000 persons per year acquire infection in the United States, and if they were infectious with a negative antibody test for 3 months each, then at any given time there would be 10,000 infected persons in the United States with a negative test. This would represent only 1% of the estimated 1,000,000 HIV-infected persons, and only 0.004% of all people in the United States.

Learning a partner's HIV antibody status depends on the partner having an antibody test. Many infected persons still do not know that they are infected, and many others at risk do not know that they are uninfected. Moreover, uninfected persons who continue to engage in unprotected intercourse with a high-risk partner should undergo additional HIV testing intermittently because they are at risk of seroconverting. Once tested, a person should discuss the test results with potential partners. In one cohort of gay men, 23% had asked partners about their HIV status.[16] Only 8 (12%) of 63 heterosexuals who had been previously tested in a Miami STD clinic had ever asked a partner about his or her HIV status.[17]

Test results must be understood. One study found that five (3%) of 146 subjects who ''knew'' they had a negative test had actually tested positive.[16] More effective HIV counseling after the positive tests may have avoided this misperception. ELISA-type test kits for HIV for home use are now technologically possible. If marketed, they would facilitate repeated testing and the sharing of results with a potential sex partner.

Avoiding Transmission

HIV risk can be further reduced by choosing sexual activities carefully (Table 23–2). Although this approach is theoretically not as effective as choosing partners carefully, in practice it may be more realistic. In addition, changes in types of sexual activities can complement more careful partner selection.

Unprotected anal receptive sex is the most efficient way of acquiring HIV infection from an infected sex

Table 23–2. Factors Influencing the Risk of Sexual Transmission of HIV

Characteristic	Estimated Relative Risk
Type of sexual intercourse	
Manual receptive*	1 (referent)
Oral receptive[78] *	10
Vaginal receptive	100
Anal receptive[19–21]	300
Use of condoms	
Condom used[34]	1 (referent)
Condom not used	50
Genital ulcer	
No ulcer	1 (referent)
Genital ulcer[26]	5

* Estimate based on anecdotal information on the risk of HIV transmission associated with manual or oral sex.

partner.[18] Studies of female partners of infected men suggest that women who had anal sex with their infected partner were two to four times more likely to be infected than women who had only vaginal sex.[19–21] Oral sex appears to be less risky than anal or vaginal sex, but no studies exist of infection rates in persons who report only oral sex. Oral sex is not risk free, but we can only guess what the relative risk might be. Some men have acquired infection after oral sex with men,[22,23] and some women appear to have acquired infection after oral sex with women.[24] Mutual masturbation is probably even less risky because skin is more impervious to viruses than are the mucous membranes. However, some persons have acquired infection after getting infected blood on their skin, so infected semen or cervical secretions could theoretically transmit infection during manual sex as well.[25]

When breaks in the skin or mucous membranes occur, the risk of transmitting or acquiring infection increases. For example, in a cohort study in Kenya, men with genital ulcers were 4.7 times more likely to seroconvert than men with urethritis.[26] The relative risk of acquiring HIV following a single exposure to an infected partner may be much higher. A subgroup of these men reported having only a single sexual contact with prostitutes; six (16%) of 37 with ulcers seroconverted, compared with none (0%) of 36 with urethritis.[26] Other activities that may increase the risk of development of traumatic ulcers and HIV infection include ''dry'' sex or the use of desiccants in the vagina; these may contribute to the high rates of transmission in Africa.[27] Non-ulcerative STDs may also facilitate the transmission of HIV by increasing the amount of virus in an area, or by inflaming the mucosa.[28] Avoiding sex when either partner has an STD would reduce transmission from an infected partner. Because some ulcers are not painful, ideally careful genital examination would precede sexual intercourse with any partner.[29]

Uncircumcised men are more likely to be seropositive.[26] The protective effect of circumcision has biologic plausibility; the foreskin is a vascular tissue that may be more likely to have breaks in the epithelium. Moreover, other studies have suggested that circumcision protects from other STDs such as genital ulcer diseases.[30] Therefore, circumcision may have an important role to play in preventing HIV transmission. However, controlled studies are needed to demonstrate the efficacy of circumcision as a prevention method.

Barriers to HIV transmission may be physical or chemical. Several studies have shown that HIV will not pass through intact latex condoms.[31,32] Natural-membrane condoms contain pores that could theoretically allow passage of intact virus, so they are considered less protective than latex condoms.[33] Condoms are unlikely to be 100% effective because they do not protect uncovered areas. This would be particularly important if either partner has an ulcer that was not covered. In addition, condoms may break or slip off. However, most condom failures are due to inconsistent use. The estimated failure rate of condoms when used consistently for pregnancy prevention is 2 per 100 couple-years of use.[34] A typical pregnancy rate is 12 per 100 couple-years, primarily because couples relying on condoms occasionally have intercourse without them.[34] How these pregnancy rates would translate to infection rates when condoms are used to prevent disease is not clear. Cross-sectional and case-control studies have suggested that condom users are protected from infections, but the magnitude of protection varies, with most studies showing a relative risk of 0.3 to 0.8.[35] These studies included people who used condoms inconsistently.

The efficacy of condoms may be different for anal intercourse. For example, a postal questionnaire in London found a breakage rate of 4.7%, commonly attributed to powerful thrusting, insufficient lubrication, and prolonged intercourse. However, in brothels in Sydney, Australia, only three (0.5%) of 664 condoms used for anal intercourse and five (0.8%) of 605 used for vaginal intercourse broke.[36] These low breakage rates were attributed to user experience, good-quality condoms, accurate counts of the number used, and the observation that commercial sex usually lasts for a shorter time than "amateur" sex.[37]

Condom breakage decreases with experience and can be reduced by recognizing the likely causes. Breakage is more common when the vagina is not well lubricated, leading to the suggestion that couples spend more time engaging in foreplay.[38] Water-based lubricants (contraceptive gel, K-Y jelly) can also decrease breakage, but oil-based lubricants (petroleum jelly, shortening) weaken the latex and should not be used. Newer condoms have been designed for anal sex and are less likely to break than condoms designed for contraception.[39] Condoms are relatively sturdy but should not be stored in hot cars or wallets for extended periods of time. This presents a dilemma because, in practice, condom failure is most often due to not having one when you need it.

Spermicides act as chemical barriers by killing sperm and, as a side benefit, some infectious agents. Several studies have suggested that spermicides may be effective in preventing STDs other than HIV infection. Case-control, cross-sectional, and experimental studies found relative risks of 0.13 to 0.90 for infections such as gonorrhea in spermicide users compared to nonusers.[35] Although they have been shown to kill viruses, including HIV, in the laboratory, spermicides have not protected against HIV *in vivo*. A placebo-controlled study in female commercial sex workers in Nairobi found similarly high seroconversion rates in those using nonoxynol-9–impregnated contraceptive sponges (55%) and in those using placebo vaginal suppositories (45%).[40]

Some women are sensitive to certain spermicides. In one study, nine (38%) of 24 commercial sex workers who used condoms lubricated with nonoxynol-9 reported vaginal irritation,[41] which might actually facilitate HIV transmission by disrupting the vaginal mucosa. This high rate of irritation may not be seen in women who use spermicides less frequently. However, because no data exist to substantiate the potential benefits of spermicides in preventing HIV transmission, recommending a combination of condoms plus spermicides is based on hypothetical considerations, unless vaginal irritation develops owing to the spermicides. Spermicides alone, without condoms, seem inadequate to protect against this deadly virus.

A sensible approach to personal protection against HIV infection would be to use condoms consistently with all new partners. Unprotected intercourse could be considered after HIV testing. This would be most important for persons who had practiced high-risk behavior in the past, but it should also be considered by persons living in areas of high HIV prevalence, even when a sex partner has no apparent risk for infection.

Decreasing the number of sexual partners will decrease the risk of infection only if it decreases exposure to infected partners. Because most people with sexually acquired HIV have had many sexual partners, a one-time "pickup" may be more likely to be infected than a person interested in a long-term relationship. If so, limiting anonymous or casual sex would reduce the risk of having sex with infected partners. Avoiding situations in which high-risk sexual encounters can occur seems prudent. For example, a person who is trying to cut down on anonymous sex should not go to singles bars. Drugs or alcohol may play an important role by clouding decisions on safe sex.[42] Sexual drives are increasingly strong as arousal increases, so planning for protection is best done early.

HEALTH CARE PROVIDERS

Health care providers can decrease HIV transmission by helping their patients avoid infection. This requires identifying persons who are most likely to benefit from

HIV prevention information, providing that information in a supportive way, and reinforcing the message. Treating HIV-infected persons improves their quality of life, provides an opportunity for reinforcing prevention messages, and may reduce HIV transmission by decreasing viral load. Prompt, effective treatment of other STDs may also reduce HIV transmission.

Health care providers have a responsibility to counsel their patients about important health risks. Many people who do not consider themselves health care providers can also contribute to HIV prevention. For example, schoolteachers, clergy, and community outreach workers interact with people who are (or should be) concerned about HIV infection in situations where exchange of information would be appropriate.

How can a counselor help clients to decrease the sexual transmission of HIV? Counselors must provide not only appropriate information about AIDS and HIV infection, but also realistic options for personal protection. A routine sexual history may indicate the need for a discussion of HIV. Anyone who has practiced risky behaviors, develops an illness that may be associated with HIV, or has an STD or unintended pregnancy should be counseled about HIV. Men should be asked directly if they have ever had sex with men. Teens tend to experiment with sex and should be offered guidance on how to do it safely.

Ultimately, HIV testing is the only way to identify infected persons who can both benefit from therapeutic intervention and also be provided with counseling on how to avoid transmitting HIV to others. HIV testing should be offered to any asymptomatic person with a history of any HIV risk behaviors. In addition, testing should also be offered to all people with STDs, or even, depending on the HIV prevalence in the area of a medical practice, to all people who are sexually active. HIV testing is relatively inexpensive and is highly sensitive and specific when done with a confirmatory test.[43]

People infected with HIV need follow-up for the medical and psychological aspects of their infection, as is true for many other medical conditions such as diabetes or heart disease. However, the psychological needs may be greater because HIV infection still carries a major social stigma. Support groups and other social services are frequently available in urban areas, and people who offer HIV testing should be familiar with community resources available to help patients with positive tests.

People who learn they are infected with HIV apparently change their sexual behavior more than those who do not learn their test results.[43a] Most studies of behavior change have involved gay men who agreed to be in cohort studies of AIDS. In Brisbane, Australia, a cross-sectional study found that condom use was more common among seropositive men who knew their antibody status (5 of 11) than among seropositive men who did not know that they were infected (1 of 10), but no differences existed among seronegative men based on knowing their HIV antibody status.[44] In a cohort in Boston, infected and uninfected persons changed most of their behaviors in similar ways, whether or not they chose to learn their test results.[45] However, men who learned they were infected decreased unprotected anal insertive intercourse more than those who did not know they were infected. In the Netherlands, seropositive homosexual men changed behavior more than seronegative men. The mean number of sexual partners in the previous 6 months decreased from 22 to 10 for HIV-positive persons and from 15 to 12 for HIV-negative persons.[46] Findings from these studies may not be generalizable to other groups. Many people in these studies had changed their behavior even before the HIV test.[45,47] Moreover, before testing, infected persons had higher levels of risky sexual practices than uninfected persons. This makes it difficult to identify changes by comparing people who test positive with people who test negative.

Less is known about the effectiveness of counseling people who are tested for HIV as part of a diagnostic evaluation or screening program. In a Baltimore STD clinic, clients who tested HIV positive continued to acquire new STDs; 122 (20%) of 612 returned with a possible or definite new STD 6 to 23 months after being told they were HIV infected.[48] The expected reinfection rate had they not been tested for HIV is not clear. Regardless, the repeat STD rate among HIV-infected persons was high. In Miami, persons who tested HIV positive developed new gonorrhea infections at a lower rate (4.5% in 6 months) than they had prior to HIV testing (6.3% in 6 months). This decrease was greater than that seen for seropositive persons who did not learn their test results (5.7% before vs. 6.2% after HIV testing).[49]

People who test HIV negative may have different changes in their behavior than those who test positive. For example, a negative test might disinhibit risky behavior, because it suggests that risky behavior did not lead to HIV infection. Gonorrhea infection rates actually increased for patients attending a Miami STD clinic after they learned they had a negative HIV test.[49] Thus, appropriate counseling of individuals with negative HIV tests may be particularly important.

Notifying partners of an HIV-infected person that they have been exposed is an essential component of HIV testing.[50] Although concerns have been raised about the cost-effectiveness of efforts to notify partners,[51] few question the ethical responsibility. Our society currently emphasizes the need to notify persons of past exposures to other hazards even when no prevention benefits are possible. Health care providers should directly discuss partner notification with HIV-infected persons to determine how it will be done, and what will be said. Some persons may prefer that health care workers notify their partners in order to maintain confidentiality or to avoid confrontation.

Because other STDs facilitate transmission of HIV, and because multiple infections often coexist, health care providers must recognize and treat all these conditions. Information about symptoms of other STDs and the need for patients to seek and obtain therapy should be included in any HIV-related counseling messages. Prompt notification and treatment of sex partners is important for other STDs as well.[52]

PUBLIC HEALTH DEPARTMENTS

Health departments must coordinate the multifaceted response to AIDS in their jurisdictions. Surveillance of both AIDS and HIV infection helps to assess the size of the problem and identifies transmission patterns for persons living in the area. Health departments educate the general public, persons at risk, and policy-makers *via* community information campaigns, partner notification, and other innovative methods. STD control efforts could also have an important impact on HIV.

Health departments are responsible for monitoring the epidemic. Surveillance allows anticipation of future health care needs and provides the health care worker and patient with information about how infection is being transmitted in their community, and what precautions should be taken. Even today, 10 years after the first case of AIDS was reported and 6 years after the HIV antibody test became widely available, important questions still remain about the current prevalence of infection in various subgroups of the population. Moreover, most persons infected with HIV are still unaware of their infection status.[53]

Health departments also define what additional interventions should be undertaken to slow the HIV epidemic. Interventions to change behavior are not easy. However, a new therapy or vaccine alone may not control HIV or eliminate AIDS. In 1990, half a century after the discovery of penicillin, more than 50,000 reported cases of primary and secondary syphilis occurred in the United States.[3] Hepatitis B has been vaccine-preventable for over 10 years but even now is apparently increasing among heterosexuals.[54]

Many health departments established clinics for HIV counseling and testing soon after the test was available. In 1989–1990, an estimated 2.2 million HIV tests were done by health departments. Most of these programs offer only a single post-test counseling session and refer HIV-infected persons to other sites for follow-up care. Evaluation of more intensive counseling in ways to avoid HIV transmission, and of the clinical and public health effect of therapy for those who are infected, is urgently needed.[28]

Health departments also have responsibility for educating the public. Effective educational campaigns and high media interest have combined to reach a wide audience.[55] By June 1990, 98% of adults aged 18 to 49 years knew that the AIDS virus could be transmitted by sexual intercourse, by sharing needles, and from a pregnant woman to her baby.[1] Condom sales increased 20% between 1986 and 1988, with most of the increase following the Surgeon General's 1986 Report on AIDS, but this increase was far short of that needed to protect people from HIV and other STDs.[56] Mass media campaigns by themselves have not generally been effective in changing behaviors; they must be part of a broader effort that includes more individualized attention.

Additional efforts are needed to reach the populations at risk. Gay men have made important changes in sexual practices,[57] with resultant decreases in the rates of syphilis and gonorrhea.[6] However, increases in pharyngeal gonorrhea in some areas suggest that a relapse to risky sexual behavior may be occurring.[58] Men who have sex with men but who do not identify themselves as gay may not have changed sexual behaviors as much. Finally, syphilis rates among black heterosexuals have more than doubled between 1985 and 1989, suggesting that their sexual behavior has not become safer in response to the HIV epidemic.[59]

Sex partner notification has been a useful public health strategy to identify individuals at highest risk of STDs and thus to interrupt the chain of community transmission. In theory, partner notification should work best for curable diseases with a sufficient latent time to allow delivery of treatment to potentially infected partners before they are able to transmit infection. Syphilis is the prototype STD most amenable to this strategy. Although no well-controlled study has documented the effectiveness of this strategy, many community syphilis outbreaks and several epidemics of resistant gonorrhea have been controlled by intensive (though costly) partner notification efforts.[52]

Partner notification for HIV infection has been pursued actively by many health departments. The name of the infected index patient is never revealed to the partners who are located. Sex partners are advised to be tested for HIV and are encouraged to use condoms with potentially infected partners. HIV infection rates are higher among known partners of HIV-infected persons than among other counseling/testing clients. Moreover, in South Carolina, partner notification efforts increased condom use from none to four (80%) of five seropositive partners and from none to 25 (69%) of 36 seronegative partners.[60] Although some have suggested the partner notification programs are unwanted, all persons who were notified appreciated the efforts of the health department.[61]

Many homosexual men have modified their sexual practices to avoid HIV infection. The majority of these changes resulted from active efforts initiated by members of the gay community to educate themselves and facilitate the safer sexual behaviors that needed to be made. Health departments need to learn how to facilitate similar community-based changes in other groups at risk of acquiring HIV infection. Unfortunately, low-income, minority, heterosexual communities at risk are not as cohesive, have little political clout, have few resources, and have many other high-priority social problems in addition to AIDS.

Only a few well-controlled studies on community intervention programs to reduce HIV risk behaviors have been reported to date. In one small Mississippi city, opinion leaders were recruited to act as behavior change "endorsers" for their gay peers.[62] They were trained in social skills for modifying behaviors and used these skills to persuade friends and acquaintances about the benefits of safer sex. Surveys of behavior in gay bars were compared before and after the intervention. Before the intervention, unprotected receptive anal intercourse was reported by 27% of respondents in the intervention city and 31% in the comparison cities. Three to 6 months after the intervention, a greater reduction was seen in the intervention city (−8.1%) than in the comparison cities (−3.7%).

Behavior change is often a slow process. The Surgeon General's report on the dangers of cigarette smoking was issued over 25 years ago, and still 26.5% of adults continue to smoke.[63] The fundamental nature of sexual behavior means it is even more complex and probably more difficult to change than smoking. No easy interventions should be expected.

At a community level, controlling high rates of STDs could substantially decrease the risk of HIV transmission in some areas.[10] The interactions of other STDs and HIV are difficult to untangle.[64] Because they are both sexually transmitted, associations might easily be attributed to the shared route of transmission. However, there is increasingly convincing evidence that HIV prolongs infectivity and therefore increases the prevalence of several STDs, and that these STDs in turn facilitate the transmission of HIV, creating an "epidemiologic synergy" that can lead to explosive increases in both conditions.[10,65]

The clinical effect of HIV on STDs is most dramatic in genital herpes; chronic mucocutaneous herpes is an AIDS-defining condition. HIV has a less dramatic influence on the natural history of other conditions, but an increased severity of disease or resistance to standard therapy has been reported for chancroid,[66] syphilis,[67] and human papillomavirus infections.[68] Many STDs facilitate HIV transmission. Evidence is strongest for genital ulcer diseases. Men with positive syphilis tests were more likely to be HIV seropositive than patients with other STDs (adjusted odds ratio, 3.3).[69] In one prospective study, men who had a genital ulcer were 4.7 times more likely to acquire HIV than men who did not.[26] These studies may underestimate the true impact of genital ulcer disease because they compare ulcers with other STDs such as gonorrhea or *Chlamydia,* which have also been associated with HIV transmission (odds ratios of 3–5).[10]

STD control as a means of reducing HIV incidence will have the greatest impact in African countries where the prevalence of genital ulcer disease is high and the prevalence of HIV infection is rising rapidly. If studies of the relative risk associated with genital ulcer disease are accurate,[64] a sizable proportion of HIV infection in Africa is attributable to genital ulcer disease. Because genital ulcers are treatable and the prevalence of ulcers could be reduced by a nationwide therapy campaign, investments in STD control might slow the HIV epidemic enough to allow people time to work through the steps needed to change sexual behavior.

In the United States as a whole, STDs are less prevalent than in Africa. However, targeted control activities in certain communities could have an important impact because STDs and HIV infection are concentrated in the same groups. For example, Miami had a syphilis rate that exceeded 0.2% for the whole city,[70] but this rate would be much higher among 20- to 34-year-olds in certain parts of the city. The HIV prevalence among STD clinic attendees in Miami was 11%.[71] Interventions aimed at reducing syphilis in these groups might successfully reduce HIV transmission. Unfortunately, many STD clinics in the United States are overburdened and underfunded. During the AIDS epidemic, syphilis rates have increased to levels not seen since 1949,[59] and chancroid has reemerged at levels not seen since 1952.[72]

SOCIETY

Society as a whole has a responsibility for addressing the AIDS epidemic. Society finances health departments, supports health care workers, and sets the environment for persons at risk for infection. Society also determines how much money should be spent on AIDS research, and what services should be made available to persons with HIV infection.

Society must learn to confront human sexuality in a more open and supportive way. For example, condoms could not even be advertised until the mid-1980s. Following the Surgeon General's Report on AIDS, which recommended using condoms, most of the condom publicity consisted of a debate about whether or not condom ads should be permitted.[56] It has been suggested in one small study that erotic instructions for condom use produce more positive attitudes.[73] But while our society is willing to use sex to sell beer, it is reluctant to mention sex when selling condoms. Even medical journals are reluctant to publish questionnaires that have been used without censoring words like "fucking."[74]

Barriers to care for HIV infection and other STDs must be removed. Confidentiality must be maintained and unfair discrimination eliminated. Fear of discrimination can influence decisions to seek counseling about HIV.[75] A supportive environment, conducive to behavior change, must be established for HIV-infected persons, men who have sex with men, drug users, and inner-city youth. The epidemic will not wait.

REFERENCES

1. Fitti JE, Cynamon M: AIDS knowledge and attitudes for April–June 1990: Provisional data from the National Health Interview Survey, advance data from Vital and Health Statistics, Publication No. 195. Washington, DC, National Center for Health Statistics, 1990
2. Centers for Disease Control: Human immunodeficiency virus infection in the United States: A review of current knowledge. MMWR 36(suppl 6):1, 1987

3. Centers for Disease Control, Center for Prevention Services, 1990 Division of STD/HIV Prevention: Annual Report. U.S. Department of Health and Human Services, Public Health Service, 1991

4. Centers for Disease Control: Premarital sexual experience among adolescent women—United States, 1970–1988. MMWR 39:929, 1991

5. DeBuono BA, Zinner SH, Daamen M, McCormack WM: Sexual behavior of college women in 1975, 1986, and 1989. N Engl J Med 322:821, 1990

6. Hessol NA, O'Malley P, Lifson A et al: Incidence and prevalence of HIV infection among homosexual and bisexual men, 1978–1988 (abstr M.A.O.27). Presented at the V International Conference on AIDS, Montreal, June 1989

7. Hearst N, Hulley SB: Preventing the heterosexual spread of AIDS: Are we giving our patients the best advice? JAMA 259:2428, 1988

8. Cochran SD, Mays VM: Sex, lies, and HIV. N Engl J Med 322:774, 1990

9. Padian N: Female partners of bisexual men. Presented at the CDC Workshop in Bisexuality and AIDS, Atlanta, October 1989

10. Wasserheit JN: Epidemiological synergy: Inter-relationships between HIV infection and other STDs. Presented at the International Workshop on AIDS and Reproductive Health, Bellagio, Italy, April 1990

11. Rolfs RT, Goldberg M, Sharrar RG: Risk factors for syphilis: Cocaine use and prostitution. Am J Public Health 80:853, 1990

12. Marx R, Aral SO, Rolfs RT et al: Crack, sex, and STD. Sex Transm Dis 18:92, 1991

13. Gwinn M, Pappaioanou M, George JR et al: Prevalence of HIV infection in childbearing women in the United States: Surveillance using newborn blood samples. JAMA 265:1704, 1991

14. St. Louis ME, Rauch KJ, Petersen LR et al: Seroprevalence rates of human immunodeficiency virus infection at sentinel hospitals in the United States. N Engl J Med 323:213, 1990

15. Goedert JJ: What is safe sex? Suggested standards linked to testing for human immunodeficiency virus. N Engl J Med 316:1339, 1987

16. Wiktor SZ, Biggar RJ, Melbye M et al: Effect of knowledge of human immunodeficiency virus infection status on sexual activity among homosexual men. J AIDS 3:62, 1990

17. Kamb ML, Otten MW, Guerena F et al: Extensive HIV seropositivity among heterosexuals in an STD clinic (abstr) W.C.99. Presented at the VII International Conference on AIDS, Florence, Italy, June 1991

18. Kingsley LA, Detels R, Kaslow R et al: Risk factors for seroconversion to human immunodeficiency virus among male homosexuals. Lancet 1:345, 1987

19. Steigbigel NH, Maude DW, Feiner CJ et al: Heterosexual transmission of HIV infection (abstr 4057). Presented at the IV International Conference on AIDS, Stockholm, Sweden, June 1988

20. Sion FS, Morais de Sa CA, Rschid de Lacerda MC et al: The importance of anal intercourse in transmission of HIV to women (abstr 4007). Presented at the IV International Conference on AIDS, Stockholm, Sweden, June 1988

21. European Study Group: Risk factors for male to female transmission of HIV. Br Med J 298:411, 1989

22. Mayer KH, DeGruttola V: Human immunodeficiency virus and oral intercourse. Ann Intern Med 107:428, 1987

23. Lifson AR, O'Malley PM, Hessol NA et al: HIV seroconversion in two homosexual men after receptive oral intercourse with ejaculation: Implications for counseling concerning safe sexual practices. Am J Public Health 81:1509, 1991

24. Marmor M, Weiss LR, Lyden M et al: Possible female-to-female transmission of human immunodeficiency virus. Ann Intern Med 105:969, 1986

25. Centers for Disease Control: Update: Human immunodeficiency virus infections in health-care workers exposed to blood of infected patients. MMWR 36:285, 1987

26. Cameron DW, Simonsen JN, D'Costa LJ et al: Female to male transmission of human immunodeficiency virus type 1: Risk factors for seroconversion in men. Lancet 2:403, 1991

27. Mann JM, Nzilambi N, Piot P et al: HIV infection and associated risk factors in female prostitutes in Kinshasa, Zaire. AIDS 2:249, 1988

28. Francis DP, Anderson RE, Gorman ME et al: Targeting AIDS prevention and treatment toward HIV-1–infected persons: The concept of early intervention. JAMA 262:2572, 1989

29. Stone KM, Grimes DA, Magder LS: Primary prevention of sexually transmitted diseases: A primer for clinicians. JAMA 255:1763, 1986

30. Aral SO, Holmes KK: Epidemiology of sexual behavior and sexually transmitted diseases. In Holmes KK, Mardh P-A, Sparling PF et al (eds): Sexually Transmitted Diseases, p 31. New York, McGraw-Hill, 1990

31. Hicks DR, Martin LS, Getchell JP et al: Inactivation of HTLV-III/LAV-infected cultures of normal human lymphocytes by nonoxynol-9 in vitro. Lancet 2:1422, 1985

32. Rietmeijer CAM, Krebs JW, Feorino PM, Judson FN: Condoms as physical and chemical barriers against human immunodeficiency virus. JAMA 259:1851, 1988

33. Van de Perre P, Jacobs D, Sprecher-Goldberger S: The latex condom, an efficient barrier against sexual transmission of AIDS-related viruses. AIDS 1:49, 1987

34. Trussell J, Hatcher RA, Cates W Jr et al: Contraceptive failure in the United States: An update. Studies Fam Plan 21:51, 1990

35. Stone KM, Grimes DA, Magder LS: Personal protection against sexually transmitted diseases. Am J Obstet Gynecol 155:180, 1986

36. Richters J, Donovan B, Gerofi J, Watson L: Low condom breakage rate in commercial sex. Lancet 2:1489, 1988

37. Golombok S, Sketchley J, Rust J: Condom failure among homosexual men. J AIDS 2:404, 1989

38. Albert AE, Hatcher RA, Graves W: Condom use and breakage among women in a municipal hospital family planning clinic. Contraception 43:167, 1991

39. Wigersma L, Oud R: Safety and acceptability of condoms for use by homosexual men as a prophylactic against transmission of HIV during anogenital sexual intercourse. Br Med J 295:94, 1987

40. Kreiss J, Ruminjo I, Ngugi E et al: Efficacy of nonoxynol-9 in preventing HIV transmission (abstr M.A.O.36). Presented at the V International Conference on AIDS, Montreal, Canada, June 1989

41. Rekart ML, Barnett JA, Manzon LM et al: Nonoxynol 9: Its adverse effects (abstr S.C.36). Presented at the VI International Conference on AIDS, San Francisco, USA, June 1990

42. Stall R, McKusick L, Wiley J et al: Alcohol and drug use during sexual activity and compliance with safe sex guidelines for AIDS: The AIDS behavioral research project. Health Educ Q 13:359, 1986

43. Burke DS, Brundage JF, Redfield RR et al: Measurement of the false positive rate in a screening program for human immunodeficiency virus infections. N Engl J Med 319: 961, 1988

43a. Higgins DL, Galavotti, C, O'Reilly KR et al: Evidence for the effects of counseling and testing on risk behaviors. JAMA 266:2419, 1991

44. Frazer IH, McCamish M, Hay I, North P: Influence of human immunodeficiency virus antibody testing on sexual behavior in a "high-risk" population from a "low-risk" city. Med J Aust 149:365, 1988

45. McCusker J, Stoddard AM, Mayer KH et al: Effects of HIV antibody test knowledge on subsequent sexual behaviors in a cohort of homosexually active men. Am J Public Health 78:462, 1988

46. van Griensven GJP, de Vroome EMM, Tielman RAP et al: Impact of HIV antibody testing on changes in sexual behavior among homosexual men in the Netherlands. Am J Public Health 78:1575, 1988

47. Fox R, Odaka NJ, Brookmeyer R, Polk BF: Effect of HIV antibody disclosure on subsequent sexual activity in homosexual men. AIDS 1:241, 1987

48. Zenilman JM, Erickson B, Fox R et al: Incidence of sexually transmitted diseases (STD) in a population previously diagnosed with HIV-1 and post-test counseled (PTC) (abstr 686). Presented at the Interscience Conference on Antimicrobial Agents and Chemotherapy, Atlanta, October 1990

49. Otten M, Zaidi A, Wroten J, et al: Effect of HIV post-test counseling on sexually transmitted disease (STD) reinfection for patients attending a STD clinic (abstr). M.C.103 Presented at the VII International Conference on AIDS, Florence, Italy, June 1991

50. Potterat JJ, Spencer NE, Woodhouse DE, Muth JB: Partner notification in the control of human immunodeficiency virus infection. Am J Public Health 79:874, 1989

51. Rutherford GW, Woo JM: Contact tracing and the control of human immunodeficiency virus infection. JAMA 259: 3609, 1988

52. Rothenberg RB, Potterat JJ: Strategies for management of sex partners. In Holmes KK, Mardh P-A, Sparling PF et al (eds): Sexually Transmitted Diseases, p 1081. New York, McGraw Hill, 1990

53. Centers for Disease Control: Publicly funded HIV counseling and testing—United States, 1985–1989. MMWR 39: 137, 1990

54. Alter MJ, Hadler SC, Margolis HS et al: The changing epidemiology of hepatitis B in the United States: Need for alternative vaccination strategies. JAMA 263:1218, 1990

55. AIDS education—a beginning. Population Reports 1989, Series L, No. 8. Washington, DC, US Government Printing Office, 1989

56. Moran JS, Janes HR, Peterman TA, Stone KM: Increase in condom sales following AIDS education and publicity, United States. Am J Public Health 80:607, 1990

57. Becker MH, Joseph JG: AIDS and behavioral change to reduce risk: A review. Am J Public Health 78:394, 1988

58. Centers for Disease Control: Trends in gonorrhea in homosexually active men—King County, Washington, 1989. MMWR 38:762, 1989

59. Rolfs RT, Nakashima AK: Epidemiology of primary and secondary syphilis in the United States, 1981 through 1989. JAMA 264:1432, 1990

60. Wykoff RF, Heath CW, Hollis SL et al: Contact tracing to identify human immunodeficiency virus infection in a rural community. JAMA 259:3563, 1988

61. Jones JL, Wykoff RF, Hollis SL et al: Partner acceptance of health department notification of HIV exposure, South Carolina. JAMA 264:1284, 1990

62. Kelly JA, StLawrence JS, Diaz YE et al: HIV risk behavior reduction following intervention with key opinion leaders of population: An experimental analysis. Am J Public Health 81:168, 1991

63. Office on Smoking and Health, Centers for Disease Control: Smoking and Health: A National Status Report, 2nd ed, p 21. A Report to Congress. DHHS Publication No. 87-8396. Washington, DC, US Government Printing Office, 1990

64. Mertens TE, Hayes RJ, Smith PG: Epidemiological methods to study the interaction between HIV infection and other sexually transmitted diseases. AIDS 4:57, 1990

65. Piot P, Laga M, Ryder R et al: The global epidemiology of HIV infection: Continuity, heterogeneity, and change. J AIDS 3:403, 1990

66. Schmid GP: Treatment of chancroid, 1989. Rev Infect Dis 12(S6):S580, 1990

67. Zenker PN, Rolfs RT: Treatment of syphilis, 1989. Rev Infect Dis 12(S6):S590, 1990

68. Palefsky JM, Gonzales J, Greenblatt RM et al: Anal intraepithelial neoplasia and anal papillomavirus infection among homosexual males with group IV HIV disease. JAMA 263:2911, 1990

69. Quinn TC, Glasser D, Cannon RO et al: Human immunodeficiency virus infection among patients attending clinics for sexually transmitted diseases. N Engl J Med 318:197, 1988

70. Centers for Disease Control: Sexually Transmitted Disease Statistics, 1987, p 136. US Department of Health and Human Services, Public Health Service, Centers for Disease Control. Washington, DC, US Government Printing Office, 1988

71. Centers for Disease Control: National HIV Seroprevalence Serosurveys: Summary of Results. Data from Serosurveillance Activities Through 1989. US Department of Health and Human Services, Public Health Service, Centers for Disease Control. Washington, DC, US Government Printing Office, 1990

72. Schmid GP, Sanders LLJr, Blount JH, Alexander ER: Chancroid in the United States: Reestablishment of an old disease. JAMA 258:3265, 1987

73. Tanner WM, Pollack RH: The effect of condom use and erotic instructions on attitudes toward condoms. J Sex Res 25:537, 1988

74. Peterman TA, Aral SO: Re: exact reproduction of survey instrument. Am J Epidemiol 129:1310, 1989

75. Fehrs LJ, Fleming D, Foster LR et al: Trial of anonymous versus confidential human immunodeficiency virus testing. Lancet 2:379, 1988

76. Peterman TA, Lui KJ, Lawrence DN, Allen JR: Estimating the risks of transfusion-associated acquired immunodeficiency syndrome and human immunodeficiency virus infection. Transfusion 27:371, 1987

77. Lederman MM, Ratnoff OD, Evatt BL, McDougal JS: Acquisition of antibody to lymphadenopathy-associated virus in patients with classic hemophilia (factor VIII deficiency). Ann Intern Med 102:753, 1985

78. Detels R, English P, Visscher BR et al: Seroconversion, sexual activity, and condom use among 2915 HIV seronegative men followed for up to 2 years. J AIDS 2:77, 1989

24

AIDS Among Drug Injectors: The First Decade

Samuel R. Friedman   *Don C. Des Jarlais*   *Alan Neaigus*

As of December 31, 1990, over 60,000 cases of acquired immunodeficiency syndrome (AIDS) among drug injectors had been reported from more than 25 countries. Among those affected were 34,398 heterosexual and 10,557 homosexual or bisexual drug injectors in the United States, as well as 14,808 heterosexual and 905 homosexual or bisexual drug injectors from Europe. Drug injectors accounted for a majority of reported AIDS cases in Italy and Spain, as well as a majority of human immunodeficiency virus (HIV)–infected persons in Scotland and Thailand.

SOCIAL ORGANIZATION OF DRUG INJECTION

Because there are very few formal organizations of drug injectors, there is a common misperception that they are not organized. Nonetheless, a multi-billion-dollar illicit drug trade, which includes many dealers and distributors who themselves inject drugs, does not persist over time without social organization. Sociologists and anthropologists have conceptualized the organization of drug injectors as a ''deviant subculture''[1-3] with shared values, a common argot, and rules for allocating status. The primary value is ''getting high,'' and a primary basis for high status within the group is the ability to obtain and use large quantities of high-quality drugs while minimizing adverse social, legal, and health consequences of such drug use.

There is strong, often brutal, competition within the drug injector subculture. There is competition for customers among persons distributing illicit drugs for

An earlier version of this chapter appeared in ''AIDS Care.''

injection, and competition between dealers and customers over the price and quality of the drugs sold. Among drug injectors there is competition for the money needed to purchase drugs, for access to the limited supply of drugs, and sometimes even for the equipment needed to inject the drugs. The illegal status of the drugs keeps prices high, reinforcing economic competition and often leading to a reliance on illegal methods of obtaining money to purchase drugs. The illegal nature of drug injection also leads to a reliance on threatened or actual violence as a means for resolving disputes.

The drug injector subculture would not be able to persist over time without positive social relationships to balance these mistrusting, often violent interactions. A common identity as persons allied against ''straight'' (conventional) society encourages the sharing of information about drug availability, police actions, and new developments that affect the group. This sharing of information is almost wholly oral, with very little communication through written or broadcast material, although the Dutch drug users' unions have used leaflets and newsletters as a means of communication. The oral information network often spreads inaccurate news, but it is efficient enough to maintain the substantial economic scale of drug injection in the United States, Europe, and several developing countries.

The primary positive social relationship within the drug injecting subculture is the small friendship group. The high price and the limited supply of drugs make it effective for drug injectors to work together in pairs or small groups to obtain money and drugs. Teamwork provides more opportunities for obtaining money and self-protection. Sharing resources among friends also provides a greater likelihood that an individual drug injector will be able to obtain drugs on any given day.

The social structure of this subculture promotes the sharing of equipment for injecting drugs in two ways. The ethic of cooperation within small friendship groups is applied to the sharing of equipment for injecting drugs. To refuse to share drug injection equipment within the small friendship group (without a socially legitimated reason) would call into question the reliability of the person with respect to other cooperative actions.

Limited supplies of drug injection equipment can also lead to sharing among casual acquaintances or complete strangers. Legal restrictions on the sale of needles and syringes, refusal of pharmacists to sell them even when they are permitted to do so, and laws against the possession of narcotics paraphernalia all serve to reduce the availability of sterile equipment for injecting illicit drugs. Even where there are no legal restrictions on drug injection equipment, sterile equipment often is not available when and where drug injectors want to inject. Persons who have drugs to inject but who lack injection equipment may borrow equipment from acquaintances, sometimes in trade for a small quantity of the drug. Such sharing contains elements of both social solidarity and economic cooperation.

Widespread sharing occurs through the use of "shooting galleries" or "house works." Shooting galleries are places where one can rent drug injection equipment for a small fee (typically $1 or $2 in New York City). After use, the equipment is returned to the proprietor of the shooting gallery for rental to the next customer. The needle and syringe may be used until they become clogged, or the needle too dull for further use. Thus, HIV or another virus can be transmitted among large numbers of drug injectors who do not know each other. This breaks the limited antiviral protection afforded by sharing only within friendship groups. Shooting galleries are typically located in or near "copping areas" (places where illicit drugs can be easily purchased). Shooting galleries, as a specialized economic activity, are most often found in areas that have very large numbers of drug injectors, although there is some evidence that shooting galleries have declined in number during the AIDS epidemic.

Areas with relatively few intravenous (IV) drug users generally cannot support shooting galleries, but these areas will usually have a functional equivalent to shooting galleries with respect to HIV transmission. "House works" are an extra set of drug injection equipment that a small-scale "dealer" (drug distributor) maintains for lending to customers. After use, the works are returned to the dealer for lending to the next customer who wants to borrow them.

Another characteristic of drug injectors' social relationships should be mentioned. Many drug injectors maintain close social relationships with persons who do not inject drugs. In a study of more than 1,100 street-recruited drug injectors in New York City, we found that 93% maintained close social relationships with noninjectors. The average sample member interacted with a close noninjector about twice a day. Furthermore, close contact with noninjectors was associated with lower levels of sharing injection equipment.

RISK FACTORS FOR HIV EXPOSURE

A number of the behaviors in which drug injectors commonly engage have been associated with exposure to HIV infection. These include (1) drug injection frequency (especially cocaine injection in some U.S. studies), (2) sharing injection equipment with friends or others, and (3) injecting in shooting galleries. Some studies have also found sexual behaviors to be significant risk factors.[4-15]

In addition to these drug injection and sexual transmission behaviors, a number of studies have identified life-style factors associated with HIV exposure among drug injectors. Social and biographic risk factors that have been reported include a prior history of syphilis, socioeconomic status, race/ethnicity, years of injection, and imprisonment.[4-18]

It is not clear how the relationships between these life-style factors and HIV exposure should be interpreted. These factors by themselves clearly do not transmit HIV. One possibility is that the life-style factors correlate with the actual transmission behavior(s) and that measurement error is obscuring the true relationships. Most measurements of transmission behaviors (*e.g.,* frequency of sharing injection equipment) have considerable measurement error, while most of the life-style factors (*e.g.,* race or number of years of injecting drugs) involve comparatively little measurement error. Alternatively, the life-style factors may be indicators of higher HIV seroprevalence among the persons with whom the index subject is sharing injection equipment or having sex.

CHANGES IN SEROPREVALENCE OVER TIME

Table 24–1 lists data for seroprevalence over time in drug injectors in 20 localities. (Although the data come from a number of disparate studies, with varying numbers of subjects, and their comparability and representativeness are not high, they nevertheless suffice to give a broad outline of the development of the epidemic.) Even before the first published report of AIDS, HIV infection was widespread among drug injectors in New York City, and present among those in Milan and Padua. It had spread to South America by 1983 (to Sao Paulo by 1983,[19] to Rio de Janeiro by 1986),[20] to Australia by 1985,[21,22] and to Asia by 1987 (to Bangkok by 1987,[23] to Manipur by late 1989).[24]

One particularly disturbing aspect of the spread of HIV in the last several years has been the rapid transmission of HIV in South American and Asian countries. The once hard distinction among "consumer," "trans-

(*Text continues p. 456*)

Table 24–1. Time-Series Data on HIV Seroprevalence in Intravenous Drug Users, by City and Year, 1977–1991

City	1977	1978	1979	1980	1981	1982	1983	1984	1985	1986	1987	1988	1989	1990	1991
New York	0	9	26	38		50		57		55				50	
Sardinia		0	0	0	1	10	18	32	43	57					
San Francisco										7	12	12	11		
Rio de Janeiro										4				20	37
Bangkok											1	43			
Bologna			0	0	9	7.5	39	37							
Milan I—hepatitis		0	7	8	8	23	43	39	43						
Milan II—MMTP					11	28	61	67	69	73					
Padua I—hepatitis		0	0	3	2	1	15	18	23	20					
Padua II—detox.							20	28	65	50					
Rome									34	42	33	31	32		
Geneva I—outpatients					6	29	38	30				37			
Geneva II—hospital					7		27		52						
Berlin I–drug deaths									31	49	49	45			
Berlin II—treatment									27	24	35				
Hamburg I—drug deaths									0	23	16	13			
Hamburg II—treatment									9	10	11				
Vienna										7	12	30	28	24	
Edinburgh						0	14	42	37						
Bilbao								42	42		44	45	27	30	
Tours						0	0	15	17						
Amsterdam										33	31	31	34		
London									5	6	4	5			
Manipur (India)										0	0	0		54	
Detroit									13		16		16		

shipping," and "producer" countries for illicit drugs has broken down. HIV transmission is now occurring among large numbers of drug injectors in countries that previously produced large amounts of drugs or served as transshipping points without having a large number of local users.

In a broad perspective, the rate of HIV spread has varied among localities. Figure 24–1 presents data on seroprevalence in the year before seroprevalence reached 10%, and then data for the year in which this figure was reached. Seroprevalence in this second year is thus an indicator of the speed with which HIV spread among drug injectors. In half of the cities, seroprevalence remained at 15% or less, and sampling error makes it uncertain whether there was indeed an increase in seroprevalence between the 2 years in any one of these cities. On the other hand, seroprevalence in the second year reached over 35% in Bangkok, Bologna, Edinburgh, and Manipur. The reasons for these variations in rate of spread have not been fully determined, and additional research into this question is greatly needed. One common factor that may have characterized cities that experienced explosive or very rapid transmission of HIV is that the drug injectors in these cities did not perceive AIDS as a local threat. (The World Health Organization is presently sponsoring studies in cities in Asia, Australia, Europe, North America, and South America that may help us better understand this phenomenon.) Particularly puzzling is that all four of the localities that reached a 35% or greater seroprevalence in the second year are places where most drug injection involves heroin, yet individual risk-factor studies in San Francisco and New York indicate that, in cities where both drugs are widely used, cocaine injection is a greater risk factor than heroin injection.[5,7] It is possible, however, that there may be cocaine-dominant cities in Latin America in which similar rates of spread have occurred without full documentation.

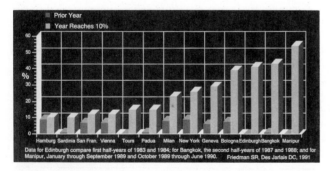

Figure 24–1. Seroprevalence among drug injectors in the year before and the year in which seroprevalence reached 10%. □ Prior year. ■ Year in which seroprevalence reached or exceeded 10%. Data for Edinburgh, compare first half-years of 1983 and 1984; for Bangkok, the second half-years of 1987 and 1988; and for Manipur, January through September 1989 and October 1989 through June 1990.

In a number of cities, seroprevalence in IV drug users seems to have plateaued, although at different levels: about 12% in San Francisco, 32% in Amsterdam, and 50% in New York. The reasons for the different levels of stabilization have not been determined, but probably include a combination of (1) differences in prevention program effects, (2) varying degrees of autonomous (individual and group) risk-reduction efforts by drug injectors, (3) differences in the stage of the epidemic at which widespread risk reduction began among drug injectors in various localities, and (4) variations in drug injectors' preexisting behaviors or network structures. The first three of these possible causes may have been affected by the extent to which diagnosed AIDS had previously become widespread among local gay men.

RISK REDUCTION AMONG DRUG INJECTORS

Considerable risk reduction has been reported, both in surveys and in ethnographic studies of drug injectors. There have been large-scale increases in the illicit sale of sterile syringes, reductions in the sharing of used works, a reduction in the sharing of syringes during initiation into drug injection, increases in syringe cleaning, and, albeit to a lesser degree, a reduction in the numbers of sexual partners and an increase in condom use.[25-30] In general, however, these changes must be seen as risk reduction rather than risk elimination, and maintenance of these gains remains problematic. Risk reduction has been greatest among those whose peer-group norms support risk reduction,[25,28,31-33] and among those with close social ties to noninjectors.[34,35]

HIV PREVENTION PROGRAMS

A brief theoretical discussion may help focus our understanding of programs aimed at reducing the transmission of HIV from one drug injector to others, or to their sex partners. A good starting point is understanding that most HIV transmission entails some form of interaction between two or more persons, and that individuals engage in such risky interactions as the result of a series of social relationships. Attempts to reduce risky interaction can focus on (1) the individual drug injector, (2) the dyads (or larger groups) that share injection equipment or have sex with each other, (3) the wider drug injection subculture, or (4) the larger social processes or structures, including both the relationships between drug injectors and the larger society and the cumulative social forces that may influence some persons to inject drugs in high-risk settings.

To date, most AIDS prevention projects have focused primarily on the drug injector as an individual. Health education, antibody testing and counseling, drug abuse treatment, providing physical means (syringes, bleach, condoms) to individuals to facilitate risk reduction, and skills training programs to teach individuals how to handle interactions so that they are more likely to avoid risk all focus on the individual user. Only a few projects have focused on changing drug user subcultures, and almost none have targeted the relationship between the larger society and drug users, even though doing so may be a prerequisite for successful implementation of harm-reduction strategies in some countries. Addressing the surrounding social relationships or structures, such as racism, gender inequality, or poverty, is as important but much more difficult.

A second consideration that should guide our understanding of prevention programs involves the nature of the agent of intervention, and the different kinds of social relationships that different modes of intervention entail. The great majority of projects have involved "outside" agencies intervening for the good of the drug injectors. Often these agencies have been health departments or drug abuse treatment agencies; others have involved unofficial interventions by activist groups. A smaller number have involved drug users themselves setting up groups to respond to the epidemic in their own ways. (Such self-organization against AIDS has been more widespread, and more successful, among gay men in many cities.) These two approaches—outside intervention versus self-organization—can be viewed as opposite poles of a continuum, with programs varying in the extent to which drug users are approached as objects to be acted upon or as subjects who can contribute ideas and actions on their own.

Within this theoretical perspective, we will review specific assessments of the major interventions to date.

Drug Abuse Treatment Programs

Drug abuse treatment has provided individuals who remain in it with some protection against HIV infection[12,36,37] and has led to a reduction in HIV risk behaviors.[38,39] To date, drug abuse treatment is the only type of AIDS prevention program whose participants have statistically significant lower rates of HIV exposure than nonparticipants. The studies showing these results, however, typically were based on samples of persons who had been in treatment for many years, so that the protective effect of participation in a drug abuse treatment program can be considered moderate rather than strong and immediate. There is also the economic question of whether or not sufficient numbers of drug injectors could be accommodated in drug abuse treatment programs to prevent an epidemic of HIV among drug injectors in any given locality.

HIV Testing

HIV testing has been implemented on a wide scale under the assumption that people who learned they were carrying the virus would act to prevent its transmission to others. Studies have generally shown that both seropositive and seronegative subjects do reduce high-risk behavior after HIV testing.[40] The strongest case for the utility of HIV testing comes from Sweden, where an unusually high percentage of the drug injectors in the country have been tested and where a new norm of social interaction has developed in which seropositive drug injectors warn others against borrowing injection equipment, and seroprevalence has stabilized.[41]

Despite the generally positive results from studies of HIV testing of drug injectors, much remains to be learned about the potential role of testing in reducing HIV transmission. First, the causal mechanisms through which testing might lead to risk reduction have not been determined. Counseling is generally considered to be an essential part of HIV testing, yet very little research has been done to identify the criteria for good HIV counseling. Second, individuals vary widely in respect to reducing HIV-transmitting risk behaviors following HIV counseling and testing, but the reasons for such varied responses have not been identified. Third, with the availability of treatment to slow the development of HIV-related disease among seropositive subjects, drug injectors at risk may have a more casual attitude toward HIV testing.

Physical Means for Reducing Risks

The provision of physical means to reduce the risk of HIV transmission is a major emphasis of many projects. These projects, frequently operating on the streets or in storefront clinics, distribute risk-reduction materials to drug injectors both for educational purposes and as an immediate way to reduce the probability that HIV will be transmitted owing to the lack of noncontaminated injection equipment or of a condom. The most widespread of these projects, perhaps, are syringe exchanges, which, along with deliberately increased over-the-counter sales of syringes, have emerged as a major new approach to reducing the spread of HIV in almost all developed countries. Syringe exchanges were initiated in the Netherlands at the instigation of drug users' organizations and have often been started, in various cities, by unofficial bodies or by individual clinics. In several cities in the United States, syringe exchanges function on a quasi-legal or illegal but tolerated basis. Syringe exchange programs vary in the extent to which they insist on participants' returning used syringes in order to get potentially infectious materials off the streets, and also in terms of the number of syringes that can be exchanged at one time. Syringe exchanges that exchange large numbers of syringes (a hundred or more at a time) are in effect recruiting some drug injectors to serve as satellite exchange staff for their friends. In most cases, syringe exchanges have functioned as fixed-site, indoor activities, although efforts have been made to distribute syringes to dealers' houses or other places where drug injectors gather. Although most are conducted by outside groups, some have been conducted by drug users' organizations.

Evaluations of syringe exchanges have found that (1) exchangers reduce high-risk behavior more than nonexchangers, (2) in some cases, the exchangers may be persons who had reduced their risk prior to coming to the exchange, but who rely on the exchange to enable them to maintain their reduced risk, (3) exchanges can reduce the number of used syringes left lying in the streets, (4) the presence of an exchange in a city does not lead to any increase in the number of persons who begin to take (or inject) drugs, and (5) in Amsterdam, Tacoma, Washington and San Francisco, the start-up or expansion of an exchange has been followed by a decline in seroconversion rates for both HIV and hepatitis B virus (HBV).[42-50]

Educational Outreach

Educational outreach by persons who can function effectively on the streets has been the major nontreatment AIDS prevention approach for drug injectors in the United States. Although some projects have used only ex-users as outreach workers, there is some evidence that some ex-users may be less effective than was originally thought.[51] Current users have been incorporated in outreach efforts conducted by drug users' unions and other groups in the Netherlands and elsewhere.[52] In most cases, outreach programs in the United States have involved the distribution of bleach and condoms, although state or local government policies have sometimes prevented this, while outreach in the Netherlands (and in some local efforts in the United States) has included syringe distribution or exchange. Although these projects have usually focused on individual education, in San Francisco, Chicago, and some other locations they have also attempted to influence the drug user subculture so that it incorporates bleach use as normative. A considerable reduction in drug-related risk and some reduction in unsafe sex practices have been reported in evaluations of outreach projects,[35,53-56] although there is also a general belief that education alone results in relatively little behavior change, and that it is important to provide the physical means for behavior change at the same time as the educational effort.

Self-Organization

In the early 1980s, there was an outburst of collective self-organization by drug users in the Netherlands who wanted acceptance and better treatment by society. The *junkiebonden* that were formed became involved in AIDS education and the distribution of syringes to drug injectors. These organizations, however, remained limited in size and tended to vary over time in their effectiveness, with periods of high activity interspersed with periods in which little was done.[57] In the last 2 years there has been renewed self-organization, particularly in Germany, where at least 25 cities now have chapters of JES (Junkies, Ex-users, Substitutionists), and in Australia, where organizations in several cities combine the efforts of current and former drug injectors. In the United States, efforts have been made to organize drug injectors against AIDS in New York City and in Minneapolis-

St. Paul.[58] The New York City effort has met with only moderate success in establishing organization, but an evaluation study indicates that considerable risk reduction has resulted among drug injectors in the neighborhood,[59] including one third of them reporting that they always use condoms during sex.[60]

In sum, then, available data indicate that a wide range of interventions can lead to risk reduction by many drug injectors, and the leveling off of seroprevalence in San Francisco, New York, Amsterdam, and other cities may indicate that these efforts have limited the spread of HIV. However, some seroconversions continue to be reported in these cities. Hence, further work will be needed to find ways to broaden and deepen the impact of interventions so that they produce a greater degree of drug-related and sex-related risk avoidance that lasts for a lifetime.

It is our opinion that such changes would necessarily require changes in the subculture of drug use and in the larger society, not just individual change. Even more immediately, they will require a greater density of existing efforts. Bleach use has become much more widespread in San Francisco, which has had about 50 outreach workers for about 15,000 drug injectors, than in New York, which has never had more than 100 outreach workers for 200,000 drug injectors. The availability of drug abuse treatment programs is also generally inadequate for preventing epidemics of HIV transmission among drug injectors. Thus, continued development of new approaches to intervention are needed at the same time as considerable increases in the scale of existing programs.

SOCIOPOLITICAL ISSUES AND THE FUTURE OF THE EPIDEMIC

In some localities, HIV seroprevalence has stabilized with a moderate rate of new infections in a dynamic population of drug injectors. In other areas the rate of new infections is high and seroprevalence is increasing rapidly. In still other areas, the virus has not yet—or has only recently—been introduced into the local population of drug injectors, and the rate of new infections cannot yet be determined. Nonetheless, there is by now a sufficient scientific knowledge base to greatly reduce the numbers of new HIV infections among drug injectors. Whether this knowledge base will be utilized is primarily a political question.

In the 10 years of the AIDS epidemic, most official responses to AIDS prevention among drug injectors have been disappointing, in the United States and elsewhere. The epidemic spread for several years after it was identified before any sizable programs began. Then, although there was some willingness to experiment with new approaches (such as outreach programs and syringe exchanges), simply doing the same or more of what was previously being done about the local "drug problem" has been the more common response. Even when innovative approaches were adopted, the funding for these programs remained woefully inadequate in many cities with large concentrations of drug injectors.

The 10 years of the AIDS epidemic have been marked by the crystallization of two broad political approaches to issues of drug use. One of these is the harm-reduction approach, which advocates a public health paradigm that aims to minimize the damage that drug users do to themselves, other persons, and society by working *with* users. The other, far more politically influential approach has been the "war on drugs" in the United States and elsewhere. This approach advocates the punishment and stigmatization of drug users through a "zero tolerance" approach, and many of its proponents view harm minimization (through bleach or syringe distribution) as sending the wrong message. Advocates of the war-on-drugs approach have succeeded in obstructing many AIDS initiatives that could prevent the spread of HIV. Los Angeles County, for example, forbade distribution of condoms or bleach (much less syringes) in its AIDS programs, and a small experimental syringe exchange in New York City was first severely limited in scope, then ended. These limitations on, and terminations of, programs were imposed without consideration of any data on the actual effects of the program. Indeed, in the United States there is a ban on the use of federal money to operate syringe exchanges or even to conduct research on the effectiveness of those funded by other sources.

Although some (but not all) opponents of projects like syringe exchanges or the distribution of bleach or condoms favor an expansion of drug abuse treatment, the actual extent of such expansion has been somewhat limited. In the United States, for example, National Institute on Drug Abuse data indicate that the October patient census increased between 1982 and 1987 from about 160,000 to about 260,000: from 71,000 to 81,000 for methadone clients, from 74,000 to 144,000 for other outpatients, from 15,000 to 27,000 for residential treatment patients, and from 3,000 to 11,000 for special in-hospital programs.[61] Yet this increase of 100,000 is comparatively small in light of the estimated total of 5.5 million persons who need treatment, including approximately 1 million drug injectors in the United States.[62] The increase is even smaller if we exclude the 70,000 increase in "other outpatients." In New York City, the epicenter of the HIV epidemic among drug injectors, the number of persons in treatment increased only from 30,535 in 1981 to 35,192 in 1991 (New York State Division of Substance Abuse Services, unpub. data).

One situation in which a punitive law-enforcement approach may dramatically *increase* HIV risk behavior among drug injectors arises when there are large numbers of persons taking heroin or cocaine by noninjection routes. Increased law enforcement can greatly increase the cost of drugs, and if sufficient treatment facilities are not available, heavy users may switch to injecting simply because it is a highly cost-efficient method of using drugs. This scenario occurred in the United States when law enforcement against opium smoking led many users to switch to injecting heroin in the 1920s and 1930s.[63] Because of the number of developing and developed countries in which smoking (without injecting) of cocaine or heroin is practiced by a large part of the population, this scenario could be repeated many times, with greatly increased HIV transmission a likely consequence.

One aspect of the response to the AIDS epidemic among drug injectors that has been disappointing in almost all countries has been the lack of a concerted effort to reduce the numbers of persons who start injecting drugs. There may be a common assumption that knowledge of AIDS will in itself reduce the number of persons who start to inject illicit drugs, but so far there has been no evidence that this has happened.[64] The United States, the United Kingdom, and Australia have all conducted mass media antidrug campaigns since AIDS was discovered among drug injectors. However, these campaigns have been against illicit drug use in general, and have merely included AIDS as one reason not to use drugs, without emphasizing AIDS or drug *injecting* as such. Evaluation of the campaign in the United States has shown an association between the amount of media campaign exposure and more negative attitudes toward illicit drugs across different geographic areas.[65] Whether these negative attitudes in the population as a whole will affect the number of persons who begin injecting illicit drugs remains to be determined.

A comprehensive campaign to reduce the number of persons who begin to inject drugs would have to include changes in the socioeconomic and social structure factors that have led to the concentration of drug injection among economically disadvantaged groups in many countries. Whether the threat of AIDS among drug injectors will lead to programs at this level remains to be seen, but very little has even been proposed at this level of intervention. Indeed, the international AIDS community has been too slow to suggest programs to target these ills. In the early years of the epidemic, this disregard could be defended on the grounds that efforts had to be concentrated on programs to spread the word about AIDS and how it is transmitted to drug injectors and their sexual partners. Ten years into the epidemic, however, we need to find ways to combine short-term urgency (and projects directly targeting AIDS risk behaviors and interactions) with other, longer term programs that aim to end some of the social roots of drug injection and needle sharing.

Acknowledgment: Research was supported by grants DA 03574, DA 05283, and DA 06723 from the National Institute on Drug Abuse.

REFERENCES

1. Des Jarlais DC, Friedman SR, Strug D: AIDS among intravenous drug users: A sociocultural perspective. In Feld-

man D, Johnson T (eds): The Social Dimensions of AIDS: Methods and Theory. New York, Praeger, 1986

2. Agar MH: Ripping and Running: A Formal Ethnography of Urban Heroin Addicts. New York, Seminar Press, 1973

3. Johnson BD, Goldstein PJ, Preble E et al: Taking Care of Business: The Economics of Crime by Heroin Abusers. Lexington, Mass, DC Heath & Co, 1985

4. Caussy D, Weiss SH, Blattner WA et al: Exposure factors for HIV-1 infection among heterosexual drug abusers in New Jersey treatment programs. AIDS Res Hum Retroviruses 6:1459, 1990

5. Chaisson RE, Baccheti P, Osmond D et al: Cocaine use and HIV infection in intravenous drug users in San Francisco. JAMA 261:561, 1989

6. D'Aquila RT, Peterson LR, Williams AB, William AE: Race/ethnicity as a risk factor for HIV-1 infection among Connecticut intravenous drug users. J AIDS 2:503, 1989

7. Friedman SR, Rosenblum A, Goldsmith D et al: Risk factors for HIV-1 infection among street-recruited intravenous drug users in New York City (abstr). Presented at the V International Conference on AIDS, Montreal, June 1989

8. Marmor M, Des Jarlais DC, Cohen H et al: Risk factors for infection with human immunodeficiency virus among intravenous drug abusers in New York City. AIDS 1:39, 1987

9. Muga R, Tor J, Llibre J et al: Risk factors for HIV-1 infection in parenteral drug users. AIDS 4:259, 1990

10. Page JB, Smith PC, Kane N: Shooting galleries, their proprietors, and implications for prevention of AIDS. Drugs Society 5:69, 1990

11. Sasse H, Salmaso S, Conti S et al: Risk behaviors for HIV-1 infection in Italian drug users: Report from a multicenter study. J AIDS 2:486, 1989

12. Schoenbaum EE, Hartel D, Selwyn PA et al: Risk factors for human immunodeficiency virus infection in intravenous drug users. N Engl J Med 321:874, 1989

13. Van den Hoek JAR, Coutinho A, van Haastrecht HJA et al: Prevalence and risk factors of HIV infections among drug users and drug-using prostitutes in Amsterdam. AIDS 2:55, 1988

14. Vlahov D, Muñoz A, Anthony JC et al: Association of drug injection patterns with antibody to human immunodeficiency virus type 1 among intravenous drug users in Baltimore, Maryland. Am J Epidemiol 132:847, 1990

15. Williams ML: HIV seroprevalence among male IVDUs in Houston, Texas. Am J Public Health 80:1507, 1990

16. De Rossi A, Bortolotti F, Cadrobbi P, Chieco-Bianchi L: Trends of HTLV-1 and HIV infections in drug addicts. Eur J Cancer Clin Oncol 24(2):279, 1988

17. Friedman SR, Des Jarlais DC, Neaigus A et al: AIDS and the new drug injector. Nature 339:333, 1989

18. Lewis DK, Watters JK: HIV seroprevalence and needle sharing among heterosexual intravenous drug users: Ethnic/gender comparisons. Am J Public Health 78:1499, 1988

19. Secretaria de Estado da Saude: AIDS no Estado de Sao Paulo. Sao Paulo, Brazil, Centro de Vigilancia Epidemiologica, September 1990

20. Bastos FI, Lima ES et al: Perfil de usarios de drogas: I. Estudo de caracteristicas de pacientes do NEPAD/UERJ, 1986–87. Rev ABP/APAL 10(2):47, 1988

21. Arachne J, Ball A: AIDS and IV drug users: The situation in Australia. Austr Drug Alcohol Rev 5:175, 1986

22. Blacker P, Tindall B, Wodak A, Cooper D: Exposure of intravenous drug users to AIDS retrovirus, Sydney, 1985. Aust NZ J Med 16:686, 1986

23. Phanuphak P, Poshyachinda V, Un-eklabh T, Rojanapithayakorn W: HIV transmission among intravenous drug abusers (abstr). Presented at the V International Conference on AIDS, Montreal, June 6, 1989.

24. Naik TN, Sarkar S, Singh HL et al: Intravenous drug users—a new high-risk group for HIV infection in India. AIDS 5:117, 1991

25. Friedman SR, Des Jarlais DC, Sotheran JL et al: AIDS and self-organization among intravenous drug users. Int J Addict 22:201, 1987

26. Des Jarlais DC, Friedman SR, Hopkins W: Risk reduction for the acquired immunodeficiency syndrome among intravenous drug users. Ann Intern Med 103:755, 1985

27. Neaigus A, Friedman SR, Stepherson B et al: Declines in syringe sharing during the first drug injection (abstr). Presented at the VII International Conference on AIDS, Florence, Italy, June 1991

28. Abdul-Quader AS, Tross S, Friedman SR et al: Street-recruited intravenous drug users and sexual risk reduction in New York City. AIDS 4:1075, 1990

29. Power R, Hartnoll R, Daviaud E: Drug injecting, AIDS, and risk behaviour: Potential for change and intervention strategies. Br J Addict 83:649, 1988

30. Chitwood DD, Comerford M: Drugs, sex, and AIDS risk: Cocaine users versus opiate users. Am Behav Sci 33:465, 1990

31. Magura S, Grossman JI, Lipton DS et al: Determinants of needle sharing among intravenous drug users. Am J Public Health 79:459, 1989

32. Huang KHC, Watters JK, Case P: Predicting compliance with HIV risk reduction behaviors among heterosexual intravenous drug users: Relative contributions of health beliefs and situational factors (abstr). Presented at the V International Conference on AIDS, Montreal, June 1989

33. Huang KHC, Watters JK, Lorvick J: Relationship characteristics of heterosexual IV drug users. Presented at a meeting of the American Public Health Association, Chicago, 1989

34. Klee H, Faugier J, Hayes C et al: Factors associated with risk behaviour among injecting drug users. AIDS Care 2:133, 1990

35. Neaigus A, Sufian M, Friedman SR et al: Effects of outreach intervention on risk reduction among intravenous drug users. AIDS Educ Prevent 2:253, 1990

36. Abdul-Quader AS, Friedman SR, Des Jarlais DC et al: Methadone maintenance and behavior by intravenous drug users that can transmit HIV. Contemp Drug Probl 14:425, 1987

37. Blix O, Gronbladh L: AIDS and IV heroin addicts: The preventive effect of methadone maintenance in Sweden (abstr). Presented at IV International Conference on AIDS, Stockholm, June 1988

38. Hartel D, Schoenbaum EE, Selwyn PA et al: Low HIV seroconversion and change in high risk behaviour in intravenous drug users from 1985–88 in the Bronx, NYC. Presented at the V International Conference on AIDS, Montreal, June 1989

39. Ball JC, Lange WR, Myers CP, Friedman SR: Reducing the risk of AIDS through methadone maintenance treatment. J Health Soc Behav 29:214, 1988

40. Higgins DL, Galavotti C, Johnson R et al: The effect of HIV antibody counseling and testing on risk behaviors: Are the studies consistent? (abstr). Presented at the VI International Conference on AIDS, San Francisco, June 1990

41. Kall K, Olin R: HIV status and changes in risk behavior among intravenous drug users in Stockholm 1987–88. AIDS 4:153, 1990

42. Des Jarlais DC, Hagan H, Purchase D et al: Safer injection among participants in the First North American Syringe Exchange Program (abstr). Presented at the V International Conference on AIDS, Montreal, June 1989

43. Fuchs D, Unterweger B, Hinterhuber H et al: Successful preventive measures in a community of IV drug addicts (abstr). Presented at the IV International Conference on AIDS, Stockholm, June 1988

44. Hagan H, Des Jarlais DC, Purchase D et al: Drug use trends among participants in the Tacoma Syringe Exchange (abstr). Presented at the V International Conference on AIDS, Montreal, June 1989

45. Hartgers C, Buning EC, van Santen GW et al: The impact of the needle and syringe-exchange programme in Amsterdam on injecting risk behavior. AIDS 3:571, 1989

46. Ljungberg B, Andersson B, Christensson B et al: HIV prevention among injecting drug users: Three years of experience from a syringe exchange program in Sweden. J AIDS 4:890, 1991

47. Oliver K: Evaluation of the Portland, Oregon, syringe exchange. Presented at the North American Syringe Exchange Convention, Tacoma, Washington, 1990

48. Stimson GV, Alldritt LJ, Dolan KA et al: Injecting Equipment Exchange Schemes: Final Report. London, Monitoring Research Group, Goldsmith's College, 1988

49. Van Haastrecht HJA, van den Hoek JAR, Coutinho RA: No trend in yearly HIV-seroprevalence rates among IVDU in Amsterdam: 1986–1988 (abstr). Presented at the V International Conference on AIDS, Montreal, June 1989

50. Wolk WS, Wodak A, Guinan JJ et al: HIV seroprevalence in syringes of intravenous drug users using syringe exchanges in Sydney, Australia, 1987 (abstr). Presented at the IV International Conference on AIDS, Stockholm, June 1988

51. Rivera-Beckman J, Friedman SR, Clatts MC, Curtis R: "Inside"—"Outside": Social process in AIDS outreach. In: Proceedings of the Second National AIDS Demonstration Research Conference. Rockville, Md, National Institute on Drug Abuse (in press)

52. De Jong W: Het Betrekken van Druggebruikers bij de Uitvoering van het AIDS-Beleid. Amsterdam, Nationale Commissie AIDS-Bestrijding, 1991

53. Feldman H, Biernacki P, Knapp T, Margolis E: Modification of needle use in out-of-treatment intravenous drug users (abstr). Presented at the V International Conference on AIDS, Montreal, June 1989

54. Moss AR, Chaisson R: AIDS and intravenous drug use in San Francisco. AIDS Public Policy 3:37, 1988

55. Wiebel W, Fritz R, Chene D: Description of intervention procedures utilized by the AIDS Outreach Intervention Projects—University of Illinois at Chicago, School of Public Health. In: Proceedings of the Community Epidemiology Work Group, Chicago, June 1989, vol III, p 68. Rockville, Md, National Institute on Drug Abuse, 1989

56. Wiebel W: Identifying and gaining access to hidden populations. In: The Collection and Interpretation of Data from Hidden Populations. NIDA Research Monograph No. 98. Rockville, Md, Department of Health and Human Services, 1990

57. Friedman SR, de Jong WM, Des Jarlais DC: Problems and dynamics of organizing intravenous drug users for AIDS prevention. Health Educ Res 3:49, 1988

58. Carlson G, Needle R: Sponsoring addict self-organization (Addicts Against AIDS): A case study. Presented at the First Annual National AIDS Demonstration Research Conference, Rockville, Md, 1989

59. Friedman SR, Neaigus A, Jose B et al: Behavioral outcomes of organizing drug injectors against AIDS. In: Proceedings of the Second National AIDS Demonstration Research Conference. Rockville, Md, National Institute on Drug Abuse (in press)

60. Jose B, Friedman SR, Neaigus A et al: Condom use among drug injectors in an organizing project neighborhood. In: Proceedings of the Second National AIDS Demonstration Research Conference. Rockville, Md, National Institute on Drug Abuse (in press)

61. Gerstein DR, Harwood HJ (eds): Treating Drug Problems. Washington, DC, National Academy Press, 1990

62. Spencer BD: On the accuracy of current estimates of the numbers of intravenous drug users. In: Turner CF, Miller HG, Moses LE (eds): AIDS: Sexual Behavior and Intravenous Drug Use. Washington, DC, National Academy Press, 1989

63. Des Jarlais DC, Courtwright DT, Joseph H: The transition from opium smoking to heroin injection in the United States. AIDS Public Policy 6:88, 1991

64. Des Jarlais DC, Friedman SR: Intravenous cocaine, crack, and HIV infection. JAMA 259:1945, 1988

65. Black G: The Partnership for a Drug-Free America attitude tracking study. Presented at the National Institute on Drug Abuse Conference on Drug Abuse Research and Practice, Washington, DC, 1991

25

The Safety of Blood and Blood Products

Susan Aoki　　*Paul Holland*

Approximately 12 million units of whole blood or packed red cells are transfused in the United States each year, as well as 2 million units of plasma and 6 million units of platelet concentrates.[1] In 1982 epidemiologic evidence began to accumulate that a new illness, acquired immunodeficiency syndrome (AIDS), that initially occurred in sexually active homosexual men and intravenous (IV) drug users could also be transmitted by transfusion of blood and blood derivatives.[2-4] Since then the details of transmission by transfusion have been well documented, and a multi-element program is in place at all U.S. blood banks to markedly reduce the risk of transmission of human immunodeficiency virus (HIV) by blood and blood products. Major parts of the HIV prevention program are the enormous changes in donor recruitment, donor education, and donor eligibility requirements. However, a most important element of the program to prevent HIV transmission by blood products is the use of reliable assays to test every unit of blood and plasma for antibody to HIV. These assays for antibody to HIV became licensed and available in 1985. The additional screening of blood for other diseases that have similar transmission modes as HIV has indirectly contributed to reducing the risks of transfusion-related HIV transmission. The great strides in blood transfusion safety are due to the blood banking community's own efforts as well as to the Food and Drug Administration's (FDA) regulation of blood collection agencies, plasma collection centers, and blood product manufacturing companies. At this time the risk of acquiring HIV infection from a whole blood transfusion is less than the risk of anaphylaxis from penicillin therapy.

EVIDENCE FOR TRANSMISSION BY TRANSFUSION

When AIDS was first described in 1981, it was identified in homosexual men with multiple sex partners and in IV drug users. Many theories were initially developed as to the cause of AIDS. Among these theories, the idea that AIDS was due to a novel infectious agent was debated for several years while epidemiologic studies sought to define modes of transmission. With the discovery of the AIDS virus, evidence began to accumulate showing that HIV was the etiologic agent of AIDS and that transmission by blood transfusion occurred.[5]

The initial indications that the agent of AIDS could be transmitted by blood products were the presence of *Pneumocystis carinii* pneumonia in several hemophiliacs who had received many clotting factor concentrates and the development of AIDS in an infant with no apparent risk factors who had received multiple transfusions at birth, including one from someone who later developed AIDS.[2-5] Laboratory and epidemiologic evidence has essentially fulfilled Koch's postulates: when HIV recovered from one person is injected into another person, it causes HIV infection and frequently leads to AIDS. This was initially verified by an experiment in which human plasma from a patient with AIDS was injected into a chimpanzee, resulting in HIV infection in the animal.[6]

The largest study to document human-to-human transmission of HIV *via* blood (and the separated components of blood, such as platelets and plasma) is the Transfusion Safety Study. Frozen samples from units of blood donated and transfused early in the HIV epidemic

463

were saved and later tested when the HIV antibody test became available. Recipients of the anti-HIV reactive units were traced and enrolled in a follow-up study.[7] Of 124 persons without other risk factors, 90% became anti-HIV reactive after transfusion with components that were later found to be reactive for HIV antibody. The infectious components were both liquid and cellular and included whole blood, red cells, platelets, cryoprecipitate, and frozen plasma. Infectivity rates for HIV were 95% to 96% for fresh blood, platelets, and cryoprecipitate but only 50% for red cell components kept refrigerated more than 3 weeks.[8] Infection rates were not influenced by a recipient's age, sex, reason for the transfusion, or the presence of other illnesses.

HIV INFECTION FROM BLOOD TRANSFUSION

Only 3% of the reported cases of AIDS in the United States were acquired from blood products. As of January 31, 1991, the number of reported U.S. cases of AIDS due to infection acquired from blood products was 5,543.[9] As shown in Figure 25–1, the number of blood product–related cases reported each year stopped rising and began to decline in 1989. Because of the delay from the time of HIV infection to the development of clinical AIDS, the multiple measures to prevent transmission through transfusion of blood or plasma products have finally been shown to have an effect. Deaths due to AIDS reported between 1981 and 1990 included 1,019 persons with hemophilia and 2,943 transfusion recipients.[10] Estimates of the number of persons currently infected with HIV acquired from blood products range as high as 15,000[11,12]; all but a handful became infected before the spring of 1985, when anti-HIV testing became routine in blood banks and plasma centers.

Hemophilia

Approximately 27% of the AIDS cases acquired through transfusion of blood products have occurred in patients with hemophilia. The prevalence of HIV infection among persons with severe hemophilia A (factor VIII deficiency) is estimated to be 76%; among those who received fewer units of blood and plasma products, such as those with less severe hemophilia A or those with hemophilia B (factor IX deficiency), the prevalence is 25% to 46%.[13] Patients with hemophilia represent a special population of blood recipients because they received not just single-donor components, such as red cells and cryoprecipitates, but also plasma derivatives, which are produced by pooling thousands of donors' plasma and processing it to concentrate the antihemophilic factor. Pooled plasma derivatives contain plasma from as many as 25,000 different donors in a single dose.[14] Out of all the "manufactured products" derived from pooled plasma, only clotting factor concentrates have been implicated in AIDS transmission. However, newer manufacturing processes may entirely eliminate the risk of HIV transmission by clotting factor concentrates. Human albumin, purified protein fraction, γ-globulin IM or IV, and the various hyperimmune globulins, such as hepatitis B immune globulin (HBIG), have never transmitted HIV (Table 25–1).

Transfusion Recipients

Disease progression has been similar in persons who acquired HIV infection through a blood transfusion and in persons who acquired infection by other modes of transmission. Recipients may report an acute febrile illness within 8 weeks of transfusion-associated HIV seroconversion.[15] For many transfusion recipients, the first indication of illness was AIDS itself. In persons acquiring HIV infection through blood transfusion, the cumulative probability of developing AIDS after an anti-HIV reactive transfusion is 13% at 3 years.[7] Several studies suggest that progression to AIDS is more rapid in infants, in persons immunocompromised at the time of transfusion, or in persons over 35 years of age.[13,16] Initial data from the AIDS epidemic suggested that if the donor progressed rapidly to AIDS, the recipient

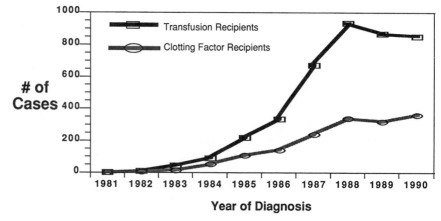

Figure 25–1. Number of AIDS cases acquired from transfusion or clotting factor concentrates, by year of diagnosis, as reported to the Centers for Disease Control.

Table 25–1. Blood Components and Derivatives Reported as Capable of Transmitting HIV

Liquid components: Whole blood, packed red cells, washed red cells, platelets, white cells	Yes
Frozen components: Plasma, red cells, cryoprecipitate	Yes
Plasma derivatives:	
Serum albumin, plasma protein fraction	No
Human immune serum γ-globulin, IM or IV	No
Hyperimmune globulins such as CMV (CMVIG), hepatitis B (HBIG), varicella-zoster (VZIG), RH(D) factor (RhIG), rabies (RIG)	No
Factor VIII concentrate (dry heated)	Yes
Factor IX complex (II, VII, IX, and X) (heated)	Yes

might also progress rapidly to AIDS[17]; however, further data have shown that the progression rate to AIDS in the donor does not affect the progression rate in the recipient.[18] In hemophiliac patients, the rate of progression from HIV infection to AIDS appears to be similar to the progression rate in persons of similar age but who acquired the infection by other routes.[19]

PREVENTION MEASURES

Beginning in 1983, a variety of measures were instituted to reduce the risk of transfusion-associated AIDS. Measures to prevent transmission by transfusion include (1) preventing donations by those at risk for HIV infection, (2) testing of all blood donations for anti-HIV (plus testing for other transfusion-transmitted infections), (3) developing physicochemical virucidal treatments of blood products, (4) stressing the use of transfusion therapy for appropriate indications, and especially the use of fewer homologous blood transfusions, and (5) the use of autologous (patient's own) blood where feasible. Additional measures include (6) donor deferral registries, (7) a confidential unit exclusion system, and (8) provision of alternative test sites for those wishing to be tested for anti-HIV.

Donor eligibility requirement changes have reflected the changing Centers for Disease Control (CDC) definition of risk groups and risk factors with respect to HIV transmission. In early 1983, persons known to be at increased risk for AIDS included those with symptoms of AIDS, homosexually active men with multiple sexual partners, IV drug abusers, persons with hemophilia, immigrants from Haiti, and sexual partners of persons at increased risk for AIDS. Symptoms of AIDS or AIDS-related complex (ARC) included night sweats; unexplained weight loss; persistent cough, fever, or diarrhea; enlarged lymph nodes; and skin or mucous membrane lesions suggestive of Kaposi's sarcoma. All these persons at increased risk were no longer recruited or were asked to defer themselves as blood or plasma donors. These initial approaches to donor exclusion had measurable effects. For example, in New York City, the number of men aged 21 to 35 years who donated blood dropped by 12%.[20] In San Francisco, results of a retrospective study suggest that donor self-deferral led to an 80% decrease in donations from persons at risk for AIDS (Fig. 25–2).[21]

Over the years, the FDA and the blood banking organizations have added more stringent eligibility requirements to exclude donors with a history of behaviors or factors associated with high risk for HIV infection. Thus, in addition to those factors mentioned above, individuals are now permanently ineligible if they have a history of a positive test for HIV, are males who have had sex with another male even once since 1977, or are persons who have engaged in prostitution since 1977. Blood donation is not permitted for 1 year after blood transfusion, acupuncture, ear piercing, tattooing, or

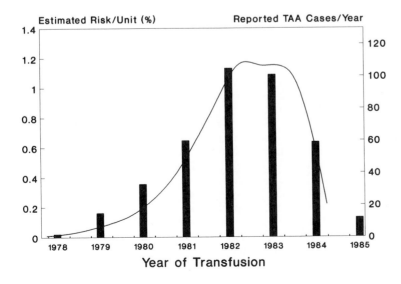

Figure 25–2. Effects of education efforts and self-deferral by donors on the reduction in AIDS high-risk donations in San Francisco (*line*) prior to the initiation of HIV testing by the blood center in 1985. Distribution of 250 reported transfusion-associated AIDS (TA-AIDS) cases by year(s) of implicated transfusions (*solid bars*). (Reproduced with permission from Busch MP et al: Risk of human immunodeficiency virus (HIV) transmission by blood transfusions before the implementation of HIV-1 antibody screening. Transfusion 31:4, 1991.)

needlestick exposure to a patient's blood. (The 1-year deferral reflects the longer period for seroconversion to hepatitis C virus, but also allows more than enough time for seroconversion to HIV.) Tables 25–2 and 25–3 summarize the reasons for permanent or temporary deferral of potential blood and plasma donors at risk of exposure to HIV.

Blood banks had to help educate the general public about the symptoms of AIDS, methods of transmission, and the activities that place people at risk for AIDS. Correcting false information has also been important. Continuous campaigns were necessary to inform people that one can *never* get AIDS by *donating* blood. Currently, donors are given an information sheet to read, and trained interviewers privately ask the donor directly about HIV risk factors and symptoms as well as about hepatitis and other diseases. Any reward for donating is seen as possibly influencing a donor's answers on the eligibility questions, so volunteer (unpaid) donors giving altruistically and without pressure (from family, work, and the like) are preferred. Since the 1970s, most blood banks in the United States have not paid donors, and inducements to donate such as T-shirts, pens, and mugs are now being phased out. (Plasma centers that collect plasma for further manufacturing processes are a separate system, and almost all pay their donors.)

To discourage blood donation for the purpose of obtaining a free HIV test, some states have offered free, rapid, anonymous HIV testing at sites other than blood banks.[22] To make donating blood a less attractive method of getting a free HIV test, some states restrict blood banks from releasing HIV testing results to the donor for a period of time after donation. Certain states have laws making it a felony for a person known to have a positive test for HIV to donate blood. Others require reporting of all individuals found to have a reactive test for HIV antibody.

Pressure from friends or family (patient-selected or patient-designated donations) may "force" some unsuitable high-risk donors to donate blood anyway. In January 1984, blood banks began using systems to allow donors to confidentially declare that their blood is not suitable for transfusion. A "confidential unit exclusion" method was developed to allow donors to indicate privately at the time of donation that their blood should not be transfused. Before alternative HIV antibody testing sites were available, it appeared that those who confidentially excluded their blood from transfusion were more likely to have laboratory tests reactive for blood-transmissible agents. In October 1986, the FDA recommended that all blood centers give donors the opportunity for confidential unit exclusion. Unfortunately, studies suggest that confidential unit exclusion is *not* effective, because the vast majority of HIV-positive blood donors designate that their units be transfused.[23] Only the anti-HIV test can prevent such units, from HIV-infected donors who do not self-exclude, from being transfused.[24]

Deferred donor registries and exclusion lists play an important role in blood safety, too. Registries (local, state, or the national Red Cross program) contain the names of all donors with positive tests for infections such as hepatitis or HIV. Lists (usually maintained by individual blood drawing centers) may also contain the names of donors reporting risk factors for AIDS or having positive laboratory results. In some states, all persons with AIDS or with positive HIV or HBsAg tests reported to public health departments may be added to statewide donor deferral lists, even if they have not been blood or plasma donors in the past.

To discover cases of HIV due to prior transfusions and to prevent secondary spread of the disease, blood banks use a variety of "lookback" procedures. The major type of lookback procedure identifies patients who received blood in the past from a donor who now tests positive for HIV antibody. When a donor is found through testing or reporting to be infected with HIV, blood banks are required to notify the recipients of previous donations. These recipients are notified of their risk, and testing for HIV antibody is strongly recommended; the lookback procedure may be terminated when two consecutive transfusion recipients are found to be anti-HIV negative. Testing and counseling of these recipients is performed to limit the spread of HIV by unsuspecting asymptomatic transfusion recipients.[25] Other lookback procedures have involved searching for implicated donors of blood or components received by patients with apparent transfusion-transmitted AIDS and matching the names of patients with AIDS against donor lists of area blood banks.[26] A broader approach is to test

Table 25–2.   Reasons (Risk Factors for AIDS) for Permanent Deferral of Blood and Plasma Donors

1. AIDS or AIDS-related complex, or a positive test for HIV antibody
2. Symptoms of AIDS or ARC
3. Male who had sex with another male, even once, since 1977
4. Illegal IV drug use
5. Engaged in prostitution since 1977
6. Hemophilia (and received clotting factor concentrates)
7. Residence in sub-Saharan Africa or the islands off the coast of Africa (unless a test for anti-HIV-2 is being used)
8. Sexual contact with any of the persons listed above

Table 25–3.   Reasons for 1-Year Deferral of Blood and Plasma Donors

1. Blood or component transfusion
2. Tattoo, ear piercing or acupuncture, unless sterile disposable equipment was used
3. Needlestick exposure in a health care setting
4. Sexual contact with a prostitute

everyone who received a transfusion between 1977 and 1985. In San Francisco, some hospital programs sent letters to all patients who received transfusions between 1978 and April 1985 notifying them of the risk of HIV from transfusion and offering free anti-HIV testing. In one such study, of over 700 patients tested (only 4% of those notified who responded), 13 were anti-HIV reactive.[27] Thus, in an area of the United States with a high prevalence of HIV infection, broad notification was not a very effective method of detecting transfusion-associated HIV, especially that which had not been identified by other means. Physicians should suggest HIV testing for patients who received many transfusions between 1978 and early 1985 or who were given clotting factor concentrates made from the plasma of thousands of donors.

BLOOD TESTING

Blood tests for HIV antibody were licensed by the FDA in March 1985. Blood banks and plasma centers began routinely testing all donations shortly thereafter with the enzyme-linked immunoassay (ELISA) and discarding those with a positive test. Like any screening test that attempts to detect an infection present in less than 5% of a population, the anti-HIV ELISA has a very large false-positive rate when applied to blood and plasma donations. Thus, although the ELISA for anti-HIV is 99% sensitive and 99% specific, the vast majority of positive ELISA tests in blood donors do not represent HIV infection. For each reactive ELISA for anti-HIV in a blood or plasma donor, a confirmatory test, such as the Western blot, is required to verify actual HIV infection as the reason for the ELISA result.[28] Causes of false-positive ELISA results include antibodies to lymphocytes (in which HIV is grown; cellular material may be present along with the virus), rheumatoid factor, elevated globulins, and nonspecific proteins.[29]

Indeterminate results, such as the presence of antibody to the p24 band on the Western blot, may identify a small subgroup of donors who are in the process of seroconverting to HIV. These donors should be retested at a later date (3 to 6 months later), as some are infected with HIV, even though the vast majority are not. Causes of indeterminate Western blot test results include reactions to the reagents used in the test, or antibody to other (not retro) viruses.[30]

Notification, counseling, and referral of donors with reactive HIV tests for further medical care is another roll blood banks have taken on. When blood donors are found to have a confirmed anti-HIV result, efforts are made to identify how the persons may have been infected, if they knew they were at risk, and their motives for donating. Using this information, blood banks attempt to refine their recruiting and donor screening procedures to avoid drawing blood or plasma from in-

dividuals who are infected with HIV and capable of transmitting it, but are not as yet reactive on the HIV antibody test.

Following infection with HIV, the antibody test may not become positive for 2 to 6 months; during this "window" period, a donor may be negative on HIV antibody testing but still able to transmit HIV infection. The p24 HIV antigen test has been evaluated extensively to see if it would decrease the risk of HIV transmission during the window period. To date there has been only one report of a blood donor with HIV who might have been identified at an earlier date by HIV antigen testing.[31] However, since p24 antigen testing in 1989 of over 500,000 volunteer donors across the United States and 8,600 samples from 1984–85 donations by young males residing in neighborhoods with a high prevalence of AIDS did not detect HIV infection earlier than with the HIV antibody test, most blood banks do not screen donors with the HIV antigen test.[32,33]

An elegant research method has been tried to detect donors in the window period. Polymerase chain reaction (PCR) techniques were applied to pooled samples from anti-HIV antibody negative volunteer blood donors in San Francisco. Even in an area of the country with a high prevalence of HIV-infected individuals, only one in 43,650 donations testing HIV antibody negative was PCR positive.[34] PCR is a very labor-intensive procedure, requires a very specialized laboratory, and has many false-positive results, so it is not practical for use as a routine assay in the blood bank setting.

HIV-2, a virus very similar to and that cross-reacts with HIV-1, was discovered in west Africa in 1985.[35] By 1990, only one U.S. citizen was reported to be infected with HIV-2, in addition to several imported cases from Africa.[36] Current anti-HIV-1 ELISA methods detect HIV-2 carriers in 60% to 100% of attempts.[37] In an effort to identify HIV-2 reactive donors in the United States, samples from 24,826 HIV-1 reactive blood donors were evaluated with a specific anti-HIV-2 assay; not one HIV-2 reactive donor was found.[36] At this time, deferral of all donors who have lived in HIV-2 endemic areas of Africa appears to make it unnecessary to specifically test for anti-HIV-2, despite the availability of such a test. Combination ELISA antibody tests for both HIV-1 and HIV-2, along with specific Western blots for both HIV-1 and HIV-2, will nonetheless be implemented because HIV-2 has spread outside west Africa.

Screening blood donations for diseases such as hepatitis and syphilis that are spread by modes of transmission similar to those of HIV may lead to rejection of donors at risk for HIV. Prior to the availability of a test for AIDS, it was known that some of the populations at high risk for hepatitis B were also at risk for non-A, non-B hepatitis. "Surrogate" tests were suggested to reduce the transmission of non-A, non-B viral hepatitis because no specific test was available at that time. Anti-HBc (antibody to the hepatitis B core) and ALT (alanine aminotransferase level), the surrogate tests chosen, have also likely had some impact on reducing the transmission of HIV, as well as hepatitis B and hepatitis C.

PHYSICIANS' EFFORTS

Limiting exposure of patients to the blood of homologous donors will diminish the risk of transmission of infections such as HIV. Such measures would include appropriate indications for blood and components, the use of single-donor components when possible, the use of autologous blood in some form or another, and prescribing of erythropoietin if indicated. The practice of having patients select their own donors, patient-designated donors, has not been shown to result in safer blood, however.

Surgeons have reduced the number of units routinely transfused to patients in the perioperative period.[38] The level of hemoglobin that can be tolerated by most patients has been recommended to be lower than the arbitrary level of 100 g/L (10 g/dl).[39] Many patients undergoing elective surgery can donate blood during the month before surgery for their own transfusion (autologous) needs at surgery. Another approach to using the patient's own blood is the intraoperative salvage of blood lost from the wound; red blood cells are washed and then returned intravenously. Additional techniques to use a patient's own blood include intraoperative phlebotomy with hemodilution and postoperative wound drainage/salvage for retransfusion if there is no evidence of infection. For many presurgical and nonsurgical anemic patients, the use of synthetic erythropoietin has eliminated the need for transfusions. Erythropoietin is especially useful in patients with anemia from renal failure and in those who cannot donate sufficient blood before surgery. Hospitals have established transfusion committees to monitor the use of blood and to keep physicians informed of appropriate indications for transfusion of blood and blood components.

PLASMA PRODUCTS

Therapeutic products derived from blood plasma include albumin, globulins, clotting factor concentrates, and plasma protein fraction. The degree of safety of these products is related to their various manufacturing processes. Because the first step in manufacturing all of these products is the pooling of the plasma of thousands of donors, one or more infected individual donors can contaminate many doses of the product. Currently, 80% of the plasma used in the manufacture of blood derivatives is collected from paid donors at commercial plasma centers. Plasma centers are a separate system from the community volunteer blood banks. Regardless of the type of collection facility, donors with risk factors

for AIDS are deferred and the donated blood or plasma is screened for HIV antibody.

In the past, factor VIII (antihemophilic factor, AHF) and factor IX complex clotting factor concentrates were not treated to remove or inactivate viruses and were responsible for the transmission of HIV as well as hepatitis B, C, and D (delta agent). Attempts in the early 1980s to inactivate virus while sparing the very heat-labile factor VIII entailed the application of "dry heat" to the lyophilized product. The dry heat reduced but did not eliminate viral transmission, so that process has been discarded. Pasteurization (wet heat), a combined treatment with solvent and detergent, and factor VIII monoclonal antibody absorption are three methods of preparation currently in use that are considered free of HIV risk. Manufacturers sometimes combine more than one treatment. It will take several years for these new coagulation products to prove their safety, but to date several have no evidence of HIV transmission.[40,41] Unfortunately, the production of completely safe factor IX complex products has been slower. Two recombinant factor VIII products (not derived from plasma, and thus HIV free) have been developed and should become generally available.[42] These improvements in coagulation factor products have greatly increased the medical treatment costs for patients with hemophilia, but the margin of safety should be worth the cost to the individual and to the health care system.

It is important to note that serum albumin, purified protein fraction and the various immunoglobulin preparations have never been shown to transmit HIV. Despite being pooled products, their manufacturing method removes or inactivates most viruses. Albumin and purified protein solution for IV use are first alcohol fractionated from plasma and then undergo heating at 60° C for 10 hours. Immunoglobulin preparations, although not heated, are manufactured by the Cohn-Oncley process, which appears to remove or inactivate HIV, owing to the ethanol in various parts of the separation process.

CURRENT RISK OF HIV TRANSMISSION BY TRANSFUSIONS

At this time, only 2% of new AIDS cases are due to transfusions and virtually all are due to transfusion before 1985. However, the number of AIDS cases due to transfusion certainly has not abated, as there are many asymptomatic HIV-infected persons who are yet to be counted among the AIDS cases. It is estimated that up to 15,000 people in the United States have been infected by transfusion of blood or blood products, and most will likely develop AIDS.[12]

On the other hand, the number of persons acquiring HIV infection by blood transfusion peaked before anti-HIV antibody testing was initiated in 1985 and has fallen to practically zero. Current estimates for the risk of contracting HIV infection, and thus AIDS, through a blood transfusion vary from 1 per 153,000 units[43] to the worst case of 1 per 36,000 units.[44] The risk is additive with each unit transfused. Between 1985 and 1989, only 38 cases of transfusion-associated HIV have been detected despite millions of transfusions having been performed. The donors responsible for these HIV transmissions appear to have donated during the window period between infection with HIV and the production of a detectable level of HIV antibody. Almost 100% of donations made in the window period are made by persons who on later questioning admit to AIDS high-risk behavior.[45] Efforts in the future will be directed primarily toward better interviewing and screening techniques rather than toward the development of even more sensitive tests for HIV.[46]

The current risk of HIV infection from the newer clotting factor concentrates is difficult to measure, because the patients who use these products have a lifetime of exposures. The institution of stricter donor screening and HIV testing by plasma centers, along with improved manufacturing processes, appears to have been very effective, however.[47]

Physicians should explain the reasons for, and the risks and benefits of, transfusions and alternative treatments to their patients.[39] Informed consent before the use of blood, blood components, and blood derivatives should be provided, just as is done when drugs are prescribed or therapeutic procedures are suggested. The estimated risks for infections or other complications of blood transfusions are listed in Table 25–4 and are compared with the risks of sustaining a fatal accident in common daily activities. The risk of acquiring an infection from blood transfusion will never be zero, but it has never been lower. Viral inactivation procedures hold promise for eliminating infections from blood and blood components, but this has not been realized yet.[48]

Table 25–4. Risks Associated with Blood or Blood Component Transfusion

Reaction, Infection, or Fatal Accident	Risk From Transfusion (ca. 1990), per Unit
Febrile or allergic (hives) reaction	1:100
Hemolytic reaction	1:6,000
Fatal hemolytic reaction	1:100,000
Infection	
HIV	1:36,000–1:153,000
Hepatitis B	1:1,300
Hepatitis C	1:500–1:1,000
Risk of fatal automobile accident, per year*	1:5,000
Risk of fatal accident at home*	1:12,500

* Source: Statistical Abstract of the United States, 107th ed, 1987.

REFERENCES

1. Surgenor DM, Wallace EL, Hao SHS, Chapman RH: Collection and transfusion of blood in the United States, 1982–88. N Engl J Med 322:1646, 1990
2. Centers for Disease Control: Possible transfusion-associated acquired immune deficiency syndrome (AIDS)—California. MMWR 31:644, 1982
3. Centers for Disease Control: *Pneumocytis carinii* pneumonia among persons with hemophilia A. MMWR 31:365, 1982
4. Centers for Disease Control: Update on acquired immune deficiency syndrome (AIDS) among patients with hemophilia A. MMWR 31:644, 1982
5. Groopman JE, Salahuddin SZ, Sarngadharan MG et al: Virologic studies in a case of transfusion associated AIDS. N Engl J Med 311:1419, 1984
6. Alter HJ, Eichberg JW, Masur H et al: Transmission of HTLV-III infection from human plasma to chimpanzees: An animal model for AIDS. Science 226:549, 1984
7. Donegan E, Stuart M, Niland JC et al: Infection with human immunodeficiency virus type 1 (HIV-1) among recipients of antibody-positive blood donations. Ann Intern Med 113:733, 1990
8. Donegan E, Lenes BA, Tomasulo PA, Mosley JW: Transfusion Safety Study Group: Transmission of HIV-1 by component type and duration of shelf storage before transfusion. Transfusion 30:851, 1990
9. Centers for Disease Control: HIV/AIDS Surveillance Report, February 1991
10. Centers for Disease Control: Mortality attributable to HIV infection/AIDS—United States, 1981–1990. MMWR 40:41, 1991
11. Kalbfleisch JD, Lawless JF: Estimating the incubation time, distribution and expected number of cases of transfusion-associated acquired immune deficiency syndrome. Transfusion 29:672, 1989
12. Centers for Disease Control: Update: Acquired immunodeficiency syndrome—United States, 1989. MMWR 39:81, 1990
13. Goedert JJ, Kessler CM, Aledort LM et al: A prospective study of human immunodeficiency virus type 1 infection and the development of AIDS in subjects with hemophilia. N Engl J Med 321:1141, 1989
14. Madhok R, Forbes CD: HIV-1 infection in haemophilia. Baillieres Clin Haematol 3:79, 1990
15. Boiteux F, Vilmer E, Girot R et al: Lymphadenopathy syndrome in two thalassemic patients after LAV contamination by blood transfusion. N Engl J Med 312:648, 1985
16. Blaxhult A, Granath F, Lidman K, Giesecke J: The influence of age on the latency period to AIDS in people infected by HIV through blood transfusion. AIDS 4:125, 1990
17. Ward JW, Bush TJ, Perkins HA et al: The natural history of transfusion-associated infection with human immunodeficiency virus. N Engl J Med 321:947, 1989
18. Samson S, Busch M, Salk S et al: HIV progression in recipients according to donor type. (abstr C.636). Presented at the VI International Conference on AIDS, San Francisco, 1990
19. Jason J, Kung-Jong L, Ragni MV et al: Risk of developing AIDS in HIV-infected cohorts of hemophilic and homosexual men. JAMA 261:725, 1989
20. Pindyck J, Waldman A, Zang E et al: Measures to decrease

the risk of acquired immunodeficiency syndrome transmission by blood transfusion. Transfusion 25:3, 1985

21. Busch MP, Young MJ, Samson SM et al: Risk of human immunodeficiency virus (HIV) transmission by blood transfusions before the implementation of HIV-1 antibody screening. Transfusion 31:4, 1991

22. Snyder AJ, Vergeront JM: Safeguarding the blood supply by providing opportunities for anonymous HIV testing. N Engl J Med 319:374, 1988

23. Busch MP, Perkins HA, Holland PV et al: HIV-1 blood donor study: Questionable efficacy of confidential unit exclusion. Transfusion 30:668, 1990

24. Leitman SF, Klein HG, Melpolder JJ et al: Clinical implications of positive tests for antibodies to human immunodeficiency virus type 1 in asymptomatic blood donors. N Engl J Med 321:917, 1989

25. Centers for Disease Control: Human immunodeficiency virus infection in transfusion recipients and their family members. MMWR 36:137, 1987

26. Samson S, Busch M, Ward J et al: Identification of HIV-infected transfusion recipients: The utility of cross-referencing previous donor records with AIDS case reports. Transfusion 30:214, 1990

27. Donegan E, Johnson D, Remedios V, Cohen S: Mass notification of transfusion recipients at risk for HIV infection. JAMA 260:922, 1988

28. Dodd RY, Fang CT: The Western immunoblot procedure for HIV antibodies and its interpretation. Arch Pathol Lab Med 114:240, 1990

29. Hunter JB, Menitove JE: HLA antibodies detected by ELISA HTLV-III antibody kits. Lancet 2:397, 1985

30. Kleinman S: The significance of HIV-1 indeterminate Western blot results in blood donor populations. Arch Pathol Lab Med 114:298, 1990

31. Irani MS, Dudley AW, Lucco LJ: Case of HIV-1 transmission by antigen-positive, antibody-negative blood. N Engl J Med 325:1174, 1991

32. Alter HJ, Epstein JS, Swenson SG et al: Prevalence of human immunodeficiency virus type 1 p24 antigen in U.S. blood donors: An assessment of the efficacy of testing in donor screening. N Engl J Med 323:1312, 1990

33. Busch MP, Taylor PE, Lenes BA et al: Screening of selected male blood donors for p24 antigen of human immunodeficiency virus type 1. N Engl J Med 323:1308, 1990

34. Busch MP, Eble BE, Khayam-Boshi H et al: Evaluation of contemporary screened blood donors for HIV-1 infection using pooled cell culture and DNA amplification techniques. N Engl J Med 325:1, 1991

35. Centers for Disease Control: Update: HIV-2 infection—United States. MMWR 38:572, 1989

36. Centers for Disease Control: Surveillance for HIV-2 infection in blood donors—United States, 1987–89. MMWR 39:829, 1990

37. George JR, Rayfield MA, Phillips S et al: Efficacies of U.S. Food and Drug Administration–licensed HIV-1-screening enzyme immunoassays for detecting antibodies to HIV-2. AIDS 4:321, 1990

38. Goodnough LT, Shuck JM: Risks, options, and informed consent for blood transfusion in elective surgery. Am J Surg 159:602, 1990

39. National Institutes of Health: Perioperative red blood cell transfusion. JAMA 260:2700, 1988

40. Pierce GF, Lusher JM, Brownstein AP et al: The use of purified clotting factor concentrates in hemophilia. JAMA 261:3434, 1989

41. Epstein JS, Fricke WA: Current safety of clotting factor concentrates. Arch Pathol Lab Med 114:335, 1990

42. Schwartz RS, Abildgaard CF, Aledort LM et al: Human recombinant DNA-derived antihemophilic factor (factor VIII) in the treatment of hemophilia A. N Engl J Med 323:1800, 1990

43. Cumming PD, Wallace EL, Schorr JB, Dodd RY: Exposure of patients to human immunodeficiency virus through the transfusion of blood components that test antibody-negative. N Engl J Med 321:941, 1989

44. Donahue JG, Nelson KE, Munoz A et al: Transmission of HIV by transfusion of screened blood. N Engl J Med 323:1709, 1990

45. Ward JW, Holmberg SD, Allen JR et al: Transmission of human immunodeficiency virus (HIV) by blood transfusions screened as negative for HIV antibody. N Engl J Med 318:473, 1988

46. Menitove JE: Current risk of transfusion-associated human immunodeficiency virus infection. Arch Pathol Lab Med 114:330, 1990

47. Gjerset GF, Mosley JW: Safety of factor VIII. Ann Intern Med 114:171, 1991

48. Horowitz B, Williams B, Rywkin S et al: Inactivation of viruses in blood with aluminum phthalocyanine derivatives. Transfusion 31:102, 1991

26

Perinatal Transmission of HIV

Herbert B. Peterson   Martha F. Rogers

The human immunodeficiency virus (HIV) epidemic in the United States is taking an increasing toll on women and infants. As of September 1990, 9.5% of all reported cases of acquired immunodeficiency syndrome (AIDS) were among women, and 1.7% were among children less than 13 years of age. However, on the basis of cases reported in 1988 and 1989, women and perinatally infected children are the fastest growing groups affected by the epidemic. From 1988 to 1989, cases among women increased by 23% and cases among perinatally infected children increased by 34%; by contrast, cases among men increased by 13%. Currently, HIV/AIDS ranks among the ten leading causes of death in women of reproductive age in the United States and, if current trends continue, it will be one of the five leading causes of death by the end of 1991. Although the current number of AIDS cases reported among children is just over 2,800, an estimated 1,500 to 1,700 infants infected with HIV were born in 1990 alone. Thus, the number of children with AIDS is expected to increase dramatically in the 1990s.

Most women with HIV infection in the United States are of childbearing age. Now that transfusions of blood and blood products are an exceedingly unlikely cause of HIV infection among infants and children, nearly all new cases of pediatric AIDS in the United States will result from transmission by an infected mother. Pregnancy, therefore, is the obvious link between the health of the mother and the health of the infant. For the sake of both women and infants, the primary prevention of HIV among women is paramount. This report, however, focuses on preventing perinatal (vertical) transmission of HIV from women already infected to their infants.

MECHANISMS OF PERINATAL TRANSMISSION

Mother-to-infant transmission of HIV may occur by three mechanisms: (1) *in utero* transmission by transplacental passage of HIV, (2) exposure to infectious maternal blood and vaginal secretions during labor and delivery, and (3) post partum, through breast-feeding. The relative percentage of perinatal transmission attributable to each mechanism is unknown.

Evidence for *in utero* transmission is based on isolated reports of HIV identified in fetal tissue[1] and amniotic fluid.[2] Whether *in utero* transmission usually occurs early in gestation or in the third trimester is unclear, although HIV has been identified in a 15-week-gestation fetus.[3]

Intrapartum transmission through exposure to infectious maternal blood and vaginal secretions is assumed to occur because the transmission patterns of HIV are similar to those of hepatitis B virus (HBV). The ability to document transmission by this mechanism is limited by a lack of precise laboratory methods to diagnose infant infection. Studies to date suggest that delivery by cesarean section does not protect against perinatal transmission.[4–6]

Transmission of HIV *via* breast-feeding is now clearly documented among women who became infected with HIV post partum through blood transfusion or sexual transmission.[7,8] Further support for this mechanism has been provided by isolation of HIV from breast milk.[8] The relative likelihood of transmission through breast-feeding remains unclear; available data from follow-up studies conflict. Two studies, a perinatal study from Zaire[9] and a report from the European Collaborative Study,[5] found no increased risk among breast-fed infants, but two others, reports from the Italian Multicentre Study[6] and the French Collaborative Study Group,[4] identified increased risks (although in the former study the increase in risk was not statistically significant).

Authorities in the United States and other developed countries have recommended that women with HIV infection refrain from breast-feeding. The risk of transmission through breast-feeding in developing countries must be considered in context, however. Because formula may be too expensive or safe water unavailable for reconstituting formula, the World Health Organization (WHO) has recommended that breast-feeding continue as the preferable method of infant feeding in most developing countries.[8]

RATE OF PERINATAL TRANSMISSION

Prospective studies of mother-to-infant transmission report transmission rates of 25% to 40%,[4-6,10] although the most recent report from the European Collaborative Study found a rate of 13%.[11] Most women in those studies were asymptomatic during pregnancy. Preliminary data suggest that women who are in later stages of HIV disease and women with CD4 counts below 400 cells/mm^3 may be more likely to transmit infection.[10]

Questions remain regarding why perinatal transmission occurs in some instances but not in most. Three studies, based on small numbers of mother-infant pairs, found that the presence of antibody to certain epitopes of gp120 is associated with reduced rates of transmission,[12-14] but the involved epitopes varied among studies. Others were not able to confirm a relationship between the presence of antibody and reduced transmission.[15] A better understanding of the determinants of perinatal transmission would permit better counseling and also provide the basis for possible therapeutic intervention.

RESEARCH STRATEGIES FOR PREVENTION

No means for interrupting mother-to-infant transmission of HIV currently exists. The potential effectiveness of various prevention strategies is difficult to assess because the timing of transmission remains uncertain. Clinical trials evaluating the effectiveness of antiviral therapy in preventing perinatal transmission will be initiated soon. Although research strategies hold some promise, available data permit only cautious optimism regarding the availability of effective interventions in the near future.

PREVENTION OF PERINATAL TRANSMISSION

At present, with no effective means to prevent *in utero* and intrapartum transmission of HIV from an infected mother to her infant, existing strategies for preventing HIV infection among infants rely on primary prevention of HIV infection among women of reproductive age. The paramount importance of this focus warrants emphasis. Once a fertile woman becomes infected with HIV, strategies necessarily shift to prevention of unintended pregnancy. If prevention of unintended pregnancy is unsuccessful and the infected woman so chooses, pregnancy termination is an option. Neither of these options permits a woman infected with HIV to bear children, and both may be unacceptable to her. Therefore, choosing one or both of them may represent an additional and possibly extreme hardship in an already difficult life. We must not oversimplify the complexity of decision-making regarding pregnancy and the intensity of the impact of these choices. Further, because most women with HIV infection are unaware that they are infected, efforts to prevent perinatal transmission must also focus on women at high risk for infection. Thus, a large number of women are faced with making complex and difficult choices. Certainly, prevention strategies that offer infected women more options should be urgently pursued. Because these are not currently available, however, we will explore the limited existing options in some detail.

In a prospective study of intravenous (IV) drug users in a methadone program in New York City,[16] approximately 44% of pregnant women known to be seropositive chose to terminate the pregnancy. However, a woman's knowledge of HIV serostatus appeared to have little or no influence on her decision to undergo abortion, as 32% of women known to be uninfected in the same population also had the procedure. A study in Atlanta[17] found that 17% of women requesting antenatal care for pregnancy subsequently requested induced abortion after finding that they were HIV positive through routinely encouraged antenatal HIV testing. In that report, a high percentage (40%) of seropositive women were first tested for HIV after 24 weeks of gestation, and thus were not eligible for pregnancy termination in the study institution.

We will not discuss the ethical and moral issues surrounding induced abortion in general, or its use for preventing birth of infants infected with HIV in particular. Clearly, however, induced abortion is not an acceptable alternative for many women with HIV infection. Further, concern has been expressed by some that women with HIV infection may be pressured into seeking induced abortions. Others have expressed concern that some women infected with HIV who choose induced abortion may experience difficulty in obtaining one. A 1988 survey of abortion providers in New York City found that women who reported themselves as infected with HIV were frequently excluded from access to abortion services.[18]

These questions and the profound individual and societal concerns regarding abortion underscore the appropriateness of focusing strategies on the prevention of *unintended* pregnancy, which may be more acceptable at both individual and societal levels. The term "unintended" is paramount, for it indicates the importance of individual choice regarding the decision to become pregnant and implies the objective that choices are informed. Focusing on preventing unintended pregnancy, however, does not eliminate considerations regarding induced abortion, because some sincere efforts to prevent unintended pregnancy may fail.

Prevention of Unintended Pregnancy

Successful strategies for preventing unintended pregnancy in women infected with HIV require understanding the determinants of decision-making regarding pregnancy, the appropriateness and safety of various alternatives for preventing pregnancy, and the means to ensure access to those alternatives for persons who choose to use them.

Determinants of Decision-Making Regarding Pregnancy

An estimated 80,000 U.S. women of reproductive age are currently infected with HIV. The great majority of these women do not know that they are infected. Most of these women are living in poverty and are women of color, IV drug users, or the sexual partners of IV drug users. The life circumstances of these women, aside from HIV status, are likely to have profound implications for decision-making regarding reproduction. How HIV infection complicates this picture is unclear. Some women infected with HIV indicate that childbearing would be inappropriate for them; others suggest that having children offers an element of hope in a life otherwise dominated by despair. Between these extremes, we have little understanding of the determinants of childbearing among women who are infected with HIV or at high risk for infection. We know even less about the impact of HIV-related illness or knowledge of HIV serostatus on decision-making regarding pregnancy.

One of the few reports to study how knowledge of HIV status affects decisions about pregnancy found that knowledge of status had little or no influence on the likelihood of undergoing induced abortion.[16] In that study, however, 44% of women infected with HIV did choose to undergo abortion. Further, how knowledge of serostatus influences decisions to become pregnant may be very different from how it influences decisions to terminate an existing pregnancy. The Institute of Medicine[18] has noted that

[a]lthough knowledge of HIV infection status alone may not fundamentally alter fertility-related behavior, this information must still be regarded as germane to reproductive counseling and planning. . . . A woman's knowledge of her own HIV infection may be a potentially empowering tool in evaluating her current and future reproductive options, even if such knowledge does not change her final decision. As more information accumulates regarding the effect of pregnancy on maternal disease progression and the impact of HIV infection on pregnancy outcome, learning of one's infection may become increasingly important for women facing reproductive decisions.

The potential usefulness of knowing one's HIV serostatus for making an informed decision regarding pregnancy is one argument for offering prenatal screening for HIV infection. Although a detailed discussion of prenatal HIV screening is beyond our scope, we note that a recent Institute of Medicine report was opposed to any mandatory newborn or prenatal HIV screening program but also concluded "that screening pregnant women for the purpose of early diagnosis and treatment is both an achievable and compelling objective." The Institute of Medicine report recommended offering voluntary HIV screening for all pregnant women in high HIV-prevalence geographic areas.[18]

Successful prevention strategies will depend not only on better understanding of what influences a woman's decision-making regarding pregnancy but also on clarifying obstacles to implementing decisions to prevent pregnancy. The National Survey of Family Growth conducted by the National Center for Health Statistics indicated that almost 60% of pregnancies among United States women in 1984–1988 were unintended; in 1988, 82% of pregnancies among teenagers were unintended.[19] Insofar as safe and effective methods of contraception are available in the United States, why are unintended pregnancy rates so high? Issues regarding the acceptability of available contraceptive methods and access to contraceptive services need to be explored, as do determinants of consistent and correct use of chosen contraceptive methods. Uncertainties regarding these issues need to be resolved if we are to help women infected with HIV who decide to prevent pregnancy to do so successfully.

Safety and Efficacy of Contraceptive Choices

The goals of primary prevention of HIV among reproductive-age women and the prevention of unintended pregnancy among women with HIV infection and women at high risk overlap when contraceptive choices are considered. Two methods of contraception—condoms and spermicides, often used together for the prevention of pregnancy—have also been encouraged for the prevention of sexually transmitted infections, including HIV infection. Some of the other currently available methods of contraception (discussed below) may also affect HIV transmission or disease progression. In general, any concerns remain theoretical; data to address potential relationships are scant or absent. The etiologic relationships between contraceptive use and HIV infection must be defined to permit sound recommendations regarding which alternatives for preventing pregnancy among women with HIV infection and women at high risk for infection are appropriate.

CONDOMS

Condoms undeniably afford protection against both pregnancy and HIV transmission. Although the degree of protection has been questioned, latex condoms clearly are a highly effective mechanical barrier to both spermatozoa and HIV. Several *in vitro* studies have found that latex condoms are impermeable to HIV.[20,21] An additional *in vitro* study found that latex condoms are impermeable to hepatitis B surface antigen (22 nm in diameter), which is appreciably smaller than HIV (120 nm in diameter).[22] A study using scanning electron microscopy on 50 samples of stretched and unstretched latex condoms found no pores in any condoms even at 2000× magnification (unpublished study sponsored by the National Institute of Child Health and Human Development). How well natural membrane condoms work as a mechanical barrier to HIV is uncertain. Because pore sizes in lamb cecum vary, some pore sizes may be large enough to allow passage of HIV; the limited *in vitro* data available to address this issue are inconsistent. At present, therefore, we must consider natural membrane condoms to be a less effective barrier to HIV than latex condoms.

Although latex condoms are an effective barrier to both HIV and spermatozoa (3,000 nm in diameter) *in vitro,* clinical studies typically report that condoms fail to prevent pregnancy in 10% to 15% of users per year of use (Table 26–1). The discrepancy between *in vitro* and clinical efficacy appears to be largely attributable to characteristics of the condom user. Although condom breakage may account for some failures, two surveys of condom breakage during vaginal intercourse found breakage rates of less than 1%.[23,24] The apparently low breakage rate of condoms during vaginal intercourse suggests that the major determinants of condom effectiveness are the consistency and correctness of condom use.

A report from the United Kingdom quantified the user's role in determining the effectiveness of condoms for preventing pregnancy and, by inference, for preventing HIV transmission.[25] In that study of married women using condoms to prevent pregnancy, pregnancy rates varied from less than 1 per 100 woman-years of use to about 15 per 100 woman-years of use, depending on selected user characteristics. Older women, women of low parity, and women who had used condoms for more than 4 years had the lowest rates. These data support the estimates of others (see Table 26–6) that a rate of 2 pregnancies per 100 woman-years of use can be achieved when condoms are consistently and correctly used. By analogy, properly used condoms should also yield high rates of clinical effectiveness for preventing HIV transmission.

The behavioral determinants of proper condom use are poorly understood. Clearly, consistency of use requires high motivation, acceptance of use by both sex partners, and the availability of condoms with each act of intercourse. The misperception that condoms are unreliable (when used properly) may be a self-fulfilling prophecy. The misperception may reduce motivation, which in turn reduces the likelihood of proper use and increases the likelihood of failure. Even highly motivated users may experience failures, however, if condoms are not used correctly. The Centers for Disease Control has published instructions for correct condom use.[26]

CONDOMS AND SPERMICIDES

Although latex condoms can serve as an effective barrier to HIV transmission, the role of spermicides, used in combination with condoms, remains unclear. Spermicides, including nonoxynol-9, are highly effective at inactivating HIV *in vitro.*[21,27,28] Reported *in vitro* data are limited, however, to cell-free HIV; the effectiveness of spermicides against cell-associated HIV is uncharacterized. Further, studies of clinical effectiveness are limited and inconsistent. To be clinically effective, spermicides would have to be present in sufficient concentration over all areas (presumably the entire vagina and cervix) of potential contact with HIV.[29] Whether the relatively small amount of spermicide present in a lubricated condom is sufficient for this purpose is unknown.

Questions have recently been raised regarding the safety of spermicides that are used with condoms for HIV prevention. Skin irritation caused by sensitivity or allergy is the most common side-effect of spermicide use.[30] The frequency and severity of irritation may be related to the frequency of application. In one small study of female commercial sex workers in British Columbia, 38% of women reported that condoms lubricated with nonoxynol-9 caused vaginal irritation; 16% reported that they had stopped using spermicidally lubricated condoms because of irritation.[31] By causing vaginal irritation and thereby producing inflammatory cells, and possibly by causing micro-ulceration, spermicides could potentially enhance the likelihood of HIV transmission. This concern is only a theoretical one at present.

Table 26–1. Contraceptive Method Failure Rates During the First Year of Use, United States

Method	% of Women Experiencing Accidental Pregnancy During First Year of Use		
	*Lowest Expected**	*Typical†*	*Lowest Reported‡*
Condom	2	12	4.2
Spermicides	3	21	0.0
Diaphragm	6	18	2.1
Oral contraceptives			
Combined	0.1	—	0.0
Progestin only	0.5	—	1.1
IUD			
Progestasert	2.0		1.9
Copper-T 380A	0.8		0.5
Norplant	0.04	0.04	0.0
Female sterilization	0.2	0.4	0.0
Male sterilization	0.1	0.15	0.0
Chance	85	85	43.1

* As estimated by Trussel et al[46] based on consistent, correct, and continuous use during the first year use.
† Among typical couples who start use (not necessarily for the first time) and continue use during the first year.
‡ Based on a literature review by Trussel et al.[46]
Adapted with permission from Trussel J, Hatcher RA, Cates W Jr et al: Contraceptive failure in the United States. Stud Fam Plann 21:51, 1990.

Whether spermicides have any beneficial or harmful impact on HIV transmission warrants further evaluation. In the meantime, it is appropriate to view the use of condoms and spermicides as separate HIV prevention strategies. The U.S. Food and Drug Administration (FDA) has approved the use of spermicides without condoms for preventing pregnancy but has given no such approval for using them without condoms to prevent sexually transmitted diseases (STDs), including HIV. Spermicides used alone for preventing pregnancy, however, are associated with high failure rates (the typical reported failure rate is 21% during the first year's use, see Table 26-1). Thus, most family planning professionals recommend that spermicides be used in combination with other barriers, including condoms.

At present, no justification exists for using spermicides alone to prevent HIV transmission. Because the clinical effectiveness of spermicides for preventing HIV transmission may depend on both the concentration and amount used, some recommend a separate intravaginal application of spermicides when spermicides are employed (*versus* the relatively small amount of spermicide present in lubricated condoms).[26] The comparative safety and effectiveness of these approaches are untested.

OTHER BARRIER METHODS

Vaginal diaphragms and cervical caps are used in combination with spermicides for pregnancy prevention, with lowest expected and typical failure rates of 6% and 18%, respectively (see Table 26-1). Whether these methods protect against HIV transmission is uncertain. Both methods provide barrier protection of the cervix, but the extent to which the cervix contributes to HIV uptake in the female genital tract is uncertain. Because the stratified squamous epithelium of the adult vagina is several layers thick and because the cervical epithelium includes both squamous epithelium and a single layer of columnar cells, the cervix may be a more likely site of infection than the vagina.[29] One study of four seropositive women found that all four had immunohistochemical evidence of HIV infection in cervical biopsy specimens; none had immunohistochemical markers of HIV infection in the vaginal tissue.[32] Although theoretical considerations and those limited data suggest that the cervix may be a key site for HIV entry into the female genital tract, experimental studies of genital tract transmission of simian immunodeficiency virus (SIV) in rhesus monkeys after hysterectomy suggest that the presence of a cervix is not required for SIV transmission to occur in monkeys (N. J. Alexander, pers. commun.). Until we better understand the role of the cervix in HIV transmission, the degree of protection afforded by barriers such as vaginal diaphragms and cervical caps will remain unclear. At present, because the vagina is presumably acceptable to HIV, using a diaphragm or cervical cap cannot be considered an appropriate alternative to using a condom for preventing HIV transmission. Further research on the role of mechanical and chemical barriers in preventing HIV infection should focus on developing prevention strategies that women can control.

The contraceptive vaginal sponge warrants special mention because one report has identified an increased risk of HIV seroconversion associated with the use of nonoxynol-9–impregnated sponges among commercial sex workers in Nairobi.[33] In that study, women who used sponges were more likely than those who did not to have genital ulcers and ulcer-associated HIV seroconversion. Whether using contraceptive sponges was causally associated with an increased risk of HIV infection is uncertain. Trauma inflicted by the sponge, use of spermicides, or both could potentially have influenced transmission.

INTRAUTERINE DEVICES

Two IUDs are currently marketed in the United States, the Copper-T 380A (ParaGard) and the progesterone-releasing IUD (Progestasert). Both are highly effective contraceptives (see Table 26–1); although the progesterone-releasing IUD is considered to be effective for only 1 year, the Copper-T 380A is approved by the FDA for 6 to 8 years of continuous use.

Although IUDs offer the advantage of not requiring specific action at the time of coitus and requiring less motivation for use than oral contraceptives, they are not appropriate for all potential users. IUDs are best suited for women at low risk for STDs. Women using IUDs in mutually monogamous relationships appear to be at little or no increased risk for pelvic inflammatory disease relative to women who do not use IUDs.[34] Women at high risk for STDs, however, are at substantially increased risk for pelvic inflammatory disease in general. Thus, IUD use cannot be recommended for most women at high risk for any STD, including HIV infection.[35] Further, there are theoretical concerns and limited data[36] suggesting that pelvic inflammatory disease in women infected with HIV may be clinically more severe than in uninfected women.

No reason exists to believe that IUDs protect against HIV transmission, and theoretical concerns have been raised regarding IUD-associated trauma and increased risks of HIV transmission. At any rate, if risks of STDs, including HIV, exist, condoms should be used by the partners of women wearing IUDs for pregnancy prevention.

ORAL CONTRACEPTIVES

Oral contraceptives, like IUDs, are highly effective for preventing pregnancy (see Table 26–1) and provide no apparent protection against HIV transmission. A study of female commercial sex workers in Nairobi raised concerns regarding a possible increased risk of transmission,[37] but data remain limited and inconsistent on this question.[38–41] Because oral contraceptives increase the likelihood of cervical ectopy (an increased percentage of the surface of the cervix covered by single-layered columnar epithelium), a harmful effect is biologically plausible, depending on the importance of the cervix for HIV transmission. In contrast, the effect of oral contraceptives on cervical mucus decreases the risk that some STDs will ascend into the upper genital tract. To the extent that the upper genital tract is important in HIV transmission, it is reasonable to speculate that oral contraceptives could potentially confer a protective effect. The impact, if any, of oral contraceptives on the risk of HIV transmission is uncertain. Regardless, women who are using oral contraceptives to prevent pregnancy and who are at risk for HIV should be advised that condom use is important, in addition, for the prevention of sexually transmitted infection.

Theoretical questions have been raised regarding the influence of oral contraceptives on HIV disease progression. Although sex steroid hormones, including oral contraceptives, have regulatory effects on immune function,[42] the clinical impact, if any, of those effects relative to HIV disease is unknown. Oral contraceptives produce opposite effects on two autoimmune conditions in women: they reduce inflammation among some women with rheumatoid arthritis but worsen the clinical course of some women with systemic lupus erythematosus. In theory, immunologic changes attributable to oral contraceptives could be either harmful or beneficial relative to HIV disease. The theoretical considerations noted do not currently warrant any changes in prescribing practice or the use of oral contraceptives.

NORPLANT

Oral contraceptives are highly effective for preventing pregnancy but require daily motivation for correct use. A new FDA-approved contraceptive, Norplant, is now available in the United States. Norplant delivers levonorgestrel (a progestin frequently used in oral contraceptive preparations) through a system of six Silastic rods. The system is implanted in the skin of the upper arm and is highly effective (see Table 26–1) for at least 5 years. The implant is inserted and removed on an outpatient basis and under local anesthesia. The expense of the system will likely limit its availability. The current cost estimate for the system alone is $350, to which are added physicians' fees for insertion and removal.

No studies of the relationship between Norplant and HIV transmission or HIV disease progression have been reported, although some of the same theoretical issues raised in regard to oral contraceptives (those that relate to the progestin component) pertain. In addition, one major side-effect of Norplant is irregular menstruation. The effect of menstrual blood on HIV transmission is not known.[35] Though such issues merit evaluation, the potential usefulness of Norplant to prevent unintended pregnancy is already evident.

Concerns that women infected with HIV may be coerced to use Norplant have generated controversy. Certainly, Norplant offers women an important new contraceptive option. However, all women, including those infected with HIV, must have ready access to medical service for both inserting and removing the implant, and both procedures must be voluntary and performed only after informed consent has been obtained.

STERILIZATION

Like steroid hormone contraceptives and IUDs, male and female sterilizations are highly effective (see Table 26–1); unlike those methods, however, sterilization is intended to be permanent. Although sterilizations may be surgically reversed in some circumstances,[43] it is often not possible to do so, and surgical restoration of fertility or *in vitro* fertilization is expensive and often unavailable, particularly to persons with limited financial resources.[44] Persons who decide to undergo sterilization rather than to use temporary methods of contraception should be certain that they accept the permanence of their decision not to bear children. In-depth counseling before sterilization helps ensure that individuals have carefully considered such a decision and understand its permanence. Studies have reported that the rate of regret after sterilization may be high.[44] Persons infected with HIV may consider sterilization to prevent perinatal transmission even if ambivalence regarding future childbearing exists. Thus, it is particularly important that regret after sterilization be minimized by careful presterilization counseling.

Concerns have been raised that persons infected with HIV, particularly women of reproductive age, may be strongly encouraged or even coerced to undergo sterilization. Although sterilization is clearly a potentially useful although not foolproof option for preventing perinatal HIV transmission (see Table 26–1), it should be part of a range of contraceptive options and reserved for those who have completed childbearing and desire the procedure after informed consent is obtained.

No known biologic relationship exists between sterilization and HIV transmission. Vasectomy decreases the number of leukocytes in semen and prevents epididymal components from entering the ejaculate.[29] Although these factors could theoretically reduce HIV infectiousness, vasectomy does not influence the efficiency of retrovirus transmission in mice.[29] At present, couples using sterilization to prevent pregnancy should be counseled to also use condoms for preventing HIV infection if either partner is at risk.[35]

Service Programs

Although a detailed description of family planning service delivery to persons infected with HIV and persons at high risk is beyond the scope of this report, it is noteworthy that a relatively small portion of individuals infected with HIV attend family planning clinics. Blinded serosurveys of women attending family planning clinics indicate a low prevalence of HIV infection, even in cities where surveys among childbearing women indicate a relatively high prevalence of infection.[45] Most women infected with HIV are poor and IV drug users or are the sexual partners of IV drug users. To effectively serve these women, providers must make their services available at low cost and in a manner sensitive to the life circumstances of infected individuals. Improved access to family planning services will require provision of those services in nontraditional settings such as drug treatment facilities, prisons, and shelters for the homeless. Further, outreach efforts will be necessary to ensure that persons infected with HIV and persons at high risk are aware that family planning services are available.

Family planning providers have an excellent opportunity to prevent HIV transmission. The overwhelming majority of clients are women who are sexually active and thus potentially at risk for acquiring STDs, including HIV infection, as well as becoming pregnant. Further, many clients have few other interactions with health care providers that might help them to prevent HIV infection. Proper counseling and support for changes in behavior that reduce the risks of acquiring infection can help women protect themselves. The consistent and correct use of contraception can prevent perinatal transmission of HIV by preventing unintended pregnancy. Condoms protect against both infection and pregnancy, but other contraceptive methods may not. Family planning providers should be particularly able to address the relationship between contraception and HIV transmission, thereby helping all clients to prevent infection and helping those who so choose to prevent pregnancy as well.

REFERENCES

1. Jovaisas E, Koch MA, Schafer A et al: LAV/HTLV-III in 20-week fetus. Lancet 2:1129, 1985
2. Mundy DC, Schinazi RF, Gerber AR et al: Human immunodeficiency virus isolated from amniotic fluid. Lancet 2:459, 1987
3. Sprecher S, Soumenkoff G, Puissant F, Degueldre M: Vertical transmission of HIV in a 15-week fetus. Lancet 2:288, 1986
4. Blanche S, Rouzioux C, Moscato MG et al: A prospective study of infants born to women seropositive for human immunodeficiency virus type 1. N Engl J Med 320:1643, 1989
5. European Collaborative Study: Mother-to-child transmission of HIV infection. Lancet 2:1039, 1988
6. Italian Multicentre Study: Epidemiology, clinical features, and prognostic factors of paediatric HIV infection. Lancet 2:1043, 1988
7. Hira FK, Mangrola UG, Mwale C et al: Apparent vertical transmission of human immunodeficiency virus type 1 by breast-feeding in Zambia. J Pediatr 117:421, 1990
8. Oxtoby MJ: Human immunodeficiency virus and other viruses in human milk: Placing the issues in broader perspective. Pediatr Infect Dis J 7:825, 1988
9. Manzila T, Baende E, Kabagabo U et al: Inability to demonstrate a dose-response effect between receipt of mother's milk and perinatally-acquired infection (PI) in a cohort of 114 infants born to HIV(+) mothers (abstr 4004). Presented at the IV International Conference on AIDS, Stockholm, June 1988
10. Ryder R, Nsa W, Behets F et al: Perinatal HIV transmission in two African hospitals: One-year follow-up (abstr 4128). Presented at the IV International Conference on AIDS, Stockholm, June 1988
11. European Collaborative Study: Children born to women with HIV-1 infection: Natural history and risk of transmission. Lancet 337:253, 1991
12. Devash Y, Calvelli TA, Wood DG et al: Vertical transmission of human immunodeficiency virus is correlated with the absence of high-affinity/avidity maternal antibodies to the gp120 principal neutralizing domain. Proc Natl Acad Sci USA 87:3445, 1990
13. Goedert JJ, Mendez H, Drummond JE et al: Mother-to-infant transmission of human immunodeficiency virus type 1: Association with prematurity or low anti-gp120. Lancet 2:1352, 1989
14. Rossi P, Moschese V, Broliden PA et al: Presence of maternal antibodies to human immunodeficiency virus 1 envelope glycoprotein gp120 epitopes correlates with the uninfected status of children born to seropositive mothers. Proc Natl Acad Sci USA 86:8055, 1989
15. Parekh BS, Shaffer N, Pau C-P et al: Lack of correlation between maternal antibodies to V-3 loop peptides of gp 120 in perinatal HIV-1 transmission. Unpublished manuscript, 1991
16. Selwyn PA, Schoenbaum EE, Davenny K et al: Prospective study of human immunodeficiency virus infection and pregnancy outcomes in intravenous drug users. JAMA 261:1289, 1989
17. Lindsay MK, Peterson HB, Feng TI et al: Routine antepartum human immunodeficiency virus infection screening in an inner-city population. Obstet Gynecol 74:289, 1989
18. Institute of Medicine, Hardy LM (ed): HIV Screening of Pregnant Women and Newborns. Washington, DC, National Academy Press, 1991
19. Forrest JD, Singh S: The sexual and reproductive behavior of American women, 1982–1988. Fam Plan Perspect 22:206, 1990
20. Van de Perre P, Jacobs D, Sprecher-Goldberger S: The latex condom, an efficient barrier against transmission of AIDS-related viruses. AIDS 1:49, 1987
21. Rietmeijer CAM, Krebs JW, Feorino PM, Judson FN: Condoms as physical and chemical barriers against human immunodeficiency virus. JAMA 259:1851, 1988
22. Minuk GY, Bohme CE, Bowen TJ: Condoms and hepatitis B virus infection. Ann Intern Med 104:584, 1986
23. Consumers Union: Consumer Reports, March 1989, p 135
24. Richters J, Donovan B, Gerofi J, Watson L: Low condom breakage rate in commercial sex. Lancet 2:1489, 1988
25. Vessey MP, Villard-Mackintosh L, McPherson K, Yeates D: Factors influencing use-effectiveness of the condom. Br J Fam Plann 14:40, 1988
26. Centers for Disease Control: Condoms for prevention of sexually transmitted diseases. MMWR 37:133, 1988
27. Hicks DR, Martin LS, Getchell JP et al: Inactivation of HTLV-III/LAV-infected cultures of normal human lymphocytes by nonoxynol-9 *in vitro* (letter). Lancet 2:1422, 1985

28. Voeller B: Nonoxynol-9 and HTLV-III (letter). Lancet 1: 1153, 1986

29. Alexander NJ: Sexual transmission of human immunodeficiency virus: Virus entry into the male and female genital tract. Fertil Steril 54:1, 1990

30. Hatcher RA, Stewart F, Trussell J et al: Contraceptive Technology, 1990–1992, 15th rev ed. New York, Irvington, 1990

31. Rekart ML, Barnett JA, Manzon LM et al: Nonoxynol-9: Its adverse effects (abstr S.C.36). Presented at the VI International Conference on AIDS, San Francisco, June 1990

32. Donegan SP, de la Monte S, Steger KA et al: HIV-1 infection of the lower female genital tract (abstr F.C.750). Presented at the VI International Conference on AIDS, San Francisco, June 1990

33. Kreiss J, Ruminjo I, Ngugi E et al: Efficacy of nonoxynol-9 in preventing HIV transmission (abstr M.A.O.36). Presented at the VI International Conference on AIDS, Montreal, June 1989

34. Lee NC, Rubin GL, Borucki R: The intrauterine device and pelvic inflammatory disease revisited: New results from the Women's Health Study. Obstet Gynecol 72:1, 1988

35. World Health Organization: AIDS Prevention: Guidelines for MCH/FP programme managers. I. AIDS and family planning. Geneva, World Health Organization, June 1990

36. Hoegsberg B, Abulafia O, Sedlis A et al: Sexually transmitted diseases and human immunodeficiency virus infection among women with pelvic inflammatory disease. Am J Obstet Gynecol 163:1135, 1990

37. Plummer F, Cameron W, Simonsen N et al: Cofactors in male-female transmission of HIV. J Infect Dis 163:223, 1991

38. Darrow WW, Bigler W, Deppe D et al: HIV antibody in 640 United States prostitutes with no evidence of intravenous drug abuse (abstr 4054). Presented at the IV International Conference on AIDS, Stockholm, June 1988

39. Mati J, Maggwa A, Chewe D et al: Contraceptive use and HIV infection among women attending family planning clinics in Nairobi, Kenya (abstr Th.C.99). Presented at the VI International Conference on AIDS, San Francisco, June 1990

40. Musicco M, the Italian Partners' Study: Oral contraception, IUD, condom use and man to woman sexual transmission of HIV infection (abstract Th.C.584). Presented at the VI International Conference on AIDS, San Francisco, June 1990

41. Goedert JJ et al: Rate of heterosexual HIV transmission and associated risk with HIV antigen (abstr 4019). Presented at the IV International Conference on AIDS, Stockholm, June 1988

42. Grossman CJ, Roselle GA, Meadenhall CL: Sex steroid regulation of autoimmunity. J Steroid Biochem (in press)

43. Peterson HB, Huber DH, Belker AM: Vasectomy: An appraisal for the obstetrician-gynecologist. Obstet Gynecol 76:568, 1990

44. Wilcox LS, Chu SY, Peterson HB: Characteristics of women who considered or obtained tubal reanastomosis: Results from a prospective study of tubal sterilization. Obstet Gynecol 75:61, 1990

45. Allen DM, Lee NC, Schulz SL et al: Determining HIV seroprevalence among women in women's health clinics. Public Health Rep 105:130, 1990

46. Trussell J, Hatcher R, Cates W Jr et al: Contraceptive failure in the United States. Stud Fam Plann 21:51, 1990

27

AIDS Vaccines

Dani P. Bolognesi

Despite overwhelming obstacles that stand before it, the search for a vaccine against human immunodeficiency virus (HIV) is now a full-fledged target goal of the biomedical research establishment. Much as experience with azidothymide has demonstrated that antiviral agents can be effective and has opened the field of anti-AIDS drugs, successful trials in animal models with candidate immunogens have established the all-important first step of feasibility and paved the way for the development of candidate vaccines, several of which are already being evaluated in man. In this chapter, progress with both simian immunodeficiency virus (SIV) and HIV vaccine research is reviewed and balanced against the many challenges that still lie ahead.

PROGRESS IN SIV VACCINE RESEARCH

The AIDS-like disease that develops in certain small subhuman primates following infection with SIV, a virus that is quite similar to HIV, establishes this as a most attractive model for development of an AIDS vaccine. Susceptible animals remain generally plentiful, the time courses for infection and disease are relatively brief, and a number of diverse SIV isolates exist that can be evaluated as both immunogens and challenge stocks. Most of the vaccine trials have used whole inactivated virus or infected cell preparations, although more recent studies have employed peptides, envelope subunits, recombinant vectors, or combinations thereof.

Inactivated Vaccines

The first attempts at vaccination with killed virus preparations were carried out by Desrosiers and colleagues[1] at the New England Primate Center with the SIVmac251 strain in rhesus macaques. A number of experiments

were conducted with different immunization and challenge protocols, with the ultimate result that two of six vaccinated monkeys were protected long term against infection. Serologic measurements included overall antibody levels and neutralizing antibody titer. Neither appeared to correlate with protection, except that an anamnestic antibody response was detected in vaccinates that became infected but was absent in protected animals.

These promising results were followed rapidly by a report from Murphey-Corb *et al*[2] at the Delta Primate Center, where eight of nine animals were protected following immunization with a formalin-fixed whole virus vaccine. In this study a virus isolate from a sooty mangabey, SIVsm Delta B670, was employed, albeit at a significantly lower dose than used by Desrosiers *et al.*[1] Again, however, protection failed to correlate with the overall level of vaccine-induced antibodies, nor were significant titers of neutralizing antibodies detected.

Parallel studies were also carried out at the California Primate Center at Davis by Carlson *et al*,[3] who used SIVmac251 inactivated by β-propiolactone. In this experiment, animals received the immunogen with different adjuvants and the challenge dose was similar to the one used at the Delta Primate Center. Again, long-term protection was achieved, the efficiency of which appeared to be dependent on the adjuvant used. In these studies there was partial correlation between protection and the prechallenge titers of neutralizing antibody.[3] However, when the same neutralization assay was applied to the animals in the New England Primate Center experiment, such a correlation was not apparent (A. J. Langlois, unpubl. observ.).

Protection against virus infection was also achieved by immunization with SIVmac251–infected cells fixed with glutaraldehyde.[4] Before challenge, prominent humoral and cellular responses were detectable, including cytotoxic T-cell responses to the SIV *gag* protein, although sera from the immunized animals failed to demonstrate neutralizing activity against the challenge virus pool.[5]

Taken together, these results indicate that vaccination with certain combinations of immunogen, adjuvant, and challenge virus dose can effectively prevent experimental infection with SIV. These achievements pave the way for determining the nature of the protective response and the essential components of the immunogen(s) against which it is elicited. Moreover, recent advances in SIV vaccine research indicate that animals vaccinated with preparations derived from one strain can resist infection from a divergent isolate.[6,7] From such models, one should be able to approach the all-important barrier of cross-protective immunity and the mechanisms involved.

Component Specific Vaccines

To date, studies along this line have employed virus envelope and core proteins in various configurations. In the main, the results thus far with such approaches have not been as consistent as those obtained with inactivated vaccines. No protection was achieved using a vaccinia recombinant expressing the SIVmac251 *env* gene alone or in combination with the *gag* gene.[8] These immunizations produced significantly higher titers of neutralizing antibodies than were obtained with whole killed virus preparations in comparable studies.[8] In contrast, experiments carried out by Hu and colleagues[9] at the Seattle Primate Center, in which a full *env*-expressing vaccinia vector was used to prime the immune response and was followed by a booster immunization with the envelope subunit produced in a baculovirus expression system, have provided long-term protection against infection of cynomolgus monkeys with SIV from *macaca menestrina* (SIVmne). Neutralizing titers were achieved in the vaccinated animals that compared favorably with those observed in persistently infected animals.

Two separate studies have been conducted with viral subunits. Detergent-disrupted virus preparations were fractionated over lentil-lectin columns and the bound (envelope-enriched) and unbound (core-enriched) materials were used to immunize animals.[10] Partial protection (two of four animals) was achieved with the envelope fraction; no protection was evident with the core material. Neutralizing antibodies were either low or absent with the assays employed.

Attempts at vaccination using purified envelope subunits produced by recombinant expression systems have also failed to induce protection against infection (Planelles *et al,* in prep.; L. D. Giodovini *et al,* in prep.; S. Putney *et al,* unpubl. observ.), even when significant titers of neutralizing antibodies were present (A. J. Langlois, unpubl. observ.).

Peptides representing conserved domains within both the external and transmembrane glycoproteins have induced a different form of protection against infection.[11] Immunized animals, although not completely resisting infection, appeared capable of suppressing virus replication to a considerable degree. In these studies, there appeared to be some correlation between antibody titers, particularly titers of neutralizing antibodies, and the degree of virus suppression observed.

Correlates of Protection in the SIV Model

From the information outlined above it is apparent that little is known about the nature of the immune functions responsible for the protection achieved. A common interpretation of the results is that protection does not correlate with neutralizing antibody titers. This general observation is punctuated by contrary instances in which protection was achieved despite the absence of detectable neutralizing antibodies to the challenge virus,[5] as well as instances in which neutralizing antibodies were clearly present but no protection was observed.[8] It would appear at first that other forms of immunity are responsible, the most likely being that associated with the cellular arm of the immune response. The demonstration that *gag*-specific cytotoxic lymphocytes (CTL) were present in animals immunized with glutaraldehyde-fixed infected cells points to cellular immunity as a possible candidate mechanism.[5]

The issue, however, is far from clear. If cellular immunity is responsible, what forms could be involved when the immunogen is a nonreplicating virus particle? Are such particles capable of efficient induction of class I major histocompatibility complex (MHC)–restricted CTL, considered to be the prevalent mechanism for virus clearance? Such cells are thought to be induced most efficiently by antigens that are synthesized *de novo* within antigen-presenting cells. Do such particles have properties akin to lipid-derived peptides[12] or subunit/adjuvant combinations,[13] which apparently can enter the cell in such a manner as to be recognized as endogenously synthesized antigens? In the same context, it is likely that class II MHC–restricted CTL are induced by these particles,[14] and this cell may also play a role in protection,[15] although no clear precedent exists in a vaccine setting. Another mechanism that should be mentioned has to do with antibody-armed killer cells (usually of the natural killer [NK] cell lineage), which have been shown to be present in HIV-infected individuals[16] and are likely to be present in SIV-infected animals.[17] Although no clear role for antibody-dependent cellular cytotoxicity (ADCC) has been established in viral diseases, it nevertheless deserves consideration at this stage of vaccine development.

The experiments conducted thus far with live recombinant vaccinia vectors should also help resolve these questions, although the results obtained are quixotic. Vaccinia *env* or vaccinia *env* plus *gag* did not protect against infection but did induce neutralizing antibodies.[8] In a separate study a vaccinia *env* vector did not induce neutralizing antibodies, but good titers became evident after a boost with a recombinant envelope subunit.[9] When animals in the latter study were challenged after the boost with the subunit, protection was achieved. Why the difference between these two experiments, particularly if cellular immunity is favored as the protective response? Might there have been protection in the latter study before the booster, possibly induced by a superior vaccinia vector? Did the subunit booster enhance CTL activity, which is protective, or is a combination of cellular and humoral (neutralizing antibodies) responses an important feature of protection? Note that in the prime/boost study,[9] only envelope components were involved, which would tend to obviate an obligatory need for other viral gene products. Again, until the critical measurements are made one can only hypothesize as to the possible significance of these studies.

Some caveats exist with regard to the use of neutralizing antibodies as an index of immunity. First and foremost, the assays used to measure these activities vary markedly from laboratory to laboratory, depending on their respective configurations. Thus, titer differences are very difficult to evaluate from study to study, particularly if they are not related to a standard reference serum to neutralizing antibody levels in an infected animal or to a common virus stock (some SIV isolates are very difficult to neutralize). There is clearly a need for a common set of assays that would allow these activities to be evaluated side by side and appropriately standardized. With regard to cellular immunity, it is also evident that functional assays must be established within the SIV model that can measure MHC-restricted CTL in SIV-susceptible monkeys, as recently shown by Letvin and colleagues.[18]

No less important to a resolution of the above issues are considerations such as challenge dose, virus host combinations, immunization schedules, and the nature of the adjuvants used. The studies to date are quite disparate in these regards,[5] and insofar as such factors are clearly integral to the question of what determines protective immunity, some standardization will be required before we can understand both the successes and the failures of the vaccine trials.

Impact of SIV Vaccines on Disease

In several of the vaccine studies, even though protection against infection was not uniformly observed, some of the preparations induced an immune response that significantly delayed the onset of disease.[1,19,20] The immunogens that gave such results included killed virus,[1] live attenuated virus,[19] and possibly peptides.[11] In addition, a distinct but close relative of SIV, HIV-2, which is nonpathogenic in monkeys, also induced a protective response against disease[20] but not against infection. In general, the observations in such cases indicate that the vaccinated animals appear able to control virus replication and possibly virus spread much more efficiently than nonvaccinated animals. On the other hand, vaccination of already infected animals has had no demon-

strable effect on either viremia or disease,[21,22] indicating that once the virus has established residence, it may be very difficult to alter on its pathogenic course.

At present, the mechanism whereby vaccination aids the host in suppressing the virus is not understood. One hypothesis is that vaccination reduces the infectious dose to a level that is more manageable by the immune system. More important to determine, however, is whether vaccine-induced immunity is superior at controlling the virus than the immune response that is naturally generated in response to infection.

HIV VACCINE DEVELOPMENT

To date, HIV-1 is known to infect only man and the chimpanzee. It follows that testing of vaccines for efficacy can proceed only in these two species, which places rather severe limitations on vaccine development. Nonetheless, vaccine studies in both systems have been encouraging.

Trials of HIV-1 Candidate Vaccines in Chimpanzees

The chimpanzee HIV-1 model differs from SIV in a number of respects. First, HIV-1 infection in chimpanzees does not lead to disease. Second, the number of chimpanzees available for research is dwindling, which dictates that experiments be limited to a few animals. Third, safety restrictions are similar to those applied to man, making it difficult to incorporate promising experimental adjuvants or carriers or other developmental vaccinology tools.

Between 1985 and 1989 a number of vaccine-related studies were conducted in chimpanzees. As with the SIV model, the immunogens used were derived principally from the HIV-1 envelope and included killed virus, subunits, peptides, and vaccinia recombinants.[23] None of these approaches protected against infection; but, importantly, at the time of challenge only low or no neutralizing antibodies and relatively weak cellular immunity were measurable.

The poor immunogenicity of these preparations led other groups to take different tacts. Girard and colleagues[24] at Pasteur Vaccins employed the prime/boost approach and tried several combinations of whole killed virus, vaccinia recombinant vectors bearing the HIV-1 envelope, *env* and *gag* viral subunits, and even nonstructural viral proteins. In the main, none of these combinations produced strong immunity. However, when animals were boosted with peptides representing the principal neutralizing determinant (PND) of the virus,[25] substantial neutralizing antibodies appeared. The animals were therefore challenged with virus, and protection was achieved.

Berman and colleagues[26] at Genentech focused instead on the properties of the immunogen and the immunization scheme. Using a highly pure preparation of gp120, a new immunization schedule, and a lower virus challenge dose, they succeeded in protecting chimpanzees against infection, reversing their own prior failed experiment.[27] In the successful study, the titer of neutralizing antibodies, particularly antibodies directed to the PND, at the time of challenge appeared to be the best correlate of protection. Of particular significance, this study employed immunogens formulated with aluminum hydroxide, an adjuvant that is suitable for use in man.

The apparent correlation between protection and the presence of neutralizing antibodies to the PND in two separate and different studies stands out and is consistent with study findings that identify this domain as the primary target of neutralizing antibodies *in vitro.*[25] In an effort to demonstrate that *in vitro* neutralization is significant *in vivo,* Emini and colleagues[28] mixed virus with neutralizing antibodies to the PND and gave the mixture to chimpanzees, with the result that no infection resulted. These studies have recently been extended to a *bona fide* passive immunization experiment with monoclonal antibodies to the PND; complete protection against infection was present at the 6-month time point (E. Emini, pers. commun.). It would thus appear that neutralizing antibodies to the PND are sufficient for protection against experimental infection with the homologous virus, which strengthens the notion that the correlation of protection with anti-PND antibodies in the vaccine studies mentioned in the previous section was probably meaningful. However, the fact that the PND also embodies CTL[29] and ADCC epitopes (K. Weinhold, unpubl. observ.) dictates that these activities also be evaluated (Fig. 27–1).

Characteristics of the HIV-1 PND

The existence of a PND in HIV-1 was established by several independent but complementary approaches. One investigative team[30] followed the reductionist approach, beginning with the entire envelope and used progressively smaller fragments until they eventually narrowed down the neutralizing antibody–inducing region to a 24-amino acid fragment within the exterior envelope glycoprotein. Importantly, not only was this fragment capable of generating neutralizing antibody activity equivalent to that induced by the whole envelope, but its presence in the neutralization reaction resulted in the abrogation of neutralizing activity of all anti-*env* antibodies, hence its designation as the PND. The very same region was uncovered by approaches that sought to identify the neutralizing antibody–inducing capability of predicted B-cell epitopes consisting of hydrophilic domains possessing strong B turns.[31] Finally, overlapping peptides covering the entire *env* gene generated only one fragment that induced neutralizing antibodies, which was localized to the same region.[32]

The PND is now known to be situated within third variable domain of the exterior gp120 glycoprotein. It

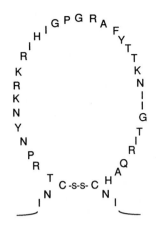

Domains of the V3 Loop

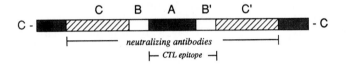

A = group specific (conserved)
B = class specific (semi-conserved)
C = type specific (variable)

Figure 27–1.   Schematic of the HIV-1 principal neutralizing domain (PND) amino acid sequence of the HIVmn isolate. A high percentage of sera from HIV-1–infected individuals from North America recognize this sequence. Variation within this domain occurs primarily at the sides of the loop; the crown and the regions near the cysteines are much less divergent from isolate to isolate. Neutralizing antibodies are principally targeted to the sides (isolate-restricted) or crown (cross-neutralizing). In addition, a CTL epitope has been mapped within this region, and evidence has been obtained that antibodies to the PND can also mediate antibody dependent cellular cytotoxicity.

is contained within a disulfide-linked loop (cysteine 303 to cysteine 337)[33] and represents a uniquely hypervariable region. This variability is apparently responsible for the predominantly isolate-specific neutralizing antibodies that result from immunization or in response to natural infection.[34] The variation in this region is extensive among naturally occurring HIV-1 isolates,[35] and significant variation occurs even within the population of viruses within a single individual.[36,37] This extensive variation, coupled with the apparent immunodominant nature of the variable domains, presents an overwhelming obstacle for vaccine development insofar as this epitope is concerned.

However, not all portions of the PND fall into the variable category, particularly regions representing the crown of the loop (see Fig. 27–1). In some instances immunization with peptides representing the PND resulted in neutralizing antibodies that recognized the semiconserved regions (the GPGRAF motif), and such sera were indeed able to cross-neutralize divergent HIV-1 isolates that possessed this sequence of amino acids within their PND.[38] To what extent this subdomain of the PND can be used to raise meaningful cross-protective immunity however remains to be determined.

The relative efficiency of anti-PND antibodies, in comparison with antibodies to other sites, in neutralizing HIV-1 suggests that this region may represent an important functional domain of the virus. Indeed, if the loop is deleted from an infectious molecular clone of the virus, infectivity is lost (S. Putney and F. Wong-Staal, pers. commun.). Similarly, amino acid substitutions at certain sites within the crown of the loop result in noninfectious viruses[39] or govern target cell preference.[40] Yet other amino acid changes appear to selectively affect the ability of HIV-1–infected cells to fuse with uninfected counterparts.[41] When this latter observation is considered in conjunction with the demonstration that anti-PND monoclonal antibodies selectively inhibit cell-cell fusion as well as virus infection at a step following binding of the envelope to the CD4 receptor,[42,43] it would appear that this domain is probably involved in the multistep process of virus entry, most likely associated with the fusion event. One hypothesis is that cleavage of the PND by proteases on the surface of the target cell represents the "trigger" for fusion. The critical cleavage sites have been proposed to reside within the semiconserved loop crown.[44,45] However, while cleavage of the PND has been observed in preparations of gp120 isolated from virions, infected cells, or mammalian expression systems (CHO cells), evidence that such cleavage occurs during the processes of infection or cell-cell fusion is lacking. Finally, it has also been suggested that the PND may contribute to the target-cell specificity of HIV-1,[46,47] perhaps through amino acid substitutions that affect its susceptibility to cleavage by different cell surface proteases.

Whatever the precise function(s) of the PND in virus entry may be, it is most likely that its conserved domains play a critical role in the process. At the same time, variation at other sites may well contribute to conformational features of the loop that are important for both function and susceptibility to immune attack, particularly by neutralizing antibodies. It is widely believed that this variability is one of the means by which the virus can escape from host immune defenses. Other factors may be represented by changes in distinct sites of the envelope, which would affect the conformation or accessibility of the PND.[48] It would thus appear that an intricate balance exists between variation, structure-function, and immune recognition in this unique structure.

Cross-Reactive Immune Responses Among Diverse HIV-1 Isolates

Experimental immunizations with HIV envelope subunits, fragments, or peptides primarily generate strain-specific neutralizing antibodies to the PND. This extends to experiments with vaccinia *env* recombinant vectors[49] and, most important, to HIV-1 infections in chimpanzees[48] and man[50] with HIV-1. The latter observations with live HIV-1 pertain to the initial neutralizing responses to the virus, which remain strain-specific for at least 1 year and perhaps longer. Thereafter the neutralizing response progressively broadens to include other isolates. This shift in responsiveness is accompanied by two important correlates: (1) recognition of other PNDs, and (2) the emergence of antibodies that block binding of gp120 and/or virus to CD4. In addition, it is likely that other potential targets are being recognized, including both linear and conformational epitopes, which for unknown reasons are occult in experimental immunizations and during the initial phases of infection. Whatever their identity, it would be important to determine their role in control of virus replication and their potential role in protection against infection. Two studies have been performed that begin to approach these questions.

In one, Prince and colleagues[51] selected sera from HIV-1–seropositive individuals on the basis of their ability to effectively cross-neutralize divergent HIV-1 isolates. The IgG fraction from the pooled sera was isolated and passively administered to chimpanzees so as to achieve circulating levels of neutralizing antibodies approaching those found in the donor pool. Two animals were then challenged with a prototypic HIV-1(IIIB) isolate and monitored for infection. Not only was infection not prevented, but no evidence was obtained that it was even retarded to a significant degree. Thus, the cross-neutralizing antibodies contained within the complex natural humoral response to HIV-1 failed to prevent HIV-1 infection. A number of possibilities have been offered to explain this result, including (1) the challenge dose may have overwhelmed the neutralizing antibody threshold, on the one hand in fact, when lower doses of challenge virus were administered, protection was achieved,[52] and (2) the presence of enhancing antibodies in the IgG preparation may have negated its neutralizing potential, on the other hand.[53] On the positive side, however, it was possible to identify high levels of circulating antibodies in the chimpanzees that blocked binding of gp120 to CD4 (T. Matthews, unpubl. observ.) and very high levels of ADCC antibodies.[51] Conspicuously missing were antibodies to the PND of the challenge virus (T. Matthews, unpubl. observ.). This was to be expected, because the HIV-1(IIIB) isolate is very rare in the population, and the outcome might have been different had a more common isolate been used.[35] These negative results with cross-neutralizing antibodies stand out sharply when compared to the studies of Emini and colleagues (described above), which demonstrated the protective capability of strain-specific anti-PND neutralizing antibodies administered passively.

In a distinct but relevant set of experiments, Fultz and colleagues[54] asked the question if preexisting immunity to infection with one HIV-1 isolate could prevent infection with a different isolate. In reciprocal studies with two divergent virus isolates, superinfection occurred in both instances despite the presence of antibody and proliferative T-cell responses specific to both strains. Although anti-PND antibodies were not analyzed, it is likely that these were only present in response to the PND of the initial infecting virus. Therefore, one interpretation of this failure by one virus to protect against challenge with a significantly different isolate after the original infection had been established is that nonprotection may be linked to the absence of anti-PND neutralizing antibodies to the superinfecting virus. This study also raises the question of the role of other forms of antiviral immunity, including those associated with the cellular arm, in protection. Indeed, almost nothing is known with regard to HIV CTL in chimpanzees.

VACCINE TRIALS IN MAN WITH HIV-1

A number of candidate immunogens are currently in the initial phases of testing in man.[55,56] To date, such trials have been carried out both in normal volunteers and in individuals already infected with HIV-1. The purpose of the trials in normal volunteers is to investigate the immunogenicity and toxicity of the preparations in a small number of subjects as an obligatory first step toward undertaking larger trials in high-risk individuals, in whom vaccine efficacy might be evaluated. The goals of the postexposure trials are to determine if vaccination is of benefit to the already infected individual, while at the same time serving as a testing ground for vaccine immunogenicity and safety. With the exception of immunogens belonging to the category of inactivated or attenuated preparations of virus or infected cells, the candidate immunogens being evaluated in normal volunteers generally mirror those undergoing animal testing in both SIV and HIV models. Thus, several envelope subunits, recombinant vaccinia bearing the HIV-1 envelope, recombinant particles with HIV-1 gene products prepared in yeast expression systems, and peptides representing portions of the p17 shell protein of the virus have been introduced in man.[55] A multitude of other virion components in various configurations are under development and consideration for clinical testing.[57]

In general, the results to date of these trials have been unremarkable from the point of view of immunogenicity testing, but neither have the immunogen and adjuvant preparations generated untoward reactions. Both aspects, however, may change as doses are esca-

lated. Indeed, it appears as if considerable quantities of certain immunogens, particularly viral subunits, may be a determining factor in the production of biologically relevant antibodies. Very little if any neutralizing activity has been detected at the lower dose ranges (up to 100 μg), and to what extent this reflects the immunogen or the carriers and adjuvants used remains unresolved.[58] One of the more interesting studies carried out used two approaches in a prime/boost configuration; a limited number of individuals initially received a gp160 envelope recombinant vaccinia vector, followed by a boost with a gp160 recombinant envelope subunit.[59] Considerable synergy was observed in both the cellular and humoral compartments. When peripheral blood mononuclear cells (PBMC) from vaccinees receiving the individual immunogens alone and in combination were introduced into SCID mice, only animals receiving PBMC from the combination resisted challenge with infectious HIV-1.[60] Whether a humoral, cellular, or combinatorial mechanism is responsible for protection remains to be determined.

Postexposure vaccination has produced results that, while puzzling, are of considerable interest. Three separate studies have been carried out employing killed virus,[61] envelope subunits,[62] and recombinant vaccinia vectors in combination with viral subunits and peptides.[63] Salk and colleagues performed studies with inactivated viral vaccines in patients already experiencing AIDS symptoms. Even though only limited immune responses specific to the vaccine were detected, some patient benefits were reported, such as stabilization of the CD4 decline and weight loss. Clinical improvement along similar lines was reported by Zagury and colleagues[63] in AIDS patients who received their own cells transformed by vaccinia recombinant vectors bearing *env, gag,* and *pol* genes of HIV-1, with the added benefit that the number of opportunistic infections was markedly reduced in comparison to the group not receiving the vaccine. Similar clinical benefits were observed by Redfield and colleagues[62] using a recombinant gp160 envelope subunit, but in that study, the immunogen used provoked novel immune responses not generally recognized in infected individuals.

To date, it has not been possible to determine the mechanism by which postexposure immunization brings about the clinical benefits observed. The hoped-for outcome is that these approaches will improve on the natural immune response, resulting in better control of the virus and its pathogenic course.[62] On the other hand, the effect may not be due to novel immune responses to the virus but may instead result from a general immune stimulation that enhances natural host defense mechanisms.[63] Both are possible, and they are not mutually exclusive. Clearly, more studies are warranted along these lines in both human and animal models, particularly with SIV, as the results with inactivated vaccines in this setting have not as yet produced the expected results.

SUMMARY AND DISCUSSION

At the heart of the issue of how best to develop an effective vaccine is an understanding of what constitutes protective immunity and how to elicit it through vaccination. To date, only fragmentary information has been obtained from SIV, chimpanzee, or human experiments as to what such immunity might entail. Moreover, insofar as most of the experiments carried out in the animal models were in the nature of feasibility studies, even if the protective elements could be defined therein, they might not necessarily apply to the more complex situations that obtain during natural transmission. Otherwise stated, immunity that is effective against experimental inocula with a given laboratory strain may not be effective against a highly divergent isolate or a mixture of natural isolates, and is even less likely to be effective against inocula consisting of both virus and infected cells. Similarly, the protective levels of immunity were achieved soon after a booster immunization, and it is not apparent to what extent these levels must be sustained in order for the vaccine to be effective in a practical sense. A dramatic illustration of these issues has been provided by studies carried out by Gardner and colleagues[64] in which it was shown that vaccine-induced immunity that produced some protection against intramuscular challenge with SIV failed to prevent infection when the virus was introduced by the mucosal route. This implies that systemic immunity may not be sufficient to protect against several modes of natural transmission that involve mucosal surfaces. Hence, although the initial protection trials in the animal models are an all-important first step, the remaining issues of how to raise cross-protective immunity that will be effective against the existing swarm of HIV-1 isolates under natural modes of transmission will require that major gaps in the current knowledge base be filled. These include basic issues such as how to correlate virus variation with biologic issues such as antigenicity, escape from immune defenses, viral transmission, tissue tropism, and pathogenesis. Equally important is the need for new insights into vaccinology principles that would address the unprecedented variability of HIV-1 and how to elicit secretory immunity in the setting of comprehensive systemic immunity.

Such considerations dictate that relevant animal models be available for extensive testing. Because of the obvious limitations on testing chimpanzees, one must look very hard in the direction of other lentiretrovirus models, particularly SIV. This leads immediately to the question of relevancy, and to what extent investigators can translate study results directly from one model to another. It appears that there may well be fundamental differences in what constitutes protective immunity against SIV in monkeys *versus* HIV-1 in chimpanzees. Thus, correlation of protection against SIV with neutralizing activity is at best weak, whereas neutralizing antibodies to the PND are currently thought to be the best correlate of protection against HIV-1 in chimpanzees. This difference is punctuated by the apparent absence of a PND within the cognate region of SIV. Indeed, the corresponding SIV domain is relatively conserved between divergent isolates,[65] and, when used as an immunogen, it induces little or no neutralizing antibody (T. Palker, unpubl. observ.).[66] Instead of a linear PND, current evidence suggests that anti-SIV neutralizing antibodies are directed at conformational determinants.[66] It remains to be determined whether this region of SIV is involved in virus entry and which variable domains of the SIV envelope are important for immune escape.[65] It is therefore possible that SIV and HIV-1 have different strategies for establishing persistent infection.

It is not clear what other aspects of the SIV model cannot be directly translated to HIV-1, and *vice versa,* but one outstanding property of SIV that is lacking in the chimpanzee HIV-1 model is the ability to induce disease very similar to human AIDS. The absence of this feature is considered a severe limitation of the chimpanzee model in relation to development of a vaccine for man. On the other hand, a better understanding of why the chimpanzee is better able to control the virus could provide fundamental clues to the development of a vaccine. The fact remains that the model can only be used to evaluate the capability of a vaccine to prevent infection, which is certainly the most relevant issue but at the same time the most difficult to achieve. Most of the viral vaccines in use protect against disease while allowing varying degrees of infection to occur. The immune response induced by the vaccine, although not sufficient to block infection entirely, reduces the virus burden sufficiently that the host can eventually clear the infection. It is not known if vaccines can be designed to completely prevent infection.

This argument raises the issue of how to set criteria for vaccines against HIV. Should one aim only for the ideal vaccine, which would guarantee blockade against infection, or is it reasonable to consider more than one type of vaccine for different applications? For instance, a vaccine designed to prevent infection would demand the highest criteria for efficacy, whereas vaccines designed to affect disease or transmission may require less rigid criteria. In this regard the lessons from the SIV model are of particular significance in that they may provide information on what one can expect if varying amounts of virus are allowed to establish residence in a susceptible host. Similarly, animals that are better able to control virus replication may be less likely to transmit the virus to other animals or to their offspring. Understanding how to affect transmission through vaccination would be of great importance for the growing problem of mother-to-infant infection in the human population.

Preventive vaccines that are capable of inducing sterilizing immunity against HIV-1 are not in sight, but that may not be the case for vaccines that may have a significant impact on the course of infection, disease onset, or disease severity. It is possible that vaccines

Table 27–1. Possible Applications of HIV Vaccines

1. Vaccines that prevent infection
2. Vaccines that affect disease without completely blocking infection
3. Vaccines that are able to curb virus transmissions
4. Vaccines that are therapeutic in nature

might be more rapidly developed for situations where virus transmission could be reduced. In this regard, vaccines applied postexposure for therapeutic purposes are already being evaluated, as discussed earlier.

It may therefore be worthwhile to consider developing several vaccines with varying criteria for efficacy and safety (Table 27–1). Were this to take place, the design of clinical trials would face several additional challenges. How many vaccines can reasonably be tested in humans, particularly in the efficacy phase? Given the low incidence of HIV infection in the general population, with notable exceptions in highly endemic areas, and the long and variable latent period between infection and the onset of disease, several parameters are expected to constrain the structure of clinical trials (such as size, geography, end point measurements, *etc.*). Fortunately, the infrastructure for conducting clinical trials with AIDS vaccines has been established and many of the initial obstacles have been overcome.[55]

In conclusion, although much remains to be accomplished before vaccines for AIDS become realities, the significant progress made has stimulated considerable interest and commitment on the part of the federal government, academia, and private industry toward this end. If this trend continues and research produces answers to the key scientific questions that remain, the prospects will become much brighter.

REFERENCES

1. Desrosiers RC, Wyand MS, Kodama T et al: Vaccine protection against simian immunodeficiency virus infection. Proc Natl Acad Sci USA 86:6353, 1989
2. Murphey-Corb M, Martin LN, Davison-Fairburn B et al: A formalin-inactivated whole SIV vaccine confers protection in macaques. Science 246:1293, 1989
3. Carlson JR, McGraw TP, Keddie E et al: Vaccine protection of rhesus macaques against simian immunodeficiency virus infection. AIDS Res Hum Retroviruses 6:1239, 1990
4. Stott EJ, Shan WL, Mills KM et al: Protection of cynomolgus macaques against simian immunodeficiency virus by whole fixed cell vaccine. Lancet 336:1538, 1990
5. Gardner MB, Stott J: Progress in the development of simian immunodeficiency virus vaccines: A review. AIDS 4(suppl 1):S137, 1990
6. Murphey-Corb M, Gardner M, Davison-Fairburn B et al: Immunization with an inactivated whole SIV vaccine blocks viral infection and/or replication after challenge with a genetically distinct strain of virus (abstr). Presented at the Third Annual Meeting of the National Cooperative Vaccine Development Groups for AIDS, Clearwater, Fla, October 1–5, 1990
7. Cranage MP, Cook N, Thompson A et al: Protection of rhesus macaques from infection with SIVmac using a formalin inactivated whole virus preparation (abstr). Presented at the MRC AIDS Directed Programme Annual Workshop, September 24–26, 1990
8. Desrosiers RC, Sehgal P, Kodama T et al: Use of simian immunodeficiency virus for AIDS vaccine research. Presented at the 21st Congress of AIDS, Annecy, France, 1989
9. Hu S-L, Abrams K, Barber G et al: Protection of macaques against homologous SIV infection by immunization with live recombinant vaccinia virus followed by recombinant-made SIVmne gp160 (abstr). Presented at the VII International Conference on AIDS, Florence, Italy, June 16–21, 1991
10. Murphey-Corb M, Martin L, Davison-Fairburn B et al: A formalin-killed whole SIV vaccine, but not DOC-disrupted glycoprotein and gag subunit preparations, protects rhesus monkeys following challenge with a 10 ID dose of live virus (abstr). Presented at the 21st Congress of AIDS, Annecy, France, 1989
11. Shafferman A, Jahrling P, Benveniste R et al: Inhibition of SIV infection in macaques preimmunized with several SIV env peptides presented as B-galactosidase fusion proteins (abstr S.A.74). In: Final Program and Abstracts, VI International Conference on AIDS, San Francisco, June 1990, vol 3, p 114
12. Rotzschke O, Falk K, Deres K et al: Isolation and analysis of naturally processed viral peptides as recognized by cytotoxic T cells. Nature 348:252, 1990
13. Takahasi H, Takeshita T, Morein B et al: Induction of CD8+ cytotoxic T cells by immunization with purified HIV-1 envelope protein in ISCOMs. Nature 344:873, 1990
14. Bolognesi D: Fresh pathways to follow. Nature 344:818, 1990
15. Orentas RJ, Hildreth JEK, Obah E et al: Induction of CD4+ human cytolytic T cells specific for HIV-infected cells by a gp160 subunit vaccine. Science 248:1234, 1990
16. Tyler DS, Lyerly HK, Weinhold KJ: Minireview: Anti-HIV-1 ADCC. AIDS Res Hum Retroviruses 5:557, 1989
17. Vowels BR, Gershwin ME, Gardner M et al: Natural killer cell activity of rhesus macaques against retrovirus-pulsed CD4+ target cells. AIDS Res Hum Retroviruses 6:905, 1990
18. Shen L, Chen ZW, Miller MD et al: Recombinant virus vaccine-induced SIV-specific CD8+ cytotoxic T lymphocytes. Science 252:440, 1991
19. Marthas ML, Sutjipto S, Higgins J et al: Immunization with a live, attenuated simian immunodeficiency virus (SIV) prevents early disease but not infection in rhesus macaques challenged with pathogenic SIV. J Virol 64:3694, 1990
20. Biberfeld G, Putkonen P, Thorstensson R et al: Protection against HIV-2 in vaccinated cynomolgus monkeys (abstr S.A.78). In: Final Program and Abstracts, VI International Conference on AIDS, San Francisco, June 1990, vol 3, p 115
21. Murphey-Corb M, Davison-Fairburn B, Ohkawa S et al: Immunization of healthy SIV-infected macaques with a formalin inactivated whole virus vaccine has no apparent effect on disease progression and survival (abstr). In: Proceedings of the 8th Annual Symposium on Non-Human Primate Models for AIDS, New Orleans, 1990, p 55
22. Gardner MB, Jennings M, Carlson JR et al: Postexposure

immunotherapy of simian immunodeficiency virus (SIV) infected rhesus with an SIV immunogen. J Med Primatol 18:321, 1989

23. Girard MP, Eichberg JW: Progress in the development of HIV vaccines. AIDS 4(suppl 1):S143, 1990

24. Girard M, Kieny M-P, Pinter A et al: Immunization of chimpanzees confers protection against challenge with human immunodeficiency virus. Proc Natl Acad Sci USA 88:542, 1991

25. Javaherian K, Langlois AJ, Silver S et al: Principal neutralizing domain of HIV-1 envelope protein. Proc Natl Acad Sci USA 86:6768, 1989

26. Berman PW, Gregory TJ, Riddle L et al: Protection of chimpanzees from infection by HIV-1 after vaccination with recombinant glycoprotein gp120 but not gp160. Nature 45:622, 1990

27. Berman PW, Groopman JE, Gregory T et al: Human immunodeficiency virus type 1 challenge of chimpanzees immunized with recombinant envelope glycoprotein gp120. Proc Natl Acad Sci USA 85:5200, 1988

28. Emini EA, Nara PL, Schleif WA: Antibody-mediated in vitro neutralization of human immunodeficiency virus type 1 abolishes infectivity for chimpanzees. J Virol 64:3674, 1990

29. Takahashi H, Cohen J, Hosmalin A et al: An immunodominant epitope of the human immunodeficiency virus envelope glycoprotein gp160 recognized by class I major histocompatibility complex molecule–restricted murine cytotoxic T lymphocytes. Proc Natl Acad Sci USA 85:3105, 1988

30. Rusche JR, Javaherian K, McDanal C et al: Antibodies that inhibit fusion of human immunodeficiency virus-infected cells bind a 24-amino acid sequence of the viral envelope, gp120. Proc Natl Acad Sci USA 85:3198, 1988

31. Palker TJ, Clark ME, Langlois AJ et al: Type-specific neutralization of the human immunodeficiency virus with antibodies to env-encoded synthetic peptides. Proc Natl Acad Sci USA 85:1932, 1988

32. Kenealy WR, Matthews TJ, Ganfield M et al: Antibodies from human immunodeficiency virus–infected individuals bind to a short amino acid sequence that elicits neutralizing antibodies in animals. AIDS Res Hum Retroviruses 5:173, 1989

33. Leonard CK, Spellman MW, Riddle L et al: Assignment of intrachain disulfide bonds and characterization of potential glycosylation sites of the type 1 recombinant human immunodeficiency virus envelope glycoprotein (gp120) expressed in chinese hamster ovary cells. J Biol Chem 265:10373, 1990

34. Putney SD, McKeating JA: Antigenic variation in HIV. AIDS 4(suppl 1):S129, 1990

35. LaRosa GJ, Davide JP, Weinhold KJ et al: Conserved sequence and structural elements in the HIV-1 principal neutralizing determinant. Science 249:932, 1990

36. Simmonds P, Balfe P, Ludlam C et al: Analysis of sequence diversity in hypervariable regions of the external glycoprotein of human immunodeficiency virus type 1. J Virol 64:5840, 1990

37. Balfe P, Simmonds P, Ludlam C et al: Concurrent evolution of human immunodeficiency virus type 1 in patients infected from the same source: Rate of sequence change and low frequency of mutations. J Virol 64:6221, 1990

38. Javaherian K, Langlois AJ, LaRosa GJ et al: Broadly neutralizing antibodies elicited by the hypervariable neutralizing determinant of HIV-1. Science 250:1590, 1990

39. Ivanoff LA, McDanal C, Morris J et al: Biological analysis of HIV-1 proviruses containing mutations in the envelope V3 domain (abstr). AIDS Res Hum Retroviruses 7:169, 1991

40. Ivanoff LA, Looney DJ, McDanal C et al: Alteration of HIV-1 infectivity and neutralization by a single amino acid replacement in the V3 loop domain. AIDS Res Hum Retroviruses 7(7):595, 1991

41. Freed EO, Myers DJ, Risser R: Mutational analysis of the cleavage sequence of the human immunodeficiency virus type 1 envelope glycoprotein precursor gp160. J Virol 63:4670, 1989

42. Hattori T, Koito A, Takatsuki K et al: Involvement of tryptase-related cellular protease(s) in human immunodeficiency virus type 1 infection. FEBS Lett 248:48, 1989

43. Clements GJ, Price-Jones MJ, Stephens PE et al: The V3 loops of the HIV-1 and HIV-2 surface glycoproteins contain proteolytic cleavage sites: A possible function in viral fusion? AIDS Res Hum Retroviruses 7:3, 1991

44. Linsley PS, Ledbetter JA, Kinney-Thomas E et al: Effects of anti-gp120 monoclonal antibodies on CD4 receptor binding by the env protein of human immunodeficiency virus type 1. J Virol 62:3695, 1988

45. Skinner MA, Langlois AJ, McDanal CB et al: Neutralizing antibodies to an immunodominant envelope sequence do not prevent gp120 binding to CD4. J Virol 62:4195, 1988

46. O'Brien WA, Koyanagi Y, Namazie A et al: HIV-1 tropism for mononuclear phagocytes can be determined by regions of gp120 outside the CD4-binding domain. Nature 348:69, 1990

47. Shioda T, Levy JA, Cheng-Mayer C: Macrophage and T cell-line tropisms of HIV-1 are determined by specific regions of the envelope gp120 gene. Nature 349:167, 1991

48. Nara PL, Smit L, Dunlop N et al: Emergence of viruses resistant to neutralization by V3-specific antibodies in experimental human immunodeficiency virus type 1 IIIB infection of chimpanzees. J Virol 64:3779, 1990

49. Earl PL, Robert-Guroff M, Matthews TJ et al: Isolate- and group-specific immune responses to the envelope protein of human immunodeficiency virus induced by a live recombinant vaccinia virus in macaques. AIDS Res Hum Retroviruses 5:23, 1989

50. Bolognesi DP: Prospects for prevention of and early intervention against HIV. JAMA 261:3007, 1989

51. Prince AM, Horowitz B, Baker L et al: Failure of a human immunodeficiency virus (HIV) immune globulin to protect chimpanzees against experimental challenge with HIV. Proc Natl Acad Sci USA 85:6944, 1988

52. Prince AM, Horowitz B, Shulman RW et al: Apparent prevention of HIV infection by HIV immunoglobulin given prior to low dose HIV challenge. In Brown F et al (eds): Vaccines 90: Modern Approaches to New Vaccines, Including Prevention of AIDS, p 347. Cold Spring Harbor, New York, Cold Spring Harbor Laboratory, 1990

53. Robinson WE Jr, Mitchell WM: Neutralization and enhancement of in vitro and in vivo HIV and simian immunodeficiency virus infections. AIDS 4(suppl 1):S151, 1990

54. Fultz PN, Srinivasan A, Greene CR et al: Superinfection of a chimpanzee with a second strain of human immunodeficiency virus. J Virol 61:4026, 1987

55. Koff WC, Schultz AM: AIDS vaccines 1990: A brief update. AIDS 4(suppl 1):S179, 1990

56. Cohen J: AIDS Vaccine Conference: Is "more" better? Science 250:369, 1990

57. Karn J, Almond JW, Tyrrell DAJ: Research strategies for AIDS vaccine development and evaluation: The MRC Programme. AIDS 4(suppl 1):S167, 1990

58. Dolin R, Graham BS, Greenberg SB et al: The safety and immunogenicity of a human immunodeficiency virus type 1 (HIV-1) recombinant gp160 candidate vaccine in humans. Ann Intern Med 114:119, 1991

59. Gorse GJ, Belshe RB, Tsai CC et al: Analysis of anti-HIV antibody responses by flow cytometric indirect immunofluorescence assay (FIFA) following rgp160 immunization (abstr). In: Final Program and Abstracts, VII International Conference on AIDS, Florence, Italy, June 16–21, 1991, p 140

60. Mosier DE, Gulizia RJ, MacIsaac PD et al: Evaluation of HIV-1 vaccines in hu-PBL-SCID mice (abstr). In: Final Program and Abstracts, VII International Conference on AIDS, Florence, Italy, June 16–21, 1991, p 139

61. Levine A, Henderson BE, Grushea S et al: Immunization of HIV-infected individuals with inactivated HIV immunogen: Significance of HIV-specific cell-mediated immune response (abstr). In: Final Program and Abstracts, VI International Conference on AIDS, San Francisco, June 1990, p 204

62. Redfield R, Polonis BD, Davis V et al: Active immunization of recombinant produced gp160 in patients with early HIV infection: Phase I trial immunogenicity and toxicity (abstr). AIDS Res Hum Retroviruses 7:136, 1991

63. Picard O, Giral P, Defer MC et al: AIDS vaccine therapy: Phase I trial. Lancet 336:179, 1990

64. Sutjipto S, Pedersen NC, Miller CJ et al: Inactivated simian immunodeficiency virus vaccine failed to protect rhesus macaques from intravenous or genital mucosal infection but delayed disease in intravenously exposed animals. J Virol 64:2290, 1990

65. Burns PW, Desrosiers RC. Selection of genetic variants of SIV in persistently infected rhesus monkeys. J Virol 65:1843, 1991

66. Putney S, Langlois A, LaRosa G et al: The principal neutralization determinant of SIV is different than HIV-1 (abstr). Presented at the VII International Conference on AIDS, Florence, Italy, June 16–21, 1991

28

A Human Rights Framework for Evaluating AIDS Policies: Consent, Confidentiality, and Antidiscrimination

Lawrence Gostin

Just as the human immunodeficiency virus (HIV) epidemic has challenged scientists and public health officials, it has challenged lawyers, ethicists, and health policy experts to find ways to minimize the stigma, breach of privacy, and discrimination inherent in the epidemic. As governments have tried to stem the spread of transmission through powers of testing, reporting, partner notification, and personal control measures, the subjects of those powers have seen their rights to confidentiality, autonomy, and freedom infringed. As private employers, schools, and public accommodations have tried to exclude persons with HIV infection or the acquired immunodeficiency syndrome (AIDS), cases of discrimination have become as serious a concern as the epidemic itself. In some countries, like the United States, the sheer volume of litigation[1] and legislation[2] provoked by the epidemic is unprecedented.

There are no easy legal or ethical rules that can reconcile these dilemmas. This is particularly true when a global approach is adopted because laws, cultures, and mores are so different around the world that there is seldom a "correct" policy.

The best I can do, then, is to define the legal and ethical conflicts, provide a set of human rights principles that can be used to balance public health and ethical perspectives, and draw attention to particular laws or practices that can provide useful models for adoption.

Human rights provides a critical perspective in the evaluation of AIDS policies, whether it be case finding, the research and distribution of pharmaceuticals or vaccines, or personal control measures. In this chapter I address a few core human rights principles: informed consent, confidentiality, and antidiscrimination. This, at least, will provide a legal and ethical framework for evaluation of AIDS policies and practices in place in many countries throughout the developed and developing worlds.

INFORMED CONSENT

The complex doctrine of informed consent developed in the United States has by no means been adopted throughout the world. Even the highest court in a developed country like Great Britain has explicitly rejected the U.S. doctrine of informed consent.[3] Nonetheless, the legal concept of consent (and the parallel ethical concept of respect for persons or autonomy) has universal application. The doctrine holds that an individual cannot be made to participate in research, testing, medical examination, or treatment without his or her agreement. The elements of consent are (1) the person must be informed of the nature, purpose, and risks of the treatment, (2) the person is competent to understand, and (3) the person agrees to participate, without duress or coercion.

The concept of consent or respect for persons is reflected in a wide number of international declarations ranging from research accords such as those established in Nuremberg,[4] Helsinki,[5] and Geneva[6] to modern human rights agreements such as the Universal Declaration of Human Rights and the European Convention of Human Rights. Certainly, the very concept of respect for persons as individuals may be at variance "with more relational definitions of the person found in other societies . . . which stress the embeddedness of the individual within society and define a person by his or her relations to others."[7] For example, in the Indian subcontinent and west Africa, great deference may be given to clinicians, healers, or elders in making decisions for individuals. While respect for cultural difference is essential, it does not provide a justification for dispensing entirely with the right of the individual to be involved in a decision that intimately affects his or her life.

Testing and Screening

Many public health and medical practitioners argue that widespread testing for HIV is essential to impede the spread of the epidemic. Some countries require mandatory testing for certain groups involved in "high-risk" behavior, such as intravenous (IV) drug users,[8] sex workers, or prisoners,[9] or require testing for the purposes of travel and immigration.[10] Other countries are contemplating routine testing of large numbers of hospitalized patients because of the significant number of unrecognized HIV infections among patients entering health care facilities.[11]

Informed consent should be viewed as a process that not only protects human rights, but also incorporates the best professional standards. The process involves pre- and post-test counseling during which the health care professional engages in a discussion with the patient, informing her of the significance of the test and the public health and clinical ramifications.

Should the doctrine of informed consent be applied to HIV testing even in the face of the public health emergency confronting much of the world? Mandatory screening programs may seem intuitively obvious, because no public health strategy can be effective unless cases of HIV can be identified. Case finding, it is argued, is the first line of defense in curbing the epidemic. Although compulsory screening may seem obvious, if examined logically it can be seen as ineffective and possibly counterproductive. Several possible justifications for compulsory screening are presented.

First, a person can be expected to make more rational decisions about behavior change if she is informed about her serologic status. This is an assumption that has yet to be demonstrated. There is still insufficient behavioral research to prove whether knowledge of seropositivity influences behavior, and if so, in what direction. The appropriate precautions in personal conduct to reduce the spread of HIV are already well known. Knowledge of seropositivity may be helpful to some in modifying their behavior. However, to others education and counseling will be the critical factors, regardless of test results.

Even if it could be demonstrated that knowledge of a positive test result does significantly influence behavior, it does not necessarily follow that *compelling* a person to take an antibody test will produce voluntary changes in behavior. The spread of HIV can be reduced only through the willingness of individuals to avoid unsafe sexual and needle-sharing behavior. The introduction of compulsory screening may have the reverse effect of causing persons vulnerable to HIV to avoid coming forward for testing, counseling, and treatment. If the public health strategy is to encourage as many people as possible to receive education and counseling, then the use of measures that can be regarded as controlling or punitive might be counterproductive.

A second argument in support of mandatory screening is that it provides an early indicator of disease status so that the person can come in for prompt treatment.[12] Knowledge of seropositivity cannot be used to alleviate an infectious condition, because there is currently no vaccine for prevention or cure of HIV infection. HIV is unlike venereal disease, in which the chain of infection can be broken by simple antibiotic treatment.[13] Thus, even with early knowledge of a person's serologic status, medicine cannot alter the cycle of infection.

Knowledge of seropositivity does enable a person to seek early treatment with antiviral medications and prophylaxis against *Pneumocystis.* The prospect of early therapeutic intervention is an important reason for being tested. Some physicians argue that there is no need for informed consent for an HIV test because no physical harm results from a serologic test and because therapeutic benefits can result from early treatment. However, the doctrine of informed consent is not obviated by these potential benefits; patients have always had the right to refuse consent for even the most efficacious medical procedures. It is for the patient to assess the purposes, benefits, and risks of a medical procedure. Consent to an HIV test is particularly critical because of the personal and social significance of HIV infection in all societies. As with many medical tests that predict grave or fatal diseases, some patients prefer to know the information, others do not. Some patients would find a positive HIV test result tò be an intolerable psychological burden.[14]

A third argument in support of mandatory screening is that it will assist public health officials in gaining a truer epidemiologic picture of the spread of HIV. Mandatory screening programs would not necessarily accomplish this epidemiologic objective because many jurisdictions still require reporting of only CDC-defined AIDS (not HIV positive test results) and most testing programs would be likely to contain biased samples. A better epidemiologic understanding of infection patterns can be obtained through blind epidemiologic research. Blind epidemiologic research poses ethical problems in some countries. Yet anonymous research safeguards privacy by not maintaining a list of patient names. It is also more likely to produce an accurate epidemiologic understanding than mandatory testing and reporting.

A fourth argument for mandatory testing is that it

will protect health care professionals and others who may come into contact with a person's blood in the workplace. Physicians engaging in invasive procedures are particularly concerned that they may contract the AIDS virus from their patients. Although the risk is exceedingly low, it is not zero. Health care professionals could legitimately claim a "right to know" if it could be demonstrated that mandatory testing of patients would significantly lower their occupational risks. It is unlikely, however, that professionals could alter their practices in a way that both provided optimal care for patients and lowered their own occupational risks. The best way to reduce occupational risk is to assume that all patients are infected, and adopt universal precautions. Although the argument favoring universal precautions may appear glib, it is nonetheless more likely to be effective than selective precautions based on a test result. A health care professional who relies on a negative test result may actually be increasing her risk of injury because of the possibility of a false-negative outcome in patients who are recently infected with HIV. Thus, whereas health care professionals may feel safer if patients are compulsorily tested, no empirical evidence exists that there would be any reduction in occupational risk. Testing of patients for the sake of the physician's health and safety violates the patient's human rights without achieving a significant public health benefit.

This argument, of course, runs the other way. Testing of health care professionals to protect the patient from contracting HIV violates the professional's human rights to privacy and autonomy. I can envision a health care system in which there is mutual mistrust between patients and their doctors, each asserting the right to know the health status of the other. This will generate substantial economic costs and human rights burdens.

The public health benefit of mandatory screening, therefore, is likely to be marginal or counterproductive, for four reasons: (1) there is no evidence that the use of compulsion would lead to voluntary changes in behavior; (2) patients cannot be compelled to comply with medical advice, even for their own benefit; (3) epidemiologic information can be gathered in a less intrusive manner by blind research; and (4) testing will not lower the occupational risks of health care professionals. Balanced against this marginal public health benefit is the potential for substantial harm to those screened. Each person screened, whether seropositive or not, must submit involuntarily to the taking of a blood sample and the collection of sensitive health care information.

Moreover, collection of information creates a demand for its use. Unauthorized disclosure of that information could result in opprobrium among family and friends and discrimination in employment, housing, and insurance. The adverse consequences of screening are serious enough for those with true-positive tests, even though the great majority are likely to be asymptomatic. In addition, there will be a small number of individuals who test positive on the ELISA and supplementary tests, but who do not harbor the virus. The risk of a false-positive result grows when low-seroprevalence populations are screened, such as in premarital screening.[15] The price of screening includes the potential for stigma and discrimination of the false-positive population.

Widespread screening has public resource as well as personal implications. Screening requires the administration and interpretation of the ELISA together with supplementary procedures. This entails significant expense for the administration of laboratories, test equipment, and personnel. Moreover, screening only indicates if a person is seropositive at a particular point in time. Thus, to be certain of identifying all infected cases, periodic retesting would be required. The substantial costs of investing in a screening program must be measured against similar levels of expenditures needed for research, education, and counseling.

One of the first principles of law and ethics is that government should adopt the least restrictive measure necessary to achieve a legitimate public health objective. Thus, if there is a less restrictive way to achieve a public health goal as well, or better, that less restrictive alternative should be adopted. The objective of mandatory screening programs can be achieved in a more effective and less restrictive way through a comprehensive voluntary program of public health education and professional testing and counseling services. Those inclined to seek treatment and behavior control are likely to respond to cost-free, readily available education and services. Such a voluntary program would achieve the same public health advantages as a mandatory program without the significant detriments of the widespread use of compulsion.

CONFIDENTIALITY VERSUS THE "RIGHT TO KNOW"

Individuals infected with HIV are concerned with maintaining the confidentiality of their health status. HIV infection is associated with sexual practice and drug use, universally regarded as sensitive activities. Consequently, the process of case identification *per se* triggers a concern with confidentiality. The majority of people infected with HIV in Pattern I countries are also members of groups subject to persistent prejudice and discrimination. Unauthorized disclosure of a person's serologic status can lead to social opprobrium among family and friends and to loss of employment, housing, and insurance. There are public health pressures to obtain detailed, sensitive information through medical surveillance and contact tracing, such as intrusive observation and disclosure of sexual partners.

Persons at risk of HIV infection, therefore, have strong grounds for desiring personal privacy and confidentiality of medical information. Their cooperation with public health authorities and treatment centers is dependent on expectations of confidentiality. Efforts to control the spread of AIDS in most countries currently rely on voluntary restraint of behaviors likely to spread HIV. Therefore, the public health objective should be to influence the behavior of those infected with HIV.

Trust in and compliance with public health programs depend on the maintenance of confidentiality.

Many countries, particularly in the developed world, provide statutory or common law protections of confidentiality. If a health care professional discloses to a third party that a patient is infected with HIV, the patient may be able to recover damages. Whether the disclosure is intentional or negligent, the patient may be compensated for the loss of a job or psychological harm resulting from the breach of confidentiality.[16] A growing number of courts in the United States have awarded damages for disclosure of a person's HIV status by health care professionals, police officers, prison guards, and others.[17]

The Duty to Warn

The decision to maintain strict confidentiality of a person's HIV status, however, may have direct consequences for the health of his sexual or needle-sharing partners. Is a person's right to confidentiality so absolute that it would prevent disclosure to persons who have a significant risk of contracting the infection?

Most liberal conceptions of "rights" hold that a person's rights yield at the point where they pose a significant risk of injury to others. A person living with HIV or AIDS has a strong, but not absolute, right to confidentiality. That privacy right could be breached only where necessary to prevent a clear, prospective harm. Thus, public health professionals who have clear evidence that an HIV-infected person is having an ongoing relationship with a sexual or needle-sharing partner may be entitled to protect the health of the partner by providing a warning. Before doing so the professional should advise the patient himself or herself to make the disclosure. It is only when no other means are available to protect the partner that an ethical justification to disclose would arise.

In the United States, the *Tarasoff* doctrine holds that a health care professional may have a *duty* to inform third parties in imminent danger.[18] Failure to protect the third party may render the health care professional liable in tort. The *Tarasoff* case involved a psychologist at the University of California who was informed by his patient that he would murder his girlfriend when she returned from a trip abroad. The psychologist took his patient's threat seriously and informed the campus police, but not the woman or her family. When the woman returned home she was murdered. The question arose whether the psychologist had a duty to protect her from harm. The court held that the psychologist was liable. The special relationship the psychologist had with his patient extended to the patient's partner, so that the psychologist had a duty to protect her.

It is interesting that in *Tarasoff* the psychologist did not relieve himself from liability by notifying the campus police. By analogy, a health care professional may not be protected simply because she notifies the public health department that her patient is HIV positive pur-

suant to a state reporting requirement. The fact that a public health department may have a contact tracing program in place may not be enough to protect the professional from liability. The *Tarasoff* doctrine appears to place the individual responsibility on the health care professional to protect third parties at risk.

The elements of the *Tarasoff* doctrine, which has been followed by many states in America, are as follows. A health care professional has a duty to warn a third party if (1) the professional knows the identity of the third party (simply knowing the patient has an unnamed partner at risk is insufficient), (2) the professional believes that the partner is in imminent danger, and (3) there is no other way to protect the partner other than by disclosing the danger to her.

It is conceivable that a court would apply the reasoning of the *Tarasoff* doctrine to protect the sexual or needle-sharing partners of a person living with HIV or AIDS. This places the health care professional in a dilemma between the duty to protect confidentiality and the duty to warn. If the professional breaches confidentiality she may be liable in damages, and if she fails to warn she may be liable.

The following proposal provides a model for resolving this dilemma. Persons living with HIV or AIDS should receive strong statutory protection against a breach of confidentiality. The law would create a narrow exception where the health care professional has a power, not a duty, to disclose the information to partners only in the following narrow circumstances: (1) the health care professional has clear evidence of a significant risk of harm to an ongoing sexual or needle-sharing partner who is named, (2) the professional is unable to convince the patient to disclose the information, and (3) the disclosure to the partner is made in a confidential and sensitive manner, offering a full opportunity for counseling and testing. By giving the health care professional a power, not a duty, to warn it means that the professional has discretion to breach confidentiality in the *narrow* circumstances indicated above. If a sexual partner is warned under these narrow circumstances, the professional would not be liable for breach of confidentiality. The professional also would avoid liability under the *Tarasoff* doctrine if she chose not to disclose the risk.

The "Right to Know"

Many groups argue that they have a "right to know" the HIV status of their clients or patients, even though the occupational risks are negligible. Groups claiming a right to know include a wide range of workers such as police, prison guards, emergency medical workers, and funeral workers.

In the United States, many states have granted these and other workers a "right to know." In some states, the list of groups with a right to know is so extensive that the exceptions swallow up the rule of confidentiality. This so-called "right to know" works differently depending on the particular state. In some states the worker has an automatic right to be informed if the person is HIV positive. In other states the worker must first sustain an ''exposure'' to the source person's blood before he has a right to know. In some states the source can even be tested for HIV without consent.

To what extent, if any, should workers have the right to know if their client is HIV positive? It is important to begin with the principle that a person's right to confidentiality holds a high ethical and legal value that should not be diminished without a compelling justification. The need to avert a clear and serious danger to a sexual or needle-sharing partner certainly represents a transcending value. But the chance that a worker will contract HIV from his client is negligible. Giving workers a right to know the client's HIV status invites discrimination and does not decrease the worker's occupational risk. The onus is on the worker to demonstrate that she has a significant risk of contracting HIV in the workplace and that knowing the person's HIV status would reduce that risk. It is unlikely that most workers could meet this ethical test for disclosure.

Workers may argue that this test is too stringent. They point to other occupational standards that require even remote risks of environmental hazards to be disclosed. The difference, however, is that when an employer is forced to disclose an environmental risk, no one is harmed. When an employer is forced to disclose a person's HIV status, that individual forgoes a deeply personal right to privacy. An individual should not be forced to make that disclosure unless it is necessary to avert a real danger.

A more troubling case arises when a worker sustains a percutaneous exposure to a patient's blood. The risk of transmission following a needlestick from an HIV-infected patient is in the range of 1 in 250, which is well within the range that justifies concern and action. Clearly, the patient has an ethical obligation to inform the worker. The question arises whether the patient should be compelled to disclose against her will. Compelling the patient to be tested will not avert a future harm, since the harm, if any, has already occurred. The disclosure, however, could significantly reduce the psychological worry of the worker. (Of course, if the source patient tests HIV positive, the worker's worry will only increase.) The worker's psychological burden is real and may affect her sexual relationships, as well as her decision to take azidothymidine as a prophylactic measure. Some states in the United States force patients to be tested for HIV and to disclose their serologic status to a professional who has sustained a percutaneous exposure. Most patients will agree to be tested if a health care professional is stuck with a needle. Whether it is sensible policy to compulsorily test the few who will not consent depends on what weight is given to the respective rights of patients and professionals. Are the patient's rights to autonomy and privacy more important than the worker's right to know? That is a value judgment which policy-makers will have to ponder.

ANTIDISCRIMINATION

Times of epidemic are also times of social tension. Fears exacerbate already extant divisions, revealing and deepening social fault lines. Discrimination against persons with HIV infection has become a worldwide phenomenon. The AIDS virus has divided nations, ethnic, cultural, and sexual groups, and individuals.[19] The potential for greater division is ever present.

HIV infection has been used as a rationale to exclude children and adults from education, jobs, housing, and insurance. All too frequently children with HIV are turned away from schools, employees are dismissed from their jobs and turned down for life or health insurance, and patients are denied appropriate treatment.

Discrimination based on an infectious condition can be as inequitable as discrimination based on other morally irrelevant grounds such as race, gender, or disability. The U.S. Supreme Court has recognized that ''society's accumulated myths and fears about disability and disease are just as handicapping as are the physical limitations that flow from actual impairment. Few aspects of handicap give rise to the same level of public fear and misapprehension as contagiousness.''[20]

A critical difference exists between discrimination based on race or gender and discrimination based on disease status. An infection is potentially transmissible and can affect a person's abilities to perform certain tasks. A decision to exclude an HIV-infected person from certain activities because of a real risk of transmission or genuine performance criteria would be understandable and would not breach antidiscrimination principles. But denying such persons rights, benefits, or privileges where health risks are only theoretical or very low and when performance is adequate is morally intolerable. Because the risk of transmission of HIV in most settings is remote, and because persons with HIV infection may function normally when not experiencing serious symptoms, no morally acceptable grounds exist for discrimination.

Irrational fears of AIDS are typically at the root of HIV-related discrimination. Public opinion surveys reveal that a consistent minority harbor anxieties about and antipathies toward those with HIV infection. On a wide variety of questions some one fourth of the public believe people with HIV should be excluded from schools, workplaces, and other public settings. Such findings have been replicated in many regions of the world.[21] Fueling both anxieties and antipathies is often a visceral hostility to those groups linked to AIDS—gay men, drug users, and prostitutes.

Not only is discrimination against persons living with HIV or AIDS morally wrong, it can also be counterproductive from a public health perspective. The World Health Organization[22] has called discrimination against persons living with HIV or AIDS unjustifiable and inimical to the goal of public health.

Fears of a breach of confidentiality and subsequent discrimination discourage individuals from cooperating with vital public health programs and treatment for sexually transmitted diseases and drug dependency. These fears also mobilize opposition to routine voluntary testing and counseling among people with high-risk behaviors. Such resistance to testing might well melt away if individuals believed they were strongly protected by the law.

Remarkably few countries have enacted legal protections against discrimination of persons living with HIV or AIDS. Even developed countries with a body of civil rights law for racial minorities and women have not extended their laws to protect persons living with HIV or AIDS. The Americans with Disabilities Act of 1990, enacted in the United States, provides a model of antidiscrimination legislation. The Act makes it unlawful to discriminate against qualified persons with a disability. Courts have consistently found that all stages of HIV disease, including AIDS, ARC, and asymptomatic HIV infection, are disabilities under the Act.[23] A person is protected if she is perceived to be disabled, even if there is no actual infection or incapacity at all. Thus, an individual who has engaged in high-risk behavior but who is not actually infected with HIV is protected under the Act.

A person with a disability must be "qualified," which means that he or she is capable of meeting all of the performance criteria for the particular position, service, or benefit. The Act, moreover, creates an affirmative obligation to provide "reasonable accommodation" if it would enable the person to meet the performance criteria. Accommodation is not reasonable if it either imposes undue financial and administrative burdens or requires fundamental alteration in the nature of the program.

Courts and human rights commissions in the United States have upheld the right of persons living with HIV or AIDS to attend schools, jobs, housing, nursing homes, and public accommodations.[23] The American judiciary has taken a firm position prohibiting pernicious discrimination against persons living with HIV or AIDS. Discrimination, however, is not always based on myths, fears, or bigotry. Discrimination in the health care setting is much more subtle, often founded on real, albeit low, risks of occupational exposure to HIV, or the genuine exercise of clinical judgment.

The Health Care Provider's Duty to Treat

Health care professionals have an ethical duty to provide treatment for persons living with HIV or AIDS. The training, licensure, and professional purpose of health care providers require that decisions be based on a good faith clinical assessment of benefit and harm to the patient, and not on the patient's disability. The risks to health care professionals who take rigorous precautions against contracting infection, moreover, are remote and do not justify deviation from this professional obligation not to discriminate. Certainly, the vast majority of health care professionals provide dedicated and equal treatment for all of their patients. Many cases, however, have been reported in which treatment was withheld from patients living with HIV or AIDS.

The Americans with Disabilities Act applies to virtually all health care providers. The Act prohibits discrimination against persons living with HIV or AIDS in the treatment they receive. Thus, health care providers cannot turn away a person living with HIV or AIDS because of their prejudices or fears. Practitioners, however, are defending their decisions not to treat, or to refer, patients with HIV infection by arguing that this is an exercise of clinical judgment and does not constitute discrimination, and that restricting the physician's right to decide whom to treat or when to refer is to dictate the practice of medicine. To be sure, the Act's acceptance of selection criteria that are "necessary for the provision of services" appears to authorize the exercise of legitimate clinical judgment based on the practitioner's areas of skill and specialization. Thus, the Act does not prohibit a practitioner from providing the most appropriate medical treatment in her judgment or from referring a person with a disability to another practitioner when clinically appropriate and when the same referral would be made for an individual without a disability. For example, a physician who specializes in treating burn victims could not refuse to treat the burns of a person because she has AIDS; but she could refuse to provide other types of medical treatment outside of her area of specialty unless she provides that treatment to nondisabled individuals.

Such fine distinctions may be hard to make in practice, particularly when the disability is directly related to the condition being treated.[24] Is denial of orthopedic surgery justified when the surgeon claims that the insertion of a pin in an immunocompromised patient infected with HIV would be contraindicated? Would denial of a kidney transplant to a person in an advanced state of AIDS deny equal opportunities?[25] The Act provides no easy answers.

The physician's exercise of clinical judgment cannot render all treatment refusals or referrals immune from review if there is evidence that they were motivated by prejudice or irrational fear. Primary practitioners such as general internists or dentists cannot claim that they possess insufficient expertise to treat *any* person living with HIV or AIDS. The courts increasingly are looking beyond the mantle of clinical judgment and are examining patterns of discriminatory behavior that unveil disguised prejudice.

Another reason for refusing to treat patients with dangerous infectious conditions is a concern about occupational hazards. Practitioners may be ethically required to endure reasonable risks when the treatment is necessary to save or prolong life. But some practitioners take a different view when the treatment is elective, even cosmetic. The question then becomes whether patient *X* should receive treatment different from that of patient *Y*, not because of clinical differences but because of a perceived occupational risk. Courts, however, are unlikely to accept occupational risks as a justification for discrimination: the risk is exceedingly low and can be kept low through the "reasonable accommodation" of strict adherence to infection control procedures; and health care professionals will probably be expected to accept some level of risk in carrying out the essential functions of their jobs, in the same way that fire fighters or police officers cannot excuse themselves from particularly dangerous assignments.

The Americans with Disabilities Act does not guarantee access to health care, but merely requires that the refusal to provide equal access cannot be based on a person's disability. A provider's health care decisions may be based, in part, on cost. Providing health services of inferior quality, or not providing services at all, because of a person's inability to pay may be unethical, but it is not necessarily unlawful in the United States. The Act does not set out to interfere in the purely financial decisions of providers. Yet a financial decision that impacts unequally and unfairly upon persons with disabilities may be challengeable. Numerous gray areas exist, such as a cost-benefit decision to limit access to *P. carinii* prophylaxis or antiviral medication, that may directly discriminate against persons living with HIV or AIDS.

Discrimination based on an immutable condition like infection should be so repugnant in society that it is unconscionable to allow it to occur. It may be argued that laws can never erase bigoted attitudes or uncaring feelings. That may be so. But laws can change *behaviors* that deny people equal opportunities based on their disabilities. The experience of civil rights laws also suggests that, if the public is imbued with the understanding that discrimination is unacceptable, as behaviors begin to change, changes in attitudes and feelings will follow.

CONCLUSION

Public health policies in the AIDS epidemic cannot be evaluated simply through a sterile calculation of scientific efficacy, adverse effects, and economic costs. Human rights burdens of the policy are as essential to measure as the scientific merits. The three human rights principles of consent, confidentiality, and antidiscrimination emerge as powerful forces in the HIV epidemic. They help define the epidemic, and the social response to persons living with HIV or AIDS, and the policies that governments adopt. Combating the negative social response to persons living with HIV or AIDS through legislation and education will take as much planning, effort, and resources as the scientific battle to confront the epidemic itself.

REFERENCES

1. Gostin L: The AIDS Litigation Project: Parts 1 and 2. JAMA 263:1961, 2086, 1990
2. Gostin L: Public health strategies for confronting AIDS: Legislative and regulatory policy in the United States. JAMA 261:1621, 1990
3. *Sidaway* v *Bethlem Royal Hospital Governors* [1985] A.C. 871
4. Nurenberg Code 1947, printed in Trials of War Criminals Before the Nurenberg Military Tribunals Under Control Council Law No. 10, vol ii, p 181. Washington, DC, US Government Printing Office, 1949
5. World Medical Association Declaration of Helsinki: Recommendations Guiding Medical Doctors in Biomedical Research Involving Human Subjects, adopted by the 18th World Medical Assembly, Helsinki, Finland, revised in 1975 and 1983
6. Council of International Organizations of Medical Sciences: Proposed International Guidelines for Biomedical Research Involving Human Subjects. Geneva, 1982
7. Christakis NA: The ethical design of an AIDS vaccine trial in Africa. Hastings Center Rep 18:31, 1988
8. Gostin L: The interconnected epidemics of drug dependency and AIDS. Harvard CR-CL Law Rev 2(6):113, 1991
9. Hammett T: AIDS in correctional facilities: Issues and options. Washington, DC, National Institute of Justice, 1986
10. Gostin LO, Cleary PD, Mayer KH et al: Screening immigrants and international travelers for the human immunodeficiency virus. N Engl J Med 322:1743, 1990
11. St Louis ME, Rauch BA, Petersen LR et al, for the Sentinel Hospital Surveillance Group: Seroprevalence rates of human immunodeficiency virus infection at sentinel hospitals in the United States. N Engl J Med 323:213, 1990
12. Rhame M: The case for wider use of testing for HIV infection. N Engl J Med 320:1248, 1989
13. Brandt A: No Magic Bullet: A Social History of Venereal Disease in the United States Since 1880. New York, Oxford University Press, 1987
14. Marzuk, Tierny, Tardiff et al: Increased risk of suicide in persons with AIDS. JAMA 259:1333, 1988
15. Cleary P, Barry M, Brandt A et al: Compulsory premarital screening for the human immunodeficiency virus: Technical and public health considerations. JAMA 258:1757, 1987
16. Dickens B: Confidentiality and the duty to warn. In Gostin L (ed): AIDS and the Health Care System. New Haven, Yale University Press, 1990
17. Gostin L, Porter L, Sandomire H: AIDS Litigation Project. Washington, DC, US Government Printing Office, 1990
18. *Tarasoff* v *Regents of the University of California,* 551 P2d 347 (1976)
19. Sabatier R: Blaming Others: Prejudice, Race and Worldwide AIDS. London, Panos Institute, 1988
20. *School Board of Nassau County, Fla* v *Arline,* 107 S Ct 1123 (1987)
21. Blendon R, Donelan K: Discrimination against people with AIDS: The public's perspective. N Engl J Med 319:1022, 1988
22. World Health Organization, Global Programme on AIDS: Progress Report No. 3, WHO/GPA/GEN/88.1. Geneva, World Health Organization, 1988
23. Gostin L: The AIDS Litigation Project: Part II. Discrimination. JAMA 263:2086, 1990
24. *United States* v *University Hospital,* 729 F2d 144 (2d Cir 1984)
25. Parmet WE: Discrimination and disability: The challenges of the ADA. Law Med Health Care 18:32, 1990

29

Technical Successes and Social Failures: Approaching the Second Decade of the AIDS Epidemic

Bruce G. Gellin   David E. Rogers

The word plague had just been uttered for the first time. Everybody knows that pestilences have a way of recurring in the world; yet somehow we find it hard to believe in ones that crash down on our heads from a blue sky. There have been as many plagues as wars in history; yet always plagues and wars take people equally by surprise. . . . Our townsfolk were not more to blame than others, they forgot to be modest, that was all, and thought that everything was still possible for them; which presumed that pestilences were impossible. . . . They fancied themselves free and no one will ever be free so long as there are pestilences.

> Albert Camus
> *The Plague,* 1948[1]

In a very real sense AIDS is a metaphor—the only really new things about the HIV epidemic are the virus itself and the pressure of the burgeoning members of young adults needing sustained care. All the rest of the problems we face are old ones that we have ignored or patched or minimized beyond all common sense.

> J. E. Osborn
> "The New England Journal of Medicine," 1986[2]

The initial report in 1981 of a small cluster of deaths from *Pneumocystis carinii* pneumonia and Kaposi's sarcoma in homosexual men announced the arrival of the global acquired immunodeficiency syndrome (AIDS) pandemic.[3] The breathtaking progress in the biomedical sciences made in the 20 years preceding the 1980s supported a cascade of powerful advances in the basic and applied sciences of molecular biology, virol-

ogy, immunology, epidemiology, and the clinical understanding of human immunodeficiency virus (HIV) infection and the syndromes it produces. Because of those efforts, this plague has been characterized better than any that preceded it. Further, although we have not yet achieved the ultimate successes—a vaccine and a cure—we have learned enough about the human immunodeficiency retrovirus and its *modus operandi* to know how to protect against it and prevent its spread.

The HIV epidemic has been fostered by the confluence of three features of modern society: the sexual revolution of the preceding three decades, the ease of international travel, and the invention of the hollow-bore needle and the availability of potions to push through it. To these features we add a fourth: lack of collective agreement, or of national will, to educate and change the behaviors of people sufficiently to prevent transmission and acquisition of this infection. That HIV infection has continued to spread in the face of knowledge about its transmission and how to prevent it focuses a glaring spotlight on our inadequate and often inappropriate social responses to this crisis. Indeed, that inadequate response has become part of the problem.

Our failures in this sector have several root causes that deserve examination: first, the expectation that a technological fix would bail us out and allow us to continue with business as usual; second, the fact that the epidemic first emerged in two groups already disliked and stigmatized by the larger society—homosexual men and intravenous (IV) drug users—who were initially resistant to acknowledging their role in the spread of disease; third, the focal and circumscribed geographic nature of the epidemic in the United States; and last, the primitive nature of our knowledge about how to promote behavioral changes and our difficulties in translating and communicating the clear lessons of science and epidemiology to multiple groups. Fierce clashes between social values, mores, and science have added conflict and confusion to all the above.

WAITING FOR A MAGIC BULLET

Ours is a society that has come to expect science to apply a quick technical fix to clear-cut health or safety problems. Until the technologies of effective immunization and curative agents for HIV infection are developed, we are forced to rely on the laborious and far more grueling efforts aimed at changing the behaviors that put people at risk of acquiring HIV infection. This requires that we actively and aggressively engage in explicit discussions of the many private behaviors inherent in sexual practices and illicit drug use that, when linked to HIV, have had such devastating social consequences. It also demands that we examine the broader social context in which HIV infection occurs and look more squarely at some of our most embarrassing and disturbing social problems: poverty, issues of race, drug use, the dissolution of families, crime, homelessness, and lack of access to medical care. All of these have become tangled in the web of AIDS and our response to it.

SCAPEGOATS AND LEPERS: JUST ANOTHER PLAGUE?

The reactions to all epidemics of recorded human history have been a result of the play of many forces—rumors, social values, religious beliefs, local mores, the political tenor of the times, and, more recently, science-based knowledge.[4] So too with our response to AIDS. As with other plagues, it was quite clear from the start that AIDS was not just a medical problem. In this instance the tone of our response was significantly tempered by the fact that it first emerged in homosexual men and IV drug users—groups already disliked and disapproved of by most of U.S. society. To many, AIDS was primitive justice: "they" were getting what they deserved, and their fate was a direct result of their immoral and illegal activities. The wider fear arose from their perceived threat to the rest of society. As one medical historian has written, "When medicine stands ineffective in the face of a dread disease, the temptation to explain disease in cultural terms is pervasive and overwhelming. Society gains comfort and hope in feeling that outsiders or socially disapproved groups are in some way responsible for the outbreak of diseases. If those groups can be placed beyond the pale of society—via stigmatization, isolation, quarantine, or genocide—the epidemic might be brought under control."[5]

It is not surprising, then, that the initial reaction of mainstream America was dominated by distaste and fear. This was fueled by the media's early use of the acronym "GRID" (gay-related immune deficiency), and it was driven by anger stemming from the lack of clear recognition by the gay community that their behavior was accelerating transmission early in the course of the epidemic in the United States. After years of fighting for their rights, sexual freedom had become a political statement for homosexual activists. Yet despite mounting evidence that anal receptive intercourse greatly facilitated person-to-person transmission of the AIDS virus, and that the more sexual partners one had, the swifter the dissemination of the epidemic, moves to reduce indiscriminate sexual contact by closing bath houses and sex clubs were interpreted by many in the gay community as threats to liberty rather than as efforts to protect the public's health. Dr. Stephen Joseph, former Commissioner of Health of New York City, stated at the Seventh Cornell Conference on Health Policy, "For some the AIDS epidemic has been viewed as a civil rights crisis with public health implications. It is not. It is a public health crisis with civil rights implications."

THE SYMBIOSIS OF AIDS AND DRUGS

The angers and concerns of the public were heightened as the disease moved into another ostracized population. Almost from the outset, the AIDS epidemic in the United States involved IV drug users, a group already dually stigmatized. This group primarily comprised black or Hispanic sectors of the urban poor. In the view of much of society, these groups had "proved" their moral failings by falling susceptible to drugs. For some, the acquisition of HIV infection was "justice" for immoral and illegal acts. Indeed, the more vengeful saw the emergence of AIDS in drug users as a form of social Darwinism, i.e., this was nature's way of eliminating both this group and reducing some of the social ills often associated with drug users—crime, homelessness and sexually transmitted diseases.

The spread of infection in these individuals was accelerated by the lack of sufficient treatment programs to accommodate all of those using drugs but not yet infected by HIV. This failure to make swift treatment available to drug users on demand has underscored one of the more egregious deficiencies in our health care system. Thus, by 1988, 55% of all new cases of AIDS in New York City occurred among heterosexual IV drug users. More than 80% of heterosexually transmitted cases of AIDS in New York in 1990 involved transmission from a male IV drug user to a non-drug-injecting female partner, and 77% of pediatric AIDS cases in New York occurred among children of IV drug users.[6]

GEOGRAPHIC HOT SPOTS ARE WARMING THE COUNTRYSIDE

The well-demarcated and geographically selective nature of the AIDS epidemic in the United States to date has also been a serious impediment to national action. That approximately 1 million Americans have been estimated to be infected with HIV should be enough to command a massive federal response.[7] However, because nearly two thirds of all AIDS cases to date have been reported from major cities in just five states (New York, California, Florida, Texas, and New Jersey[8]), policy-makers from nonendemic areas have avoided supporting costly HIV-related legislative initiatives that would take funds and programs away from the quite different needs of their constituencies. This was highlighted recently by the way the Comprehensive AIDS Resources Emergency (CARE) Act (the "Ryan White" bill) played out. This legislative initiative, which directed emergency funding to areas hardest hit by the AIDS epidemic, was passed overwhelmingly by Congress with great fanfare. Yet by the time funds were finally appropriated, more than 75% of the initial $875 million pledge had vanished.

Although the current burden of AIDS continues to fall most heavily on urban areas, it is increasingly clear that HIV does not recognize geographic boundaries. In the past year, rural areas saw a 37% increase in documented AIDS cases, while there was only a 5% increase in cases in urban areas during the same period.[9,10] AIDS has become a national disease.

A FAILURE TO COMMUNICATE

Perhaps the most important reason for our failure to halt the spread of HIV infection has been our singular inability to impart information about how to prevent transmission in ways that will effect the profound behavioral changes necessary to stop its spread. Part of this is simple ignorance. Our behavioral science knowledge is far less advanced than our biomedical skills. We know how to get to the moon and how to sequence the genome, but we do not know how to get a teenager to predictably refuse experimentation with mind-altering drugs, to use condoms with absolute consistency, or to sharply reduce his or her number of sexual partners.

Four additional components conspire to leave those at greatest risk the least informed. First, we are not conducting the research that might help make us more effective communicators; second, attempts to provide more explicit educational messages to the public have often been blocked by those who feel that such messages condone offensive or immoral behaviors; third, the messages that are transmitted are often confusing and incomplete; and fourth, the messages are not reaching those most in need of them.

What You Don't Know Won't Hurt You

More troublesome than our ignorance has been the frequent failure to use the educational methods at hand or to encourage behavioral research in order to discover how to do it more effectively. We know quite precisely the way that the AIDS virus is transmitted. But without knowing more about the behaviors of those at risk, and without appropriate intervention techniques, our current strategies are largely shots in the dark. The important research needed to better aim our risk reduction campaigns and programs has been subverted at all levels of government. The recent review of the government's AIDS research program by the Institute of Medicine[11] focused on the continued neglect of research that could provide a fuller understanding of the high-risk sexual and drug-using behaviors that contribute to continued transmission. The National Institute of Child Health and Human Development has prepared a national survey of health and AIDS risk prevalence, yet the Department of Health and Human Services has blocked its release, claiming "concerns about its scope and content." Thus, the much-outdated Kinsey Report remains our principal source of information on our most intimate behaviors—the behaviors that allow the spread of HIV infection to continue. To know which interventions may be most appropriate we need to better understand "the behaviors relevant to the transmission of HIV, including but not limited to human sexual development and practices and drug addiction and abuse."[11]

Just Say No?

There is abundant evidence that arguments of moral persuasion, with appeals for abstinence from sex and drugs, do not work. They are not the serious and sustained programs that are urgently needed. Although efforts to develop well-targeted, unequivocal, and explicit educational messages designed to promote behavioral change have gradually improved over the decade, they remain tangled in a morass of moral arguments. Although it has been reasonably documented that access to contraceptive services does not influence adolescents' decisions to become sexually active[12] and that access to clean needles does not foster drug use,[13,14] many of our elected and appointed officials and a number of religious leaders fear that making such services widely available will be interpreted as a policy condoning offensive sexual acts and drug use. Thus the use of federal funds for educational materials that are directed at homosexuals or that do not emphasize monogamous heterosexual marriage and abstinence from IV drug use is legislatively prohibited. Research on the effectiveness of a needle exchange program cannot be funded by the National Institute of Drug Abuse because of laws that restrict the possession of drug paraphernalia. As a result, the community-based programs designed to reduce HIV exposure by making clean needles available to drug users are forced to operate illegally.[15]

Mixed Messages Are Bad Messages

Because of these clashes between taste and science, many of the messages about HIV transmission and infection have been contradictory and incomplete and have allowed HIV transmission and discrimination against HIV-infected individuals to persist.

It is disquieting to realize that science is not necessarily the driver of health and social policies. Although Dr. Louis Sullivan, Secretary of the Department of Health and Human Services, has stated that "Any policy based on fear and misconceptions about HIV only complicates and confuses disease control efforts without adding any protection to the public health,"[16] reality doesn't always hold up to this credo.

As an example, although the United States has long been a source of HIV infection to the rest of the world, in 1987 the U.S. Congress imposed international travel restrictions on HIV-infected foreign visitors *to* the United States who were applying for visas, and HIV infection was added to the list of "dangerously contagious diseases."[16] It took 3 years for this misleading policy to be corrected.

Despite the clear statement of the commitment to include HIV-infected persons under the protective umbrella of the Americans with Disabilities Act (ADA) of 1990, an amendment that specifically excludes HIV-infected food handlers is maintained in this legislation. This kind of schizophrenia has tended to perpetuate unwarranted fears and the kinds of discrimination that the ADA is designed to end.[16]

That HIV testing sites and AIDS hot-lines were overrun in the weeks following the recent revelation of the HIV infection of a celebrity athlete, Magic Johnson, is testimony that the barrage of information that has been broadcast on "risky" behaviors may not have been received by those whose behaviors place them at highest risk. And, while knowledge of explicit tasks may not be enough to prevent unwanted behaviors, solid information on how you *don't* catch AIDS—subtracting the few well-identified high-risk behaviors from the wide range of quite intimate human activities that do not transmit HIV infection—is also important. This deserves more attention, for it has become increasingly evident that those who know not only how HIV infection is transmitted but, equally important, it is *not* transmitted, seem better able to deal with the issue; they are more tolerant of and tend to be less discriminatory toward people with AIDS.[17-19]

Lastly, one of the very real educational problems in getting across clear and well-understood messages is that the terminology of epidemiology does not translate very well. "Casual contact" was intended to be distinguished from a "true exposure," but the phrase is not clear enough. As long as there remains sufficient doubt about the lack of transmission by casual contact, the movement for *no* contact, driven by fear of the unknown, will persist. In his 1986 report on AIDS,[20] Surgeon General Koop's pronouncement couldn't have been clearer: "Shaking hands, hugging, social kissing, coughing, or sneezing will not transmit the AIDS virus. Nor has AIDS been contracted from swimming pools or bathing in hot tubs or from eating in restaurants. . . . AIDS is not contracted from sharing bed linens, towels, cups, straws, dishes, or any other eating utensils. You cannot get AIDS from toilets, doorknobs, telephones, office machinery,

or household furniture." Although these facts are no longer unknown, the message has not been adequately received and understood by many. It needs to be sharpened and broadcast along with explicit risk-reduction messages.

Reaching the Target Audience: Trees Falling in the Woods Are Not Heard

Although many feel that most IV drug users are extraordinarily difficult to reach, an increasing body of evidence demonstrates that appropriately tailored educational and risk-reduction messages may substantially reduce the proportion of IV drug users who share needles and syringes.[21,22] To date, concerns about "taste" or worries about offending moral sensibilities have too often blocked the production and broadcast of potentially lifesaving messages. Perhaps the most striking example of this remains television's consistent refusal to use that powerful medium to help to fight this epidemic. Except for the courage of a few local television producers and owners in inner cities who acknowledged that "the risk of AIDS was worse than the risk of angering viewers,"[23] it was only in the shadow of the announcement of the HIV infection of Magic Johnson that major television networks have considered running condom advertisements.

BEGINNING THE SECOND DECADE

Where has this left us in late 1991? Clearly, in trouble. This epidemic is far from over. It has already claimed more American lives than the Vietnam War, and it is the leading cause of death in persons 25 to 44 years of age. In recent years the epidemic has shifted into the decaying urban centers and is increasingly associated with IV drug users and their sexual partners. Thus it is now having its greatest impact on the black and Hispanic communities, especially adolescents, women, and children—traditionally the medically disenfranchised, for whom access to adequate health care was a problem long before HIV.

Within the urban community most affected by AIDS, health systems are overstressed, understaffed, and underfunded. As acute care hospitals assume the care of increasing numbers of persons with AIDS, city hospital systems are approaching a medical gridlock, often so overloaded that they are having difficulty caring for those with any kind of acute medical problem. In cities already hardest hit by this epidemic there are increasing numbers of reports of patients who wait for days in emergency departments before hospital beds become available, and elective admissions are often difficult to arrange. The severe and growing shortage of long-term-care beds and nursing home facilities for AIDS patients is approaching crisis proportions in the Northeast. This has resulted in prolonged stays in expensive acute care facilities and prevents those hospitals from fulfilling their appropriate role.

Stresses on hospitals translate to stresses on hospital personnel. Health professionals at all levels are unhappy and discouraged by the increased case load of complicated patients to whom they are able to offer only limited treatments.[24] Coupled with these pressures, the magnified fears of contagion from HIV-infected patients have contributed to staffing shortages at all levels, and these appear likely to get worse.

TAKING STOCK AND TAKING CHARGE

How can we better cope with this public health emergency of our times? Given the accumulating knowledge about the virus, we have some clear and obvious strategies that should be pursued more aggressively. Further, despite the problems recounted, our social response to AIDS has been significantly better than was the case in earlier plagues in history. The difference is *data*. The knowledge that the virus is actually not very contagious, and that the modes of its transmission are clear-cut, that humans are the sole reservoir, and that person-to-person transmission requires considerable intimacy has permitted control of the kinds of hysteria that characterized responses in the past. Application of this information has provided the rationale for keeping HIV-infected children in the schoolroom, HIV-infected adults in the workplace, and for removing HIV infection from the list of dangerously contagious diseases. The same data were the basis for including the HIV-infected among those protected from discrimination by the Americans with Disabilities Act of 1990. Condoms, once a public unmentionable, are now sold in grocery stores and are now marketed to women, who increasingly bear the brunt of this illness. With the recognition of the potential explosion of this epidemic into the adolescent community, school districts that have long wrestled with issues of sex education and teenage pregnancies have made some significant and courageous decisions. There is no more clear statement of intent than the recent decision of the New York City School Board to allow the distribution of condoms in public schools.

WHERE DO WE GO FROM HERE?

Clearly, much more is required if we are to make full use of what we know both to reduce the spread of HIV infection and to make life more bearable for those already infected. Most needed is for those in leadership positions at all levels—federal, state, and local—to publicly acknowledge that we have a devastating epidemic on our hands. This simple recognition, coupled with messages about the importance of nondiscriminatory and compassionate care for those already infected, the need for appropriate education to prevent further spread, and the vital importance of further research to develop definitive solutions to HIV infection, would do much to set the proper steps in motion.

Perhaps most powerful would be the establishment of an AIDS epidemic control unit within the highest level of government. Such a unit should be allotted the resources and authority to act decisively to deal with the HIV crisis. The various measures might include, but would not be limited to, the following:

1. Development of a comprehensive national HIV plan with the full participation of involved federal agencies and with input from national organizations representing various levels of government to identify priorities and resources necessary for preventing and treating HIV disease.
2. Offer disaster relief for regions or cities most seriously affected by AIDS.
3. Improving access to care for all HIV-infected persons.
4. Assuring more equity in entry into drug treatment trials, particularly for women, children, drug users, and those with HIV infection housed in U.S. jails and prisons.
5. Promoting expansion of drug treatment programs to include all who request such treatment, and coupling these programs with appropriate HIV prevention and treatment services.
6. Encourage Congress to remove government restrictions that have been imposed on the use of funds for HIV education, services, and research.
7. Give greater priority and funding to behavioral, social science, and health services research.
8. Speeding the development of clear, explicit, culturally appropriate educational programs about prevention and protection for use in places where adolescents and young adults gather, including schools, social clubs, movie theaters, "shooting galleries," and on regular commercial television programs.
9. Taking steps to address the growing shortage of health professionals who treat HIV-infected people.
10. Addressing the increasing need for out-of-hospital housing, nursing home beds, and day care services for those with HIV infection, and the respite services needed by their caretakers.
11. Encouraging and supporting the myriad community-based organizations that have been in the forefront of the efforts to combat AIDS, to mute discrimination, and to care for those infected.

In the minds of many, over time our society will be judged by how well we deal with some of the social problems of our times. HIV infection and its resultant, AIDS, is embedded in many of those problems. The biomedical sciences are providing an increasingly clear view of what is needed to prevent further devastation by this virus. We can only hope that further scientific advances will ultimately permit us to cure those already infected and to prevent illness from occurring at all. But until that time we must be more effective in using present knowledge to effect the social and behavioral changes required to halt this epidemic. We can if we decide it is important enough.

REFERENCES

1. Camus A: The Plague [transl Stuart Gilbert]. New York, Alfred A Knopf, 1983
2. Osborn JE: The AIDS epidemic: Multidisciplinary trouble. N Engl J Med 314:779, 1986
3. Centers for Disease Control: Kaposi's sarcoma and pneumocystis pneumonia among homosexual men in New York City and California. MMWR 30:305, 1981
4. Ron A, Rogers DE: AIDS in the United States: Patient care and politics. Daedalus 118:41, 1981
5. Ludmerer KM: Patients beyond the pale: A historical view. In Rogers DE, Ginzberg E (eds): Public and Professional Attitudes Toward AIDS Patients: A National Dilemma. Boulder, Colo, Westview Press, 1989
6. State of New York, Department of Health: AIDS—New York's response: A five year interagency plan. State of New York, 1989
7. Centers for Disease Control: HIV prevalence estimates and AIDS case projections for the United States: Report based upon a workshop. MMWR 39(RR-16):1, 1990
8. Centers for Disease Control: HIV/AIDS Surveillance Report. Atlanta, Centers for Disease Control, March 1991
9. National Commission on AIDS: Report No. Three: Research, the Workforce, and HIV Epidemic in Rural America, August 21, 1990
10. Verghese A, Berk SL, Sarubbi F: Urbs in rure: Human immunodeficiency virus infection in rural Tennessee. J Infect Dis 160:1051, 1989
11. Institute of Medicine: The AIDS research program of the National Institutes of Health: Report of a study committee of the Institute of Medicine AIDS activities. Washington, DC, National Academy Press, 1991
12. National Research Council: Risking the Future. Washington, DC, National Academy Press, 1987
13. Hartgers C, Buning EC, van Santen GW et al: The impact of the needle and syringe exchange programme in Amsterdam on injecting risk behaviors. AIDS 3:571, 1981
14. Purchase D, Hagan H, DesJarlais DC et al: Historical account of the Tacoma syringe exchange (abstr Tb.D.P.74). Poster presentation at V International Conference on AIDS, Montreal, June 1989
15. Goldstein A: Clean needle programs for addicts proliferate. Washington Post, April 23, 1991
16. National Commission on AIDS: Annual Report to the President and the Congress, August 1990. No. 274-550-814/20762. Washington, DC, US Government Printing Office, 1990
17. Friedland G, Kahl P, Saltzman B: Additional evidence for lack of transmission of HIV by close interpersonal (casual) contact. AIDS 4:639, 1990
18. Gershon RRM, Vlahov D, Nelson KE et al: The risk of transmission of HIV-1 through non-percutaneous, non-sexual modes: A review. AIDS 4:645, 1990
19. Dab W, Moatti JP, Bastide ST et al: Misconceptions about transmission of AIDS and attitudes toward prevention in the French general public. AIDS 3:443, 1989
20. Koop CE: Surgeon General's Report on Acquired Immunodeficiency Syndrome. Washington, DC, US Government Printing Office, 1986
21. DesJarlis DC, Friedman S: The psychology of preventing AIDS among intravenous drug users: A social learning conceptualization. Am Psychol 48:865, 1988
22. Stephens RC, Feucht TE, Roman SW: Effect of an intervention program on AIDS-related drug and needle behavior among intravenous drug users. Am J Public Health 81:568, 1991
23. Osborn JE: Public health and the politics of AIDS prevention. Daedalus 118:123, 1981
24. Bosk CL, Frader JE: AIDS and its impact on medical work: The culture and politics of the shop floor. Millbank Q 68(suppl 2):257, 1990
25. National Commission on AIDS: Report No. One: Failure of United States Health Care System To Deal with HIV Epidemic, December 5, 1989

VI

HIV Infection and the Health Care Worker

30

Occupational Risk of HIV Infection in Health Care Workers

Ruthanne Marcus   *David M. Bell*

Instances of occupationally acquired human immuno-deficiency virus (HIV) infection among health care workers are well documented and substantial data are available on the risk of infection after a single exposure to HIV-infected blood. However, data remain limited on the epidemiology of blood contact among health care workers, risk factors for HIV transmission after an exposure to infected blood, the cumulative risk of infection among health care workers who may have multiple and possibly unrecognized exposures, and the efficacy of specific preventive measures. The risk to an individual health care provider over a lifetime career depends on several factors, including (1) the risk of HIV transmission after a single contact, (2) the number of HIV-infected patients treated by the worker, and (3) the number and types of blood contact experienced by the worker. This chapter reviews available data on occupationally acquired HIV infection in health care workers and discusses available information on determinants of risk.

OCCUPATIONALLY ACQUIRED HIV INFECTION IN HEALTH CARE WORKERS

No single source of information adequately summarizes the occupational risk of HIV infection in health care workers. Review of multiple sources of data is required, including data from the Centers for Disease Control's (CDC) AIDS/HIV case surveillance system, individual case reports, and epidemiologic studies.

Data are collected on the CDC's AIDS case report form on a history of employment in a clinical laboratory or health care setting. As of March 31, 1991, the CDC had received reports of 135,617 persons with AIDS for whom occupational information was available. Of these persons, 6,436 (4.8%) had been employed in health settings; 94% were within one or more well-recognized nonoccupational transmission categories, three (<1%) seroconverted and subsequently developed AIDS after a documented occupational exposure to HIV-infected blood, and 6% had an undetermined risk. In contrast, 3% of the non-health care workers with AIDS have an undetermined risk. Of the 336 health care workers in the undetermined risk category, 57% are still under investigation to determine risk, 22% have either died, refused to be interviewed, or are unavailable for follow-up, and 73 (20%) could not be reclassified into a known transmission category after follow-up investigation (C. Ciesielski, CDC, pers. commun.).[1]

Of these 73 workers, none had had a documented exposure to blood or other body fluids of a patient with AIDS or HIV infection, and approximately 40% did not recall exposure to blood or body fluids of any patient in the 10 years before the diagnosis of AIDS. Compared with the 6.9 million health care workers in the United States, these 73 workers were more likely to be men (73% *vs.* 23%) and more likely to be black (30% *vs.* 13%). Therefore, these health care workers are more similar to other persons with AIDS than to other health care workers without AIDS. The occupations of these workers included aide/attendant (14), physician (11), hospital maintenance worker (11), technician (9), nurse (8), paramedic (4), dental worker (3), embalmer (3), therapist (2), surgeon (1), and 7 in other job categories. The proportion of these workers who acquired infection due to occupational exposure cannot be determined (C. Ciesielski, CDC, pers. commun.).

In a separate surveillance project, CDC also collects information on persons reported by state health departments as having occupationally acquired HIV infection. As of September 30, 1991, the CDC had received reports of 28 health care workers in the United States who had seroconverted to HIV after well-documented percutaneous, mucous membrane, or skin exposures to HIV: 12 (43%) were laboratory workers, 11 (39%) were nurses, 3 (11%) were physicians, and 2 were health care workers had other occupations. Twenty-three (82%) of the workers had percutaneous exposures, 4 (14%) had mucocutaneous exposures, and 1 had both a percutaneous and a mucocutaneous exposure; 27 of the 28 were exposed to HIV-infected blood, and the remaining worker was exposed to concentrated virus.[2]

In addition, the CDC is aware of 18 other cases of HIV infection among health care workers without non-occupational risk behaviors for HIV infection but for whom data to document seroconversion after a known occupational exposure were not obtained (C. Ciesielski, CDC, pers. commun.). In some of these cases baseline serologic testing was not performed; in other cases the worker had a history of exposure to blood but the HIV serostatus of the source patient was not known.

At least 12 additional cases have been reported from outside the United States; ten of these cases involved percutaneous exposures, one was a mucous membrane exposure to HIV-infected blood, and in another case a woman providing health care to a neighbor with HIV became infected.[3-14] With the exception of one case, in which a nurse was exposed to bloody pleural fluid,[8] documented transmission of HIV in a clinical setting has always been due to occupational exposure to blood.

PROSPECTIVE STUDIES

Several prospective cohort studies of the risk to health care workers of HIV infection have been conducted. In these studies health care workers with percutaneous, mucous membrane, or skin contact with blood of HIV-infected patients are prospectively followed with serologic testing at the time of the exposure and periodically thereafter.[15-27] The results of these various studies have been consistent, demonstrating that the risk of acquiring HIV infection after a percutaneous exposure (i.e., needlestick or cut with a sharp object) is approximately 0.3% (upper limit of 95% confidence interval [CI] = 0.6%).[23,24,26] This risk represents an average of many types of percutaneous exposures from source patients in various stages of infection. There are insufficient data to accurately stratify the risk of infection based on the size (large- vs. small-gauge) or type (hollow- vs. solid-bore) of needle, the depth or severity of exposure, or the volume of blood involved. *In vitro* studies, con-ducted to attempt to answer some of these questions, have found that the volume of blood transferred in a needlestick injury is apparently greater with increased depth of penetration, is somewhat greater for hollow-bore than for solid-bore needles, and is reduced at least 50% with glove use.[28]

Details of several of the larger prospective studies of health care workers ongoing in the United States are provided here. In the CDC prospective surveillance of health care workers exposed to HIV-infected blood, as of June 30, 1991, 1,548 health care workers with percutaneous, mucous membrane, and nonintact skin contact were tested at least 6 months after exposure. Of the 1,366 workers with percutaneous exposures, three seroconverted to HIV (0.22%; upper limit of 95% CI = 0.57%). An additional health care worker with a needlestick injury was seropositive when first tested for HIV 10 months after exposure; however, this worker had a nonoccupational risk (a sexual partner infected with HIV). Of the 182 health care workers with mucous membrane or nonintact skin exposure, none seroconverted to HIV (0%; upper limit of 95% CI = 1.62%).[29]

Henderson and colleagues have followed health care workers at the Clinical Center, National Institutes of Health (NIH), after exposure to HIV-infected blood.[26] Of 179 workers with percutaneous exposures, one seroconverted (1/179 = 0.56%; upper limit of 95% CI = 3.06%), while none among 346 with mucous membrane exposures seroconverted (0/346 = 0%; upper limit of 95% CI = 0.86%) and none among 2,712 with cutaneous exposures seroconverted (0/2,712 = 0%; upper limit of 95% CI = 0.11%).

In a similar study at San Francisco General Hospital, one of 189 health care workers with a cumulative 273 needlestick exposures to HIV seroconverted (1/273 = 0.37% per exposure).[24] In Canada, as of March 31, 1991, 397 health care workers with documented percutaneous or mucous membrane exposures to HIV infection have been followed; none has seroconverted (Health and Welfare Canada, Federal Centre for AIDS, unpubl. data).

Although HIV transmission after a mucous membrane or cutaneous exposure to infected blood has been reported,[2,6,10,30] no such seroconversions have occurred in health care workers enrolled in prospective studies.[23,24,26] The risk of HIV infection due to these types of exposures is not precisely known, but it is lower than that from percutaneous exposures. At NIH, Fahey *et al* conducted a retrospective questionnaire survey before and after staff training in the use of universal precautions. Of 559 initial respondents, 136 (24.3%) estimated 6,528 cutaneous blood contacts with HIV-infected blood. After training in universal precautions, 33 (12.3%) of 269 of these health care workers self-reported 1,428 contacts. No health care worker who reported contact with HIV-positive blood was seropositive for HIV when tested at least 6 months after the last reported contact (upper bound of the 95% CI for first survey = 0.05%; for second survey = 0.21%).[31]

To address concerns about the possibility of delayed seroconversion after exposure, several investigators have used polymerase chain reaction (PCR) techniques to examine specimens from HIV-antibody negative health care workers more than 6 months after exposure to HIV-infected blood.[24,26,32,33] Of 237 seronegative workers, only three were seropositive by PCR, all in one study. However, in these three cases, enzyme-linked immunosorbent assays (ELISA) and Western blot antibody studies, p24 antigen assays, and viral cultures were negative. Subsequently, PCR testing on two of these workers was negative,[24] casting additional doubt on the significance of the initial positive test. The remaining positive health care worker has continued to be positive by the PCR but has no other laboratory evidence of HIV infection. The significance of this isolated positive PCR result is unknown. These data, combined with data on several hundred health care workers who have remained seronegative when tested 2 or more years after exposure,[23,24,26] suggest that seroconversion (if it occurs) more than 6 months after occupational exposure is likely to be uncommon.

Some health care workers with occupational exposures to HIV-infected blood have elected to take zidovudine (AZT) as attempted postexposure prophylaxis. In January 1990 the U.S. Public Health Service published recommendations for the management of exposures to HIV and considerations for the use of AZT.[34] Because of the lack of data on AZT efficacy and toxicity, these recommendations do not encourage or discourage the use of AZT for this purpose, but provide physicians and workers with guidance in their decision to begin treatment. Considerations include the risk of HIV infection after exposure and the factors that have been postulated to influence this risk, the apparent need to begin prophylaxis promptly if prophylaxis is given, the limitations of current knowledge of the efficacy and toxicity of AZT, and the need for postexposure follow-up, regardless of whether AZT is taken.

In several prospective studies of exposed health care workers, investigators have collected data on the use and short-term toxicity of AZT; similar data have been collected by other institutions using their own protocols.[35] In the CDC health care worker surveillance project, 166 (26%) of 630 health care workers enrolled from October 1988 through June 1991 elected to initiate a course of AZT postexposure prophylaxis. The number of workers starting AZT increased from 5% of new enrollees during the period of October through December 1988 to 46% of new enrollees during the period of January through March 1991. Of the 133 health care workers who had completed at least 6 weeks of follow-up, 96 (72%) reported side-effects: nausea in 59, malaise and/or fatigue in 43, and headache in 27. Thirty percent of the 133 workers discontinued therapy before completing the prescribed course.[29]

Similar results have been found at the NIH Clinical Center,[36] San Francisco General Hospital,[37] and in studies in Italy[38] and Canada.[39] Burroughs-Wellcome Company initiated a prospective, randomized, double-blind, placebo-controlled trial to evaluate AZT postexposure use in health care workers; however, this trial was terminated prematurely because of low enrollment.[40] Of 84 health care workers enrolled in the trial, 49 received AZT and 35 received placebo. None of the participants in either group experienced serious drug toxicity requiring discontinuation of therapy. Additional data are needed on the short- and long-term side-effects of postexposure AZT use.

No health care worker has seroconverted in any prospective study after taking AZT, although this is not unexpected, insofar as the risk of seroconversion after percutaneous exposure to HIV-infected blood has been estimated as approximately 0.3%. HIV seroconversion, despite AZT use, has been reported in at least seven cases. Five of the cases involved intravenous injection of a large inoculum of HIV-infected blood, which may explain the failure of AZT to prevent infection. One of the five cases involved a transfusion of HIV-infected blood[34]; two involved an attempted suicide and an assault of several ml of infected blood,[41,41a] and the remaining two occurred during nuclear medicine procedures in patients who were inadvertently injected with a syringe of blood from a patient with HIV infection.[42]

In two additional cases, AZT failed in health care workers who sustained needlestick injuries with the blood of HIV-infected patients. One of the workers began AZT use within 6 hours after a deep needlestick injury at a dosage of 250 mg every 6 hours, which was continued for 8 weeks,[14] and the other began AZT 8 hours after an intramuscular injury from a 16-gauge needle, at a dosage of 1,000 mg/day for 1 week (C. Ciesielski, CDC, pers. commun.).

Assessment of AZT efficacy in lowering the risk of infection after an occupational exposure will require a prospective trial involving many thousands of exposed workers. The discontinuation of the Burroughs-Wellcome trial after 1 year owing to enrollment of only 84 workers suggests that assessment of efficacy will have to be based on additional laboratory and animal studies[43] rather than on a clinical trial.

SEROPREVALENCE SURVEYS IN HEALTH CARE WORKERS

Cross-sectional studies of HIV seroprevalence in groups of health care workers provide additional information for evaluating the risk of occupationally acquiring HIV infection (Table 30–1). Such studies must be interpreted carefully, taking into account whether the enrolled health care workers are representative of the population being studied, and whether information is available to assess the likelihood of occupational and nonoccupational exposure to HIV.

In March 1991 the CDC, in cooperation with the American Academy of Orthopaedic Surgeons (AAOS), conducted a voluntary, anonymous seroprevalence sur-

Table 30–1.   HIV Seroprevalence in Selected Groups of Health Care Workers

Worker Group	No. Tested	No. (%) Positive	No. Positive With Community Risk	% Prevalence, Excluding Seropositives With Community Risk	Reference
Orthopedic surgeons	3,420	2 (0.06)	2	0.00	44
Medical personnel in U.S. Army					
Reserve	58,394	138 (2.37)	N.A.	N.A.	45
Dentists					
San Francisco	304†	0 (0)	—†	0	47
Sacramento	89	0 (0)	0	0	46
USA 1986 annual meeting, and New					
York City	1,132†	1 (0.09)	—†	0.09	50
USA—1987 annual meeting	1,195	0 (0)	0	0	48
USA—1988 annual meeting	1,165	1 (0.09)	0	0.09	49
USA—1989 annual meeting	1,480	0 (0)	0	0	49
Denmark	961	0 (0)	0	0	51
Dental assistants (New York City and					
Sacramento)	176	0 (0)	0	0	46, 50
Dental hygienists (New York City and					
Sacramento)	167	0 (0)	0	0	46, 50
Hemodialysis staff (New York, Paris,					
Chicago, Brussels, Florence)	356	0 (0)	0	0	53–57
Blood donors, USA—20 urban					
regions	39,220*	19 (0.05)	10	0.02	58

* Estimated number of blood donors who were health care workers.
† Persons with community risk not included.

vey at the AAOS annual meeting.[44] Of the 3,420 orthopedic surgeons who participated, 2 (0.06%; upper limit of 95% CI = 0.18%) were positive for HIV antibody and one had an indeterminate result. The two seropositive surgeons were among 108 who reported nonoccupational risks for HIV infection (HIV seroprevalence 1.8%; upper limit of 95% CI = 5.7%). In comparison, among the 3,267 participants who did not report nonoccupational risks for HIV infection, none was HIV seropositive (upper limit of 95% CI = 0.092%). Of the 45 participants who did not respond to the question on risk factors, none was HIV positive. The one surgeon whose serum tested indeterminate for HIV antibody did not report a nonoccupational risk.

Both of the HIV-positive participants were men and reported having performed surgery on patients with risk factors for HIV infection. One of the two surgeons reported performing surgery on patients with known HIV infection or AIDS. Although both had sustained percutaneous injuries in the previous year, neither reported an injury from a sharp object contaminated with the blood of a patient known to have HIV infection or AIDS. The surgeon with an indeterminate result, a man who had retired from clinical practice, reported never having operated on a patient with known HIV infection or AIDS or on a patient with known risk factors for HIV or AIDS.

Although participants in this serosurvey may not be representative of all orthopedic surgeons, preliminary analyses suggest that the likelihood of occupational HIV

exposure among participants was comparable to the exposure of over 10,000 orthopedic surgeons in the United States and Canada who responded to a mailed questionnaire survey conducted by the AAOS. Compared with the questionnaire survey respondents, serosurvey participants were more likely to be in residency or fellowship training (18% *vs.* 14%), to have trained or practiced in one or more areas of high AIDS incidence since 1977 (75% *vs.* 69%), to have operated on one or more patients with known infection (49% *vs.* 43%), to have had a patient's blood contact their skin in the previous month (87% *vs.* 83%), and to have sustained a percutaneous injury from a sharp object contaminated with a patient's blood in the previous month (39% *vs.* 34%). Thus, although these results may not be applicable to all orthopedic surgeons, no evidence was found to suggest a high rate of previously undetected HIV infection among a large group of orthopedic surgeons, including those who train or practice in areas of high HIV/AIDS incidence.

Other seroprevalence surveys conducted among various groups of health care workers have been useful for identifying previously undetected HIV infection, but they are limited in their ability to estimate the occupational and nonoccupational risks for HIV infection. Cowan and colleagues at Walter Reed Army Medical Center tested members of the U.S. Army Reserve, who spend about 90% of their time working in civilian life, for HIV antibody.[45] Of those workers employed in a medical field, 2.37 per 1,000 tested were seropositive for HIV (138/58,349 = 2.37; 95% CI = 2.02–2.83). In contrast, 925 of 619,112 (1.49 per 1,000 tested; 95% CI = 1.41–1.60) nonmedical personnel were HIV positive. The higher rate of HIV infection in medical workers was found primarily among never-married men who may not have acquired infection occupationally.

Several seroprevalence surveys of dental personnel have been conducted.[46–52] In the largest published study, Klein *et al* tested 1,309 dental workers, including 1,132 dentists and 177 dental hygienists and assistants, more than half of whom practiced in areas of the United States reporting a large number of AIDS cases.[50] Fifteen percent of the participants had treated patients with AIDS and 72% had treated patients at risk for HIV infection. One dentist without behavioral risks for HIV infection tested seropositive (1/1,309 = 0.08%). This dentist worked in an area of the United States with a high prevalence of HIV infection. He did not report treating any patients with AIDS, but did report treating those at increased risk for infection.[50] Several other surveys of dental workers have also found low rates of infection.[46–52]

Workers in hemodialysis units have also been studied because of the recognized high risk of hepatitis B virus (HBV) infection in such workers in the past. In several small studies, none of 356 dialysis workers tested for HIV have been seropositive.[53–57]

Chamberland and colleagues have studied blood donors who work in health care settings as part of a larger study of blood donors at 20 urban regional centers in the United States. Between March 1990 and May 1991, an estimated 39,220 health care workers donated blood in these centers. Of these, 19 (0.05%) were positive for HIV antibody. Upon interview, 10 (53%) reported community risk factors for HIV infection. Excluding these 10 health care workers, the seroprevalence was 0.02%.[58]

With a few exceptions,[59–61] studies of health care workers' exposure and infection risk have not been conducted in developing countries, where the HIV seroprevalence among patients is high and resources for infection control are limited. In the few studies that have been conducted in these countries, rates of HIV infection in medical workers and in the community were similar.

HIV SEROPREVALENCE IN PATIENTS

The likelihood that a health care worker will be exposed to the blood of a patient with HIV infection depends in part on the prevalence of HIV in the patient population. In the United States, data are available from numerous seroprevalence surveys among hospitalized patients and among outpatients at hospital emergency departments, hemodialysis centers, and at clinics for sexually transmitted diseases,[62] drug treatment,[63] women's health,[64,65] tuberculosis,[66] college students,[67] and primary care outpatients.[68]

In the CDC sentinel hospital study, in which blinded HIV antibody testing is conducted on selected leftover blood specimens at a group of voluntarily participating hospitals in the United States, from January 1988 to June 1989, St. Louis *et al* found seroprevalence rates ranging from 0.1% to 7.8%, depending on hospital location, among 89,547 specimens tested at 26 hospitals.[69] Specimens were not tested if they came from patients admitted for diagnoses that may be associated with HIV infection, such as certain infectious diseases, unexplained fever, neuropsychiatric conditions, neoplasms, and gunshot or knife wounds. This study demonstrated that the rate of HIV infection was quite high in some areas.

Of 616 serial hospital admissions in a Department of Veterans Affairs Hospital in Washington, DC, 23 (3.7%) were positive for HIV antibody.[70] Only eight of the 23 were already known to be infected, including four who had been diagnosed with AIDS.

Several studies of HIV seroprevalence have been conducted in emergency department patients.[71–81] In a CDC study, blinded HIV antibody testing was conducted on leftover blood specimens of emergency department patients in one inner-city and one suburban hospital in each of three cities in the United States with a high AIDS incidence. Seroprevalence rates per 100 patient visits were 4.1 to 8.9 in the inner-city emergency departments, 6.1 in one suburban emergency department, and 0.2 and 0.7 in the other two suburban hospitals. Rates were highest among patients in the 15- to 44-year-old age group, in men, in blacks, and in patients presenting with pneumonia. The percentage of patients whose HIV infection was unknown ranged from 66% to 70% for inner-city emergency departments, 40% in the suburban emergency department with a higher seroprevalence, and 76% and 91% in the other two suburban emergency departments.[71]

In a study conducted in several hospitals in Portland, Oregon, two (0.45%) of 444 emergency department patients tested in a 48-hour period were HIV seropositive.[78] In 1987, Kelen *et al* at Johns Hopkins Hospital in Baltimore found 5.2% (119/2,302) of patients presenting to the emergency department to be infected with HIV[73]; by 1989, the rate had increased to 6.0% (152/2,544).[74] At Charity Hospital in New Orleans, 11 (2%) of 534 emergency department patients' sera were seropositive for HIV antibodies.[76] Schweich and colleagues identified HIV antibody in ten (1.6%) of 607 pediatric patients who underwent phlebotomy; all but one child had known risk factors for HIV infection.[79] In a community emergency department in the Midwest, one (0.76%) of 262 trauma patients was seropositive.[77]

Numerous studies have been conducted on the prevalence of HIV among hemodialysis patients.[53–57,82–87] In these studies rates have ranged from 0% to 39%, depending on the city where the dialysis unit was located and the patient population treated. For example, centers that treated a large proportion of IV drug users had higher rates of HIV infection among the patients.

Collectively these patient seroprevalence studies demonstrate that the prevalence of HIV infection varies with geographic area and patient diagnosis, as well as with patient's age, sex, and race/ethnicity, and that the infection status of many patients is often unknown. The results of these studies emphasize the need for observing universal precautions.

EPIDEMIOLOGY OF BLOOD CONTACT

To better understand the epidemiology of blood contact in health care workers, researchers have conducted observational studies of the nature and frequency of blood contact (defined as percutaneous, mucous membrane, or skin contact) during procedures performed in hospital operating and delivery rooms and emergency departments. These studies, which have added to information obtained in questionnaire surveys,[88-91] are useful for defining risk factors for blood contact and for devising preventive measures. The reported rates of blood contact and sharps injuries may vary in these studies owing to differences in study methodology, the definition of blood contact, procedures observed, and the use of infection control precautions.

A summary of several studies conducted in operating rooms is provided in Table 30–2. At San Francisco General Hospital, Gerberding *et al* evaluated instances of blood contact among surgical personnel during consecutive procedures in all specialties for a 2-month period. Blood contact was observed in 84 (6.4%) of 1,307 surgical procedures; percutaneous exposures occurred in 1.3% of the procedures.[92] Factors affecting the risk of blood contact were the length of the procedure, the volume of blood loss, and if the operation involved major vascular or intra-abdominal gynecologic surgery. The risk of exposure was not influenced by the surgeon's prior knowledge of the patient's serostatus or risk of HIV infection. The authors concluded that the use of barrier protection (such as double gloves, waterproof garments, and face shields) protects against mucous membrane and cutaneous blood contact, and that preoperative screening for HIV infection does not reduce the risk of blood contact.

Three CDC studies have provided additional data on blood contact frequency and preventability. In a study conducted at Grady Memorial Hospital in Atlanta, trained observers were present in the operating room during surgeries on the general surgery, trauma, orthopedics, burn, gynecology, and plastics services. At least one blood contact was observed during 62 (30.1%) of 206 surgical procedures.[93] Each procedure was performed by a team of several health care workers, for a total of 1,828 person-procedures; of these, 96 (5.3%) involved 147 blood contacts (133 skin contacts, ten percutaneous injuries, and four eye splashes). Of 110 blood contacts among surgeons, 81 (74%) were potentially preventable with the use of additional barrier precautions, such as face shields and fluid-resistant gowns.

Obstetric personnel are also at risk for occupational exposure to blood-borne pathogens. In a CDC observational study of 202 vaginal and 28 cesarean deliveries, 112 blood contacts were observed in 74 (32.2%) procedures, including the following: 106 skin contacts, four needlesticks, and two mucous membrane splashes.[94] The four needlesticks occurred during vaginal deliveries and during performance or repair of an episiotomy or laceration. Knowledge that the woman had or was at risk for HIV infection did not prevent the likelihood of blood or amniotic fluid exposure. Over half of the obstetricians' contacts might have been prevented with the use of barrier precautions such as face shields, impervious gowns, and impervious shoe covers; half of the midwives' contacts might have been prevented with the use of gowns.

Tokars *et al* observed blood contact during operations in two pairs of hospitals, one inner city and one suburban, in New York and Chicago.[97] General, orthopedic, gynecologic, cardiac, and trauma surgeries were observed. At least one blood contact was recorded in 644 (46.6%) of the 1,382 surgical procedures observed (95 procedures resulted in percutaneous injuries,

Table 30–2.   Selected Prospective Studies of Blood Contact Among Operating and Delivery Room Personnel

Location	No. of Procedures	% of Procedures With One or More Blood Contacts	% of Procedures With One or More Sharp Injuries	Reference
United States				
New York and Chicago	1,382	46.6	6.9	97
San Francisco	1,307*	6.4	1.3	92
Albuquerque	684*	27.8	3.1	95
Milwaukee	234	50.4	15.4	96
Atlanta (surgery)	206	30.1	4.9	93
(obstetrics)	230	32.2	1.7	94
Outside United States				
Saudi Arabia	2,016	N.A.	5.6	88

* Includes endoscopic procedures.

28 procedures resulted in mucous membrane contacts, and 585 procedures resulted in blood-skin contacts). Of 99 percutaneous injuries that occurred in the 95 surgical procedures, 76 (80%) were caused by suture needles. In 24 of the injuries, the sharp was held by a co-worker. Many of the 99 injuries appeared to be potentially preventable: 46 were associated with the use of fingers rather than an instrument to hold tissue being sutured, and 63% affected the nondominant hand, primarily the distal forefinger. Injuries occurring on this portion of the hand might be prevented by the use of a barrier such as a thimble.

Popejoy and Fry in Albuquerque, New Mexico, observed a blood contact in 190 (27.8%) of 684 consecutive surgical procedures.[95] In Milwaukee, Telford and Quebbeman identified at least one blood contact in 50.4% of 234 surgical procedures.[96] In Saudi Arabia a survey was conducted of eight general surgeons, four orthopedic surgeons, two urologists, and four surgical residents. These physicians reported 112 accidental injuries (5.6%) during 2,016 operations (including 107 needlestick injuries, four knife cuts, and one diathermy burn).[88]

In another study focusing on cardiac surgery, Pate studied blood exposure during 50 coronary bypass operations and 17 cardiac valve replacements performed in Memphis, Tennessee; he reported 0.4 to 1.5 skin punctures, lacerations, or eye splashes per operation.[98]

The frequency of blood contact among hospital emergency department workers has also been studied prospectively.[71,74,99] In a CDC study in six hospitals, blood contact varied by procedure observed; for example, blood contacts were observed in 63% of 19 thoracotomies, 5% of 1,499 incidents of wound care, 4% of 2,697 IV line insertions, and 2% of 2,493 phlebotomy procedures. It was estimated that an individual emergency department physician or nurse would experience 0.37 percutaneous blood contacts annually and 31.81 cutaneous blood contacts with current glove use. Gloves significantly reduced the frequency of blood contact. With 100% glove compliance the annual frequency of cutaneous blood contact for an emergency department physician or nurse could be reduced to 12.73. The relative risk of blood contact for ungloved *versus* gloved emergency department workers was 19.8 for obtaining arterial blood, 13.0 for inserting an IV line, and 5.4 for phlebotomy.

Wong and colleagues conducted a prospective study using a daily questionnaire to study blood contact and barrier precaution use among 277 physicians on a medical service.[100] Before implementation of universal precautions, the number of blood and body fluid contacts was 5.07 per physician per patient care month; the number decreased to 2.66 after the implementation of precautions. During the 9-month study period, the physicians sustained 1,553 blood and body fluid contacts, including 1,379 skin contacts with blood and 49 needlesticks. Eighty-nine percent of the exposures occurred during procedures that involved the insertion or manipulation of needles or catheters.

Based in part on studies such as these, several researchers have estimated the cumulative risk to health care workers of HIV infection.[71,92,101–106] For example, Gerberding *et al* have estimated that one worker at San Francisco General Hospital will become infected with HIV every 8 years.[92] Howard developed a model to predict that 47 of the approximately 18,000 Fellows of the American College of Surgeons would become infected with HIV during their surgical career.[102] Such calculations are most likely to be accurate when the prevalence of HIV infection in the patient population is well defined, the frequency of blood contact, especially sharps exposures, is established, and the use of infection control practices is ascertained.

AEROSOLS

Some health care workers have expressed concern about the potential occupational risk of HIV transmission from aerosolized blood and body fluids generated by high-speed equipment such as drills, lasers, and electrocautery devices. Aerosols are not droplets but tiny, invisible particles called droplet nuclei, which, unlike droplets, remain suspended in the air for extended periods of time. Although inspired particles 10 to 100 μm in diameter may be deposited in the upper airway or in bronchi, true respirable aerosols capable of reaching the alveoli consist of particles less than 5 to 10 μm in diameter. There are no known cases of transmission of a blood-borne pathogen by aerosols in a clinical setting. In studies conducted in dental operatories and in hemodialysis units, HBsAg was not detected in the air during treatment of patients infected with HBV.[107] Aerosolized HIV has been detected in laboratory studies,[108] although these studies should not be interpreted to mean that HIV is aerosolized in a clinical setting or that HIV is transmitted *via* this route. Until further research is conducted, the possibility of occupational transmission of HIV through aerosolized blood should be considered theoretical.

FUTURE NEEDS

A better understanding of the factors that result in occupational transmission of HIV is essential for the development of preventive measures. Additional research is needed to further identify the factors that result in seroconversion after exposure to HIV, to better quantify the risk of HIV transmission after cutaneous or mucous membrane contact with HIV-infected blood, and to better define the frequency and preventability of occupational blood contacts. Surveillance of health care workers with occupationally acquired HIV infection or AIDS and studies on the prevalence and incidence of HIV infection in health care workers with frequent blood contact will assist in assessing these risks by providing data on the factors affecting infection. Studies are also needed to assess the effect of preventive measures, including new or improved medical devices,[109–111] work practices, and personal protective equipment,[92,112] in preventing blood contact without adversely affecting patient care.

REFERENCES

1. Ciesielski C, Gooch B, Hammett T, Metler R: Dentists, allied professionals with AIDS. J Am Dent Assoc 122:42, 1991
2. Metler R, Ciesielski C, Marcus R, Berkelman R: Occupationally-acquired HIV infection, United States (abstr W.D.4178). Presented at the VIIth International Conference on AIDS, Florence, Italy, June 16–20, 1991
3. Bygbjerg IC: AIDS in a Danish Surgeon (Zaire, 1976) (letter). Lancet 1:925, 1983
4. [N.A.]: Acquired immune deficiency syndrome (AIDS): Update. Weekly Epidemiol Rec 59:382, 1984
5. [N.A.]: Needlestick transmission of HTLV-III from a patient infected in Africa (letter). Lancet 2:1376, 1984
6. Grint P, McEvoy M: Two associated cases of the acquired immune deficiency syndrome (AIDS). PHLS Commun Dis Rep 42:4, 1985
7. Neisson-Vernant C, Arfi S, Mathez D et al: Needlestick HIV seroconversion in a nurse (letter). Lancet 2:814, 1986
8. Oksenhendler E, Harzic M, Le Roux J-M et al: HIV infection with seroconversion after a superficial needlestick injury to the finger (letter). N Engl J Med 315:582, 1986
9. Michelet C, Cartier F, Ruffault A et al: Needlestick HIV infection in a nurse (abstr 9010). Presented at the IV International Conference on AIDS, Stockholm, Sweden, June 12–16, 1988
10. Gioannini P, Sinicco A, Cariti G et al: HIV infection acquired by a nurse. Eur J Epidemiol 4:119, 1988
11. Lima G, Traina C: [Remarks on a case of AIDS-related syndrome (ARC/LAS) in a nurse.] [In Italian.] Minerva Med 79:141, 1988
12. Ponce de Leon S, Sanchez-Mejorada G, Zaidi-Jacobson M: AIDS in a blood bank technician in Mexico City (letter). Infect Control Hosp Epidemiol 9:101, 1988
13. Serra MA, Nogueira JM, Garcia-Lomas J, Rodrigo JM: Un caso de transmision por virus de la inmunodeficiencia humana tipo 1 tras puncion accidental en personal sanitario. Med Clin 47:475, 1988
14. Looke DFM, Grove DI: Failed prophylactic zidovudine after needlestick injury (letter). Lancet 1:1280, 1990
15. Hirsch MS, Wormser GP, Schooley RT et al: Risk of nosocomial infection with human T-cell lymphotropic virus III (HTLV-III). N Engl J Med 312:1, 1985
16. Weiss SH, Saxinger WC, Rechtman D et al: HTLV-III infection among health care workers: Association with needle-stick injuries. JAMA 254:2089, 1985
17. McCray E, The Cooperative Needlestick Surveillance Group: Occupational risk of the acquired immunodeficiency syndrome among health care workers. N Engl J Med 314:1127, 1986
18. McEvoy M, Porter K, Mortimer P et al: Prospective study of clinical, laboratory, and ancillary staff with accidental exposures to blood or body fluids from patients infected with HIV. Br Med J 294:1595, 1987
19. Joline C, Wormser GP: Update on a prospective study of health care workers exposed to blood and body fluids of acquired immunodeficiency syndrome patients (abstr). Am J Infect Control 15:86, 1987

20. Weiss SH, Goedert JJ, Gartner S et al: Risk of human immunodeficiency virus (HIV-1) infection among laboratory workers. Science 239:68, 1988
21. Hernandez E, Gatell JM, Puyuelo T et al: Risk of transmitting the HIV to health care workers (HCW) exposed to HIV infected body fluids (abstr 9003). Presented at the IV International Conference on AIDS, Stockholm, Sweden, June 12–16, 1988
22. Pizzocolo G, Stellini R, Cadeo GP et al: Risk of HIV and HBV infection after accidental needlestick (abstr 9012). Presented at the IV International Conference on AIDS, Stockholm, Sweden, June 12–16, 1988
23. Marcus R, Cooperative Needlestick Surveillance Group: Surveillance of health care workers exposed to blood from patients infected with the human immunodeficiency virus. N Engl J Med 319:1118, 1988
24. Gerberding JL, Littell C, Brown A, Ramiro N: Cumulative risk of HIV and hepatitis B (HBV) among health care workers (HCW): Longterm serologic followup & gene amplification for latent HIV infection (abstr 959). In: Program and Abstracts of the Interscience Conference on Antimicrobial Agents and Chemotherapy, Atlanta, 1990
25. Ramsey KM, Smith EN, Reinarz JA: Prospective evaluation of 44 health care workers exposed to human immunodeficiency virus-1, with one seroconversion (abstr). Clin Res 36:22A, 1988
26. Henderson DK, Fahey BJ, Willy M et al: Risk for occupational transmission of human immunodeficiency virus type 1 (HIV-1) associated with clinical exposures: A prospective evaluation. Ann Intern Med 113:740, 1990
27. Puro V, Ranchino M, Profili F: Occupational exposures to blood and risk of HIV transmission in a general hospital (1986–88). Eur J Epidemiol 6:67, 1990
28. Mast SM, Gerberding JL: Factors predicting infectivity following needlestick exposure to HIV: An in vitro model. Clin Res 39:58A, 1991
29. Marcus R, Tokars JI, Culver DH et al, for the Cooperative Needlestick Surveillance Group: Zidovudine use after occupational exposure to HIV-infected blood (abstr 979). In Program and Abstracts of the Interscience Conference on Antimicrobial Agents and Chemotherapy, Chicago, September 29–October 2, 1991
30. Centers for Disease Control: Update: Human immunodeficiency virus infections in health-care workers exposed to blood of infected patients. MMWR 36:285, 1987
31. Fahey BJ, Koziol DE, Banks SM, Henderson DK: Frequency of nonparenteral occupational exposures to blood and body fluids before and after universal precaution training. Am J Med 90:145, 1991
32. Wormser GP, Joline C, Bittker S et al: Polymerase chain reaction for seronegative health care workers with parenteral exposure to HIV-infected patients. N Engl J Med 321:1681, 1989
33. Henry K, Campbell S, Jackson B et al: Long-term followup of health care workers with work site exposure to human immunodeficiency virus. JAMA 263:1765, 1990
34. Centers for Disease Control: Public Health Service statement on management of occupational exposure to human immunodeficiency virus, including considerations regarding zidovudine postexposure use. MMWR 39(No. RR-1):1, 1990
35. Henderson DK, Gerberding JL: Prophylactic zidovudine after occupational exposure to the human immunodeficiency virus: An interim analysis. J Infect Dis 160:321, 1989

36. Fahey BJ, Beekmann SE, Schmitt J et al: Assessment of risk for occupational HIV-1 infection in health-care workers (HCW) and safety of zidovudine (AZT) administered as postexposure chemoprophylaxis for occupational exposures (abstr 960). In: Program and Abstracts of the Interscience Conference on Antimicrobial Agents and Chemotherapy, Atlanta, October 21–24, 1990

37. Gerberding JL, Wugofski L, Berkvan G et al: Facilitated surveillance and post-exposure AZT prophylaxis for health care workers (HCW): The San Francisco General Hospital model (abstr 961). In: Program and Abstracts of the Interscience Conference on Antimicrobial Agents and Chemotherapy, Atlanta, October 21–24, 1990

38. Puro V, Ippolito G, the Italian Study Group on Occupational Risk of HIV Infection: AZT prophylaxis after occupational exposure to HIV in health care workers (abstr W.D.4151). Presented at the VIIth International Conference on AIDS, Florence, Italy, June 16–21, 1991

39. Papillon M, Houle L, Lebel F: Zidovudine prophylaxis for health care workers following occupational HIV exposure (abstr W.D.4182). Presented at the VIIth International Conference on AIDS, Florence, Italy, June 16–21, 1991

40. LaFon SW, Mooney BD, McMullen JP et al: A double-blind, placebo-controlled study of the safety and efficacy of Retrovir (zidovudine, ZDV) as a chemoprophylactic agent in health care workers exposed to HIV (abstr 489). In: Program and Abstracts of the Interscience Conference on Antimicrobial Agents and Chemotherapy, Atlanta, October 21–24, 1990

41. Durand E, Le Jeunne C, Hugues FC: Failure of prophylactic zidovudine after suicidal self-inoculation of HIV-infected blood. N Engl J Med 324:1062, 1991

41a. Jones PD: HIV transmission by stabbing despite zidovudine prophylaxis. Lancet 338:884, 1991

42. Lange JMA, Boucher CAB, Hollak CEM et al: Failure of zidovudine prophylaxis after accidental exposure to HIV-1. N Engl J Med 322:1375, 1990

42a. Poldes JA, Bell DM, Rutherford GW, et al: (abstr M.C.3324). Presented at the VIIth International Conference on AIDS, Florence, Italy, June 16–21, 1991

43. Shih CC, Kaneshima H, Rabin L et al: Postexposure prophylaxis with zidovudine suppresses human immunodeficiency virus type 1 infection in SCID-hu mice in a time-dependent manner. J Infect Dis 163:625, 1991

44. Centers for Disease Control: Preliminary analysis: HIV serosurvey of orthopedic surgeons, 1991. MMWR 40:309, 1991

45. Cowan DN, Brundage JF, Pomerantz RS et al: Human immunodeficiency virus infection among members of the U.S. Army Reserve Components with medical and health occupations. JAMA 265:2826, 1991

46. Flynn NM, Pollet SM, Van Horne JR et al: Absence of HIV antibody among dental professionals exposed to infected patients. West J Med 146:439, 1987

47. Gerberding JL, Nelson K, Greenspan D et al: Risk to dental professionals from occupational exposure to human immunodeficiency virus: Follow-up (abstr 698). In: Program and Abstracts of the Interscience Conference on Antimicrobial Agents and Chemotherapy, New York, October 4–7, 1987

48. Siew C, Gruninger SE, Hojvat S: Screening dentists for HIV and hepatitis B. N Engl J Med 318:1400, 1988

49. Gruninger SE, Siew C, Chang SB et al: Hepatitis B, C, and HIV among dentists (abstr 2131). J Dent Res 70, 1991

50. Klein RS, Phelan JA, Freeman K et al: Low occupational risk of human immunodeficiency virus infection among dental professionals. N Engl J Med 318:86, 1988

51. Ebbesen P, Melbye M, Scheutz F et al: Lack of antibodies to HTLV-III/LAV in Danish dentists (letter). JAMA 256:2199, 1986

52. Harper S, Flynn N, Van Horne J et al: Absence of HIV antibody among dental professionals, surgeons, and household contacts exposed to persons with HIV infection (abstr THP.215). Presented at the III International Conference on AIDS, Washington, DC, June 1–5, 1987

53. Goldman M, Liesnard C, Vanherweghem J-L et al: Markers of HTLV-III in patients with end stage renal failure treated by haemodialysis. Br Med J 293:161, 1986

54. Peterman TA, Lang GR, Mikos NJ et al: HTLV-III/LAV infection in hemodialysis patients. JAMA 255:2324, 1986

55. Comodo N, Martinelli F, De Majo E et al: Risk of HIV infection on patients and staff of two dialysis centers: Seroepidemiological findings and prevention trends. Eur J Epidemiol 4:171, 1988

56. Assogba U, Ancelle Park RA, Rey MA et al: Prospective study of HIV 1 seropositive patients in hemodialysis centers. Clin Nephrol 29:312, 1988

57. Chirgwin K, Rao TKS, Landesman SH: HIV infection in a high prevalence hemodialysis unit. AIDS 3:731, 1989

58. Chamberland ME, Petersen L, Munn V et al: Health-care workers who donate blood: Surveillance for occupationally-acquired HIV-1 infection (abstr 7). In Program and Abstracts of the Interscience Conference on Antimicrobial Agents and Chemotherapy, Chicago, September 29–October 2, 1991

59. Mann JM, Francis H, Quinn TC et al: HIV seroprevalence among hospital workers in Kinshasa, Zaire: Lack of association with occupational exposure. JAMA 256:3099, 1986

60. N'Galy B, Ryder RW, Bila K et al: Human immunodeficiency virus infection among employees in an African hospital. N Engl J Med 319:1123, 1988

61. Lu S-L, Sow I, Coll E et al: HIV-1, HIV-2, and HBV serologic status among Dakar hospital workers (abstr 9009). Presented at the IV International Conference on AIDS, Stockholm, Sweden, June 12–16, 1988

62. McCray E, Onorato IM, and State and Local Health Departments: HIV seroprevalence in clients attending sexually transmitted disease (STD) clinics in the United States, 1988–90 (abstr F.C.44). Presented at the VIth International Conference on AIDS, San Francisco, June 20–24, 1990

63. Allen DM, Onorato IM, Sweeney PA, and State and Local Health Departments: Seroprevalence of HIV infection in intravenous drug users (IVDUs) in the United States (U.S.) (abstr F.C.551). Presented at the VIth International Conference on AIDS, San Francisco, June 20–24, 1990

64. Sweeney PA, Allen D, Onorato I, and State and Local Health Departments: HIV seroprevalence among women of reproductive age seeking clinic services, United States, 1988–1990 (abstr F.C.568). Presented at the VIth International Conference on AIDS, San Francisco, June 20–24, 1990

65. Stricof RL, Nattell TC, Novick LF: HIV seroprevalence in clients of sentinel family planning clinics. Am J Public Health 81(suppl):41, 1991

66. Hnath R, McCray E, Onorato IM, and State and Local Health Departments: HIV seroprevalence in patients attending tuberculosis clinics in the United States, 1988–

90 (abstr Th.C.726). Presented at the VIth International Conference on AIDS, San Francisco, June 20–24, 1990

67. Gayle HD, Keeling RP, Garcia-Tunon M et al: Prevalence of the human immunodeficiency virus among university students. N Engl J Med 323:1538, 1990

68. Petersen LR, Engel R, Herring N: Sentinel surveillance for HIV infection in primary care outpatients in the United States (abstr Th.C.754). Presented at the VIth International Conference on AIDS, San Francisco, June 20–24, 1990

69. St. Louis ME, Rauch KJ, Petersen LR et al, for the Sentinel Hospital Surveillance Group: Seroprevalence rates of human immunodeficiency virus infection at sentinel hospitals in the United States. N Engl J Med 323:213, 1990

70. Gordin FM, Gibert C, Hawley HP, Willoughby A: Prevalence of human immunodeficiency virus and hepatitis B virus in unselected hospital admissions: Implications for mandatory testing and universal precautions. J Infect Dis 161:14, 1990

71. Marcus R, Bell D, Culver D, Cooperative Emergency Department Study Group: Contact with blood of patients infected with HIV among emergency care providers (ECPs) (abstr Th.C.604). Presented at the VIth International Conference on AIDS, San Francisco, June 4–9, 1990

72. Baker JL, Kelen GD, Sivertson KT, Quinn TC: Unsuspected human immunodeficiency virus in critically ill emergency patients. JAMA 257:2609, 1987

73. Kelen GD, Fritz S, Qaqish B et al: Unrecognized human immunodeficiency virus infection in emergency department patients. N Engl J Med 318:1645, 1988

74. Kelen GD, DiGiovanna T, Bisson L et al: Human immunodeficiency virus infection in emergency patients: Epidemiology, clinical presentations, and risk to health-care workers. The Johns Hopkins experience. JAMA 262:516, 1989

75. Kelen GD, Fritz S, Qaqish B et al: Substantial increase in human immunodeficiency virus (HIV-1) infection in critically ill emergency patients: 1986 and 1987 compared. Ann Emerg Med 18:378, 1989

76. Risi GF, Gaumer RH, Weeks S et al: Human immunodeficiency virus: Risk of exposure among health care workers at a southern urban hospital. South Med J 82:1079, 1989

77. Zeman MG, Mayhue FE: Human immunodeficiency virus (HIV) seropositivity in a midwestern community trauma population (abstr 62). Ann Emerg Med 17:409, 1988

78. Jui J, Modesitt S, Fleming D et al: Multicenter HIV and hepatitis B seroprevalence study. J Emerg Med 8:243, 1990

79. Schweich PJ, Fosarelli PD, Duggan AK et al: Prevalence of human immunodeficiency virus seropositivity in pediatric emergency room patients undergoing phlebotomy. Pediatrics 89:660, 1990

80. Soderstrom CA, Furth PA, Glasser D et al: HIV infection rates in a trauma center treating predominantly rural blunt trauma victims. J Trauma 29:1526, 1990

81. Rhee KJ, Albertson TE, Kizer KW et al: The HIV-1 seroprevalence rate of injured patients admitted through California emergency departments. Ann Emerg Med 20:969, 1991

82. Marcus R, Favero MS, Banerjee S et al: Prevalence and incidence of human immunodeficiency virus among patients undergoing long-term hemodialysis. Am J Med 90:614, 1991

83. Baltimore-Boston Collaborative Study Group: Human immunodeficiency virus infection in hemodialysis patients. Arch Intern Med 148:617, 1988

84. Morrison AJ, Freer CV, Poole CL et al: Prevalence of human T-lymphotropic virus type-III antibodies among patients in dialysis programs at a university hospital. Ann Intern Med 104:805, 1986

85. Neumayer H-H, Wagner K, Kresse S: HTLV-III antibodies in patients with kidney transplants or on haemodialysis (letter). Lancet 1:497, 1986

86. Perez GO, Ortiz C, De Medina M et al: Lack of transmission of human immunodeficiency virus in chronic hemodialysis patients. Am J Nephrol 8:123, 1988

87. Johnston BL, Poole CL, Zito DR et al: Cohort study of human immunodeficiency virus (HIV) antibody testing among patients receiving long-term dialysis at a university hospital. Am J Infect Control 16:235, 1988

88. Hussain SA, Latif ABA, Choudhary AAAA: Risk to surgeons: A survey of accidental injuries during operations. Br J Surg 75:314, 1988

89. Mangione CM, Gerberding JL, Cummings SR: Occupational exposure to HIV: Frequency and rates of underreporting of percutaneous and mucocutaneous exposures by medical housestaff. Am J Med 90:85, 1991

90. Lowenfels AB, Wormser GP, Jain R: Frequency of puncture injuries in surgeons and estimated risk of infection. Arch Surg 124:1284, 1989

91. Willy ME, Dhillon GL, Loewen NL et al: Adverse exposures and universal precautions practices among a group of highly exposed health professionals. Infect Control Hosp Epidemiol 11:351, 1990

92. Gerberding JL, Littell C, Tarkington A et al: Risk of exposure of surgical personnel to patients' blood during surgery at San Francisco General Hospital. N Engl J Med 322:1788, 1990

93. Panlilio AL, Foy DR, Edwards JR et al: Blood contacts during surgical procedures. JAMA 265:1533, 1991

94. Panlilio A, Welch B, Foy D et al: Blood and amniotic fluid contact during obstetrical procedures (abstr Th.C.603). Presented at the VI International Conference on AIDS, San Francisco, June 20–24, 1990

95. Popejoy SL, Fry DE: Blood contact and exposure in the operating room. Surg Gynecol Obstet 172:480, 1991

96. Telford GL, Quebbeman EJ: Risk of injury and blood exposure in the operating room environment. Presented at the American College of Surgeons Clinical Congress, San Francisco, October 1990

97. Tokars J, Bell D, Marcus R et al: Percutaneous injuries during surgical procedures (abstr Th.D.108). Presented at the VIIth International Conference on AIDS, Florence, Italy, June 16–21, 1991

98. Pate JW: Risks of blood exposure to the cardiac surgical team. Ann Thorac Surg 50:248, 1990

99. Henry K, Collier P, O'Boyle-Williams CA, Campbell S: Observed and self-reported compliance with universal precautions among emergency department personnel at two suburban community hospitals (abstr M.D.58). Presented at the VIIth International Conference on AIDS, Florence, Italy, June 16–21, 1991

100. Wong ES, Stotka JL, Chinchilli VM et al: Are universal precautions effective in reducing the number of occupational exposures among health care workers? A prospective study of physicians on a medical service. JAMA 265:1123, 1991

101. Hagen MD, Meyer KB, Kopelman RI, Pauker SG: Human immunodeficiency virus infection in health care workers: A method for estimating individual occupational risk. Arch Intern Med 149:1541, 1989

102. Howard RJ: Human immunodeficiency virus testing and the risk to the surgeon of acquiring HIV. Surg Gynecol Obstet 171:22, 1990

103. Orient JM: Assessing the risk of occupational acquisition of the human immunodeficiency virus: Implications for hospital policy. South Med J 83:1121, 1990

104. Schiff SJ: A surgeon's risk of AIDS. J Neurosurg 73:651, 1990

105. Wears RL, Vukich DJ, Winton CN et al: An analysis of emergency physicians' cumulative career risk of HIV infection. Ann Emerg Med 20:749, 1991

106. McKinney WP, Young MJ: The cumulative probability of occupationally-acquired HIV infection: The risks of repeated exposures during a surgical career. Infect Control Hosp Epidemiol 11:243, 1990

107. Petersen NJ: An assessment of the airborne route in hepatitis B transmission. Ann NY Acad Sci 353:157, 1980

108. Johnson GK, Robinson WS: Human immunodeficiency virus-1 (HIV-1) in the vapors of surgical power instruments. J Med Virol 33:47, 1991

109. Jagger J, Hunt EH, Brand-Elnagger J, Pearson RD: Rates of needle-stick injury caused by various devices in a university hospital. N Engl J Med 319:284, 1988

110. Diaz-Buxo JA: Cut resistant glove liner for medical use. Surg Gynecol Obstet 172:312, 1991

111. Jagger J, Pearson RD: Universal precautions: Still missing the point on needlesticks. Infect Control Hosp Epidemiol 12:211, 1991

112. Beck WC, Meyer KK: Barrier protection technology. In Howard RJ (ed): Infectious Risks in Surgery, p 125. Norwalk, Conn, Appleton & Lange, 1991.

31

Safety Precautions for Health Care Workers

General Precautions to Prevent the Transmission of Blood-Borne and Aerosolized Pathogens

Kathleen McMahon Casey

The clinical emergence of human immunodeficiency virus (HIV) infection early in 1981 increased the overall concern about blood-borne pathogens and transmission to health care providers. Although hepatitis has long been a factor infections acquired (or transmitted) by health care workers, the case-fatality rate of HIV elevated the perceived risk in the minds of most people. The conjunction of HIV and hepatitis B virus (HBV) with the emerging risk of tuberculosis transmission has led to new scrutiny of possible aerosolized transmission of infective agents. This chapter focuses on the general safety precautions that providers and health care agencies can employ to prevent the transmission of blood-borne and aerosolized pathogens.

BLOOD-BORNE PATHOGENS

HIV-1

HIV has been isolated from blood,[1-3] semen,[4] tears,[5] saliva,[6] breast milk,[7] epithelial cells,[8] cervical and vaginal secretions,[8-10] urine,[6] and brain tissue and cerebrospinal fluid (CSF)[11] of infected persons. Transmission has occurred through sexual contact with infected individuals, through infusion of contaminated blood products, through sharing of contaminated needles, through infected mother-to-child perinatal contact, and, rarely, through needlestick accidents and the exposure of open skin and mucous membranes to infected blood. At present, the exact method of transmission is unknown. Because of the similar modes of transmission of HIV and

HBV, HBV precautions (hepatitis/enteric precautions) were introduced[12] for managing the HIV-seropositive individual. These blood and body fluid precautions rely on the use of protective barriers and attire. Gloves are worn when hand exposure to blood or body fluids is anticipated; masks and protective eyewear are worn if blood or body fluid splashes to the face and mouth are anticipated. Specimen labels identify the type of precautions indicated. Soiled lines and equipment are separately contained, and blood or body fluid spills are thoroughly disinfected.

Several studies[12-28] and case reports[29-39] have addressed the risk to health care providers of HIV transmission. This literature supports the recommendations of the Centers for Disease Control (CDC).[12,29,40-49] In addition, secondary findings and interpretative comments by the researchers are beneficial in evaluating infection control measures. This literature reaffirms that the risk of acquiring HIV through contact with patients or their biologic specimens is slight but not negligible.

Hepatitis

Viral hepatitis is the second most common reportable infectious disease in the United States, with HBV accounting for about 45% of all cases.[50] Although 25,000 cases are reported to the CDC yearly, it is estimated that 300,000 cases occur annually. The case rate has been rising since 1980 despite the availability of a safe and effective vaccine since 1982.

It is frequently presumed that hepatitis is not a fatal

illness, and, compared to the AIDS case-fatality rate, the mortality from hepatitis is low. However, the risk of acquiring an infection when jabbed by a needle with hepatitis-infected blood is very high. Because of the high virus titer in infected persons (10^6 to 10^9 virus particles/ml of blood), the health care provider has a 10% to 35% chance of acquiring an infection, as opposed to a 0.4% chance following exposure to HIV-infected blood.[37,51]

Reported cases of HBV-infection underestimate the true incidence because of subclinical infection and underreporting. About one third of infected adults are completely asymptomatic, one third have a flulike illness, and one third develop the classic signs of jaundice, dark urine, fatigue, anorexia, and abdominal pain. Chronic carriers of HBV are at high risk for chronic persistent hepatitis, cirrhosis, chronic active hepatitis, and hepatocellular carcinoma.

Hepatitis is the major infectious occupational hazard to health care workers. Approximately 12,000 providers become infected yearly (as opposed to possibly zero to 15 who become infected by HIV).[37] Only 30% to 40% of providers have been vaccinated.[50,52] Commonly cited reasons for refusing vaccination include lack of financing of vaccination by the employer, fear of contracting AIDS from the vaccine, workers' belief that they are not at sufficient risk of HBV infection to warrant vaccination, and a nonspecific fear of adverse reactions to the vaccine.[53]

As with HIV, the major modes of HBV transmission are sexual, parenteral, or exposure to blood and blood-containing body fluids. HBV is not transmitted by casual contact, by fecal-oral or airborne routes, or by ingestion of contaminated food or drinking water.

ASSESSING THE RISK OF HIV TRANSMISSION

Casual Contact

Research on the risk to household associates of a patient with AIDS or ARC reaffirms the lack of casual transmission. Because in many respects health care workers and fellow patients assume the role of household contacts of hospitalized HIV-seropositive patients, a review of the studies performed on household contacts of patients with AIDS or ARC patients is beneficial. In a study by Fischl and associates[54] evaluating household contacts of adults with AIDS, contact included personal contact such as hugging, kissing, and sharing kitchen and bathroom facilities. Further evidence supporting the lack of transmission to household contacts came from work by Jason,[55] Redfield,[56] Friedland[57] and their colleagues. The contact included sharing of household items such as drinking glasses, eating plates, nail clippers, and eating utensils. Contact also involved sharing household facilities such as the toilet, bath or shower, kitchen, and beds, and washing items used by the patient, such as dishes, the bath, toilet, and clothes. Interactions with the patient included hugging, kissing on the cheek, shaking hands, and kissing on the lips. Other less frequent contacts such as helping to bathe, sharing razors, toothbrushes, and sharing clothes were also reported. Despite this close contact, only one of the 101 household contacts studied was HIV seropositive.[57] This was a child who had had signs and symptoms of HIV infection since infancy and was probably infected perinatally by her mother, who had AIDS.

The absence of horizontal transmission of HIV is in sharp contrast to the apparent horizontal transmission of HBV infection in households[58,59] and dental and surgical practices.[60-63] Therefore, even though HIV, like HBV, is present in saliva and blood, horizontal transmission of HIV by casual contact appears to be minimal to nonexistent. These activities of sharing other body fluids *in small amounts* do involve HBV, however. Therefore, a case finding of HBV infection is very important.

Needlestick Injuries

Based on documented case reports of occupationally acquired HIV infection, needlestick injuries and other percutaneous exposures are by far the most common route of transmission. These injuries include superficial injuries, inadvertent injection of blood, and intramuscular (IM) injections. Nurses account for 80% of health care workers infected occupationally. So far, there are 19 documented cases of occupationally related acquisition of HIV by health care workers; in 16 cases needles were incriminated.[37]

Needles have posed a risk for transmission of disease as long as they have been used. Recommendations for needle handling include advice not to manipulate them in any way or to recap them. One reason frequently given for recapping needles is the discomfort of carrying an exposed, used needle to the syringe container.[64] This discomfort has been alleviated with the installation of puncture-resistant containers close to areas where sharps or needles are used.

However, this misses the point on the vast majority of needlestick injuries.[65] The National Academy of Science's Committee on Trauma Research[66] reports that "the most successful injury-prevention approaches have involved improved product designs and changes in the man-made environment. . . ." This contradicts the general opinion that employees cause needlesticks by their own carelessness[67,68] or dangerous behavior. Rather, employees may be viewed as victims of the inherently dangerous devices they are required to handle under difficult circumstances. Another key factor is the widespread underreporting (approximately 40%) of injuries.[24,67,69] Reasons include the fear of jeopardizing current or future employment, being labeled as a careless employee, insufficient encouragement from peers and supervisors to report accidents, lack of time to initiate paperwork and occupational health follow-up, inability to accept the reality of an exposure, denial, lack of awareness that exposure occurred, difficulty in negotiating the employee health service, fear of blame, and not wanting to deal with the consequences. The cost of documenting an exposure has been high, the benefit low.

Case Reports

To highlight the special risk of needlesticks, illustrative case reports of injuries follow.

NEEDLESTICK EXPOSURES

Seroconversion of a Female Health Care Worker after a Contaminated Needlestick Accident[31]

During an emergency procedure, the nurse sustained a deep IM needlestick. The large-bore (1.67-mm diameter), visibly contaminated needle and syringe unit had been used on an AIDS patient. The health worker was enrolled in the CDC's surveillance study.

After 48 hours, skin tests for mumps and *Candida* were strongly positive. Fourteen days later fever, chills, myalgias, and arthralgias developed, necessitating hospital admission on the following day. The patient had fever to 40.3° C, an enlarged right axillary lymph node, and persistent erythema and induration at the skin test site. Within a few days an abdominal rash appeared. Epstein-Barr virus (EBV) and cytomegalovirus (CMV) tests were negative. The diagnosis was a viral syndrome of undetermined etiology.

A month later rehospitalization was required for continued abdominal cramping and pain. Because *Clostridium* was detected in the patient's stool, she began a course of oral vancomycin, which alleviated the symptoms. Subsequently she has suffered mild, intermittent oral candidiasis, persistent enlargement of a postcervical lymph node, and transient enlargement of suboccipital and inguinal lymph nodes.

On day 9 after the original needlestick accident the nurse was seronegative. However, she tested positive on days 184 and 239. Viral cultures were negative on day 239, as was her husband's HIV test. The nurse had no other known risk factors.

Seroconversion of a Female Nurse after a Contaminated Needlestick Injury[32]

While resheathing a needle used to draw blood from the arterial line of an AIDS patient, a nurse in Britain accidentally struck herself. Thirteen days after the injury she experienced a severe flulike illness that included mild sore throat, headache, myalgia, and facial neuralgia. Seventeen days later a rash developed on the trunk and chest, spreading to the neck and face; it was not associated with antibiotic use. General malaise persisted, with severe arthralgias and pyrexia up to 39° C for 20 days. The generalized lymphadenopathy resolved and recovery was uneventful. The nurse tested negative for EBV, CMV, parvovirus, and rubella virus.

The nurse was HIV seronegative on day 27 after the injury. On days 49 and 57, she was found to be HIV seropositive. No other risk factors were identified.

Seroconversion of a Female Nurse after a Needlestick Injury[33]

During a thoracentesis performed on a patient with a pleural infusion who had persistent generalized lymphadenopathy and was seropositive for HIV and HBsAg, a nurse suffered a superficial needlestick injury to her finger while recapping a needle contaminated with bloody pleural effusion fluid. She received specific immunoglobulins and hepatitis B vaccine at that time.

Twenty-five days later she developed fatigue, fever, and vomiting. On day 26 her temperature was 39.4° C. On day 53 an acute anicteric hepatitis developed. On day 181, CMV, EBV, and hepatitis B and A assays were negative but the tuberculin skin test was positive.

The patient was HIV seronegative on days 1 and 13 but seropositive on days 68, 82, and 151. Her serum viral HIV culture was negative on days 103 and 181. Her husband was HIV seronegative on day 110. No other risk factors were determined.

Seroconversion of a Female Nursing Student After a Needlestick Accident[34]

A nursing student pricked the fleshy part of her index finger with a needle used to draw blood from an AIDS patient. There was no apparent injection of blood.

A month later she was HIV seronegative. Subsequently a fever and rash developed. Within 4 months the nursing student was HIV seropositive. Her husband was HIV seronegative. No other risk factors were identified.

NONNEEDLESTICK EXPOSURES

A few case reports have identified apparent transmission *via* blood-splattering accidents[29] during dialysis procedures, the holding of an arterial puncture site, and phlebotomy blood collection tube transfer procedures. Despite numerous other reported episodes of similar exposures, no other seroconversions have been documented. Universal safeguards and protective attire will reduce the risk involved.

UNIVERSAL PRECAUTIONS

The CDC's universal precautions to protect health care workers were first published in August 1987. Hitherto, disease-specific or category-specific isolation precautions were standard. The universal precautions were introduced "since medical history and examination cannot reliably identify all patients infected with HIV and other blood-borne pathogens."[49] This ushered in the era of using blood and body fluid precautions in contacts with *all* patients.

The CDC's endorsement was further strengthened

by the October 1987 joint advisory notice of the Department of Health and Human Services and the Department of Labor.[70] This guide outlined the protective mechanisms and barriers to be implemented: engineering controls, altered work practices, and the use of protective equipment.

In June 1988, the CDC published a report meant to clarify and supplement the earlier one.[48] It stratified body fluids into categories: those to which universal precautions applied and those to which they did not apply (Table 31A–1). Universal precautions were meant to supplement, not replace, recommendations for routine infection control. Implementation then did not eliminate the need for category- or disease-specific isolation precautions, such as enteric precautions for infectious diarrhea, as had been widely thought since August 1987. Additionally, strict precautions for certain clinical and laboratory areas were delineated (including invasive procedures,[71] dentistry,[72] autopsies or mortician's services,[69] dialysis,[45] and clinical and research laboratories[12]).

As a response to this development, the body substance isolation system is gaining ground as an alternative to the two-tier, disease-specific program. The development of various isolation precautions in the course of the HIV epidemic is summarized in Table 31A–2.

BODY SUBSTANCE ISOLATION SYSTEM

The body substance isolation (BSI) system[73,74] was developed initially for two purposes: to reduce the risks to patients from cross-transmission of organisms, usually *via* the hands of personnel, and to reduce the risks to

Table 31A–1. Applicability of Universal Precautions to Various Body Fluids

Universal Precautions Apply	Universal Precautions Do Not Apply (Unless Visible Blood Is Present in the Fluid)
Blood	Saliva
Other body fluids	Feces
Semen	Nasal secretions
Vaginal secretions	Sputum
Tissue	Sweat
Other:	Tears
Synovial	Urine
Pleural	Vomitus
Peritoneal	Human breast milk
Pericardial	
Amniotic	

Adapted from Centers for Disease Control: Update: Universal precautions for prevention of transmission of human immunodeficiency virus, hepatitis B, and other bloodborne pathogens in health care settings. MMWR 37(4), 1988

Table 31A–2. The Development of Isolation Precautions in the HIV Epidemic

Year	Activity
1980	Blood precautions for arthropod-borne viral fever, viral hepatitis, malaria
	Protective isolation for immunocompromised patients
	Other disease- or category-specific precautions (*e.g.*, respiratory, strict, enteric)
	Routine care
1981	First clinical cases of GRIDS (AIDS) appear and are recognized
1983	Protective isolation discontinued
	Blood and body fluid precautions initiated
1984	First report of occupationally acquired case (British nurse infected by a patient)
1985	HIV antibody testing became commercially available
1986	Health care worker studies: three occupationally acquired infections from puncture injuries
1987 (May)	CDC reported three occupationally acquired infections from splashes
1987 (August)	Universal precautions initiated
1987 (October)	Joint notice (Labor Department, Health and Human Services Department)—OSHA regulations instituted
1988 (April)	CDC's summary of health care worker acquired cases: 15/22 needlesticks or puncture injuries; 7/22 nonintact skin or mucous membrane contact with skin
1988 (June)	Revision of universal safeguards to reflect applicability
	Advisement that category- or disease-specific isolation can also apply (hospitals develop their own)
1989–1991*	Body substance isolation system, which is interaction-driven and calls for judgment, gains momentum
1990	Engineering controls initiated
1991	Tuberculosis prevention and containment arise as a prominent concern

* First registered nurse who went public with her occupationally acquired HIV illness dies.
First patient known to have become HIV infected from her health care provider (dentist) dies.

health care workers of becoming infected by organisms harbored by patients. This design is fundamentally different from disease-driven or category-driven ones in that intervention (hand washing, gowns, *etc.*) is based on the interaction with the patient, not the diagnosed or suspected disease. It has a value-added feature in that it is in place before diagnoses are made, when transmission is likely to occur. One study[73] clearly demonstrated a decreased nosocomial infection rate of marker illness such as *Serratia* infections and amikacin-resistant gram-negative baccillary infections after implementation of the BSI system.

Main Elements of the BSI System

Hand washing for 10 seconds with soap, running water, and friction is performed when hands are visibly soiled and between most patient contacts. An exception might be when the same provider is doing the same task for a series of patients and has contact with only dry, intact skin (*e.g.,* measuring weights or blood pressures).

Gloves are needed when contact with mucous membranes, moist body substances and fluids, or non-intact skin is anticipated. They are worn only when the worker has contact, not necessarily for the entire patient interaction. If the patient has multiple open skin sites with which the provider expects to come in contact, multiple glove changes may be necessary; hand washing is not necessarily needed between changes.

Protective clothing is needed when the worker expects to be in contact with soiled items, moist body substances, or large, open wounds, or anticipates splattering of his or her own mucous membranes with the patient's moist body fluids. Protective clothing includes aprons, gowns, mask, goggles, hats, and shoe coverings. Paper masks such as health workers used for respiratory isolation are inadequate. A water-resistant type is needed and possibly one that is resistant to particles, mist, and dust.

Needles are not recapped by hand and are discarded in a rigid, puncture-resistant container with the syringe or tubing attached. If recapping cannot be avoided, a recapping device or at least the "scooping" method is used. Due care is taken with all needled or sharp-edged devices.

Trash and linen are bagged so as not to leak. State and local jurisdiction regulations supersede infection control standards and must be followed.

Laboratory specimens need not be specifically labeled. Workers take care through protective clothing and approach to prevent contact with moist body fluids.

Room selection is based on the patient's self-care and hygienic abilities. Only patients with aerosolized droplet-borne infections specifically need a private room. These rooms are identified on the outside in some manner, traditionally through the use of a stop sign with a message alert.

Factors That Impede Use of the BSI System

Public Relations People in the community often would rather not share a hospital room with anyone who has a known infection. This attitude is heightened with HIV. The perceived or actual public relations threat often leads to the adoption of a "private room only for HIV" policy. This policy can be discriminatory, es-

pecially when no private rooms are available. In general, such rooms are medically unnecessary.

Time in Retraining Providers who have been familiar with category- and disease-specific plans may be rigidly opposed to change. A period of change always creates the need for change agents, instruction, monitoring, teaching, and problem-solving.

Fear of Not Meeting OSHA Standards Because institutions are assessed fines and penalties for failing to comply adequately with universal safeguards, agencies are gunshy about being creative in this realm.

Problem Areas in Universal Safeguards

Sharp Object Injuries in the Health Care Setting There continues to be a high level of needlesticks, scalpel cuts, lancet injuries, and surgical accidents despite the admonishment not to recap and to use caution when handling sharp instruments. Universal precautions are not universally adhered to,[13,14,16-18,28,37,68,75,76] and acceptance is limited.[21,67] Sources of resistance vary[77,78] but may include all of the following:

1. Workers are more likely to resist changes they believe will affect them adversely, particularly changes that affect their work habits, prestige, and power in the work setting or their perceived control over the environment.
2. Workers who have been trained to exercise professional judgment are likely to resist changes that limit their discretionary powers.
3. Workers' perceptions of top-level commitment to the change will in turn affect their own commitment.
4. Workers will resist change if they do not understand or agree with the goals and expected outcomes of the change.
5. Workers must have confidence that the proposed change will actually contribute to the stated goals.
6. Workers must believe that management will rigorously evaluate and, if necessary, modify the program to meet new circumstances.

The institution of general organizational measures to prevent the transmission of infectious organisms must involve the health care providers themselves. Table 31A–3 lists activities from an organizational change perspective.

Safe Needled Devices and Sharp Instruments A significant reduction in needlestick injuries is not likely to occur if prevention efforts are limited to needle-handling practices. Clearly, alternative approaches are indicated. Engineering controls are being added to these efforts.

Changes in Needle-Handling Practices With the advent of HIV, health care providers must unlearn old behaviors and learn new ones. With respect to needle-handling, it was common practice to remove the needle and detach the syringe, which was then deposited in

Table 31A–3. Organizational Change Concepts

1. Plan for active and passive resistance
2. Plan for long-term commitment, not short-term compliance
3. Request survey feedback
4. Structure educational campaign: initial and continuous
5. Ensure employee involvement
6. Ensure a genuine top-level commitment
7. Provide incentives and deterrents
8. Devise monitors, evaluations, and modifications

Adapted with permission from Kearns KP, Hagg M: Universal precautions: Employee resistance and strategies for planned organizational change. Hosp Health Services Admin 33(4):521, 1988.

the nearest garbage bin. Currently it is requested that needles and syringes not be disconnected but be placed unaltered into a collection device. Having puncture-proof containers close to the user of needled equipment has contributed to a reduced rate of needlestick injuries in most settings but not in all.

It was common practice for nurses to assist physicians during procedures by handing them needled syringes with medication premixed in the syringe, taking collected specimens, covering and labeling them appropriately, and cleaning up the used items from the work site. All of these practices have changed so that the user of the equipment cleans up after himself or herself.

Cardiac arrest and other emergencies continue to plague health providers with a heightened degree of risk. Multiple studies have shown that providers do not adhere to infection control principles mainly out of haste and the perceived loss of critical time to stabilize the patient.[21,26,28] It is clear that improved methods of control are required, such as the redesign of needled devices and ease and access to protective attire.

Needle recapping or manipulation is frequently cited as a major culprit in occupational exposures. The practice of not recapping needles was introduced in 1983. Some reasons why providers do recap needles with "safety covers" are the perception that covered needles are inherently safer than exposed ones (true), the perception that workers might put colleagues or themselves at risk if accidentally stuck by an uncovered sharp object (true), and the lack of a nearby needle receptacle (possibly true).[77]

Other problems inherent in device handling[79,80] include difficulty in handling sharp equipment such as scalpels and needles in small spaces during surgery, disassembly of the protective cover from the scalpel or blade when it is removed from the handle, visual difficulty in determining which side of the scalpel has the edge, passing sharp medical equipment from one person to the other, placing one's hand into scissors soaking in disinfectant, slipping of sharp equipment due to moist body fluid on the surface of the instrument, accidents sustained while handling lancets of the tiny spring-

loaded fingerstick devices, and breaking open glass ampules while preparing medication.

The injuries show the relationship between equipment design and hazard. Interventions that would improve the safety of sharp instruments are listed in Table 31A–4. Needled products that incorporate the latest design in medical equipment are shown in Figures 31A–1 through 31A–2. Featured are needle-less systems and automatic needle sheathing devices. Each piece of equipment needs to be individually evaluating in the various clinical settings in which it may be adopted. Designs, flaws, or size differences matter a great deal. The user can test devices serially for suitability.

Additionally, practices that require health care workers to use needles must be reexamined. One study that investigated the value of switching needles in the attempt to obtain a sterile blood specimen found it to be an unnecessary step.[81] Methods of obtaining a sterile urine specimen by catheterization, central venous catheter flushing, route of medication delivery (oral *versus* parenteral), and other clinical procedures can be similarly addressed.

Use of Mechanical Barriers and Other Protective Attire

Gloves The OSHA mandate on the number of valuable barrier precautions has greatly increased the use of protective barrier attire, especially gloves. Initially, vinyl gloves were suspected of not providing the high level of safety from virus protection that latex gloves were thought to provide. It has been determined, however, that the primary benefits of vinyl gloves may be in comfort, fit, better manual dexterity, heat conduction, and having more "give." In the clinical setting, latex

Table 31A–4. Equipment Design to Improve the Safety of Sharp Instruments

Equipment or Task	Point
Needle holders	Automatic pickup features that avoid pulling needle through tissue
Scalpel blades	Bright colors to alert user to sharp edge; automatic covers
Needled device	Automatic sheaths; redesign to needle-less systems
Surgical gloves	Use of materials that resist punctures and cuts
Lances from fingerstick devices	Design of release feature or automatic resheathing feature after use
Handing sharp objects	Sterile passing plate or tray; replacing glass

Some data from Jagger J, Hunt EH, Pearson ED: Sharp object injuries in the hospital: Causes and strategies for prevention. Am J Infect Control 18:230, 1990.

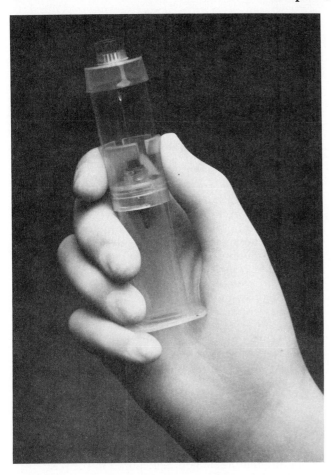

Figure 31A–1. Needle adaptor: Safe designs prevent needle-stick injuries (photo of SAF-T CLIK Shielded Blood Needle Adaptor, courtesy of Ryan Medical, Inc, Brentwood, TN).

gloves are necessary for the safe handling of any chemotherapeutic agents or waste.

Gloves are worn when exposure to blood and body fluids containing blood is expected.[49] They are used also when the health care provider has a cut, scratch, or dermatologic lesion. Double gloving may prevent some exposures, particularly during hazardous invasive procedures such as surgery in which multiple punctures are expected.[82,83]

Newer gloves are meant to resist punctures (Fig. 31A–3). One study evaluated the use of gloves in the context of body substance isolation.[73] The most prevalent situations in which gloves were justifiably required were those involving contact with the insertion site of an indwelling medical device, including oral and nasal endotracheal tubes, chest tubes, surgical drains, and central lines. The second most prevalent situation involved care of the patient's mouth or oral cavity.

Protective Eyeware Protective eyewear is not generally necessary unless splashing or splattering is expected. Form-fitting attire and combination goggles/mask (whole face mask) are commercially available.

Resuscitation Full infection control practice in emergency situations is a goal, not a reality. Ambu bags and airway devices are kept readily available in places where arrests may occur. A retrospective project that details the locations of previous arrests may be indicated to identify sites for placement of emergency gear. Identifying methods of assisting first responders into protective attire is a critical management goal.

Gowns Gowns protect clothes from splatters or spills. A disposable apron worn beneath the gown affords more protection. In general, however, gowns are not strikeproof.

Blood and Body Fluid Spills The management of blood and body fluid spills is handled elsewhere in this book, in the discussion of disinfection procedures.

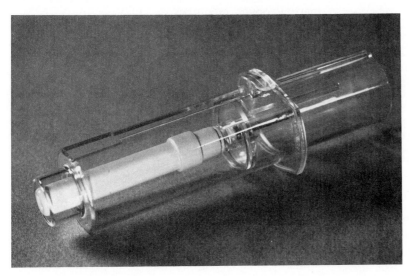

Figure 31A–2. Shielded needle on blood collection unit: Retracting shielded needle systems impact on primary prevention methods (photo courtesy of Medical Safety Products, Inc., Denver, CO).

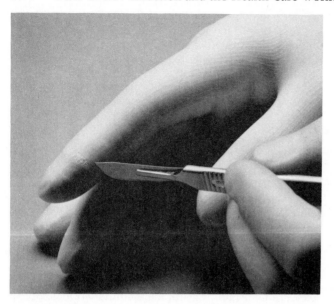

Figure 31A–3. Tougher, reusable gloves: Manual dexterity needs to be maintained, but a more durable, protective design is required to prevent cuts and slashes in surgery (photo courtesy of Smith & Nephew Perry, Massillon, OH).

Trash Color-coded, waterproof, labeled bags containing potentially infectious waste are disposed of according to state regulations. Double bagging is necessary if contamination of the outside may have occurred. Blood and body fluids can be safely flushed down a drain or toilet connected to a sanitary sewer.

Linen Soiled linen is placed in an impervious labeled bag and considered potentially infectious. Care is taken not to aerosolize the material while handling it. Double bagging may be necessary.

Staff Development and Occupational Health Risks

Currently, Joint Commission Accreditation and State Department of Health inspectors require orientation and yearly mandatory review of educational interventions about blood-borne pathogens and other occupational health risks, such as chemotherapy and the presence and handling of biohazardous material. It is estimated that 70% of all health care providers are women. Nurses sustain the great majority of infections from blood-borne pathogens because they administer drugs and blood and work in close proximity to patients' fluids. Education usually relies on in-service education sessions, which may be difficult for staff to attend because of workload or a perceived poor education design. Programs must be planned at convenient hours and should be frequently repeated. HBV vaccination should be easy to obtain. Focus groups can help employee health de-

partments identify the best plans to reach most providers with blood or body fluid contact.

AEROSOLIZED PATHOGENS

Mycobacterium tuberculosis

The United States experienced a significant decrease in the number of tuberculosis cases reported from 1953, when 84,000 cases were reported, to 1984, when 22,000 cases were reported.[84] This had led to a common belief among care providers that *Mycobacterium tuberculosis* was no longer a threat. Since 1984, however, the long-term decline in the number of cases ceased and then reversed itself, with the greatest tuberculosis-related morbidity now seen in HIV-infected individuals.[85,86] Outbreaks of tuberculosis on AIDS units have been reported, and resistant disease has been documented.[87] This led to the publication of guidelines to prevent tuberculosis transmission.[84,87–92]

M. tuberculosis is an aerobic, acid-fast bacillus that spreads by the respiratory route and by person-to-person spread. Infection is acquired by inhalation of droplet nuclei aerosolized by the infected person in the course of talking, coughing, and sneezing. A cough can produce 3,000 infectious droplet nuclei, and talking for 5 minutes can produce the same. Particles stay suspended in the air for a long time. Prolonged exposure to these aerosolized droplets is usually necessary for infection to develop. In HIV-infected patients,[90] infection can be acquired in this manner or as a result of reactivation of latent tuberculosis infection acquired in the past.

The characteristic clinical features of tuberculosis include fever, weight loss, fatigue, night sweats, and pulmonary symptoms (cough, hemoptysis, chills, and chest pain). These characteristic symptoms vary with the extent of immunosuppression. Up to 75% of AIDS patients with tuberculosis may have a nonpulmonary form of the disease that affects the lymph nodes, bone marrow, bones, meninges, and kidneys.

Early diagnosis and intensive case findings are critical to disease management and the prevention of further spread, particularly in institutional settings. Not all infected persons develop disease. Approximately 5% of persons with newly acquired infection do so within the first year or two, and an additional 5% develop disease later in life. These patients (infected but without the disease) cannot spread the infection. They are not considered to represent "tuberculosis cases" usually having a positive tuberculin skin test but no clinical symptoms or evidence on chest radiographs. The infection does remain viable and can be reactivated. Conditions besides HIV that are associated with progression from infection to active disease include old, untreated tuberculosis, substance abuse, silicosis, diabetes mellitus, prolonged corticosteroid therapy, immunosuppressive therapy, leukemias and Hodgkin's disease, end-stage renal disease, and chronic malabsorption syndromes.

There are three tools for the diagnosis of tuberculosis: the Mantoux tuberculin skin test, chest radiography, and sputum culture. Screening and case findings involve Mantoux skin tests for at-risk groups (IV drug users, correctional facilities inmates, HIV-infected persons), follow-up, and therapy or preventative treatment under observation.

Infection Control Measures for Tuberculosis

Patients with pulmonary or laryngeal tuberculosis are most infectious before diagnosis and treatment. Most patients are noninfectious after the first several weeks of drug therapy. An average of 25% of close contacts of a patient with pulmonary tuberculosis will have positive results on the tuberculin skin test.

The following action and precautions should be taken to prevent airborne transmission of *T. mycobacterium:*[93]

1. All patients with HIV and undiagnosed pulmonary disease should be suspected of having infectious tuberculosis. Respiratory precautions should be implemented until they are deemed unnecessary.
2. Procedures that stimulate coughing, forceful exhalation (such as sputum collection or induction), suctioning, aerosolized pentamidine treatments, and bronchoscopy should be performed in special rooms or booths with negative air pressure in relation to adjacent rooms or hallways, or rooms in which air is exhausted directly to the outside (Fig. 31A–4).
3. Ensure a well-ventilated environment.
4. Patients should cover their mouth and nose when coughing or sneezing.
5. Use of properly installed and maintained special ultraviolet light fixtures.

The prolonged exposure ordinarily necessary to acquire infection makes it more difficult to assign risk status to certain activities. In the prechemotherapy era, Riley estimated it took nursing students 18 months of exposure to become infected.[94] In the 1990 Florida clinic case of 17 infections,[95] the two greatest risk factors were found to be (1) working 40 hours or more per week, and (2) being in the room where aerosolized pentamidine treatments were given. Spread of infection within the building and area is aided by ventilation systems.

The ordinary surgical masks that providers wear for airborne infections are insufficient for tuberculosis prevention. Tight-fitting industrial particulate respirators that filter out particles in the droplet nucleus size range (1–5 μm) are much more suitable (Fig. 31A–5). These disposable respirators may be most beneficial when ventilation is inadequate, the patient's symptoms suggest a high potential for infectiousness, the patient is un-

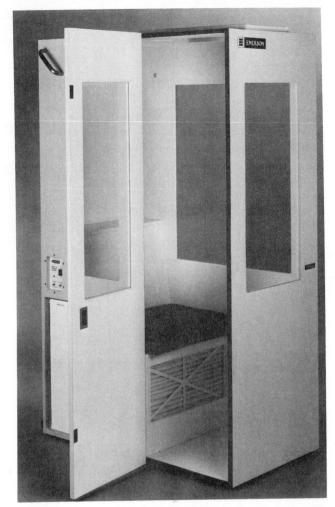

Figure 31A–4. Aerosol safety: High air-exchange rates, alarms, and self-contained air space allows for less occupational health risks (photo courtesy of JH Emerson Company, Cambridge, MA).

dergoing a procedure that increases infectiousness, or the patient cannot cover his or her mouth.[84] Patients may also wear these masks to prevent exhalation of tuberculosis bacilli. The mask should not have a valve that releases expired air to the outside. Comfort can be a problem with these devices. Generally, the more efficient they are, the greater the work of inhaling through them.

Table 31A–5 summarizes infection control standards for the prevention of tuberculosis transmission.

AEROSOLIZED PENTAMIDINE

Aerosolized pentamidine became widely used in the 1980s to reduce the occurrence of *Pneumocystis carinii* pneumonia in AIDS patients. With the Fisoneb device

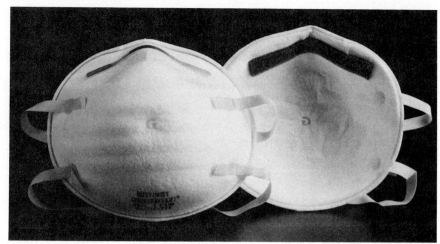

Figure 31A–5. Prevention of tuberculosis transmission: Serious attention to special micron filtration masks (photo courtesy of Louis M. Gerson Co, Inc, Middleboro, MA).

(Lymphomed), which provided an "on demand" inhalation-stimulus stream of mist, there were rarely any complaints except for taste and coughing. With the increased use of the Respirgard II nebulizer, which provides a constant stream, there are reports of breathing difficulties, rashes, headaches, and tearing eyes on the part of nurses and respiratory therapists who administer the drug.[96–99]

Table 31A–5. Prevention of Tuberculosis: Recommendations for Infection Control

Avoid unnecessary bronchoscopies
  Sputum induction with hypertonic saliva preferred
Screen for tuberculosis
  At diagnosis of HIV and yearly if patient is taking
    aerosolized pentamidine
  Initiate preventive drug therapy
  Screen health care workers annually
Masks
  Particulate respirators
Environmental controls
  Fresh, nonrecirculated air
  Annual consultation with engineers regarding heating,
    ventilating, and air conditioning systems
  Add ultraviolet light (UV) wherever possible
  Add UV and high-energy filters to ventilation ductwork
  Assess air flow, discharge site, and intake source for
    potential risk to patients, visitors, and staff
Source control
  Provide specially constructed booth to perform sputum
    inductions and provide aerosolized pentamidine
    treatments
  Pretreat patients with bronchodilators to prevent cough
  Ensure tight-fitting mask delivery system for pentamidine
  Implement respiratory isolation for suspected tuberculosis
    patients
  Teach patients to cover their mouths when sneezing or
    coughing

Data reproduced with permission from Nardell EA: Dodging droplet nuclei (editorial). Am Rev Respir Dis 142:501, 1990.

A recent study examined the long half-life of aerosolized pentamidine excreted *via* the lungs. There was a correlation between the lung level and the urinary level of pentamidine. The investigator then studied the potential effect on health care workers and was able to detect pentamidine in the urine of 50%. In two patients who received a single 300-mg dose of Pentam *via* the Respirgard II inhaler, the drug was detectable in the urine 3 weeks later (G. Smoldone, pers. commun.). This crucial research provides us with the first tool for measuring occupational exposures to pentamidine *via* aerosol administration.

CONCLUSION

Infection control practices are generally adequate to avoid transmission of infection to and from health care providers. New advances in equipment design, engineering controls, and technical support will make needled devices more user friendly.[100] HBV vaccination programs must be taken seriously by providers and administrators.

Numerous studies show a consistent underreporting of needlestick injuries.[101] Rates vary from 40% to 50%, and a large percentage of health care providers have sustained needlesticks. Lack of reporting has been linked to lack of resources available to workers, anxiety, denial, fear of occupational stress, time constraints, and lack of viable alternatives. Lack of reporting, in conjunction with overall laxness in adhering to universal precautions under certain conditions, speaks to the lack of progress made in many key areas.

A decreased patient risk of infection will be the likely outcome of a generic body substance isolation program.[102] Such plans will become more important as the CDC and governmental legislative bodies decide on the issue of the infected health care worker and invasive procedures.[103] Infection control is a strong component of any responsible practice.

REFERENCES

1. Gallo RC, Salahuddin SZ, Popovic M et al: Frequent detection and isolation of cytopathic retroviruses (HTLV-III) from patients with AIDS and at risk for AIDS. Science 224:500, 1984
2. Barre-Sinoussi F, Chermann JC, Rey F et al: Isolation of a T-lymphotropic retrovirus from a patient at risk for acquired immunodeficiency syndrome (AIDS). Science 220: 868, 1983
3. Levy JA, Hoffman AD, Kramer SM et al: Isolation of lymphocytopathic retroviruses from San Francisco patients with AIDS. Science 225:840, 1984
4. Zagny D, Bernard J, Liebowitz J et al: HTLV-III in cells cultured from semen of two patients with AIDS. Science 226:449, 1984
5. Fujikawa LS, Salahuddin SZ, Palestine AG et al: Isolation of human T-lymphotropic virus type III from tears of a patient with acquired immunodeficiency syndrome. Lancet 2:529, 1985
6. Groopman JE, Salahuddin SZ, Sarngadharan MG et al: HTLV-III in saliva of people with AIDS-related complex and healthy homosexual men at risk for AIDS. Science 226:447, 1984
7. Thiry L, Sprecher-Goldberger S, Jonckheer T et al: Isolation of AIDS virus from cell free breast milk of three healthy virus carriers (letter). Lancet 2:891, 1985
8. Vogt MW, Witt DJ, Craven DE et al: Isolation patterns of the human immunodeficiency virus from cervical secretions during the menstrual cycle of women at risk for the acquired immunodeficiency syndrome. Ann Intern Med 106:380, 1987
9. Wofsy C, Cohen JB, Haver LB et al: Isolation of AIDS-associated retrovirus from genital secretions of women with antibodies to the virus. Lancet 1:527, 1986
10. Vogt MW, Witt DJ, Craven DE et al: Isolation of HTLV-III/LAV from cervical secretions of women at risk for AIDS. Lancet 1:525, 1986
11. Levy JA, Shimabukuro J, Hollander H, et al: Isolations of AIDS-associated retroviruses from cerebrospinal fluid and brain of patients with neurological symptoms. Lancet 2: 586, 1985
12. Centers for Disease Control: Acquired immune deficiency syndrome (AIDS): Precautions for clinical and laboratory staffs. MMWR 31:575, 1982
13. Henderson DK, Saah AJ, Zak BJ et al: Risk of nosocomial infection with human T-cell lymphotropic virus type III/lymphadenopathy associated virus in a large cohort of intensively exposed health care workers. Ann Intern Med 104:644, 1986
14. Moss A, Osmond D, Bacchetti P et al: Risk of seroconversion for acquired immunodeficiency syndrome (AIDS) in San Francisco health workers. J Occup Med 28:821, 1986
15. McCray E, Cooperative Needlestick Surveillance Group, Centers for Disease Control: Special report: Occupational risk of the acquired immunodeficiency syndrome among health care workers. N Engl J Med 314:1127, 1986
16. Baker JL, Kelen GD, Sivertson KT et al: Unsuspected human immunodeficiency virus in critically ill emergency patients. JAMA 257:2609, 1987
17. Gerner HM, Ivey FD, Lane TW: Follow-up and education of employees exposed to a patient with HIV antibodies and massive bleeding. Am J Infect Control 17:349, 1989
18. Gerberding JL, Bryant-LeBlanc CE, Nelson K et al: Risk of transmitting the human immunodeficiency virus, cytomegalovirus and hepatitis B virus to health care workers exposed to patients with AIDS and AIDS-related conditions. J Infect Dis 156:1, 1987
19. Gerberding JL, Littell C, Tarkington A et al: Risk of exposure of surgical personnel to patients' blood during surgery at San Francisco General Hospital. N Engl J Med 322:1788, 1990
20. Gergert B, Maguire BT, Hulley SB et al: Physicians and acquired immunodeficiency syndrome. JAMA 262:1969, 1989
21. Nwanyanwu OC, Tabasuri TH, Harris GR: Exposure to and precautions for blood and body fluids among workers in the funeral home franchises of Fort Worth, Texas. Am J Infect Control 17:208, 1989
22. Willy ME, Dhillon GL, Loewen NL et al: Adverse precautions practices among a group of highly exposed health professionals. Infect Control Hosp Epidemiol 11:351, 1990
23. Becker CE, Cone JE, Gerberding J: Occupational infection with human immunodeficiency virus (HIV). Ann Intern Med 110:653, 1989
24. Jones DB: Percutaneous exposure of medical students to HIV. JAMA 264:1188, 1990
25. Evans R, Shanson DC: Serological studies on health care workers caring for patients with human immunodeficiency virus. J Hosp Infect 12:85, 1988
26. Kelen GD, DiGiovanna T, Bisson L et al: Human immunodeficiency virus infection in emergency department patients: Epidemiology, clinical presentations, and risk to health care workers. The Johns Hopkins experience. JAMA 262:516, 1989
27. Marcus R: Surveillance of health care workers exposed to blood from patients with human immunodeficiency virus. N Engl J Med 319:1118, 1988
28. Hammond JS, Eckes JM, Gomez GA et al: HIV, trauma, and infection control: Universal precautions are universally ignored. J Trauma 30:555, 1990
29. Centers for Disease Control: Update: Human immunodeficiency virus infection in health care workers exposed to blood of infected patients. MMWR 36:285, 1987
30. Pear R: Three health workers found infected by blood of patients with AIDS. New York Times, May 20, 1987, p 1, col B12
31. Stricof RL, Morse DL: HTLV-III/LAV seroconversion following a deep intramuscular needlestick injury (letter). N Engl J Med 314:1115, 1986
32. [N.A.]: Needlestick transmission of HTLV-III from a patient infected in Africa. Lancet 2:376, 1984
33. Oksenhendler E, Harzic M, LeRoux J et al: HIV infection with seroconversion after a superficial needlestick injury to the finger (letter). N Engl J Med 315:582, 1986
34. Neisson-Vernant C, Arfi S, Mathez D et al: Needlestick HIV seroconversion in a nurse (letter). Lancet 2:814, 1986
35. Centers for Disease Control: Apparent transmission of human T-lymphotrophic virus type III/lymphadenopathy associated virus from a child to a mother providing health care. MMWR 35:76, 1986
36. Grint P, McEvoy M: Two associated cases of the acquired immune deficiency syndrome (AIDS). PHLS Commun Dis Rep 42:4, 1986
37. Gerberding JL: Current epidemiologic evidence and case reports of occupationally acquired HIV and other blood-borne diseases. Infect Control Hosp Epidemiol 11(suppl): 588, 1990
38. Durand E, LeJeunne C, Hugues FC: Failure of prophylactic

zidovudine after suicidal self-inoculation of HIV-infected blood (letter). N Engl J Med 15:1062, 1991

39. Gioannini P, Sinicco A, Gariti G et al: HIV infection acquired by a nurse. Eur J Epidemiol 4:119, 1988
40. Centers for Disease Control: Acquired immunodeficiency syndrome (AIDS): Precautions for health care workers and allied professionals. MMWR 32:450, 1983
41. Centers for Disease Control: Summary: Recommendations for preventing transmission of infection with human T-lymphotropic virus type III/lymphadenopathy associated virus in the workplace. MMWR 36:285, 1985
42. Centers for Disease Control: Update: Evaluation of HTLV III/LAV infection in health care personnel—United States. MMWR 34:577, 1985
43. Centers for Disease Control: Recommended additional guidelines for HIV antibody counseling and testing in the prevention of HIV infection and AIDS, April 30, 1987
44. Centers for Disease Control: Recommendations for preventing transmission of infection with human T-lymphotropic virus type III/lymphadenopathy-associated virus during invasive procedures. MMWR 35:221, 1986
45. Centers for Disease Control: Recommendations for preventing possible transmission of human T-lymphotropic virus type III/lymphadenopathy-associated virus from tears. MMWR 34:533, 1985
46. Centers for Disease Control: Recommendations for assisting in the prevention of perinatal transmission of human T-lymphotropic virus type III/lymphadenopathy associated virus and acquired immunodeficiency syndrome. MMWR 34:721, 1985
47. Centers for Disease Control: Recommendations for providing dialysis treatment to patients infected with human T-lymphotropic virus type III/lymphadenopathy associated virus. MMWR 35:376, 1986
48. Centers for Disease Control: Update: Universal precautions for prevention of transmission of human immunodeficiency virus, hepatitis B virus, and other bloodborne pathogens in health-care settings. MMWR 37:377, 1988
49. Centers for Disease Control: Recommendations for prevention of HIV transmission in health-care settings. MMWR 36:35, 1987
50. Kane MA, Alter MJ, Hadler SC et al: Hepatitis B infection in the United States—recent trends and future strategies for control. Am J Med 87(suppl 3a):3a, 1989
51. Gerberding JL, Hopewell PC, Kaminsky LS et al: Transmission of hepatitis B without transmission of AIDS by accidental needlestick. N Engl J Med 312:56, 1985
52. Centers for Disease Control: Protection against viral hepatitis. MMWR 39:3, 1990
53. Sienko DG, Anda RF, McGee HB et al: Hepatitis B vaccination programs for hospital workers: Results of a statewide survey. Am J Infect Control 16:193, 1988
54. Fischl MA, Dickinson GM, Scot GB et al: Evaluation of heterosexual partner, children and household contacts of adults with AIDS. JAMA 257:640, 1987
55. Jason JM, McDougal JS, Dixon G et al: HTLV-III/LAV antibody and immune status of household contacts and sexual partners of persons with hemophilia. JAMA 255:212, 1986
56. Redfield RR, Markham PD, Salahuddin SZ et al: Frequent transmission of HTLV-III among spouses of patients with AIDS-related complex and AIDS. JAMA 253:1571, 1985
57. Friedland GH, Saltzman BR, Rogers MF et al: Lack of transmission of HTLV-III/LAV infections to household

contacts of patients with AIDS or AIDS-related complex with oral candidasis. N Engl J Med 314:344, 1986
58. Bernier RH, Sampliner R, Gerety R et al: Hepatitis B infection in households of chronic carriers of hepatitis B surface antigen: Factors associated with prevalence of infection. Am J Epidemiol 116:119, 1982
59. Szmuness W, Price AM, Hirsh RL et al: Familial clustering of hepatitis B infection. N Engl J Med 289:1162, 1973
60. Lane MA, Lettau LA: Transmission of HBV from dental personnel to patients. J Am Dent Assoc 110:634, 1985
61. Hadler SC, Sorley DL, Acree KH et al: An outbreak of hepatitis B in a dental practice. Ann Intern Med 95:133, 1981
62. Carl M, Blakey DL, Francis DP et al: Interruption of hepatitis B transmission by modification of a gynaecologist's surgical technique. Lancet 1:731, 1982
63. Centers for Disease Control: Nosocomial transmission of hepatitis-B virus associated with a spring-loaded finger-stick device—California. MMWR 39:610, 1990
64. Jagger J, Hunt EH, Pearson RD: Recapping used needles: Is it worse than the alternative? (letter). J Infect Dis 162:784, 1990
65. Jagger J, Pearson RD: A view from the cutting edge (editorial). Infect Control 8:51, 1987
66. National Academy of Science, Committee on Trauma Research: Injury in America: A Continuing Public Health Problem. Washington, DC, National Academy Press, 1985
67. Jackson MM, Dechairo DC, Gardner DF: Perceptions and beliefs of nursing and medical personnel about needle-handling practices and needlestick injuries. Am J Infect Control 14:1, 1986
68. [N.A.]: Reported needlesticks increase three-fold despite sharps boxes. Hosp Infect Control 17:131, 1990
69. Beekman SE, Fahey BJ, Gerbending JL et al: Risky business: Using necessarily imprecise casualty counts to estimate occupational risks for HIV-1 infection. Infect Control Hosp Epidemiol 11:371, 1990
70. Department of Labor and Department of Health and Human Services: Joint Advisory Notice: Protection against occupational exposure to hepatitis B virus (HBV) and human immunodeficiency virus (HIV). Fed Reg 52:418118, 1987
71. Centers for Disease Control: Recommendation for preventing transmission of infection with human T-lymphotropic virus type III/lymphadenopathy-associated virus during invasive procedures. MMWR 35:221, 1986
72. Centers for Disease Control: Recommended infection control practices for dentistry. MMWR 35:237, 1986
73. Lynch P, Cummings MJ, Roberts P et al: Implementing and evaluating a system of generic infection precautions: Body substance isolation. Am J Infect Control 18:1, 1990
74. Jackson MM, Lynch P: Infection prevention and control in the era of the AIDS/HIV epidemic. Semin Oncol Nurs 5:236, 1989
75. Miramontes H: Progress in establishing safety protocols on CDC and OSHA recommendations. Infect Control Hosp Epidemiol 11(suppl):561, 1990
76. De Laune S: Risk reduction through testing, screening and infection control precautions—with special emphasis on needlestick injuries. Infect Control Hosp Epidemiol 11(suppl):563, 1990
77. Becker MH, Janz NK, Band J et al: Noncompliance with universal precautions policy: Why do physicians and nurses recap needles? Am J Infect Control 18:232, 1990

78. Kearns KP, Hogg M: Universal precautions: Employee resistance and strategies for planned organizational change. Hosp Health Serv Admin 33:521, 1988

79. Jagger J, Hunt EH, Pearson RD: Sharp object injuries in the hospital: Causes and strategies for prevention. Am J Infect Control 18:227, 1990

80. Jagger J, Hunt EH, Brand-Elnaggar J et al: Rates of needlestick injury caused by various devices in a university hospital. N Engl J Med 319:284, 1990

81. Krumholz HM, Cummings S, York M: Blood culture phlebotomy: Switching needles does not prevent contamination. Ann Intern Med 113:290, 1990

82. McLeod GG: Needlestick injuries at operations for trauma: Are surgical gloves an effective barrier? J Bone Joint Surg 71:489, 1989

83. Church J, Sanderson P: Surgical glove punctures. J Hosp Infect 1:84, 1980

84. Centers for Disease Control: Guidelines for preventing the transmission of tuberculosis in health-care settings, with special focus on HIV-related issues. MMWR 39(RR-17):1, 1990

85. Department of Health and Human Services: HIV-Related Tuberculosis, p. 4. Atlanta, DHHS, 1990

86. Sunderam G, McDonald RJ, Maniatis T et al: Tuberculosis as a manifestation of the acquired immunodeficiency syndrome (AIDS). JAMA 256:362, 1986

87. Centers for Disease Control: Update: Tuberculosis elimination—United States. MMWR 39:153, 1990

88. [N.A.]: TB outbreaks warrant new attention to old disease. Hosp Infect Control 17:125, 1990

89. Department of Health and Human Services: Tuberculosis Elimination Plan, U.S.A. Atlanta, DHHS, 1990

90. Division of Tuberculosis Control, Centers for Disease Control and the American Thoracic Society: National tuberculosis training initiative: Core curriculum on tuberculosis. New York, American Lung Association, 1990

91. Bureau of Tuberculosis Control, New York City Department of Health: Tuberculosis At-a-Glance. New York, NYC Department of Health, 1990

92. Des Prez RM, Heim CR: Mycobacterium tuberculosis. In Mandell GL, Douglas Jr RG, Bennett JE (eds): Principles and Practices of Infectious Diseases, 3rd ed, p 1877. New York, Churchill Livingstone, 1990

93. Nardell EA: Dodging the droplet nuclei. Am Rev Respir Dis 142:501, 1990

94. Riley RL: The hazard is relative. Am Rev Respir Dis 96:623, 1967

95. Centers for Disease Control: Mycobacterium tuberculosis transmission in a health clinic—Florida 1988. MMWR 38:256, 1989

96. Montgomery AB, Corkery KJ, Brunette ER et al: Occupational exposure to aerosolized pentamidine. Chest 98:386, 1990

97. Stranberg RW: Guidelines to prevent employee exposure to aerosolized pentamidine (letter). CAI/OSHA Information Bulletin, California Department of Industrial Relations. San Francisco, 1990

98. Kacmarek RM: Ribavirin and pentamidine aerosols: Caregiver beware! (letter). Respir Care 35:1034, 1990

99. Scott F: Pentamidine experts take a hard look at side effects of treatment. Respir Care Adv 3(39):1, 1990

100. [N.A.]: Hot line increases needlestick reporting, rapid prophylaxis. Hosp Infect Control 17:101, 1990

101. [N.A.]: One-third of needlesticks go unreported at hospital. Hosp Infect Control 17:107, 1990

102. Hopkins CC: Implementation of universal blood and body fluids precautions. Infect Dis Clin North Am 3(4):747, 1989

103. Transcript of the proceedings: Open meeting on the risk of transmission of bloodborne pathogens to patients during invasive procedures, Feb 21–22, 1991, Atlanta, GA. Rockville, MD, CDC National AIDS Clearinghouse (in press)

Special Considerations for Surgeons

31B

Daniel R. Benson

Concern over the exposure of health care workers to blood and other bloody body fluids has increased recently. Health care workers, including surgeons, are often exposed to bloody fluids of human immunodeficiency virus (HIV)–infected patients. As of December 31, 1990, 24 cases of seroconversion to HIV-antibody-positive status following occupational exposure had been reported to the Centers for Disease Control (CDC). In another 16 health care workers seroconversion was thought to be occupationally acquired but a specific incident could not be documented.[1] Eleven additional cases of occupationally acquired HIV infection have been reported from countries other than the United States.[2] Some of these seroconversions occurred in surgeons.

Several prospective studies indicate that the risk of HIV transmission to a health care worker following a single percutaneous exposure to HIV-infected blood is 0.3%.[3,4] Transmission of HIV after mucous membrane or skin exposure to HIV-infected blood has been reported,[5] but the risk of transmission by these means is less well known.

Surgeons who perform or assist in surgical procedures may sustain skin or mucous membrane contamination by either splash or gown soak-through. The use of needles and other sharp instruments, particularly in deep, poorly exposed areas, puts the surgeon at particular risk for percutaneous injury. Certain specialists, such as oral surgeons and orthopedic surgeons, face the additional risk of skin penetration by sharp bone fragments.

Further, the use of oscillating saws and drills creates a splatter of blood droplets well away from the wound. In six prospective studies, the percentage of cases in which at least one surgical team member experienced a percutaneous injury ranged from 1.3% to 15.4%.[6-10] In a more recent CDC study, preliminary data indicated that percutaneous injuries occurred during 96 (6.9%) of 1,382 operative cases on general surgery, gynecology, orthopedic surgery, cardiac surgery, and trauma surgery services.[11] Skin contamination occurs even more often. In a study at Grady Memorial Hospital, Atlanta, trained observers monitored a sample of operations performed on six surgical services. In 62 (30.1%) of 206 operations, at least one blood contact was observed. Of 1,828 operating room person-procedures observed, 96 (5.3%) involved 147 blood contacts (133 skin contacts, ten percutaneous injuries, and four eye splashes). The risk factors for a surgeon contacting patient blood were (1) performing a trauma, burn, or orthopedic procedure, (2) patient blood loss greater than 250 ml, and (3) being in the operating room longer than 1 hour. Of 110 blood contacts among surgeons, 81 (74%) were thought to be potentially preventable with the use of additional barrier precautions, such as face shields and fluid-resistant gowns.[12]

The resistance of gown fabrics to fluid penetration varies considerably. In a study conducted at Duke University, 13 of 17 commercially available gowns examined did not prevent HIV-1 penetration. Visible soak-through of blood was the most obvious feature, but virus penetration without visible soak-through also occurred. The investigators suggested that until more is known about the mechanics of fluid micropenetration of barrier materials, surgeons and other health care workers should consider wearing more fluid-impervious gowns, particularly when caring for high-risk patients.[13] For example, a plastic apron or supplemental sleeve protection would help to prevent soak-through to the skin. Latex glove material is not impervious to perforation during the operative procedure. The difficulty of the case and length of the procedure both contribute to an increased incidence of perforation. In one study, the overall perforation rate for surgeons' and scrub nurses' gloves was 48.2% and 42.5%, respectively. Only 38.9% of the glove perforations were known by the surgeon at the time of their occurrence.[14] The health care workers most at risk are those likely to sustain needlesticks, cuts, and skin tears in the presence of contaminated body fluids. The risk of percutaneous injury appears to be equal among surgeons and the scrub team.[12] All of these findings emphasize the need for special care and precautions when operating.

PREVENTING HIV TRANSMISSION IN THE OPERATING SUITE

The chief defense against HIV transmission is the prevention of transmission. The CDC has issued a series of recommendations, known as universal precautions, designed to prevent transmission in the health care setting.[15] The basis for the CDC recommendations is that health care workers should consider blood and body fluids containing visible blood from all patients as potentially capable of transmitting blood-borne infection, and that universal precautions should be observed. The CDC's universal precautions apply to blood and other body fluids that contain visible blood as well as to semen, vaginal secretions, cerebrospinal fluid, pleural fluid, peritoneal fluid, pericardial fluid, and amniotic fluid. The universal precautions do not apply to feces, saliva, nasal secretions, sputum, sweat, tears, or vomitus unless they are visibly contaminated with blood. Although HIV and hepatitis B virus have been detected in these fluids, epidemiologic studies have not shown such fluids to transmit HIV.[16] These recommendations were developed because most of the serologic tests used for the detection of HIV depend on the formation of antibody by the infected patient. There is, however, a window of time during the patient is infectious with virus but anti-HIV antibodies have not yet appeared. Therefore, even an HIV-seronegative patient might carry HIV. Additionally, other blood-borne infections such as HBV, HCV, and HTLV-I, can be transmitted if the surgeon does not protect adequately against contamination.

Studies of patients seen in the emergency room have shown that increasing numbers are HIV positive. This is particularly true in inner-city hospitals in areas of high HIV prevalence. In a study at Johns Hopkins Hospital in Baltimore, patients who had sustained penetrating trauma had an HIV prevalence of 13.6%. Many patients did not know their HIV status or failed to reveal it.[17,18] An accurate history might uncover risk potential, but necessarily many patients will enter the operating room without serodiagnosis. The surgical team usually operates on trauma patients without any knowledge of the patient's HIV status.

The surgeon risks infection if the patients' infected blood enters through an open wound such as a needlestick or contaminates exposed skin or mucous membranes. The goal of the health care team is to prevent needlesticks, cuts, or any skin contamination in the operating room, the clinic, or the hospital ward. There has been some discussion of the possibility that hot-smoke fumes from electrocautery or surgical power instruments could create an aerosolization of the virus.[19] To date, however, there are no epidemiologic data to suggest that HIV transmission occurs by this route. Two large studies, one done in dentists[20] and the other done in orthopedic surgeons,[21] have shown the prevalence of anti-HIV antibodies to be lower than that expected in the general population. Many of the subjects worked in high-prevalence areas with high-speed instruments and electrocautery. If in fact the virus were spread by aerosolization, one would expect a higher than normal prevalence in these health care workers. Compared to HBV, HIV seems to be relatively difficult to transmit from patient to health care worker. Barrier precautions have been shown to decrease the transmission of HBV. This suggests that universal precautions are an effective means of preventing HIV transmission.

BARRIER PRECAUTIONS FOR OPERATING PERSONNEL

The barrier precautions recommended for orthopedic surgeons to prevent skin contamination have been presented in a monograph published by the American Academy of Orthopaedic Surgeons, *Recommendations for the Prevention of Human Immunodeficiency Virus (HIV) Transmission in the Practice of Orthopaedic Surgery.*[22] The following recommendations have been taken, in part, from that monograph.

In the operating room, do not hurry. Excessive speed may result in an injury. If the patient is known to be HIV positive, or if the team is highly suspicious of the patient's HIV status, then the most experienced operating staff should be responsible for the surgical procedure. Consideration should be given to excusing less experienced members of the surgical team, such as medical students, interns, and junior residents, from difficult HIV-infected cases.

The surgeon and the operating team should wear the best available surgical garb that offers protection against contact with blood. This surgical garb may include:

1. Knee-high, waterproof surgical shoe and leg covers if considerable blood or fluid is expected to leave the operation site. The knee-high covers should be supplemented with routine shoe covers to prevent slipping on the wet operating room floor (Fig. 31B–1).
2. Water-impervious gowns. If none are available, a waterproof apron can be worn under the gown. Not all surgical gowns will prevent soak-through or virus penetration.[13]

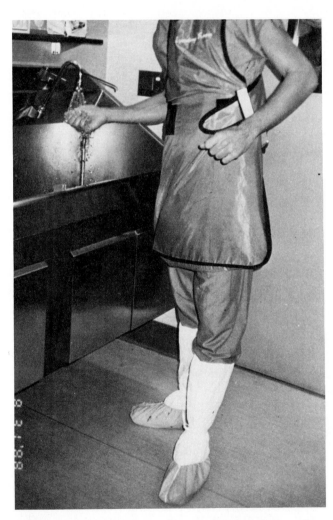

Figure 31B–1. While performing a surgical procedure where a great deal of blood or fluid is expected to contaminate the floor or sheets, the health-care worker should wear knee-high, fluid-impervious boots. The surgeon in this photograph has knee-high boots, which are supplemented by usual shoe covers to prevent slipping on the fluid-covered floor.

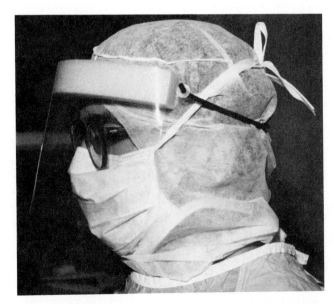

Figure 31B–2. Eye protection is important to prevent splatter of the eyes. Full glasses or goggles are good, but a face shield is better. The welder's-type mask used by this surgeon will prevent splatter to the face, particularly if a high-speed drill or saw is being used. Additionally, the head cover should enclose the lower portion of the face and the neck. The standard nurse's cap is not adequate to cover exposed skin.

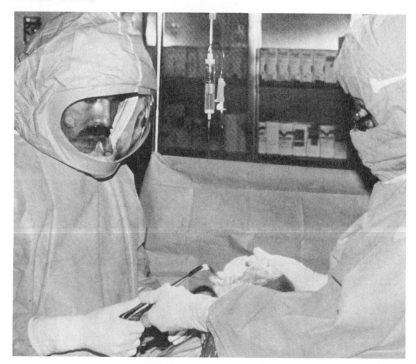

Figure 31B–3. The best possible protection is a total body or space suit, such as the surgeons in this picture are wearing. These suits include an inflow/outflow air system, which prevents respiratory contamination from the surgeon to the patient's wound and prevent contamination of the surgeon from the vapors created by electrocautery smoke or high-speed drilling.

3. Double latex gloves. If sharp bony fragments are involved or multiple wires are being used for fixation, the surgeon should consider placing a glove made of cloth or Kevlar (a puncture-resistant material) between the latex gloves. These materials will prevent some skin penetration, particularly by wires or bone, but will not prevent a needlestick.

4. A head cover that maximizes head and skin coverage, ideally a hat that extends down to protect the neck and lower portion of the face (Fig. 31B–2).

5. Protective eyewear, at least full glasses if not goggles. It is better if a face shield is worn (see Fig. 31B–2). Most protective is the total body suit with an inflow/outflow air supply (Fig. 31B–3).

6. Standard surgical mask. If the mask is splattered or moist it should be changed. If splatter is expected, a face shield should prevent the mask from contamination (see Fig. 31B–2).

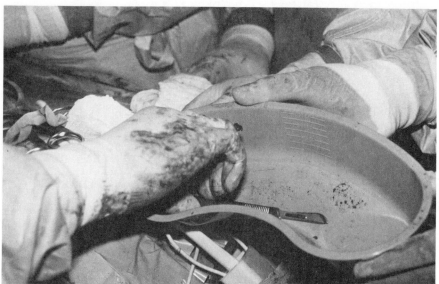

Figure 31B–4. When asking for sharp instruments, such as a scalpel, the surgeon should request them orally. An announcement should be made by the scrub personnel that the sharp instrument is being passed. The use of an intermediate tray, such as this basin, protects the surgeon or his team members from being cut as the instrument is being passed across the field.

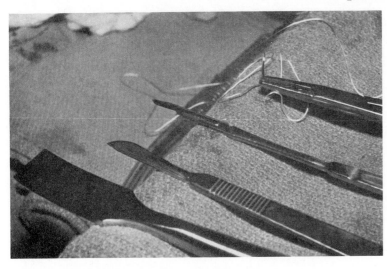

Figure 31B–5. Sharp instruments, such as osteotomes and scalpels, should be protected on the Mayo stand. If they are left hanging over the edge, as illustrated in this example, accidental skin penetration is likely to occur. Additionally, suture needles should not be loaded and placed on the Mayo stand in an upright position before they are needed. If a member of the operating team should accidently place a hand or an arm on the Mayo stand, skin penetration is possible.

To avoid skin penetration during a surgical procedure, the surgeon and team should observe the following precautions:

1. Be aware and cautious at all times. Before a long and difficult case, or if HIV infection is suspected, the case should be discussed before the procedure is begun. The discussion should include the entire operating team (surgeons, nurses, technicians, and anesthesiologists). The potential for glove penetration or skin contamination for that specific operative case should be the basis for the team's instruction.
2. Before sharp instruments are passed, an oral announcement should be made. The surgeon should request the scalpel and the scrub nurse or technician should respond with the statement that the scalpel is being passed. It might be best to pass these on an intermediate tray (Fig. 31B–4).
3. Sharp instruments should be protected on the Mayo stand to prevent accidental wounds when the surgeon reaches for them or if someone leans on the stand. This includes suture needles, which should not be loaded and left upright until the surgeon is ready to use them (Fig. 31B–5).
4. In closing wounds, instrumentation or other non-touch suturing techniques should be used. The surgeon should not tie with the needle in the hand (Fig. 31B–6). If it is necessary to do a manual tie, the suture needle should be removed to prevent accidental sticks.
5. Two surgeons should avoid simultaneously suturing the same wound. (One wound, one surgeon.)
6. The surgeon should take extra care when digitally examining sharp fracture fragments (Fig. 31B–7) or working with sharp instruments or wires (Fig. 31B–8).
7. The surgical team should check periodically (hourly) to evaluate whether blood has contam-

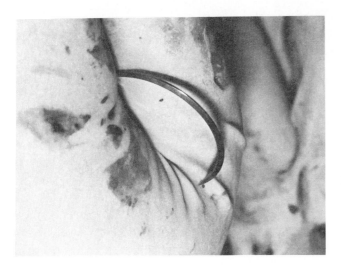

Figure 31B–6. When tieing suture, instrument-tie, or other no-touch techniques should be used if possible. If hand ties are necessary, the needle should be removed from the suture before tying. Tying with the needle in hand, such as demonstrated here, is dangerous and unnecessary.

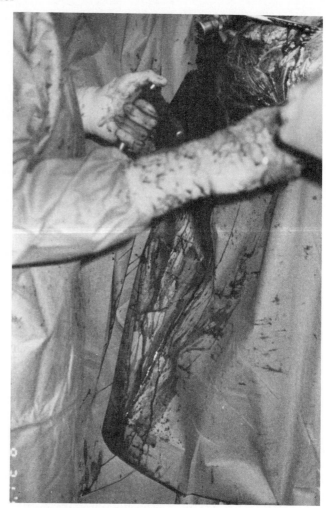

Figure 31B–7. When probing deep wounds where sharp bony fragments are present, the surgeon should be careful not to puncture his glove and skin. The use of a cloth or Kevlar glove between the two layers of latex gloves may help to prevent skin puncture in cases such as this.

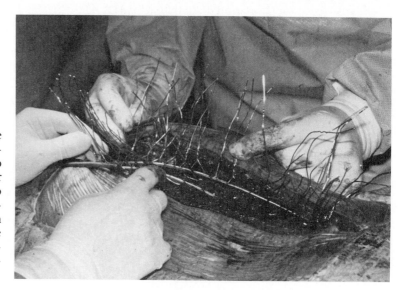

Figure 31B–8. In cases that involve the use of a large number of wires or other sharp instrumentation, great care must be taken to prevent skin puncture. The use of cloth or Kelvar gloves is also helpful in these cases, to prevent accidental sticks. In this case—a patient with spinal curvature—a Luque rod with multiple wires is being used to secure the spine to a rod. With this number of wires present, members of the surgical team can accidentally puncture their gloves and skin.

inated the surgical gowns or shoe protectors, particularly if a large amount of blood has been lost or the procedure is lengthy.

8. Exposed wires and pins should be covered with pieces of catheter tubing or cork to prevent accidental skin penetration during the remainder of the operative procedure.

When an incident or a contamination occurs, the following steps should be implemented:

1. If the blood contaminates intact skin, the area should be immediately washed with a soap and water solution. If it is not possible for the surgeon or a member of the surgical team to leave the operating room to wash at the scrub sink, the cir-

culating nurse can wash the area on an emergency basis (Fig. 31B–9).

2. If the skin is cut or punctured, the gloves should be immediately removed and the wound bled. The wound is then washed with surgical soap, or 70% isopropyl alcohol can be poured directly on the wound.

3. If allowed by law, or if the patient consents, blood should be drawn to confirm HIV status. This is not necessary when the patient is known to be HIV positive. HBV and HCV status should also be checked.

4. The incident should be reported to the facility's occupational health unit.

5. The health care worker's HIV and HBV status should be immediately confirmed by serotesting. If the patient is HIV positive, the health care

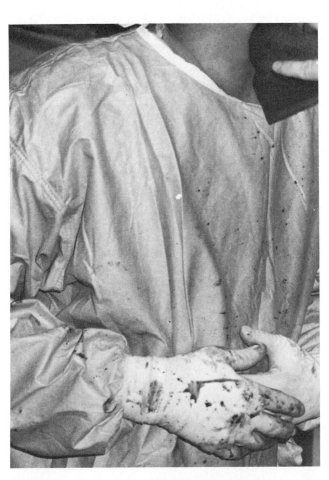

Figure 31B–9. If the skin is left unprotected, and splatter causes contamination, the bloody fluid should immediately be washed with soap and water. If the surgeon cannot leave the case to do this at the scrub sink, the circulating nurse or technician can wipe off the contamination with a wet towel or with 70% isopropyl alcohol. In this case, the surgeon should have protected his neck with proper head gear.

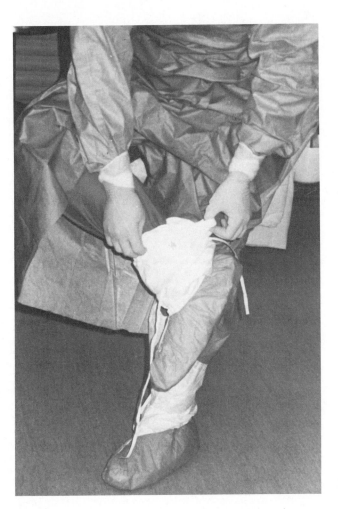

Figure 31B–10. This example demonstrates the surgeon properly removing his shoe covers while still wearing gloves. The shoe covers in this case have not been contaminated with visible blood, but the technique is correct.

worker should undergo repeated HIV testing at 3 months, 6 months, and 1 year. Regardless of whether the test is negative or positive, counseling should be sought from a qualified individual.

6. If stuck with a needle in a case of known or suspected HIV infection, the surgical team member should consider a 6-week course of zidovudine. If decided, it should be started within the hour of the stick.[23] (*Caution:* Zidovudine has side-effects, and the recipient should be advised of them by a knowledgeable person.)

During the course of a surgical procedure, other individuals may enter the operation. In these cases the scrub personnel should put on clean gloves before gloving and gowning the newly arrived team members. This measure is designed to prevent skin contamination by blood or bloody fluids that may be on the gloves of the scrub personnel.

At the completion of the case, the following precautions should be considered:

1. Bloody outer gloves are removed before the patient's wound is washed and a dressing applied. If necessary, the surgeon dons a clean pair of gloves to apply the dressing.
2. The boots should be removed before the gloves are taken off (Fig. 31B–10).
3. The surgical team members should remove all blood-contaminated clothing in a manner that avoids contact with blood (Fig. 31B–11). The gown and gloves should be removed as a unit and

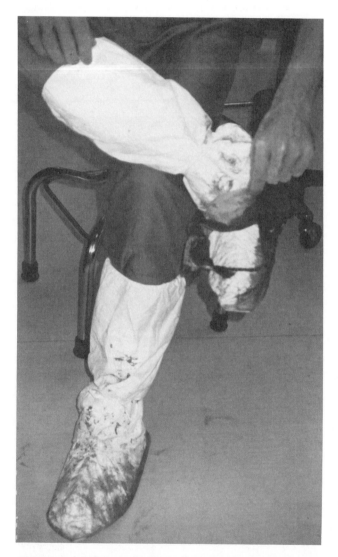

Figure 31B–11. Bloody shoewear or gowns should not be removed with bare hands, as the surgeon demonstrates in this case. The gloves should be left on until all contaminated materials have been removed. Additionally, bloody boots and gowns should be removed before leaving the operating room. Surgical team members should not walk through surgical corridors with bloody boots, because of the risk of contamination.

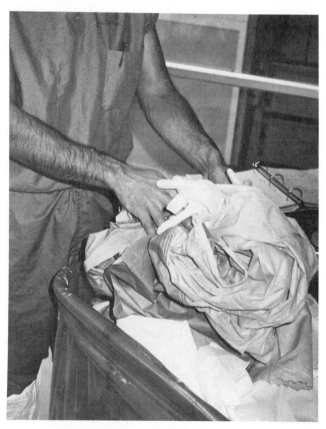

Figure 31B–12. The surgical gown and gloves should be removed as a unit, keeping the contaminated, bloody side rolled within, and should then be placed in proper containers for infectious waste. These are usually colored red or yellow, depending on your hospital.

discarded in disposable infectious waste containers (Fig. 31B–12).

4. The surgical team members should wash hands, forearms, and face with antiseptic soap at the surgical scrub sink. The surgeon should not leave the operating room with blood-soaked shoe covers.

5. Before removing bloody gloves, the surgical team members should not touch anything (*e.g.,* telephone or cabinets).

HIV TRANSMISSION IN BONE ALLOGRAFTS

There has been one reported case of a bone graft causing HIV seroconversion. The donor's hip was removed for a total joint replacement. A previous history of a significant risk factor (lymphadenopathy in a previous acute viral illness) either was not obtained or was disregarded. The donor did not undergo HIV testing prior to the donation, but subsequently died of AIDS.[24] If a surgeon elects to use allograft bone, the methods of donor selection and allograft excision and preparation should be known. To this end, surgeons may consult the guidelines of organizations dealing with bone tissue banking, such as the American Federation of Clinic Tissue Banks, the South-Eastern Organ Procurement Foundation, and the American Association of Tissue Banks.[25,26]

In deciding whether to use frozen bone allograft, the orthopedic surgeon must bear in mind that the possibility of transporting bone allograft from a donor infected with HIV, although remote, does exist. The bone bank should combine rigorous donor selection, screening for HIV antigen and antibody, and histopathologic studies of donor tissues. With living donors not all of these precautions are possible, but a repeated determination of HIV antibody and antigen levels at 3 months will probably result in an equal degree of safety.

CONCLUSION

By observing the precautions outlined here, the surgical team can avoid unnecessary contamination or skin penetration. This will greatly decrease the chance of transmission of HIV or other viruses from the patient to the health care worker. Better materials for glove and gown construction are being developed by industry. Although none of these techniques will reduce the likelihood of contamination to zero, they will greatly reduce its incidence.

REFERENCES

1. Henderson DK: HIV-1 in the health care setting. In Mandell GL, Douglas RG Jr, Bennett JE (eds): Principles and Practice of Infectious Disease, 3rd ed. New York, Churchill Livingstone

2. Marcus R, Kay K, Mann J: Transmission of human immunodeficiency virus (HIV) in health-care settings world wide. Bull WHO 67:577, 1989

3. Henderson DK, Fahey BJ, Willy M et al: Risk for the occupational transmission of human immunodeficiency virus type-1 (HIV-1) associated with clinical exposure: A prospective evaluation. Ann Intern Med 113:740, 1990

4. Marcus R, CDC Cooperative Needle Stick Study Group: Surveillance of health care workers exposed to blood from patients infected with the human immunodeficiency virus. N Engl J Med 319:1118, 1988

5. Centers for Disease Control: Update: Human immunodeficiency virus infections in health-care workers exposed to blood of infected patients. MMWR 36:285, 1987

6. Gerberding JL, Littell C, Tarkington A et al: Risk of exposure of surgical personnel to patients' blood during surgery at San Francisco General Hospital. N Engl J Med 322:1788, 1990

7. Panlilio AL, Foy DR, Edwards JR et al: Blood contacts during surgical procedures. JAMA 265:1533, 1991

8. Popejoy S, Fry D: Blood exposure to surgical staff and frequency of exposure reporting (abstr 3192). Presented at the 6th International Conference on AIDS, San Francisco, 1990

9. Hussain SA, Latid AB, Choudhary AA: Risk of surgeons: A survey of accidental injuries during operating. Br J Surg 75:341, 1988

10. Telford GL, Quebbeman EJ: Risk of injury and blood exposure in the operating room environment (abstr). Presented at the American College of Surgeons Annual Clinical Congress, San Francisco, October 1990

11. Centers for Disease Control: Draft: Estimates of the risk of endemic transmission of hepatitis B virus and human immunodeficiency virus to patients by the percutaneous route during invasive surgical and dental procedures. Published as an abstract by Tokars JI, Marcus R, Culver DH, Bell DM, for the Cooperative Study Group: Blood contact during surgical procedures (abstr 958). Presented at the 30th Interscience Conference on Antimicrobial Agents and Chemotherapy, Atlanta, October 1990

12. Panlilio AL, Foy DR, Edwards JR et al: Blood contacts during surgical procedures. JAMA 265:1533, 1991

13. Shadduck PP, Tyler DS, Lyerly HK et al: Commercially available surgical gowns do not prevent penetration by HIV-1. Surg Forum 41, 1990

14. Brough SJ, Hunt TM, Barrie WW: Surgical glove perforations. Br J Surg 75:317, 1988

15. Centers for Disease Control: Recommendations for prevention of HIV transmission in health-care settings. MMWR 36(suppl 25):3S, 1987

16. Centers for Disease Control: Acquired immunodeficiency syndrome (AIDS): Precautions for clinical and laboratory staffs. MMWR 36(suppl 31):577, 1982

17. Kelen GD, DiGiovanna T, Bisson L et al: Human immunodeficiency virus in emergency department patients. JAMA 262:516, 1989

18. Kelen GD, Fritz S, Qaqish B et al: Unrecognized human immunodeficiency virus infection in emergency department patients. N Engl J Med 318:1645, 1988

19. Johnson GK, Robinson WS: Human immunodeficiency virus-1 (HIV-1) in the vapors of surgical power instruments. J Med Virol 33:47, 1991

20. Klein RS, Phelan JA, Freeman K et al: Low occupational risk of human immunodeficiency virus among dental professionals. N Engl J Med 381:86, 1988

21. Centers for Disease Control: Preliminary analysis: HIV serosurvey of orthopaedic surgeons. MMWR 40:309, 1991

22. American Academy of Orthopaedic Surgeons: Recommendations for the Prevention of Human Immunodeficiency Virus (HIV) Transmission in the Practice of Orthopaedic Surgery. Park Ridge, Ill, American Academy of Orthopaedic Surgeons, 1989

23. Centers for Disease Control: Public health service statement on management of occupational exposure to human immunodeficiency virus, including considerations regarding zidovudine post exposure use. MMWR 39:1, 1990

24. Centers for Disease Control: Transmission of HIV through blood transplantation: Case report and public health recommendations. MMWR 37:597, 1988

25. South-Eastern Organ Procurement Foundation: Guidelines and Standards for the Excision, Preparation, Storage and Distribution of Human Tissue Allograft for Transplantation. Richmond, Va, South-Eastern Organ Procurement Foundation, 1988

26. American Association of Tissue Banks: Standards for Bone Banking. Arlington, Va, American Association of Tissue Banks, 1987

Special Considerations for Dentists

31C

David Archibald

The recent reporting by the Centers for Disease Control (CDC) of the apparent transmission of human immunodeficiency virus (HIV) from a dentist to three of his patients[1,2] has reinforced concerns about infection control procedures for oral health care workers. Almost all areas of modern dental practice involve the use of sharp instruments, including burs, needles, scalpels, scalers, or orthodontic wires that can cause bleeding in the oral cavity or accidental puncture wounds to practitioners. To a certain degree, some of the exposures of dental personnel to HIV-infected blood *via* accidental puncture wounds may be unavoidable. However, epidemiologic data indicate that the risk of a practitioner or a patient acquiring HIV infection during dental procedures is exceedingly low. Moreover, the volume of blood encountered in most dental procedures is less than that encountered in most other types of surgical procedures.

Dental personnel face the same infection control situations as other health care workers who perform invasive procedures with sharp instruments, except that dental treatment is usually performed outside of the hospital or operating room setting. Strict adherence to sterile techniques is usually more easily achieved in institutional settings than in private dental offices. However, general infection control precautions for all health care workers apply to dental personnel as well. This chapter examines the special aspects of treatment of the oral cavity that may affect safety precautions for the oral health care worker when dealing with HIV-seropositive patients.

RISKS OF VIRAL TRANSMISSION IN DENTISTRY

Because HIV and hepatitis B virus (HBV) are transmitted by similar modes, it is important to recognize that dental personnel are at increased risk for acquiring HBV infection[3] and are responsible for several outbreaks of HBV infection among dental patients. In one reported case, a dentist in rural Indiana who did not wear gloves was the probable source of nine symptomatic and 15 asymptomatic cases of HBV infection.[4] Two of the symptomatic patients died. The dentist was reported to be an assiduous hand scrubber. This practice could have caused microlesions in his skin that allowed both exit and entry of the virus. Transmission from an infected patient to the dentist *via* nongloved hands and then from the dentist to the other patients was the presumed route of the virus.[4] The titer of HBV is much greater than the titer of HIV in blood and other fluids, and analyses of needlestick injuries have shown that the risk of infection following a wound with HIV-infected blood is much less than with HBV-infected blood. However, it is not unreasonable that episodes similar to those seen with HBV transmission could also occur with HIV, and one such event may have occurred in Florida.

Four individuals who were patients of a dentist with acquired immunodeficiency syndrome (AIDS) have been reported to be infected with HIV.[1,2] Two of the individuals had no known risk factors for HIV infection. The third patient had a history of multiple heterosexual partners and of non-intravenous (IV) drug use, and the fourth had a known behavioral risk factor for HIV infection. All of the patients denied sexual contact with the dentist or with other patients in the practice. The first three patients all underwent at least one invasive dental procedure after the dentist's initial diagnosis of AIDS. Sequence analysis of the V3 regions of gp120 of viral isolates from the dentist and the first three patients revealed a 3.4% average nucleotide difference. The nucleotide differences between the V3 regions of viral isolates derived from control non-patient infected individuals from the same geographic area and from the three patients and the dentist were 13%. The fourth patient's viral isolates appeared to be unrelated to isolates from the other three patients or the dentist. Nucleotide sequence analyses of the V4-C3-V5 region of gp120 revealed an average difference from the three patients and the dentist of 1.8%, *versus* a 4.8% difference from the local controls. The differences in the control *versus* the patient/dentist sequences were highly significant and strongly implicated the dentist as the common source of the viruses isolated from the three patients. Further, there was a signature amino acid sequence in the V3 regions of isolates from the three patients and the dentist that was not seen in any other North American isolate.[2] Recently, two additional HIV-infected patients of the dentist have been identified who have similar nucleotide sequences.[5]

The route of transmission has not been established in this case. The dentist had known behavioral risk factors for HIV infection and so probably was not infected by contact with a patient. Infection control procedures, including routine gloving, masking, and autoclaving of all instruments, had been instituted in 1987, before two of the patients were treated by the dentist. Two of the three patients received dental treatment only after the dentist had been diagnosed with AIDS, when his CD4+ cell count probably would have been below 200 cells/mm³ and the viral titers might have been higher.[2] The most likely route of transmission was blood-blood contact. During an invasive procedure such as suturing, a puncture wound in the dentist's hand could have allowed his blood to contact intact or nonintact oral mucosal tissue. However, the use of instruments or equipment contaminated with blood or saliva from the dentist cannot be ruled out as a possible mode of transmission. The dentist did have dental prophylaxes carried out on his own teeth by a hygienist in his office during the time he was known to be infected. A retrospective study of infection control procedures in the office did not reveal any unusual practices, however. Other epidemiologic studies of patients treated by health care workers, including dentists, with AIDS are in progress, and these studies may yield more information on the risks and modes of HIV transmission.[2]

Klein *et al* examined the risk of dental personnel acquiring HIV infection from patients by assaying 1,309 dental professionals, including 1,132 dentists, 131 hygienists, and 46 assistants, for anti-HIV antibody.[6] Half of the subjects practiced in urban areas of the United States where many cases of AIDS have been reported, and 72% reported having treated patients with AIDS or behavioral risk factors for AIDS. Ninety-four percent of the dental personnel recalled one or more accidental punctures of their skin with instruments while treating patients in the 5 years preceding the study. Further, the use of gloves and other infection control practices was inconsistent among the practitioners. Even with all the aforementioned factors likely to increase the chance of transmission, only one dentist without a behavioral risk factor for AIDS had serum antibodies to HIV.[6]

HIV IN SALIVA

Only rarely has HIV been cultured from the saliva of HIV-infected individuals. Ho *et al* isolated HIV from only one of 83 saliva samples collected from 71 symptomatic and asymptomatic HIV-infected individuals.[7] Levy and Greenspan detected infectious virus in three of 55 whole saliva samples from HIV-infected individuals.[8] Estimates are that greater than 10^5 infectious HBV virions per milliliter are present in the saliva of chronically infected individuals,[9] whereas it is estimated that only one infectious HIV virion per milliliter is found in the saliva of HIV-infected individuals.[8] HIV nucleic acids have been detected in saliva samples[10,11] in the absence of infectious virus.[10] There have been case reports in which saliva or oral sexual contact was considered the mode of HIV transmission. However, it is difficult to segment different sexual practices on a retrospective basis and attribute the transmission solely to contact with HIV-infected saliva.

Whole saliva from the majority of people contains varying amounts of serum or whole blood.[9,12] Activities that abrade the oral mucosa may increase the quantity of detectable blood in the oral cavity. Further, individuals with symptomatic HIV infection are more likely to have oral mucosal or gingival lesions, which should increase the serum or whole blood content in their saliva.

It has been demonstrated that both toothbrushing and passionate kissing markedly increased the percentage of individuals who have detectable hemoglobin in their salivas.[12] Also, these practices increased the hemoglobin concentration in the saliva of individuals who were already hemoglobin positive. This may indicate that breaks in the integrity of the oral mucosa are generated from rubbing. Therefore, any manipulation of the oral mucosa may lead to an increase in the amount of blood in the mouth and thereby increase the possibility of viral transmission. The presence of blood or serum transudate in saliva has not, however, led to verifiable reports of HIV transmission through saliva.

Besides low virus titers, there may be other reasons for the lack of infectivity of saliva. Some *in vitro* data suggest that saliva may inhibit the infectivity of HIV. Fultz *et al* were unable to infect a chimpanzee by topical application of cell-free HIV to the oral mucosa.[13] Fultz speculated that saliva might be inhibitory to the virus, so she incubated HIV with normal human and chimpanzee salivas, filtered the mixtures, and then attempted to culture the virus *in vitro* on peripheral white blood cells.[14] Infectivity was inhibited if the virus was incubated with saliva for a minimum of 30 minutes. Fox *et al* carried out further studies that showed that inhibitory activity was present in whole and submandibular saliva collected from women, children, and HIV-infected and HIV-uninfected men.[15,16] In these assays the virus-saliva mixtures were filtered before addition to cell cultures; thus, nonspecific binding of the mixtures to filters may have accounted for the observed effect. A subsequent study showed that the inhibitory effect was due to the artifact of binding of virus-saliva mixtures to filters. However, HIV inhibitory activity independent of this cause was also present in salivas.[17] The activity, which could be removed with the use of 0.45-μm filters, was detected at moderate levels in submandibular/sublingual and minor salivary gland saliva and at higher levels in whole saliva. Aggregation of virus with high molecular weight salivary mucins or interactions between salivary glycolipids and viral envelope proteins are two of many possible mechanisms that might account for this phenomenon. Antibodies to HIV have been detected in the saliva of asymptomatic and symptomatic individuals infected with HIV.[18] Whether these antibodies affect transmission is not known at present.

The mucosae of the oral cavity have been reported to contain HIV-infected cells. Becker *et al* demonstrated the presence of viral antigens in two of 26 biopsies of oral tissue using immunohistochemistry.[19] The infected cells, found in the gingiva and tongue, were assumed to be infected mononuclear cells. Other investigators found evidence of HIV-infected mononuclear cells in the tonsillar tissues of patients with AIDS at autopsy by using an anti-gp41 monoclonal antibody.[20] Dental pulp tissue from a patient with AIDS has been reported to contain HIV proviral DNA when assayed by polymerase chain reaction techniques.[21] The determination of the cell type in this case was not possible. However, these reports reinforce the need for dental personnel to treat all oral soft tissues from HIV-infected patients with proper infection control procedures.

PRECAUTIONS FOR DENTAL PERSONNEL

Not all dental patients with HIV or other infectious diseases will be identified through history, physical examination, or a laboratory test. HBV survives well on environmental surfaces, attains high virus titers in blood, and has been transmitted in the dental setting. Therefore, infection control procedures effective for the prevention of HBV infections should apply to all dental patients and should be adequate for preventing HIV transmission. The CDC recommendations for prevention of HIV transmission in dental settings are described below.[22–24]

1. Obtain an up-to-date medical history from all patients and include questions about medications, current illnesses, hepatitis, unintentional weight loss, lymphadenopathy, oral soft tissue lesions, or other infections. A medical consultation may be indicated if a history of active infection or systemic disease is elicited.

2. Because blood, saliva and gingival fluid from all patients should be considered infective, gloves must be worn by all personnel when examining all oral lesions. All work should be completed on one patient, when possible. Hands should be washed and regloved before performing procedures on another patient.

3. Surgical masks and protective eyewear or chin-length plastic face shields must be worn when splashing or spattering of blood, saliva, or gingival fluids is likely. Rubber dams, high-speed suction, and proper patient positioning when appropriate should be used to minimize generation of aerosols, droplets, and splatter. Reusable or disposable gowns, lab coats, or uniforms must be worn when clothing is likely to be soiled with blood or saliva.

4. Impervious-backed paper, aluminum foil, or clear plastic wrap may be used to cover surfaces such as light handles or x-ray unit heads and buttons that are difficult or impossible to disinfect. The coverings should be removed (while the dental health care worker's hands are gloved), discarded, and replaced (after ungloving) with clean material between patients, Figures 31C–1 through 31C–3 illustrate the use of clear plastic wrap on such surfaces.

5. Sharp instruments should be handled with extraordinary care to prevent unintentional injuries. Recapping of needles increases the risk of needlestick injuries. Therefore, during dental procedures that require multiple injections of anesthetic or other medications from a single syringe, it is recommended that the unsheathed needle be placed on a sterile field between injections without recapping.

6. Instruments that normally penetrate soft tissues or bone (*e.g.,* forceps, scalpels, bone chisels, files, sur-

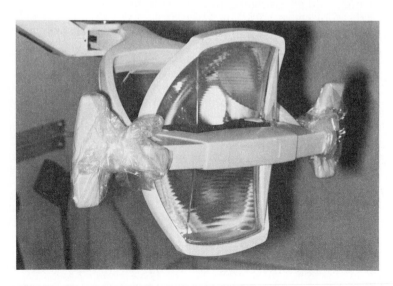

Figure 31C–1. Dental light with easily applied and easily removed clear plastic bags on handles.

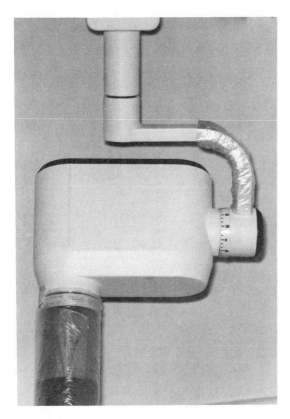

Figure 31C–2. X-ray head with clear plastic wrap applied to areas handled by dental personnel.

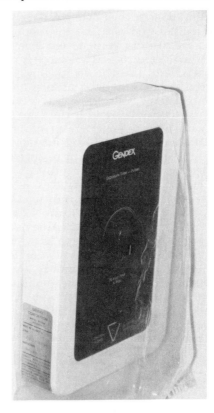

Figure 31C–3. X-ray unit control panel sheathed in easily removable clear plastic wrap.

gical burs) should be sterilized after each use. Instruments that come into contact with oral tissues but do not penetrate bone or soft tissues (*e.g.,* amalgam condensers, plastic instruments and burs) should be sterilized after each use if possible; otherwise they should receive high-level disinfection.

7. Before high-level disinfection or sterilization, instruments should be cleaned to remove debris with a thorough scrubbing with soap and water or a detergent or with a mechanical device (*e.g.,* ultrasonic cleaner). Persons involved in cleaning or disinfecting instruments should wear heavy-duty rubber gloves to prevent hand injuries.

(*Sterilization*—Metal and heat stable dental instruments should be routinely sterilized between uses by autoclaving, dry heat, or chemical vapor. The adequacy of sterilization should be verified by the periodic use (weekly for most dental practices) of spore-testing devices. Heat and steam-sensitive chemical indicators may be used on the outside of each pack to ensure that it has been exposed to a sterilizing cycle.

Heat-sensitive instruments may require up to 10 hours' exposure in a liquid chemical agent registered by the U.S. Environmental Protection Agency (EPA) as a disinfectant/sterilant. This should be followed by rinsing with sterile water.

High-level disinfection may be achieved by immersing the instrument in boiling water for at least 10 minutes or in an EPA-registered disinfectant/sterilant chemical for the exposure time recommended by the chemical's manufacturer.)

8. Environmental surfaces such as countertops that have been contaminated with blood or saliva should be wiped with absorbent toweling and then disinfected with a suitable germicide such as 5,000 ppm sodium hypochlorite (a 1:10 dilution of household bleach).

9. Laboratory supplies and materials, such as impressions and bite registrations, should be thoroughly cleaned of blood and saliva and disinfected before being handled, adjusted, or sent to a dental laboratory. The same processes should be repeated when the materials are returned from the laboratory and before they are placed in the patient's mouth. Because of the ever-increasing variety of dental materials, dental personnel are advised to consult with manufacturers about the stability of specific materials relative to disinfection procedures. A chemical germicide that is registered with the EPA as a "hospital disinfectant" and that has a label claim for mycobactericidal activity is preferred.

10. Care of nonsterilizable equipment: Handpieces, ultrasonic scalers, and air or water syringes that cannot be sterilized or receive high-level disinfection should

be treated in the following manner to reduce the risk of disease transmission. After use, the handpiece should be flushed for 20 to 30 seconds and then thoroughly scrubbed with a detergent and water to remove adherent material. It should then be thoroughly washed and wiped with absorbent material saturated with a chemical germicide registered with the EPA as a "hospital disinfectant" and mycobactericidal. The solution must remain in contact with the handpiece for the time specified by the disinfectant's manufacturer. After the disinfection process, the disinfectant should be removed by rinsing with sterile water.

12. Because water retraction valves within the dental units may aspirate infective materials back into the handpiece and water line, check valves should be installed with the dental units to reduce the risk of transfer of infected matter. It is prudent to allow water to be discharged from the unit for 20 to 30 seconds at the end of its use on each patient. This process should be repeated for several minutes at the beginning of each day to flush out bacteria that may have accumulated overnight. Sterile saline or water should be used as a coolant/irrigator when performing surgical procedures involving the cutting of soft tissue or bone with a handpiece.

REFERENCES

1. Centers for Disease Control: Possible transmission of human immunodeficiency virus to a patient during an invasive dental procedure. MMWR 39:489, 1990
2. Centers for Disease Control: Update: Transmission of HIV infection during an invasive dental procedure—Florida. MMWR 40:21, 1991
3. Ahtone J, Goodman RA: Hepatitis B and dental personnel: Transmission to patients and prevention issues. J Am Dent Assoc 106:219, 1983
4. Shaw FE, Barrett CL, Hamm R et al: Lethal outbreak of hepatitis B in a dental practice. JAMA 255:3260, 1986
5. McCann D: Two more Acer patients test HIV-positive. ADA News 22(12):1, 1991
6. Klein RS, Phelan JA, Freeman K et al: Low occupational risk of human immunodeficiency virus infection among dental professionals. N Engl J Med 318:86, 1988
7. Ho DD, Byington RE, Schooley RT et al: Infrequency of isolation of HTLV-III virus from saliva in AIDS. N Engl J Med 313:1606, 1985
8. Levy JA, Greenspan D: HIV in saliva. Lancet 2:1248, 1988
9. Jenison SA, Lemon SM, Baker LN, Newbold JE: Quantitative analysis of hepatitis B virus DNA in saliva and semen of chronically infected homosexual men. J Infect Dis 156:299, 1987
10. O'Shea S, Cordery M, Barrett WY et al: HIV excretion patterns and specific antibody responses in body fluids. J Med Virol 31:291, 1990
11. Goto Y, Yeh C-K, Notkins AL et al: Detection of proviral sequences in saliva of patients infected with human immunodeficiency virus type 1. AIDS Res Human Retroviruses 7:343, 1991
12. Piazza M, Chirianni A, Picciotto L et al: Passionate kissing and microlesions of the oral mucosa: Possible role in AIDS transmission. JAMA 261:244, 1989
13. Fultz PN, McClure HM, Daugharty H et al: Vaginal transmission of human immunodeficiency virus (HIV) to a chimpanzee. J Infect Dis 154:896, 1986
14. Fultz PN: Components of saliva inactivate human immunodeficiency virus. Lancet 2:1215, 1986
15. Fox PC, Wolff A, Yeh C-K et al: Saliva inhibits HIV-1 infectivity. J Am Dent Assoc 116:635, 1988
16. Fox PC, Wolff A, Yeh C-K et al: Salivary inhibition of HIV-1 infectivity: Functional properties and distribution in men, women and children. J Am Dent Assoc 118:709, 1989
17. Archibald DW, Cole GA: In vitro inhibition of HIV-1 infectivity by human salivas. AIDS Res Hum Retroviruses 6:1425, 1990
18. Archibald DW, Zon L, Groopman JE et al: Antibodies to human T-lymphotropic virus type III (HTLV-III) in saliva of acquired immunodeficiency syndrome (AIDS) patients and in persons at risk for AIDS. Blood 67:831, 1986
19. Becker J, Ulrich P, Kunze R et al: Immunohistochemical detection of HIV structural proteins and distribution of T-lymphocytes and Langerhans cells in the oral mucosa of HIV infected patients. Virchows Archiv [A] Pathol Anat 412:413, 1988
20. Smith SK, Lewis G, Archibald D: Immunohistochemical detection of HIV-1 antigens in oropharyngeal tissues. J Dent Res 70:436, 1991
21. Glick M, Trope M, Pliskin ME: Detection of HIV in the dental pulp of a patient with AIDS. J Am Dent Assoc 119:649, 1989
22. Centers for Disease Control: Recommendations for preventing transmission of infection with human T-lymphotropic virus type III/lymphadenopathy-associated virus during invasive procedures. MMWR 35:221, 1986
23. Centers for Disease Control: Recommended infection control practices for dentistry. MMWR 35:237, 1986
24. Centers for Disease Control: Recommendations for prevention of HIV transmission in health-care settings. MMWR 36:3S, 1987

Special Considerations for Emergency Personnel

31D

Gabor D. Kelen

EPIDEMIOLOGY OF HIV-1 AS IT RELATES TO EMERGENCY MEDICINE

In the United States alone there are more than 500,000 allied emergency personnel: physicians, nurses, prehospital care providers (not including ancillary staff, fire fighters, or police).[1] Emergency medicine is a procedure- and intervention-oriented specialty. Its very nature implies frequent patient contact and potential exposure to blood and body fluids in uncontrolled or poorly controlled circumstances. By most estimates, approximately 1 million residents of the United States are infected with human immunodeficiency virus type 1 (HIV-1),[2] and a large proportion are unaware of their infection. Because there are 90 million emergency department patient visits a year in the United States,[1] with approximately 10% of these involving prehospital care providers, the potential for exposure of emergency personnel to HIV-1 is considerable.

The implications of the acquired immunodeficiency syndrome (AIDS) epidemic were not well appreciated by emergency personnel until spring 1987, when much publicity was given to two reports. The first was a report by the Centers for Disease Control (CDC) describing the first known cases of occupational transmission of HIV-1 following nonparenteral exposures.[3] One of those transmissions occurred during a resuscitation attempt in an emergency department setting. Two weeks later a publication from the Johns Hopkins emergency department revealed that six (3.0%) of 203 critically ill and injured patients had unsuspected HIV-1 infection.[4] All six patients had been transported by ambulance and required procedures in the prehospital setting; all six were bleeding on arrival in the emergency department and required invasive procedures. Thus, with these two reports, the potential impact of the AIDS epidemic for emergency personnel began to be widely appreciated.

Despite the heightened awareness of HIV-1 among emergency personnel following those two reports, many practitioners interpreted the emergency department–based study as implying that the potential for occupational exposure to HIV-1 was restricted to contact with a narrowly defined cohort of patients. All six HIV-1 seropositive patients in that study were young black men between the ages of 25 and 34 years who presented with trauma; five of the six had sustained penetrating trauma.[4] It was our observation that many emergency personnel took precautions only when dealing with such patients.

Although it was realized that occult HIV-1 infection among patients was not likely to be so confined, subsequent emergency department–based studies were aimed at determining whether it was possible to identify patients with unrecognized HIV-1 infection based on ascertainable features in the clinical setting. It was thought that such identification would aid practitioners in determining under what selective circumstances precautions were necessary.

A large follow-up serosurvey conducted at Johns Hopkins in 1987 revealed that 119 (5.2%) of 2,302 general emergency department patients were HIV-1 seropositive. Seventy-seven percent of those seropositive, or 4% of the general emergency department population, were unaware of their infection.[5] The restricted associations with HIV-1 infection seen in the first study did not hold. Although occult HIV-1 infection predominated among young black men in the follow-up study also, HIV-1 infection was widely distributed across all races, both sexes, and a wide age range. Further, unlike the situation delineated in the initial study, HIV-1 infection was not limited to patients with certain clinical conditions but was present in significant proportions (2.8% to 16.7%) in patients in all categories of presenting problems. A third general emergency department serosurvey conducted in 1988 at Johns Hopkins demonstrated that even rigorous risk factor assessment in the emergency department failed to identify 27% of those with unrecognized HIV-1 infection.[6] The data from these latter two studies imply that patients harboring HIV-1 infection cannot be readily identified in an emergency department setting from ascertainable variables such as demographics, clinical condition, and even risk factor assessment. That patients with HIV-1 infection are not readily identified is a finding common to all emergency department–based HIV-1 serosurveys.[7-12]

Although the Johns Hopkins emergency department population is the best-defined study population, a few emergency department or trauma center serosurveys have been reported from other parts of the country (Table 31D–1). Investigators at Henry Ford Hospital recently presented data showing a 4.7% rate of HIV-1 infection in 1988 among critically ill and injured patients arriving in their emergency department.[7] Zeman and Mayhue reported a 0.38% seroprevalence in 1987 among trauma patients from a hospital that serves as the regional trauma center in Peoria, Illinois.[8] Zalut and associates reported 7.15% and 0.4% seroprevalence rates in 1988 from Chicago inner-city and suburban hospital emergency departments, respectively.[9] A CDC cooperative multicenter study undertaken in 1989 revealed HIV-1 seroprevalence rates of 4.2% to 8.9% in three northeastern United States hospital-based inner-city emer-

Table 31D–1. Hospital Emergency Department (ED)–Based HIV-1 Serosurveys

Location	*Facility*	*Patient Population*	*Year*	*Seroprevalence*	*Reference*
Baltimore	Inner city	Critically ill and injured	1986	3.0%	Baker *et al*[4]
Baltimore	Inner city	General ED patients	1987	5.2%	Kelen *et al*[5]
Peoria	Urban	ED trauma	1987	0.38%	Zeman and Mayhue[8]
Baltimore	Inner city trauma center	Trauma patients	1987–88	1.1%–6.0%	Soderstrom *et al*[12]
Baltimore	Inner city	General ED patients	1988	6.0%	Kelen *et al*[6]
Detroit	Inner city	Critically ill and injured	1988	4.7%	Lewandowski *et al*[7]
Chicago	Inner city	General ED patients	1988	7.15%	Zalut *et al*[9]
	Suburban	General ED patients	1988	0.4%	Zalut *et al*[9]
Northeastern cities (three)	Inner city	General ED patients	1989	4.2%–8.9%	Marcus *et al*[10]
	Suburban	General ED patients	1989	0.4%–6.4%	Marcus *et al*[10]
Minneapolis	City	General ED patients	1989	1.32%	Strum[11]

gency departments and 0.4% to 6.4% among corresponding suburban hospital emergency departments in the same cities.[10] In another 1989 serosurvey, Strum reported a 1.32% seroprevalence rate among emergency department patients seen at a Minneapolis hospital.[11] Soderstrom and associates reported an HIV-1 seroprevalence rate among trauma victims predominantly transported from rural areas to a Baltimore trauma center to be 1.67%, with significantly higher rates among assault victims (5.99%) and those who lived in the city (3.81%).[12] Although these studies do not provide a comprehensive description of seroprevalence rates among emergency department patients in the United States, they do indicate that HIV-1 seroprevalence among emergency department patients is highest in inner cities, but not negligible in suburban centers and locations within the country that have not to date been associated with the HIV-1 epidemic.

Regardless of the specific HIV-1 infection rates among emergency departments patients today, emergency departments will experience increasing visits by patients with known and occult HIV-1 infection. The number of AIDS cases is expected to increase fourfold to fivefold by 1992 from the time these studies were undertaken.[13] The 3.0% seroprevalence rate among critically ill and injured patients in the initial Johns Hopkins Hospital emergency department study, conducted in 1986,[4] rose to 7.8% 1 year later.[14] Among the general patient population in that department, the rate rose from 5.2% in 1987[5] to 6.0% in 1988[6] to 8.9% in 1989.[10] The increase in emergency department visits by symptomatic HIV-1-infected patients is increasing in dramatic proportions in our institution. Whereas in 1988 there were one or two such patient visits per day,[15] by mid-1991 there were several (two to five) such patients present in the emergency department during any given 8-hour shift (Kelen, unpubl. observ.).

Currently, emergency practitioners in suburban and nonendemic areas may be the most complacent regarding the risk of occupational transmission of blood-borne infections. However, some cases of occupational transmission have occurred in settings with HIV-1 infection

rates as low as 2.5 per 1,000.[16] Also, the continued increase in emergency department visits by HIV-infected patients will not be restricted to inner-city facilities in AIDS-endemic areas. In recent years, new AIDS cases have been decreasingly concentrated in regions of the country previously recognized for a high prevalence of AIDS.[17]

POTENTIAL OCCUPATIONAL MODES OF OCCUPATIONAL TRANSMISSION

HIV-1 has now been isolated from blood,[18] serum,[19] semen,[20] vaginal secretions,[21] saliva,[22] breast milk,[23] tears,[24] urine,[25] CSF,[26] synovial fluid,[27] amniotic fluid,[28] alveolar fluid,[29] bone marrow,[30] and brain.[30] However, transmission has been documented only from blood and blood products,[31] semen[32] and vaginal secretions,[31] *in utero* and possibly from breast milk or breast-feeding,[33] and from transplanted tissue and organs.[34–36] Although one early report suggested possible transmission from saliva,[37] current evidence indicates that this is a highly unlikely mode of transmission, and no documented cases have been forthcoming. It is clear that casual contact is not a mode of transmission,[38] and thus it should not be a concern for medical practitioners.

Most occupational transmissions of HIV-1 are from needlestick injuries or other mishaps with sharp instruments. Initially it was thought that infiltration or injection of infected blood was necessary to transmit the virus.[39,40] However, there have been cases of superficial needlestick injuries[41,42] and nonparenteral exposures[2,43] that have resulted in nosocomial transmission. One of the more recent cases of occupational transmission occurred in a laboratory worker who worked with concentrated virus but had no known percutaneous, direct skin or mucous membrane exposures.[44] Although there were minor breaks in compliance with Biosafety Level 3 precautions, he routinely wore gloves and gown. Whether or not appropriate precautions were taken, the case illustrates that it is possible to become infected with HIV-1 without realizing that an exposure has taken place—a situation of certain concern for emergency practitioners.

Blood has been the predominant infectious medium in occupational transmission. There is at least one case reported in which another body fluid was involved—needlestick injury following pleurocentesis—but even this transmission medium was described as having been bloody.[42]

ASSESSMENT OF RISKS TO EMERGENCY HEALTH CARE WORKERS

The risk of occupational transmission of HIV-1 can be assessed from data that fall into three categories: data on health care workers with AIDS,[45] estimates from surveillance studies,[46-52] and case reports.[3,16,39-44,47,48,52-56] These are covered in detail elsewhere in this volume. The modes of transmission of HIV-1 are similar to those for hepatitis B virus (HBV). Emergency department personnel have been shown to have among the highest rates of occupational exposures to HBV.[57,58]

At the time of this writing, the CDC has reported 40 cases of occupationally acquired HIV-1 in health care providers in the United States.[59] Of these, 24 are documented by seroconversion. The remaining 16 occurred under significantly compelling circumstances that even though documentation of seroconversion was not possible, alternative explanations are not readily apparent. Most of these 40 cases are associated with percutaneous exposure with contaminated sharp instruments. Some of the occupational transmissions occurred during emergencies or procedures commonly performed in emergency departments.[3,40,46]

The risk of occupational transmission of HIV-1 following percutaneous exposure from a blood-contaminated sharp instrument is generally accepted to be approximately 0.35% (95% CI: 0.12–0.84; Poisson distribution).[60] This figure is derived from meta-analysis of several surveillance studies. To date, only six of the reported cases of occupationally related seroconversions in the United States have been uncovered in surveillance studies.[46,47,48,52]

The numbers of health care providers with occupationally acquired HIV-1 infection are surely underestimated. A recent study by Tandberg and associates revealed significant underreporting of needlestick injuries in a cohort of emergency department providers in the greater Albuquerque area.[61] Emergency department physicians in this group reported less than one eighth of their needlesticks, whereas nurses and prehospital providers reported two thirds of such exposures. Skin contacts are probably underreported to an even greater extent. If this behavior is prevalent, it could be a major problem for emergency providers, as all emergency department studies to date demonstrate that the vast majority of HIV-infected patients are those whose infection remains undiagnosed.[4-7,10,14,62]

Exposures

Some 80% to 90% of the documented nosocomial transmissions occurred through needlesticks or sharp instruments.[31] Forty percent of injuries with sharp instruments are considered preventable, and many are due to inferior device design.[63] Many of these exposures occur during recapping of needles. A large proportion of needlestick injuries and exposures are related to disposal of sharp objects and instruments, while only a few occur during actual patient management.[63-65] There are data to indicate that new workers are at the greatest risk of sustaining sharp instrument injuries.[65]

Little information is available regarding exposures during emergency procedures or patient care. An early Johns Hopkins emergency department study reported circumstances under which potential exposure to unanticipated HIV-1 infection may occur, and associated patient seroprevalence rates (Table 31D–2).[5] In a later study, Johns Hopkins researchers reported 32 instances of unprotected emergency health care provider exposures to blood and 16 instances of unprotected exposures to other body fluids during a 6-week, 'round-the-clock direct observational study.[6] Precautions taken were not generally assessed. However, an investigation in the same emergency department conducted at the same time assessed providers' compliance with universal precautions during the care of critically ill or injured patients. Overall, glove use rate was 64% to 85% in situations where skin exposure to blood was a possibility.[66] In the CDC multicenter emergency department study, observers noted a 4% aggregate rate of blood exposures,

Table 31D–2. Exposure of Health Care Workers to Unrecognized HIV in 2,275 Emergency Department Patients With Unknown HIV Status

Exposure	Seropositivity Rate No. (%) Seropositive
Patients bleeding on arrival	268 (6.0)
Exposure to patients' body fluids	1892 (4.3)
Performance of major emergency invasive procedure*	99 (5.0)
Placement of intravenous lines before arrival at hospital	239 (3.8)
Patients with altered level of consciousness at presentation	291 (5.8)
Patients admitted to hospital	854 (4.1)
Patients admitted to operating suite directly from emergency room	65 (4.6)

* Central line placement, venous cutdown, thoracotomy, thoracostomy tube placement, intubation, transvenous or transthoracic pacing, or pericardiocentesis.
Reproduced with permission from Kelen GD et al: Unrecognized human immunodeficiency virus infection in emergency department patients. N Engl J Med 318:1645, 1988.

of which 98% were skin contacts.[46] Exposure during arterial blood sampling was 20 times higher during ungloved procedures as during gloved procedures, demonstrating the efficacy of using gloves for such procedures.

One study examined the epidemiology of needlesticks among prehospital emergency personnel, drawing their sample from the St. Louis (Missouri) EMS system.[65] That study found an incidence of 145 injuries per 1,000 employee-years, with most injuries (43%) reported by personnel who had been employed for less than a year.

UNIVERSAL PRECAUTIONS APPLIED TO EMERGENCY MEDICINE

In 1983 the CDC recommended that precautions be taken with patients with known or suspected infection with blood-borne pathogens.[67] Two years later the CDC advanced the concept of universal precautions,[68] according to which "all patients should be assumed to be infectious for HIV-1 and other blood-borne pathogens." In 1987, a few months following the CDC's report of seroconversion in three health care workers with non-parenteral exposures to HIV-1 and the appearance of Johns Hopkins emergency department seroprevalence data, the CDC consolidated its universal precautions recommendations.[55] More recently, recommendations that included situations specific to prehospital care workers and public-safety workers (fire fighters, law enforcement officers, correctional facility workers) have been made.[45]

Although initially the CDC recommended that all patients' bodily fluids be considered infectious,[68] a recent revision recommends that only potential contact with blood and certain fluids need be of concern.[69] Precautions are recommended for personnel who might come in contact with bodily fluids from which HIV-1 or HBV transmission could occur. These fluids include blood, amniotic fluid, pericardial fluid, peritoneal fluid, synovial fluid, cerebrospinal fluid, semen, and vaginal secretions, or any bodily fluid visibly contaminated with blood. Occupational transmission of HIV-1 has been documented from blood,[3,16,39–41,43,47,48,52–56] bloody pleural fluid,[42] and concentrated virus,[44] while semen

and vaginal secretions have been implicated in the sexual transmission of HIV-1 but not in nosocomial transmission. HBsAg has been detected in synovial fluid,[70] amniotic fluid,[71] and peritoneal fluid.[72] Other bodily fluids (feces, nasal secretions, sputum, sweat, tears, urine, vomitus, breast milk, saliva) are not considered infectious because of lack of epidemiologic evidence of transmission, even though HIV-1 has been isolated from some of these fluids.[22,24,25] Saliva is considered a potentially infectious medium for dentists, owing to frequent contamination with blood.[45] Although not specifically stated, this caveat should also hold for emergency practitioners, because oral conditions and procedures frequently involve blood.

There are two potential limitations to following infection control recommendations in a discriminatory manner in the emergency setting. One is of general concern and the other is specific to emergency practice. First, documentation of transmission from bodily fluid exposures is difficult at best, and in our experience such exposures are even less likely to be reported[61] and may even go unrecalled. Thus, it may be too early to conclude that certain bodily fluids are not infectious. Second, emergency practitioners cannot always know in advance if bodily fluids will be tainted with visible blood. In recognition of this point, the CDC issued a specific caveat advocating following universal precautions "under uncontrolled emergency circumstances," during which all bodily fluids should be treated as potentially infectious.[45] In the prehospital or emergency department setting, few circumstances involving major procedures can be considered controlled. In patients with serious illness or injury, a relatively benign situation can instantaneously change to an uncontrolled situation in which the patient either begins to bleed profusely or requires immediate intervention in the form of major procedures. Thus, emergency providers frequently cannot anticipate exposure to body fluids or blood.

Accordingly, based on the CDC guidelines, we have made the following recommendations regarding barrier precautions in emergency settings (Table 31D–3).[66] The recommendations are based on the reasonable possibility of the procedure or intervention resulting in exposure to blood or blood-tinged bodily fluids, or on the degree of active bleeding by the patient from injuries

Table 31D–3. Precautions Expected Under Given Circumstances

	Clinical Situation				
Intervention*	No Bleeding	Active Bleeding	Profuse Bleeding	Major Trauma	Resuscitation
Examination	—	Gloves	All†	All	All
Minor	Gloves	Gloves	All	All	All
Major	All	All	All	All	All

* See text for definitions.
† All = gloves, gown, mask, and eye protection.

or from iatrogenically induced bleeding from previous procedures. Procedures have been classified as examination, minor, or major on the basis of potential extent of exposure as a result of the procedure itself (Table 31D–4).[66] Thus, major procedures are so designated not because of inherent invasiveness but rather because of the reasonable possibility that they will generate profuse bleeding, spray, or aerosolization of blood or bloody bodily fluids. For example, placing a nasogastric tube is not considered a major procedure. However, practitioners of emergency medicine will easily recall many instances in which the procedure induced nasal bleeding along with severe coughing and sneezing, resulting in the wide spray of blood. All major trauma cases, patients critically ill, and all resuscitations by definition are opportunities for significant exposure to blood, and thus maximum barrier precautions should be followed regardless of what intervention or procedure is contemplated.

Unfortunately, even as the risks in emergency settings become better defined and recognized, initial assessments of compliance with universal precautions (particularly barrier precautions) have not been encouraging. In one northeastern inner-city emergency department–based study in which universal precautions were strictly applied, appropriate (barrier) precautions were followed only 44% of the time during management of patients with critical illness or injury.[66] The rate of compliance was only 19% for interactions with profusely bleeding patients, and only 16% during the performance of major procedures. Other studies applying less stringent criteria have reported even lower rates of compliance. Hammond *et al* found that surgical residents at the University of Miami/Jackson Memorial Medical Center were in compliance with strict universal precautions only 16% of the time during trauma resuscitations.[73] Baraff and Talan at the University of California–Los Angeles Medical Center emergency department[74,75] and Campbell and associates at the St. Paul–Ramsey Medical Center emergency department in Minneapolis[76] found similar lack of compliance. A survey of emergency medicine residencies revealed that barrier attire was available in 82% of responding programs but was consistently used in only 16%.[77] Reasons for failure to comply have been sought. Emergency care providers have indicated that barrier protection is time-consuming to put on and interferes with the skillful performance of procedures.[66,73] Others have indicated lack of familiarity with protocols.[73]

Only two studies have been reported to date that

Table 31D–4. Classification of Interventions for Appropriate Barrier Attire

Examination	*Minor*	*Major*
Physical examination	Phlebotomy	Arterial canalization
Pelvic examination*	Venous cannulation	Central venous catheter placement
Splinting	Arterial sampling	Swan-Ganz catheter placement
Casting	IM injection	Cricothyroidotomy
Fracture/dislocation reduction	Foley catheter placement	Culdocentesis
Ocular tonometry	Local anesthesia	Nasogastric tube placement
Electrocardiogram lead placement	Nerve blocks	Endotracheal suctioning
Spinal immobilization	Arthrocentesis	Tracheal intubation (oral or nasal)
CPR†	Lumbar puncture	Foreign body removal
Cardioversion‡	Thoracentesis	Gastric lavage
Defibrillation§	Pericardiocentesis	Incision and draining‖
External cardiac pacing	Paracentesis	Nasal packing
Patient extrication	Intraosseous catheter placement	Peritoneal lavage
		Internal temporary cardiac pacing (transthoracic/transvenous)
		Wound repair¶
		Wound irrigation
		Cutdown
		Sigmoidoscopy
		Precipitous vaginal delivery
		Thoracostomy
		Thoracotomy

* If patient complains of bleeding or if bleeding could possibly be encountered, all precautions should be taken.
† CPR is categorized as an exam, but since it always implies a resuscitation effort, risk of blood exposure from other providers activities or a bleeding patient is considerable. Therefore all precautions are required.
‡ Cardioversion of itself is a benign procedure. However, a reasonable expectation under emergency conditions is that it may fail, requiring a resuscitation effort. Therefore, all precautions would be prudent.
§ Implies a resuscitation effort.
‖ Requires irrigation.
¶ Requires high-pressure irrigation, resulting in spray.

have evaluated methods to improve compliance with barrier precautions in an emergency setting. A recent study from a university teaching hospital that has an HIV-1 seroprevalence rate of approximately 1% found that intensive educational efforts were associated with only moderate or insignificant increases in compliance.[75] Researchers at Johns Hopkins Hospital reported a substantial increase in compliance with universal precautions among emergency department staff following implementation of a policy with a monitoring component.[78] Overall compliance improved from 44% to 73%, with rates of compliance reaching 80% for personnel under the emergency department's control. The type and implementation of policy that drove the improvement are similar to the expected elements in the final regulations to be issued by OSHA.[79]

Adherence to barrier universal precautions is not inexpensive,[80] and it is legitimate to question its effectiveness *vis-à-vis* costs.[81] This is especially true insofar as much of the cost is for disposable items that protect only against nonparenteral exposures. However, the greater problem is from needlestick exposures. The value of barrier protection beyond wearing gloves may prove minimal.

On the other hand, the greatest portion of the cost entailed by adequate barrier protection is for gloves.[80] Also, HIV-1 is just one of the important transmissible infections that providers confront in the workplace. Other agents such as hepatitis B and C viruses, HTLV and other retroviruses, Epstein-Barr virus, cytomègalovirus, and perhaps others are just as important, and in some cases (*e.g.,* HBV) easier to transmit.[45] (In fact, HBV vaccine is considered an important adjunct to universal precautions).[69,82] Johns Hopkins researchers reported that in 1988, almost 25% of the general emergency department patient population were infected with either HIV-1, HBsAg, or HCV.[83] A general dictum followed in emergency practice is to assume the worst until proven otherwise, and proceed from there. In a similar vein, it would seem prudent to strictly observe all aspects of universal precautions, including barrier protection, until they are demonstrated to be of low utility.

Emergency providers with possible exposure to HIV-1 should follow the guidelines set forth by the CDC[45] and local institutional policy. Management of postexposure HBV infection should be undertaken independently.[84]

In summary, the impact of the AIDS epidemic for emergency personnel will continue to grow and will not be restricted to large urban centers. Accordingly, the potential risk of occupational acquisition of HIV-1 will grow. Even though the risk of seroconversion following parenteral exposure to HIV-1 is probably less than 1%, as the seroprevalence of HIV-1 in patient populations increases, the number of exposures will likely increase. Currently, the best protection against HIV-1 and other blood-borne pathogens is to observe universal precautions. However, industry must address the problems inherent in current barrier technology and device design.

REFERENCES

1. American Hospital Association: Hospital Statistics. Chicago, American Hospital Association, 1990
2. Centers for Disease Control: HIV prevalence estimates and AIDS case projections for the United States: Report based on a workshop. MMWR 39(RR-16):5, 1990
3. Centers for Disease Control: Update: Human immunodeficiency virus infections in health-care workers exposed to blood of infected patients. MMWR 36:285, 1987
4. Baker JL, Kelen GD, Sivertson KT, Quinn TC: Unsuspected human immunodeficiency virus in critically ill emergency patients. JAMA 257:2609, 1987
5. Kelen GD, Fritz S, Qaqish B et al: Unrecognized human immunodeficiency virus infection in emergency department patients. N Engl J Med 318:1645, 1988
6. Kelen GD, DiGiovanna T, Bisson L et al: Human immunodeficiency virus infection in emergency patients: Epidemiology, clinical presentations, and risk to health care workers. The Johns Hopkins experience. JAMA 262:516, 1989
7. Lewandowski D, Ognjan A, Rivers E et al: HIV-1 and HTLV-1 seroprevalence in critically ill resuscitated emergency department patients (abstr Th.A.P.9.142). Presented at the Vth International Conference on AIDS, Montreal, 1989
8. Zeman MG, Mayhue FE: Occupational risk of HIV infection (letter). Ann Emerg Med 18:798, 1989
9. Zalut T, Cooper MA, Wainstein J et al: Prevalence of HIV-positive patients in multiple emergency department settings (abstr). Ann Emerg Med 19:611, 1990
10. Marcus R, Bell DM, Culver DH, Cooperative Emergency Department Study Group: Frequency of emergency care providers' contact with blood of patients infected with human immunodeficiency virus (abstr). Ann Emerg Med 19:454, 1990
11. Strum JT: HIV prevalence in a midwestern emergency department. Ann Emerg Med 20:272, 1991
12. Soderstrom CA, Furth PA, Glasser D et al: HIV infection rates in a trauma center treating predominantly rural blunt trauma victims. J Trauma 29:1526, 1989
13. Centers for Disease Control: Quarterly report to the Domestic Policy Council on the prevalence and rate of spread of HIV and AIDS—United States. MMWR 37:551, 1988
14. Kelen GD, Fritz S, Qaqish B et al: Substantial increase in human immunodeficiency virus (HIV-1) infection in critically ill emergency patients: 1986–87 compared. Ann Emerg Med 18:378, 1989
15. Kelen GD, Johnson G, DiGiovanna TA et al: Profile of patients with human immunodeficiency virus infection presenting to an inner-city emergency department. Ann Emerg Med 19:963, 1990
16. Wallace MR, Harrison WO: HIV seroconversion with progressive disease in health care worker after needlestick injury. Lancet 1:1454, 1988
17. Centers for Disease Control: AIDS and human immunodeficiency virus infection in the United States: 1988 update. MMWR 38:S-4, 1989
18. Gallo RC, Salahuddin SZ, Popovic M et al: Frequent detection and isolation of cytopathic retroviruses (HTLV-III) for patients with AIDS and at risk for AIDS. Science 224:500, 1984

19. Michaelis B, Levy JA: Recovery of human immunodeficiency virus from serum. JAMA 257:1327, 1987

20. Levy JA, Hoffman AD, Kramer SM et al: Isolation of lymphocytopathic retroviruses from San Francisco patients with AIDS. Science 226:449, 1984

21. Vogt MW, Witt DJ, Craven DE et al: Isolation of HTLV-III/LAV from cervical secretions of women at risk for AIDS. Lancet 1:525, 1986

22. Groopman JE, Salahuddin SZ, Sarngadharan MG et al: HTLV-III in saliva of people with AIDS-related complex and healthy homosexual men at risk for AIDS. Science 226:447, 1984

23. Thiry L, Sprecher-Goldberger S, Jonckheer T et al: Isolation of AIDS virus from cell-free breast milk of three healthy virus carriers (letter). Lancet 2:981, 1985

24. Fujikawa LS, Salahuddin SZ, Palestine AG et al: Isolation of human T-lymphotropic virus type III from the tears of a patient with the acquired immunodeficiency syndrome. Lancet 2:529, 1985

25. Levy JA, Kaminski LS, Morrow WJW et al: Infection by the retrovirus associated with the acquired immunodeficiency syndrome. Ann Intern Med 103:694, 1985

26. Levy JA, Shimabukuro J, Hollander H et al: Isolation of AIDS-associated retroviruses from cerebrospinal fluid and brain of patients with neurological symptoms. Lancet 2:586, 1986

27. Withrington RH, Cornes P, Harris JRW et al: Isolation of human immunodeficiency virus from synovial fluid of a patient with reactive arthritis. Br Med J 294:484, 1987

28. Mundy DC, Schinazi RF, Gerber AR et al: Human immunodeficiency virus isolated from amniotic fluid. Lancet 2:459, 1987

29. Ziza J-M, Brun-Vezinet F, Venet A et al: Lymphadenopathy-associated virus isolated from bronchoalveolar lavage fluid in AIDS-related complex with lymphoid interstitial pneumonitis. N Engl J Med 313:183, 1985

30. Salahuddin SZ, Markham PD, Popovic M et al: Isolation of infectious human T-cell leukemia/lymphotropic virus type III (HTLV-III) from patients with acquired immunodeficiency syndrome (AIDS) or AIDS-related complex (ARC) and from health carriers: A study of risk groups and tissue sources. Proc Natl Acad Sci USA 82:5530, 1985

31. Centers for Disease Control: Update: Acquired immunodeficiency syndrome and human immunodeficiency virus infection among health care workers. MMWR 37:229, 1988

32. Stewart GJ, Tyler JPP, Cunningham AL et al: Transmission of human T-cell lymphotropic virus type III (HTLV-III) by artificial insemination by donor. Lancet 2:581, 1985

33. Ziegler JB, Cooper DA, Johnson RD, Gold J: Postnatal transmission of AIDS-associated retrovirus from mother to infant. Lancet 1:896, 1985

34. Centers for Disease Control: Transmission of HIV through bone transplantation: Case report and public health recommendations. MMWR 37:597, 1988

35. Centers for Disease Control: Human immunodeficiency virus infection transmitted from an organ donor screened for HIV antibody—North Carolina. MMWR 36:306, 1987

36. Quarto M, Germinario C, Fontana A, Barbuti S: HIV transmission through kidney transplantation from a living related donor. N Engl J Med 320:1754, 1989

37. Salahuddin SZ, Groopman JE, Markham PD et al: HTLV-III in symptom-free seronegative persons. Lancet 2:1418, 1984

38. Friedland GH, Saltzman BR, Rogers MF et al: Lack of transmission of HTLV-III/LAV infection to household contacts of patients with AIDS or AIDS-related complex with oral candidiasis. N Engl J Med 314:344, 1986

39. N.A.: Needlestick transmission of HTLV-III from a patient infected in Africa. Lancet 2:1376, 1984

40. Stricof RL, Morse DL: HTLV-III/LAV seroconversion following a deep intramuscular needlestick injury (letter). N Engl J Med 314;1115, 1986

41. Neisson-Vernant C, Arfi S, Mathez D et al: Needlestick HIV seroconversion in a nurse (letter). Lancet 2:814, 1986

42. Oksenhendler E, Harzic M, Le Roux JM et al: HIV infection with seroconversion after a superficial needlestick injury to the finger (letter). N Engl J Med 315:582, 1986

43. Gioannini P, Sinicco A, Cariti G et al: HIV infection acquired by a nurse. Eur J Epidemiol 4:119, 1988

44. Weiss SH, Goedert JJ, Gartner S et al: Risk of human immunodeficiency virus infection among laboratory workers. Science 239:68, 1988

45. Centers for Disease Control: Guidelines for prevention of transmission of human immunodeficiency virus and hepatitis B virus to health-care and public-safety workers. MMWR 38:S-6, 1989

46. Marcus R, CDC Cooperative Needlestick Surveillance Group: Surveillance of health care workers exposed to blood from patients infected with the human immunodeficiency virus. N Engl J Med 319:1118, 1988

47. Gerberding JL, Bryant-Leblanc CE, Nelson K et al: Risk of transmitting the human immunodeficiency virus, cytomegalovirus, and hepatitis B virus to health care workers exposed to patients with AIDS and AIDS-related conditions. J Infect Dis 156:1, 1987

48. Henderson DK, Fahey BJ, Saah AJ et al: Longitudinal assessment of risk for occupational/nosocomial transmission of human immunodeficiency virus, type 1 in health care workers (abstr 634). Presented at the Intersciences Conference on Antimicrobial Agents and Chemotherapy, Los Angeles, 1988

49. Kuhls TL, Viker S, Parris NB et al: Occupational risk of HIV, HBV and HSV-2 infections in health care personnel caring for AIDS patients. Am J Public Health 77:1306, 1987

50. McEvoy M, Porter K, Mortimer P et al: Prospective study of clinical, laboratory, and ancillary staff with accidental exposures to blood or body fluids from patients infected with HIV. Br Med J 294:1595, 1987

51. Health and Welfare Canada: National surveillance program on occupational exposures to HIV among health-care workers in Canada. Can Med Assoc J 138:31, 1988

52. Ramsey KM, Smith EN, Reinarz JA: Prospective evaluation of 44 health care workers exposed to human immunodeficiency virus-1, with one seroconversion (abstr). Clin Res 36:22A, 1988

53. Michelet C, Cartier F, Ruffault A et al: Needlestick HIV infection in a nurse (abstr). Presented at the Fourth International Conference on AIDS, Stockholm, June 12–16, 1988

54. Centers for Disease Control: Update: Acquired immunodeficiency syndrome and human immunodeficiency virus infection among health care workers. MMWR 37:229, 1988

55. Centers for Disease Control: Recommendations for prevention of HIV transmission in health care settings. MMWR 36(suppl 2S):1S, 1987

56. Centers for Disease Control: Apparent transmission of human T-lymphotropic virus type III/lymphadenopathy-associated virus from a child to a mother providing health care. MMWR 35:76, 1986

57. Dienstag JL, Ryan DM: Occupational exposure to hepatitis

B virus in hospital personnel: Infection or immunization? Am J Epidemiol 115:26, 1982

58. Kunches LM, Craven DE, Werner BG, Jacobs LM: Hepatitis B exposure in emergency medicine personnel: Prevalence of serologic markers and need for immunization. Am J Med 75:269, 1982

59. State of Maryland: Occupational exposure to human immunodeficiency virus: A review of current management. Commun Dis Bull, December 1990

60. Henderson DK: HIV-1 in the health care setting. In Mandell GL, Gordon DR, Bennet JE (eds): Principles and Practice of Infectious Diseases, 3rd ed. New York, Churchill-Livingstone, 1990

61. Tandberg D, Stewart KK, Doezema D: Under-reporting of contaminated needlestick injuries in emergency health care workers. Ann Emerg Med 20:66, 1990

62. Apprahamian C, Walker SB, Quebbeman JE et al: Use of medical center facilities by human immunodeficiency virus (HIV)–positive patients. J Trauma 30:745, 1990

63. Jagger J, Hunt EH, Brand-Elnaggar J, Pearson RD: Rates of needle-stick injury caused by various devices in a university hospital. N Engl J Med 319:284, 1988

64. Wormser GP, Joline C, Duncanson F: Needle-stick injuries during the care of patients with AIDS. N Engl J Med 310:1461, 1984

65. Hochreiter MC, Barton LL: Epidemiology of needlestick injury in emergency medical service personnel. J Emerg Med 6:9, 1988

66. Kelen GD, DiGiovanna TA, Celentano DD et al: Adherence to universal (barrier) precautions during interventions on critically ill and injured emergency department patients. J AIDS 3:987, 1990

67. Garner JS, Simmons BP: Guideline for isolation precautions in hospitals. Infect Control 4:245, 1983

68. Centers for Disease Control: Recommendations for preventing transmission of infection with human T-lymphotropic virus type III/lymphadenopathy-associated virus in the workplace. MMWR 34:681, 1985

69. Centers for Disease Control: Universal precautions for prevention of transmission of human immunodeficiency virus, hepatitis B and other blood borne pathogens in health-care settings. MMWR 37:377, 1988

70. Onion DK, Crumpacker CS, Gilliland BC: Arthritis of hepatitis associated with Australia antigen. Ann Intern Med 75:29, 1971

71. Lee AKY, Ip HMH, Wong VCW: Mechanisms of maternal-fetal transmission of hepatitis B virus. J Infect Dis 138:668, 1978

72. Bond WW, Petersen NJ, Gravelle CR, Favero MS: Hepatitis B virus in peritoneal dialysis fluid: A potential hazard. Dialysis Transplant 11:592, 1982

73. Hammond JS, Eckes JM, Gomez GA, Cunningham DN: HIV, trauma and infection control: Universal precautions are universally ignored. J Trauma 30:555, 1990

74. Baraff LJ, Talan DA: Compliance with universal precautions in a university hospital emergency department. Ann Emerg Med 18:654, 1989

75. Talan DA, Baraff LJ: Effect of education on the use of universal precautions in a university hospital emergency department. Ann Emerg Med 19:1322, 1990

76. Campbell S, Maki M, Henry K: Compliance with universal precautions among emergency department personnel (abstr), Book 2, p 99. Presented at the VIth International Conference on AIDS, San Francisco, 1989

77. Huff JS, Basala M: Universal precautions in emergency medicine residencies (letter). Ann Emerg Med 18:654, 1989

78. Kelen GD, Green G, Fortenberry C et al: Substantial improvement in adherence to universal precautions in an emergency department following administrative changes (abstr). Ann Emerg Med 19:481, 1990

79. Office of Occupational Health and Safety: Occupational exposure to blood borne pathogens: Proposal rule and notice of hearing. Fed Reg 54:23042, 1989

80. Doebbeling BD, Wenzel RP: The direct costs of universal precautions in a teaching hospital. JAMA 264:2083, 1990

81. Bartlett JG: Panel: AIDS and hepatitis B: Can we make the workplace safe? Response. In: Proceedings from the 3rd National Forum on AIDS and Hepatitis B, p 3. Bethesda, MD, National Foundation for Infectious Diseases, 1989

82. Immunization Practices Advisory Committee: Recommendations for protection against viral hepatitis. MMWR 34:313, 1985

83. Kelen GD, Chan DW, Green GB et al: Seroprevalence of HIV, HTLV, HCV and HBV among emergency department patients and potential risk to health care workers (abstr). Presented at the VIIth International Conference on AIDS, Florence, Italy, June 19–20, 1990

84. Centers for Disease Control: Protection against viral hepatitis: Recommendations of the Immunization Practices Advisory Committee (ACIP). MMWR 39(No. RR-2):1, 1990

Postexposure Management of Health Care Workers Occupationally Exposed to HIV

31E

Julie Louise Gerberding

The number of health care workers seeking care following accidental occupational exposures to human immunodeficiency virus (HIV) will no doubt increase as the acquired immunodeficiency syndrome (AIDS) epidemic progresses. Despite implementation of universal precautions and the availability of safer products and techniques, accidental exposure to HIV is a potential consequence of employment in a health care facility for many individuals. Although aggressive efforts to decrease the frequency of such exposures must remain the highest priority for occupational health programs, provision of postexposure care is also important.

A comprehensive postexposure program for HIV must include prompt access to efficient postexposure care, confidential supportive counseling and testing, and risk reduction education. With the widespread availability of zidovudine as a licensed antiretroviral agent, postexposure chemoprophylaxis with zidovudine or other drugs has gained in popularity. Although the use of zidovudine cannot yet be recommended, many health care workers choose to receive this experimental treatment.[1-3]

DECONTAMINATION

Little information is available with which to develop the most effective strategy for decontaminating exposures to HIV. However, common sense and knowledge of the molecular structure of HIV suggest that simply washing cutaneous wounds with soap and water is the most appropriate approach. Established first aid treatment for puncture wounds and lacerations need not be altered by concerns about HIV contamination. The use of bleach, iodofors, or other disinfectant agents has not been shown to be more efficacious than cleaning with soap and water alone, and at present their use is not recommended. Mucous membrane splashes with material that might contain HIV should be flushed with water. If the eye is involved in a splash, it should be rinsed with sterile water or eye irrigant. If none is available, clean tap water is an acceptable alternative.

EXPOSURE HISTORY

Eliciting an accurate history of occupational exposure may be difficult because health care workers may perceive a much greater or much lesser degree of exposure than actually occurred. The exposure history is helpful in documenting that an actual exposure to blood or other body fluid occurred, and for identifying the severity of the accident, which may be useful in assessing transmission risk.[4]

The infectivity of an exposure may depend on the amount of virus inoculated, which in turn is dependent on the volume of inoculum and the HIV titer. Large-bore hollow needles, intramuscular exposures, actual injections of blood, and exposure to concentrates of HIV are factors that appear more commonly among reports of needlestick transmission of HIV than among routine needlesticks.[5-8] Whether these factors will prove to be predictive of infectivity remains to be seen, but common sense suggests that large-volume exposures are apt to be more hazardous.

The history of an accidental needlestick exposure should reflect the following information: needle size, depth of penetration, bodily fluid involved, presence or absence of an actual injection of blood, time elapsed before the wound was decontaminated, location of the wound, and whether the wound bled spontaneously

Table 31E–1. Needlestick History Intake Form

SOURCE PATIENT

HIV risk assessment
   Known HIV-infected
      CD4 count
      H/O zidovudine use
   HIV risk factors evident
   HIV risk not evident
HBV Risk assessment
   Known HBsAg/HBeAg positive
   Clinical hepatitis/etiology unknown
   HBV risk factors evident
   HBV risk not evident

EXPOSURE DETAILS

Body fluid involved
Exposure details
   Depth of penetration
   Injection volume (if any)
   Type of device
   Needle gauge
   Intended use
   Mechanism of injury
   Needle passed through gloves?
Time to decontamination
Decontamination used

(Table 31E–1). It is also useful to document the purpose for which the needle was being used and the exact mechanism by which the injury occurred. Because preliminary data indicate that the use of gloves may reduce the volume of blood transferred during a needlestick exposure, the use of gloves and whether the needle passed through gloves *en route* to the skin are also important components of the needlestick history.[9]

The factors influencing infectivity during mucosal exposures have not been established. However, it is possible that mucocutaneous exposures involving large volumes of blood and prolonged contact with a portal of entry may be associated with a higher risk of transmission than when these factors are not present. In delineating a history of a mucosal exposure it is important to specify the site of exposure, the volume of blood involved, the duration of contact, and the mechanism used for decontamination. In the case of skin contact it is important to determine if there was an obvious disruption in the integrity of the skin as well. The mechanism of the accident that resulted in the exposure, the use or nonuse of protective equipment, and any other aspects of the accident that may have a bearing on future risk reduction intervention should be identified.

SOURCE PATIENT ASSESSMENT

The virus titers in HIV-infected individuals increase as the disease progresses.[10] Those who are in the process of acute seroconversion transiently may have titers in excess of 10^4/ml, which then fall by 2 or more logs.[11]

As symptoms of HIV illness appear, virus titers increase, and by the time full-blown AIDS has developed, titers may be in excess of 10^4/ml.[10] Although these values represent population averages, identification of the clinical stage of illness in the source patient may be an important component of risk analysis in the occupational setting. Therefore, when source patients are known to have HIV infection, it is important to ascertain the clinical stage of illness and, if possible, a CD4 count.

When the HIV status of the patient is unknown, it is appropriate to evaluate the individual clinically and epidemiologically for the presence or absence of risk behaviors for HIV infection.[3] In most centers, if HIV infection is not deemed extraordinarily unlikely, the source patient will be asked to consent to testing for HIV infection. In some states, when the source patient cannot consent, either because of illness or incompetence, proxy consent is allowed. In the absence of proxy consent, some states allow testing by administrative proxy. In other states, consent is not required at all for source patient testing, and the results may or may not be divulged to the source patient.

Whatever mechanism for source patient testing is followed, the information should be regarded as confidential and managed in a way that minimizes any harm accruing to the source. When the source patient refuses HIV testing, the exposed health care worker can be managed as if the source were positive, especially if risk behaviors associated with HIV infection are noted in the source patient. If the source patient is HIV negative and the pretest probability of infection is low, the health care worker can be reassured that HIV transmission is extremely unlikely. Because seroconversion may be delayed in some patients with HIV infection, a single negative test does not rule out infection in a source.[12,13] However, for purposes of managing the exposed health care worker, routine follow-up testing of the source patient is not recommended, and case management should be individualized.

Because of the conflict of interest, the source patient should not be directly approached by the exposed health care worker for HIV testing. A trained counselor who serves as an advocate for the source patient should be involved in the counseling and the decision to test, in a manner that does not inflict any sense of guilt or responsibility for the accident. In most centers source patient test results are handled as are other HIV test results. They are communicated to the exposed health care worker and to the clinicians directly involved in providing care to the exposed health care worker, and in addition to the clinicians responsible for the source patient's care.

POSTEXPOSURE PROPHYLAXIS FOR HIV

Provision of postexposure interventions designed to prevent transmission of infectious agents once exposure has occurred is not a new concept and has long been the approach to managing hepatitis B virus (HBV) exposures when previous immunization was not accomplished. Indeed, all personnel exposed to blood-borne pathogens should receive adequate HBV immunoprophylaxis, regardless of HIV concerns.[14] Postexposure immunoprophylaxis for HIV is not yet a realistic goal. However, postexposure chemoprophylaxis with zidovudine or other antiretroviral drugs is a promising strategy. Because zidovudine is licensed and widely available, it is currently the drug of choice for postexposure chemoprophylaxis in centers that have elected to provide this experimental therapy.[1-3] As new antiretroviral therapies are developed, alternative approaches will emerge.

Zidovudine acts by inhibiting reverse transcriptase, a step of virus infection that occurs after the virus has already entered cells. Because the pathogenesis of transcutaneous infection such as occurs in health care worker exposure is unknown, it is not clear whether zidovudine therapy is a rational choice in this situation. The cutaneous target cell, the time that elapses before the virus becomes irreversibly integrated into the host cell chromosome, and the extent of early virus dissemination to distant sites are unknown at this time. Ideally, a postexposure agent should act very quickly and should prevent virus from being taken up and incorporated into target cell genome. If zidovudine is to be effective in this setting it must be swallowed, absorbed, distributed, taken up by target cells, phosphorylated, and available to inhibit reverse transcriptase.[15]

There is evidence from murine, feline, and SCID-hu mouse models that postexposure zidovudine chemoprophylaxis can be efficacious.[16-19] However, in primate systems, neither pre-exposure nor postexposure chemoprophylaxis has been shown to be effective.[20-22] The data from primate studies are difficult to interpret, however, because relatively large inocula of virus (titers that are likely to exceed by several logs the amount of virus present in a typical needlestick injury) are used.

Three case reports in the literature describing failure of zidovudine to protect against the development of HIV infection following exposure are consistent with the primate experience. In the first published study, a relatively large volume of blood was inoculated intravenously.[23] Although the exposed individual started zidovudine immediately after the exposure and took a large dose of drug, the time to achieve therapeutic drug levels may have been prolonged because the patient had been in the hospital for bowel surgery and the integrity of the absorptive process was unclear. In the second case, zidovudine treatment was delayed for 6 hours after a severe exposure, and the source patient had been taking zidovudine for several months prior to the accident, which raises the possibility of drug resistance.[24,25] In the third case a very large volume of HIV-infected blood was intentionally self-inoculated in a suicide attempt. Zidovudine was started after the fact but failed to protect.[26]

These anecdotal case reports may indicate that zidovudine has no efficacy at all in providing postexposure protection, or that it is not likely to protect in situations where transmission is most likely, *i.e.,* a large-inoculum exposure. However, it is also true that without denominator data one cannot ascertain the efficacy of zidovudine, because only failures are apt to be published in the literature, and successful courses of treatment cannot be recognized. If it were possible to design a clinical trial comparing zidovudine chemoprophylaxis with no therapy or with other therapy, we might be able to ascertain whether this drug offers any advantage to exposed health care workers. However, such a trial would require several thousand participants and is not likely to be feasible. In fact, the only trial of this magnitude that was attempted was stopped because of low subject accrual.[27] In the meantime, most institutions have been left with the awareness that zidovudine treatment is requested by many informed health care workers. When such treatment is provided it must be considered experimental and offered under protocols that monitor for evidence of toxicity and seroconversion.

Such an interim treatment protocol has been developed by investigators at the University of California, the Clinical Centers of the National Institutes of Health, and the Centers for Disease Control (CDC), and has been implemented at selected study sites. The study protocol provides 4 weeks of zidovudine treatment to exposed health care workers, who are monitored biweekly for toxicity. Initially, 1,200 mg/day (200 mg every 4 hours) of zidovudine is provided. After 72 hours the dosage is reduced to 1,000 mg/day by eliminating the 4 A.M. dose. Clinicians also may elect to treat with only 500 mg/day. When toxicity is observed, the drug dosage is reduced or the drug is discontinued altogether, depending on the degree of toxicity noted.

At San Francisco General Hospital, where a similar protocol has been in place for more than 2 years, the experience has been generally favorable. Fifty percent of health care workers eligible for protocol treatment have elected therapy. No serious toxic effects have been noted, although subjective symptoms of a flu-like illness that respond to dose reduction or discontinuation are relatively common. Relative neutropenia may also appear but has not been clinically important to date. Thus, it appears that zidovudine does not produce short-term toxic effects that would contraindicate therapy, and until the drug is established as an efficacious agent or better drugs are found, it is likely that such interim protocols will remain in effect.

Most experts agree that the single most important aspect of any zidovudine treatment protocol is prompt administration of the drug, as soon as possible after the exposure. Data from animal experiments strongly suggest that delayed treatment, especially beyond 24 hours, is much less likely to have a beneficial effect in the recipient animal.[16,17,19] In most centers the goal is to provide zidovudine immediately after the accidental exposure. This in turn requires concerted efforts on the part of the institution to provide prompt access to a reporting and treatment program.

REPORTING OF OCCUPATIONAL EXPOSURES

Traditionally, most occupational exposures have been reported in the emergency department or in the employee health service during normal business hours. HIV issues have changed this approach, for two main reasons: (1) the desire to provide prompt access to zidovudine therapy has necessitated a more efficient response system, and (2) the special fears and stresses inherent in sustaining an HIV exposure make access to immediate counseling and supportive information essential.

In large institutions where exposures are relatively common, a "needlestick hotline" mechanism is one solution to this issue. A hotline program that provides expert consultation 24 hours a day is optimal in this setting. Such a program has been in effect at San Francisco General Hospital for the past 2 years and is staffed by expert clinicians who can provide immediate expert consultation and advice.[2] More important, these experts are trained to recognize the psychological trauma associated with an HIV needlestick and can provide initial crisis intervention and arrange for follow-up care.

In settings where HIV or other blood-borne exposures are relatively uncommon, hotlines may be too expensive and too labor intensive to be practical. Solutions that have been adopted in these situations include link-ups with larger institutions that have a program in place, provision of needlestick management protocols that are readily accessible in the emergency department, or assigning an individual in the institution to provide the initial intervention and then to provide follow-up care as indicated in the employee health service or other clinical setting.

Whatever mechanism is provided to facilitate reporting of exposures, confidentiality must be respected. Concerns about punitive aspects of having sustained an exposure, peer pressure or concerns about stigmatization in the work setting, and concerns about HIV testing and risk-behavior analysis are legitimate worries that can interfere with the incentive to report accidental injuries.[28] Because reporting is important to ensure access to appropriate medical and psychological care, these obstacles must be addressed directly and overcome, with sensitive and sensible provisions to ensure worker confidentiality.

HIV TESTING

Baseline testing for HIV and other blood-borne infectious agents is recommended after any exposure in which transmission of a blood-borne agent is suspected. Documentation of baseline status allows the worker to ascertain in the future that the accidental exposure was temporally related to seroconversion or the acquisition of symptomatic infection. Moreover, such testing affords the opportunity to conduct risk educational intervention that may have a bearing on nonoccupational risk behaviors and general HIV awareness. Health care workers who elect to defer initial testing should be strongly advised to have serum banked, so that it may be recovered and tested at a later date if indicated for medical workers compensation or for psychological reasons.

When HIV transmission is a possibility, testing of the health care worker for HIV infection is generally recommended.[3] Such testing may be performed periodically, typically at baseline and again at 6 weeks, 3 months, and 6 months. Testing beyond 6 months is not recommended, because to date all health care worker infections have been documented prior to the 6-month follow-up visit. However, some centers continue to follow individuals for a full year after exposure, particularly if zidovudine therapy has been elected.[2] Experience at San Francisco General Hospital has indicated that many workers cope fairly well during the postexposure interval until the time that follow-up testing is due. Access to a trained counselor or a sensitive clinician in the postexposure interval is helpful in reassuring the health care worker that such follow-up testing is routine, and in addition promotes establishment of a positive educational and risk reduction intervention.

Because the majority of health care workers who have seroconverted after occupational exposures have evidenced symptoms of the acute retroviral illness, it is important to remind health care workers that should a febrile illness consistent with HIV seroconversion develop, they should seek care from their provider as soon as possible. If the HIV antibody test is negative at this time, an HIV p24 antigen test should be encouraged if HIV infection is suspected.

Currently there is no role for polymerase chain reaction (PCR) (gene amplification) technology in diagnosing seroconversion in health care workers. In the one case in which gene amplification was reported in a seroconverting health care worker, the PCR test was negative at a time when the antigen and Western blot assays were positive.[29] Similarly, no evidence of seronegative latent infection in those undergoing prolonged follow-up has been detected by PCR.[30,31]

RISK REDUCTION INFORMATION

Risk reduction education during the follow-up interval after exposure encompasses two main topics: (1) behavior modification designed to prevent HIV transmission to persons at risk during the interval when the health care worker could be incubating HIV, and (2) assessment and risk reduction interventions designed to prevent future occupational exposures. The CDC recommends that individuals exposed to HIV practice safe sex and avoid pregnancy for 6 months after the exposure.[2] In addition to these interventions, many author-

ities recommend that breast-feeding be avoided and that blood donation be deferred during the follow-up interval. These recommendations may seem ludicrous for individuals who have sustained very trivial accidental exposures in which the risk of HIV transmission is deemed extremely unlikely. However, the most conservative approach would be to recommend that these practices be adopted and to help the health care workers make individual decisions about how best to implement them in their situations.

Risk reduction interventions designed to prevent similar occupational exposures in the future must be handled in a tactful manner lest the health care worker perceive that he or she is being blamed for his accident. In many cases the health care worker will already have formulated some idea on why the accident occurred, and specifically on what could be done in the future to prevent a similar occurrence. In some cases the interventions will require facilitating changes in job design or changes that must be negotiated through the supervisor.

If a careful history of the occupational exposure has been obtained, it may be possible to collate this information to provide good surveillance of the overall pattern of injuries and accidents within a given institution. When systematic problems appear, it is then possible to implement interventions with supervisors or administrators that will not necessitate disclosure of the health care worker's identity during this problem-solving process.

RECORD KEEPING AND DOCUMENTATION

As with all other aspects of postexposure management, protecting the confidentiality of the involved worker is of paramount importance. Creative efforts are needed to develop a system for maintaining adequate documentation of the exposure and follow-up so that the worker can recover workers compensation benefits or other entitlements, should they be indicated, and to protect the confidentiality of the worker and prevent untoward disclosures of sensitive information. One solution to this problem is to maintain exposure management records in a file that is kept separate from employee health records or routine hospital records. This may be difficult when postexposure care is provided in the emergency department, and it is one good reason for bypassing the emergency room all together and allowing postexposure care to occur in a setting where confidentiality can be maximally protected.

At San Francisco General Hospital a coded system is used to protect the confidentiality of the exposed individual. Exposure records are collated by code rather than by personal identifiers, and the link between the individual's identity and the numeric code is kept in a locked file separate from all aspects of the medical records department. If a worker later requires disclosure of the documents or consents to have them released to outside agencies, the numeric code can be replaced with personal identifiers.

REFERENCES

1. Henderson DK, Gerberding JL: Prophylactic zidovudine after occupational exposure to the human immunodeficiency virus: An interim analysis. J Infect Dis 160:321, 1989

2. Gerberding JL, Wugofski L, Berkvam G et al: Facilitated surveillance and post-exposure AZT prophylaxis for health care workers (HCW): The San Francisco General Hospital model (abstr 961). Presented at the 30th Interscience Congress on Antimicrobials and Chemotherapy, Atlanta, October 21–24, 1990

3. Centers for Disease Control: Public Health Service statement on management of occupational exposure to human immunodeficiency virus, including considerations regarding zidovudine use. MMWR 39:1, 1990

4. Beekman SE, Fahey B, Gerberding JL, Henderson DK: Is casualty count the best method for assessing the risks for occupational HIV-1 infection? Infect Cont Hosp Epidemiol 11:371, 1990

5. Centers for Disease Control: Update: Acquired immunodeficiency syndrome and human immunodeficiency virus infection among health care workers. MMWR 37:229, 1988

6. Stricof RL, Morse DL: HTLV-III/LAV seroconversion following a deep intramuscular needlestick injury (letter). N Engl J Med 314:1115, 1986

7. [N.A.]: Needlestick transmission of HTLV-III from a patient infected in Africa. Lancet 2:1376, 1984

8. Weiss SH, Goedert JJ, Gartner S et al: Risk of human immunodeficiency virus (HIV-1) infection among laboratory workers. Science 239:68, 1988

9. Mast S, Gerberding JL: Factors influencing infectivity during accidental needlestick exposure to HIV: An in vitro model (abstr). Clin Res 1991 39(1)

10. Ho DD, Moudgil TM, Alam M: Quantitation of human immunodeficiency virus type 1 in the blood of infected persons. N Engl J Med 321:1621, 1989

11. Daar ES, Moudgil T, Meyer RD, Ho DD: Transient high levels of viremia in patients with primary human immunodeficiency virus type 1 infection. N Engl J Med 324: 961, 1991

12. Imagawa DT, Lee MH, Wolinsky SM et al: Human immunodeficiency virus type 1 infection in homosexual men who remain seronegative for prolonged periods. N Engl J Med 320:1458, 1989

13. Pezella M, Rossi P, Lombardi V et al: HIV viral sequences in seronegative people at risk detected by in situ hybridization and polymerase chain reaction. Br Med J 298:713, 1989

14. Centers for Disease Control: Protection against viral hepatitis: Recommendations of the Immunization Practices Committee. MMWR 39:1, 1990

15. Gerberding JL: Prevention of HIV infection during the 1990's: Criteria for postexposure prophylaxis for health care providers sustaining occupational exposure to HIV. In Sande MA, Root RK (eds): Contemporary Issues in Infectious Disease, p 227. New York, Churchill Livingstone, 1991

16. Tavares L, Roneker C, Johnston K et al: 3'-azido-3'-deoxythymidine in feline leukemia virus–infected cats: A model for therapy and prophylaxis of AIDS. Cancer Res 47:3190, 1987

17. Ruprecht RM, OBrien LG, Rossoni LD, Nusiniff-Lehrman S: Suppression of mouse viraemia and retroviral disease by 3'-azido-3'-deoxythymidine. Nature 323:467, 1986

18. McCune JM, Namikawa R, Shih CC et al: 3'-azido-3'-deoxythymidine suppresses HIV infection in SCID-hu mouse. Science 247:564, 1990

19. Shih CC, Kaneshima H, Rabin L et al: Post-exposure prophylaxis with zidovudine suppresses human immunodeficiency virus type 1 infection in SCID-hu mice in a time-dependent fashion. J Infect Dis 163:625, 1991

20. McClure HM, Anderson DC, Fultz P et al: Prophylactic effects of AZT following exposure of macaques to an acutely lethal variant of SIV (SIV/SMM/PBj-14) (abstr). Presented at the V International Conference on AIDS, Montreal, June 4–9, 1989

21. Lundgren B, Hedstrom KG, Norrby E et al: Inhibition of early occurrence of antigen in SIV-infected macaques as a measurement of antiviral efficacy (abstr). Presented at the Symposium on Non-human Primate Models for AIDS, November 1988

22. Gerberding JL, Marx P, Gould R et al: Simian model of retrovirus chemoprophylaxis with constant infusion zidovudine ± interferon alpha (abstr) 31st Interscience Congress on Antimicrobial Agents and Chemotherapy, Chicago, Oct 1991

23. Lange JMA, Boucher CAB, Hollak CEM et al: Failure of zidovudine prophylaxis after accidental exposure to HIV. N Engl J Med 322:1375, 1990

24. Looke DFM, Grove DI: Failed prophylactic zidovudine after needlestick injury (letter). Lancet 335:1280, 1990

25. Larder BA, Kemp SD: Multiple mutations in HIV-1 reverse transcriptase confer high-level resistance to zidovudine (AZT). Science 246:1155, 1989

26. Durand E, LeJeunne C, Hugues FC: Failure of prophylactic zidovudine after suicidal self-inoculation of HIV-infected blood. N Engl J Med 324:1062, 1991

27. LaFon SW, Nusinof-Lehrman S, Barry D: Prophylactically administered Retrovir in health care workers potentially exposed to the human immunodeficiency virus. J Infect Dis 158:503, 1988

28. Mangione C, Gerberding JL, Cummings S: Occupational exposure to HIV: Frequency and rates of underreporting of percutaneous and mucocutaneous exposures by medical housestaff. Am J Med 90:85, 1991

29. Henderson DK, Fahey BJ, Willy M et al: Risk for occupational transmission of human immunodeficiency virus type 1 (HIV-1) associated with clinical exposures. Ann Intern Med 113:740, 1990

30. Gerberding JL, Littell C, Sande M: Longterm followup of health care workers with polymerase chain reaction and antibody testing to detect delayed seroconversion (abstr Th.C.601). Presented at the VI International Conference on AIDS, San Francisco, June, 1990

31. Wormser GP, Joline C, Bittker S et al: Polymerase chain reaction for seronegative health care workers with parenteral exposure to HIV-infected patients. N Engl J Med 321:1681, 1989

Sterilization, Disinfection, and Environmental Control

31F

Martin S. Favero

This chapter describes the general procedures used in health care facilities to sterilize or disinfect instruments or to decontaminate items, devices, and environmental surfaces. These standard procedures have been devised using relatively stringent criteria and are more than adequate for sterilizing or disinfecting instruments, devices, and other items contaminated with blood or other body fluids from persons infected with blood-borne pathogens, including human immunodeficiency virus (HIV) and hepatitis B virus (HBV).

The effective use of antiseptics, disinfectants, and sterilization procedures helps to prevent hospital-acquired infections. Historically, steam autoclaves and dry heat sterilizers have been used for sterilizing devices, equipment, and supplies in hospitals. Ethylene oxide gas is used for sterilizing heat-sensitive items. Recently several alternatives to ethylene oxide have been developed, including hydrogen peroxide vapor and plasmas as well as formulations containing hydrogen peroxide and/or peracetic acid. Liquid chemical germicides used as cold sterilants have also been on the market for many years in the United States but are used to disinfect rather than to sterilize medical devices.[1]

The choice of which procedure or method or specific chemical germicide to use for sterilization, disinfection, or environmental sanitization depends on a great many factors. No single chemical germicide or agent or procedure is adequate for all purposes. Factors that should be considered in the selection of a specific sterilization or disinfection procedure include (1) the degree of microbiologic inactivation required for the particular device, (2) the nature and physical composition of the device being treated, and (3) the cost and ease of using a particular procedure.[1-3]

REGULATION OF CHEMICAL GERMICIDES

The primary agency in the United States government that is involved with disinfection and sterilization procedures is the Environmental Protection Agency (EPA). The EPA approves sterilizers such as steam autoclaves and ethylene oxide gas sterilizers, as well as chemical germicides formulated as sterilants and disinfectants (germicides used on devices or environmental surfaces). The EPA requires manufacturers of chemical germicides formulated as general disinfectants, hospital disinfectants, and disinfectants applied to other environments to test these formulations using specific and standardized protocols for microbicidal efficacy, stability, and toxicity to humans.[1]

The Food and Drug Administration (FDA) regulates chemical germicides that are formulated as antiseptics, preservatives, or drugs to be used on or in the human body or as preparations to be used to inhibit or kill microorganisms on the skin. The FDA has an advisory panel that reviews nonprescription antimicrobial drug products. Manufacturers of such formulations voluntarily submit data to the panel, which in turn categorizes the products for their intended use: antimicrobial soaps, health care personnel handwashes, patient preoperative skin preparations, skin antiseptics, skin wound cleansers, skin wound protectants, and surgical hand scrubs. General chemical germicides for each use are further divided into three categories: category I, safe and efficacious; category II, not safe or efficacious; and category III, insufficient data to categorize.[4,5]

Chemical germicides formulated as antiseptics are categorized basically by use and efficacy and are not regulated or registered in the same fashion that the EPA regulates and registers a disinfectant. Currently, many of the antimicrobial antiseptic formulations on the market are in category III, which means that health care workers must make decisions based on information derived from the manufacturer or from studies published in the scientific literature.

The Centers for Disease Control (CDC) does not approve, regulate, or test chemical germicides formulated as sterilants, disinfectants, or antiseptics. Rather, the CDC recommends broad strategies for the use of sterilants, disinfectants, and antiseptics to prevent transmission of infections in the health care environment.[2]

The definitions of sterilization, disinfection, antisepsis, and other related terms, such as decontamination and sanitization, are generally accepted in the scientific community, but some of these terms are misused. It is important to understand the definition and inferred capabilities of each term and the related procedure.

Sterilization

The term *sterilization* is one that students and professionals have memorized and recited seemingly forever. It can be the simplest or the most complex concept, depending on how it is viewed and how it is applied. The definition of sterilization can change depending on the vantage point from which it is viewed. I choose to view this term somewhat as a hologram and will define it in the context of the *state* of sterilization, the *procedure* of sterilization, and the *application* of sterilization.

An item, device, or solution is considered to be sterile when it is completely free of all living microorganisms. This *state* of sterility is the objective of the sterilization procedure, and in this context the definition, for all practical purposes, is a categorical and absolute one—an item is either sterile or it is not.

A sterilization *procedure* is one that kills all microorganisms, including high numbers of bacterial endospores. Sterilization can be accomplished by heat, ethylene oxide gas, radiation (in industry), and by a number of liquid chemical germicides, notably those approved by the EPA as cold sterilants. A sterilization procedure from an operational standpoint is defined as a process following which the probability of a microorganism surviving on an item is less than 1 in a million (10^{-6}). This approach is used by the medical device industry to sterilize large quantities of medical devices.

The application of sterilization process principles in industry is much more sophisticated and controlled than are sterilization procedures used in health care facilities. However, steam autoclaves, ethylene oxide sterilizers, and dry heat sterilization ovens used in health care facilities have operational protocols that are verified by the manufacturer to accomplish sterilization, and all the variables that control for the inactivation of microorganisms are either automated or built into simple controls in the devices.

The *application* of the sterilization process involves the strategy associated with a particular medical device or solution and the context of its exposure to humans. Almost 30 years ago, Spaulding[6] proposed that the nature of device and equipment sterilization and disinfection could be understood more readily if medical devices, equipment, and surgical materials were divided into three categories based on the risk of infection involved in their use. Briefly, devices that are exposed to sterile areas of the body, such as blood, require sterilization; devices that touch mucous membranes may be either sterilized or disinfected; and devices or items that touch skin or environmental surfaces can be sanitized with a low-level disinfectant or simply cleaned with soap and water.

In the context of these categorizations, Spaulding also classified chemical germicides by activity level. The activity levels are listed in Table 31F–1 and are as follows.

HIGH-LEVEL DISINFECTION

This procedure kills vegetative microorganisms but not necessarily high numbers of bacterial spores. Chemical germicides used in this procedure are, by Spaulding's definition, capable of accomplishing sterilization, that is, they kill all microorganisms, including a high number of bacterial spores, when the contact time is relatively long (6 to 10 hours). As high-level disinfectants, however, they are used for a relatively short period of time (10 to 30 minutes). These chemical germicides are registered with the EPA as sterilant/disinfectants.

INTERMEDIATE-LEVEL DISINFECTION

This procedure kills vegetative microorganisms, including *Mycobacterium tuberculosis,* all fungi, and most viruses. These chemical germicides often correspond to EPA-approved "hospital disinfectants" that are also "tuberculocidal."

LOW-LEVEL DISINFECTION

This procedure kills most vegetative bacteria except *M. tuberculosis,* some fungi, and some viruses. These chemical germicides usually are ones approved by the EPA as "hospital disinfectants" or "sanitizers."

The relation between EPA's system of classification and the CDC's recommendation for strategies of sterilization and disinfection is shown in Table 31F–2.

Decontamination

This procedure renders a device, items, or material safe to handle, *i.e.,* safe in the sense of reasonably free of the probability of transmission of infection. The decontamination process sometimes is a sterilization procedure such as steam autoclaving. Often this may be the most cost-effective procedure for decontaminating a device or an item. On the other hand, simply cleaning with soap and water may be equally effective. When chemical germicides are used for decontamination, they can range in activity from sterilant/disinfectants, which might be used to decontaminate spills of highly infectious agents in research or clinical laboratories, to low-level disinfectants or sanitizers, which might be used to decontaminate environmental surfaces.

Table 31F–1. Levels of Germicidal Action

| Level | Bacteria | | | Fungi | Viruses | |
	Vegetative Bacteria	Tubercle Bacillus	Spores		Lipid and Medium-sized	Nonlipid and Small
High	+	+	+	+	+	+
Intermediate	+	+	±	+	+	±
Low	+	−	−	±	+	−

Table 31F–2. Centers for Disease Control and Environmental Protection Agency Classification Schemes for Sterilants, Disinfectants, and Sanitizers

EPA Product Classification	Type of Device or Surface	CDC Process Classifications
Sterilant/disinfectant	Critical (surgical instruments, catheters, implants)	Sterilization (sporicidal chemical, prolonged contact time)
	Semicritical (some endoscopes, endotracheal tubes, laryngoscopes)	High-level disinfection (sporicidal chemical, short contact time)
Hospital disinfectant (with label claim for tuberculocidal activity)	Noncritical (large blood spills, contaminated control knobs of dialysis machines, blood pressure cuffs)	Intermediate-level disinfection
Hospital disinfectant; sanitizer	Noncritical (exterior of machines, bed pans, floors)	Low-level disinfection or soap and water

Antiseptics

An antiseptic is a substance that has antimicrobial activity and is formulated to be used on or in living tissue to inhibit or destroy microorganisms. Quite often the distinction between an antiseptic and a disinfectant is not made; however, the differences are great and applications are substantially different. A disinfectant is a chemical germicide that is formulated for use solely on medical devices, instruments, or environmental surfaces. An antiseptic is a chemical germicide that is formulated for use solely on or in living tissues. Some chemical germicidal agents, such as iodophors, can be used as active ingredients in disinfectants as well as in antiseptics. However, the precise formulations are significantly different, they are used differently, and the germicidal efficacy of each formulation differs substantially. Consequently, disinfectants should never be used as antiseptics, and *vice versa*.

HIV and HBV

Viruses can be inactivated by a variety of chemical germicides. Studies on inactivation of HBV and HIV have shown that neither virus is unusually resistant. In 1977 it was proposed that the resistance level of HBV be considered to be between that of the tubercle bacillus and bacterial spores, but nearer that of the former.[8] At that time, this type of rationale appeared reasonable, and it was believed that the most conservative approach would be to recommend at least high-level disinfection for all types of medical devices known or thought to be contaminated with HBV. Subsequently, two studies employing direct chimpanzee inoculation with disinfectant-treated human serum with high titers of HBV showed that a variety of intermediate- to high-level disinfectant chemicals (two commercial glutaraldehyde-based products, 500 mg/L free chlorine from sodium hypochlorite, an iodophor product, 70% isopropanol, 80% ethanol, and dilutions of glutaraldehyde as low as 0.1%) were effective inactivators of the virus in relatively short exposure times and at low temperatures.[9,10]

HIV is relatively unstable in the environment[11] and is rapidly inactivated after being exposed to commonly used chemical germicides at concentrations much lower than those used in practice.[12–15] When considered in the context of environmental conditions in health care facilities, the demonstrated sensitivity of HIV to germicides, in addition to low viral titers in blood of infected patients (*ca.* 100 to 10,000 HIV/ml), has resulted in no changes in currently recommended strategies for sterilization, disinfection, or housekeeping. Although the EPA has recently approved specific HIV label claims for a large number of proprietary germicidal formulations (mostly those germicides used for housekeeping purposes), the presence or absence of such a claim should not be the major criterion in the selection of germicidal products.

ENVIRONMENTAL CONSIDERATIONS

Environmental surfaces such as walls, floors, and other surfaces are not associated with transmission of infections to patients or health care workers.[1–3] Therefore, extraordinary attempts to disinfect or sterilize these environmental surfaces are not necessary. However, cleaning should be done routinely.

Disinfectant-detergent formulations registered by the EPA can be used for cleaning environmental surfaces, but the actual physical removal of microorganisms by scrubbing is probably at least as important as any antimicrobial effect of the germicidal agent used.

No hospital protocol dealing with sterilization, disinfection, and housekeeping procedures needs to be changed because of concerns about contamination with HIV or HBV.[1,7] Thus, if an EPA-registered nontuberculocidal quaternary ammonium disinfectant-detergent is being used for housekeeping purposes, it can continue to be used.

As was pointed out earlier, decontamination is defined as a process that renders contaminated material, devices, and surfaces safe to handle, *i.e.*, the risk of infection transmission is eliminated or reduced significantly. For decontaminating spills of blood and other body fluids, the CDC recommends the use of chemical germicides that are approved for use as hospital disinfectants and are tuberculocidal when used as recommended.[7] This is a special protocol applicable to sites within health care facilities or laboratories that have become *significantly* contaminated with blood or body fluids. This strategy is relatively conservative and requires common-sense judgment in assessing risk levels, including the size and location of the blood or body fluid spill. Because the CDC does not recommend specific commercial products, the EPA system of classification for label claim registration has been used for guidance on product selection (*i.e.,* hospital disinfectant with claim of tuberculocidal activity; see Table 31F–2). In essence, that results in the user choosing chemical germicides that have intermediate to high levels of germicidal activity (*e.g.,* sodium hypochlorite bleach, iodophors, and phenolics) rather than low levels of activity (*e.g.,* quaternary ammonium compounds). A product with tuberculocidal activity is indicated because mycobacteria are unusually resistant to chemical germicides, not because of a concern for the transmission of *M. tuberculosis* from environmental surfaces.

Protocols for housekeeping, laundry, sanitization, disinfection, and sterilization used in health care facilities are relatively conservative and need not be changed because of a concern for HIV or HBV contamination.

Infectious Waste

The CDC has published recommendations for the identification, handling, transport, storage, and disposal of infectious waste.[2,7] However, there is no evidence to suggest that most hospital waste is any more infective than residential waste, and there is no epidemiologic evidence that hospital waste has caused disease in the community as a result of improper disposal. Therefore, identifying wastes for which special precautions are indicated is largely a matter of judgment about the relative risk of disease transmission. The most practical approach to the management of infectious waste is to identify those wastes with the potential for causing infection during handling and disposal and for which some special precautions appear prudent. Hospital wastes for which special precautions appear prudent include microbiology laboratory waste, pathology waste, needles and sharp instruments, and blood specimens or blood products.

Although any item that has had contact with blood, exudates, or secretions may be potentially infective, it is not usually considered practical or necessary to treat all such waste as infective. In general, infectious waste should either be incinerated or should be decontaminated before disposal in a sanitary landfill. Bulk blood, suctioned fluids, excretions, and secretions may be carefully poured down a drain connected to a sanitary sewer. Other infectious wastes may be ground and flushed into a sanitary sewer. Universal precautions[7] are not intended to alter these basic recommendations for waste management.

REFERENCES

1. Favero MS, Bond WW: Sterilization, disinfection and antisepsis in the hospital. In: Manual of Clinical Microbiology, p 183. Washington, DC, American Society for Microbiology, 1991
2. Garner JL, Favero MS: Guidelines for handwashing and hospital environment control. HHS Publication No. 85-1117. Atlanta, Centers for Disease Control, 1985
3. Rutala WA: Guideline for selection and use of disinfectants. Am J Infect Control 18:99, 1990
4. Bruch MK, Larson E: Regulation of topical antimicrobials: History, status and future perspective. Infect Control Hosp Epidemiol 10:505, 1989
5. Zanowiak P, Jacobs MR: Topical anti-infective products. In: Handbook of Nonprescription Drugs, 7th ed, p 92. Washington, DC, American Pharmaceutical Association, 1982
6. Spaulding EH: Chemical disinfection and antisepsis in the hospital. J Hosp Res 9:5, 1972
7. Centers for Disease Control: Recommendations for prevention of HIV transmission in health-care settings. MMWR 36(No. 2S):1, 1987
8. Bond WW, Petersen NJ, Favero MS: Viral hepatitis B: Aspects of environmental control. Health Lab Sci 14:235, 1977
9. Bond WW, Favero MS, Petersen NJ, Ebert JW: Inactivation of hepatitis B virus by intermediate- to high-level disinfectant chemicals. J Clin Microbiol 18:535, 1983
10. Kobayashi H, Tsuzuki M, Koshimizu K et al: Susceptibility of hepatitis B virus to disinfectants and heat. J Clin Microbiol 20:214, 1984
11. Resnik L, Veren K, Salahuddin SF et al: Stability and inactivation of HTLV-III/LAV under clinical and laboratory environments. JAMA 255:1887, 1986
12. McDougal JS, Cort SP, Kennedy MS et al: Immunoassay for the detection and quantitation of infectious human retrovirus, lymphadenopathy-associated virus (LAV). J Immunol Methods 76:171, 1985
13. Martin LS, McDougal JS, Loskoski SL: Disinfection and inactivation of the human T lymphotrophic virus type III lymphadenopathy-associated virus. J Infect Dis 152:400, 1985
14. Spire B, Barre-Sinoussi F, Montagnier L, Chermann JC: Inactivation of lymphadenopathy associated virus by chemical disinfectants. Lancet 2:899, 1984
15. Spire B, Barre-Sinoussi F, Dormont D et al: Inactivation of lymphadenopathy-associated virus by heat, gamma rays, and ultraviolet light. Lancet 1:188, 1985

32

Management of Health Care Workers Infected With HIV or Other Blood-Borne Pathogens

David K. Henderson

The appearance of the acquired immunodeficiency syndrome (AIDS) and human immunodeficiency virus (HIV) infection in the United States in 1981[1] had a profound impact on virtually every aspect of society. This unique sexually transmitted and blood-borne infectious disease almost immediately grasped the attention of both scientists and the public. Beginning in 1981, the health care workplace began to feel the effects of AIDS; by 1991, the impact of HIV infection on health care was staggering. Perhaps no venue felt the impact of AIDS more fully than the health care workplace. As early as 1983 the risk of occupational or nosocomial transmission of HIV became apparent.[2] Subsequent investigations have at least partially quantified the risk for occupational infection in the health care setting.[3-5] Initially, the risk for occupational infection was associated purely with parenteral exposures to blood from HIV-infected patients.[2,6] Subsequent documentation of occupational infections resulting from nonparenteral exposures[7] forced the U.S. Public Health Service's Centers for Disease Control (CDC) to reconsider its existing infection control recommendations. The CDC's universal precautions[8] were issued as a result of these deliberations. These thoughtful recommendations revitalized the approach to infection control in virtually every hospital in the country.

The issue of the management of health care workers infected with HIV was discussed tangentially in several places prior to 1990[9-12]; however, the first instances of documented HIV transmission from a health care provider to a patient[13,14] produced a flurry of interest in this difficult topic. Concerns about HIV transmission from infected providers to their patients rekindled interest in the similar risks for provider-to-patient transmission of hepatitis B virus (HBV) as well. Anecdotal reports of provider-to-patient transmission of HBV, including several clusters of cases,[15-34] prompted similar concerns as early as the 1970s.[35,36] Soon after provider-to-patient transmission of HBV was identified, the need for quantitation of the risk of such transmission was emphasized.[36] Subsequently, investigators acknowledged that, for a variety of reasons, including the small magnitude of risk for provider-to-patient transmission of HBV, prospective studies attempting to quantitate this risk were not practical.[37] These same experts suggested in 1975[36] and again in 1981[37] that "the implications of removing trained personnel from patient contact are too broad, the number too great, and the psychosocial effect too devastating to base decisions on any but conclusive data." Ultimately, the U.S. Public Health Service issued recommendations suggesting that HBV-infected practitioners need not be restricted from practice unless they were shown to transmit infection.[29,38,39] The CDC also recommended that practitioners who were found to transmit infection be allowed to return to practice as long as (1) the practitioners followed CDC and state recommendations regarding informed consent and (2) an ongoing surveillance program was in place to detect additional instances of HBV transmission.[29] Subsequently the CDC reversed its position on HBV transmission, noting that "[a] worker who is HBsAg positive and who has transmitted hepatitis B virus to another individual during the performance of his or her job duties should be excluded from the performance of those job duties which place other individuals at risk for acquisition of hepatitis B infection."[40]

A risk of provider-to-patient transmission of HIV was suggested very early in the epidemic, primarily because of the striking epidemiologic similarities between HIV infection and HBV. As early as 1985, the CDC[9,10] and others[11] suggested that provider-to-patient transmission of the agent responsible for AIDS was at least a theoretical possibility. In the October 1985 recommendations, the CDC noted that the difficult issues related to the management of HIV-infected health care workers who perform invasive procedures (including recommendations for the serologic testing of these health care providers) would be addressed in a subsequent guideline.[10] The invasive procedure guidelines, issued in April 1986, concluded that "routine serologic testing for evidence of [HIV] infection is not necessary for HCW's who perform or assist in invasive procedures or for patients undergoing invasive procedures, since the risk of transmission in this setting is so low."[12] These guidelines also advocated that health care workers with illnesses that might compromise their ability to perform invasive procedures adequately or safely be evaluated medically to determine physical and mental competence for performing invasive procedures.[12] Thus was born the "case-by-case" management concept for HIV-infected health care workers. In July 1991, the CDC issued new guidelines recommending that health care workers who perform "exposure-prone" invasive procedures be aware of their HIV and HBV serologic status.[41] The guidelines also recommended that HIV-infected or HBeAg-positive infected health care workers voluntarily refrain from performing exposure-prone invasive procedures or seek the counsel of an expert review panel to determine which of these procedures, if any, could be performed safely.[41] Finally, the guidelines recommended that an infected provider who had been approved for an exposure-prone invasive procedure by the expert review panel should notify the patient of his or her infection prior to the procedure.[41] Management of infected health care workers was problematic in 1985 and remains so today. This chapter addresses several of the difficult issues regarding the management of HIV-infected health care providers and attempts to provide a framework for further consideration of these difficult questions.

MAGNITUDE OF RISK OF PROVIDER-TO-PATIENT TRANSMISSION OF HIV

Data on the magnitude of risk of provider-to-patient transmission of HIV are most relevant to a discussion of the appropriate management of HIV-infected health care workers. If the risks of provider-to-patient transmission associated with invasive procedures were extraordinary, everyone would agree that practice restrictions would be necessary. Although establishing a consensus as to the "tolerable" level of risk would be extremely difficult, everyone would agree that some level is unacceptable. Because the primary risk for transmission of blood-borne pathogens occurs through exposure of the patient's bloodstream to blood from the infected provider, invasive procedures (*i.e.,* surgical or dental procedures) represent the major risk for provider-to-patient transmission of blood-borne pathogens. Most authorities agree that routine patient care activities pose no measurable risk of transmission.[8,10,11] One could argue that the only scientific reason for making a recommendation restricting the practices of HIV- or HBV-infected providers is that the risk of infection associated with infected practitioners performing invasive procedures is unacceptable, an argument that has been proffered by some.[42,43] Nonetheless, 10 years into the HIV epidemic, the magnitude of the risk of provider-to-patient transmission of HIV remains unknown. Some professional societies or organizations established positions regarding the management of HIV-infected health care providers prior to the documentation of the first instance of provider-to-patient HIV transmission.[44–51] Each of these proposals acknowledged a theoretical risk of provider-to-patient transmission of HIV. A few recommended that HIV-infected providers voluntarily restrict themselves from the practice of invasive procedures.[47,49,50] Only one recommended routine serologic screening of practitioners.[46] Others advocated the case-by-case management strategy.[46,48]

The first documented instances of practitioner-to-patient transmission[13,14] resulted in substantial publicity in the lay press and considerable controversy in the health care community. The molecular epidemiologic assessment of this epidemic[14] provided solid confirmation that transmission of HIV from the dentist to his patients had, in fact, occurred. The precise mechanisms responsible for the epidemic transmission of infection in the dentist's office, however, remain obscure. To date, this epidemic remains the only instance in which transmission of HIV from a provider to a patient has been documented.

The documentation that HIV transmission had occurred in a practice setting prompted the American Medical Association (AMA),[52] the American Dental Association (ADA),[53] and ultimately the CDC[41] to modify their positions to recommend that HIV-infected health care providers who perform invasive procedures voluntarily restrict their practices. Other organizations have taken an intermediate position, arguing that voluntary restrictions be recommended for only the small subset of invasive procedures that have been epidemiologically implicated as representing a clear risk of transmission.[54]

The concept of *primum, non nocere* is the cornerstone of the positions of the organizations that have recommended across-the-board restrictions.[47,49,52,53] In some respects this position is ironic, as many health care organizations have opposed similar interventions that have been recommended to reduce the probability of harm to patients (*e.g.,* drug or alcohol testing, mandatory competency review, and so forth). Based on the estimated prevalences of drug abuse, alcohol abuse, and hypocompetence among practitioners, these latter interventions would likely have a much more profound influence on patient outcomes than a recommendation for practice restrictions for HIV- or HBV-infected providers.

Gostin has eloquently argued that the approach taken by professional health care organizations and societies to issues such as alcohol and drug abuse is also appropriate for the management of HIV-infected health care providers.[42,43] Gostin notes that most professional societies have standards and rules that prevent providers from performing procedures on patients while under the influence of alcohol or drugs, while emphasizing that few of these societies (and few health care institutions) have attempted to initiate drug or alcohol screening programs. Such an approach—*i.e.,* voluntary restriction of infected providers, at the discretion of the provider, from invasive procedures, with professional (and the obvious threat of legal) sanctions for those who violate the standard[43]—represents perhaps the most reasonable approach to practice restriction. Such an approach is not without problems, however. In point of fact, most professional organizations preclude *all,* not selected aspects of, patient care activities for providers under the influence of alcohol or drugs. Others may argue that professional standards for alcohol and drug use and professional competence are ineffective and that more stringent rules (including drug or alcohol testing) are in fact appropriate. In addition, from a 1991 societal perspective, alcohol use (perhaps even social drug use) and HIV infection do not represent level playing fields. Whereas alcohol and, to a lesser extent, casual drug use has become somewhat or well tolerated by society, HIV infection continues to be associated with substantial social stigma. Because of the social and political overtones associated with HIV infection, one might reasonably anticipate that HIV-related standards, recommendations, or guidelines would receive a different intensity of scrutiny—from health care institutions, professional organizations, and society at large. An essential component of the approach to restrictions advocated by Gostin[43] is defining which "seriously invasive procedures" represent "significant risks" to the patient.[55] The concept of significant risk is important, because the U.S. Supreme Court adopted "significant risk" as its standard in the landmark *School Board* v. *Arline* case.[56] In that case the court held that a teacher who was disabled (because she had a chronic infectious disease) could not be discharged from her job because she did not present a "significant" risk for transmission.[56] Barnes and colleagues emphasize that the U.S. Congress has twice affirmed this approach, first in the Civil Rights Restoration Act of 1988 (Public Law 100-259,134, Congressional Record H.587–8) and later in the Americans with Disabilities Act of 1990 (Public Law 101-336, 104 Stat. 327).[55] Feldblum[57,58] has argued that the new CDC guidelines[41] may, unfortunately, be used by the courts to redefine "significant risk" to encompass risks, such

as the risk of provider-to-patient transmission of HIV, that are below our ability to measure them. Further, she argues that such an inappropriate redefinition may undercut the Americans with Disabilities Act, possibly rendering it relatively ineffective to prevent discrimination against employees with many kinds of disabilities.[57,58]

Because of differences in technique or skill, a procedure associated with substantial risk of provider-to-patient blood exposure for one surgeon may be associated with virtually no risk for a second surgeon. Trying to achieve consensus from health care societies regarding a standard definition of "significant risk" is likely to be equally problematic.[55,57,58] Finally, a policy recommending voluntary restriction that is not accompanied and supported by a serologic screening program may actually encourage infected providers to be less than honest regarding their personal risks for infection and their own serostatus. In a restrictive environment, a surgeon who develops jaundice and icteric sclerae might conclude that he or she would be well-advised to avoid medical counsel (and serologic testing) for the illness and simply assume that he or she had acquired hepatitis A from consuming shellfish, as opposed to having acquired hepatitis B from an occupational exposure. Gostin has argued that disincentives for honest reporting would likely disappear as practice restrictions become better accepted as the ethical standard for the health care professions.[43] In such a restrictive environment, acceptance from health care providers may be slow in coming.

Curiously, society has apparently tolerated the long-held CDC recommendation that HBV-infected health care professionals be allowed to practice until they have been shown to transmit infection.[29,38,39] Though now reversed,[40] the earlier recommendations went further, recommending that individuals found to transmit infection be allowed to resume practice if they followed appropriate infection control guidelines and did not continue to transmit infection.[29,38,39,59]

In February 1991, the CDC convened an official meeting to address the risks of transmission of blood-borne pathogens during invasive procedures. The notice for the meeting was published in both the "Federal Register"[60] and "Morbidity and Mortality Weekly Report."[14] At this meeting the CDC distributed a draft risk-assessment document.[61] This document attempted to estimate the magnitude of risk of provider-to-patient transmission of HIV and HBV by constructing a risk-assessment model, based on the limited data available in the medical literature. In this model, the risk of HIV seroconversion associated with a patient undergoing a single invasive procedure performed by an HIV-infected surgeon was estimated to be between 2.4 and 24 per 1 million procedures.[61] The risk of HBV infection associated with a patient undergoing a single invasive procedure performed by an HBV-infected surgeon was estimated to be approximately 1 in 420 procedures.[61]

The draft risk-assessment model has several limitations, most of which are clearly spelled out in the document itself. Data from several small studies in the literature were used to estimate the magnitude of risk of patient-to-provider transmission of HBV. Data from one small observational study performed in operating rooms in four hospitals[62] and data from prospective studies assessing the risk of patient-to-provider transmission of HIV[3-5] were used in combination to try to estimate the risk of provider-to-patient transmission of HIV. Thus, only scant data are directly or indirectly relevant to the assessment of the magnitude of risk of provider-to-patient transmission of HIV. Previously published estimates of the risk of provider-to-patient transmission of HIV have ranged from one infection per 130,000 procedures[42] to one to 2.4 infections per 1 million procedures.[59,61,63] A few additional studies have provided either prospective or retrospective assessment of the risk of HBV[18,64-66] or HIV[67-70] transmission from infected practitioners to patients. In each of the HIV-related investigations, patients of infected health care practitioners were retrospectively evaluated serologically after the health care worker's HIV serologic status became known. None of these investigations identified instances of probable provider-to-patient HIV transmission. Only one infected patient was identified in these studies; that patient was known to have community-based risks for HIV infection.[67]

The estimate of the risk of provider-to-patient transmission of HBV in the CDC draft[61] is also problematic. Data from several studies (some representing unpublished CDC observations) were combined to yield some measure of the risk of provider-to-patient transmission. Not all of these studies are directly comparable; many were published prior to the beginning of the HIV epidemic.[15-20] The entry of HIV into the health care workplace resulted in the broad-based implementation of universal precautions and increased attention to the details of the appropriate biosafety precautions. Whereas compliance with universal precautions is by no means complete, these recommendations, and the presence of HIV in the health care workplace, have resulted in behavior modification in the health care setting. Nonetheless, transmission of HBV to a patient from a provider who is aware of his or her infection status and who has been counseled about appropriate prevention techniques is a rare event. CDC investigators found only a few such cases in their exhaustive review.[18,26,29,61]

Restricting infected practitioners is not the only or even the most effective way to reduce the risk of provider-to-patient transmission. Determining the factors associated with a risk of patient-to-provider and provider-to-patient blood exposures during invasive procedures is a first step.[71-73] In addition, professional societies should carefully evaluate invasive procedures performed by their members for features of those procedures associated with an increased risk of patient-to-provider and provider-to-patient blood exposures. Historically, biosafety considerations have not been a major concern for device manufacturers. Creative advances in technology and instrumentation may substantially reduce the risks of provider or patient exposure. These types of prevention-oriented interventions are likely to have a much more profound impact on the transmission of these and other blood-borne pathogens in the health care setting.

From these limited data, several preliminary conclusions can be drawn: (1) Based on the epidemiology and known routes of transmission of HIV and HBV, there is risk of provider-to-patient transmission of these and other blood-borne pathogens. (2) Inadequate data are available to assess the magnitude of the risk of provider-to-patient transmission of either of these viruses. (3) The existing limited data suggest that these risks are likely to be extremely small and quite difficult to measure with precision. (4) Obtaining data to provide a more accurate assessment of these risks, while of paramount importance, will be extremely difficult.

SOCIETY'S WILLINGNESS AND ABILITY TO TOLERATE RISK OF PROVIDER-TO-PATIENT TRANSMISSION OF HIV

Ten years' experience with the HIV epidemic in the United States has taught most investigators that the public's perceptions of risks in society are uneven at best. Society simply does not measure all risks in a similar fashion. Members of society are willing to accept substantial risks they perceive as "voluntary" (*i.e.,* someone chooses to drive a car, smoke cigarettes, consume alcohol, and the like) but are much less willing to accept "involuntary" risks, almost irrespective of their magnitudes. Thus, the same society that tolerates an extraordinary number of tobacco- or alcohol-related deaths annually may be less willing to accept any level of risk of provider-to-patient transmission of HIV. Similarly, the same health care professionals who blithely dismissed or ignored the 200 annual deaths related to occupational infections with HBV and who have offered only indifferent acceptance of the HBV vaccines were terrorized by the identification of risk of occupational infection with HIV. Thus, society's willingness to accept some level of risk of provider-to-patient transmission of blood-borne pathogens remains a major obstacle to the development of any policy on the management of HIV-infected health care workers.

From the beginning of the epidemic in the United States, AIDS and HIV infection have been shrouded in mystery and accompanied by anxiety. The attitudes of the general public[74-77] and of health care professionals[78,79] have reflected this anxiety, rather than the factual evidence about the transmission and transmissibility of HIV that has been systematically developed in the past decade.

Virtually every decision that we make, whether consciously or unconsciously, involves risk assessment.

The distinction between ''voluntary'' and ''involuntary'' risk is artificial. Although one can ''elect'' some risks; one cannot avoid all risk. All of us accept ''involuntary'' risks (many of which are likely to be of a magnitude quite similar to the estimates of the magnitude of risk of provider-to-patient transmission of HIV) every day in our lives without giving these risks much thought. Although we ''control'' our cars, we cannot voluntarily control the car on the other side of the street being driven by someone who has elected a higher level of risk by consuming an excessive amount of ethanol. In homes and workplaces, one finds asbestos, polychlorinated bromphenyls, and other toxic substances. Even lying in bed, motionless, behind locked doors, is associated with risk (pulmonary embolism, osteoporosis). To manage risks effectively in our lives, we are forced to compare risks with others that we know and understand. Thus, lying in bed is perceived as safe, when in fact it is only safer than some other activity. Assessing comparative risks and ordering risks in perspective allows us to make appropriate choices in our own lives and for our society.

Irrespective of whatever policy regarding the management of HIV-infected health care providers is ultimately implemented, some risk of provider-to-patient transmission will remain for patients in the health care setting. This risk, like all related transmission risks, can never be reduced to zero. Because the magnitude of risk of provider-to-patient transmission of HIV—even in the absence of practice restrictions—is so small that it has eluded measurement, determining the efficacy or the specific impact on the rate of provider-to-patient HIV transmission of a policy restricting infected health care providers will be problematic. The only valid scientific reason for making such a recommendation is that the risk associated with infected practitioners performing ''invasive'' procedures is ''significant''[43,55,57,58] and therefore unacceptable. As noted above, attempting to determine a level of risk that is acceptable to society (and therefore not ''significant''[55,57,58]) is likely to be quite difficult. Recommending practice restrictions for HIV-infected health-care workers in the context of the *primum non nocere* may suggest to some individuals that society should try to achieve zero risk with respect to this socially sensitive question. In my own opinion, such a position may be dangerous, since zero risk can never be achieved and because such a position runs counter to virtually every other HIV prevention guideline or recommendation published to date. At the very least, we should try to educate the public about risk perception, risk management, and ''significant'' risk.

Current U.S. Public Health Service Guidelines

The CDC issued revised guidelines in July 1991 entitled, ''Recommendations for preventing transmission of human immunodeficiency virus and hepatitis B virus to patients during exposure-prone invasive procedures.''[41] These revised guidelines recommend that:

health-care workers who perform exposure-prone procedures should know their HIV antibody status. Health-care workers who perform exposure-prone procedures and who do not have serologic evidence of immunity to HBV from vaccination or from previous infection should know their HBsAg status, and, if that is positive, should also know their HBeAg status. Health-care workers who are infected with HIV or HBV (and are HBeAg positive) should not perform exposure-prone invasive procedures unless they have sought counsel from an expert review panel and have been advised under what circumstances, if any, they may continue to perform these procedures. Such circumstances would include notifying prospective patients of the health-care worker's seropositivity before they undergo exposure-prone invasive procedures.

The revised guidelines fall short of defining exposure-prone procedures; however, they do provide characteristics of procedures that might be categorized as exposure-prone[41]:

Characteristics of exposure-prone procedures include digital palpation of a needle tip in a body cavity or the simultaneous presence of a health-care worker's fingers and a needle or other sharp instrument or object in a poorly visualized or highly confined anatomical site. Performance of exposure-prone procedures presents a recognized risk of percutaneous injury to the health care worker, and—if such an injury occurs—the health-care worker's blood is likely to contact the patient's body cavity, subcutaneous tissues, and/or mucous membranes.

OPTIONS FOR MANAGING INFECTED PROVIDERS

Most aspects of patient care are associated with virtually no risk of provider-to-patient transmission of blood-borne pathogens; only ''invasive procedures'' (and specifically those invasive procedures characterized as ''exposure-prone''[41]) are thought to be associated with a potential for ''significant'' risk. HIV- or HBV-infected providers who do not perform invasive procedures need not be restricted from practice.[8,12,40] The issue of the appropriate management of infected health care providers who perform invasive procedures, and therefore pose a risk for the transmission of blood-borne pathogens to patients, is without question among the most difficult that health care workers have had to face since HIV and AIDS appeared in the workplace and society. This difficulty is compounded by the complex political and social baggage associated with HIV infection. As is the case for all controversial issues in society, no single approach or answer will satisfy everyone. Historically, science has provided the foundation for deciding about such issues. The fact that only limited scientific data are available that directly address the risks of infection makes this particular decision even more problematic. Clearly, additional data are needed to provide solid footing for recommendations or guidelines for HIV- or HBV-infected health care workers. In order to provide clear, science-based recommendations, several difficult questions must be answered, among them: (1) What is the magnitude of risk of provider-to-patient transmission of HIV? (2) What magnitude of risk of provider-to-patient transmission will society accept? (3) How can the public be educated about relative risk and risk perception? (4) How should infected health care workers who wish to perform invasive procedures be managed until we know the answers to the first three questions?

Advantages of Recommending Practice Restrictions

Recommending practice restriction for providers infected with these blood-borne pathogens would, in the current social climate, likely be perceived by society as affording protection to patients. Such a decision is also likely to be politically popular, in light of the public misperceptions and anxieties regarding risks of HIV transmission.[74-77] In addition, such recommendations have been viewed by some as consonant with the *primum non nocere* principle. Practice restrictions could be either mandatory or voluntary. While mandatory restriction (clearly entailing mandatory participation in a periodic screening program) might be viewed as appropriate by some[80] and as unnecessarily and inappropriately intrusive by others,[81] voluntary restriction (as advocated by the AMA,[52] the ADA,[53] and more recently by the CDC[41] might be viewed as acceptable by society and might be more easily accepted by practitioners. Some have argued that voluntary restrictions might be implemented without required participation in a serologic screening program[41,43]; others have expressed the opinion that a recommendation for restricting HIV-infected practitioners from invasive procedures will result in mandatory screening programs for all providers who perform such procedures.[55]

Recommending restrictions might improve the specificity of what have been perceived as vague U.S. Public Health Service recommendations.[55] Restrictive recommendations might also compel professional societies to consider all invasive procedures in order to identify those associated with a risk of provider-to-patient transmission of infection. As professional societies evaluate procedures, they are likely to consider aspects of these procedures that might be altered to make them safer, both for patients and for providers. Thus, implementing practice restrictions might force professional societies to give serious thought to biosafety considerations.

Finally, recommending practice restrictions would, in all likelihood, prevent some instances of provider-to-patient transmission of infection. Based on limited available data, the CDC hypothesized that 13 to 128 pa-

tients may have been infected by providers during the first 10 years of the HIV epidemic in the United States.[61] Because of the paucity of relevant data, this estimate was received with considerable skepticism; nonetheless, these estimates do provide a loose framework for considering these difficult issues. Some, but certainly not all, of the 13 to 128 cases might have been preventable through practice restrictions. Some individuals might argue that prevention of even a single case of infection would be worth the considerable costs (both human and financial) of implementing practice restrictions.

Disadvantages of Recommending Practice Restrictions

Practice restrictions are likely to be viewed as intrusive by some health care workers. Deciding what level of risk is significant[55,57,58] and which procedures are associated with significant risk is likely to be an extremely difficult and contentious process. The potential exists for these issues to be handled unevenly by different professional societies or institutions. Eventually such restrictions are likely to be challenged in the courts. Recommending practice restrictions for a perceived risk of 2.4 per 100,000 to 2.4 per 1 million procedures[61] may inappropriately fuel public anxiety, and may result in an unfortunate redefinition of "significant risk."[57,58] Recommending practice restrictions may be viewed as consonant with the zero-tolerable-risk position. Such a recommendation is inconsistent with the recent (and currently applicable) U.S. Public Health Service's decision to discontinue HIV-1–related "geographic deferrals" for blood donors from Pattern II countries (countries in which heterosexual spread is the major route of HIV transmission). Estimates suggested that allowing immigrant donors from these countries to donate blood would be associated with three to ten cases of transfusion-associated HIV infection annually (a case accrual rate either analogous to, or in excess of, what might reasonably be anticipated from a "no-restrictions-for-infected-providers" guideline). Some (but presumably not all) of these cases could be prevented by maintaining geographic deferrals for Pattern II countries. Other sensitive U.S. Public Health Service HIV guidelines that could theoretically fall prey to the zero-tolerable-risk position include the recommendation that HIV-infected children be allowed to attend schools. Admittedly, the risk of classmate-to-classmate transmission is likely to be less than the risk of provider-to-patient transmission during invasive procedures; nonetheless, even this risk will not be zero.

Implementing practice restrictions for invasive procedures may result in the removal of infected personnel from all patient care activities. In one published account, on learning of a dental student's HIV seropositivity, an *ad hoc* committee recommended that the student be "permanently removed from patient care activities."[82] According to the report, although the student is still enrolled in dental school and options for the student's gaining clinical experience are being explored, including the possibility of the student providing dental care for a group of HIV-positive patients, the student apparently remains restricted from all patient care activities.[82] Implementing practice restrictions for invasive procedures may also result in decreased access to care for HIV-infected patients, and may result in decreased access to care for all patients living in high-HIV-prevalence areas. Recommending even voluntary practice restrictions may provide a legitimate lever for insurers and health care institutions to require mandatory testing of all providers performing significantly invasive procedures. Recommending practice restrictions will undoubtedly adversely affect the careers of many health care providers, many of whom have been plying their trades successfully, and without harm to patients, under the auspices of the currently existing CDC guidelines. The precise number of providers who will be affected is unknown; nonetheless, the number is likely to be substantial.[55,63,81]

Advantages of Recommending Against Practice Restrictions

A formal recommendation that practice restrictions are not needed might transmit an important message to society about relative risk and might help educate society about significant risk.[55] If such a recommendation were made as part of an integrated approach to educating society about risk and relative risk, the recommendation, in itself, might help alleviate inappropriate fears and anxieties regarding the transmission and transmissibility of HIV. Because the risk of provider-to-patient transmission of HIV and HBV is so small that it has as yet eluded measurement or even precise estimation, a recommendation that infected providers need not be restricted would allow such providers to continue to provide care, ensuring their own careers and ensuring that medical care is available to their patients. Removing "career jeopardy" would also likely improve access to care for patients who harbor blood-borne infections. Such a recommendation might also improve access to care for all patients living in areas with high prevalences of HIV and might provide indirect encouragement for young people to enter the health care professions. Such a recommendation would also likely be viewed as consistent with existing U.S. Public Health Service HIV and HBV guidelines.

Disadvantages of Recommending Against Practice Restrictions

Recommending that restrictions are not necessary might result in infected providers assuming that the risk of transmission is trivial. If this were to happen, infected personnel might be less motivated to adhere to recommended infection control procedures. Because of the current social and political climates surrounding HIV-related issues, the public might interpret such a

recommendation as representing insensitivity on the part of the U.S. Public Health Service to issues of patient protection. Professional societies that have positions based on the *primum non nocere* principle might view such a recommendation as a violation of this principle. If so, such a recommendation might be associated with substantial sociopolitical fallout. Politicians may attempt to pass legislation mandating a different approach. Finally, and perhaps most important, a recommendation that practice restrictions are not necessary would likely result in a small number of cases of provider-to-patient transmission of HBV and HIV, some percentage of which might have been prevented by voluntary or mandatory practice restrictions.

Advantages of Deferring the Decision Regarding Practice Restrictions

Until July 1991,[41] U.S. Public Health Service recommendations had suggested that HIV-infected providers be managed on a case-by-case basis, but not necessarily be excluded from performing invasive procedures.[12] Thus, the new guidelines are substantially different from the older ones.

U.S. Public Health Service recommendations for practitioners infected with HBV have also been somewhat confusing. Earlier publications from the CDC suggested that HBV-infected individuals could perform invasive procedures without obtaining informed consent, as long as they did not transmit infection.[29,38,39] A 1989 recommendation states that providers who have transmitted infection should not perform invasive procedures,[40] while the 1982,[38] 1986,[29] and 1990[39] recommendations advocate allowing the individual to perform invasive procedures as long as patients are informed, consent is obtained, and a mechanism for detecting subsequent transmission is in place. The 1991 guidelines have more clearly delineated U.S. Public Health Service recommendations for practitioners infected with HBV.[41]

The new recommendations were made on the basis of extremely limited data. Deferring the decision regarding formal guidelines might have allowed scientists to gather more information about the risk of transmission of these blood-borne pathogens, perhaps providing a more complete scientific base for future guidelines or recommendations. Allowing local autonomy for institutions would have allowed thoughtful, reasonable, regional management of these problems. Deferring the decision until additional information is available is consistent with the cautious and eloquent recommendations of Alter and Chalmers[36] made 16 years ago regarding the management of chronic HBV carriers.

Disadvantages of Deferring the Decision Regarding Practice Restrictions

Because some experts found prior U.S. Public Health Service recommendations vague,[55] deferring the decision about practice restrictions would likely have prevented issuance of more definitive guidelines. As with recommending against practice restrictions, in the current sociopolitical climates, the public might have interpreted *status quo* recommendations as a "do-nothing" position, suggesting that the U.S. Public Health Service is insensitive to patient risks. Professional societies that have positions based on the *primum non nocere* principle might view such a recommendation as a violation of this principle. Again, such a recommendation might be associated with substantial political fallout and perhaps with legislation mandating testing or restrictions. Indeed, such legislation has already been proposed and, at the time of this writing, has been passed by the U.S. Senate and is pending in the House of Representatives. In addition, a separate amendment has been proposed that would essentially elevate the July 1991 CDC guidelines[41] to law.

THE IMPACT OF GUIDELINES RECOMMENDING PRACTICE RESTRICTIONS FOR HEALTH CARE WORKERS CHRONICALLY INFECTED WITH BLOOD-BORNE PATHOGENS

Implementing a restrictive policy for infected health care providers may have substantial effects on health care in the United States. The impact of such a recommendation may well be felt by institutions, by health care providers, and ultimately by society.

Institutional Impact

The introduction of restrictive guidelines into the health care workplace may have substantial impact on institutions. Since, under the Americans with Disabilities Act, HIV infection is presumed to represent a handicap, any change in a health care worker's practice would have to be accomplished within the context of "reasonable accommodation." Terminating the employment of the health care worker would be a violation of the law. Because certain of the health care occupations most likely to be affected (*e.g.,* cardiovascular surgeon, orthopedic surgeon, gynecologic surgeon) are somewhat unique, what represents a truly "reasonable accommodation" for an infected individual in any of these occupations remains a matter of conjecture.

Although many organizations and individuals have argued that voluntary restrictions for infected health care workers could be accomplished without mandatory screening programs,[41,43] others have suggested that an official recommendation that infected health care workers not perform some procedures would result in the mandatory screening of all individuals who perform those procedures.[55] Such a position would most likely be advanced by those who have financial and risk management concerns in the institution and would almost certainly be welcomed, if not championed, by malprac-

tice insurers. Thus, the likelihood that some form of serologic screening program would accompany official recommendations to restrict the practices of HIV-infected health care providers seems likely.[55] In that context, another problem for health care institutions involves the management of health care workers identified as prevalent positives in a screening program. If, as a result of guidelines, recommendations, or insurance requirements, institutions began screening employees who perform invasive procedures for markers of infectivity for HBV or HIV, prevalent positive employees would be identified. Determining, for worker's compensation purposes, the source of an individual employee's infection (*i.e.,* occupational *vs.* nonoccupational) may be virtually impossible. Some have argued that proof of causation should not be a precondition for the awarding of worker's compensation[83]; such a position seems appropriate, in that most health care workers have willingly accepted these risks to provide care for all patients. Whether those making compensation determinations have a similar view of these issues remains to be determined. Nonetheless, should guidelines be implemented recommending practice restrictions (thereby resulting in the implementation of institutional screening programs), institutions may wish to establish a policy regarding the management of practitioners identified as prevalent positives before implementing the screening program.

A particularly thorny issue for institutions attempting to implement a serologic screening/practice restriction program is that of protecting the privacy of the infected health care worker and the confidentiality of test results. Maintaining the privacy of a dynamic surgeon may be difficult if the surgeon is precipitously removed from the operating suite and suddenly becomes part of the hospital administration, especially if some institution-based individuals know the reason for the career change. Other aspects of the management information regarding co-workers' privacy and the confidentiality of information are equally complex. Who in the hospital administration really "needs to know" about the employee, and how can those who know appropriately shepherd this information? With respect to AIDS and HIV infection, history has painfully demonstrated the difficulties of maintaining an infected health care worker's privacy.[83,84]

Finally, institutions will have to support screening programs with financial resources as well, and the costs of implementing and maintaining such a program will not be trivial. The cost of implementing a screening/practice restriction program at one major academic medical center has been estimated to be in excess of $830,000.[85] These are staggering costs in the absence of a clearly measurable benefit.

Impact on Health Care Providers

Either voluntary self-restriction or participation in a mandatory screening/practice restriction program is clearly associated with career jeopardy for health care providers who routinely perform invasive procedures.[82] Implementation of restrictions will unquestionably result in the virtual eradication of careers of individuals who may have been productive and dedicated members of the medical community—individuals whose loss from medicine will be felt. Although intended to restrict such individuals from the practice of invasive procedures, a recommendation for any practice restrictions may result in the removal of infected individuals from *all* aspects of clinical care.[82] Some health care workers may envision required participation in such a program as an invasion of privacy. One might anticipate seeing one or more of these cases tested in the courts.

Restrictive guidelines may cause some health care workers to become reluctant to treat patients known to have blood-borne infections. Does the concept of career jeopardy influence a health care worker's moral and ethical obligation to provide care for all patients? Such questions never have easy answers; nonetheless, the presence of either voluntary or mandatory screening/practice restrictions provides an altered context within which these issues must be considered.

In the long run, money and financial concerns will considerably influence the management of health care workers who pose a risk for provider-to-patient transmission of blood-borne pathogens. Malpractice insurers could, for example, require a guarantee that health care providers doing invasive procedures be noninfectious for HBV and HIV. Alternatively, insurers could offer premium advantages to institutions who voluntarily screen personnel who perform invasive procedures and voluntarily restrict those found to be infected with HIV and HBV from performing invasive procedures.

Impact on Health Care Delivery

The implementation of practice restrictions could have substantial short- and long-term effects on health care delivery. Provision of adequate health care for HIV-infected patients may become even more problematic than it is in 1991. Access to care has already been identified as a significant problem for many HIV-infected patients. In addition, one might anticipate problems with the delivery of a variety of types of health care in areas in which the prevalence of HIV infection is high. One might hypothesize that HIV seroprevalence data might be given serious consideration by young surgeons, invasive cardiologists, invasive diagnostic radiologists and dentists as they choose where to establish their practices.

One could also postulate that recruitment and retention of high-quality individuals into the health care professions, especially those involving invasive procedures, may be adversely affected by an official recommendation for practice restrictions for personnel who acquire blood-borne infections. Intelligent young people who understand that not all risks can be avoided in the health care environment may elect to get an MBA or a law degree.

CONCLUSION

Many important questions regarding the management of providers infected with blood-borne pathogens remain unanswered. The new U.S. Public Health Service guidelines have raised as many questions as they have answered. Each of the options for management discussed in this chapter is associated with problems in implementation. Regardless of recommendations for the management of infected practitioners, health care professionals and their professional societies need to take a fresh look at infection control standards for invasive procedures.[41,73] Substantial risk reduction can likely be achieved through identifying factors associated with a risk for blood-to-blood exposures, modification of procedures associated with such risks, and through technological advances that may reduce such risks.[41,73]

Whereas these are difficult, complex issues, both science and society can benefit from the prescient advice of Alter and Chalmers.[36,37] The morbidity and mortality risks associated with HIV- or HBV-infected practitioners performing invasive procedures must be managed in perspective, in the context of the myriad risks present in the health care setting. Based on currently available evidence, and in the absence of data documenting a science-based, society-embraced "significant" level of risk, the consequences of restricting the practices of providers infected with these blood-borne pathogens are likely to substantially outweigh the potential benefit to the public health.

Note Added in Proof

The Centers for Disease Control (CDC) held a meeting in November, 1991 to attempt to determine which invasive medical, surgical, and dental procedures should be categorized as exposure prone. At this meeting, the representatives of virtually every major dental, medical, and surgical society in attendance stressed that such a classification was not feasible—primarily because of practitioner-to-practitioner variation in technique. An exposure-prone procedure for one surgeon frequently would not be exposure-prone for another. Perhaps more importantly the representatives of these organizations and societies emphasized their almost universal displeasure with the July CDC guidelines. At the time this chapter is going to press, CDC representatives have stated publicly that the July 1991 guidelines are being "revisited." Further, these same individuals have indicated a willingness, and perhaps even a desire, to modify the guidelines to align them more closely with the views of the major professional societies and organizations. Reports in the major newspapers have suggested that the guidelines are being modified; however, as yet, no formal revisions have been issued. Because of the legal, social, and political complexity of these issues, these problems are likely to be extraordinarily difficult to resolve, and it is unclear (in December 1991) when or whether the July 1991 CDC guidelines will be revised.

REFERENCES

1. Centers for Disease Control: *Pneumocystis* pneumonia. MMWR 30:250, 1981
2. [N.A.]: Needlestick transmission of HTLV-III from a patient infected in Africa. Lancet 2:1376, 1984
3. Marcus R: The Cooperative Needlestick Surveillance Group: Surveillance of health care workers exposed to blood from patients infected with the human immunodeficiency virus. N Engl J Med 319:1118, 1988
4. Gerberding JL, Bryant-LeBlanc CE, Nelson K et al: Risk of transmitting the human immunodeficiency virus, cytomegalovirus, and hepatitis B virus to health care workers exposed to patients with AIDS and AIDS-related conditions. J Infect Dis 156:1, 1987
5. Henderson DK, Fahey BJ, Willy M et al: The risk for occupational/nosocomial transmission of HIV-1 associated with clinical exposures: A prospective evaluation. Ann Intern Med 113:740, 1990
6. Weiss SH, Saxinger WC, Rechtman D et al: HTLV-III infection among health care workers: Association with needle-stick injuries. JAMA 254:2089, 1985
7. Centers for Disease Control: Update: Human immunodeficiency virus infections in health-care workers exposed to blood of infected patients. MMWR 36:285, 1987
8. Centers for Disease Control: Recommendations for prevention of HIV transmission in health-care settings. MMWR 36(suppl 2S):1S, 1987
9. Centers for Disease Control: Update: Evaluation of human T-lymphotropic virus type III/Lymphadenopathy-associated virus infection in health-care personnel—United States. MMWR 34:575, 1985
10. Centers for Disease Control: Summary and recommendations for preventing transmission of infection with human T-lymphotropic virus type III/lymphadenopathy-associated virus in the workplace. MMWR 34:681, 1985
11. Gerberding JL, Henderson DK: Design of rational infection control policies for human immunodeficiency virus infection (HIV). J Infect Dis 156:861, 1987
12. Centers for Disease Control: Recommendations for preventing transmission of infection with human T-lymphotropic virus type III/lymphadenopathy-associated virus during invasive procedures. MMWR 35:221, 1986
13. Centers for Disease Control: Possible transmission of human immunodeficiency virus to a patient during an invasive dental procedure. MMWR 39:489, 1990
14. Centers for Disease Control: Update: Transmission of HIV infection during an invasive dental procedure—Florida. MMWR 40:21, 1991
15. Levin ML, Maddrey WC, Wands JR et al: Hepatitis B transmission by dentists. JAMA 228:1139, 1974
16. Grob P, Moeschlin P: Risk to contacts of a medical practitioner carrying hepatitis B. N Engl J Med 293:197, 1975
17. Snydman DR, Hindman SH, Wineland MD et al: Nosocomial viral hepatitis B: A cluster among staff with subsequent transmission to patients. Ann Intern Med 85:573, 1976
18. Goodwin D, Fannin SL, McCracken BB: An oral surgeon–related hepatitis B outbreak. Calif Med, vol 14, 1976
19. Rimland D, Parkin WE, Miller GB et al: Hepatitis B outbreak traced to an oral surgeon. N Engl J Med 296:953, 1977
20. Collaborative study by the central public health laboratories: Acute hepatitis B associated with gynaecological surgery. Lancet 1:1, 1980
21. Haeram JW, Siekbe JC, Ulstrup J et al: HBsAg transmission from a cardiac surgeon incubating hepatitis B resulting in chronic antigenemia in four patients. Acta Med Scand 210:389, 1981
22. Hadler S, Sorley D, Acree K et al: An outbreak of hepatitis B in a dental practice. Ann Intern Med 95:133, 1981
23. Grob P, Bischof B, Naeff F: Cluster of hepatitis B transmitted by a physician. Lancet 2:1218, 1981
24. Reingold AL, Kane MA, Murphy EL et al: Transmission of hepatitis B by an oral surgeon. J Infect Disease 145:262, 1982
25. Goodman RA, Ahtone JL, Finton RJ: Hepatitis B transmission from dental personnel to patients: Unfinished business. Ann Intern Med 96:119, 1982
26. Coutinho RA, Albrecht-vanLent P, Stoutdesjijk L et al: Hepatitis B from doctors. Lancet 1:345, 1982
27. Carl M, Blakey D, Francis D et al: Interruption of hepatitis B transmission by modification of a gynaecologist's surgical technique. Lancet 1:731, 1982
28. Ahtone J, Goodman RA: Hepatitis B and dental personnel. JADA 106:219, 1983
29. Lettau LA, Smith JD, Williams D et al: Transmission of hepatitis B with resultant restriction of surgical practice. JAMA 255:934, 1986
30. Shaw FE, Barrett CL, Hamm R et al: Lethal outbreak of hepatitis B in a dental practice. JAMA 255:3261, 1986
31. A District Control of Infection Officer: Acute hepatitis B following gynaecological surgery. J Hosp Infect 9:34, 1987
32. Centers for Disease Control: Outbreak of hepatitis B associated with an oral surgeon—New Hampshire. MMWR 36:132, 1987
33. Welch J, Webster M, Tilzey A et al: Hepatitis B infections after gynaecological surgery. Lancet 1:205, 1989
34. Flower AJ, Prentice M, Morgan G et al: Hepatitis B infection following cardiothoracic surgery (abstr). Presented at the International Symposium on Viral Hepatitis, Houston, 1990
35. Alter HJ, Seeff LB, Kaplan PM et al: Type B hepatitis: The infectivity of blood positive for e antigen and DNA polymerase after accidental needlestick exposure. N Engl J Med 295:909, 1976
36. Alter HJ, Chalmers TC, Freeman BM et al: Health-care workers positive for hepatitis B surface antigen: Are their contacts at risk? N Engl J Med 292:454, 1975
37. Alter HJ, Chalmers TC: The HBsAg positive health worker revisited. Hepatology 1:467, 1981
38. Centers for Disease Control: Hepatitis surveillance report number 48. Atlanta, CDC, 1982
39. Hadler SC: Hepatitis B virus infection and health care workers. Vaccine 8(suppl):S24, 1990
40. Centers for Disease Control: Guidelines for prevention of transmission of human immunodeficiency virus and hepatitis B virus to health-care and public-safety workers. MMWR 38(suppl 6):1, 1989
41. Centers for Disease Control: Recommendations for preventing transmission of human immunodeficiency virus

and hepatitis B virus to patients during exposure-prone invasive procedures. MMWR 40:1, 1991

42. Gostin L: HIV-infected physicians and the practice of seriously invasive procedures. Hastings Center Rep 19(1): 32, 1989

43. Gostin L: The HIV-infected health care professional: Public policy, discrimination, and patient safety. Law Med Health Care 18:303, 1990

44. American Medical Association: Ethical issues in the growing AIDS crisis: Council on Ethical and Judicial Affairs. JAMA 259:1360, 1988

45. American Medical Association: Ethical issues in the growing AIDS crisis: The HIV-positive practitioner. JAMA 260: 790, 1988

46. American Academy of Pediatrics Task Force on Pediatric AIDS: Pediatric guidelines for infection control of human immunodeficiency virus (acquired immunodeficiency virus) in hospitals, medical offices, schools, and other settings. Pediatrics 82:801, 1988

47. American Academy of Orthopaedic Surgeons Task Force on AIDS and Orthopaedic Surgery: Recommendations for the Prevention of Human Immunodeficiency Virus (HIV) Transmission in the Practice of Orthopaedic Surgery. Park Ridge, Ill, American Academy of Orthopaedic Surgeons, 1989

48. American Hospital Association: Management of HIV Infection in the Hospital, 3rd ed. Chicago, American Hospital Association, 1988

49. Committee on Ethics, American College of Obstetricians and Gynecologists: Human immunodeficiency virus infection: Physicians' responsibilities. Obstet Gynecol 75: 1043, 1990

50. Department of Health and Social Security [England]: AIDS: HIV-Infected Health Care Workers. Report of the Recommendations of the Expert Advisory Group on AIDS. London, Her Majesty's Stationery Office, 1988

51. Speller DEC, Shanson DC, Ayliffe GAJ, Cooke EM: Acquired immunodeficiency syndrome: Recommendations of a Working Party of the Hospital Infection Society. J Hosp Infect 15:7, 1990

52. Dickey N, American Medical Association: Statement of the American Medical Association to the Centers for Disease Control regarding HIV transmission during invasive procedures. Presented at an open meeting on the risks of transmission of bloodborne pathogens to patients during invasive procedures, Atlanta, January 30, 1991

53. Neidle E, American Dental Association: Estimates of the risk of endemic transmission of hepatitis B virus and human immunodeficiency virus to patients by the percutaneous route during invasive surgical and dental procedures. Presented at an open meeting on the risks of transmission of bloodborne pathogens to patients during invasive procedures, Atlanta, January 30, 1991

54. Association for Practitioners in Infection Control, Society of Hospital Epidemiologist of America: Position Paper: The HIV-infected health care worker. Infect Control Hosp Epidemiol 11:647, 1990

55. Barnes M, Rango NA, Burke GR, Chiarello L: The HIV-infected health care professional: Employment policies and public health. Law Med Health Care 18:311, 1990

56. *School Board* v. *Arline.* 480 U.S. 273, 1987

57. Feldblum C: A reply to Gostin. Law Med Health Care, 1991 (in press)

58. Feldblum C: Disability anti-discrimination laws and HIV testing of health-care providers. Courts Health Sci Law, 1991 (in press)

59. Gramelspacher GP: Uncertainty, accountability, and HIV-infected physicians. Hastings Center Rep 20:52, 1990

60. Department of Health and Human Services: Open meeting on the risks of transmission of bloodborne pathogens to patients during invasive procedures. Fed Reg 56:2527, 1991

61. Centers for Disease Control: Draft–Estimates of the risk of endemic transmission of hepatitis B virus and human immunodeficiency virus to patients by the percutaneous route during invasive surgical and dental procedures. Presented at an open meeting on the risks of transmission of bloodborne pathogens to patients during invasive procedures, Atlanta, January 30, 1991

62. Tokars J, Marcus R, Culver DH, Bell DM: Blood contacts during surgical procedures (abstr 958). In: Program and Abstracts of the 30th Interscience Conference on Antimicrobial Agents and Chemotherapy, Atlanta, 1990, p 246

63. Rhame FS: The HIV-infected surgeon. JAMA 264:507, 1990

64. Williams SV, Pattison CP, Berquist KR: Dental infection with hepatitis B. JAMA 232:1231, 1975

65. Meyers JD, Stamm WE, Kerr MM, Counts GW: Lack of transmission of hepatitis B after surgical exposure. 240: 1725, 1978

66. LaBreque DR, Mubs JM, Lutwick LL et al: The risk of hepatitis B transmission from health-care workers to patients in a hospital setting: A prospective study. Hepatology 6: 205, 1986

67. Mishu B, Schaffner W, Horan J et al: A surgeon with AIDS: Lack of evidence of transmission to patients. JAMA 264: 467, 1990

68. Porter JD, Cruickshank JG, Gentle PH et al: Management of patients treated by surgeon with HIV infection. Lancet 113, 1990

69. Armstrong FP, Miner JC, Wolfe WH: Investigation of a health care worker with symptomatic human immunodeficiency virus infection: An epidemiologic approach. Milit Med 152:414, 1988

70. Sacks JJ: AIDS in a surgeon. N Engl J Med 313:1017, 1985

71. Gerberding JL, Littell C, Tarkington A et al: Risk of exposure of surgical personnel to patients' blood during surgery at San Francisco General Hospital. N Engl J Med 322:1788, 1990

72. Panlilio AL, Foy DR, Edwards JR et al: Blood contacts during surgical procedures. JAMA 265:1533, 1990

73. Gerberding JL, Schecter WP: Surgery and AIDS: Reducing the risk. JAMA 265:1572, 1991

74. Blendon RJ, Donelan K: Discrimination against people with AIDS. N Engl J Med 319:1022, 1988

75. Gerbert B, Maguire BT, Hulley SB, Coates TJ: Physicians and acquired immunodeficiency syndrome: What patients think about human immunodeficiency virus in medical practice. JAMA 262:1969, 1989

76. Marshall PA, O'Keefe P, Fisher SG et al: Patients' fear of contracting the acquired immunodeficiency syndrome from patients. Arch Intern Med 150:1501, 1990

77. Lee BJ III: Attitudes: Physicians, AIDS, and the American public. Arch Intern Med 150:29, 1990

78. Somogyi AA, Watson-Abady JA, Mandel FS: Attitudes toward the care of patients with acquired immunodeficiency syndrome: A survey of community internists. Arch Intern Med 150:50, 1990

79. Taylor KM, Eakin JM, Skinner HA et al: Physicians perception of personal risk of HIV infection and AIDS through occupational exposure. Can Med Assoc J 143:493, 1990

80. Cloren M: A call for mandatory HIV testing and restriction of certain health professionals. St Louis Univ Public Law Rev 9:412, 1990

81. Isaacman SH: The other side of the coin: HIV-infected health care workers. St Louis Univ Public Law Rev 9:439, 1990

82. Comer RW, Myers DR, Steadman CD et al: Management considerations for an HIV positive dental student. J Dent Educ 55:187, 1991

83. Aoun H: When a house officer gets AIDS. N Engl J Med 321:693, 1989

84. Gramelspacher GP, Miles SH, Cassel CK: When the doctor has AIDS. J Infect Dis 162:534, 1990

85. Gerberding JL: Expected costs of implementing a mandatory human immunodeficiency virus and hepatitis B virus testing and restriction program for health-care workers performing invasive procedures. Infect Control Hosp Epidemiol 12:443, 1991

Index

ISBN 0-397-51229-5